FIFTH EDITION

COMMUNITY HEALTH NURSING

CONCEPTS AND PRACTICE

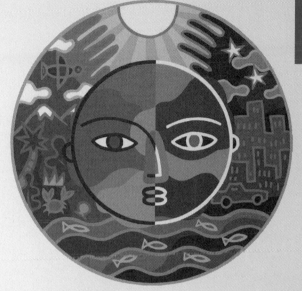

Judith Ann Allender, RN,C, MSN, EdD

Professor
Department of Nursing, College of Health and
Human Services
California State University
Fresno, California

Barbara Walton Spradley, RN, MN

Associate Professor, Emerita
School of Public Health
University of Minnesota
Minneapolis, Minnesota

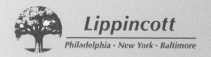

Lippincott
Philadelphia · New York · Baltimore

Acquisitions Editor: Margaret Zuccarini
Editorial Assistant: Hilarie Surrena
Senior Project Editor: Tom Gibbons
Senior Production Manager: Helen Ewan
Production Coordinator: Pat McCloskey
Art Director: Carolyn O'Brien
Manufacturing Manager: William Alberti
Indexer: Alexandra Nickerson
Compositor: Peirce Graphic Services, Inc.
Printer: Courier-Kendalville
Cover Illustration: José Ortega

5th Edition

9 8 7 6 5 4 3 2

Library of Congress Cataloging-in-Publication Data

Allender, Judith Ann.
    Community health nursing / Judith Ann Allender, Barbara Walton Spradley.—5th ed.
        p. cm.
    Fourth ed. has Spradley first on t.p.
    Includes bibliographical references and index.
    ISBN 0-7817-2122-9 (cloth : alk. paper)
        1. Community health nursing. 2. Public health nursing.   I. Spradley, Barbara Walton.
    II. Title.

RT98 S68 2000
610.73'43—dc21   00-061819

Care has been taken to confirm the accuracy of the information presented and to describe generally accepted practices. However, the authors, editors, and publisher are not responsible for errors or omissions or for any consequences from application of the information in this book and make no warranty, express or implied, with respect to the content of the publication.

The authors, editors, and publisher have exerted every effort to ensure that drug selection and dosage set forth in this text are in accordance with the current recommendations and practice at the time of publication. However, in view of ongoing research, changes in government regulations, and the constant flow of information relating to drug therapy and drug reactions, the reader is urged to check the package insert for each drug for any change in indications and dosage and for added warnings and precautions. This is particularly important when the recommended agent is a new or infrequently employed drug.

Some drugs and medical devices presented in this publication have Food and Drug Administration (FDA) clearance for limited use in restricted research settings. It is the responsibility of the health care provider to ascertain the FDA status of each drug or device planned for use in his or her clinical practice.

To our husbands, Gil and Neil,
with love and thanks

Contributors

Carmen Adams, DNSc, RN,C
Assistant Professor, Department of Nursing
Quinnipiac College
Hamden, Connecticut

Tina Bayne, MS, RN, CS
Associate Professor, Intercollegiate Center for
    Nursing Education
Washington State University
Spokane, Washington

Derryl Block, MPH, RN, PhD
Assistant Professor
University of Minnesota, School of Nursing
Minneapolis, Minnesota

Dorothy Brockopp, PhD, RN
Assistant Dean for Undergraduate Studies
Professor of Nursing
College of Nursing
University of Kentucky
Lexington, Kentucky

Nancy Clark, RN, MSN, MPA, EdD Candidate
Professor and Chair, Department
    of Nursing
California State University, Stanislaus
Turlock, California

Pamela Dole, EdD, MPH, FNP
Hunter College School of Nursing
New York, New York

Laura N. Harris, MA
Environmental Specialist
Harris Consulting Associates
Bozeman, Montana

Donald C. Johnson, DrPH
Adjunct Professor, Department of Nursing
California State University, Stanislaus
Turlock, California
Chief of Health Education (Retired)
World Health Organization
Geneva, Switzerland

LaVohn Josten, PhD, RN
Associate Professor
University of Minnesota, School of Nursing
Minneapolis, Minnesota

Kathy Y. Karsting, MPH, RN,C
Health Services Coordinator
Lincoln Public School District
Lincoln, Nebraska

Tamara McKinnon, RN, MSN
Lecturer, Department of Nursing
California State University, San Jose
San Jose, California

Terry W. Miller, PhD, RN
Dean and Professor, School of Nursing
Pacific Lutheran University
Tacoma, Washington

Paula Milone-Nuzzo, RN, PhD, FAAN, FHHC
Professor
Associate Dean for Academic Affairs
Yale University School of Nursing
New Haven, Connecticut

Barbara A. Moynihan, PhD, APRN, CS
Director of the Masters of Science in Forensic Nursing
    Program
Quinnipiac College
Hamden, Connecticut

Cherie Rector, RN,C, PhD
Professor, Department of Nursing
California State University, Bakersfield
Bakersfield, California

Elaine Saline, RN, MPH
Education Specialist
University of Minnesota
School of Nursing
Minneapolis, Minnesota

Sonia Sandhaus, RN,C, MSN, FNP
Staff Nurse
Moses Taylor Hospital
Scranton, Pennsylvania

Cindy Tait, RN, MPH, PHN
President, Center for Healthcare Education, Inc.
Adjunct Faculty
Loma Linda University
Riverside, California

Pamela Thul-Immler, MPH, RN,C
Thul-Immler, Inc.
Psychiatric Consulting
Woodruff, Wisconsin

Joyce V. Zerwekh, RN, EdD
Associate Professor, College of Nursing
Florida Atlantic University
Boca Raton, Florida

Contributors to Previous Editions

Sara T. Fry, RN, PhD

Michele Hadeka, RN, MS

Elaine Richard, RN, MS

Reviewers

Glenda Avery, RN, MSN, CS, ANP
Assistant Professor
Clayton College and State University
Morrow, Georgia

Nettie Birnbach, RN, EdD, FAAN
Professor Emeritus
College of Nursing
State University of New York at Brooklyn
Brooklyn, New York

Mary Ann Boyd, PhD, DNS, RN, CS
Professor, Graduate Faculty
Coordinator, Undergraduate Psychiatric Nursing
School of Nursing
Southern Illinois University
Edwardsville, Illinois

Christine Brosnan, DrPH, RNC
Assistant Professor
School of Nursing
University of Texas—Houston Health Science Center
Houston, Texas

Nancy J. Clark
Nursing Professor
California State University
Stanislaus, California

Helen Cox, RN,C, EdD, FAAN
Executive Associate Dean and Professor
Texas Tech University Health Sciences Center
School of Nursing
Lubbock, Texas

Bonnie Faherty, FNP, PhD, CS
Associate Professor
Department of Health Sciences
California State University
Northridge, California

Valerie Grossman, BSN, CEN
Director of Medical-Surgical Services
Viahealth of Wayne
Newark, New York
Consultant, Triage First, Inc.
Rochester, New York

June Helberg-Albright, EdD, RN, C, GNP
Associate Professor of Clinical Nursing
University of Rochester
School of Nursing
Rochester, New York

Eleanor Howell, RN, PhD
Associate Dean and Associate Professor
Creighton University, School of Nursing
Omaha, Nebraska

Linda Johanson, RN, MS, EdD
Academic Advisor and Lecturer
Department of Adult Health
University of North Carolina at Charlotte
Charlotte, North Carolina

Nancy Michela, RN,C, MS
Associate Professor
Department of Nursing
The Sage Colleges
Troy, New York

Kathleen M. Nokes, PhD, RN, FAAN
Professor
Hunter-Bellevue School of Nursing
CUNY Hunter College
New York, New York

Linda Sawyer, RN, MS, PhD
Assistant Clinical Professor
Community Health Systems, School of Nursing
University of California, San Francisco
San Francisco, California

Beverly Siegrist, RN, MSN, EdD
Associate Professor
Department of Nursing
Western Kentucky University
Bowling Green, Kentucky

Preface

The fifth edition of *Community Health Nursing: Concepts and Practice* represents a continuing effort to capture the essence and clarify the practice of community health nursing. It is written to share the authors' enthusiasm for a field whose dynamic nature calls for nursing creativity, leadership, and innovation with you, the student community health nurse. The potential for community health nurses to protect and enhance the health of at risk populations and to influence the quality of health services poses exciting challenges and opportunities.

As a basic text, the fifth edition, like the other four, is designed to give you, the undergraduate nursing student, a comprehensive introduction to the field of community health nursing. It is also designed to be a professional resource in order to enlarge the vision and enhance the impact of practicing community health nurses.

With a continuing and escalating demand for nurses to practice in the community, it is important that the meaning of community health nursing as a specialized field of nursing practice be clearly understood. The challenge for the nurse who wishes to practice community health nursing lies in incorporating public health principles with nursing knowledge and skills to offer preventive, health-promoting, and protective services that benefit aggregates and populations. As a beginning practitioner in this field, you may have limited impact on aggregates, but an aggregate or population-based orientation must be germane to your practice. With experience and advanced preparation in public health, you can become a specialist in public or community health.

The fifth edition of this text continues to use the term *community health nurse* to describe a practitioner in the community whose work incorporates public health philosophy, theory, and skills with an emphasis on aggregates and populations.

ABOUT THE FIFTH EDITION

This edition of *Community Health Nursing: Concepts and Practice* continues to be written with you, the undergraduate nursing student, in mind. It is "user friendly" with many mini-case studies woven throughout the text in order for you to more easily apply the information with your clients. The text is comprehensive and incorporates the impact of the global health status. We are a small planet with big health problems that impact each person's health and the role of the community health nurse now and in the future. As a nation, we have a new and continuing health agenda through *Healthy People 2010* that gives direction to our work. These new goals and objectives are incorporated throughout the text. Finally, the text format is designed to provide you with the comprehensive, globally sensitive information and skills you need to be an effective practitioner with aggregates, groups, and individuals in the community.

Organization of the Text

In this edition the text has been expanded by nine additional chapters and is organized into seven units. Unit titles as well as most chapter titles have been reworded to include more descriptive language, provide greater continuity for the reader, and expand the work with specific populations.

Unit I, Foundations of Community Health Nursing, introduces you to the conceptual and historical bases for practice in this field. Seven chapters compose this unit, describing first the basic concepts of community and health that provide the opportunities and challenges in the field of community health nursing (Chapter 1); history and nature of community health nursing (Chapter 2); its structure and functions (Chapter 3); the economic considerations that influence community health practice (Chapter 4); and the roles and settings for practice (Chapter 5). The unit concludes with two broader chapters providing the context for community health nursing practice: the values and ethical decision-making that influence community health nursing (Chapter 6) and the impact of culture on health and community health nursing practice (Chapter 7).

Unit II, Tools of Community Health Nursing, provides you with an understanding of the tools needed for practice in this field and how to develop and use them. The unit has six chapters that encompass the specific tools the community health nurse must develop to be effective with community aggregates. The unit focuses on communication and collaboration, two essential skills of the community health nurse (Chapter 8); health promotion through education (Chapter 9); leadership and management responsibilities (Chapter 10); examples of nursing research and discussion of practicing nurses' involvement in and use of research (Chapter 11); and promoting quality in health care services through quality measurement and improvement (Chapter 12). Finally, Chapter 13 describes the ways in which community health nurses can influence the health care system through leadership, power, effecting change, policy-making, and advocacy for the health of the community.

Unit III, Public Health Principles in Community Health Nursing, contains three very important chapters embracing essential elements of public health practice germane to community health nursing. It begins with the principles of epidemiology as the foundation for prevention and control of negative health consequences (Chapter 14). Next is a comprehensive chapter on communicable disease control (Chapter 15). The unit concludes with environmental health and safety concerns (Chapter 16). Throughout the unit the role of the community health nurse is emphasized.

Unit IV, Community as Client, is the first of two units that follow a similar nursing process organizational format. This five-chapter unit begins with the theoretical basis for the practice of community health nursing (Chapter 17). Next, the assessment of communities (Chapter 18) and the planning, intervention, and evaluation of health care in communities (Chapter 19) are discussed. Treatment of communities in crisis (Chapter 20) is expanded in this edition to include communities suffering disasters, group violence, and terrorism. The final chapter in this unit is new and focuses on the global community, exploring international health concerns (Chapter 21).

Unit V, The Family as Client, is a four-chapter unit. It begins with the theoretical basis for promoting family health (Chapter 22), followed by the assessment of families (Chapter 23). The planning, intervention, and evaluation of health care to families follow (Chapter 24). The unit concludes with examination of families in crisis and those experiencing domestic violence and abuse (Chapter 25). These chapters were organized under different units in previous editions. Although nurses work with individual families in the community, this text also supports the need to view clusters of families as aggregates for community health nursing intervention.

Unit VI, Aggregates With Developmental Needs, examines client populations based on age-appropriate needs. In this unit you are helped to understand their needs and how to intervene with each population group. The five chapters in this unit emphasize promoting and protecting the health of populations in each major life cycle stage. First is maternal, perinatal, and newborn populations (Chapter 26), and then infants, toddlers, and preschool populations (Chapter 27). The next chapter, on school-age children and the adolescent population (Chapter 28), is expanded from previous editions and emphasizes the role of the school nurse and school-based health care services. Adult men and women and the working population (Chapter 29) is also expanded from previous editions, with occupational health nursing presented in more detail. Finally, Chapter 30 describes the older adult population and the need to compress the years of morbidity and extend the years of wellness.

Unit VII, Vulnerable Aggregates, has seven chapters, six of which are entirely new to this fifth edition. Because community health nurses are expected to work more frequently with vulnerable populations, this unit focuses on specific groups you may encounter in the community. First, the rural populations at-risk for health care accessibility are discussed (Chapter 31). Next we examine the needs of clients living in poverty and the homeless (Chapter 32), in addition to the complex and often unmet needs of migrant populations (Chapter 33). Many clients in the community with unmet mental health needs are described (Chapter 34), as well as the needs of clients with various addictions, such as substance abuse, eating disorders, or gambling (Chapter 35). Many of the clients we serve in the community live high-risk lifestyles often bringing them in contact with law enforcement and the corrections/incarceration systems in the country. Clients in correctional facilities and the needs of their families are explored (Chapter 36). Finally, we examine the role of the community health nurse working with clients and their families through home care services, long-term care, and hospices (Chapter 37).

New Chapters

To keep abreast of changes in vulnerable populations' needs and delivery of health services, this edition introduces many new topics and expands on numerous others. Seven chapters (Chapters 21 and 31 to 36) are completely new to this edition; two chapters (Chapters 9 and 11) from the fourth edition have been rolled into the new and expanded Chapter 19 on planning, intervening and evaluating health care in the community; and Chapter 37 discusses more fully clients receiving home care, those with long-term care needs, and those involved with hospices. One of the new chapters on global health concerns (Chapter 21) enlarges the view of community and addresses the globalization of public health.

We expand the emphasis on at-risk populations from one chapter in the fourth edition to seven chapters in this edition. Models have been provided to assist you with understanding the causes of vulnerability, client needs, and nursing interventions. Most chapters have been expanded, and all have been updated to include the latest research and information on populations' needs and delivery of services.

Key Features

The fifth edition of *Community Health Nursing: Concepts and Practice* includes key features from previous editions as well as new features.

Features continued from previous editions include:
- An emphasis on aggregate-level nursing and the community health nurse's opportunity and responsibility not only to serve individuals and families but also to promote and protect the health of communities and populations.
- An emphasis on health promotion, health protection, and illness prevention. This, in addition to the aggregate emphasis, reflects the view set forth in this text that community health nursing is the amalgamation of nursing science with public health science. Public health philosophy, values, knowledge, and skills are an essential part of community health nursing practice.
- A balance of theory with application to nursing practice. The fifth edition continues the presentation of theoretical and conceptual knowledge to provide you with an understanding of human needs and a rationale for nursing actions. At the same time the text presents practical information on how you can use theory to undergird practice.
- A summary of highlights at the end of each chapter provides you with an overview of material covered and serves as a review for study.
- References and Selected Readings at the end of each chapter provide you with classic sources, current research, and a broad base of authoritative information for furthering knowledge on each chapter's subject matter.
- A student-friendly writing style has been a hallmark of this text since the first edition. Topics are expressed and concepts explained to enhance your understanding and capture your interest. Writing style remains consistent throughout the text (including contributed chapters) to promote an uninterrupted flow of ideas for your learning.
- Learning Objectives and Key Terms sharpen your focus and provide a guide for learning the chapter content.
- Activities to Promote Critical Thinking at the close of each chapter are designed to challenge you, promote critical-thinking skills, and encourage your active involvement in solving community health problems. They are enhanced in this edition to include activities using the Internet.
- Recurring displays throughout the text highlight important content and create points of interest for student learning.
  - Levels of Prevention boxes address a chapter topic, describe nursing actions at each of the three levels of prevention, and are unique to this text.
  - Research: Bridge to Practice boxes describe a current public health or nursing research study related to the chapter subject matter.
  - The Global Community boxes emphasize an international perspective on chapter topics.
  - New art has been added throughout the text to clarify important concepts and enhance your interest in and understanding of material.
  - A Glossary and Appendices provide definitions of all key terms highlighted throughout the text, plus other important resources for student learning and community health nursing practice.

Features New to This Edition

Additional recurring displays new to this edition include:
- Voices From the Community—in these displays clients, practicing nurses, and students share their feelings about the topic presented in the chapter in which they appear. This personalizes the material and lets you feel what the person is expressing.
- Clinical Corner—17 case studies have been incorporated in key chapters throughout the text. Each Clinical Corner includes a case study and concludes with questions for critical thinking. These cases do not always get easily solved, just as in the real world of community health nursing, and give you a "real" picture of the community.
- Bridging Financial Gaps—these displays explore examples from practice and the nursing literature where services are more easily and clearly delivered to clients. They demonstrate innovative approaches to "cutting red tape" that often impedes clients from getting services.
- At the end of most chapters there are Internet sites appropriate to the content and 800 numbers to assist with accessing services for clients.
- Additional Assessment Tools—this edition is greatly enhanced by the inclusion of many assessment tools. There are tools for assessing communities, families, cultures, diets, teens and others for substance abuse and other addictive behaviors, gang involvement, home and neighborhood safety, and geriatric medication and fall prevention safety. These tools enhance your ability to assess client needs and serve the community.

Ancillary Teaching-Learning Services

A complete supplemental teaching-learning service is available to students and faculty on the Internet. This innovative feature is provided through Lippincott Williams & Wilkins' website, called *Connection,* and includes both student and faculty features.

STUDENT FEATURES

The student-focused *Connection* website includes several features found in the text that are updated regularly and are designed to be companion learning tools for the student:

- Clinical Corner—regularly updated interactive case studies designed to enhance your application of the pedagogic material in the text.
- Research: Bridge to Practice—regularly updated summaries of public health and public health nursing research that has an impact on practice.
- Bridging Financial Gaps—regularly updated information about the latest ways the government, local communities, or neighborhood programs are bridging financial gaps for clients.
- Voices From the Community—input from professionals, peers, and clients in the community regarding their feelings about current public health issues.

The following features are also included:

Interactive Exercises. The website includes interactive exercises based on key concepts recurring throughout the text. For example, an interactive exercise may focus on your role as a community health nurse in eliminating a communicable disease in a particular community. In order to accomplish this you may need to access resources to conduct a community assessment, explore issues related to school-age children, use principles of epidemiology, and update yourself on communicable disease control. The exercise takes you to four chapters in the text and may necessitate your accessing other Internet resources, which encourages you to integrate information from a variety of sources in order to solve the problem, just as community health nurses must do.

Chapter Outlines. These outlines are designed to assist you with organizing your thoughts about each chapter. They can be used as highlights for studying material to prepare you for testing.

Sample Test Questions. Sample test questions are included. An analysis is given for each distractor chosen and why it is the best answer or why it is not a good answer choice. This will help you understand community health nursing content and should prepare you better for the NCLEX.

FACULTY FEATURES

The ancillary Internet teaching package for faculty includes the following:

Chapter Outlines. These outlines will assist you in your classroom planning and weighing numbers and types of test items you will use.

Overhead Transparencies. A set of about 75 overhead transparencies is provided as a companion to the text. They are available for faculty use to enhance classroom discussion and promote student learning.

Suggested Classroom Activities. Approximately 100 suggested classroom activities are provided to enhance discussion and student learning. They will assist you in creating a more active learning environment.

Testbank. Test questions for each chapter are included. There are approximately 200 NCLEX-style multiple-choice questions and a key is provided for all questions with rationale for the correct answers and distractors.

Judith Ann Allender, RN,C, MSN, EdD
Barbara Walton Spradley, RN, MN

Acknowledgments

We are grateful to many individuals for their assistance in completing this fifth edition. To acknowledge them all would be impossible, given the limitations of space and memory. Many have unwittingly enriched the writing by sharing their experiences and expertise. Others have directly provided ideas, criticism, encouragement, and support. To all we offer our sincere gratitude.

Many individuals have made important new contributions to this fifth edition. Sixteen chapters were written in whole or in part by contributing authors. These experts in the field were sought out specifically for their expertise and currency in the area explored in their chapters. Many are faculty members in universities and colleges around the country. Some are in practice and teach part-time. All have contributed excellent information to enhance this edition of *Community Health Nursing: Concepts and Practice*. We wish to thank the contributors to past editions whose work, in many cases, is still entwined in the chapters of this edition. We are grateful to each of them.

We wish to thank our faculty colleagues for their ideas and encouragement. In particular, we are grateful to Ben Cuellar and Mariamma Mathai at California State University, Fresno.

Others have made a variety of contributions to this fifth edition. First, we want to thank our students for assistance with research, stimulation, and support, especially Vera Ko-valenkov, Noemi Loeffel, Susan Viola, and Khoua Yang. We are also grateful to the many community colleagues in both nursing and other fields who have supported and contributed to our efforts.

We would like to thank the many people who provided their suggestions and assistance as reviewers throughout the revision process.

Many people at Lippincott Williams & Wilkins have provided invaluable assistance. We are grateful to Susan Glover, our editor for most of this revision, for her direction, support, and patience, and to Margaret Zucarrini, who inherited this project and guided us in a professional manner to completion. Special thanks also go to Laura Bonazzoli, developmental editor, for her outstanding vision and editorial critique; to Bridgett Blateau and especially Hilarie Surrena for their editorial assistance; and to Tom Gibbons for excellent production editing. We arc grateful to all the other helpful people at Lippincott Williams & Wilkins.

Finally, we are grateful to the many friends and family members who provided essential encouragement and assistance. We especially wish to thank Beth Allender for her research efforts. Thanks to our families for encouragement and inspiration. Most importantly, we are grateful to our husbands, Gil Allender and Neil Kittlesen, for their unflagging support, interest, and encouragement. Their lives in our lives make the effort worthwhile.

Contents

UNIT VI Aggregates With Developmental Needs   513

Opportunities and Challenges of Community Health Nursing

KEY TERMS

- Aggregate
- Biostatistics
- Collaboration
- Common-interest community
- Community
- Community health
- Community health nursing
- Community of solution
- Continuous needs
- Epidemiology
- Episodic needs
- Evaluation
- Geographic community
- Health
- Health continuum
- Health promotion
- Illness
- Population
- Population-focused
- Primary prevention
- Public health
- Public health nursing
- Rehabilitation
- Research
- Secondary prevention
- Self-care
- Self-care deficit
- Tertiary prevention
- Wellness

LEARNING OBJECTIVES

Upon mastery of this chapter, you should be able to:
- Define community health and distinguish it from public health.
- Explain the concept of community.
- Describe three types of communities.
- Diagram the health continuum.
- Differentiate between the three levels of prevention.
- Analyze six components of community health practice.
- Describe eight characteristics of community health nursing.

On entering the new millennium, the opportunities and challenges in nursing are boundless. New biotechnologies offer opportunities not experienced before: women can give birth to eight living babies in one delivery; multiple defective organs can be replaced; and aged astronauts can spend days in space. However, challenges abound, since millions of people die each year from wars, drought, and starvation; preventable ancient, new, and reemerging infectious diseases; and unhealthy lifestyle choices. In addition, opportunities and challenges confront the nurse personally and professionally. It seems that on completing a professional degree in nursing, the complexity of career decisions would become more simple. This is not the case, since the choices are confounded by the expanding arenas in which nurses practice.

As a specialty in nursing practice, community health nursing offers unique challenges and opportunities. For the nurse entering this field, there is the challenge of understanding and the opportunity for enriching the heritage of early public health nursing efforts. There is the challenge of expanding nursing's focus from the individual and family to encompass communities, and the opportunity to impact the health status of populations. There also is the challenge of determining the needs of populations at risk and the opportunity for designing interventions to address their needs. There is the challenge of learning the complexities of the health care system and the opportunity to shape its service delivery. Community health nursing is community based and, most importantly, it is population focused. Operating within an environment of rapid change and increasingly complex challenges, this field of nursing holds the potential for positively shaping the quality of community health services and improving the health of the general public.

You have provided nursing care in familiar acute care settings with the very ill, both young and old, with other professionals at your side. You worked as part of a team, in close proximity, to welcome a new life, reestablish a client's health, or comfort someone toward a peaceful death. Now, you are being asked to leave the familiarity of the acute care setting and go out into the community—into homes, schools, recreational facilities, the work setting, and other environments that are familiar to clients and unfamiliar to you. Here, there are minimal or no monitoring devices, charts full of laboratory data, or professional and allied health workers at your side to assist you. You will be asked to use the nontangible skills of listening, assessing, planning, teaching, coordinating, evaluating, and referring. Often, your practice will be solo and you will need to combine creativity, ingenuity, and resourcefulness along with the above-mentioned skills. You will be providing care not only to individuals but also to families and other groups in a variety of settings within the community. Talk about boundless opportunities and challenges! But perhaps, just perhaps, you might find this a rewarding kind of nursing—one that constantly challenges you, interests you, and allows you to use your skills holistically with clients of all ages, at all stages of illness and wellness; one that absolutely demands the use of your critical-thinking skills. And you may decide, when you finish your community health nursing course, that you have found your career choice; finding out begins with understanding the concepts of community and health.

This chapter provides an overview of the basic concepts of the terms *community* and *health,* the components of community health practice, and the salient characteristics of contemporary community health nursing practice so that you can enter this field of nursing in concert with its intentions. The opportunities and challenges of community health nursing will become even more apparent as the chapter progresses. The discussion of the concepts and theories that make community health nursing an important specialty within nursing begins with the broader field of community health, which provides the context and essential content for community health nursing practice.

COMMUNITY HEALTH

Human beings are social creatures. All of us, with rare exception, live out our lives in the company of other people. An Eskimo lives in a small, tightly knit community of close relatives; a rural Mexican lives in a small village with hardly more than 200 members. In contrast, a New Yorker might be a member of many overlapping communities such as professional societies, a political party, religious group, neighborhood, and city. Even those who try to escape community membership always begin their lives in some type of group and usually continue to depend on groups for material and emotional support. Communities are an essential and permanent feature of the human experience.

The communities in which we live and work have a profound influence on our collective health and well-being. Here are three examples:

- Research has established that both smoking and passive exposure to tobacco smoke are directly associated with negative health effects (Andrews, 1998). More states, communities, and organizations (including hospitals, schools, restaurants, and airlines) have developed regulatory approaches to smoking. They include removing cigarette vending machines, prohibiting televised commercials, increasing cigarette taxes, and restricting smoking in public places. Such community rules protect nonsmokers, promote the potential for reduced heart and lung disease on a community-wide basis, and have contributed to the downward trend in cigarette smoking in the last three decades (McDermott et al., 1998). Community-wide efforts to identify causative lifestyle factors followed by appropriate interventions to reduce chronic diseases are ongoing in several countries (Jeffery & French, 1998; Nusselder et al., 1996; Spake, 1998).
- In the early 1990s Vanderbilt University and Medical Center in Nashville, Tennessee, initiated a comprehensive health promotion program, called HEALTH Plus. It included lifestyle change interventions delivered through seminars, behavior change programs, fitness testing, aerobics, and strength and flexibility conditioning. It received the Tennessee Governor's Council on Physical Fitness and Health Award as the top work site health promotion program in the state during 1992. Cholesterol levels of 397 high-risk employees dropped from 231 to 218 mg/dL; more than 50% of 11,000 employees participated in at least one health promotion activity; and after only 1 year of operation, a 22% difference in costs from health care claims was observed between participants and nonparticipants (Cavanaugh & Price, 1993). In this instance, collective health was influenced by the community in which these people worked.
- On a larger scale, state laws that require using a seat belt and child restraints and that severely penalize the combination of drinking and driving protect motorists and reduce the risk of vehicular crashes, injuries, and death.

Just as a whole is greater than the sum of its parts, the health of a community is more than the sum of the health of its individual citizens. A community that achieves a high level of wellness is composed of healthy citizens, functioning in an environment that protects and promotes health. Community health, as a field of practice, seeks to provide organizational structure, a broad set of resources, and the collaborative activities needed to accomplish the goal of an optimally healthy community.

In acute care, the health of an individual is the primary focus. Community health broadens that focus to concentrate on families, populations, and the community at large. The community becomes the recipient of service, and health becomes the product. Viewed from another perspective, community health is concerned with the interchange between population groups and their total environment, and with the impact of that interchange on collective health.

Although many believe that health and illness are individual issues, evidence indicates that they also are community issues. Spread of the HIV pandemic, nationally and internationally, is a dramatic and tragic case in point (U.S. Agency for International Development, 1997). Other community and national concerns are the rising incidence and prevalence of sexually transmitted diseases, substance abuse, tuberculosis, teen pregnancy, family and teen violence, terrorism, and pollution-driven environmental hazards. Communities can influence the spread of disease, provide barriers to protect members from health hazards, organize ways to combat outbreaks of infectious disease, and promote practices that contribute to individual and collective health (Nossal, 1998; Sourtzi et al., 1996; Stockhausen, 1994).

Many different professionals work in community health to form a complex team. The city planner designing an urban renewal project necessarily becomes involved in community health. The social worker counseling on child abuse or the use of chemical substances among adolescents is involved in community health. A physician treating clients affected by a sudden outbreak of hepatitis and seeking to find the source is engaged in community health practice. Prenatal clinics, meals for the elderly, genetic counseling centers, and educational programs for the early detection of cancer all are part of the community health effort.

The professional nurse is an integral member of this team, a linchpin and a liaison between physicians, social workers, government officials, and law enforcement officers. Community health nurses work in every conceivable kind of community agency from a state public health department to a community-based advocacy group. Their duties range from examining infants in a well-baby clinic or teaching elderly stroke victims in their homes, to carrying out epidemiologic research or engaging in health policy analysis and decision-making. Despite its breadth, however, community health nursing is a specialized practice. It combines all of the basic elements of professional, clinical nursing with public health and community practice. This text examines the unique contribution made by community health nursing to our health care system.

Community health and public health share many features. Both are organized community efforts aimed at the promotion, protection, and preservation of the public's health. Historically, as a field of practice, public health mostly has been associated with official or government efforts—for example, federal, state, or local tax-supported health agencies that target the whole range of health issues. In contrast, private health efforts, such as the American Lung Association or the American Cancer Society, work toward solving selected health problems. The latter augments the former. Currently, public health practice encompasses both and works collaboratively with all health agencies and efforts, public or private, concerned with the public's health. In this text, community health practice refers to a focus on specific, designated communities. It thus is a part of the larger public health effort and recognizes the fundamental concepts and principles of public health as its birthright and foundation for practice.

Winslow's classic 1920 definition of public health still holds true and forms the basis for our understanding of community health in this text:

> **Public health is the science and art of preventing disease, prolonging life, and promoting health and efficiency through organized community efforts for the sanitation of the environment, the control of communicable infections, the education of the individual in personal hygiene, the organization of medical and nursing services for the early diagnosis and preventive treatment of disease, and the development of the social machinery to insure everyone a standard of living adequate for the maintenance of health, so organizing these benefits as to enable every citizen to realize his birthright of health and longevity (Pickett & Hanlon, 1990, p. 5).**

Turnock (1997) offers a more concise definition of public health and states that it includes "activities that society undertakes to assure the conditions in which people can be healthy. This includes organized community efforts to prevent, identify, and counter threats to the health of the public (p. 375)."

Given this understanding of public health, the concept of community health can be defined. **Community health** is the identification of needs and the protection and improvement of collective health within a geographically defined area.

One of the challenges community health practice faces is to remain responsive to the community's health needs. As a result, its structure is complex; numerous health services and programs are currently available or will be developed. Examples include health education, family planning, accident prevention, environmental protection, immunization, nutrition, early periodic screening and developmental testing, school programs, mental health, occupational health, and the care of vulnerable populations.

Community health practice, a part of public health, sometimes is misunderstood. Even many health professionals think of community health practice in limiting terms such as sanitation programs, clinics in poverty areas, or massive campaigns to prevent communicable disease. Although these are a part of its ever-broadening focus, community health practice is much more. To understand the nature and significance of this field, it is necessary to more closely examine the concept of community and the concept of health.

THE CONCEPT OF COMMUNITY

The discussion now focuses on the concepts of community and health. Together, these concepts provide the foundation for understanding community health. Broadly defined, a community is a collection of people who share some important feature of their lives. In this text, the term **community** refers to a collection of people who interact with one another and whose common interests or characteristics form the basis for a sense of unity or belonging. It can be a society of people holding common rights and privileges, as citizens of a town, or sharing common interest, as a community of farmers, or living under the same laws and regulations, as a prison community. The function of any community includes its members' collective sense of belonging, as well as shared identity, values, norms, communication, and common interests and concerns (Baldwin et al., 1998; Clark, 1999). Some communities, such as a tiny village in Appalachia, are composed of people who share almost everything. They live in the same location, work at a limited number of jobs, attend the same churches, and make use of the single health clinic with its visiting physician and nurse. Other communities, such as Mothers Against Drunk Driving or the community of professional nurses, are large, scattered, and composed of individuals who share only a common interest and involvement in a certain goal. Although most communities of people share many aspects of their experience, the following criteria provide a useful framework for identifying three types of communities that have relevance to community health practice: geography, common interest, and health problem.

Geographic Community

A community often is defined by its geographic boundaries and thus is called a **geographic community.** A city, town, or neighborhood is a geographic community. Consider the community of Hayward, Wisconsin. Located in northwestern Wisconsin, it is set in the north woods environment, far removed from any urban center and in a climatic zone characterized by extremely harsh winters. With a population of approximately 2000, it is considered a rural community. The population has certain identifiable characteristics, such as age and sex ratios, and its size fluctuates with the seasons: summers bring hundreds of tourists and seasonal residents. Hayward is a social system as well as a geographic location. The families, schools, hospital, churches, stores, and government institutions are linked in a complex network. This community, like others, has an informal power structure. It has a communication system that includes gossip, the newspaper, the "co-op" store bulletin board, and the radio station. In one sense, then, a community consists of a collection of people located in a specific place and is made up of institutions organized into a social system.

Local communities such as Hayward vary in size. A few miles south of Hayward lie several other communities, including Northwoods Beach and Round Lake; these three, along with other towns and isolated farms, form a larger community called Sawyer County. If a nurse worked for a health agency serving only Hayward, that community would be of primary concern; however, when working for the Sawyer County Health Department, this larger community would be the focus. A community health nurse employed by the State Health Department in Madison, Wisconsin, would have an interest in Sawyer County and Hayward, but only as one small part of the larger community of Wisconsin.

Frequently, a single part of a city can be treated as a community. In Seattle, for example, the district near the waterfront forms a community of many transient and homeless people. In New York, the neighborhood called Harlem is a community, as is the Haight-Ashbury district of San Francisco.

In community health, it is useful to identify a geographic area as a community. A community demarcated by geographic boundaries, such as a city or county, becomes a clear target for analysis of health needs. Available data, such as morbidity and mortality figures, can augment assessment studies to form the basis for planning health programs. Media campaigns and other health education efforts can readily reach intended audiences. Examples include distributing educational information on safe sex, self-protection, the dangers of substance abuse, or where to seek shelter from abuse and violence. A geographic community is easily mobilized for action. Groups can be formed to carry out intervention and prevention efforts that address needs specific to that community. Such efforts might include more stringent policies on day care, shelters for battered women, work site safety programs in local hazardous industries, or improved sex education in the schools. Furthermore, health actions can be enhanced through support of politically powerful individuals and resources present in a geographic community.

On a larger scale, the world can be considered as a global community. Indeed, it is becoming increasingly important to view the world this way. Borders of countries change with political revolution. Communicable diseases are not aware of arbitrary political boundaries. A person can travel around the world in 24 hours, and so can diseases. Children starving in Africa can and do affect persons living in the United States. The world is one large community that needs to work together to ensure a healthy today and a healthier tomorrow. "As part of renewing the health-for-all policy for the 21st century, the World Health Organization proposes that governments will need to work together to develop a broader base for international relations and collaborative strategies that will place greater emphasis on international health security" (Yach & Bettcher, 1998, p. 736).

Common-Interest Community

A community also can be identified by a common interest or goal. A collection of people, although they are widely scattered geographically, can have an interest or goal that binds the members together. This is called a **common-interest community.** The members of a church in a large metropolitan area, the members of a national professional organization, or women who have had mastectomies are all common-interest communities. Sometimes, within a certain geographic area, a group of people become a community by promoting their common interest. Disabled individuals scattered throughout a large city may emerge as a community through a common interest in promoting adherence to federal guidelines for wheelchair access, parking spaces, toilet facilities, elevators, or other services for the disabled. The residents in an industrial community may develop a common interest in air or water pollution issues, whereas others who work but do not live there may not share that interest. Communities form to protect the rights of children, stop violence against women, clean up the environment, promote the arts, preserve historical sites, protect endangered species, develop a smoke-free environment, or provide support after a crisis. The kinds of shared interests that lead to the formation of communities are widely varied.

Common-interest communities whose focus is on a health-related issue become a useful medium for change. The group's single-minded commitment is a mobilizing force for action. Many successful prevention and health promotion efforts, including improved services and increased community awareness of specific problems, have resulted from the work of common- interest communities.

Community of Solution

A type of community encountered frequently in community health practice is a group of people who come together to solve a problem that affects all of them. The shape of this community varies with the nature of the problem, the size of the geographic area affected, and the number of resources needed to address the problem. Such a community has been called a **community of solution** (National Commission on Community Health Services, 1967). A water pollution problem may involve several counties whose agencies and personnel must work together to control upstream water supply, industrial waste disposal, and city water treatment. This group of counties forms a community of solution around a health problem. In another instance, several schools may collaborate with law enforcement and health agencies, as well as legislators and policy makers, to study patterns of students' substance abuse and design possible preventive approaches. The boundaries of this community of solution form around the schools, agencies, and political figures involved. Figure 1–1 depicts some communities of solution related to one city.

Recently, communities of solution have formed in many cities to attack the spread of HIV infection. Public health agencies, social service groups, schools, and media personnel have banded together to create public awareness of the dangers present and to promote preventive behaviors. A community of solution is an important medium for change in community health.

Populations and Aggregates

The three types of communities just discussed underscore the meaning of the concept of community: in each instance, a collection of people choose to interact with one another be-

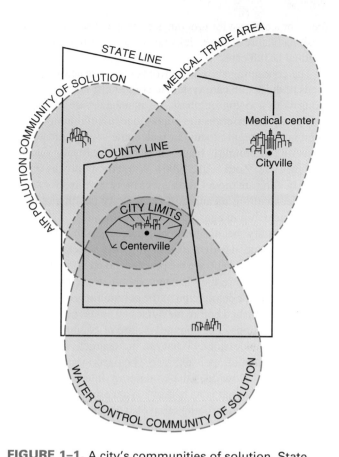

FIGURE 1–1. A city's communities of solution. State, county, and city boundaries (shown in solid lines) may have little or no bearing on health solution boundaries.

cause of common interests, characteristics, or goals. The concept of population has a different meaning. In this text, the term **population** refers to all of the people occupying an area, or all those sharing one or more characteristics. A population, in contrast to a community, is made up of people who do not necessarily interact with one another and who do not necessarily share a sense of belonging to that group. A population may be defined geographically, such as the population of the United States or a city's population. This designation of a population is useful in community health for epidemiologic study and for collecting demographic data for purposes such as health planning. A population also is defined by common qualities or characteristics, such as the elderly population or the homeless population. In community health, this meaning becomes useful when targeting intervention with a specific group of people, such as the homeless, whose common characteristics, such as their homelessness with its health-related problems, become a major focus of the intervention.

In this text, an **aggregate** refers to a mass or grouping of distinct individuals who are considered as a whole and who are loosely associated with one another. It is a broader term, encompassing many different-sized groups. Both communities and populations are types of aggregates. Thus, the aggregate focus, or a concern for groupings of people, becomes a distinguishing feature of community health practice in contrast to individual health care.

The continuing shift away from acute care settings as the focus of the health care system to community-based services, along with a rising emphasis on managed care of populations, only underscores the importance of community health nursing's aggregate focus. In fact, some say it validates the focus of community health nursing over many decades (Smith, 1998; Zotti et al., 1996). With community as central to the health care model, it becomes more essential for nurses to understand the meaning of community health and to assume leadership in aggregate level health care.

Community health workers, including the community health nurse, need to define the community targeted for study and intervention: Who are the people who compose the community? Where are they located and what are their characteristics? A clear delineation of the community or population must be established before the nurse can assess needs and design interventions. The complex nature of communities also needs to be understood. What are the characteristics of the people in terms of age, sex, race, socioeconomic level, and health status? How does the community interact with other communities? What is its history? What are its resources? Is the community undergoing rapid change, and if so, what are the changes? These questions, as well as the tools needed to assess a community for health purposes, are discussed in detail in Chapter 18.

THE CONCEPT OF HEALTH

Health in the abstract refers to a person's physical, mental, and spiritual state; it can be positive (as being in good health) or negative (as being in poor health). The World Health Organization defines health positively as "a state of complete physical, mental, and social well-being and not merely the absence of disease or infirmity" (Thomas, 1997, p. 845). Our understanding of the concept of health builds on this classic definition. **Health,** in this text, refers to a holistic state of well-being, which includes soundness of mind, body, and spirit. Community health practitioners value a strong emphasis on **wellness,** which includes the definition of health just mentioned but incorporates the capacity to develop a person's potential to lead a fulfilling and productive life, one that can be measured in terms of quality of life (Harper & Lambert, 1994). They also are beginning to understand the relationship of health to environment.

This is not a new concept. Almost a century and a half ago, Florence Nightingale explored the health and illness connection with the environment. She believed that a person's health was greatly influenced by ventilation, noise, light, cleanliness, diet, and a restful bed. She laid down simple rules about maintaining and obtaining "health," which were written for lay women caring for family members to "put the constitution in such a state as that it will have no disease" (Nightingale, 1859, preface).

In some cultures, health is viewed differently. Some see it as the freedom from and the absence of evil. Illness, to some, is seen as punishment for being bad or doing evil (Spector, 2000). Many nurses may come from or know families in which health and illness beliefs are heavily influenced by superstition, folk beliefs, or "old wives tales." This is not unusual, and encountering such beliefs when working with various groups in the community is common. Chapter 4 explores these beliefs more thoroughly for a better understanding of how health beliefs influence every aspect of a person's life.

Although health is widely accepted as desirable, the nature of health often is ambiguous. Consumers and providers often define health and wellness in different ways. To clarify the concept for nurses who are considering community health practice, the distinguishing features of health are briefly characterized; the implications of this concept for professionals in the field can then be examined more fully.

The Health Continuum: Wellness–Illness

Society suggests a polarized or black-and-white way of thinking about health: people are either well or ill. Yet wellness is a relative concept, not an absolute, and **illness** is a state of being *relatively* unhealthy. There are many levels and degrees of wellness and illness, from a robust 70-year-old woman who is fully active and functioning at an optimal level of wellness, to a 70-year-old man with end-stage renal disease. Someone recovering from pneumonia may be mildly ill, whereas a teenaged boy with limitations in functioning because of episodic depression may be described as mildly well. Because health involves a range of degrees from optimal health at one end to total disability or death at the other (Fig. 1–2), it often is described as a continuum. This **health continuum** applies not only to individuals but also to families and communities. A nurse might speak of a dysfunctional family, meaning they are experiencing a relative degree of illness; or a healthy family might be described as one that exhibits many wellness characteristics such as effective communication and conflict resolution, as well as the ability to work together and use resources appropriately. Likewise, a community, as a collection of people, may be described in terms of degrees of wellness or illness.

A healthy community, first described by Cottrell (1976) as a competent community, is one in which the various organizations, groups, and aggregates of people making up the community do at least four things:

1. They collaborate effectively in identifying the problems and needs of the community.
2. They achieve a working consensus on goals and priorities.
3. They agree on ways and means to implement the agreed-on goals.
4. They collaborate effectively in the required actions.

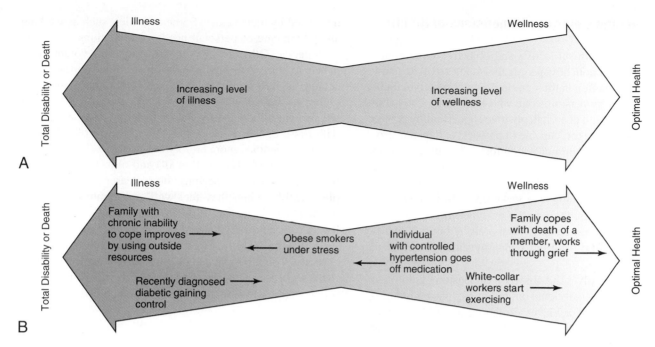

FIGURE 1–2. A. The wellness–illness continuum. The level (degree) of illness increases as one moves toward total disability or death; the level of wellness increases as one moves toward optimal health. This continuum shows the relative nature of health. At any given time a person can be placed at some point along the continuum. **B.** Dynamic nature of the wellness-illness continuum. A person's relative health is usually in a state of flux, either improving or deteriorating. This diagram of the wellness–illness continuum shows several examples of people in changing states of health.

The health of an individual, family, group, or community moves back and forth along this continuum throughout life.

By thinking of health relatively, as a matter of degree, the scope of nursing practice can be broadened to focus on preventing illness or disability and promoting wellness. Traditionally, most health care has focused on treatment of acute and chronic conditions at the illness end of the continuum. Gradually, the emphasis is shifting to focus on the wellness end of the continuum (U.S. Department of Health and Human Services, 2000). Community health practice ranges over the entire continuum; it always works to improve the degree of health in individuals, families, groups, and communities. In particular, community health practice emphasizes the promotion and preservation of wellness and the prevention of illness or disability (Hudson-Rodd, 1994).

Health as a State of Being

Health refers to a state of being including many different qualities and characteristics. An individual might be described in terms such as energetic, outgoing, enthusiastic, beautiful, caring, loving, and intense. Together, these qualities become the essence of a person's existence; they describe a state of being. Similarly, a specific geographic community, such as a neighborhood, has many characteristics. It might be characterized by the terms congested, deteriorating,

unattractive, dirty, and disorganized. These characteristics suggest diminishing degrees of vitality. A third example might be a population, such as workers involved in a massive layoff who band together to provide support and share resources to effectively seek new employment. This community shows signs of healthy and positive coping.

Health involves the total person or the total community. All of the dimensions of life affecting everyday functioning determine an individual's or a community's health, including physical, psychological, spiritual, economic, and sociocultural experiences. All of these factors must be considered when dealing with the health of an individual or community. The approach should be holistic. Thus, clients' placement on the health continuum can be known only if the nurse considers all facets of their lives, including not only their physical status but also the status of home, family, and work.

When considering an aggregate or group of people in terms of health, it becomes useful for intervention purposes to speak of the "health of a community." With aggregates as well as individuals, health as a state of being does not merely involve that group's physical state but also includes psychological, spiritual, and socioeconomic factors. The health of south central Los Angeles after the riots in the early 1990s is an example. Extensive damage from interracial fighting, burning, and looting left the community totally devastated. This community's health was at a dangerously low point and in need of healing and restoration.

Subjective and Objective Dimensions of Health

Health involves both subjective and objective dimensions; that is, it involves both how people feel (subjective) and how well they can function in their environment (objective). Subjectively, a healthy person is one who feels well, who experiences the sensation of a vital, positive state. Healthy people are full of life and vigor, capable of physical and mental productivity. They feel minimal discomfort and displeasure with the world around them. Again, people experience varying degrees of vitality and well-being. The state of feeling well fluctuates. Some mornings we wake up feeling more energetic and enthusiastic than we do on other mornings. How people feel varies day by day, even hour by hour; nonetheless, how they feel overall is a strong indicator of their state of health.

Health also involves the objective dimension of ability to function. A healthy individual or community carries out necessary activities and achieves enriching goals. Unhealthy people not only feel ill but are limited, to some degree, in their ability to carry out daily activities. Indeed, levels of illness or wellness are measured largely in terms of ability to function (Hoeymans et al., 1997). A person confined to bed is labeled sicker than an ill person managing self-care. A family that meets its members' needs is healthier than one that has poor communication patterns and is unable to provide adequate physical and emotional resources. A community actively engaged in crime prevention or policing industrial wastes shows signs of healthy functioning. Degree of functioning is directly related to state of health (see Voices from the Community).

The ability to function can be observed. A man dresses and feeds himself and goes to work. Despite financial exigencies, a family nourishes its members through a supportive emotional climate. A community provides adequate resources and services for its members. These performances, to some degree, can be regarded as indicators of health status. Some community health agencies assess clients' ability to function as a measure of client progress and nursing care effectiveness (Bultema et al., 1996; Wilson, 1998).

The actions of an individual, family, or community are motivated by their values. Some activities, such as walking and taking care of personal needs, are functions valued by most people. Other actions (eg, bird watching, volunteering to help a charity, or running) have more limited appeal. In assessing the health of individuals and communities, the community health nurse can observe people's ability to function but also must know their values, which may contrast sharply with those of the professional. The influence of values on health is examined more closely in Chapter 5.

Subjective (feeling well or ill) and objective (functioning) dimensions together provide a clearer picture of people's health. When they feel well and demonstrate functional ability, they are close to the wellness end of the health continuum. Even those with a disease such as arthritis or diabetes may feel well and perform well within their capacity. These people can be considered healthy or closer to the wellness end of the continuum. Figure 1–3 depicts the relationships between the subjective and objective views of health.

Continuous and Episodic Health Care Needs

Community health practice encompasses populations in all age groups with birth-to-death developmental health care needs. These **continuous needs** may include parents needing assistance with providing a toddler-proof home, establishing positive toilet-training techniques, effectively dealing with the progressive emancipation of their preteens and teenagers, anticipatory guidance for reducing and managing the stress associated with retirement, or coping with the death of an aged parent. These are developmental events experienced by most people and represent typical life occurrences. The community health nurse has the skills to work at the individual, family, and group level to meet these needs. On an individual and family level, a home visit may be the appropriate place for intervention. If the nurse sees that the community has many young and growing families, and several families have similar developmental issues, a class for mothers and babies, parents and teenagers, or preretirement adults may be formed to meet weekly at the library or health clinic waiting room. In these instances, the nurse works with groups ranging from small to large.

In addition, populations may have one-time, specific, negative health events, such as an illness or injury, that are not an expected part of life. These **episodic needs** might include couples giving birth to infants with Down syndrome, teenagers incurring head injuries from an automobile crash, or adults diagnosed with HIV/AIDS.

In a given day, the community health nurse may interact with clients having either or both continuous and episodic health care needs. For example, when can parents expect children with Down syndrome to begin toilet training? How do middle-aged adults, planning their retirement and preparing for the death of an aged parent, deal with their adult child's AIDS diagnosis? Complex situations such as these

Voices from the Community

"I never thought much about being healthy or not, now that you ask. I keep busy, I cook like I'm expecting company, I have a good appetite. I really think all these so-called healthy things people suggest are fads, just so someone can get rich—like tofu and low fat this and that. Don't give me margarine, only butter, . . . and skim milk, it's like drinking water! I work in my garden, I read, and I eat fresh foods, and don't talk to me about my smoking, it's the one pleasure I have left."

—Bettie, age 81

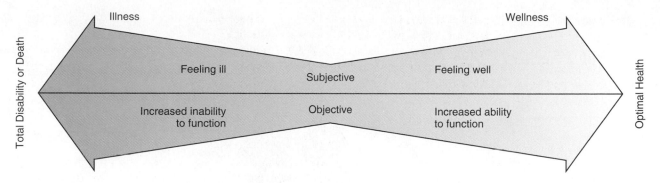

FIGURE 1–3. Subjective and objective views of the wellness–illness continuum.

may be positively influenced by the interaction with and services of the community health nurse.

COMPONENTS OF COMMUNITY HEALTH PRACTICE

Community health practice can best be understood by examining six basic components, which, when combined, encompass its services and programs: (1) promotion of health, (2) prevention of health problems, (3) treatment of disorders, (4) rehabilitation, (5) evaluation, and (6) research.

Promotion of Health

Promotion of health is recognized as one of the most important components of public health and community health practice (Sourtzi et al., 1996; U.S. Department of Health and Human Services, 1998). **Health promotion** includes all efforts that seek to move people closer to optimal well-being or higher levels of wellness. Nursing, in particular, has a social mandate for engaging in health promotion (Erickson, 1996; Pender, 1996). Health promotion programs and activities include many forms of health education such as teaching the danger of drug use, demonstrating healthful practices like regular exercise, and providing more health-promoting options like heart-healthy menu selections. Community health promotion, then, encompasses "the development and management of preventive or primary health care systems responsive to community health needs" (Erickson, 1996, p. 168). Wellness programs in schools and industry are an example and are useful when accompanied by desire, opportunity, and resources that encourage more healthful practices (Luepker et al., 1996; Wong et al., 1996). Demonstration of such healthful practices as eating nutritious foods, either vegetarian (Fig. 1–4) or nonvegetarian (Fig. 1–5), and exercising more regularly often is performed and promoted by individual health workers. In addition, groups and health agencies that support a smoke-free environment, encourage physical fitness programs for all ages, or demand that food products be properly labeled underscore the importance of these practices and create public awareness.

The goal of health promotion is to raise levels of wellness for individuals, families, populations, and communities. Community health efforts accomplish this goal through a three-pronged effort to:

1. Increase the span of healthy life for all citizens
2. Reduce health disparities among population groups
3. Achieve access to preventive services for everyone

Specifically, in the 1980s, the U.S. Public Health Service published the Surgeon General's report, *Healthy People,* and continued with *Promoting Health, Preventing Disease: 1990 Health Objectives for the Nation* and *Healthy People 2000.* The Surgeon General's report provided vision and an agenda for significantly reducing preventable death and disability nationwide, enhancing quality of life, and greatly reducing disparities in the health status of populations. It emphasized the need for individuals to assume personal responsibility for controlling and improving their own health destiny. It challenged society to find ways to make good health available to vulnerable populations whose disadvantaged state placed them at greater risk for health problems. Finally, it called for an intensified shift in focus from treating preventable illness and functional impairment to concentrating resources and targeting efforts that promote health and prevent disease and disability (Allison et al., 1999; U.S. Department of Health and Human Services, 1998). In the late 1990s, the U.S. Public Health Service outlined 28 priority areas for intervention in its publication *Healthy People 2010* (2000) (Display 1–1). Under each of the 28 areas, *Healthy People 2010* outlines several objectives, stated in measurable terms, that specify targeted incidence and prevalence changes and that address age, gender, and culturally vulnerable groups along with improvement in public health systems. Healthy people make healthy communities and a healthy society.

The implications of this national agenda for health have far-reaching consequences for persons engaged in health care. For centuries health care has focused on the illness end of the health continuum, but health professionals can no longer justify concentrating most of their efforts exclusively on treating the sick and injured. We now live in an

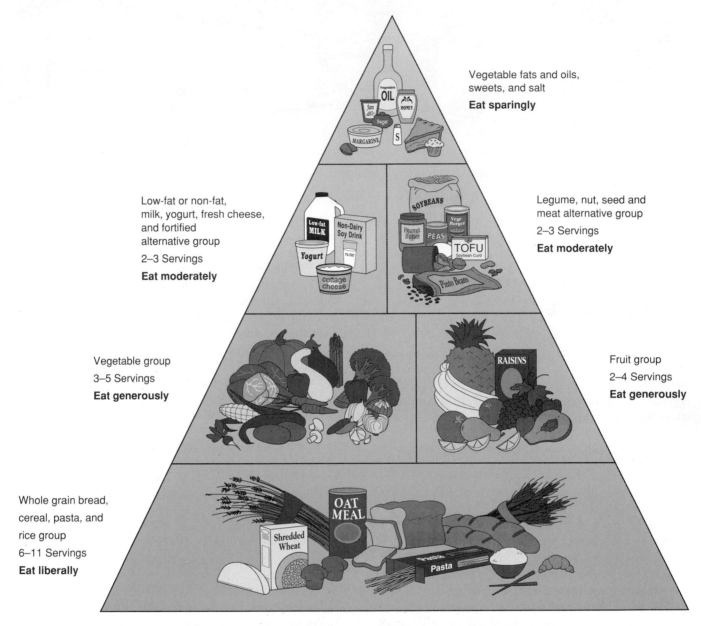

FIGURE 1–4. The vegetarian food pyramid. (Adapted from the Vegetarian Resource Group of the American Dietetic Association, The Health Connection.)

age when it is not only possible to promote health and prevent disease and disability, but our mandate and responsibility is to do so (U.S. Department of Health and Human Services, 2000).

Prevention of Health Problems

Prevention of health problems constitutes a major part of community health practice. Prevention means anticipating and averting problems or discovering them as early as possible to minimize possible disability and impairment. It is practiced on three levels in community health: (1) primary prevention, (2) secondary prevention, and (3) tertiary prevention (see Levels of Prevention) (Neuman, 1995; Turnock, 1997; Williams & Torrens, 1999). These concepts recur throughout this text, since they are basic to community health nursing. Once the differences among the levels of prevention are recognized, a sound foundation on which to build additional community health principles can be developed.

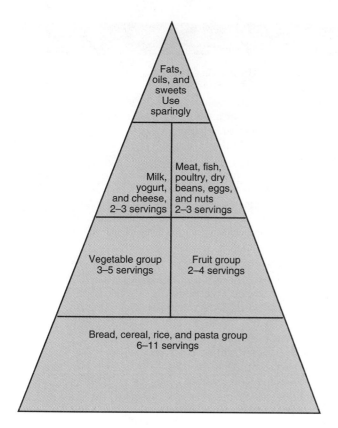

FIGURE 1–5. The Food Pyramid. In April of 1992, the U.S. Department of Agriculture replaced the old four food groups, in use since 1946, with the food pyramid. It emphasizes grains, fruits, and vegetables as the basis of a healthy diet. Recommended daily servings in each group are noted.

Primary prevention obviates the occurrence of a health problem; it includes measures taken to keep illness or injuries from occurring. It is applied to a generally healthy population and precedes disease or dysfunction. Examples include a community health nurse who encourages elderly people to install and use safety devices, such as grab bars by bathtubs or hand rails on steps, to prevent injuries from falls, and the nurse who teaches young adults healthy lifestyle behaviors so that they can adopt changes for a lifetime, for themselves and their children. Local health departments help to control and prevent communicable diseases such as rubeola or poliomyelitis by providing regular immunization programs. Primary prevention involves anticipatory planning and action on the part of community health professionals who must project themselves into the future, envision potential needs and problems, and then design programs to counteract them so that they never occur. A community health nurse who instructs a group of overweight individuals on how to follow a well-balanced diet while losing weight is preventing the possibility of nutritional deficiency. Educational programs that teach safe-sex practices or the dangers of smoking and substance abuse are other examples of primary prevention. In addition,

when the community health nurse serves on a fact-finding committee exploring the effects of a proposed toxic waste dump on the outskirts of town, the nurse is concerned about primary prevention. The concepts of primary prevention and planning for the future are foreign to many social groups who may resist on the basis of conflicting values. The Parable of the Dangerous Cliff (Display 1–2) illustrates such a value conflict.

Secondary prevention involves efforts to detect and treat existing health problems at the earliest possible stage when disease or impairment already exist. Hypertension or cholesterol screening in many communities helps to identify high-risk individuals and encourages early treatment to prevent heart attacks or stroke. Other examples are teaching breast and testicular self-examination, encouraging regular mammograms and Pap smears for early detection of possible cancer, and providing skin testing for tuberculosis when infants are 1 year of age and periodically throughout life, with increasing frequency for high-risk groups. Secondary prevention attempts to discover a health problem at a point when intervention may lead to its control or eradication. This is the goal behind water and soil testing for contaminants and hazardous chemicals in community environmental health. It also prompts community health nurses to watch for early signs of child abuse in a family, emotional disturbances in a group of widows, or alcohol and drug abuse among adolescents.

Tertiary prevention attempts to reduce the extent and severity of a health problem to its lowest possible level to minimize disability and restore or preserve function. Examples include treatment and rehabilitation of persons after a stroke to reduce impairment, postmastectomy exercise programs to restore functioning, and early treatment and management of diabetes to reduce problems or slow their progress. The persons involved have an existing illness or disability whose impact on their lives is lessened through tertiary prevention. In broader community health practice, tertiary prevention is used to minimize the effects of an existing unhealthy community condition. Examples of such prevention are insisting that people provide wheelchair access, warning urban residents about the dangers of a chemical spill, and recalling a contaminated food or drug product. When a community experiences a disaster such as an earthquake or a tornado, preventing injuries among the survivors or volunteers during rescue is another example of tertiary prevention—eliminating additional injury to those already experiencing a tragedy.

Health assessment of individuals, families, and communities is an important part of all three levels of preventive practice. Health status must be determined to anticipate problems and select appropriate preventive measures. Community health nurses working with young parents who themselves have been victims of child abuse can institute early treatment for the parents to prevent abuse and foster adequate parenting of their children. If assessment of a community reveals inadequate facilities and activities to meet the future needs of its growing senior population, agencies and groups can collaborate to develop the needed resources.

DISPLAY 1–1. Issues in Community Health Nursing

Priority Areas for National Health Promotion and Disease Prevention

The context in which *Healthy People 2010* was developed differs from that in which Healthy People 2000 was framed—and will continue to evolve through the decade. Advances in preventive therapies, vaccines and pharmaceuticals, assistive technologies, and computerized systems will all change the face of medicine and how it is practiced. New relationships will be defined between public health departments and health care delivery organizations. Meanwhile, demographic changes in the United States—reflecting an older and more radically diverse population—will create new demands on public health and the overall health care system. Global forces—including food supplies, emerging infectious diseases, and environmental interdependence—will present new public health challenges (U.S. Department of Health and Human Services, 2000).

Its report, *Healthy People 2010,* states two broad goals: to (1) increase the quality and years of healthy life, and (2) eliminate health disparities. To accomplish these goals, measurable objectives were established under each of the following 28 priority areas:

Healthy People 2010 Focus Areas

1. Access to Quality Health Services
2. Arthritis, Osteoporosis, and Chronic Back Conditions
3. Cancer
4. Chronic Kidney Disease
5. Diabetes
6. Disability and Secondary Conditions
7. Educational and Community-Based Programs
8. Environmental Health
9. Family Planning
10. Food Safety
11. Health Communication
12. Heart Disease and Stroke
13. HIV
14. Immunization and Infectious Diseases
15. Injury and Violence Prevention
16. Maternal, Infant, and Child Health
17. Medical Product Safety
18. Mental Health and Mental Disorders
19. Nutrition and Overweight
20. Occupational Safety and Health
21. Oral Health
22. Physical Activity and Fitness
23. Public Health Infrastructure
24. Respiratory Diseases
25. Sexually Transmitted Diseases
26. Substance Abuse
27. Tobacco Use
28. Vision and Hearing

This national listing is a guide to policy makers and health planners at all levels. It provides a framework for prioritizing and addressing specific health needs in designated communities.

Health problems are most effectively prevented by maintaining healthy lifestyles and healthy environments. To these ends, community health practice directs many of its efforts to providing safe and satisfying living and working conditions, nutritious food, and clean air and water. This area of practice includes the field of preventive medicine, which is a population-focused, or community-oriented, branch of medical practice that incorporates public health sciences and principles (Barton, 1999).

Treatment of Disorders

The third component of community health practice is treatment of disorders. It focuses on the illness end of the continuum and is the remedial aspect of community health practice. This occurs by three methods: (1) direct service to people with health problems, (2) indirect service that helps people to obtain treatment, and (3) development of programs to correct unhealthy conditions. Examples of direct service include the following: a nursing center serving a homeless population provides health screening, education, and referral ser-

vices; elderly persons confined to home with disabling chronic illness obtain home visits from a nursing agency for assistance with treatment regimens, supervision of medications, and personal care; or a neighborhood health center provides an educational program and support group for people wanting to stop smoking or lose weight. Many kinds of community agencies provide direct health care or health-related services.

The second method of treating disorders is indirect service by assisting people with health problems to obtain treatment. In many instances, a community agency may not be able to provide needed care and refers the individuals or groups concerned to a more appropriate resource. A young woman with postpartum bleeding, assisted by the community health nurse, can obtain an immediate appointment with a physician at the local clinic. A social worker can help a family that is plagued by personal and economic problems to enter a family therapy and counseling program. Several community agencies provide information and referral services. An effective community health nurse works diligently to develop partnerships with health care workers in agencies that provide services to potential clients. The quality of this

LEVELS OF PREVENTION

DIETARY PRACTICES

GOAL

To avoid nutritional deficiencies and enhance community nutritional status through healthy dietary practices

PRIMARY PREVENTION

Provide educational programs, literature, and posters of the food pyramids in schools, work sites, food stores, and other public places to promote awareness. Encourage restaurants to offer healthy menu items. Teach families how to cook healthy foods, do a kitchen cupboard survey, recommend nutrition classes offered at neighborhood centers.

SECONDARY PREVENTION

Conduct community screening programs for early detection of individuals with poor eating habits among groups such as adolescents, young female workers, and the elderly. Initiate educational and incentive programs to improve dietary practices. Teach individuals and families on a one-to-one basis how to modify eating habits to promote wellness.

TERTIARY PREVENTION

Case finding in schools and work sites to diagnose those persons who have eating disorders (ie, anorexia, bulimia, compulsive eating), or other lifestyle patterns that inhibit positive dietary practices, and work with the individual, initiating treatment and incorporating other professionals as appropriate.

partnership is paramount in ensuring that clients' needs are met. It builds a bridge between the client who has a health care need and the individual or group who provides a service to meet the need. A strong relationship may make the difference between the resolution of a problem and frustration with the health care system.

The third method of treatment of disorders is the development of programs to correct unhealthy conditions. One community with a high incidence of alcoholism and drug abuse initiated a chemical dependency counseling and treatment center. In another community, the health department developed new regulations for industrial waste disposal as a result of increased pollution of the water supply. Individual community members and health workers also take corrective action to remedy situations such as a case of apparent child abuse, poor nutrition in a school lunch program, or inhumane conditions and treatment in a nursing home.

Rehabilitation

Rehabilitation, the fourth component of community health practice, involves efforts to reduce disability and, as much as possible, restore function. People whose handicaps are congenital or acquired through illness or accident, such as

DISPLAY 1–2. Parable of the Dangerous Cliff

Twas a dangerous cliff, as they freely confessed,
    Though to walk near its crest was so pleasant;
But over its terrible edge there has slipped
    A duke, and full many a peasant.
The people said something would have to be done
    But their projects did not at all tally.
Some said, "Put a fence around the edge of the cliff";
    Some, "an ambulance down in the valley."
The lament of the crowd was profound and was loud,
    As their hearts overflowed with their pity;
But the cry of the ambulance carried the day
    As it spread through the neighboring city.
A collection was made to accumulate aid
    And the dwellers in highway and alley
Gave dollars or cents
Not to furnish a fence
But "an ambulance down in the valley."
"For the cliff is all right if you're careful," they said.
"And if folks ever slip and are dropping,
    It isn't the slipping that hurts them so much
As the shock down below when they're stopping."
So for years (we have heard), as these mishaps occurred,
    Quick forth the rescuers sally,
To pick up the victims who fell from the cliff,
    With the ambulance down in the valley.
Said one in his plea, "It's a marvel to me

That you'd give so much greater attention
To repairing results than to curing the cause;
You had much better aim at prevention.
    For the mischief, of course, should be stopped at its
        source,
Come neighbors and friends, let us rally.
    It is far better sense to rely on a fence
Than an ambulance down in the valley."
"He is wrong in his head," the majority said;
    "He would end all our earnest endeavor.
He's a man who would shirk this responsible work,
    But we will support it forever.
Aren't we picking up all, just as fast as they fall,
    and giving them care liberally?
A superfluous fence is of no consequence,
If the ambulance works in the valley."
The story looks queer as we've written it here,
    But things oft occur that are stranger.
More humane, we assert, than to care for the hurt,
    Is a plan for removing the danger.
The very best plan is to safeguard the man,
    And attend to the thing rationally;
To build up the fence and try to dispense
    With the ambulance down in the valley.
Better still! Cut down the hill!
—*Author Unknown*

stroke, heart condition, amputation, or mental illness, can be helped to regain some measure of lost function or to develop new compensating skills. For example, a factory worker who lost his leg in an industrial accident received good medical and nursing care, prosthetic fittings, and physical and occupational therapy; he then retrained to assume an office job.

In community health, the need to reduce disability and restore function applies equally to families, groups, communities, and individuals. Many groups form for rehabilitation and offer support and guidance for those recuperating from some physical or mental disability. Examples include Alcoholics Anonymous, halfway houses for psychiatric patients discharged from acute care settings, ostomy clubs, or drug rehabilitation programs. Rehabilitation services often are needed and sought by whole communities, as when an inner city area desires to provide decent, safe playgrounds for its children.

As an element of community health practice, rehabilitation becomes increasingly significant when disease trends and changes in life expectancy are considered. Chronic diseases, such as cancer, heart disease, diabetes, and mental illness, are major cripplers. So, too, are accidents and injuries from many causes, including violence. Abuse of drugs, alcohol, and tobacco further adds to the list of disabling conditions. As a result, the need for rehabilitation services and long-term care has increased, stimulated further by the rising number of elderly persons with chronic health problems (Kaye et al., 1996).

Evaluation

Evaluation, the fifth component of community health practice, is the process by which that practice is analyzed, judged, and improved according to established goals and standards. Evaluation of health and health care should be an integral part of every kind of health service, from individual practice to national and international programs. Whether done on a single-case basis or at the program level, evaluation helps to solve problems and provides direction for future health care efforts. Its goals are to determine the needs and success of activities and to develop improved services. In one community, evaluation of mental health services revealed a need for more comprehensive psychiatric emergency care on a 24-hour basis. If a psychiatric crisis occurred during the night, police were the only persons available to help, and jail was the only place to take the mentally ill person. The deficiency was corrected by providing 24-hour psychiatric emergency service in the community mental health center. In other instances, evaluation of community-wide education programs targeting cardiovascular disease showed a reduction in risk factors (Stofan et al., 1998; Winkleby et al., 1996), and evaluation of school and work site health promotion programs showed their effect on program goals (McCormick et al., 1995; Resnicow et al., 1998). Evaluation studies of many types of

community health interventions exist in the literature and provide insights and direction for further community health planning.

A comprehensive discussion of evaluation is provided in Chapters 19 and 24.

Research

Research, the sixth component of community health practice, is systematic investigation to discover facts affecting community health and community health practice, solve problems, and explore improved methods of health service. Community health practitioners conduct and use scientific investigations at all levels, from federal agencies such as the U.S. Public Health Service to state and local groups conducting research. **Epidemiology** (the study of health and disease determinants and distribution in populations) and **biostatistics** (the science of statistically measuring population health conditions) are the primary public health measurement and analytic sciences underlying community health practice. Chapter 14 addresses these sciences more extensively.

Researchers in community health investigate the characteristics and patterns of illness and health. Conditions such as food poisoning, trauma, alcoholism, lung cancer, child abuse, drug dependency, and suicide are studied for possible causes and means of prevention. Health and healthful behavior are analyzed, for example, in nutrition projects and studies of normal human growth and behavior for a better understanding of ways to promote healthful living.

Community health researchers also explore ways to improve health care. For example, an experimental intervention program among 22 work sites was aimed at increasing consumption of fruits and vegetables. It was found that interventions that included work site *plus* family involvement were more successful in increasing fruit and vegetable consumption than was work site intervention alone (Sorensen et al., 1999). A review of community-based nursing research provided evidence that "community-based nursing practice includes quality services that can control costs; a focus on disease prevention and health promotion; the organization of services where people live, work, and learn; partnerships and coalitions; service to people across the life span; services to culturally diverse populations; access to services for at-risk populations; development of the community's capacity for health; work with policy makers for policy change; and efforts to make the environment healthier" (Flynn, 1998, p. 165). Other research projects focus on the effectiveness of drug treatment programs, long-term stroke rehabilitation, improved treatment approaches to obesity, or empowerment of the disenfranchised and underserved.

Chapter 11 expands on the community health nurse's role in the use and conduct of research.

Community health researchers also examine the impact of social and environmental factors on health and health services provision. For example, one study on the effects of a 25¢ cigarette tax imposed in Massachusetts revealed that it promoted quitting among adult smokers and reduced cigarette consumption among low-income teenagers (Biener et al., 1998). Other research studies identify social, environmental, and psychological factors contributing to the poor health of homeless families (Gelberg et al., 1997; Herman et al., 1997). More studies center on the needs and care of the elderly and other age-specific groups (Conn, 1998). Others investigate ways to improve health services' planning and policy development through efforts such as studying the community's needs and program utilization.

CHARACTERISTICS OF COMMUNITY HEALTH NURSING

Eight characteristics of community health nursing are particularly salient to the practice of this specialty: (1) it is a field of nursing; (2) it combines public health with nursing; (3) it is population focused; (4) it emphasizes prevention, health promotion, and wellness; (5) it promotes client responsibility and self-care; (6) it uses aggregate measurement and analysis; (7) it uses principles of organizational theory; and (8) it involves interprofessional collaboration.

Field of Nursing

The two characteristics of any specialized nursing practice are (1) specialized knowledge and skills, and (2) focus on a particular set of people receiving the service. These two characteristics are true for community health nursing. As a specialty field of nursing, community health nursing adds public health knowledge and skills that address the needs and problems of communities and aggregates and focuses care on communities and vulnerable populations.

Confusion over the meaning of "community health nursing" arises when it is defined only in terms of where it is practiced. Because health care services have shifted from the hospital to the community, many nurses in other specialties now practice in the community. Examples of these practices include home care, mental health, geriatric nursing, long-term care, or occupational health. Although community health nurses today practice in the same or similar settings as other specialties, the difference lies in applying the public health principles to large groups and communities of people (Fig. 1–6). For nurses moving into this field of nursing, it requires a shift in focus—from individuals to aggregates. Nursing and other theories undergird its practice (see Chapter 17), and the nursing process (incorporated in Chapters 18 and 19) is one of its basic tools (see Levels of Prevention discussed earlier).

Community health nursing, then, as a field of nursing, combines nursing science with public health science to formulate a community-based and population-focused practice

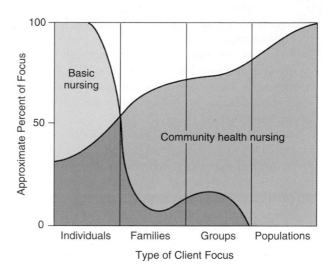

FIGURE 1–6. Difference in client focus between basic nursing and community health nursing.

(Williams, 2000). It "synthesizes the knowledge from the public health sciences and professional nursing theories" (ANA, 1999, 2000) to improve the health of communities and vulnerable populations. For instance, community health nurses are nursing when their concern for homeless individuals sleeping in a park leads to development of a program providing food and shelter for this population. Community health nurses are nursing when they collaborate to institute an AIDS education curriculum in the local school system. When they assess the needs of elderly people in retirement homes to ensure necessary services and provide health instruction and support, they are, again, nursing.

During the first 70 years of this century (1900 to 1970), community health nursing was known as **public health nursing.** The later title of community health nursing was adopted to better describe where the nurse practices, but the terms, as used here, are interchangeable.

Combines Public Health with Nursing

Community health nursing is grounded in both public health science and nursing science, which makes its philosophical orientation and the nature of its practice unique. It has been recognized as a subspecialty of both fields. Recognition of this specialty field continues with a greater awareness of the important contributions made by community health nursing to improve the health of the public (Zerwekh, 1992).

Knowledge of the following elements of public health is essential to community health nursing (ANA, 1999; Williams, 1977, 1983, 2000):

1. History and philosophy of public health, including emphasis on the greatest good for the greatest number
2. Concept of aggregates—assessing needs, planning and providing services, and evaluating services' impact on

population groups—including aggregate-level decision-making

3. Priority of preventive, protective, and health-promoting strategies over curative strategies
4. Means for measurement and analysis of community health problems, including epidemiologic concepts and biostatistics
5. Influence of environmental factors on aggregate health
6. Principles underlying management and organization for community health, since the goal of public health is accomplished through organized community efforts
7. Public policy analysis and development
8. Health advocacy and the political process

There are many ways in which community health nursing incorporates public health knowledge into its practice. For example, it is general knowledge that physical activity may contribute to important health and well-being outcomes among older adults. What has been overlooked in the literature are the determinants of and beliefs about physical activity among older women living in the community. One nurse in Columbia, Missouri, conducted a study using qualitative interviews with 30 older women (Conn, 1998). The findings, when compared with exercise among 30 similar women who took part in an episodic exercise study, revealed that the women in this study talked about physical activity as embedded in their social lives. The women in the episodic exercise study viewed exercise as separate from their daily lives. These findings of beliefs about overall physical activity suggest that a social model may be useful in planning public health interventions to increase activity among older women. This gives the community health nurse valuable information about exercise as seen by older adult women so that better programs can be planned. In another study, a group of community health nurses were part of an experimental study to test the effectiveness of a physical education program among 422 third and fourth graders. Two groups— a population-based group including all children in the classroom, and a risk-based group of children with at least two risk factors for cardiovascular disease—were selected (Harrell et al., 1998). The researchers determined that the brief intervention improved the cardiovascular disease risk profile of both groups of children and that the classroom, or population-based approach, was easier to implement and used fewer resources. This epidemiologic study combined public health and nursing practice to show that nurses can be agents for change in community health.

Population Focused

The central mission of public health practice is to improve the health of population groups. Community health nursing shares this essential feature: it is **population focused,** meaning that it is concerned for the health status of population groups and their environment. A population may consist of the elderly living throughout the community or southeast

Asian refugees clustered in one section of a city. It may be a scattered group with common characteristics, such as people at high risk of developing coronary heart disease or battered women living throughout a county. It may include all people living in a neighborhood, district, city, state, or province. Community health nursing's specialty practice serves populations and aggregates of people.

Working with individuals and families as parts of aggregates has been common for community health nursing; however, such work must expand to incorporate a population-oriented focus, a feature that distinguishes it from other nursing specialties. Basic nursing focuses on individuals and community health nursing focuses on aggregates, but the many variations in community needs and nursing roles inevitably cause some overlap (Display 1–3).

A population-oriented focus requires the assessment of relationships. When working with groups and communities, the nurse does not consider them separately but rather in context, that is, in relationship to the rest of the community. When an outbreak of hepatitis occurs, for example, the community health nurse does more than work with others to treat it. The nurse tries to stop spread of the infection, locate possible sources, and prevent its recurrence in the community.

DISPLAY 1–3. **Parable of the Trees: Population-Focused Practice**

There were once two sisters who inherited a large tract of heavily forested land from their grandmother. In her will, the grandmother stipulated that they must preserve the health of the trees. One sister studied tree surgery and became an expert in recognizing and treating diseased trees. She also was able to spot conditions that might lead to problems and prevent them. Her work was invaluable in keeping single or small clusters of trees healthy. The other sister became a forest ranger. In addition to learning how to care for individual trees, she studied the environmental conditions that affected the well-being of the forest. She learned the importance of proper ecologic balance between flora and fauna and the impact of climate, geography, soil conditions, and weather. Her work was to oversee the health and growth of the whole forest. Although she spent time walking through the forest assessing conditions, her aerial view from their small plane was equally important for spotting fires, signs of disease, or other potential problems. Together, the sisters preserved a healthy forest.

Nursing also has tree surgeons and forest rangers. Various nursing specialties, like the tree surgeons, serve the health needs of individuals and families. Community health nurses, like the forest rangers, study and address the needs of populations. Both are needed and must work together to ensure healthy communities.

As a result of their population-oriented focus, community health nurses seek to discover possible groups with a common health need, such as expectant mothers, or groups at high risk of developing a common health problem, such as potential diabetics or victims of child abuse. Community health nurses continually look for problems in the environment that influence community health and seek ways to increase environmental quality. They work to prevent health problems, such as promoting school-based education about safe sex or exercise programs for groups of seniors.

A population-oriented focus involves a new outlook and set of attitudes. Individualized care is important, but prevention of aggregate problems in community health nursing practice reflects more accurately its philosophy and benefits more people. The community or population-at-risk is the client. Furthermore, since community health nurses are concerned about several aggregates at the same time, service will, of necessity, be provided to multiple and overlapping groups.

Emphasizes Prevention, Health Promotion, and Wellness

In community health nursing, the promotion of health and prevention of illness are of first-order priority. There is less emphasis on curative care. Some corrective actions always are needed, such as cleanup of a toxic waste dump site, stricter enforcement of day care standards, or home care of the disabled; however, community health best serves its constituents through preventive and health-promoting actions (U.S. Department of Health and Human Services, 1998). These include services to mothers and infants, prevention of environmental pollution, school health programs, senior citizens' fitness classes, and "workers' right-to-know" legislation that warns against hazards in the workplace.

Another distinguishing characteristic of community health nursing is its emphasis on positive health, or wellness (McNab, 1996; Pavri, 1994). Medicine and acute care nursing deal primarily with the illness end of the health continuum. In contrast, community health nursing has a primary charge to prevent health problems from occurring and to promote a higher level of health. For example, although a community health nurse may assist a population of new mothers in the community with postpartum fatigue and depression, the nurse also works to prevent such problems among women of child-bearing age by developing health education programs, establishing prenatal classes, and encouraging proper rest, nutrition, adequate help, and stress reduction.

Community health nurses concentrate on the wellness end of the health continuum in a variety of ways. They teach proper nutrition or family planning, promote immunizations among preschool children, encourage regular physical and dental checkups, assist with starting exercise classes or physical fitness programs, and promote healthy interpersonal relationships. Their goal is to help the community reach its optimal level of wellness.

This emphasis on wellness changes the community health nursing role from a reactive to a proactive stance. It places a greater responsibility on community health nurses to find opportunities for intervention. In clinical nursing and medicine, the patients seek out professional assistance because they have health problems. As Williams put it several years ago, "patients select themselves into the care system, and the providers' role is to deal with what the patients bring to them" (1977, p. 251). Community health nurses, in contrast, seek out potential health problems. They identify high-risk groups and institute preventive programs. They watch for early signs of child neglect or abuse and intervene when any occur, often long before a request for help is made. They look for possible environmental hazards in the community, such as smoking in public places, and work with appropriate authorities to correct them. A wellness emphasis requires taking initiative and making sound judgments, which are characteristics of effective community health nursing.

Promotes Client Responsibility and Self-Care

The goal of public health, "to increase quality and years of healthy life and eliminate health disparities" (U.S. Department of Health and Human Services, 1998), requires a partnership effort. Just as learning cannot take place in schools without student participation, the goals of public health cannot be realized without consumer participation. Community health nursing's efforts toward health improvement go only so far. Clients' health status and health behavior will not change unless people accept and apply the proposals (developed in collaboration with clients) presented by the community health nurse.

Community health nurses can encourage individuals' participation by promoting their autonomy rather than permitting a dependency. For example, elderly persons attending a series of nutrition or fitness classes can be encouraged to take the initiative and develop health or social programs on their own. Independence and feelings of self-worth are closely related. By treating people as independent adults, with trust and respect, community health nurses help promote self-reliance and the ability to function independently.

Consumers frequently are intimidated by health professionals and are uninformed about health and health care. They do not know what information to seek and are hesitant to act assertively. For example, a migrant worker brought her 2-year-old son, who had symptoms resembling those of scurvy, to a clinic. Recognizing a vitamin C deficiency, the physician told her to feed the boy large quantities of orange juice but gave no explanation. Several weeks later, she returned; the child was much worse. After questioning her, the nurse discovered that the mother had been feeding the child large amounts of an orange soft drink, not knowing the difference between that and orange juice. Obviously, the quality of care is affected when the consumer does not understand and cannot participate in the health care process.

When people believe that their health, and that of the community, is their own responsibility, not just that of health professionals, they will take a more active interest in promoting it. The process of taking responsibility for developing one's own health potential is called **self-care** (Orem, 1995; Stanhope & Knollmueller, 1997), a concept discussed in Chapter 19. As people maintain their own lives, health, and well-being, they are engaging in self-care. Some examples of self-care activities at the aggregate level include a community building safe playgrounds, developing teen employment opportunities, and providing senior exercise programs.

When people's ability to continue self-care activities drops below their need, they experience a **self-care deficit.** At this point, nursing may appropriately intervene. However, nursing's goal is to assist clients to return to or reach a level of functioning where they can attain optimal health and assume responsibility for maintaining it (Orem, 1995). To this end, community health nurses foster their clients' sense of responsibility by treating them as adults capable of managing their own affairs. Nurses can encourage people to negotiate health care goals and practices, develop their own programs, contact their own resources (such as support groups or transportation services), identify and implement lifestyle changes that promote wellness, and learn ways to monitor their own health.

Uses Aggregate Measurement and Analysis

Community health nursing uses aggregate measurement and analysis. The need to collect and examine data on the entire population under study before making intervention decisions is fundamental to community health nursing in a public health practice. Analyses of health states, environmental factors, health-related services, economic patterns, and social policy are among the many foci of community health research and evaluation, described further in Chapters 11 and 19.

Uses Principles of Organizational Theory

Community health nursing uses principles from organizational theory to provide effective administration of health care services. Public health has long been defined as the protection and improvement of community health through organized community efforts. It is the organization and administration of such services that enables practitioners to ultimately address community needs. Chapter 6 elaborates on this subject.

As community health nurses carefully assess group and community needs, establish priorities, and plan, implement, and evaluate services, they are using public health management and organizational principles. For example, Redford and Whitten (1997) write about the role of communication technology in ensuring access to care and information in rural areas. They cite a variety of programs that keep clients,

students, and others in contact with needed services. For example, in Lawrence, Kansas, the Home-Based Electronic Link to Professionals allows nurses to use interactive tele-video (ITV) to monitor chronically ill patients, guide caregivers in performing tasks, and educate and support patients and families without being physically present in the home. A hospice project uses low-end ITV equipment, which runs through a patient's television over regular telephone lines, to enable hospice nurses to be available for terminally ill patients and their families. Other programs use community education courses, delivered through ITV, to enhance participation from rural students in academic course work and for consumer health education. Consumers have access to programs on diabetes, Alzheimer disease, coping with cancer, attention deficit disorders, and weight management. Also, they can interact with health care professionals hundreds of miles away from their rural homes.

Involves Interprofessional Collaboration

Community health nurses must work in cooperation with other team members, coordinating services and addressing the needs of population groups. This interprofessional **collaboration** among health care workers, other professionals, and clients is essential in establishing effective services and programs. Individualized efforts and specialized programs, when planned in isolation, can lead to fragmentation and gaps in health services. For example, without collaboration, a well-child clinic may be started in a community that already has a strong early and periodic developmental screening and testing program, yet community prenatal services may be nonexistent. Interprofessional collaboration is important in individualized practice, since nurses need to plan with the physician, social worker, physical therapist, teacher, or counselor and must keep them informed of the client's health status; however, it is a greater necessity when working with population groups (Corrigan & Udas, 1996; Hooper-Briar & Lawson, 1996).

Effective collaboration requires team members who are strong individuals with various areas of expertise and who can make a commitment to team goals. Community health nurses who think and act interdependently make a great contribution to the team effort. In appropriate situations, community health nurses also function autonomously, making independent judgments. Collaboration involves working with members of other professions on community advisory boards and health planning committees to develop needs assessment surveys and contribute toward policy development efforts.

Interprofessional collaboration requires clarification of each team member's role, a primary reason for community health nurses to understand the nature of their practice. When planning a city-wide immunization program with a community group, for example, community health nurses need to explain the ways that they might contribute to the program's objectives. They can offer to contact key community leaders, with whom they have established relationships, to build community acceptance of the program. They can share their knowledge of the public's preference about times and locations for the program. They can help to organize and give the immunizations, and they can influence planning for follow-up programs. Collaboration is discussed further in Chapter 8.

Client participation is promoted when people serve as partners on the health care team. An aim of community health nursing is to collaborate with people rather than do things for them. As consumers of health services are treated with respect and trust and, as a result, gain confidence and skill in self-care—promoting their own health and that of their community—their contribution to health programs will become increasingly valuable. The consumer perspective in planning and delivering health services makes those services relevant to consumer needs. Community health nurses encourage the involvement of health care consumers by soliciting their ideas and opinions, by inviting them to participate on health boards and committees, and by finding ways to promote their participation in decisions affecting their collective health.

SUMMARY

Community health nursing has opportunities and challenges to keep the nurse interested and involved in a community-focused career for a lifetime. Community health is more than environmental programs and large-scale efforts to control communicable disease. It is defined as the identification of needs and the protection and improvement of collective health within a geographically defined area. To comprehend the nature and significance of community health and to clarify its meaning for the specialty practice of community health nursing, it is important to understand the concepts of community and of health.

A community, broadly defined, is a collection of people who share some common interest or goal. There are three types: geographic, common-interest, and health problem-solving communities. Sometimes, a community such as a neighborhood, city, or county is formed by geographic boundaries. At other times, a community may be identified by its common interest; examples are a religious community, a group of migrant workers, or citizens concerned about air pollution. A community also is defined by a pooling of efforts by people and agencies toward solving a health-related problem.

Health is an abstract concept that can be understood more clearly by examining its distinguishing features. First, people are neither sick nor well in an absolute sense but have levels of illness or wellness. These levels may be plotted along a continuum ranging from optimal health to total disability or death. This is known as the health continuum. Thus, a person's state of health is dynamic, varying from day to day and even hour to hour.

Second, health is a state of being that includes all of the many characteristics of a person, family, or community: physical, psychological, social, and spiritual. These characteristics often indicate the degree of wellness or illness of an individual or community and suggest the presence or absence of vitality and well-being.

Third, health has both subjective and objective dimensions: the subjective involves how well people feel; the objective refers to how well they are able to function. Most often, functional performance diminishes dramatically toward the illness end.

Fourth, health care needs can be either continuing, as in developmental concerns occurring over a person's lifetime, or episodic, occurring unexpectedly once or twice in a lifetime. Community health nursing deals with continuing needs, whereas episodic needs are managed in acute care settings.

Community health practice incorporates six basic elements: (1) promotion of health, (2) prevention of health problems, (3) treatment of disorders, (4) rehabilitation, (5) evaluation, and (6) research.

The eight important characteristics of community health practice include the following: (1) it is a field of nursing; (2) it combines public health with nursing; (3) it is population focused; (4) it emphasizes prevention, health promotion, and wellness; (5) it promotes client responsibility and self-care; (6) it uses aggregate measurement and analysis; (7) it uses principles of organizational theory; and (8) it involves interprofessional collaboration.

ACTIVITIES TO PROMOTE CRITICAL THINKING

1. Identify a community of people about whom you have some knowledge. What makes it a community? What characteristics does this group of people share? Work on this activity in a group of peers or family members. Do they think like you think? Is there a difference between the views of family members versus nursing student peers?
2. Select two populations for whom you have some concern and place each group on the health continuum. What factors influenced your decision? What factors influenced where each group was placed on the continuum?
3. Describe three preventive actions (one primary, one secondary, and one tertiary) that might be taken to move each of your selected populations closer to optimal wellness.
4. Select a current, common health problem and break it down into the three levels of prevention. At each level, identify activities in which the community health nurse would engage.

5. Discuss how you might implement one health-promotion effort with your selected populations.

6. Browse the Internet for community health nursing research articles that focus on levels of prevention. Find one focusing on each level. What could you have done as a community health nurse to approach the health of those involved in the articles focusing on secondary and tertiary prevention to have kept the clients at the primary level of prevention?

7. Place yourself on the health continuum. What factors influenced your decision?

8. Using the eight characteristics of community health nursing outlined in this chapter, give examples of how a community health nurse might demonstrate meeting each characteristic.

REFERENCES

Allison, J., Kiefe, C., & Weissman, N.W. (1999). Can data-driven benchmarks be used to set the goals of Healthy People 2010? *American Journal of Public Health, 89*(1), 61–65.

American Nurses Association (1999). *Scope and standards of public health nursing practice.* Washington, D.C.: American Nurses Publishing.

American Nurses Association (2000). *Public health nursing: A partner for healthy populations.* Washington, D.C.: American Nurses Publishing.

Andrews, J. (1998). Optimizing smoking cessation strategies. *The Nurse Practitioner, 23*(8), 47–65.

Baldwin, J.H., Conger, C.O., Abegglen, J.C., & Hill, E.M. (1998). Population-focused and community-based nursing: Moving toward clarification of concepts. *Public Health Nursing, 15*(1), 12–18.

Barton, P.L. (1999). *Understanding the U.S. health service system.* Chicago: AUPHA Press.

Biener, L., Aseltine, R.H., Cohen, B., & Anderka, M. (1998). Reactions of adult and teenaged smokers to the Massachusetts tobacco tax. *American Journal of Public Health, 88*(9), 1389–1391.

Bultema, J.K., Mailliard, L. Getzfrid, M.K., Lerner, R.D., & Colone M. (1996). Geriatric patients with depression: Improving outcomes using a multidisciplinary clinical path model. *Journal of Nursing Administration. 26*(1), 31–38.

Cavanaugh, K.J. & Price, A.H. (1993, November/December). A worksite program that works. *Healthcare Forum Journal, 36*(6), 37.

Clark, M.J. (1999). The community context. In M.J. Clark (Ed.), *Nursing in the community* (3rd ed., pp. 3–11). Stamford, CT: Appleton & Lange.

Conn, V.S. (1998). Older adults and exercise: Path analysis of self- efficacy related constructs. *Nursing Research, 47*(3), 180–189.

Corrigan, D. & Udas, K. (1996). Creating collaborative child- and family-centered, education, health and human service systems. In J. Sikula, T. Buttery, & E. Guyton (Eds.), *The handbook of research on teacher education* (2nd ed., pp. 893–921). New York: Simon & Schuster Macmillan.

Cottrell, L.S., Jr. (1976). The competent community. In B.H. Kaplan, R.N. Wilson, & A.H. Leighton (Eds.), *Further explorations in social psychiatry.* New York: Basic Books.

Erickson, G.P. (1996). To pauperize or empower: Public health nursing at the turn of the 20th and 21st centuries. *Public Health Nursing, 13*(3), 163–169.

Flynn, B.C. (1998). Communicating with the public: Community-based nursing research and practice. *Public Health Nursing, 15*(3), 165–170.

Gelberg, L., Gallagher, T.C., Anderson, R. M., & Koegel, P. (1997). Competing priorities as a barrier to medical care among homeless adults in Los Angeles. *American Journal of Public Health, 87*(2), 217–220.

Harper, A.C., & Lambert, L.J. (1994). *The health of populations: An introduction* (2nd ed.). New York: Springer.

Harrell, J.S., Gansky, S.A., McMurray, R.G., Bangdiwala, S.I., Frauman, A.C., & Bradley, C.B. (1998). School-based interventions improve health in children with multiple cardiovascular disease risk factors. *Pediatrics, 102*(2), 371–380.

Herman, D.B., Susser, E.S., Struening, E.L., & Link, B.L. (1997). Adverse childhood experiences: Are they risk factors for adult homelessness? *American Journal of Public Health, 87*(2), 249–255.

Hoeymans, N., Feskens, E.J.M., van den Bos, G.A.M., & Kromhout, D. (1997). Age, time and cohort effects on functional status and self-rated health in elderly men. *American Journal of Public Health, 87*(10), 1620–1625.

Hooper-Briar, K. & Lawson, H.A. (1996). *Expanding partnerships for vulnerable children, youth, and families.* Alexandria, VA: Council on Social Work Education.

Hudson-Rodd, N. (1994). Public Health: People participating in the creating of healthy places. *Public Health Nursing, 11*(2), 119–126.

Jeffery, R.W. & French, S.A. (1998). Epidemic obesity in the United States: Are fast foods and television viewing contributing? *American Journal of Public Health, 88*(2), 277–280.

Kaye, H.S., LaPlante, M.P., Carlson, D., & Wenger, B.L. (1996). Trends in disability rates in the United States, 1970–1994. U.S. Department of Education, National Institute on Disability and Rehabilitation Research (NIDRR), 17, 1–6.

Luepker, R.V., Perry, C.L., McKinlay, S.M. et al. (1996) Outcomes of a field trial to improve children's dietary patterns and physical activity. *Journal of the American Medical Association, 275*(10), 768–776.

McCormick, L.K., Steckler, A.B., & McLery, K.R. (1995). Diffusion of innovations in schools: A study of adoption and implementation of school-based tobacco prevention curricula. *American Journal of Health Promotion, 9,* 210–219.

McDermott, S.R., Scott, K.L., & Frintner, M.P. (1998). Accessibility of cigarettes to minors in suburban Cook County, Illinois. *Journal of Community Health, 23*(2), 153–160.

McNab, C.M. (1996). The public health nursing role: An overview of future trends. *Nursing Standard, 10*(51), 44–48.

National Commission on Community Health Services. (1967). *Health is a community affair.* Cambridge: Harvard University Press.

Neuman, B. (1995). The Neuman systems model. In B. Neuman

(Ed.), *The Neuman systems model* (3rd ed.). Norwalk, CT: Appleton & Lange.

Nightingale, F. (1859). *Notes on nursing: What it is, and what it is not* [Commemorative edition, 1992]. Philadelphia: J.B. Lippincott.

Nossal, G. (1998). The biotechnology revolution and world health. *Public Health Reports, 113*(2), 122–127.

Nusselder, W.J., van der Velden, K., van Sonsbeek, J.L.A., Lenior, M.E., & van den Bos, G.A.M. (1996). The elimination of selected chronic diseases in a population: The compression and expansion of morbidity. *American Journal of Public Health, 86*(2), 187–194.

Orem, D. (1995). *Nursing concepts of practice* (5th ed.). St. Louis: Mosby–Year Book.

Pavri, J.M. (1994). Overview one hundred years of public health nursing: Visions of a better world. *Imprint, 41*(4), 43–48.

Pender, N.J. (1996). *Health promotion in nursing practice* (3rd ed.). Norwalk, CT: Appleton & Lange.

Pickett, G.E. & Hanlon, J.J. (1990). *Public health administration and practice.* (9th ed.). St. Louis: Times Mirror–Mosby.

Redford, L.J. & Whitten, P. (1997). Ensuring access to care in rural areas: The role of communication technology. *Generations, 21*(3), 19–23.

Resnicow, K., Davis, M., Smith, M., et al. (1998). Results of the teachwell worksite wellness program. *American Journal of Public Health, 88*(2), 250–257.

Smith, D.R. (1998). Public health and the winds of change. *Public Health Reports, 113*(2), 160–161.

Sorensen, G., Stoddard, A., Peterson, K., Cohn, N., Hunt, M.K., Stein, E., Palombo, R., & Lederman, R. (1999). Increasing fruit and vegetable consumption through worksites and families in the treatwell 5-a-day study. *American Journal of Public Health, 89*(1), 54–60.

Sourtzi, P., Nolan, P., & Andrews, R. (1996). Evaluation of health promotion activities in community nursing practice. *Journal of Advanced Nursing, 24,* 1214–1223.

Spake, A. (1998, December 21). The valley of death: Researchers probe a mysterious plague of heart disease. *U.S. News & World Report,* 53–54.

Spector, R.E. (2000). *Cultural diversity in health & illness* (5th ed.). Upper Saddle River, NJ: Prentice-Hall Health.

Stanhope, M. & Knollmueller, R.N. (1997). *Public and community health nurse's consultant: A health promotion guide.* St. Louis: Mosby–Year Book.

Stockhausen, L.J. (1994). Clinical strategies for health promotion. *Journal of Nursing Education, 33*(5), 232–235.

Stofan, J.R., DiPietro, L., Davis, D., Kohl, H.W., III, & Blair, S.N. (1998). Physical activity patterns associated with cardiorespiratory fitness and reduced mortality: The aerobics center longitudinal study. *American Journal of Public Health, 88*(12), 1807–1813.

Thomas, C.L. (Ed.) (1997). *Taber's cyclopedic medical dictionary* (18th ed.). Philadelphia: F.A. Davis.

Turnock, B.J. (1997). *Public health: What it is and how it works.* Gaithersburg, MD: Aspen Publishers.

U.S. Agency for International Development. (1997, December). *Accomplishments in HIV/AIDS programs* (pp. 1–16). Washington, DC: U.S. Agency for International Development.

U.S. Department of Health and Human Services. (2000). *Healthy People 2010* (conference edition, in two volumes). Washington, DC: U.S. Government Printing Office.

Williams, C. (2000). Community-based population-focused practice: The foundation of specialization in public health nursing. In M. Stanhope & J. Lancaster (Eds.), *Community health nursing: Process and practice for promoting health* (5th ed.). St. Louis: Mosby.

Williams, C.A. (1977). Community health nursing: What is it? *Nursing Outlook, 25*(4), 250–254.

Williams, C.A. (1983). Making things happen: Community health nursing and the policy arena. *Nursing Outlook, 31,* 225–228.

Williams, S.J. & Torrens, P.R. (1999). *Introduction to health services* (5th ed.) Albany: Delmar Publishers.

Wilson, A. (1998). Education is the key to understanding outcomes. *Home Healthcare Nurse, 16*(11), 785.

Winkleby, M.A., Taylor, C.B., Jatulis, D., & Fortmann, S.P. (1996). The long-term effects of a cardiovascular disease prevention trial: The Stanford five-city project. *American Journal of Public Health, 86*(12), 1773–1779.

Wong, Y., Bauman, K.E., & Koch, G.G. (1996). Increasing low income employee participation in a worksite health promotion program: A comparison of three common strategies. *Health Education Research, 11,* 71–76.

Yach, D. & Bettcher, D. (1998). Public health policy forum: The globalization of public health: I. Threats and opportunities. *American Journal of Public Health, 88*(5), 735–738.

Zerwekh, J.V. (1992). Community health nurses: A population at risk. *Public Health Nursing, 9*(1), 1.

Zotti, M.E., Brown, P., & Stotts, C. (1996). Community-based nursing versus community health nursing: What does it all mean? *Nursing Outlook 44*(5), 211–217.

SELECTED READINGS

Anderson, J. & Yuhos, R. (1993). Health promotion in rural settings: A nursing challenge. *Nursing Clinics of North America, 28*(1), 145–155, 157.

Baldwin, J.H. (1995). Are we implementing community health promotion in nursing? *Public Health Nursing, 12*(3), 159–164.

Bandura, A. (1995). Exercise of personal and collective efficacy in changing societies. In A. Bandura (Ed.), *Self-efficacy in changing societies* (pp. 1–45). New York: Cambridge University Press.

Black, D.R., Tobler, N.S., & Sciacca, J.P. (1998). Peer helping/involvement: An efficacious way to meet the challenge of reducing alcohol, tobacco, and other drug use among youth? *Journal of School Health, 68*(3), 87–93.

Castro, R.M. & Julia, M.C. (1994). *Interprofessional care and collaborative practice.* Pacific Grove, CA: Brooks–Cole Publishing Company.

Evans, R.G., Barer, M.L., & Marmor, T.R. (Eds.) (1994). *Why are some people healthy and others not? The determinants of health of populations.* Hawthorne, NY: Aldine de Gruyter.

Foege, W. (1994). Preventive medicine and public health. *Journal of the American Medical Association, 271*(21), 1704–1705.

Henry, V., Schmitz, K., Reif, L., & Rudie, P. (1992). Collaboration: Integrating practice and research in public health nursing. *Public Health Nursing, 9*(4), 218–222.

Hunt, D.L. & McKibbon, K.A. (1997). Locating and appraising systematic reviews. *Annals of Internal Medicine, 126,* 532–538.

Kiefe, C.I., Weissman, N.W., Allison, J.J., Farmer, R.M., Weaver, M., & Williams, O.D. (1998). Identifying achievable benchmarks of care (ABCs): Concepts and methodology. *International Journal of Quality Health Care, 10,* 443–447.

Martin, K. & Scheet, N. (1992). *The Omaha system: Applications for community health nursing.* Philadelphia: W.B. Saunders.

McKnight, J. & Van Dover, L. (1994). Community as client: A challenge for nursing education. *Public Health Nursing, 11*(1), 12–16.

National Center for Health Statistics. (1997). *Health, United States, 1996–1997 and injury chartbook.* Hyattsville, MD: National Center for Health Statistics.

National Institute for Nursing Research Priority Expert Panel. (1995). *Community-based health care: Nursing strategies.* Bethesda, MD: National Institute for Nursing Research.

Palmer, R.H. (1996). Quality health care. *Journal of the American Medical Association, 275*(23), 1851–1852.

Portnoy, F.L. & Dumas, L. (1994). Nursing for the public good. *Nursing Clinics of North America, 29,* 371–376.

Somerville, M.A. (1998). Making health, not war: Musings on global disparities in health and human rights. A critical commentary by Solomon R. Benatar. *American Journal of Public Health, 88*(2), 301–303.

Yankelovich, D. (1996). Trends in American cultural values. *Criterion, 35,* 2–9.

Zhu, B., Giovino G.A., Mowery, P.D., & Eriksen, M.P. (1996). The relationship between cigarette smoking and education revisited: Implications for categorizing persons' educational status. *American Journal of Public Health, 86*(11), 1582–1589.

Evolution of Community Health Nursing

KEY TERMS

■ Causal thinking
■ Community-based
  nursing
■ District nursing

LEARNING OBJECTIVES

Upon mastery of this chapter, you should be able to:
■ Describe the four stages of community health nursing's development.
■ Analyze the impact of societal influences on the development and practice of community health nursing.
■ Explore the academic and advanced professional preparation of community health nurses.

We believe that the story of the evolution of community health nursing—complete with its heroines, antagonists, battlefields, epidemics, plot twists, setbacks, and triumphs—is as exciting as any novel. And we hope that this brief overview of this fascinating story will inspire you to meet the challenges awaiting you in your own community health experience and to seize your opportunity to enrich the heritage of earlier public health nursing efforts.

This chapter examines the international roots of community health nursing as a specialty. The historical and philosophical foundations of community health nursing that undergird the dynamic nature of its practice are explored. First, the chapter traces community health nursing's historical development as a specialty practice. Next, it describes the global societal influences that shaped early and evolving community health nursing practice. Finally, the chapter describes the academic and advanced professional preparation needed of community health nurses today. Nursing's past influences its present, and both guide the future of community health nursing in the 21st century.

HISTORICAL DEVELOPMENT OF COMMUNITY HEALTH NURSING

Before the nature of community health nursing can be fully grasped or its practice defined, it is necessary to understand its roots and the factors that shaped its growth over time. Community health nursing is the product of centuries of responsiveness and growth. Its practice has adapted to accommodate the needs of a changing society, yet it has always maintained its initial goal of improved community health. Community health nursing's development, which has been influenced by changes in nursing, public health, and society, can be traced through several stages. This section examines these stages.

The history of public health nursing, since its recognized inception in Europe, and more recently in America, encompasses continuing change and adaptation (Pavri, 1994). The historical record reveals a professional nursing specialty that has been on the cutting edge of innovations in public health practice and has provided leadership to public health efforts. A summary of public health nursing made in the early 1900s still holds true:

> **It is precisely in the field of the application of knowledge that the public health nurse has found her great opportunity and her greatest usefulness. In the nationwide campaigns for the early detection of cancer and mental disorders, for the elimination of venereal disease, for the training of new mothers and the teaching of the principles of hygiene to young and old; in short, in all measures for the prevention of disease and the raising of health standards, no agency is more valuable than the public health nurse (Department of Philanthropic Information, 1938, p. 8).**

In tracing the development of public health nursing and, later, community health nursing, the leadership role clearly has been evident throughout its history. Nurses in this specialty have provided leadership in planning and developing programs, in shaping policy, in administration, and in the application of research to community health.

Four general stages mark the development of public health/community health nursing: (1) the early home care nursing stage, (2) the district nursing stage, (3) the public health nursing stage, and (4) the community health nursing stage.

Early Home Care Nursing (Before Mid-1800s)

Within the historical development of home care nursing, the prototype of **community-based nursing** can be seen; the term used to describe the setting for nursing care delivery. For many centuries, the sick were tended at home by female family members and friends. The focus of this care was to reduce suffering and promote healing (Kalisch & Kalisch, 1995). The Bible cites numerous instances of visiting the sick and extols a woman of noble character as one who "opens her arms to the poor and extends her hands to the needy" (Proverbs 31:20) and who is "a helper of many," as Phoebe was described in the New Testament (Romans 16:2).

The early roots of home care nursing began with religious and charitable groups. Medieval times saw the development of various institutions devoted to the sick, including hospitals and nursing orders. In England, the Elizabethan Poor Law, written in 1601, provided medical and nursing care to the poor and disabled. Another example was the friendly visitor volunteers organized by St. Frances de Sales in the early 1600s in France. This association was directed by Madame de Chantel and assisted by wealthy women who cared for the sick poor in their homes (Dolan, 1978). In Paris, St. Vincent de Paul started the Sisters of Charity in 1617, an organization composed of nuns and lay women dedicated to serving the poor and needy. The ladies and sisters, under the supervision of Mademoiselle Le Gras in 1634, promoted the goal of teaching people to help themselves as they visited the sick in their homes. In their emphasis on preparing nurses and supervising nursing care, as well as determining causes and solutions for clients' problems, the Sisters of Charity laid a foundation for modern community health nursing (Bullough & Bullough, 1978).

Unfortunately, the years that followed these accomplishments marked a serious setback in the status of nursing and care of the sick. From the late 1600s to the mid-1800s, the social upheaval after the Reformation caused a decline in the number of religious orders, with subsequent curtailing of nursing care for the sick poor. Babies continued to be delivered at home by midwives, most of whom had little or no training. Concern over high maternal mortality rates prompted efforts to better prepare midwives and medical students. One midwifery program was begun in Paris in 1720 and another in London by Dr. William Smellie in 1741.

The Industrial Revolution created additional problems; among them were epidemics, high infant mortality, occupational diseases and injuries, and increasing mental illness both in Europe and America. Hospitals were built in larger cities, and dispensaries were developed to provide greater access to physicians. However, disease was rampant, mortality rates were high, and institutional conditions, especially in prisons, hospitals, and "asylums" for the insane, were deplorable. The sick and afflicted were kept in filthy rooms without adequate food, water, cover, or care for their physical and emotional needs (Bullough & Bullough, 1978). Reformers like John Howard, an Englishman who investigated the spread of disease in prisons and hospitals in 1779, revealed serious needs that would not be addressed until much later.

Both Catholic and Anglican religious nursing orders, although few, continued their work of caring for the sick poor in their homes. For example, in 1812, the Sisters of Mercy organized in Dublin to provide care for the sick at home. Generally, however, with the status of women at an all-time low, often only the least respectable women pursued nursing. In 1844, in his novel *Martin Chuzzlewit*, Charles Dickens portrayed the nurse Sairy Gamp as an unschooled and slovenly drunkard, reflecting society's view of nursing at the time. It was in the midst of these deplorable conditions and in response to them that Florence Nightingale began her work.

Much of the foundation for modern community health nursing practice was laid through Florence Nightingale's remarkable accomplishments (Fig. 2–1). Born in 1820 into a wealthy English family, her extensive travel, excellent education—including training at the first school for nurses in Kaiserwerth, Germany—and determination to serve the needy resulted in major reforms and improved status for nursing. Her work during the Crimean War (1854 to 1856) with the wounded in Scutari is well documented (Woodham-Smith, 1951; Florence Nightingale Museum, 1997). Conditions in the military hospitals during the war were unspeakable. Thousands of sick and wounded men lay in filth without

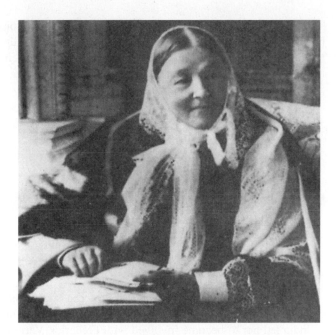

FIGURE 2–1. Florence Nightingale's concern for populations-at-risk as well as her vision and successful efforts at health reform provided a model for community health nursing today.

beds, clean coverings, food, water, or laundry facilities. Florence Nightingale organized competent nursing care and established kitchens and laundries that resulted in saving hundreds of lives. Her work further demonstrated that capable nursing intervention could prevent illness and improve the health of a population at risk—precursors to modern community health nursing practice. Her subsequent work for health reform in the military was supported by implementing another public health strategy: the use of biostatistics. Through meticulously gathered data and statistical comparisons, Miss Nightingale demonstrated that military mortality rates, even in peacetime, were double those of the civilian population because of the terrible living conditions in the barracks. This work led to important military reforms.

Miss Nightingale's concern for populations at risk included a continuing interest in the population of the sick at home. Her book *Notes on Nursing,* published in England in 1859 (Nightingale, 1992), was written to improve nursing care in the home (Bullough & Bullough, 1978).

Florence Nightingale also became a skillful lobbyist for health care reform. Her exemplary influence on English politics and policy improved the quality of existing health care and set standards for future practice. Furthermore, she demonstrated how population-focused nursing works.

In her work to help establish the first nonreligious school for nurses in 1860 at St. Thomas Hospital in London, she promoted a standard for proper education and supervision of nurses in practice known as the Nightingale Model. Principles she wrote about in *Notes on Nursing* relate directly to her early education and the notions held by Hippocrates in ancient Greece, which she had studied for years. Specifically,

THE GLOBAL COMMUNITY

Hisama, K.K. (1996). Florence Nightingale's influence on the development and professionalization of modern nursing in Japan. *Nursing Outlook, 44*(6), 284–288.

Despite Florence Nightingale's early and dramatic influence on nursing in Japan, sociocultural and geopolitical barriers have hindered the establishment of professional nursing. In 1885, Kanehiro Takagi, a navy doctor, established the first training school for nurses in Tokyo. He had studied at St. Thomas's Hospital in London and was impressed by the nurses trained there by Florence Nightingale. However, the independent thinking and careful actions, rather than unquestioned obedience, which is crucial in applying scientific knowledge, was not translated to nurses practicing in Japan. In Japan, there are three forms of nurses: *Kangofus,* educated nurses who care for the sick in small clinics and hospitals and who function almost as servants to physicians; *Hokenfus,* health nurses who have higher standards of education and a certain degree of autonomy in their nursing practice; and *Sanbas,* or midwives.

The roots of Hokenfus go back to the Kyoto Kanbyofu School, where Linda Richards, the first graduate of an American nursing school, was invited to teach in the late 1880s. Although the school was closed after operating for 11 years, the spirit of public health nursing in Japan was sustained by a handful of nurses who had studied in the United States and Canada. Kiyoshi Saito, along with other physicians who had studied in the United States, realized the importance of public health nursing.

Beginning in the 1920s, Saito helped to initiate the formal training of Hokenfus by establishing new programs for nurses. The 1937 legislation of Hokenjoho (Rules for Public Health Department) helped Hokenfus to advance their professional status. Hokenfus were community-based nurses who worked independently of physicians and focused on "health nursing" in contrast to "sick nursing," in Nightingale's terms. Notice that there were few Hokenfus compared with the number of Kangofus, and much of their autonomy was lost in postwar Japan's new government regulations.

Since World War II, there have been changes in Japanese nursing with the encouragement of the Kangofus model, hospital-based nurses (called Kangofus), and Jun-Kangofus. Their educational preparation had not been as rigorous or lengthy, which served the feudalistic medical system well. Most remain unmarried and were not involved in hospital chores but were there primarily to serve the physician, not the patient.

Currently, some Japanese nursing leaders believe that Japan could best be served by following the Hokenfu model. Japanese Hokenfus established themselves as health professionals. They marry and live and work in the community. Many nurses continue their careers by becoming Hokenfus, working in the community. Under the Hokenfu model, needlessly long hospitalization of patients would be replaced with community-based health care, a step that Japan needs to take, since they are feeling the drain on the health care dollar, caused in part by extended hospitalizations.

With the recent drive to upgrade Japanese nursing education, the pressure to reduce medical costs, the weakening of the grip of the old medical system, and the realization among Japanese women of their basic rights, the opportunity for reform and a new vision for Japanese nursing in the 21st century are within reach, and Florence Nightingale's influence again may be a driving force.

her concern with the environment of patients, the need for keen observation, the focus on the whole patient rather than disease, and the importance of assisting nature to bring about a cure all reflect Hippocrates' teachings (Nightingale, 1992; LeVasseur, 1998) (see The Global Community).

Another great nurse and healer in her own right was Mary Seacole (1805 to 1881). She has been called the "Black Nightingale." She was the daughter of a well-respected "doctress" who practiced Creole or Afro-Caribbean medicine in Jamaica. She began by helping her mother at an early age and spent many years developing her skills. She helped populations who experienced tropical diseases, especially cholera, in Central America, Panama, and the Caribbean. She attempted, through many formal channels, to join Florence Nightingale in Scutari and was rejected again and again. Undaunted, she went to the Crimea on her own to open a hotel for sick and convalescing soldiers, where she met Miss Nightingale and many of the troops she cared for in Jamaica. Many of the military commanders sought her out for her knowledge of healing, and she was affectionately known by the troops as "Mother Seacole." After the war and into her old age, she continued to provide nursing care in London and when visiting Jamaica. She focused her caregiving among high-risk clients of the day and did so in an innovative, entrepreneurial manner unique for women, especially for women of color in the 1800s (Florence Nightingale Museum, 1997).

District Nursing (Mid-1800s to 1900)

The next stage in the development of community health nursing was the formal organization of visiting nursing, or **district nursing.** In 1859, William Rathbone, an English philanthropist, became convinced of the value of home nursing as a result of private care given to his wife (Kalisch & Kalisch, 1995). He employed Mary Robinson, the nurse who had cared for his wife, to visit the sick poor in their homes and teach them proper hygiene to prevent illness. The need was so great, it soon became evident that more nurses were needed. In 1861, with Florence Nightingale's help and advice, Rathbone opened a training school for nurses connected with the Royal Liverpool Infirmary and established a visiting nurse service for the sick poor in Liverpool. Florence Lees, a graduate of the Nightingale School, was appointed first Superintendent-General of the District Nursing System (Mowbray, 1997). As the service grew, visiting nurses were assigned to districts in the city—hence the name district nursing. Subsequently, other British cities also developed district nursing training and services. An example is the Nurse Training Institution for district nurses, founded in Manchester in 1864. Privately financed, the nurses were trained and then "dispensed food and medicine" to the sick poor in their homes "and were closely supervised by various middle and upper class women who collected the necessary supplies" (Bullough & Bullough, 1978, p. 143).

Although Florence Nightingale is best remembered for her professionalization of nursing, she had a full understanding of the need for community health nursing. This has been recorded from conversations and from her writings;

> **Hospitals are but an intermediate stage of civilisation. At present hospitals are the only place where the sick poor can be nursed, or, indeed often the sick rich. But the ultimate object is to nurse all sick at home (Nightingale, 1876).**

> **The aim of the district nurse is to give first rate nursing to the sick poor at home (Nightingale, 1876 [cited in Mowbray, 1997, p. 24]).**

> **The health visitor must create a new profession for women (conversation with Frederick Verney, 1891 [cited in Mowbray, 1997, p. 25]).**

For years, Florence Nightingale studied the social and economic conditions of India. The plight of the poor and ill in India led her to become involved with Frederick Verney in a pioneering "health at home" project in England in 1892. She wrote a series of papers on the need for "home missioners" and "health visitors," endorsing the view that prevention was better than cure (Mowbray, 1997).

In the United States, the first community health nurse, Frances Root, hired by the Women's Board of the New York Mission in 1877, pioneered home visits to the poor in New York City. In 1885, district nursing associations were founded in Buffalo and, in 1886, in Boston and Philadelphia. These district associations served the sick poor exclusively because patients with enough money had private home nursing care. The English model, however, with standards for visiting nurses' education and practice established in 1889 under Queen Victoria, was not followed in the United States. Instead, visiting nursing organizations sprang up in many cities without common standards or administration. Twenty-one such services existed in the United States in 1890.

Although district nurses primarily cared for the sick, they also taught cleanliness and wholesome living to their patients, even in that early period. One example was the Boston program, founded by the Women's Educational Association, which "emphasized the teaching of hygiene and cleanliness, giving impetus to what was called instructive district nursing" (Bullough & Bullough, 1978, p. 144). This early emphasis on prevention and "health" nursing became one of the distinguishing features of district nursing and, later, of public health nursing as a specialty.

The work of district nurses in the United States focused mostly on the care of individuals. District nurses recorded temperatures and pulse rates and gave simple treatments to the sick poor under the immediate direction of a physician. They also instructed family members in personal hygiene, diet and healthful living habits, and the care of the sick. The problems of early home care patients in the United States were numerous and complex. Thousands of European and eastern European immigrants filled tenement housing in the poorest and most crowded slums of the large coastal cities during the late 1800s. Inadequate sanitation, unsafe and unhealthy working conditions, and language and cultural barriers added to poverty and disease. Nursing educational programs at that time did not prepare district nurses to cope with their patients' multiple health and social problems.

The sponsorship of district nursing changed over time. Early district nursing services in both England and the United States were founded by religious organizations. Later, sponsorship shifted to private philanthropy. Funding came from contributions and, in a few instances, from fees charged to patients on an ability-to-pay basis. Finally, visiting nursing began to be supported by public money. An early example occurred in Los Angeles where, in 1897, a nurse was hired as a city employee. Although one form of funding dominated, all three types of financing continued to exist as they still do. Although the government was beginning to assume more responsibility for the public's health, most district nursing services during this time remained private.

In England, the establishment of "health visitors" in poor areas of London began at the turn of the 19th century. These health care providers enhanced the English model of health visitor/district nurse/midwife as the backbone of the primary health care system. "The impact of early health visiting was clearly shown by the halving of infant mortality in the areas within two years. . . . " (Beine, 1996, p. 59). The main focus of the health visitor's work was giving advice to poor mothers and teaching hygiene to prevent infant diarrhea (Beine, 1996).

Public Health Nursing (1900 to 1970)

By the turn of the century, district nursing had broadened its focus to include the health and welfare of the general public, not just the poor. This new emphasis was part of a broader consciousness about public health. Robert Koch's demonstration that tuberculosis was communicable led to Johns Hopkins Hospital hiring a nurse, Reba Thelin, in 1903 to visit the homes of tuberculosis patients. Her job was to ensure that patients followed prescribed regimens of rest, fresh air, and proper diets and to prevent possible infection (Sachs, 1908). A growing sense of urgency about the interrelatedness of health conditions and the need to improve the health of all people led to an increased number of private health agencies. These agencies supplemented the often-limited work of government health departments. By 1910, new federal laws made states and communities accountable for the health of their citizens.

Specialized programs such as infant welfare, tuberculosis clinics, and venereal disease control were developed, causing a demand for nurses to work in these areas (Fig. 2–2). Bullough and Bullough comment, "Although the hospital

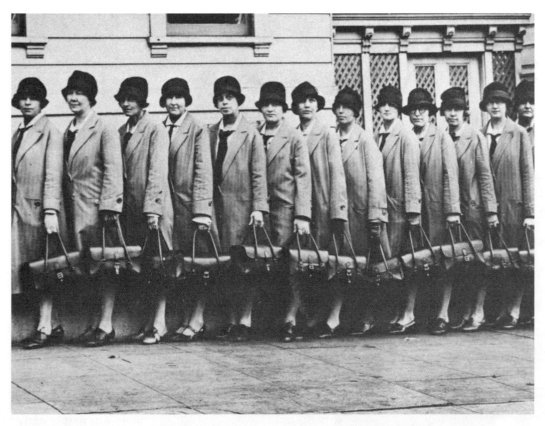

FIGURE 2–2. Public health nurses—uniforms and symbols. (Photograph courtesy of Visiting Nurses and Hospice of San Francisco.)

nursing school movement emphasized the care of the sick, a small but growing number of nurses were finding employment in preventive health care" (1978, p. 143). In 1900, there were an estimated 200 public health nurses. By 1912, that number had grown to 3000 (Gardner, 1936). "This development was important: it brought health care and health teaching to the public, gave nurses an opportunity for more independent work, and helped to improve nursing education" (Bullough & Bullough, 1978, p. 143).

The role of the district nurse expanded during this stage. Lillian D. Wald (1867–1940), a leading figure in this expansion, first used the term "public health nursing" to describe this specialty (Bullough & Bullough, 1978). District nurses, while caring for the sick, had pioneered in health teaching, disease prevention, and promotion of good health practices. Now, with a growing recognition of familial and environmental influences on health, public health nurses broadened their practice even more. Nurses working outside of the hospital increased their knowledge and skills in specialized areas such as tuberculosis, maternal and child health, school health, and mental disorders.

Lillian Wald's contributions to public health nursing were enormous. A graduate of the New York Hospital Training School, she started teaching home nursing but quickly changed to a career of social reform and nursing activism (Backer, 1993). Appalled by the conditions of an immigrant neighborhood in New York's Lower East Side, she and a nurse-friend, Mary Brewster, started the Henry Street Settlement in 1893 to provide nursing and welfare services. Her book, *The House on Henry Street,* portrays her work and views on public health nursing. Nursing visits conducted through her organization were supervised by nurses in contrast to earlier models in which nursing services were administered by lay boards and actual care was supervised by lay persons. Demonstrating that nursing could reduce illness-caused absenteeism, Wald convinced the New York City Board of Education to hire the first school nurse in the United States in 1902. Her suggestion that nurse intervention could reduce death rates resulted in the Metropolitan Life Insurance Company starting a visiting nurse service in 1909 for policy holders (Kalisch & Kalisch, 1995).

The legendary accomplishments of Lillian Wald reflect her driving commitment to serve needy populations. Through her efforts, the New York City Bureau of Child Hygiene was formed in 1908 and, later, the Children's Bureau at the federal level in 1912 (Fig. 2–3). Wald's emphasis on illness prevention and health promotion through health teaching and nursing intervention, as well as her use of epidemiologic methodology, established these actions as hallmarks of public health nursing practice. She promoted rural nursing and family-focused nursing and encouraged improved coursework at Teachers College of Columbia University (New York) to prepare public health nurses for practice. Through her work and influence with the legislature to establish health and social policies, improvements were made in child labor and pure food laws, tenement housing, parks, city recreation centers, immigrant handling, and teaching of mentally handicapped children. In 1912, she also helped to found and was

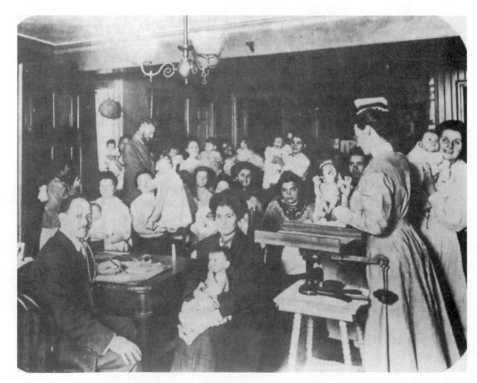

FIGURE 2–3. Examination of infants was part of early health department programs in which district nurses played a major role.

first president of the National Organization for Public Health Nursing (NOPHN), an organization that set standards and guided public health nursing's further development and impact on public health (Kalisch & Kalisch, 1995). Her exemplary accomplishments truly reflect a concern for populations at risk. They further demonstrate how nursing leadership, involvement in policy formation, and use of epidemiology lead to improved health for the public.

By the 1920s, public health nursing was acquiring a more professional stature, in contrast to its earlier association with charity. Nursing as a whole was gaining professional status as a science in addition to being an art. National nursing organizations began to form during this stage and contributed to nursing's professional growth. The first of these emphasized establishing educational standards for nursing. Called the American Society of Superintendents of Training Schools for Nurses in the United States and Canada, it was started by Isabel Hampton Robb in 1893 and later became known as the National League of Nursing Education in 1912, the forerunner of the National League for Nursing (NLN) established in 1952 (Ellis & Hartley, 1997). In 1890, a meeting of nursing leaders at the World's Fair in Chicago initiated an alumnae organization of 10 schools of nursing to form the National Associated Alumnae of the United States and Canada in 1896, created to promote nursing education and practice standards. In 1899, the group was renamed the Nurses' Associated Alumnae of the United States and Canada. Canada was excluded from the title in 1901 because New York, where the organization was incorporated, did not allow representation from two countries. In 1911, the organization went through a final name change to the American Nurses' Association (ANA), while Canadian nurses formed

their own nursing organization (Ellis & Hartley, 1997). The previously mentioned NOPHN, founded by Lillian Wald and Mary Gardner, merged with the NLN (1952). These three organizations, in particular, strengthened ties between nursing groups and improved nursing education and practice.

As nursing education became increasingly rigorous, collegiate programs began to include public health as essential content in basic nursing curricula. The first collegiate program with public health content to be accredited by the NLN began in 1944 (NOPHN, 1944). Previously, only postgraduate courses in public health nursing had been offered for nurses choosing this specialty. The first of such courses had been developed by Adelaide Nutting in 1912 at Teachers College in New York in affiliation with the Henry Street Settlement. A group of agencies met in 1946 to establish guidelines for public health nursing, and by 1963 public health content was required for NLN accreditation in all baccalaureate nursing programs. The nurse practitioner movement (NP), starting in 1965 at the University of Colorado, initially was a part of public health nursing and emphasized primary health care to rural and underserved populations. The number of educational programs to prepare NPs increased, with some NPs continuing in public health and others moving into different clinical areas.

During this period, as a result of the influence of Lillian Wald and other nursing leaders, the family began to emerge as a unit of service (Fig. 2–4). The multiple problems faced by many families impelled a trend toward nursing care generalized enough to meet diverse needs and provide holistic services. Public health nurses gradually gained more autonomy in such areas as home care and instruction of good health practices to families and community groups. Their collaborative relationships with other community health

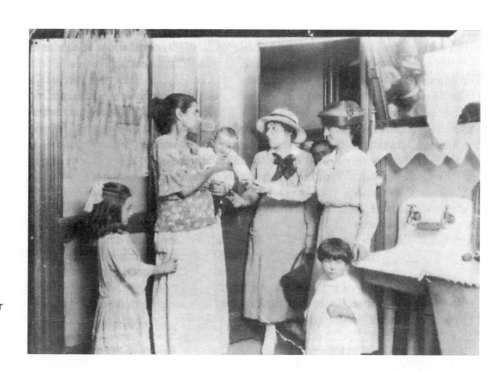

FIGURE 2–4. The public health nurse, carrying her bag of equipment and supplies, makes regular home visits to provide physical and psychological care as well as health lessons to families.

providers grew as the need to avoid gaps and duplication of services became apparent. Public health nurses also began keeping better records of their services.

Industrial nursing, another form of public health nursing, also expanded during this period (see Chapter 29). The first known industrial nurse, Philippa Flowerday Reid, was hired in Norwich, England by J. and J. Colmans in 1878. Her job was to assist the company physician and visit sick employees and their families in their homes. In the United States, the Vermont Marble Company was first to begin a nursing service in 1895; other companies followed soon after. By 1910, 66 firms in the United States employed nurses. During World War I, the number of industrial nurses greatly increased with recognition that nursing service reduced worker absenteeism (Bullough & Bullough, 1978). Early industrial nursing was the forerunner of modern occupational health nursing, which is explored in depth in Chapter 29.

During this stage, the institutional base for much of public health nursing shifted to the government. By 1955, 72% of the counties in the continental United States had local health departments. Public health nursing constituted the major portion of these local health services and emphasized health promotion as well as care for the ill at home (Scutchfield & Keck, 1997). Some of the district nursing services, known as visiting nurse associations (VNAs), remained privately funded and administered, offering their own home nursing care. In some places, city or county health departments joined administratively and financially with VNAs to provide a combination of services, such as home care of the sick and health promotion to families.

Rural public health nursing, which had already been organized around 1900 in Great Britain, Germany, and Canada, also expanded in the United States (see Chapter 31). Initially, starting in 1912, rural nursing was privately financed and largely administered through the Red Cross and the Metropolitan Life Insurance Company, but responsibility had shifted to the government by the 1940s (Bullough & Bullough, 1978). An innovative example of rural nursing was the Frontier Nursing Service (FNS), started by Mary Breckenridge in 1925 to serve mountain families in Kentucky. From six outposts, nurses on horseback visited remote families to deliver babies and provide food and nursing services. Over the years, the service has expanded to provide medical, dental, and nursing care (Tirpak, 1975). The FNS continues today in its remarkable accomplishments of reducing mortality rates and promoting health among this disadvantaged population.

The public health nursing stage was characterized by service to the public, with the family targeted as a primary unit of care. Official health agencies, which placed greater emphasis on disease prevention and health promotion, provided the chief institutional base.

Community Health Nursing (1970 to the Present)

The emergence of the term community health nursing heralded a new era. While public health nurses continued their

work in public health, by the late 1960s and early 1970s many other nurses, who were not necessarily practicing public health, were based in the community. Their practice settings included community-based clinics, doctors' offices, work sites, and schools. To provide a label that encompassed all nurses in the community, the ANA and others called them community health nurses.

This term was not universally accepted, however, and many people — including nurses and the general public — had difficulty distinguishing community health nursing from public health nursing. For example, nursing education, recognizing the importance of public health content, required course work in public health for all baccalaureate students. This meant that graduates were expected to incorporate public health principles such as health promotion and disease prevention into nursing practice, regardless of their sphere of service. Consequently, some people questioned whether public health nursing retained any unique content. Although leaders like Carolyn Williams clearly stated that community health nursing's specialized contribution lay in its focus on populations (Williams, 1977), this concept did not appear to be widely understood or practiced.

To distinguish the domains of community and public health nursing, the U.S. Department of Health and Human Services, Bureau of Health Professionals, Division of Nursing in 1984 convened a Consensus Conference on the Essentials of Public Health Nursing Practice and Education in Washington, DC (U.S. Department of Health and Human Services, Division of Nursing, 1984). This group concluded that *community health nursing* was the broader term, referring to all nurses practicing in the community, regardless of their educational preparation. *Public health nursing,* viewed as a part of community health nursing, was described as a generalist practice for nurses prepared with basic public health content at the baccalaureate level and a specialized practice for nurses prepared in public health at the masters level or beyond.

Confusion also arose around the question of whether community health nursing is a generalized or a specialized practice. Graduates from baccalaureate nursing programs were inadequately prepared to practice in public health; their education had emphasized individualized and direct clinical care and provided little understanding of applications to populations and communities. By the mid-1970s, various community health nursing leaders had identified knowledge and skills needed for more effective community health nursing practice (Roberts & Freeman, 1973). These leaders valued promoting the health of the community, but both education and practice continued to emphasize direct clinical care to individuals, families, and groups in the community (de Tornyay, 1980). Reflecting this view, the ANA's Division of Community Health Nursing developed *A Conceptual Model of Community Health Nursing* in 1980. This document distinguished generalized community health nursing preparation at the baccalaureate level and specialized community health nursing preparation at the masters or postgraduate level. The generalist was described as one who provided nursing service to individuals and groups of clients while keeping "the community perspective in mind" (ANA, 1980, p. 9).

Finally, confusion also arose over the changing roles and functions of community health nurses. Accelerated changes in health care organization and financing, technology, and social issues made increasing demands on community health nurses to adapt to new patterns of practice. Many new kinds of community health services appeared. Hospital-based programs reached into the community. Private agencies proliferated, offering home care and other community-based services. Other community health professionals assumed responsibilities that traditionally had been the domain of public health nursing. Some school counselors in Oregon, for example, began coordinating home visits previously done by school nurses, and health educators, who were part of a more recently developed discipline, took over large segments of client education. Social workers, too, provided services that overlapped with community health nursing roles. Health educators, counselors, social workers, epidemiologists, and nutritionists working in community health came prepared with different backgrounds and emphases in their practice. Their contributions were and still are important. Their presence, however, forced community health nurses to reexamine their own contribution to the public's health and incorporate stronger interdisciplinary and collaborative approaches into their practice (see Levels of Prevention).

The debate over these areas of confusion continued through the 1980s, with some issues yet unresolved. Still, the direction in which public health and community health nursing must move remains clear: to care *for*, not simply *in*, the community. Public health nursing continues to mean the synthesis of nursing and the public health sciences applied to promoting and protecting the health of populations. Community health nursing, for some, refers more broadly to nursing in the community. In this text, the term community health nursing is used synonymously with public health nursing and refers to specialized population-focused nursing practice, which applies public health science and nursing science. A possible distinction between the two terms might be to view community health nursing as a beginning level of specialization and public health nursing as an advanced level. Clarification and consensus on the meaning of these terms helps to avoid misconceptions and misuse and are explored more fully in Chapter 17. Whichever term is used to describe this specialty, the fundamental issues and defining criteria remain: (1) are populations and communities the target of practice? and (2) are the nurses prepared in public health and engaging in public health practice?

As community health nursing continues to evolve, many signs of positive growth are evident. Community health nurses are carving out new roles for themselves in primary health care. Collaboration and interdisciplinary teamwork are recognized as crucial to effective community nursing. Practitioners work through many kinds of agencies and institutions, such as senior citizen centers, ambulatory services, mental health clinics, and family planning programs. Community needs assessment, documentation of nursing

LEVELS OF PREVENTION

ENHANCING COMMUNITY HEALTH NURSING'S IMPACT

GOAL

To avoid misunderstanding and misuse of community health nursing by clarifying and enhancing its role in the delivery of health services.

PRIMARY PREVENTION

To prevent misunderstanding and misuse from occurring. Proactively develop knowledge and skills and participate in policy formation, political activism, collaborative program development, and defining community health nursing's role. Conduct research on health and nursing outcomes to ensure theory-based practice, to establish credibility in the community, and to acquire funding for programs.

SECONDARY PREVENTION

To detect early signs of misunderstanding and misuse and correct them. Identify agencies where community health nurses could more fully practice population-based nursing and have a greater impact on promoting the community's health. Develop measures to enlarge the nurses' vision and to promote aggregate-level interventions. Foster nurse involvement on community boards, in politics and policy formation, in program development, and in research and collaboration with community colleagues.

TERTIARY PREVENTION

To identify misunderstanding and misuse, minimize their impact, and improve nursing function. Identify community health nurses who lack vision or clarity of their role. Through education, staff development, or reassignment, provide opportunities for developing vision, knowledge, and skills to enlarge their role and impact on the health of populations.

outcomes, program evaluation, quality improvement, public policy formulation, and community nursing research are high priorities. This field of nursing is assuming responsibility as a full professional partner in community health.

Internationally, community nursing services are well established in England, although they may be an invisible service, since it was written in a London newspaper that "one of the possible memorials for Princess Diana might be a new nursing service based along the lines of the 'old nursing service'" (Birch, 1998, p. 19). Scandinavia, the Netherlands, and Australia have active community health services, but services are relatively underdeveloped in France and Ireland. Furthermore, there are relatively few professional nurses working in the community in central and eastern Europe and the former USSR. Volunteers, lay providers, and paraprofessionals provide the bulk of community health services in China, Africa, and India.

In 1978, a joint World Health Organization (WHO) and the United Nations Childrens' Fund International Conference in Alma-Ata, the Soviet Union, adopted a declaration on primary health care as the key to attain the goal of health

TABLE 2–1. Development of Community Health Nursing

Stages	Focus	Nursing Orientation	Service Emphasis	Institutional Base (Agencies)
Early home care (Before mid-1800s)	Sick poor	Individuals	Curative	Lay and religious orders
District nursing (1860–1900)	Sick poor	Individuals	Curative; beginning of preventive	Voluntary; some government
Public health nursing (1900–1970)	Needy public	Families	Curative; preventive	Government; some voluntary
Emergence of community health nursing (1970–present)	Total community	Populations	Health promotion; illness prevention	Many kinds; some independent practice

for all by the year 2000. At this conference, delegations from 134 governments agreed to incorporate the concepts and principles of primary health care in their health care systems to reach this goal (WHO, 1978, 1998). This was adopted by the World Health Assembly and endorsed by the United Nations General Assembly in 1981. On paper, at least, everyone acknowledged the crucial need of nurses to be involved in reaching this goal. In practice, support has not been forthcoming in many countries. Policymakers and the public still need to be educated to realize that nursing's most effective contributions to the overall health of the population are based in the community (Beine, 1996).

Table 2–1 summarizes the most important changes that have occurred during community health nursing's four stages of development. It shows these changes in terms of focus, nursing orientation, service emphasis, and institutional base.

SOCIETAL INFLUENCES ON COMMUNITY HEALTH NURSING'S DEVELOPMENT

Many factors influenced the growth of community health nursing. To better understand the nature of this field, the forces that began and continue to shape its development must be recognized. Six are particularly significant: advanced technology, progress in causal thinking, changes in education, the changing role of women, the consumer movement, and economic factors.

Advanced Technology

Advanced technology has contributed in many ways to shaping the practice of community health nursing. For example, technologic innovation has greatly improved health care, nutrition, and lifestyle and has caused a concomitant increase in life expectancy. Consequently, community health nurses direct an increasing share of their effort toward meeting the needs of the elderly population and addressing chronic con-

ditions. As another example, for many people, the advances in technology in the home have been life-altering. Online communities for older adults have been developed, bringing the elderly out of loneliness and among a community of caring others through the computer (Furlong, 1997); online interfaith programs connect homebound people with religious leaders and fellow parishioners (Gunderson, 1997); and innovative telecommunication technologies promote safety, independence, and social interaction for people of all ages with disabilities (Mann, 1997).

Advanced technology also has been a strong force behind industrialization, large-scale employment, and urbanization. We are now primarily an urban society, with approximately 75% of the world's population living in urban or suburban areas. Population density leads to many health-related problems, particularly the spread of disease and increased stress. Community health nurses are learning how to combat these urban health problems. In addition, changes in transportation and high job mobility have affected the health scene. As people travel and relocate, they are separated from families and traditional support systems; community health nurses design programs to help urban populations cope with the accompanying stress. New products, equipment, methods, and energy sources in industry also have increased environmental pollution and industrial hazards. Community health nurses have become involved in related research, occupational health, and preventive education. Technological innovation has promoted medicine's complex diagnostic and treatment procedures, thus making illness-oriented care more dramatic and desirable, as well as more costly. Community health nurses face a challenge to demonstrate the physical and economic value of technology for wellness-oriented care.

Finally, innovations in communications and computer technology have shifted America from an industrial society to an "information economy" (Brink, 1997). Our economy is built on information—the production and marketing of knowledge—making it global and around-the-clock. Community health nurses now are in the business of information distribution and use computer technologies to enhance the efficiency and effectiveness of their services. Associated with high use of technology are societal needs for "high touch" (Jorgenson,

1997). Interacting with machines creates a greater need for human contact; technological complexity, speed, and impersonality all induce stress. Stress management and interventions for other technology-induced health problems will continue to shape the future role of community health nursing.

Progress in Causal Thinking

Relating disease or illness to its cause is known as **causal thinking** in the health sciences. Progress in the study of causality, particularly in epidemiology, has significantly affected the nature of community health nursing (Finnegan & Ervin, 1997; Friedman, 1994). The *germ theory* of disease causation, established in the late 1800s, was the first real breakthrough in control of communicable disease. At that time, it was established that disease could be spread or transmitted from patient to patient or from nurse to patient by contaminated hands or equipment. Nurses incorporated the teaching of cleanliness and personal hygiene into basic nursing care. A second advance in causal thinking was initiated by the tripartite view that called attention to the interactions among a causative agent, a susceptible host, and the environment. This information offered community health nursing new ways to control and prevent health disorders. For example, nurses could decrease the vulnerability of individuals (host) by teaching them healthier lifestyles. They could instigate measles vaccination programs as a means of preventing the organism (agent) from infecting children. They could promote proper disinfection of a neighborhood swimming pool (environment) to prevent disease. Further progress in causal thinking led to the recognition that not just one single agent, but many factors—a multiple causation approach—contribute to a disease or health disorder. A food poisoning outbreak that is associated with a restaurant might be caused not only by the salmonella organism but also by improper food handling and storage, lack of adherence to minimum food preparation standards, and lack of adequate health department supervision and enforcement (see Chapter 14).

Community health nurses can control health problems by examining all possible causes and then attacking strategic causal points. Efforts to prevent AIDS provide a dramatic case in point. Contact reporting, condom use, protection of health workers serving HIV-infected patients, HIV screening, and public education about AIDS are examples of a multifaceted approach. Current causal thinking has led to a broader awareness of unhealthy conditions; in addition to disease, problems such as accidents and environmental pollution are major targets of concern. As a result, work-related stress, environmental hazards, chemical food additives, and alcohol and nicotine consumption during pregnancy are all examples of concerns in community health nursing practice.

Nursing's contribution to public health adds a further application of causal thinking. That is, nursing seeks to identify and implement the causes, or contributing factors, of wellness. Community health nurses do more than prevent illness; they seek to promote health (Morgan & Marsh, 1998). By conducting research and applying research findings, community health nurses promote health-enhancing behaviors. These include promoting healthier lifestyle practices such as eating low-fat diets, exercising, and maintaining social support systems, promoting healthy conditions in schools and work sites, and designing meaningful activities for adolescents and the elderly.

Changes in Education

Changes in education, especially those in nursing education, have had an important influence on community health nursing practice. Education, once an opportunity for a privileged few, has become widely available; it is now considered a basic right and a necessity for a vital society. When people's understanding of their environment grows, an increased understanding of health usually is involved. For the community health nurse, health teaching has steadily assumed greater importance in practice. For the learner, education has led to more responsibility. As a result, people believe that they have a right to know and question the reasons behind the care they receive. Community health nurses have shifted from planning for clients to collaborating with clients.

Education has had other effects. Scientific inquiry, considered basic to progress, has created a dramatic increase in knowledge. The wealth of information relevant to community health nursing practice means that nursing students have more content to assimilate, and practicing community health nurses have to make greater efforts to keep abreast. In contrast to earlier times when nurses were trained to work as apprentices in hospitals or health agencies and perfunctorily follow orders, today's educational programs, including continuing education, prepare nurses to think for themselves in the application of theory to practice. Community health nursing has always required a fair measure of independent thinking and self-reliance; now, community health nurses need skills in such areas as population assessment, policy making, political advocacy, research, management, collaborative functioning, and critical thinking. As the result of expanding education, community health nurses have had to reexamine their practice, sharpen their knowledge and skills, and clarify their roles.

Changing Role of Women

The changing role of women has profoundly affected community health nursing. In the last century, the women's rights movement made considerable progress; women achieved the right to vote and gained greater economic independence by moving into the labor force. Today, in the civilian work force, 71.1% of married women with children work, and 59.8% of women aged 18 years and older work, up from 51.5% 20 years earlier, compared with 75% of the men, down from 77.4% in 1980. It is projected that by 2006, these numbers will continue to show more women in the work force (61.4%), whereas there will be fewer men (73.6%) (U.S. Department of Commerce, 1998). Women today have more education and consequently more influence than before. The percentage of women in 1997 in professions such as medicine (26.2% of physicians in the United States are women), law (26.7% of lawyers and judges are women), and engineering (9.6% of engineers are women) is increasing, with these percentages nearly doubling the numbers from 1983 (U.S. Department of Commerce, 1998). Naisbitt and Aburdene described the 1990s as the "decade of women in leadership." They write, "In business and many professions women have increased from a minority as low as 10 percent in 1970 to a critical mass ranging from 30 to 50 percent in much of the business world, including banking, accounting, and computer science" (1990, p. 217). Yet women continue to be paid less than men. For example, figures from the Department of Labor Statistics show that women earn 67% of a man's salary for the same job. Women and men in management, executive, and administrative positions had a median annual salary in 1997 of $31,208 and $46,654, respectively (U.S. Department of Commerce, 1998). All of these changes mean that many more women must manage dual roles of career and family, often under disadvantaged economic conditions.

Although the diversity of career options and employment opportunities for women has been a positive factor, these gains have decreased the number of women entering nursing. As a profession, nursing's contributions and status have improved, but its ability to compete with careers offering higher pay and status remains problematic. Changes resulting from the women's movement continue. Nurses still struggle for equality—equality of recognition, respect, and autonomy, as well as job selection, equal pay for equal work, and equal opportunity for advancement in the health field. If community health nurses are to influence the field of community health, they need status and authority equal to that of their colleagues. This step requires nurses to demonstrate their competence and learn to be assertive in assuming roles as full professional partners. Although only 6.5% of registered nurses (RNs) in 1997 were men (up from 4.2% in 1983), they hold over a third of nursing administrative positions (U.S. Department of Commerce, 1998). This may be influenced by a larger proportion of women in nursing having less than full-time careers. The women's movement has contributed to community health nursing's gains in assuming leadership roles, but a need for greater influence and involvement remains.

Consumer Movement and Changing Demographics

The consumer movement also has affected the nature of community health nursing. Consumers have become more aggressive in demanding quality services and goods; they assert their right to be informed about goods and services and to participate in decisions that affect them regardless of sex, race, or socioeconomic level. This movement has stimulated some basic changes in the philosophy of community health nursing. Health care consumers are viewed as active members of the health team rather than as passive recipients of care. They may contract with the community health nurse for family care or group services, represent the community on the local health board, or act as ombudsmen by serving as representatives or advocates for their community constituents, for example, to investigate complaints and report findings to protect the quality of care in a local nursing home. This assumption of consumers' responsibility for their own health means that the community health nurse often supplements, in contrast to primarily supervising, clients' services.

Changing demographics, such as shifting patterns in immigration, numbers of births and deaths, and a rapidly increasing population of elderly persons, affect community health nursing planning and programming efforts. Monitoring these changes is essential for relevant and effective nursing services.

The consumer movement and changing demographics also have contributed to increased concern for the quality of health services, including a demand for more humane, personalized health care. Dissatisfied with fragmented services offered by an array of health workers, consumers seek more comprehensive, coordinated care. For example, senior citizens in a high-rise apartment building need more than a series of social workers, nutritionists, recreational therapists, nurses, and other callers ascertaining a variety of specific needs and starting a variety of separate programs. Community health nurses seek to provide holistic care by collaborating with others to offer more coordinated, comprehensive, and personalized services—a case management approach.

Economic Forces

Myriad economic forces have affected community health nursing practice. Unemployment and the rising cost of living, combined with mounting health care costs, have resulted in numerous people carrying little or no health insurance. With limited or no access to needed health services, these populations are especially vulnerable to health problems and further economic stress. Other economic forces affecting community health nursing are changing health care financing patterns (including prospective payment and Diagnosis-Related Groups); decreased federal, state, and local subsidy of public health programs; pressures for health care cost containment through managed care; and increased competition and managed competition among providers of health services (see Chapter 7 for further explanation of health economics).

Global economic forces also influence community health nursing practice. As the United States experiences increasing interdependence with foreign countries for trade, investments, and production of goods, the population has experienced a growing mobility and increased immigration, particularly among Hispanic and Asian groups. Under these conditions, the spread of communicable disease poses a serious threat, as do problems associated with unemployment and poverty. Furthermore, the fastest-growing sector of the job market is in technical areas, which require new or retrained workers, and these jobs frequently are accompanied by health problems related to the high level of technology and stress.

Community health nursing has responded to these economic forces in several ways. One is by assuming new roles, such as health educators in industry or case managers for government and privately sponsored programs for the elderly. Another is by directly competing with other community health service providers, particularly in such areas as ambulatory care or home care. Still another is by developing new programs and service emphases. Elder day care, respite care, senior fall-prevention programs, teen pregnancy and drug prevention projects, and programs for the homeless are a few examples of the response by community health nursing to the changing community needs created by demographic and economic forces. Yet another community health nursing response has been to develop new revenue-generating services, such as workplace wellness or health screening programs, to augment depleted budgets.

Economic factors continue to play a significant role in shaping community health nursing practice. Limited dollars for health promotion services and increased demands for home care have drawn some public health agencies into more illness-oriented than wellness-oriented services. Yet community health nurses continue to be resourceful in finding ways to foster the community's optimal health while adapting to changing economic conditions.

PREPARATION FOR COMMUNITY HEALTH NURSING

The demands of community health nursing practice are significant, as described in Chapter 1, and are elaborated in future chapters. The daily routine of the community health nurse may include organizing a flu clinic for seniors in the community, making home visits, giving a presentation on playground safety at a parent-teacher meeting, participating in a team meeting in the health department office, answering telephone calls, and charting. All of the skills learned in a basic baccalaureate nursing program are needed to effectively manage this type of day. Furthermore, this day may not represent the bigger picture of the community health nurse's role on community advisory panels, grant writing for new programs, or participation in or presentation of inservices. Academic preparation for this role and continuous professional development is necessary and must meet the requirements expected by employers for people in this specialty in nursing and, in many instances, in state regulations.

Academic Preparation

The minimum preparation for community health nurses in many states has been graduation from a baccalaureate-level nursing program, a nursing major built on 2 years of liberal arts and science courses (Ellis & Hartley, 1997). This can be achieved in a variety of ways. Some students enter a baccalaureate program as their initial higher educational experience after high school or later. Others complete an associate degree program in nursing and continue on to a university to receive the baccalaureate degree. This requires additional courses in liberal arts and sciences, along with selected nursing courses, mostly the public health nursing course and often a critical care nursing and a leadership-management course. In some programs designed to extend an RN to a Bachelor of Science in Nursing (BSN), nurses with years of experience in acute care nursing can "challenge" the two previously mentioned courses by taking a test to demonstrate clinical expertise or by presenting a portfolio of experience, or a combination of these. In several states, completing a hospital-based program prepares students in basic nursing skills in 2 to 3 years. Often, these programs already are aligned with a university and offer a step program, making a smooth transition to the baccalaureate degree. Nevertheless, whatever the initial entry into practice, a comprehensive nursing education that is rich in leadership, management, research, health maintenance and promotion, disease prevention, and community health nursing experience is needed to meet the demands of this specialty (Display 2–1).

In some states, meeting criteria for entry into practice as a public health nurse is required by some employers. In California, the State Board of Registered Nursing (BRN) has established specific criteria, including completion of specific coursework, such as child abuse and prevention information, which needs to be documented in undergraduate classes. On graduation, a school transcript, application, and fee are sent to the BRN to receive the public health nursing certificate. After passing the RN license examination (NCLEX), these nurses then can sign "RN, PHN" after their names. Only those who have completed a baccalaureate nursing program can apply for this certificate, and only people with the certificate can take jobs as community health nurses. In California, this means employment as an RN in settings such as in health departments, schools, and Native American health services, which may request a PHN certificate.

Professional Development

Completing your baccalaureate education may not be sufficient educational preparation for more demanding community health nursing settings. In addition, to maintain licensure in most states, it is mandated that nurses participate in continuing education programs and receive continuing education units. In most of the United States, courses on specific topics are offered by employers, nursing associations, nurs-

---

DISPLAY 2–1. Statement of American Public Health Association Public Health Nursing Section (October 1996)

Public health nursing practice is a systematic process by which:

1. Health and health care needs of a population are assessed to identify subpopulations, families, and individuals who would benefit from health promotion or who are at risk of illness, injury, disability, or premature death
2. A plan for intervention is developed, with the community, to meet identified needs, taking into account available resources, the range of activities that contribute to health, and the prevention of illness, injury, disability, and premature death
3. The plan is implemented effectively, efficiently, and equitably
4. Evaluations are conducted to determine the extent to which the interventions have an impact on the health status of individuals and the population
5. Results of the process are used to influence and direct the current delivery of care, deployment of health resources, and the development of local, regional, state, and national health policy and research to promote health and prevent disease.

---

ing journals, and private programs that travel to various cities. These help nurses to remain current on topics covered by the courses; however, a community health nurse may consider more lengthy and formal professional development opportunities such as advanced nursing practice programs or certification opportunities.

On finishing an undergraduate nursing program, the thought of continuing on in school may be overwhelming. However, in a few months or many years after graduation, continuing in higher education may seem right. It may take a few years to find a particular focus in nursing and to decide on specializing at an advanced level. When that time comes, a variety of course work and degree options are available. For example, short-term certificate programs specialize in a narrow focus of health care such as early recognition and prevention of child abuse, research, grant writing, or team management. These may or may not be offered for university credit, but either way, the content enhances a nurse's role in an agency. Matriculation in an NP program or a master's degree program in nursing is a longer commitment and would give the nurse greater marketability. In some health departments, NPs run well-child clinics; in schools, the school nurse with an NP license can direct a school-based clinic. Advanced practice in community health nursing can open doors into leadership positions in community health agencies. A master's degree in business, public health, education,

or epidemiology can lead to management positions, private community health agency ownership, agency teaching, or research positions. A doctoral program may be the next educational step for those wanting tenure-track university teaching, research, or upper-level administrative positions.

The American Nurses Credentialing Center (ANCC) provides other opportunities by offering nurses certification in over 45 specialty areas. There are two in community health nursing: a generalist certificate as a community health nurse, and a clinical nurse specialist certification in community health nursing. Related certifications as an NP or in nursing administration also exist. Each certification is awarded after completing a certain number of years of practice in the specialty, paying a fee, and after passing an ANCC Certification Examination. When certification is awarded, the nurse can sign RN as "RN,C." Many employers reward the initiative required for certification with promotion or a higher salary accompanied by additional responsibilities and opportunities.

SUMMARY

The specialty of community health nursing developed historically through four stages. The early home care stage (before the mid-1800s) emphasized care to the sick poor in their homes by various lay and religious orders. The district nursing stage (mid-1800s) included voluntary home nursing care for the poor by specialists or "health nurses" who treated the sick and taught wholesome living to patients. The public health nursing stage (1900 to 1970) was characterized by an increased concern for the health of the general public. The community health nursing stage (1970 to the present) includes increased recognition of community health nursing as a specialty field with focus on communities and populations.

Six major societal influences have shaped the development of community health nursing. They are advanced technology, progress in causal thinking, changes in education, the changing role of women, the consumer movement, and economic factors such as health care costs, access, limited funds for public health, and increased competition among health service providers.

Academic preparation for community health nursing begins at the baccalaureate level. However, students beginning at the diploma or associate degree level can advance to a BSN completion program and then are prepared to enter this challenging specialty in nursing. The demands of community health nursing require additional courses in liberal arts and science, along with courses in community health nursing practice at the student level. Once students complete an undergraduate degree, completing additional educational programs is required to keep current and, in most states, to maintain licensure, advance in practice opportunities, or to branch out into administration, teaching, or research.

ACTIVITIES TO PROMOTE CRITICAL THINKING

1. Select one societal influence on the development of community health nursing and explore its continuing impact. What other events are occurring today that shape community health nursing practice? Support your arguments with documentation. Use the Internet to find your documentation.

2. Using the Internet, seek out information about a historical public health nursing leader. Using this information, determine how the practitioner might deal with current population-based issues such as AIDS, sexually transmitted diseases, or child neglect and abuse.

3. Assume that you have been asked to make a home visit to a 75-year-old man living alone whose wife recently died. Besides assessing his individual needs, what additional factors should you consider for assessment and intervention that would indicate an aggregate or population-focused approach? What self-care practices might you encourage or teach?

4. Interview a community health nursing director to determine what population-based programs are offered in your locality. Explore nursing's role in the assessment, development, implementation, and evaluation of these programs. Discuss with the director how community health nurses might expand their population-focused interventions.

5. Go to the office of your university nursing college or school and locate brochures for advanced degrees in nursing and related areas. Peruse them and see if any of the programs appeal to you. Request more information from at least one of them through the mail or the Internet.

REFERENCES

American Nurses Association, Community Health Nursing Division. (1980). *A conceptual model of community health nursing* (Publication No. CH-10 2M 5/80). Kansas City, MO: Author.

American Public Health Association, Public Health Nursing Section (1996, October). *The definition and role of public health nursing: A statement of the Public Health Nursing Section.* Washington, DC: Author.

Backer, B. (1993). Lillian Wald: Connecting caring with activism. *Nursing and Health Care, 14*(3), 122–129.

Beine, J. (1996). Changing with the times. *Nursing Times, 92*(48), 59–62.

Birch, K. (1998). Speaking out. *Nursing Times, 94*(27), 19.

Brink, S. (1997). The twin challenges of information technology and population aging. *Generations, 21*(3), 7–10.

Bullough, V. & Bullough, B. (1978). *The care of the sick: The emergence of modern nursing.* New York: Neale, Watson.

Department of Philanthropic Information, Central Hanover Bank and Trust Company. (1938). *The public health nurse.* New York: National Organization for Public Health Nursing.

de Tornyay, R. (1980). Public health nursing: The nurse's role in community-based practice. *Annual Review of Public Health, 1,* 83.

Dickens, C. (1910). *Martin Chuzzlewit.* New York: Macmillan.

Dolan, J.A. (1978). *Nursing in society: A historical perspective.* Philadelphia: W.B. Saunders.

Ellis, J.R. & Hartley, C.L. (1997). *Nursing in today's world: Challenges, issues, and trends.* Philadelphia: Lippincott-Raven.

Finnegan, L. & Ervin, N.E. (1997). An epidemiological approach to community assessment. In B.W. Spradley & J. A. Allender (Eds.). *Readings in community health nursing* (pp. 186–193). Philadelphia: Lippincott-Raven Publishers.

Florence Nightingale Museum. (1997). *The Florence Nightingale Museum's School Visit Pack.* London: Florence Nightingale Museum Trust.

Friedman, G.D. (1994). *Primer of epidemiology* (4th ed.). New York: McGraw-Hill.

Furlong, M. (1997). Creating online community for older adults. *Generations, 21*(3), 33–35.

Gardner, M.S. (1936). *Public health nursing* (3rd ed.). New York: Macmillan.

Gunderson, G. (1997). Spirituality, community, and technology: An interfaith program goes online. *Generations, 21*(3), 42–45.

Jorgenson, J. (1997). Therapeutic use of companion animals in health care. *Image: Journal of Nursing Scholarship, 29*(3), 249–254.

Kalisch, P. & Kalisch, B. (1995). *The advance of American nursing* (3rd ed.). Philadelphia: J.B. Lippincott Company.

LeVasseur, J. (1998). Plato, Nightingale, and contemporary nursing. *Image: Journal of Nursing Scholarship, 30*(3), 281–285.

Mann, W.C. (1997). Common telecommunications technology for promoting safety, independence, and social interaction for older people with disabilities. *Generations, 21*(3), 28–29.

Morgan, I.S. & Marsh, G.W. (1998). Historic and future health promotion contexts for nursing. *Image: Journal of Nursing Scholarship, 30*(4), 379–383.

Mowbray, P. (1997). *Florence Nightingale museum guidebook.* London: The Florence Nightingale Museum Trust.

Naisbitt, J. & Aburdene, P. (1990). *Megatrends 2000.* New York: William Morrow.

National Organization for Public Health Nursing (1944). Approval of Skidmore College of Nursing as preparing students for public health nursing. *Public Health Nursing, 36,* 371.

Nightingale, F. Letter. The Times, London, England, April 14, 1876.

Nightingale, F. (1992). *Notes on nursing (Commemorative Edition).* Philadelphia: J.B. Lippincott Company.

Pavri, J.M. (1994). Overview one hundred years of public health nursing: Visions of a better world. *Imprint, 41*(4), 43–48.

Roberts, D. & Freeman, R. (Eds.) (1973). *Redesigning nursing education for public health: Report of the conference* (Publication No. [HRA] 75- 75). Bethesda, MD: U.S. Department of Health, Education and Welfare.

Sachs, T.B. (1908). The tuberculosis nurse. *American Journal of Nursing, 8,* 597.

Scutchfield, F.D. & Keck, C.W. (1997) *Principles of public health practice.* Albany: Delmar Publishers.

Tirpak, H. (1975). The Frontier Nursing Service: Fifty years in the mountains. *Nursing Outlook, 33*(3), 308–310.

U.S. Department of Commerce. (1998). *118th statistical abstract of the U.S., Economics and Statistics Administration, Bureau of the Census.* Washington, DC: Author.

U.S. Department of Health and Human Services, Division of Nursing. (1984). *Consensus conference on the essentials of public health nursing practice and education: Report of the conference.* Rockville, MD: U.S. Department of Health and Human Services.

U.S. Department of Health and Human Services. (2000). *Healthy people 2010* (conference edition, in two volumes). Washington, DC: Author.

Williams, C.A. (1977). Community health nursing: What is it? *Nursing Outlook, 25,* 250–254.

Woodham-Smith, C. (1951). *Florence Nightingale.* New York: McGraw-Hill.

World Health Organization (1978). *Primary health care: Report of the International Conference on Primary Health Care, Alma-Ata, USSR.* Geneva: World Health Organization.

World Health Organization. (1998). *The world health report: 1998.* Geneva: World Health Organization.

INTERNET RESOURCES

American Nurses Credentialing Center (ANCC):
http://www.nursingworld.org/ancc/accrdorg/index.htm;
http://www.nursingworld.org/ancc/approver/index.htm;
http://www.nursingworld.org/ancc/provider/index.htm;
http://www.nursingworld.org/ancc/magnet.htm

American Public Health Association (APHA):
http://www.apha.org

National Center for Health Statistics (NCHS):
http://www.cdc.gov/nchswww/products/pubs/pubd/nvsr/47-pre/47-pre.htm

SELECTED READINGS

Barnes, D., Eribes, C., Juarbe, T., Nelson, M., Proctor, S., Sawyer, L., Shual, M., & Meleis, A.I. (1995). Primary health care and primary care: A confusion of philosophies. *Nursing Outlook, 43*(7), 7–16.

Baumann, L.C. & Schmelzer, M. (1994). Writing to learn in community health nursing: The aggregate. *Public Health Nursing, 11*(4), 255–258.

Bray, M.L., & Edwards, L.H. (1994). A primary health care approach using Hispanic outreach workers as nurse extenders. *Public Health Nursing, 11*(1), 7–11.

Buhler-Wilkerson, K. (1988). Public health nursing: A photographic study. Turn-of-the-century visiting nurses. *Nursing Outlook, 36*(5), 241–43.

Calabria, M.D. & Macrae, J.A. (Eds.). (1994). *Suggestions for thought by Florence Nightingale.* Philadelphia: University of Pennsylvania Press.

Frachel, R.R. (1988). A new profession: The evolution of public health nursing. *Public Health Nursing, 5*(2), 86–90.

Hansen, B. (1997). The image and advocacy of public health in American caricature and cartoons from 1860 to 1900. *American Journal of Public Health, 87*(11), 1798–1807.

Hawkins, J.W., Veeder, N.W., & Matteson, P.S. (1995). Nurses and settlement houses: Blueprint for neighborhood clinics. *Nursing Connections, 8*(4), 58–64.

Kunitz, S.J. (1996). The history and politics of US health care policy for American Indians and Alaskan Natives. *American Journal of Public Health, 86*(10), 1464–1473.

Reinhard, S.C., Christopher, M.A., Mason, D.J., McConnell, K., Rusca, P., & Toughill, E. (1996). Promoting healthy communities through neighborhood nursing. *Nursing Outlook, 44*(5), 223–228.

Slater, V.E. (1994). The educational and philosophical influences on Florence Nightingale, an enlightened conductor. *Nursing History Review, 2,* 137–152.

Spradley, B. & Allender, J.A. (1997). *Readings in community health nursing* (5th ed.). Philadelphia: J.B. Lippincott.

Wald, L. (1971). *The House on Henry Street.* New York: Dover Publications, Inc. (reprinted from 1915 edition published by Henry Holt and Co., New York).

Roles and Settings for Community Health Nursing Practice

KEY TERMS

- Advocate
- Assessment
- Assurance
- Case management
- Clinician
- Collaborator
- Conceptual skills
- Controller
- Educator
- Evaluator
- Human skills
- Leader
- Managed care
- Manager
- Organizer
- Planner
- Policy development
- Researcher
- Technical skills

LEARNING OBJECTIVES

Upon mastery of this chapter, you should be able to:

- Identify the three core public health functions basic to community health nursing.
- Describe and differentiate among seven different roles of the community health nurse.
- Discuss the seven roles within the framework of public health nursing functions.
- Explain the importance of each role for influencing people's health.
- Identify and discuss factors that affect a nurse's selection and practice of each role.
- Describe seven settings in which community health nurses practice.
- Discuss the nature of community health nursing, and the common threads basic to its practice, woven throughout all roles and settings.
- Identify principles of sound nursing practice in the community.

Historically, community health nurses have engaged in many roles. From the beginning, nurses in this professional specialty have provided care to the sick, taught positive health habits and self-care, advocated on behalf of needy populations, developed and managed health programs, provided leadership, and collaborated with other professionals and consumers to implement changes in health services. The settings in which these nurses practiced varied, too. The home certainly has been one site for practice, but so too have clinics, schools, factories, and other community-based locations. Today, the roles and settings of professional community health nursing practice have expanded even further.

This chapter examines how the conceptual foundations and core functions of community health nursing are integrated into the various roles and the settings in which community health nurses practice. It provides an opportunity to gain greater understanding about how and where community health nursing is practiced. Furthermore, it will expand awareness of the many existing and future possibilities for community health nurses to improve the public's health.

CORE PUBLIC HEALTH FUNCTIONS

Community health nurses work as partners within a team of professionals in public health and other disciplines, nonprofessionals, and consumers to improve the health of populations. The various roles and settings for practice hinge on three primary functions of public health:

assessment, policy development, and assurance. They are foundational to all roles assumed by the community health nurse and are applied at three levels of service: to individuals, to families, and to communities (Display 3–1). Regardless of role or setting of choice, these foundational responsibilities direct the work of all community health nurses.

Assessment

An essential first function in public health, **assessment,** means that the community health nurse must gather and analyze information that will affect the health of the people to be served. The nurse and others on the health team need to determine health needs, health risks, environmental conditions, political agendas, and financial and other resources, depending on the persons, community, or population targeted for intervention. Data may be gathered in many ways; typical methods include interviewing people in the community, conducting surveys, gathering information from public records, and using research findings.

The community health nurse usually is trusted and valued by clients, agencies, and private providers. This trust typically affords a nurse access to client populations that are difficult to engage, to agencies, and to health care providers. In the capacity of trusted professional, community health nurses gather relevant client data that enable them to identify strengths, weaknesses, and needs.

At the community level, assessment is done both formally and informally as nurses identify and interact with key community leaders. With families, the nurse can evaluate family strengths and areas of concern in the immediate living environment and the neighborhood. At the individual level, people are identified within the family who are in need of services, and the nurse evaluates the functional capacity of these individuals through the use of specific assessment measures, using a variety of tools. Assessment of communities and families is described in detail in Chapters 18 and 23.

Policy Development

Policy development, defined in Display 3–1, is enhanced by the synthesis and analysis of information obtained during assessment. At the community level, the nurse provides leadership in convening and facilitating community groups to evaluate health concerns and develop a plan to address the concerns. Typically, the nurse recommends specific training and programs to meet identified health needs of target populations. This is accompanied by raising the awareness of key policy makers about factors such as health regulations and budget decisions that negatively affect the health of the community. With families, the nurse recommends new programs or increased services based on identified needs. Additional data may be needed to identify trends in groups or clusters of families so that effective intervention strategies can be used with

these families. At the individual level, the nurse assists in the development of standards for individual client care, recommends or adopts risk-classification systems to assist with prioritizing individual client care, and participates in establishing criteria for opening, closing, or referring individual cases.

Assurance

Assurance activities—the activities that make certain that services are provided—often consume most of the community health nurse's time. With the increase in programmatic funding and direct state reimbursement through Medicaid programs, community health nurses in many settings have been required to focus on direct service to individuals rather than on population-based services. Nonetheless, community health nurses perform the assurance function at the community level when they provide service to target populations, improve quality assurance activities, and maintain safe levels of communicable disease surveillance and outbreak control. In addition, they participate in research, provide expert consultation, and provide services within the community based on standards of

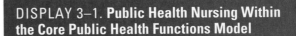

DISPLAY 3–1. Public Health Nursing Within the Core Public Health Functions Model

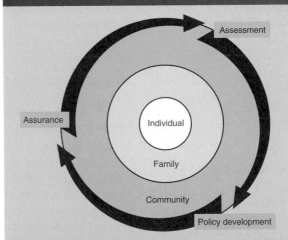

The model includes assessment, policy development, and assurance surrounding the individual, family, and community. *Assessment* is the regular collection, analysis, and sharing of information about health conditions, risks, and resources in a community. *Policy development* uses the information gathered during assessment to develop local and state health policies and to direct resources toward those policies. *Assurance* focuses on the availability of necessary health services throughout the community. It includes maintaining the ability of both public health agencies and private providers to manage day-to-day operations as well as the capacity to respond to critical situations and emergencies (Conley & Dahl, 1993).

care. Care is provided to clusters of families within a geographic setting or in one setting, such as a neighborhood clinic.

Individuals should receive nursing services based on standards developed by the American Nurses Association (ANA), such as the *Code for Nurses With Interpretive Statements* (1985), *Nursing's Social Policy Statement* (1995), *Standards of Clinical Nursing Practice* (1997), and *Scope and Standards of Public Health Nursing Practice* (1999). The community health nurse consults with other health care providers and team members regarding the individual's plan of care and participates on quality assurance teams to measure the quality of care provided (Conley & Dahl, 1993). The three core functions of assessment, policy making, and assurance are woven throughout all of the nurse's roles and the various community settings of practice.

ROLES OF COMMUNITY HEALTH NURSES

Just as the health care system is continually evolving, community health nursing practice evolves to remain effective with the clients it serves. Over time, the role of the community health nurse has broadened. This breadth is reflected in the definition of public health nursing from the American Public Health Association, Public Health Nursing Section (1996):

> **Public health nurses integrate community involvement and knowledge about the entire population with personal, clinical understandings of the health and illness experiences of individuals and families within the population. They translate and articulate the health and illness experiences of diverse, often vulnerable individuals and families in the population to health planners and policy makers, and assist members of the community to voice their problems and aspirations. Public health nurses are knowledgeable about multiple strategies for intervention, from those applicable to the entire population, to those for the family, and the individual. Public health nurses translate knowledge from the health and social sciences to individuals and population groups through targeted interventions, programs, and advocacy.**
>
> **Public health nursing may be practiced by one public health nurse or by a group of public health nurses working collaboratively. In both instances, public health nurses are directly engaged in the inter-disciplinary activities of the core public health functions of assessment, assurance and policy development. Interventions or strategies may be targeted to multiple levels depending on where the most effective outcomes are possible. They include strategies aimed at entire population groups, families, or individuals. In any setting, the role of public health nurses focuses on the prevention of illness, injury or disability, the promotion of health, and maintenance of the health of populations.**

Community health nurses wear many hats while conducting day-to-day practice. At any given time, however, one role is primary. This is especially true for specialized roles such as that of full-time manager. This chapter examines seven major roles: (1) clinician, (2) educator, (3) advocate, (4) manager, (5) collaborator, (6) leader, and (7) researcher. It then examines the factors that influence the selection and performance of those roles.

Clinician Role

The most familiar role of the community health nurse is that of clinician or care provider; however, the provision of nursing care takes on new meaning in the context of community health. The **clinician** role in community health means that the nurse ensures that health services are provided not just to individuals and families, but also to groups and populations. Nursing service still is designed for the special needs of clients; however, when those clients comprise a group or population, clinical practice takes different forms. It requires different skills to assess collective needs and tailor service accordingly. For instance, the community health nurse might visit elderly persons in a seniors' high-rise apartment building. This is an opportunity to assess the needs of that entire aggregate and design appropriate services.

For community health nurses, the clinician role involves certain emphases different from basic nursing. Three, in particular, are useful to consider here: the clinician's emphasis on holism, health promotion, and skill expansion.

HOLISTIC PRACTICE
Most clinical nursing seeks to be broad and holistic. In community health, however, a holistic approach means considering the broad range of interacting needs that affect the collective health of the "client" as a larger system (Caraher & McNab, 1996; Patterson, 1998). The client is a composite of people whose relationships and interactions with each other must be considered in totality. Holistic practice must emerge from this systems perspective. For example, when working with a group of pregnant teenagers living in a juvenile detention center, the nurse would consider the girls' relationships with one another, their parents, the fathers of their unborn children, and the detention center staff. The nurse would evaluate their ages, developmental needs, and peer influence, as well as their knowledge of pregnancy, delivery, and issues related to the choice of keeping or giving up their babies. The girls' reentry into the community and their future plans for school or employment also would be considered. Holistic service would go far beyond the physical condition of pregnancy and childbirth. It would incorporate consideration of pregnant adolescents in this community as a population-at-risk. What factors contributed to these girls' situations, and what preventive efforts could be instituted to protect other teenagers? The clinician role, as a community health nurse, involves holistic practice from an aggregate perspective.

FOCUS ON WELLNESS

The clinician role in community health also is characterized by its focus on promoting wellness (Frenn, 1996). As discussed in Chapter 1, the community health nurse provides service along the entire range of the health continuum but especially emphasizes promotion of health and prevention of illness. Nursing service includes seeking out clients at risk for poor health to offer preventive and health-promoting services, rather than waiting for them to come for help after problems arise (Caraher, 1995; Kristjanson & Chalmers, 1997). People are identified who are interested in achieving a higher level of health, and the community health nurse works with them to accomplish that goal and then sustain the behavior. The nurse may help employees of a business learn how to live healthier lives or may work with a group who wants to quit smoking. The community health nurse may hold seminars with a men's group on enhancing fathering skills or may assist several families with terminally ill members to gain strength through a support system during the death and dying process. Groups and populations are identified that may be vulnerable to certain health threats, and preventive and health-promoting programs can be designed. Examples include immunization of preschoolers, family planning programs, cholesterol screening, and prevention of behavioral problems in adolescents. Protecting and promoting the health of vulnerable populations is an important component of the clinician role and is addressed extensively in the chapters in Unit VII on vulnerable aggregates.

EXPANDED SKILLS

Many different skills are used in the role of the community health clinician. In the early years of community health nursing, emphasis was placed on physical care skills. With time, skills in observation, listening, communication, and counseling became integral to the clinician role as it grew to encompass an increased emphasis on psychological and sociocultural factors. Recently, environmental and community-wide considerations—such as problems caused by pollution, violence and crime, drug abuse, unemployment, poverty, homelessness, and limited funding for health programs—have created a need for stronger skills in assessing the needs of groups and populations and intervening at the community level. The clinician role in population-based nursing also requires skills in collaboration with consumers and other professionals, use of epidemiology and biostatistics, community organization and development, research, program evaluation, administration, leadership, and effecting change (Keller et al., 1998). These skills are addressed in greater detail in later chapters.

Educator Role

A second important role of the community health nurse is that of **educator** or health teacher. Health teaching, a widely recognized part of nursing practice, is legislated through nurse practice acts in several states and is one of the major functions of the community health nurse (Breckon et al., 1998). The educator role is especially useful in promoting the public's health for at least two reasons.

First, community clients usually are not acutely ill and can absorb and act on health information. For example, a class of expectant parents, unhampered by significant health problems, can grasp the relationship of diet to fetal development. They understand the value of specific exercises to the childbirth process, are motivated to learn, and are more likely to perform those exercises. Thus, the educator role has the potential for finding greater receptivity and providing higher yield results.

Second, the educator role in community health nursing is significant because a wider audience can be reached. With an emphasis on populations and aggregates, the educational efforts of community health nursing are appropriately targeted to reach many people. Instead of limiting teaching to one-on-one or small groups, the nurse has the opportunity and mandate to develop educational programs based on community needs that seek a community-wide impact. Community-wide antidrug use campaigns, dietary improvement programs, and improved handwashing efforts among children provide useful models for implementing the educator role at the population level and demonstrate its effectiveness in reaching a wide audience (Chou et al., 1998; Early et al., 1998; Perry et al., 1998).

One factor that enhances the educator role is the public's higher level of health consciousness. Through plans ranging from the President's Physical Fitness Program to local antismoking campaigns, people are recognizing the value of health and are increasingly motivated to achieve higher levels of wellness. When a middle-aged man, for example, is discharged from the hospital after a heart attack, he is likely to be more interested than before the attack in learning how to prevent another. He can learn how to reduce stress, develop an appropriate and gradual exercise program, and alter his eating habits. Families with young children often are interested in learning about children's growth and development; most parents are committed to raising happy, healthy children. Health education can affect the health status of people of all ages (Laflin, 1996; Niffenegger, 1997). In more businesses and industries, nurses promote the health of employees through active wellness-education and injury-prevention programs (Burton & Connerty, 1998; Kidd et al., 1997). The companies recognize that improved health of their workers means less absenteeism and higher production levels in addition to other benefits (Maes et al., 1998). Some companies even provide exercise areas and equipment for employee use and pay them for their participation.

Whereas nurses in acute care teach patients with a one-on-one focus about issues related to their hospitalization, community health nurses go beyond these topics to educate people in many areas. Community-living clients need and want to know about a wide variety of issues such as family planning, weight control, smoking cessation, and stress reduction. Aggregate level concerns also include such topics as environmental safety, sexual discrimination and harassment at school or work, violence, and drugs. What foods and additives are safe to eat? How can people organize the community to work for reduction of violence on television? What are health consumers' rights? Topics taught by community health nurses extend from personal and family health to environmental health and community organization.

As educators, community health nurses seek to facilitate client learning. Information is shared with clients both formally and informally. Nurses act as consultants to individuals or groups. Formal classes may be held to increase people's understanding of health and health care. Established community groups may be used in the nurse's teaching. For example, a nurse may teach parents and teachers at a parent-teacher meeting about signs of mood-modifying drug and alcohol abuse, discuss safety practices with a group of industrial workers, or give a presentation on the importance of early detection of child abuse to a health planning committee considering the funding of a new program. At times, the community health nurse facilitates client learning through referrals to more knowledgeable sources or through use of experts on special topics. Clients' self-education is facilitated by the nurse; in keeping with the concept of self-care, clients are encouraged and helped to use appropriate health resources and to seek out health information for themselves. The emphasis throughout the health teaching process continues to be placed on illness prevention and health promotion. Health teaching as a tool for community health nursing practice is discussed in Chapter 9.

Advocate Role

The issue of clients' rights is important in health care. Every patient or client has the right to receive just, equal, and humane treatment. The role of nurse includes client advocacy, which is highlighted in the ANA's code for nurses (1985) and *Nursing's Social Policy Statement* (1995). Our current health care system often is characterized by fragmented and depersonalized services, and many clients—especially the poor, disadvantaged, those without health insurance, and people with language barriers—frequently are denied their rights. They become frustrated, confused, degraded, and unable to cope with the system on their own. The community health nurse often acts as an **advocate** for clients, pleading their cause or acting on their behalf. Clients may need someone to explain which services to expect and which services they ought to receive, to make referrals as needed, and to write letters to agencies or health care providers written for them. They need someone to guide them through the complexities of the system, to assure the satisfaction of their needs (Snowball, 1996). This is particularly true for minorities and disadvantaged groups (Holmes & Warelow, 1997).

ADVOCACY GOALS
There are two underlying goals in client advocacy. One is to help clients gain greater independence or self-determination.

Until they can research the needed information and access health and social services for themselves, the community health nurse acts as an advocate for the clients by showing them what services are available, the ones to which they are entitled, and how to obtain them. A second goal is to make the system more responsive and relevant to the needs of clients. By calling attention to inadequate, inaccessible, or unjust care, community health nurses can influence change.

Consider the experience of the Merrill family. Gloria Merrill has three small children. Early one Tuesday morning, the baby, Tony, suddenly started to cry. Nothing would comfort him. Gloria went to a neighbor's apartment, called the local clinic, and was told to come in the next day. The clinic did not take appointments and was too busy to see any more patients that day. Gloria's neighbor reassured her that "sometimes babies just cry." For the rest of the day and night, Tony cried almost incessantly. On Wednesday, there was a 45-minute bus ride and a wait of 3½ hours in the crowded reception room, a wait punctuated by interrogations from clinic workers. Gloria's other children were restless, and the baby was crying. Finally, they saw the physician. Tony had an inguinal hernia that could have strangulated and become gangrenous. The doctor admonished Gloria for waiting so long to bring in the baby. Immediate surgery was necessary. Someone at the clinic told Gloria that Medicaid would pay for it. Someone else told her that she was ineligible because she was not a registered clinic patient. At this point, all of her children were crying. Gloria had been up most of the night. She was frantic, confused, and felt that no one cared. This family needed an advocate.

ADVOCACY ACTIONS
The advocate role incorporates four characteristic actions: (1) being assertive, (2) taking risks, (3) communicating and negotiating well, and (4) identifying resources and obtaining results. First, advocates must be assertive. Fortunately, in the Merrills' dilemma, the clinic had a working relationship with the City Health Department and contacted Tracy Lee, a community health nurse liaison with the clinic, when Gloria broke down and cried. Tracy took the initiative to identify the Merrills' needs and find appropriate solutions. She contacted the Department of Social Services and helped the Merrills to establish eligibility for coverage of surgery and hospitalization costs. She helped Gloria to make arrangements for the baby's hospitalization and the other children's care. Second, advocates must take risks—go out on a limb if need be—for the client. The community health nurse was outraged at the kind of treatment received by the Merrills: the delays in service, the impersonal care, and the surgery that could have been planned as elective rather than as an emergency. She wrote a letter describing the details of the Merrills' experience to the clinic director, the chairman of the clinic board, and the nursing director. It resulted in better care for the Merrills and a series of meetings aimed at changing clinic procedures and providing better telephone screening. Third, advocates must communicate and negotiate well by bargaining

thoroughly and convincingly. The community health nurse helping the Merrill family stated the problem clearly and argued for its solution. Finally, advocates must identify and obtain resources for the client's benefit. By contacting the most influential people in the clinic and appealing to their desire for quality service, the nurse caring for the Merrill family was able to facilitate change.

Advocacy at the population level incorporates the same goals and actions. Whether the population is homeless people, battered women, or migrant workers, the community health nurse, in the advocate role, speaks and acts on their behalf. The goals remain the same: to promote clients' self-determination and to shape a more responsive system. Advocacy for large aggregates, such as the millions with inadequate health care coverage, means changing national policies and laws (see Chapter 13). Advocacy may take the form of presenting public health nursing data to ensure that providers deliver quality services (Bushy, 1997). It may mean conducting a needs assessment to demonstrate the necessity for a shelter and multiservice program for the homeless. It may mean testifying before the legislature to create awareness of the problems of battered women and the need for more protective laws. It may mean organizing a lobbying effort to require employers of migrant workers to provide proper housing and working conditions. In each case, the community health nurse works with representatives of the population to gain their understanding of the situation and to ensure their input.

Manager Role

Community health nurses, like all nurses, engage in the role of managing health services. As a manager, the nurse exercises administrative direction toward the accomplishment of specified goals by assessing clients' needs, planning and organizing to meet those needs, directing and leading to achieve results, and controlling and evaluating the progress to ensure that goals are met. The nurse serves as a **manager** when overseeing client care as a case manager, supervising ancillary staff, managing caseloads, running clinics, or conducting community health needs assessment projects. In each instance, the nurse engages in four basic functions that make up the management process. The management process, like the nursing process, incorporates a series of problem-solving activities or functions: planning, organizing, leading, and controlling and evaluating. These activities are sequential and yet also occur simultaneously for managing service objectives (Megginson et al., 1997; Swansburg & Swansburg, 1999). While performing these functions, community health nurses most often are participative managers; that is, they participate with clients, other professionals, or both to plan and implement services.

NURSE AS PLANNER

The first function in the management process is planning. A **planner** sets the goals and direction for the organization or project and determines the means to achieve them. Specifically, planning includes defining goals and objectives, determining the strategy for reaching them, and designing a coordinated set of activities for implementing and evaluating them. Planning may be strategic, which tends to include broader, more long-range goals (Hall, 1998; Swansburg & Swansburg, 1999; U.S. Department of Health and Human Services, 2000). An example of strategic planning is setting 2-year agency goals to reduce teenage pregnancies in the county by 50%. Planning may be operational, which focuses more on short-term planning needs. An example of operational planning is setting 6-month objectives to implement a new computer system for client record keeping.

The community health nurse engages in planning as a part of the manager role when supervising a group of home health aides working with home care clients. Plans of care must be designed that include setting short-term and long-term objectives, describing actions to carry out the objectives, and designing a plan for evaluating the care given. With larger groups, such as a program for a homeless mentally ill population, the planning function is used in collaboration with other professionals in the community to determine appropriate goals for shelter and treatment and to develop an action plan to carry out and evaluate the program (Rowland & Rowland, 1997). The concept of planning with communities and families is discussed further in Chapters 19 and 24, respectively.

NURSE AS ORGANIZER

The second function of the manager role is that of **organizer.** This involves designing a structure within which people and tasks function to reach the desired objectives. A manager must arrange matters so that the job can be done. People, activities, and relationships have to be assembled to put the plan into effect (Rowland & Rowland, 1997). Organizing includes deciding the tasks to be done, who will do them, how to group the tasks, who reports to whom, and where decisions will be made (Robbins, 1997). In the process of organizing, the nurse manager provides a framework for the various aspects of service so that each runs smoothly and accomplishes its purpose. The framework is a part of service preparation. When a community health nurse manages a well-child clinic, for instance, the organizing function involves making certain that all equipment and supplies are present, that required staff are hired and are on duty, and that staff responsibilities are clearly designated. The final responsibility as an organizer is to evaluate the effectiveness of the clinic. Is it providing the needed services? Are the clients satisfied? Do the services remain cost-effective? All of these questions must be addressed by the organizer.

NURSE AS LEADER

In the manager role, the community health nurse also must act as a **leader.** As a leader, the nurse directs, influences, or persuades others to effect change to positively affect people's health and move them toward a goal. The leading function includes persuading and motivating people, directing activities, ensuring effective two-way communication, resolving conflicts, and coordinating the plan. Coordination means bringing people and activities together so that they function in harmony while pursuing desired objectives.

Community health nurses act as leaders when they direct and coordinate the functioning of a hypertension screening clinic, a weight control group, or a three-county mobile health assessment unit. In each case, the leading function requires motivating the people involved, keeping clear channels of communication, negotiating conflicts, and directing and coordinating the activities established during planning so that the desired objectives can be accomplished.

NURSE AS CONTROLLER AND EVALUATOR

The fourth management function is to control and evaluate projects or programs. A **controller** monitors the plan and ensures that it stays on course. In this function, the community health nurse must realize that plans may not proceed as intended and may need adjustments or corrections to reach the desired results or goals. Monitoring, comparing, and adjusting make up the controlling part of this function. At the same time, the nurse must compare and judge performance and outcomes against previously set goals and standards—a process that forms the **evaluator** aspect of this management function.

An example of the controlling and evaluation function is evident in a program started in several preschool day-care centers in a city in the Midwest. The goal of the project was to reduce the incidence of illness among the children through intensive physical and emotional preventive health education with staff, parents, and children. The two community health nurses managing the project were pleased with the progress of the classes and monitored the application of the prevention principles in day-to-day care. However, staff became busy after several weeks, and some plans were not being followed carefully. Preventive activities were not being closely monitored, such as ensuring that the children covered their mouths if they coughed or washed their hands after using the bathroom and before eating. Several children who were clearly sick had not been kept at home. Including the lonely children in activities sometimes was overlooked. The nurses worked with staff and parents to motivate them and get the project back on course. They held monthly meetings with the staff, observed the classes periodically, and offered one-on-one instruction to staff, parents, and children. One activity was to establish competition between the centers for the best health record with the promise of a photograph of the winning center's children and an article in the local newspaper. Their efforts were successful.

MANAGEMENT BEHAVIORS

As managers, community health nurses engage in many different types of behaviors. These behaviors or parts of the manager role were first described by Mintzberg (1973). He grouped them into three sets of behaviors: (1) decision-making, (2) transferring of information, and (3) engaging in interpersonal relationships.

Decision-Making Behaviors

Mintzburg identified four types of decisional roles or behaviors: entrepreneur, disturbance handler, resource allocator, and negotiator. A manager serves in the entrepreneur role when initiating new projects. Starting a nursing center to serve a homeless population is an example. Community health nurses play the disturbance-handler role when they manage disturbances and crises, particularly interpersonal conflicts among staff, between staff and clients, or between clients, especially when being served in an agency. The resource-allocator role is demonstrated by determining the distribution and use of human, physical, and financial resources. Nurses play the negotiator role when negotiating, perhaps with higher levels of administration or a funding agency, for new health policy or budget increases to support expanded services for clients.

Transfer of Information Behaviors

Mintzburg described three informational roles or behaviors: monitor, information disseminator, and spokesperson. The monitor role requires collecting and processing information, such as gathering ongoing evaluation data to determine whether a program is meeting its goals. In the disseminator role, nurses transmit the collected information to people involved in the project or organization. In the spokesperson role, nurses share information on behalf of the project or agency with outsiders.

Interpersonal Behaviors

While engaging in various interpersonal roles, the community health nurse may function as figurehead, leader, and liaison. In the figurehead role, the nurse acts in a ceremonial or symbolic capacity, such as participating in a ribbon-cutting ceremony to mark the opening of a new clinic or representing the project or agency for news media coverage. In the leader role, the nurse motivates and directs people involved in the project. In the liaison role, a network is maintained with people outside of the organization or project for information exchange and project enhancement.

MANAGEMENT SKILLS

What types of skills and competencies does the community health nurse need in the manager role? Three basic management skills are needed for successful achievement of goals; they are human, conceptual, and technical (Robbins, 1997). **Human skills** refer to the ability to understand, communicate, motivate, delegate, and work well with people. An example is a nursing supervisor or team leader's ability to gain the trust and respect of staff and promote a productive and satisfying work environment. A manager can accomplish goals only with the cooperation of others. Thus, human skills are essential to successfully perform the manager role. **Conceptual skills** refer to the mental ability to analyze and interpret abstract ideas for the purpose of understanding and diagnosing situations and formulating solutions. Examples are analyzing demographic data for program planning or developing a conceptual model to describe and improve organizational function. Finally,

technical skills refer to the ability to apply special management-related knowledge and expertise to a particular situation or problem. Such skills might include a community health nurse implementing a staff development program or developing a computerized management information system.

CASE MANAGEMENT

Case management has become the standard method of managing health care in the delivery systems in the United States, and managed care organizations have become an integral part of community-oriented care (Mundt, 1996; Weiss, 1997). **Case management** is a systematic process by which a nurse assesses clients' needs, plans for and coordinates services, refers to other appropriate providers, and monitors and evaluates progress to ensure that clients' multiple service needs are met in a cost-effective manner. **Managed care,** the broader umbrella under which case management exists, is a cost-containing system of health care administration (Resnick & Tighe, 1997). Managed care, as an approach to delivering health care, is discussed in detail in Chapter 7. As clients leave hospitals earlier, as families struggle with multiple and complex health problems, as more elderly persons need alternatives to nursing home care, as competition and scarce resources contribute to fragmentation of services, and as the cost of health care continues to increase, there is a growing need for someone to oversee and coordinate all facets of needed service. Through case management, the nurse addresses this need in the community (Williams & Torrens, 1999).

The activity of case management often follows discharge planning as a part of continuity of care. When applied to individual clients, it means overseeing their transition from the hospital back into the community and following them to ensure that all of their service needs are met. Case management also applies to aggregates. This involves overseeing and assuring that a group's or population's health-related needs are met, particularly those at high risk of illness or injury. For example, the community health nurse may work with battered women who come to a shelter. First, the nurse must ensure that their immediate needs for safety, security, food, finances, and child care are met. Then, the nurse must work with other professionals to provide more permanent housing, employment, ongoing counseling, and financial and legal resources for this group of women. Whether applied to families or aggregates, case management, like other applications of the manager role, uses the three sets of management behaviors and engages the community health nurse as planner, organizer, leader, controller, and evaluator.

Collaborator Role

Community health nurses seldom practice in isolation. They must work with many people, including clients, other nurses, physicians, teachers, health educators, social workers, physical therapists, nutritionists, occupational therapists, psychologists, epidemiologists, biostaticians, attorneys, secretaries, environmentalists, city planners, and legislators. As members of the health team (Gardner, 1996; Milligan et al., 1999), community health nurses assume the role of **collaborator,** which means to work jointly with others in a common endeavor, to cooperate as partners. Successful community health practice depends on this multidisciplinary collegiality and leadership (Ales, 1998; Brandon, 1996). Everyone on the team has an important and unique contribution to make to the health care effort. As on a championship ball team, the better all members play their individual positions and cooperate with other members, the more likely the health team is to win.

The community health nurse's collaborator role requires skills in communicating, in interpreting the nurse's unique contribution to the team, and in acting assertively as an equal partner. The collaborator role also may involve functioning as a consultant.

The following examples show a community health nurse functioning as collaborator. Three families needed to find good nursing homes for their elderly grandparents. The community health nurse met with the families, including the elderly members, made a list of desired features, such as a shower and access to walking trails, and then worked with a social worker to locate and visit several homes. The grandparents' respective physicians were contacted for medical consultation, and in each case the elderly member made the final selection. In another situation, the community health nurse collaborated with the city council, police department, neighborhood residents, and manager of a senior citizens' high-rise apartment building to help a group of elderly people organize and lobby for safer streets. In a third example, a school nurse noticed a rise in the incidence of drug use in her schools. She initiated a counseling program after joint planning with students, parents, teachers, the school psychologist, and a local drug rehabilitation center.

Leadership Role

Community health nurses are becoming increasingly active in the leadership role, separate from leading within the manager role mentioned earlier in this chapter. The leadership role focuses on effecting change (Chapter 10 elaborates on this role); thus, the nurse becomes an agent of change. As leaders, community health nurses seek to initiate change that positively affects people's health. They also seek to influence people to think and behave differently about their health and the factors contributing to it.

At the community level, the leadership role may involve working with a team of professionals to direct and coordinate such projects as a campaign to eliminate smoking in public areas or to lobby legislators for improved child day-care facilities. When they guide community health decision-making, stimulate an industry's interest in health promotion, initiate group therapy, direct a preventive program, and influence health policy, they assume the leadership role. For example, a community health nurse started a rehabilitation program that included self-esteem building, career counseling, and job placement to help women in a halfway house who recently were released from prison.

The community health nurse also exerts influence through health planning. The need for coordinated, accessible, cost-effective health care services creates a challenge and an opportunity for the nurse to become more involved in health planning at all levels: organizational, local, state, national, and international. A community health nurse needs to exercise leadership responsibility and assert the right to share in health decisions (Rowland & Rowland, 1997). One community health nurse determined that there was a need for a mental health program in his district. He planned to implement it through the agency for which he worked, but certain individuals on the health board were opposed to adding new programs because of cost. His approach was to gather considerable data to demonstrate the program's need and cost-effectiveness. He invited individual key board members to lunch to convince them of the need. He prepared written summaries, graphs, and charts and, at a strategic time, presented his case at a board meeting. The mental health program was approved and implemented.

A broader attribute of the leadership role is that of visionary. A leader with vision develops the ability to see what can be and leads people on a path toward that goal. A leader's vision may include long-term and short-term goals. In one instance, it began as articulating the need for stronger community nursing services to an underserved population in an inner city neighborhood served by a community health nurse. In this densely populated, tenant-occupied neighborhood, drugs, crime, and violence were commonplace. One summer, an 8-year-old boy was shot and killed. The enraged immigrant families in this neighborhood felt helpless and hopeless. Several families were visited by the nurse, and they shared their concerns with her. The nurse felt strongly about this blighted community and offered to work with the community to effect change. Volunteers from neighborhood churches were gathered by the community health nurse, and together they began to discuss the community concerns. Together they prioritized their needs and began planning to make this a healthy community. The nurse organized her work week to provide health screening and education to families in the basement of a church one morning a week. Initially, only a few families accessed this new service. In a matter of months it became recognized as a valuable community service, and it expanded to a full day with a growing volunteer group soon outgrowing the space. The community health nurse worked closely with influential community members and the families being served. They determined that many more services were needed in this neighborhood, and they began to broaden their outreach and think of ways to get the needed services.

Within a year, the group had written several grants to the city and a private corporation to expand the voluntary services. The funding that they obtained allowed them to rent vacant storefront space, hire a part-time nurse practitioner, contract with the health department for additional community health nursing services, and negotiate with the local university to have medical, nursing, and social work students placed on a regular basis. The group, under the visionary leadership of the community health nurse, has plans to add a one-on-one reading program for children, a class in English as a second language for immigrant families, a mentoring program for teenagers, and dental services. Even the police department had opened a substation in the neighborhood, making their presence more visible. This community health nurse's vision filled an immediate, critical need in the short term and developed into a comprehensive community center in the long term. Neighborhood violence and crime has diminished, and it is a place where children can play safely.

Researcher Role

In the **researcher** role, community health nurses engage in systematic investigation, collection, and analysis of data for solving problems and enhancing community health practice. But how can research be combined with practice? Although research technically involves a complex set of activities conducted by persons with highly developed and specialized skills, research also means applying that technical study to real-practice situations. Community health nurses base their practice on the evidence found in the literature to enhance and change practice as needed. The work of several researchers over 15 years supports the value of intensive home visiting to high-risk families (Kitzman et al., 1997; Olds et al., 1997). The outcomes of this research are changing practice protocol to high-risk families in many health departments.

Research is an investigative process in which all community health nurses can become involved in asking questions and looking for solutions. Collaborative practice models between academics and practitioners combine research methodology expertise with practitioners' knowledge of problems to make community health nursing research both valid and relevant (Twinn, 1997).

THE RESEARCH PROCESS

Community health nurses practice the researcher role at several levels. In addition to everyday inquiries, community health nurses often participate in agency and organizational studies to determine such matters as job satisfaction among public health nurses and organizational variables (Cumbey & Alexander, 1998). Some community health nurses participate in more complex research on their own or in collaboration with other health professionals (Raisler et al., 1999). The researcher role, at all levels, helps to determine needs, evaluate effectiveness of care, and develop theoretical bases for community health nursing practice. Chapters 11 and 14 explain community health research in greater detail.

Research literally means to *search again*—to investigate, discover, and interpret facts. All research in community health, from the simplest inquiry to the most complex epidemiologic study, uses the same fundamental process. Simply put, the research process involves the following steps: (1) identify an area of interest, (2) specify the research question or statement, (3) review the literature, (4) identify a conceptual framework, (5) select a research design, (6) collect and analyze data, (7) interpret the results, and (8) communicate the findings (see Chapter 11).

Investigation builds on the nursing process, that essential dynamic of community health nursing practice, using it as a problem-solving process (Polit & Hungler, 1999). In using the nursing process, the nurse identifies a problem or question, investigates by collecting and analyzing data, suggests and evaluates possible solutions, and selects a solution, or rejects them all and starts the investigative process over again. In a sense, the nurse is gathering data for health planning—investigating health problems to design wellness-promoting and disease-preventing interventions for community populations (see The Global Community).

ATTRIBUTES OF THE RESEARCHER ROLE

A questioning attitude is a basic prerequisite to good nursing practice. A nurse may have revisited a patient many times and noticed some change in his condition, such as restlessness or pallor. Consequently, the nurse wonders what was causing this change and what could be done about it. In everyday practice, numerous situations are encountered that challenge the nurse to ask questions. Consider the following examples:

- The newspaper reports another group of children arrested for using illegal drugs. Is there an increase in the incidence of illegal drug use in the community?
- Several day-care children appear to have excessive bruises on their arms and legs. What is the incidence of reported child abuse in this community? What could be done to promote earlier detection and improved reporting?
- Several elderly persons are living alone and without assistance in a neighborhood. How prevalent is this situation and what are this population's needs?
- While driving through a neighborhood, the nurse notices that there is not a single playground around for miles. Where do the kids play?

Each of these questions places the nurse in the role of investigator. They express the fundamental attitude of every researcher: a spirit of inquiry.

A second attribute, careful observation, also is evident in the examples just given. The nurse needs to develop a sharpened ability to notice things as they are, including deviations from the norm and subtle changes suggesting the need for nursing action. Coupled with observation is open-mindedness, another attribute of the researcher role. In the case of the bruises seen on day-care children, a community health nurse's observations suggest child abuse as a possible cause. However, open-mindedness requires consideration of other alternatives, and as a good investigator, these also are explored.

Analytic skills also are used in this role. In the example of illegal drug use, the nurse already has started to analyze the situation by trying to determine its cause-and-effect relationships. Successful analysis depends on how well the data have

THE GLOBAL COMMUNITY

Twinn, S. (1997). Methodological issues in the evaluation of the quality of public health nursing: A case study of the maternal and child health centres in Hong Kong. *Journal of Advanced Nursing, 25,* 753–759.

In response to the demand for the evaluation of the quality of client care in all nursing disciplines, this study discusses the development of a collaborative study with the Department of Health in Hong Kong to evaluate the quality of public health nursing in the maternal and child health centers.

Using both qualitative and quantitative methods of data collection, a multiple case study design was developed. The findings demonstrated implications for clinical practice and methodologic issues for the evaluation of care. The findings indicate three major issues for continued consideration. First is the cultural context of care, which includes perceptions of care such as demands on the service and expectations of care. Second is the use of health data, including both the methods of recording data and the sources of data. Third is the method of data collection, in particular, the implications of the use of language in data collection tools.

The findings suggest that both the use of professional language and the need for translation have implications for data collection methods. The researcher believed that methodologies for the evaluation of care must address culturally specific issues, especially where English was not the first language of the study subjects. In addition, the use of language in the method of data collection raises more general issues punctuated by the distortion of translation in the collection and analysis of qualitative data. Samples of three translations of the same interviewer's question and the responses given demonstrate how dramatically different the question is asked and answered by people for whom English is a second language. This has major implications both in the quality of care delivered and the validity of research conducted by the people providing care or doing the research conducted by the people providing care or doing the research using a second language.

Examples of three verbatim translations follow:
Translator 1
Question: Have you seen the bruising on children's body that alarm you for more attention or some marks of physical punishment?
Response: No, I haven't seen that. But I've seen some burning marks of the candle. But it is quite common for the boat people to use these, burning on newborn's body for they always cry.
Translator 2
Question: Have you seen any bruises that caused concern?
Response: No I haven't . . . but I have seen some burn marks resulting from joss sticks. The newborn babies of fisherman got pairs of burn marks on their trunk if they cry a lot.
Translator 3
Question: Have you ever seen some bruise marks or "bamboo stick" marks that will warrant you to do something about it?
Response: No, I have never seen one. But I did see babies burned with joss sticks. The newborn babies like to cry, and when they cry, the boat people like to use joss sticks to burn their babies on their nipples. They usually make the marks with the joss sticks and make several holes (p. 758).

been collected. Insufficient information can lead to false interpretations, so it is important to seek out the needed data. Analysis, like a jigsaw puzzle, involves studying the pieces and fitting them together until the meaning of the whole picture can be described.

Finally, the researcher role involves tenacity. The community health nurse persists in an investigation until facts are uncovered and a satisfactory answer is found. Noticing an absence of playgrounds and wondering where the children play is only a beginning. Being concerned about the children's safety and need for recreational outlets, the nurse gathers data about the location and accessibility of play areas as well as felt needs of community residents. A fully documented research report may result. If the data support a need for additional play space, the report can be brought before the proper authorities (see Research: Bridge to Practice).

SETTINGS FOR COMMUNITY HEALTH NURSING PRACTICE

The previous section examined community health nursing from the perspective of its major roles. The roles now can be

RESEARCH Bridge to Practice

Molinari, C., Ahern, M., & Hendryx, M. (1998). Gains from public-private collaborations to improve community health. *Journal of Healthcare Management, 43*(6), 498–510.

In many disciplines, theoretical and empirical evidence shows that community collaboration affects health and behaviors of the inhabitants. However, such evidence remains outside of the health care field. The researchers' contributions add to this evidence and demonstrate how public and private collaborations improve community health.

Telephone survey data were obtained from over 1800 randomly selected residents of a northwest urban county in the state of Washington during 1995. Multivariant analysis was used to assess the relationship between community quality and health status. Community quality was measured by respondents' perceptions of their community problems. Findings indicate that health is dependent on how people perceive the quality of their community.

It was found that leadership and vision can make an enormous difference in the quality of a community health system and in the cost-effectiveness of care provided. Health care leaders can develop understanding of their community and the impact of community characteristics on health through consultation with local and regional experts, input from other community leaders, and visits to the neighborhoods surrounding the service delivery sites. "Community networks can be developed with the common focus of improving the community's health. Collaborative efforts between the private health sector, the public health sector, and community members can enhance social relationships and thus promote the health of residents" (Molinari et al., p. 498).

placed in context by viewing the settings in which they are practiced. The types of places in which community health nurses practice are increasingly varied and include a growing number of nontraditional settings and partnerships with nonhealth groups. Employers of community health nurses range from state and local health departments and home health agencies to managed care organizations, businesses and industry, and nonprofit organizations. For this discussion, however, these settings are grouped into seven categories: (1) homes, (2) ambulatory service settings, (3) schools, (4) occupational health settings, (5) residential institutions, (6) parishes, and (7) the community at large.

Homes

For a long time, the most frequently used setting for community health nursing practice was the home. In the home, all of the community health nursing roles, to varying degrees, are performed. Clients discharged from acute care institutions, such as hospitals or mental health facilities, are regularly referred to community health nurses for continued care and follow-up. Here, the community health nurse can see clients in a family and environmental context, and service can be tailored to clients' unique needs.

For example, Mr. White, 67 years of age, was discharged from the hospital with a colostomy. Doreen Levitz, the community health nurse from the county public health nursing agency, immediately started home visits. She met with Mr. White and his wife to discuss their needs as a family and to plan for Mr. White's care and adjustment to living with a colostomy. Practicing the clinician and educator roles, she reinforced and expanded on the teaching started in the hospital for colostomy care, including bowel training, diet, exercise, and proper use of equipment. As part of a total family care plan, Doreen provided some forms of physical care for Mr. White as well as counseling, teaching, and emotional support for both Mr. White and his wife. In addition to consulting with the physician and social service worker, she arranged and supervised visits from the home health aide, who gave personal care and homemaker services. She thus performed the manager, leader, and collaborator roles.

The home also is a setting for health promotion. Many community health nursing visits focus on assisting families to understand and practice healthier living. They may, for example, instruct on parenting, infant care, child discipline, diet, exercise, coping with stress, or managing grief and loss.

The character of the home setting is as varied as the clients served by the community health nurse. In one day, the nurse may visit a well-to-do widow in her luxurious home, a middle-income family in their modest bungalow, and an elderly transient man in his one-room fifth-story walk-up. In each situation, the nurse can view the clients in perspective and, therefore, better understand their limitations, capitalize on their resources, and tailor health services to meet their needs. In the home, unlike most other health care settings, clients are on their own turf. They feel comfortable and secure in familiar surroundings and often are better able to understand and apply health information. Client self-respect can be promoted, since the client is host while the nurse is a guest.

Sometimes, the thought of visiting in clients' homes can cause anxiety for the nurse. This may be the first nursing experience out of the acute care, long-term care, or clinic setting. Visiting clients in their own environment can make the nurse feel uncomfortable. The nurse may be asked to visit families in unfamiliar neighborhoods, and now must walk through them to visit the client. Frequently, fear of the unknown is the real fear, which often has been enhanced by stories from previous nurses. This may be the same feeling as that experienced when caring for your first client, entering the operating room, or having a client in the intensive care unit. However, in the community there are more variables, and there are basic safety measures that should be used by all people when out in public. General guidelines for safety and making home visits are covered in detail in Chapter 23. Nevertheless, the specific instructions given during the clinical experience should be followed, and everyday, common-sense safety precautions should be used.

Changes in the health care delivery system, along with shifting health economics and service delivery (discussed in Chapter 7), are changing community health nursing's use of the home as a setting for practice. The increased demand for highly technical acute care in the home requires specialized skills best delivered by nurses with this expertise. With skills in population-based practice, community health nurses serve the public's health best by focusing on sites where they can have the greatest impact. At the same time, they can collaborate with various types of home care providers, including hospitals, other nurses, physicians, rehabilitation therapists, and durable medical equipment companies to ensure continuous and holistic service. The nurse continues to supervise home care services and engage in case management. Chapter 37 further examines the nurse's role in the home care setting.

Ambulatory Service Settings

Ambulatory service settings include a variety of places for community health nurses' practice in which clients come for day or evening services that do not include overnight stays. Community health centers are an example of an ambulatory setting. Sometimes, multiple clinics offering comprehensive services are community based or are located in outpatient departments of hospitals and medical centers. They also may be based in comprehensive neighborhood health centers. A single clinic, such as a family planning clinic or well-child clinic, may be found in a location more convenient for clients, perhaps a church basement or empty storefront. Some kinds of day-care centers, such as those for physically disabled or emotionally disturbed adults, use community health nursing services. Additional ambulatory care settings include health departments and community health nursing

agencies where clients may come for assessment and referral or counseling.

Offices are another type of ambulatory care setting. Some community health nurses provide service in conjunction with a medical practice; for example, a community health nurse associated with a health maintenance organization sees clients in the office and undertakes screening, referrals, counseling, health education, and group work. Others establish independent practices by seeing clients in community nursing centers as well as making home visits (Lockhart, 1995; Scott & Moneyham, 1995; Walker, 1994).

Another type of ambulatory service setting includes places where services are offered to selected groups. For example, community health nurses practice in migrant camps, Native American reservations, correctional facilities, children's day-care centers, through churches as parish nurses, and in remote mountain and coal-mining communities. Again, in each ambulatory setting, all of the community health nursing roles are used to varying degrees. Several special ambulatory settings are explored in detail later: children's day-care centers are discussed in Chapter 27; migrant health is explored in Chapter 33; correctional nursing is explored in detail in Chapter 36; and later in this chapter, parish nursing is discussed.

Schools

Schools of all levels make up a major group of settings for community health nursing practice. Nurses from community health nursing agencies frequently serve private schools of elementary and intermediate levels. Public schools are served by the same agencies or by community health nurses hired through the public school system. The community health nurse may work with groups of students in preschool settings, such as Montessori schools, as well as in vocational or technical schools, junior colleges, and college and university settings. Specialized schools, such as those for the developmentally disabled, are another setting for community health nursing practice.

Community health nurses' roles in school settings are changing. School nurses, whose primary role initially was that of clinician, are widening their practice to include more health education, interprofessional collaboration, and client advocacy. For example, one school had been accustomed to using the nurse as a first-aid provider and record keeper. Her duties were handling minor problems, such as headaches and cuts, and keeping track of such events as immunizations. This nurse sought to expand her practice and, after consultation and preparation, collaborated with a health educator and some of the teachers to offer a series of classes on personal hygiene, diet, and sexuality. She started a drop-in health counseling center in the school and established a network of professional contacts for consultation and referral. Community health nurses in school settings also are beginning to assume managerial and leadership roles and to recognize that the researcher role should be an integral part of their practice. The nurse's role with school-aged and adolescent populations is discussed in great detail in Chapter 28.

Occupational Health Settings

Business and industry provide another group of settings for community health nursing practice. Employee health has long been recognized as making a vital contribution to individual lives, productivity of business, and the well-being of the entire nation. Organizations are expected to provide a safe and healthy work environment in addition to offering insurance for health care. More companies, recognizing the value of healthy employees, are going beyond offering traditional health benefits to supporting health promotional efforts. Some businesses, for example, offer healthy snacks such as fruit at breaks and promote jogging during the noon hour. A few larger corporations have built exercise facilities for their employees, provide health education programs, and offer financial incentives for losing weight or staying well.

Community health nurses in occupational health settings practice a variety of roles. The clinician role was primary for many years, as nurses continued to care for sick or injured employees at work. However, recognition of the need to protect employees' safety, and later, to prevent their illness led to the inclusion of health education in the occupational health nurse role. Occupational health nurses also act as employee advocates, assuring appropriate job assignments for workers and adequate treatment for job-related illness or injury. They collaborate with other health care providers and company management to offer better services to their clients. They act as leader and manager in developing new health services in the work setting endorsing programs such as hypertension screening or weight control. Occupational health settings range from industries and factories, such as an automobile assembly plant, to business corporations and even large department store systems. The field of occupational health offers a challenging opportunity, particularly in smaller businesses where nursing coverage usually is not provided. Chapter 29 more fully describes the role of the nurse serving the working adult population.

Residential Institutions

Any facility where clients reside can be a setting in which community health nursing is practiced. Residential institutions can include a halfway house in which clients live temporarily while recovering from drug addiction, or an inpatient hospice program in which terminally ill clients live. Some residential settings, such as hospitals, exist solely to provide health care; others provide other services and support. Community health nurses based in a community agency maintain continuity of care for their clients by collaborating with hospital personnel, visiting clients in the hospital, and planning care during and af-

ter hospitalization. Some community health nurses may serve one or more hospitals on a regular basis by providing a liaison with the community, consultation for discharge planning, and periodic in-service programs to keep hospital staff updated on community services for their clients. Other community health nurses with similar functions are based in the hospital and serve the hospital community.

A long-term care facility is another example of a residential site providing health care that may use community health nursing services. In this setting, where residents usually are elderly with many chronic health problems, the community health nurse functions as advocate and collaborator to improve services. The nurse may, for example, coordinate available resources to meet the needs of residents and their families and help safeguard the maintenance of quality operating standards. Chapter 37 discusses the community health nurse's role in long-term care settings and hospices. Sheltered workshops and group homes for mentally ill or developmentally disabled adults are other examples of residential institutions that serve clients who share specific needs.

Community health nurses also practice in settings where residents are gathered for purposes other than receiving care. Health care is offered as an adjunct to the primary goals of the institution. For example, many nurses work with camping programs for children and adults offered by churches and other community agencies, such as the Boy Scouts, Girl Scouts, or the YMCA. Camp nurses practice all available roles, often under interesting and challenging conditions.

Residential institutions provide unique settings for the community health nurse to practice health promotion. Clients are a "captive" audience whose needs can be readily assessed and whose interests can be stimulated. These settings offer the opportunity to generate an environment of caring and optimal-quality health care provided by community health nursing services.

Parishes

Parish nursing finds its beginnings in an ancient tradition. The beginnings of community health nursing can be traced to religious orders (see Chapter 2), and for centuries churches, temples, mosques, and other spiritual communities were important sources of health care. In parish nursing today, the practice focal point remains a faith community and the religious belief system provided by the philosophical framework (Joel, 1998). "Church-based health promotion (CBHP) is a large-scale effort by the church community to improve the health of its members through education, screening, referral, treatment, and group support" (Ransdell & Rehling, 1996, p. 195).

In some geopolitical communities, parish nurses may be the most acceptable primary care providers. The role of the parish nurse can be broad, being defined by the needs of the members and the philosophy of the religious community. However, the goal is to enhance and extend services available in the larger community, not to duplicate them.

The ANA has written standards of care for parish nursing practice in collaboration with Health Ministries Association, Inc. (ANA, 1998). The standards act as guidelines for faith communities planning to offer or offering parish nursing services (Display 3–2). When community health nurses work as parish nurses, they enhance accessibility to available health services in the community while meeting the unique needs of the members of that religious community, practicing within the framework of the tenets of that religion. For instance, in a Roman Catholic community in which artificial forms of birth control are not acceptable, client education about family planning methods would incorporate methods approved by the clergy, and referrals to primary care providers would be limited to those with similar beliefs. Working in an ashram-based program, the nurse might be asked to teach nutrition and stress reduction based on vegetarian meals and relaxation exercises grounded in Hindu tradition, such as meditation and yoga.

Community at Large

Unlike the six settings already discussed, the seventh setting for community health nursing practice is not confined to a specific philosophy, location, or building. When working with groups, populations, or the total community, the nurse may practice in many different places. For example, a community health nurse, as clinician and health educator, may work with a parenting group in a church or town hall. Another nurse, as client advocate, leader, and researcher, may study the health needs of a neighborhood's elderly population by collecting data throughout the area and meeting with resource people in many places. Also, a nurse may work with community-based organizations such as an AIDs organization or a support group for parents experiencing the violent death of a child. Again, the community at large becomes the setting for practice of a nurse who serves on health care planning committees, lobbies for health legislation at the state capital, runs for a school board position, or assists with flood relief in another state or another country.

Although the term "setting" implies a place, remember that community health nursing practice is not limited to a specific site. Community health nursing is a specialty of nursing defined by the nature of its practice, not its location, and can be practiced anywhere (Josten et al., 1996; Williams, 2000).

SUMMARY

Community health nurses play many roles, including that of clinician, educator, advocate, manager, collaborator, leader, and researcher. Each role entails special types of skills and expertise. The type and number of roles that are practiced vary with each set of clients and each specific situation, but the nurse should be able to successfully function in each of these roles as the particular situation demands. The role of manager is one that the nurse must play in every situation because it involves assessing clients' needs, planning and organizing to meet those needs, directing and leading clients to achieve results, and controlling and evaluating the progress to ensure that the goals and clients' needs are met. A type of comprehensive management of clients has become known as case management and is an integral part of community health nursing practice.

As a part of the manager role, the nurse must engage in three crucial management behaviors: decision-making, transferring information, and relationship building. Nurses also must use a comprehensive set of management skills: human skills that allow them to understand, communicate, motivate, and work with people; conceptual skills that allow them to interpret abstract ideas and apply them to real situations to formulate solutions; and technical skills that allow them to apply special management-related knowledge and expertise to a particular situation or problem.

There also are many types of settings in which the community health nurse must practice and in which these roles are enacted. Setting does not necessarily mean a specific location or site, but rather a particular situation. These situations can be grouped into seven major categories: homes; ambulatory service settings, where clients come for care but do not stay overnight; schools; occupational health settings, which serve employees in business and industry; residential institutions such as hospitals, long-term care facilities, halfway houses, or other institutions in which people live and sleep; parishes, where care is based on the philosophy of the religious organization; and the community at large, which encompasses a variety of locations.

DISPLAY 3–2. Assuring Congregational Health and Wholeness

Functions of the Parish Nurse
1. Counselor
2. Integrator of faith and health
3. Teacher
4. Referral agent
5. Coordinator of volunteers

Accountability
1. ANA Standards of Nursing Practice (ANA, 1998)
2. Parish Nursing Standards (Djupe et al., 1994)
3. Congregational Standards (Djupe et al., 1994)
4. Institutional Standards (Djupe et al., 1994)
5. ANA Social Policy Statement (ANA, 1995)
6. Nurse Practice Act
7. Patient Rights (American Heart Association, ANA, NLN)

(American Nurses Association. [1995]. *Nursing: A social policy statement.* Washington, DC: American Nurses Association; ANA [1998]. *Parish nursing standards of practice.* Kansas City, MO: American Nurses Association; Djupe, A.M., Olson, H., Ryan, J., & Lantz, J. [1994]. *Reaching out: Parish nursing services* [2nd ed.]. Park Ridge, IL: Lutheran General Health System.)

CLINICAL CORNER | **Roles and Settings of Community Health Nurse Practice**

Scenario

You are a nurse working in the cardiac intensive care unit (CICU) in Capitol City Hospital. Your hospital recently has been purchased by a health maintenance organization. Rumors about downsizing of nursing staff are rampant among hospital employees. Realizing that many nurses have more seniority than you, you decide to make an appointment with your supervisor to discuss the rumors and assess your status with the hospital. Your supervisor advises you that layoffs are imminent and that, given your date of hire, there is a high likelihood that you are at risk of "termination."

Your situation is as follows:

You received an Associate of Arts (ADN) Degree in Nursing 10 years ago. You worked as a Registered Nurse on the medical-surgical unit for 6 years at Capitol City Hospital. Four years ago, you left your permanent position to work part-time on the evening shift to continue your education and receive a Bachelor of Science in Nursing (BSN). Your goal in returning to school was to prepare yourself for either a supervisory position in the hospital or future practice in the community setting. You completed your BSN 2 years ago and subsequently obtained your permanent position in the CICU.

During your BSN education, you studied under one of the administrators of the local managed care program and became interested in managed care. Your county has operated a managed care program for 2 years. Your preceptor encouraged you to apply for a position as a nurse liaison, but you decided to return to work at Capitol City Hospital because you believed that you lacked the necessary experience for a position in the community setting.

Recently, you were approached by a neighbor who volunteers for his daughter's school. He informed you of a vacancy in the position of school nurse. This position was appealing to you because of the proximity to your home and the flexible schedule. Once again, however, you gave it little serious consideration because of your perceived lack of experience.

Glancing in the classified section of the newspaper last Sunday, you noticed advertisements for the following nursing positions:

- Clinic nurse in the local health department
- Occupational health nurse for a computer company in Metropolis

You now have four possible community health nurse (CHN) employment avenues to pursue:

- Managed care
- School nursing
- Clinic nurse
- Occupational health nurse

Questions

1. List factors that must be considered when analyzing employment opportunities:
   Salary
   Job location
   Flexibility in hours
   Professional challenge
   Opportunity for advancement
   Personal comfort level with existing skills (versus challenge of learning new job)
   Adequacy of personal skills and knowledge base
2. Given the scenario, brainstorm about actual and potential options:
   Continue in present position and hope that position is not eliminated
   Analyze options for advancement within Capitol City Hospital
   Identify means of securing current position
   Contact your preceptor to explore employment opportunities with managed care program
   Apply for CHN position of
   School nurse
   Occupational health nurse
   Clinic nurse
3. For each of the CHN roles, identify what clients you might be serving:
   Individuals
   Aggregates
   Communities
   Disease-focused
   High-risk
   Cultural
   Ethnic
   Geographic
4. Choose one of the CHN roles along with a setting and client base. Discuss potential issues related to:
   - Ethical considerations and dilemmas
   - Benefits of this CHN role
   - Drawbacks of working in this role
   - Job stability
   - Experience and education requirements
   - Social justice
   - Developing interdisciplinary partnerships

ACTIVITIES TO PROMOTE CRITICAL THINKING

1. Discuss ways for a community health nurse to make service holistic and focused on wellness with (a)

preschool-aged children in a day-care setting; (b) a group of chemically dependent adolescents; or (c) a group of elders living in a senior high rise.

2. Select one community health nursing role and describe its application in meeting the needs of your friend or next-door neighbor.

3. Describe a hypothetical or real situation in which you, as a community health nurse, would combine the roles of leader, collaborator, and researcher (investigator). Discuss how each of these roles might be played.

4. If your community health nursing practice setting is the community at large, will your practice roles be any different from those of the nurse whose practice setting is the home? Why? What determines the roles played by the community health nurse?

5. Interview a practicing community health nurse and determine which roles are played by that nurse over 1 month of practice. Describe the ways in which each role is enacted. How many instances of this nurse's practice were aggregate focused? In which of the settings does the nurse mostly practice? If you were a public health consultant, what suggestions might you make to expand this nurse's role into aggregate-level practice?

6. Search the Internet or go to the library and find two sources of health-related information for consumers. Was the information accurate?

7. Search the Internet or go to the library and find two research articles on community health nursing. In what settings did the research take place? Did the nursing authors collaborate with interdisciplinary team members on this research? If so, how do you think this collaboration helped the research? If you were to conduct research in the community, would you conduct it with only nurses on the team, or would your team be interdisciplinary? Why? What would be the benefits or limits of each? (See Clinical Corner.)

REFERENCES

Ales, B. (1998). Community collaboration: The nursing administrator's role in implementing a child abuse prevention program. *Journal of Nursing Administration, 28*(6), 43–48.

American Nurses Association. (1985. *Code for nurses with interpretive statements*. Kansas City, MO: American Nurses Publishing.

American Nurses Association. (1995). *Nursing's social policy statement*. Washington, DC: American Nurses Publishing.

American Nurses Association. (1999). *Scope and standards of community health nursing practice*. Washington, DC: American Nurses Publishing.

American Nurses Association. (1997). *Standards of clinical nursing practice*. Washington, DC: American Nurses Publishing.

American Nurses Association. (1998). *The scope and standards of parish nursing practice*. Washington, DC: American Nurses Publishing.

American Public Health Association. (1996, March). *The definition and role of public health nursing: A statement of APHA* (Public Health Nursing Section 1–5). Washington, DC:

Author. Available at http://www.apha.org/science/sections/phnrole.html.

Brandon, R. (1996). The collaborative services movement: Implications for national policymakers. In L. Hooper-Briar & H. Lawson (Eds.), *Expanding partnerships for vulnerable children, youth and families* (pp. 322–346). Washington, DC: Council on Social Work Education.

Breckon, D.J., Harvey, J.R., & Lancaster, R.B. (1998). *Community health education: Settings, roles and skills for the 21st century* (4th ed.). Gaithersburg, MD: Aspen.

Burton, W.N. & Connerty, C.M. (1998). Evaluation of a worksite-based patient education intervention targeted at employees with diabetes mellitus. *Journal of Emergency Medicine, 40*(8), 702–706.

Bushy, A. (1997). Empowering initiatives to improve a community's health status. *Journal of Nursing Care Quality, 11*(4), 32–42.

Caraher, M. (1995). Health promotion in a changing society. *Journal of Contemporary Health, 1*(2), 53–58.

Caraher, M. & McNab, M. (1996). The public health nursing role: An overview of future trends. *Nursing Standard, 10*(51), 44–48.

Chou, C.-P., Montgomery, S., Pentz, M.A., Rohrbach, L.A., Johnson, A., Flay, B.R., & MacKinnon, D.P. (1998). Effects of a community-based prevention program on decreasing drug use in high-risk adolescents. *American Journal of Public Health, 88*(6), 944–948.

Conley, E. & Dahl, J. (1993). *Public health nursing within core public health functions: A progress report from the public health nursing directors of Washington*. Olympia: Washington State Department of Health.

Cumbey, D.A. & Alexander, J.W. (1998). The relationship of job satisfaction with organizational variables in public health nursing. *Journal of Nursing Administration, 28*(5), 39–46.

Early, E., Battle, K., Cantwell, E., English, J., Lavin, J.E., & Larson, E. (1998). Effect of several interventions on the frequency of handwashing among elementary public school children. *American Journal of Infection Control, 26*(3), 263–269.

Frenn, M. (1996). Older adults' experience of health promotion: A theory for nursing practice. *Public Health Nursing, 13*(1), 65–71.

Gardner, S. (1996). *Beyond collaboration to results: Hard choices in the future of services to children and families*. Fullerton, CA: Center for Collaboration for Children, California State University.

Hall, P.J. (1998). Planning an integrated population-based program. *Journal of Nursing Administration, 28*(10), 40–47.

Holmes, C.A. & Warelow, P.J. (1997). Culture, needs and nursing: A critical theory approach. *Journal of Advanced Nursing, 25,* 463–470.

Joel, L.A. (1998). Parish nursing: As old as faith communities. *American Journal of Nursing, 98*(8), 7.

Josten, L., Aroskar, M., Reckinger, D., & Shannon, M. (1996). *Educating nurses for public health leadership*. Minneapolis: University of Minnesota.

Keller, L.O., Strohschein, S., Lia-Hoagberg, B., & Schaffer, M. (1998). Population-based public health nursing interventions: A model from practice. *Public Health Nursing, 15*(3), 207–215.

Kidd, P., Townley, K., Cole, H., McKnight, R., & Piercy, L.

(1997). The process of chore teaching: Implications for farm youth injury. *Family Community Health, 19*(4), 78–89.

Kitzman, H., et al. (1997). Effect of prenatal and infancy home visitation by nurses on pregnancy outcomes, childhood injuries, and repeated childbearing: A randomized controlled trial. *Journal of the American Medical Association, 278*(8), 644–652.

Kristjarson, L.J. & Chalmers, K.I. (1997). Preventive work with families: Issues facing public health nurses. In B.W. Spradley & J.A. Allender (Eds.) *Readings in community health nursing* (5th ed., pp. 377–38). Philadelphia: Lippincott-Raven Publishers.

Laflin, M.T. (1996). Promoting the sexual health of geriatric patients. *Topics in Geriatric Rehabilitation, 11*(4), 43–54.

Lockhart, C.A. (1995). Community nursing centers: An analysis of status and needs. In B. Murphy (Ed.), *Nursing centers: The time is now*. New York: National League for Nursing.

Maes, S., Berhoeven, C., Kittel, F., & Scholten, H. (1998). Effects of a Dutch work-site wellness-health program: The Brabantia project. *American Journal of Public Health, 88*(7), 1037–1041.

Megginson, L.C., Mosley, D.C., & Pietri, P.H., Jr. (1997). *Management: Leadership in action* (5th ed.). New York: Harper & Row.

Mintzberg, H. (1973). *The nature of managerial work*. New York: Harper & Row.

Molinari, C., Ahern, M., & Hendryx, M. (1998). Gains from public- private collaborations to improve community health. *Journal of Healthcare Management, 43*(6), 498–510.

Mulligan, R.A., Gilroy, J., Katz, K., Rodan, M.F., & Subramanian, K.N. (1999). Developing a shared language: Interdisciplinary communication among diverse health care professionals. *Holistic Nursing Practice, 13*(2), 47–53.

Mundt, M.H. (1996). Key elements of nurse case management in curricula. In E.L. Cohen (Ed.), *Nurse case management in the twenty-first century* (pp. 48–54). St. Louis: Mosby.

Niffenegger, J.P. (1997). Proper handwashing promotes wellness in children. *Journal of Pediatric Health Care, 11*, 26–31.

Olds, D.L., et al. (1997). Long-term effects of home visitation on maternal life course and child abuse and neglect: Fifteen-year follow- up of a randomized trial. *Journal of the American Medical Association, 278*(8), 637–643.

Patterson, E.F. (1998). The philosophy and physics of holistic health care: Spiritual healing as a workable interpretation. *Journal of Advanced Nursing, 27*, 287–293.

Perry, C.L., Bishop, D.B., Taylor, G., Murray, D.M., Mays, R.W., Dudovitz, B.S., Smyth, M., & Story, M. (1998) Changing fruit and vegetable consumption among children: The 5-a-day power plus program in St. Paul, Minnesota. *American Journal of Public Health, 88*(4), 603– 609.

Polit, D.F. & Hungler, B.P. (1999). *Nursing research: Principles and methods* (5th ed.). Philadelphia: Lippincott Williams & Wilkins.

Ransdell, L.B. & Rehling, S.L. (1996). Church-based health promotion: A review of the current literature. *American Journal of Health Behavior, 20*(4), 195–207.

Resnick, C. & Tight, E.G. (1997). The role of multidisciplinary community clinics in managed care systems. *Social Work, 42*(1), 91–98.

Robbins, R. (1997). *Organizational behavior* (8th ed.). Upper Saddle River, NJ: Prentice-Hall.

Rowland, H.S. & Rowland, B.L. (1997). *Nursing administration handbook* (4th ed.). Gaithersburg, MD: Aspen.

Raisler, J., Alexander, C., & O'Campo, P. (1999). Breast-feeding and infant illness: A dose response relationship? *American Journal of Public Health, 89*(1), 25–30.

Scott, C.B. & Moneyham, L. (1995). Perceptions of senior residents about a community-based nursing center. *Image, 27*(3), 181–186.

Snowball, J. (1996). Asking nurses about advocating for patients: "reactive" and proactive accounts. *Journal of Advanced Nursing, 24*(1), 67–75.

Swansburg, R.C. & Swansburg, R.J. (1999). *Introductory management and leadership for nurses* (2nd ed.). Sudbury, MA: Jones and Bartlett Publishers.

Twinn, S. (1997). Methodological issues in the evaluation of the quality of public health nursing: A case study of the maternal and child health centres in Hong Kong. *Journal of Advanced Nursing, 25*, 753–759.

U.S. Department of Health and Human Services (1998, September 15). *Healthy people 2010 objectives: Draft for public comment*. Washington, DC: Author.

Walker, P.H. (1994). Dollars and sense in health reform: Interdisciplinary practice and community nursing centers. *Nursing Administration Quarterly, 19*(1), 1–11.

Weiss, M. (1997). The quality evolution in managed care organizations: Shifting the focus to community health. *Journal of Nursing Care Quality, 11*(4), 27–31.

Williams, C. (2000). Community-based population-focused practice: The foundation of specialization in public health nursing. In M. Stanhope & J. Lancaster (Eds.), *Community health nursing: Process and practice for promoting health* (5th ed.). St. Louis: Mosby.

Williams, S.J. & Torrens, P.R. (1999). *Introduction to health services* (5th ed.). Albany: Delmar Publishers.

SELECTED READINGS

Association of Community Health Nursing Educators Committee on Practice. (1993). *Differentiated nursing practice in community health*. Lexington, KY: Author.

Bay Area Nursing Directors. (1996, August 31). *Eight core competencies for public health nursing in California: A draft*. San Francisco: Author.

Coss, C. (1993). Lillian D. Wald: Progressive activist. *Public Health Nursing, 10*(2), 134–137.

Davis, R. (1997). Community caring: An ethnographic study within an organizational culture. *Public Health Nursing, 14*, 92–100.

Hall, R.H. (1996). *Organizations, structures, processes, and outcomes* (6th ed.). Englewood Cliffs, NJ: Prentice-Hall.

Happell, B. (1998). Student nurses' attitudes toward a career in community health. *Journal of Community Health, 23*(4), 269–279.

Hayes, J.M. (1999). Respite for caregivers: A community-based model in a rural setting. *Journal of Gerontological Nursing, 25*(1), 22–26.

Hooper-Briar, K. & Lawson, H. (1994). *Serving children, youth, families and communities through interprofessional collaboration and service integration: A framework for action*. Oxford, OH: The Institute for Educational Renewal at Miami University and the Danforth Foundation.

Hunt, R. (1998). Community-based nursing: Philosophy or

setting? *American Journal of Nursing, 98*(10), 44–47. Available at http://www.nursingcenter.com.

Koponen, P., Helio, S.-L., & Aro, S. (1997). Finnish pubic health nurses' experiences of primary health care based on the population responsibility principle. *Journal of Advanced Nursing, 26,* 41–48.

Larson, E. (1995). New rules for the game: Interdisciplinary education for health professionals. *Nursing Outlook, 43,* 180–185.

McCloskey, J.C. & Maas, M. (1998). Interdisciplinary team: The nursing perspective is essential. *Nursing Outlook, 46*(4), 157–163.

Reutter, L.I. & Ford, J.S.(1996). Perceptions of public health nursing: Views from the field. *Journal of Advanced Nursing, 24,* 7–15.

Rheinhard, S.C, Christopher, M.A., Mason, D.J., Rusca, P., & Toughill, E. (1996). Promoting healthy communities through neighborhood nursing. *Nursing Outlook, 44,* 223–228.

Williams, C. A. (1977). Community health nursing: What is it? *Nursing Outlook, 25,* 250–254.

Transcultural Nursing in the Community

KEY TERMS

- Cultural assessment
- Cultural diversity
- Cultural relativism
- Cultural self-awareness
- Cultural sensitivity
- Culture
- Culture shock
- Dominant values
- Enculturation
- Ethnic group
- Ethnicity
- Ethnocentrism
- Microculture
- Minority group
- Race
- Subcultures
- Tacit
- Transcultural nursing
- Value

LEARNING OBJECTIVES

Upon mastery of this chapter, you should be able to:

- Define and explain the concept of culture.
- Discuss the meaning of cultural diversity and its significance for community health nursing.
- Describe the meaning and effects of ethnocentrism on community health nursing practice.
- Identify five characteristics shared by all cultures.
- Contrast the health-related values, beliefs, and practices of culturally diverse populations with those of the dominant U.S. culture.
- Conduct a cultural assessment.
- Apply transcultural nursing principles in community health nursing practice.

American society values individuality. People are delighted to see children grow and develop in unique ways. We applaud an individual's creative achievements. We also respect one another's personal preferences about food, dress, or the vehicles we drive. The right to be yourself—and thereby to be different from others—is even protected by state and federal laws. Although individuality is part of the dominant culture, there are limits to the range of differences most Americans find acceptable. People whose behavior falls outside of the acceptable range are labeled as deviants or misfits. For example, the United States culture approves moderate social drinking but not alcoholism. The beliefs and sanctions of the dominant or majority culture are called **dominant values.** In the United States, the majority culture is made up largely of Anglo-Saxons whose dominant values include the work ethic, thrift, success, independence, initiative, respect for others, privacy, cleanliness, youthfulness, attractive appearance, and a focus on the future.

Dominant values are important to consider in the practice of community health nursing because they shape people's thoughts and behaviors. Why are some client behaviors acceptable to health professionals and others not? Why do nurses have such difficulty persuading certain clients to accept new ways of thinking and acting? Explanations can be found by examining the concept of culture, especially its influence on health and on community health nursing practice.

THE MEANING OF CULTURE

Culture refers to the beliefs, values, and behavior that are shared by members of a society and provide a design or "map" for living. It is culture that tells people what is acceptable or unacceptable in a given situation. It is culture that dictates what to do, say, or believe. Culture is learned. As children grow up, they learn from their parents and others around them how to interpret the world. In turn, these assimilated beliefs and values prescribe desired behavior.

Anthropologists describe culture as the acquired knowledge that people use to generate behavior and interpret experience (Spradley & McCurdy, 2000). This knowledge is more than simply custom or ritual; it is a way of organizing and thinking about life. It gives people a sense of security about their behavior; without having to consciously think about it, they know how to act. Culture also provides the underlying values and beliefs on which people's behavior is based. For example, culture determines the value placed on achievement, independence, work, and leisure. It forms the basis for the definitions of male and female roles. It influences a person's response to authority figures, dictates religious beliefs and practices, and shapes child-rearing. According to Giger and Davidhizar, "culture is a time-dependent patterned behavioral response resulting from imprinting the mind through social and religious structures and intellectual and artistic manifestations" (Dowd, Giger, & Davidhizar, 1998, p. 119).

Every community, every social or ethnic group, has its own culture. Furthermore, all of the individual members believe and act based on what they have learned within that specific culture. As anthropologist Edward Hall said, "Culture controls our lives" (1959, p. 38). Even the smallest elements of everyday living are influenced by culture. For instance, culture determines the distance to stand from another person while talking. A comfortable talking distance for Americans is at least two and a half feet, whereas Latin Americans prefer a shorter distance, often only 18 inches, for dialogue. Culture also influences people's perception of time. In American culture, when someone makes an appointment, they expect the other person to be on time or not more than a few minutes late. To keep a person waiting (or to be kept waiting) for 45 minutes or an hour is insulting and intolerable. Yet there are other cultural groups, including Native Americans and Asians, whose response to time is much more flexible; their members think nothing of waiting or keeping someone else waiting for an hour or two. Clearly, culture is the knowledge people use to design their own actions and, in turn, to interpret others' behavior (Spradley & McCurdy, 2000).

Cultural Diversity

Race refers to a biologically designated group of people whose distinguishing features, such as skin color, are inherited. An **ethnic group** is a collection of people with common origins and with shared culture and identity. A person's **ethnicity** is that group of qualities that mark his or her association with a particular ethnic group. When a variety of racial or ethnic groups join a common, larger group, cultural diversity occurs. **Cultural diversity** (also called cultural plurality) means that a variety of cultural patterns coexist within a designated geographic area. Cultural diversity occurs not only between countries or continents, but also *within* many countries, including the United States (Meleis, 1997).

Immigration patterns over the years have contributed to marked cultural diversity in the United States. Early settlers came primarily from European countries through the 1800s, peaking in numbers just after the turn of the century, with almost 9 million immigrants admitted in the first decade of the 20th century. During much of this time, especially during the late 1600s through the early 1800s, African slaves were brought to the United States against their will, mostly to southern states where they were sold to plantation owners as laborers. Immigration stayed high during the early 1900s, then dropped sharply from 1930 to 1950. Immigration from non-European countries such as India, Korea, and Chile then steadily increased. The total number of immigrants from any country in the last decade of the century may surpass 10 million people (Table 4-1).

As shown in Table 4-2, immigrants come from all countries in the world, in greater numbers from some regions than others. Of the 915,900 people immigrating in 1996, almost 18% of them came just from Mexico, with the second largest group of 116,800, or almost 13%, coming from the Caribbean (Cuba, Dominican Republic, Haiti, Jamaica, Trinidad, and Tobago) (U.S. Department of Commerce, 1998). An estimated 5 million undocumented immigrants came to the United States between 1982 and 1996, with 2.7 million of them coming from Mexico. In 1997, the foreign-born population of the United States numbered 25.8 million persons, or 9.7% of the total population. Over half of the foreign-born population in the United States were born in Central America, South America, or the Caribbean; 27% were from Asia; and 17% came from Europe (U.S. Bureau of the Census, 1998a).

There are people representing over 100 different ethnic groups living in the United States, and more than half of them are significant in size. According to the United States Census

TABLE 4-1. Immigrants Admitted to the United States in the 20th Century

Decade	Nos.
1901–1910	8,795,000
1911–1920	5,736,000
1921–1930	4,107,000
1931–1940	528,000
1941–1950	1,035,000
1951–1960	2,515,000
1961–1970	3,322,000
1971–1980	4,493,000
1981–1990	7,338,000
1991–1996 (5 y)	6,146,000

From U.S. Department of Commerce, 1998.

TABLE 4–2. Immigrants and Region of Birth (1996)	
All countries	915,900
Europe	147,600
Asia	307,800
North America	340,500
South America	61,800
Africa	52,900

From U.S. Department of Commerce, 1998.

Bureau (U.S. Department of Commerce, 1998), significant minorities include Hispanic Americans, numbering over 29 million in 1997, representing approximately 11% of the population; Asian Americans, numbering slightly more than 10 million, or approximately 3.7% of the population; and American Indians, Eskimos, and Aleuts at 0.9%. The largest ethnic group in the United States is African American, numbering 34.2 million, or about 12.8% of the population (U.S. Bureau of the Census, 1998b). By 2050, people of Hispanic origin are projected to make up 24.5% of the population, whereas African Americans will grow to only 15.4% of the population, and Asian–Pacific Islander Americans will more than double their numbers to 8.2% of the population. The American Indian, Eskimo, and Aleut will likely stay near 0.9%. These changes, primarily resulting from immigration, will make the "minority" population in 2050 total 47.2%, and European Americans may no longer be the majority. In some states, especially those bordering Mexico, such as California, Arizona, New Mexico, and Texas, and some industrialized states in the eastern United States, this change already has occurred or will occur much sooner than 2050.

Immigration patterns are strongly influenced by immigration laws established since the 1800s. The Immigration Reform and Control Act of 1986 (Public Law 99–603) and the Immigration Act of 1990 (Public Law 101–649) have new limits on the number of immigrants being admitted. Furthermore, the law's greater stringency places annual numerical ceilings on certain immigrant groups while authorizing increases among immigrants who are highly skilled workers or are family members of aliens who have been legalized recently.

"Today's immigrants and refugees are finding themselves in a more confusing social climate than did their predecessors, a climate characterized by ambivalence about whether they should be accepted and ambiguity about their status" (Meleis, 1997, p. 42). The newcomers find an environment that is both welcoming and hostile. On one hand, they may find tolerance of diversity in the United States, demonstrated by the interest in ethnic food, cultural celebrations, and sensitivity to employees from different backgrounds. On the other hand, a backlash exists, demonstrated by a rise in hate crimes, national and local policies that curb services to the undocumented immigrant, restriction in English as a second language (ESL) and bilingual education, and limits to potential class action suits that challenge some of the practices of the immigration and nationalization services (Meleis, 1997).

Although broad cultural values are shared by most large national societies, within those societies are smaller cultural groups called subcultures. **Subcultures** are relatively large aggregates of people within a society who share separate distinguishing characteristics such as ethnicity (African or Hispanic Americans), occupation (farmers or physicians), religion (Catholics or Muslims), geographic area (New Englanders or Southerners), age (the elderly or school children), or sex or sexual preference (women or the gay community). Within these subcultures are smaller groups that anthropologists call microcultures.

Microcultures are systems of cultural knowledge characteristic of subgroups within larger societies. Members of a microculture will usually share much of what they know with everyone in the greater society but will possess a special cultural knowledge that is unique to the subgroup (Spradley & McCurdy, 2000, p. 15).

Examples can range from a group of Hmong immigrants adopting selected aspects of the United States culture to a third-generation Norwegian American community whose members share unique foods, dress, and values.

The members of each subculture and microculture retain some of the characteristics of the society from which they came or in which their ancestors lived (Mead, 1960). Some of their beliefs and practices, such as the food they eat, the language they speak at home, the way they celebrate holidays, or their ideas about sickness and healing, remain an important part of their everyday life. Native American groups have retained some aspects of their traditional cultures. Mexican Americans, Irish Americans, Swedish Americans, Italian Americans, African Americans, Puerto Rican Americans, Chinese Americans, Japanese Americans, Vietnamese Americans, and many other ethnic groups have their own microcultures.

Furthermore, certain customs, values, and ideas are unique to the poor, the rich, the middle class, women, men, youth, and the elderly. Many deviant groups, such as narcotic abusers, gangs, criminals, and transient alcoholics, have developed their own microcultures. Regional microcultures, such as that of the white Appalachian people living in the hills of Kentucky, also have distinctive ways of defining the world and coping with life. Other microcultures, such as those of rural migrant farm workers and urban homeless families, acquire their own sets of beliefs and patterns for dealing with their environments. Many religious groups have their own microcultures. Even occupational and professional groups, such as nurses or attorneys, develop their own special languages, beliefs, and perspectives.

Ethnocentrism

There is a difference between a healthy cultural or ethnic identification and ethnocentrism. Anthropologists explain that "**ethnocentrism** is the belief and feeling that one's own culture is best. It reflects our tendency to judge other people's beliefs and behavior using values of our own native culture"

(Spradley & McCurdy, 2000, p. 16). It causes people to believe that their way of doing things is right and to judge others' methods as inferior, ignorant, or irrational. Ethnocentrism blocks effective communication by creating biases and misconceptions about human behavior. In turn, this can cause serious damage to interpersonal relationships and interfere with nurse effectiveness (Eliason, 1993; Leininger, 1991a).

Bennett (1991) believes that people experience a developmental progression along a continuum from ethnocentrism to ethnorelativism, or seeing all behavior in a cultural context. Some people may stop progressing and remain stagnated at one stage, whereas others may move backward on the continuum. The left side of the continuum represents the most extreme reaction to intercultural differences: denial. On the right side is the characterization of people who show the most sensitivity to intercultural differences: integration (Fig. 4–1).

CHARACTERISTICS OF CULTURE

In their study of culture, anthropologists and sociologists have made significant contributions to the field of community health. Their findings shed light on why and how culture influences behavior. Five characteristics shared by all cultures are especially pertinent to nursing's efforts to improve community health: culture is (1) learned, (2) integrated, (3) shared, (4) tacit, and (5) dynamic.

Culture Is Learned

Patterns of cultural behavior are acquired, not inherited. Rather than being genetically determined, the way people dress, what they eat, how they talk—all are learned. Spradley and McCurdy offer the following explanation:

> **At the moment of birth, we lack a culture. We don't yet have a system of beliefs, knowledge, and patterns of customary behavior. But from that moment until we die, each of us participates in a kind of universal schooling that teaches us our native culture. Laughing and smiling are genetic responses, but as infants we soon learn when to**

smile, when to laugh, and even how to laugh. We also inherit the potential to cry, but we must learn our cultural rules for when crying is appropriate (2000, p. 14).

Each person learns his or her culture through socialization with the family or significant group, a process called **enculturation.** When growing up in a given society, a child acquires certain attitudes, beliefs, and values and learns how to behave in ways appropriate to that group's definition of the female or male role; children are learning their culture.

Although culture is learned, the process and results of that learning are different for each person. Each individual has a unique personality and experiences life in a singular way; these factors influence acquisition of culture. Families, social classes, and other groups within a society differ from one another, and this sociocultural variation has important implications for planned change. Because culture is learned, parts of it can be relearned. People might change certain cultural elements or adopt new behaviors or values. Some individuals and groups are more willing than others to try new ways and thus influence change.

Culture Is Integrated

Rather than being an assortment of various customs and traits, a culture is a functional, integrated whole. As in any system, all parts of a culture are interrelated and interdependent. The various components of a culture, such as its social mores or religious beliefs, perform separate functions, coming in relative harmony with each other to form an operating and cohesive whole. In other words, to understand culture, single traits should not be described independently. Each part must be viewed in terms of its relationships to other parts and to the whole.

A person's culture is an integrated web of ideas and practices. For example, a nurse may promote consuming three balanced meals a day, a practice tied to the belief that nutrition leads to good health and that prevention is better than cure. These cultural traits, in turn, are related to the nurse's values about health. Health, the nurse believes, is essential for maximum energy output and productivity at work. Productivity is important because it enables people to reach goals. These values are linked to social or religious beliefs about hard work

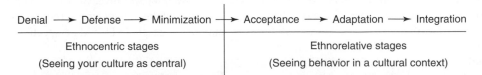

FIGURE 4–1. Bennett's stages of cross-cultural sensitivity. Describes both ethnocentric and ethnorelative stages, with the use of examples (denial, defense, minimalization, acceptance, adaptation, and integration). (Adapted from Bennet, M. [1991]. *Toward a developmental model of intercultural sensitivity.* In M. Paige [Ed.], *Education for the intercultural experience* (Chapter 1). Yarmouth, ME: Intercultural Press.)

and taboos against laziness. Thus, these ideas and beliefs about nutrition, health, economics, religion, and family all are interrelated and work to motivate behavior.

For example, parents who are Jehovah's Witnesses may refuse a blood transfusion for their child. Their actions might seem irrational or ignorant to those who do not understand their religious beliefs. However, that choice represents behavior consistent with the couple's cultural values and standards. The single behavior of refusing blood transfusions, when viewed in context, is part of a larger religious belief system and a basic component of their culture.

In some cultural groups, modesty for women may make it uncomfortable and perhaps traumatic to be examined by a person of the opposite sex. Asking certain Native American groups to comply with rigid appointment scheduling means requiring them to reframe their concept of time. It also violates their values of patience and pride. Before nurses attempt a change in a person's or group's behavior, they need to ask how that change will affect the people involved through its influence on other parts of their culture. Extra time and patience or different strategies may be needed if change still is indicated. Nurses often may find that their own practice system can be modified to preserve clients' cultural values.

Culture Is Shared

Culture is the product of aggregate behavior, not individual habit. Certainly, individuals practice a culture, but customs are phenomena shared by all members of the group. The anthropologist G. Murdock explains:

> **Culture does not depend on individuals. An ordinary habit dies with its possessor, but a group habit lives on in the survivors, and is transmitted from generation to generation. Moreover, the individual is not a free agent with respect to culture. He is born and reared in a certain cultural environment, which impinges on him at every moment of his life. From earliest childhood his behavior is conditioned by the habits of those around him. He has no choice but to conform to the folkways current in his group (1972, p. 258).**

A culture's values are among its most important elements. A **value** is a notion or idea designating relative worth or desirability. Each culture classifies phenomena "into good and bad, desirable and undesirable, right and wrong" (Foster, 1962, p. 18). When people respond in favor of or against some practice, they are reflecting their culture's values about that practice. One person may eagerly anticipate eating a steak for dinner. Another, who believes that eating meat is sacrilegious or unhealthful, will experience revulsion at the idea. Some American subcultures think that loud, vocal expressions are a necessary way to deal with pain. Others value silence and stoicism. Some have high regard for speed and efficiency, whereas others prefer patience and thoughtfulness. Either way, values serve a purpose. Shared values give

people in a specific culture stability and security; they provide a standard for behavior. From these values, members know what to believe and how to act. The normative criteria by which people justify their decisions are based on values that are more deeply rooted than behaviors and consequently more difficult to change.

Knowing that culture is shared helps nurses to understand human behavior. For example, a community health nurse tried unsuccessfully to persuade a mother to limit the amount of "catnip" tea she fed her infant. The infant was pacified with the tea and was not consuming a sufficient amount of infant formula, thus putting him at risk for developmental problems. She discovered that the mother was acting in a tradition of her rural subculture, which held that catnip promoted good health (it acts as an antispasmodic [Spector, 2000], perhaps causing relaxation and a more contented infant with fewer symptoms of "colic"). The fact that all of the other mothers in that group also used catnip with their babies proved a powerful deterrent to the change suggested by the nurse. Individual health behavior always is influenced by other people of the same culture. Thus, it becomes difficult for one person to eliminate a cultural practice when it is reinforced by other group members. Group acceptance and a sense of membership usually depend on conforming to shared cultural practices (Spradley & McCurdy, 2000).

Thus, community health nursing may need to focus on an entire group's health behavior to affect individual practices. The pattern of consuming large amounts of the tea was modified, for instance, when the nurse worked with the entire rural community. She began with a well-recognized cultural strategy: to work through formal or informal leaders. She contacted the oldest woman in the community and discussed the cultural practice. The elder shared the group's beliefs that catnip tea is vital to the well-being of infants for the first 6 months. When the nurse explained her concerns of low formula intake and low weight gain, the community leader clarified that only one or two ounces of the tea a day was needed. She shared this information among the women, and as a result, the mothers gradually reduced the amount of tea they gave their infants. The infant drank more formula and gained weight appropriately. A cultural tradition was retained while the health of the infant improved. The community health nurse can use this new information and the supportive information from the community leader to improve the health of other infants.

Culture Is Mostly Tacit

Culture provides a guide for human interaction that is mostly unexpressed and at the unconscious level, or **tacit.** Members of a cultural group, without the need for discussion, know how to act and what to expect from one another. Culture provides an implicit set of cues for behavior, not a written set of rules. Spradley and McCurdy explain that culture often is "so regular and routine that it lies below a conscious level"

(2000, p. 16). It is like a memory bank where knowledge is stored for recall when the situation requires it, but this recall process mostly is unconscious. Culture teaches the proper tone of voice to use for each occasion. It prescribes how close to stand when talking with someone or how to respond to elders. Individuals learn to make responses that are appropriate to their sex, role, and status. They know what is right and wrong. All of these attitudes and behaviors are so ingrained, so tacit, that people seldom, if ever, need to discuss them.

Because culture is mostly tacit, it is difficult to realize which of one's own behaviors may be offensive to people from other groups. It also is difficult to know the meaning and significance of other cultural practices. In some groups, such as Native American women, silence is valued but may make others uncomfortable. Offering food to a guest in many cultures is not merely a social gesture but an important symbol of hospitality and acceptance, and to refuse, for any reason, may be an insult and a rejection. Touching or calling someone by their first name may be viewed as a demonstration of caring by some but is seen as disrespectful and offensive by others. Consequently, community health nurses have a twofold task in developing cultural sensitivity; not only must they try to learn clients' culture, but they also must try to make their own culture less tacit and more explicit. Nurses bring both their professional and personal cultural history to the work place, often developing unique values not shared with others who are not in the profession (Fielo & Degazon, 1997). Cross-cultural tension can be resolved through conscious efforts at developing awareness, patience, and acceptance of cultural differences (Display 4–1).

Culture Is Dynamic

Every culture undergoes change; none is entirely static. Within every cultural group are individuals who generate innovations. More important, some members see advantages in doing things differently and are willing to adopt new practices. Each culture, including our own, is an amalgamation of ideas, values, and practices from a variety of sources. This process depends on the extent of exposure to other groups. Nonetheless, every culture is in a dynamic state of adding or deleting components. Functional aspects are retained; less functional ones are eliminated.

When this adaptation does not occur, the cultural group may face serious difficulty. For example, many Southeast Asian refugees in the United States have continued to prepare and eat food in their traditional fashion. Uncooked pork is a part of that diet. As a result, a study showed that "between 1975 and 1984, the incidence of trichinosis in the United States was 25 times greater for the Southeast Asian refugee population than for the general United States population" (Stehr-Green & Schantz, 1986, p. 1238). Other recent outbreaks of trichinosis among this population reinforce the need for further education and control measures.

DISPLAY 4–1. Culture Shock

An increasing number of immigrants and refugees from many different countries have been assimilated into American culture in recent years. Whereas they quickly adapt in many respects, learning the language and seeking housing and employment, they continue to operate within the framework of their own cultural beliefs and behaviors. The conflict between their culture and American culture often causes **culture shock**, "a state of anxiety that results from cross-cultural misunderstanding . . . and an inability to interact appropriately in the new context" (Spradley & McCurdy, 2000, p. 16). Immigrants and refugees find themselves in a strange setting with people who act in unfamiliar ways. Speaking their own language in their homes and retaining values and familiar practices all help to promote some sense of security in the new environment.

The same is true for nurses and others working overseas in unfamiliar countries. No longer are the small but important cues available that orient a stranger to appropriate behavior. Instead, a person in a different culture may feel isolated and anxious and even become dysfunctional or ill. Immersion in the culture over time and learning the new culture are the major remedies. As adjustment occurs, old beliefs and practices that are still functional in the new setting can be retained, whereas others that are not functional must be replaced.

Community health nurses need to remember the dynamic nature of culture for several reasons. Cultures and subcultures do change over time. Patience and persistence are key attributes to cultivate when working toward improving health behaviors. Another point to remember is that cultures change as their members see greater advantages in the "new ways." Discussing these advantages needs to be done in a language understood by members and in the context of their own cultural value system. This is an important reason for nurses to develop an understanding of their clients' culture (Eliason, 1993; Leininger, 1991b, 1995; Taylor, 1998). Furthermore, change within a culture is usually brought about by certain key individuals who are receptive to new ideas and able to influence their peers. These key persons can adapt the change process so that "new" practices are culturally consistent and fit with group values. Tapping this resource becomes imperative for successful change. Finally, the health care culture is dynamic, too. We Westerners are just beginning to appreciate the validity of many of the non-Western cultures' health care practices, such as acupuncture, meditation, and using various therapeutic herbs and spices (eg, turmeric, fenugreek). Nurses can learn much from their clients and their cultures (Holland & Courtney, 1998). While discovering more effective ways of working with clients, nurses may choose to modify their own practices.

SELECTED CULTURAL COMMUNITIES

An examination of the meaning and nature of culture clearly underscores the need to recognize cultural differences and understand clients in the context of their cultural backgrounds. Practically speaking, however, how can knowledge of cultural diversity be integrated into everyday community health nursing practice? Who are the diverse cultural communities served by community health nurses? What are their differences? Do they share some features? To provide insights and answers to these questions, this section describes five cultural communities. Descriptions intentionally are kept brief as a reminder that each culture is complex and unique and deserves a more comprehensive study than is possible within the scope of this chapter. Also, remember that over 100 different ethnic groups live in the United States, and only five of these are described here. Further information is provided by the references and selected readings.

Native American Indians and Alaska Natives

Native Americans and Alaska natives, the first known settlers of this continent, form a large cluster of tribal groups whose members are descendants of the original Native Americans inhabiting this country when whites settled in this land: first, the Vikings came around 1010 AD, and then Europeans "discovered" it in the 1500s (Spector, 2000). Native Americans and Alaska natives have adopted many Anglo-American values and practices, yet preserve large aspects of their own culture.

POPULATION CHARACTERISTICS AND CULTURE

Native Americans and Alaska natives, or Native American Indians, are a diverse group made up of different tribes and 400 federally recognized nations. They are scattered throughout 26 states in the United States (including Alaska and the Aleutian Islands) with many living on reservations and in rural areas; however, just as many live in cities. Eskimos, Aleuts, and Indians living in Alaska are known as Alaska natives; those living in other states are know as American Indians. Oklahoma, Arizona, California, New Mexico, North Carolina, and Alaska have the most Native Americans (West, 1993). By 2050, the census bureau estimates there will be about 4.3 million Indians, nearly double the number in 1996 (U.S. Department of Commerce, 1998). Some of this increase can be attributed to official recognition as tribal members if persons can provide information linking them to a tribe or nation. If accepted, these people can declare themselves as Native Americans. Each tribe or nation has its own distinct language, beliefs, customs, and rituals. Thus, the community health nurse cannot assume that knowledge of one group can be generalized to others. Knowledge of certain similarities (Display 4–2) among the various Native American cultures can assist nurses in working

---

DISPLAY 4–2. Similarities Among Native American Cultures

Value dignity of the individual
Value family and community
Respect for advancing age; elders are leaders
Live in harmony with nature, respect the environment
Value symbolic arts and crafts
Live in the present, little concern for the distant future
Value generosity and sharing, discourage competition
Integrate religion into everyday life
Treat body and soul as one unit
Use herbal medicines and traditional healing practices
Value rituals and ceremonies
Practice periods of silence, value thoughtful speech
Value patience

From Bell, 1994; Orque et al., 1983; and West, 1993.

---

with the members of a specific tribe (Bell, 1994; West, 1993). For many Native American groups, their large extended family networks reinforce cultural standards and expectations, as well as provide emotional support and practical assistance (Seideman et al., 1994).

HEALTH PROBLEMS

Health problems among Native Americans tend to be both chronic and socially related (West, 1993). One third of Native Americans live in abject poverty and experience the afflictions associated with poor living conditions, including malnutrition, tuberculosis (TB), and high maternal and infant death rates (Spector, 2000). The highest ranking health problems in children include dysentery, impetigo, intestinal infectious diseases, skin diseases, staphylococcal infections, respiratory disease, influenza, and pneumonia. For adults, trachomatous conjunctivitis poses a serious health threat not common in the rest of the U.S. population. Diabetes, TB, and obesity all rank higher among Native Americans than the general population. Poor sanitation, crowded housing, and low immunization levels contribute to a variety of communicable diseases. On the other hand, heart disease is lower among Indians than whites.

Alcoholism is the major health problem of Native Americans. Its destructive effects on families include a high incidence of fetal alcohol syndrome (FAS) and fetal alcohol effects (FAE), along with a high incidence of violence and injuries. Substance abuse, increasingly among children using inhalants, is prevalent among those living on reservations.

HEALTH BELIEFS AND PRACTICES

Native Americans as a group prefer traditional healing practices and folk medicine over Western medicine. As many as

"90% of Indians today still seek out a medicine man before going to a health clinic" (West, 1993, p. 231). Many of their beliefs about health and illness have supernatural explanations, and their health and dietary practices are closely tied to cultural and religious beliefs. American Indians practice purification rituals such as immersion in water and the use of sweat lodges to maintain their harmony with nature and cleanse the body and spirit. The basis of therapy lies in nature, with herbal teas, charms, and fetishes used as preventive and curative measures. Because of decades of racism and government paternalism, many Native Americans feel oppressed and dehumanized and carry considerable resentment and lack of trust toward whites. As a result, many maintain a degree of separateness from overall American culture. Nurses must overcome these barriers through patience, acceptance, and respect for their culture, as illustrated in the case study of the community health nurse, Sandra Josten, and her new client from a Native American community.

African Americans

A second cultural group is black Americans, or African Americans. Unlike Native Americans, the decedents of this group originally came to this continent as free settlers as early as 1619 (Bennett, 1962), but most of about 4 million who followed came as slaves in the 17th and 18th centuries, mostly from the west coast of Africa. Most African Americans living today were born in the United States; however, some have immigrated recently from African countries, the West Indies, the Dominican Republic, Haiti, and Jamaica, often to escape poverty or political persecution.

CLINICAL CORNER — Sandra's New Clients

As she drove up the dirt road and parked her car next to the community hall, Sandra Josten felt apprehensive. She had been alerted by the previous community health nurse about the difficulty of working with these Native American people: "This tribe is lazy and unappreciative. You can't get anywhere with them." Only through the urging of an Indian community aide, Mrs. Brown, had a group of the women reluctantly agreed to meet with the new nurse. They would see what she had to say.

Sandra's steps echoed hollowly as she walked across the wooden floor of the large room to the far corner where a group of women sat silently in a circle. Only their eyes turned; their faces remained impassive. Mrs. Brown rose slowly, greeted the nurse, and introduced her to the group. Swallowing her fear, Sandra smiled. She told them of her background and explained that she had not worked with Indian people before. There was a long silence. No one spoke. Sandra continued, "I'd like to help you if I can, maybe with problems about care of your children when they are sick or questions about how to keep them healthy, but I don't know what you need or want." Silence fell again. She would like to learn from them, she repeated. Would they help her? Again Sandra felt an uncomfortable silence.

Then one woman began to speak. Quietly, but with deep feeling, she described several bad experiences with the previous nurse and the county social worker. Then others spoke up: "They tell us what we should do. They don't listen. They say our way is not good." Seeing Sandra's interest and concern, the women continued. One of their main concerns was their children's health. Another was the high incidence of accidents and injuries on the reservation. They wanted to learn how to give first aid. Other concerns were expressed. The group agreed that Sandra could help them by teaching a first-aid class.

In the weeks that followed, Sandra taught several classes on first aid and emergency care. She then began a series of sessions on child health. Each time, she asked the women to choose a topic or problem for discussion and then elicited from them their accustomed ways of dealing with each problem; for example, how they handled toilet training or taught their children to eat solid foods. Her goal was to learn as much as she could about their culture and incorporate that information into her teaching, which preserved as many of their practices as possible. Sandra also visited informally with the women in their homes and at community gatherings. She learned about their way of life, their history, and their values. For example, patience was highly valued. It was important to be able to wait patiently, even if a scheduled meeting was delayed as much as 2 hours. It also was important for others to speak, which explained the Indian women's comfort with silences during a conversation. Other values influenced their way of life. Courage, pride, generosity, and honesty all were important determinants of behavior. These also were values by which they judged Sandra and other professionals. Sandra's honesty in keeping her promises enabled the women to trust her. Her generosity in giving her time, helping them occasionally with some household task, and arranging for child care during classes won their respect.

The women came to accept her, and Sandra was invited to eat with them and share in tribal get-togethers. The women criticized and advised her on acceptable ways to speak and act. Her openness and patience to learn and her respect for them as a people had paved the way to improving their health. At first, Sandra felt that her progress was slow, but this slowness was an advantage. She had built a solid foundation of cross-cultural trust, and in the months that followed, she saw many changes in their health practices.

POPULATION CHARACTERISTICS AND CULTURE

In 1997, African Americans numbered 34.2 million and constituted 12.8% of the U.S. population (U.S. Bureau of the Census, 1998b), with projections showing an increase to 15.4% by the year 2050 (U.S. Department of Commerce, 1998). One third of the African-American population is younger than 18 years of age. Slightly more than 8% of African Americans are older than 65, with most being women, compared with 13% who are older than 65 years in the total population. Fifty-eight percent of black children live with their mothers only, compared with 21% of white children.

Despite improvements in the legal and social climate for African Americans, great disparities exist. Average family income for African Americans is 63% of the income earned by white families. More than 26% of African Americans live in poverty, contrasted with 8.6% of whites. Although they make up 12.8% of the population, blacks make up over 50% of prison inmates. Close to 36% of African American families in households headed by women live below the poverty level. Unemployment among African Americans is 10% compared with 4.2% for whites (U.S. Department of Commerce, 1998).

Educational disparities also exist. About half of the African Americans who have less than a high school education are not in the work force, compared with 36% of whites with a similar education. However, 89% of both blacks and whites with a college degree are employed. African American women acquire more educational training than their male counterparts; however, their earnings are lower than those of black men.

Like Native Americans and Asians, there is no single African American culture; rather, this group forms a heterogeneous community. Like other large ethnic and racial groups, many factors influence their culture, and this results in much diversity within the African American population. Among the variables determining specific microcultures within the African American community are economic level, religious background, education, occupation, social class identity, geographic origin, and residence in an integrated or segregated neighborhood (Porter & Villarruel, 1993). For community health nurses, this means that specific groups of African Americans have their own unique values, character, lifestyle, and health needs.

The primary language of most African Americans is English. Recent black immigrants from Caribbean or other countries may retain the language of their country of origin but generally learn English as well. Many African Americans speak variations of soul talk, also called black English or black Creole. It evolved from pidgin spoken during the era of slavery and has become a dynamic and meaningful language of its own. For some African Americans, soul talk symbolizes racial pride and identity.

HEALTH PROBLEMS

African Americans have much higher mortality rates than whites and a life expectancy of 70.3 years contrasted with 76.8 years for whites (U.S. Department of Commerce, 1998). Their major health problems include cardiovascular disease and stroke, cancer, diabetes mellitus, cirrhosis, a high infant mortality rate (twice that of whites), homicide and accidents, and malnutrition (Display 4–3). Several factors contribute to these problems. Stress and discrimination, poverty, lack of education, high rates of teen pregnancy, inadequate housing, and inadequate insurance for health care are among the risk factors influencing the health of this population. In the last three decades, a dramatic increase in black households headed by women, single-parent births (most frequently among teens), and a limited presence of male role models has further exacerbated family vulnerability.

Mortality rates for communicable diseases, including AIDS, also are higher for blacks than whites. African Americans with AIDS made up nearly 46% of the reported cases in 1997, 80% of whom were black men (U.S. Department of Commerce, 1998). The incidence of TB among this population also is rising, with many of the cases being diagnosed in conjunction with an AIDS diagnosis (see Chapter 15).

HEALTH BELIEFS AND PRACTICES

Although African Americans have absorbed most of the dominant culture in the United States, some retain aspects of their ancestors' traditional values and practices. Some, for example, hold to traditional African beliefs about health being a sign of harmony with nature and illness being evidence of disharmony. Evil spirits, the punishment of God, or a hex placed on the person might account for this disharmony. Healers treat body, mind, and spirit. Prayer, laying on of hands, magic or other rituals, special diets, wearing of preventive charms or copper bracelets, ointments, and other folk

---

DISPLAY 4–3. Mortality Data for African Americans

- African-American men die from strokes at almost twice the rate of white men.
- Coronary heart disease death rates are higher for African-American women than for white women.
- Black men experience a higher risk of cancer than white men.
- Diabetes is 33% more common among African Americans than among whites.
- African American babies are twice as likely as white babies to die before their first birthday.
- Homicide is the most frequent cause of death for male African Americans between ages 15 and 34 years. The homicide rate for those between the ages of 25 and 34 years is seven times that for whites.
- The rate of AIDS among male African Americans is more than triple that of white males. Among women and children, the gap is even wider.

Adapted from Spector, R.E. (2000). *Cultural diversity in health and illness* (5th ed.). Stamford, CT: Appleton & Lange.

remedies sometimes are practiced. Each African American community has its own set of health beliefs and practices, which must be determined by the community health nurse before planning any interventions.

Asian Americans

A third cultural cluster is composed of immigrants and refugees from various Pacific Rim countries (Display 4–4). Coming from China, Korea, Japan, Thailand, Laos, the Philippines, Vietnam, Cambodia, and other Asian countries, some of these people recently have been transplanted from their own cultures to an entirely different culture, whereas others may have lived here many years or were born in America.

POPULATION CHARACTERISTICS AND CULTURE

In 1997, there were 10.1 million Asians and Pacific Islanders living in the United States, representing 3.8% of the total population (U.S. Bureau of the Census, 1998c). The largest groups are Chinese and Filipinos, numbering over 1.5 million persons from each country. Other fairly large groups come from Vietnam, Korea, India, Iran, Laos, and Cambodia. Each group represents a distinct culture with its own unique challenges for community health nurses, as illustrated in the case study of the Kim family (see Clinical Corner).

Whereas each Asian culture is distinct in language, values, and customs, some general traits are shared by many Asians. Traditional Asian families tend to be patriarchal (the father is the head of the household) and patrilineal (the genealogy is carried through the male line). Male members are valued over female members. Elders are respected (Hansen, 1996). The male role generally is that of provider, whereas the female role is that of homemaker. Traditional Asians value achievement because it brings honor to the family name. Saving face or preserving dignity and family pride is important. Cooperation is valued over competition.

DISPLAY 4–4. Asian-Pacific Populations

Asian refers to:	**Pacific Islander refers to:**
Chinese	Polynesian
Filipino	Hawaiian
Japanese	Samoan
Asian Indian	Tongan
Korean	Micronesian
Vietnamese	Guamanian
Laotian	Melanesian
Thai	Fijian
Cambodian	Tahitian
Pakistan	Marshallese
Indonesian	Trilese
Hmong	
Mien	

HEALTH PROBLEMS

Health problems for Asian Americans include malnutrition, TB, mental illness, cancer, respiratory infections, arthritis, parasitic infestations, and chronic diseases associated with aging. Suicide rates and stress-related illness are particularly high among Asian refugee groups who have had to flee their countries under stressful conditions. However, Asians view mental illness as shameful, and the stigma attached to it prompts them to somaticize it or hide it as long as possible.

HEALTH BELIEFS AND PRACTICES

Asian health beliefs vary among subcultures. Many Asians believe in the Chinese concepts of yin (cold) and yang (hot), which do not refer to temperature but to the opposing forces of the universe regulating normal flow of energy. A balance of yin and yang results in qi (pronounced chee), which is the desired state of harmony. Illness results when there is an imbalance in these forces. If the imbalance means an excess of yin, then "cold" foods, such as vegetables and fruits, are avoided, and "hot" foods, such as rice, chicken, eggs, and pork, are offered. Some Asians view Western medicines as "hot" and Eastern folk medicines and herbal treatments as "cold," which explains why some groups practice both for balance. The Vietnamese have a similar hot-and-cold belief but call it Am and Dong. Other Asian groups, such as the Filipinos, view illness as an act of God and pray for healing. The Khmer of Cambodia believe that illness reflects a deviation from moral standards, and the Hmong consider illness to be a visitation by spirits. All have traditional healers, who, depending on the culture, include acupuncturists, herbalists, herb pharmacists, spirit and magic experts, or a shaman. Most Asian cultures also exercise traditional self-care practices, including herbal medicines and poultices, types of acupuncture, and massage (Lin-Fu, 1991; Dehn, 1997). Southeast Asians also practice dermabrasive techniques of cupping, pinching, rubbing, and burning. These are used to relieve symptoms such as headaches, sore throats, coughs, fever, and diarrhea by bringing toxins to the skin surface or compensating for heat lost. Because these techniques leave a bruise-like lesion on the skin, they can be mistaken for physical abuse (Muecke, 1983). Each client requires careful **cultural assessment** (defined on p. 72) before implementing nursing action. This involves detailed data gathering about the client's cultural practices.

Hispanic Americans

A fourth cultural cluster comprises groups who are of Hispanic origin and have immigrated to the United States, some many generations earlier. More than half came from Mexico, followed by Puerto Rico, Cuba, Central and South America, and Spain (Spector, 2000). Those with Mexican and Central American backgrounds generally are referred to as Latinos (Holland & Courtney, 1998). Depending on the region of the country, socioeconomic status, immigra-

| CLINICAL CORNER | The Kim Family |

Armed with enthusiasm and pamphlets on pregnancy and prenatal diet, Paula Morrow, the community health nurse, began home visits to the Kim family. Paula's initial plan was to discuss pregnancy and fetal development, teach diet, and prepare the mother for delivery. Mr. Kim, a graduate student, was present to interpret since Mrs. Kim spoke little English. Their two boys, 3 years and 1½ years of age, respectively, played happily on the kitchen floor. The family offered tea to the nurse and listened politely as she explained her reasons for coming and added, "How can I be most helpful to you? What would you like from my visits?"

The Kims were grateful for this approach. Hesitant at first, they hinted at Mrs. Kim's fears of American doctors and hospitals; her first two children had been born in Korea. None of the family had any experience with Western medicine. They shared some concerns about adjustment to living in the United States. It was difficult to shop in American food stores with their overwhelming variety of foods, many of which the Kims found unfamiliar. Mrs. Kim, who had come from a family whose servants prepared the food, was an inexperienced cook. Servants also had cared for the children, and her role had been that of an aristocrat in hand-tailored silk gowns.

Listening carefully, Paula began to realize the striking differences between her own culture and that of her clients. Her care plans changed. In subsequent visits, she determined to learn about Korean culture and base her nursing intervention on that knowledge. She learned about their traditional ways of raising children, the traditional male and female roles, and practices related to pregnancy and lactation. She respected their value of "saving face" and attempted never to offend their pride or dignity. As time went on, her interest and respect for their way of life won their trust. She inquired about their cultural practices before attempting any intervention. As a result, the Kims were receptive to her suggestions. When possible, she adapted her teaching and suggestions to comply with the Kims' culture. For example, appropriate changes were made in Mrs. Kim's diet that were compatible with her food preferences and cultural eating patterns. Because she was not accustomed to drinking milk, she increased her calcium intake by learning to prepare custards (which disguised the milk flavor) and by eating more green, leafy vegetables. After 5 months, a strong, positive relationship had been established between this family and the nurse. Mrs. Kim delivered a healthy baby girl and looked forward to continued supportive visits from the community health nurse.

tion or citizenship status, or age, members of this large minority group refer to themselves as either Mexican American, Spanish American, Latin American, Latin, Latino, or Mexican (Spector, 2000).

POPULATION CHARACTERISTICS AND CULTURE

Hispanics are a fast-growing and large ethnic group in the United States, and people of Hispanic origin are predicted to number over 58 million, or 17.5% of the population, by 2025 (U.S. Department of Commerce, 1998). In 1997, this group numbered over 29 million and accounted for 11% of the U.S. population (U.S. Department of Commerce, 1998).

The Hispanic population has Spanish as their common and primary language; nonetheless, their diverse cultural and linguistic backgrounds account for diversity in dialects (Magar, 1990). Hispanic people value extended, cohesive families. Families have been patriarchal, with male members perceived as superior and female members seen as a family-bonding life force. These traditional family structures are changing with migration, urbanization, women in the work force, and social movements. Spousal roles are becoming more egalitarian (Friedman, 1990). However, vestiges of the machismo man and the self-sacrificing woman still are evident in the Hispanic culture and continue to shape behavior.

HEALTH PROBLEMS

Health problems among the Hispanic population are complicated by experiences in their countries of origin as well as socioeconomic and lifestyle factors in this country. Tuberculosis is high in this group, especially among those younger than 35 years of age. Hypertension, diabetes, and obesity are major concerns. Other problems include infectious diseases, particularly AIDS and pneumonia, parasitic infections, malnutrition, gastroenteritis, alcohol and drug abuse, accidents, and violence. Frequently, the most important health issues for Hispanics are related to the fact that the population is young and has a high birth rate. Post-traumatic stress disorder is a major problem among refugees from Central and South America who have experienced war and physical and emotional torture (Magar, 1990).

HEALTH BELIEFS AND PRACTICES

Religion plays an important part in Latino culture. For most Latinos, Catholicism is the dominant religion (95% of Mexican Americans are Catholic), but often it is "a blend of both Catholicism and pre-Cortesian Indian beliefs and ideology" (Friedman, 1990, p. 221). Latinos believe in submission to the will of God and that illness may be a form of "castigo," or punishment for sins. They cope with illness through prayers and faith that God will heal. Their religion also determines the rituals used in healing. For example, "solisto,"

TABLE 4–3. Hispanic Health Beliefs and Folk Diseases

Belief Name	Explanation/Treatment
Ataque	Severe expression of shock, anxiety, or sadness characterized by screaming, falling to the ground, thrashing about, hyperventilation, violence, mutism, and uncommunicative behavior. Is a culturally appropriate reaction to shocking or unexpected news, which ends spontaneously.
Bilis	Vomiting, diarrhea, headaches, dizziness, nightmares, loss of appetite, and the inability to urinate brought on by livid rage and revenge fantasies. Believed to come from bile pouring into the bloodstream in response to strong emotions and the person "boiling over."
Bilong (hex)	Any illness may be caused by this; proper diagnosis and treatment requires consulting with a santero or santera (priest or priestess).
Caide de mollera	A condition thought to cause a fallen or sunken anterior fontanel, crying, failure to nurse, sunken eyes, and vomiting in infants. Popular home remedies include holding the child upside down over a pan of water, applying a poultice to the depressed area of the head, or inserting a finger in the child's mouth and pushing up on the palate. (Note: According to Western medicine, these symptoms are indicative of dehydration and can be life-threatening. The community health nurse's role is imperative—to promoting hydration and definitive health care.)
Empacho	Lack of appetite, stomach ache, diarrhea, and vomiting caused by poorly digested food. Food forms into a ball and clings to the stomach, causing pain and cramping. Treated by strongly massaging the stomach, gently pinching and rubbing the spine, drinking a purgative tea (*estafiate*), or by administering *azarcon* or *greta,* medicines that have been implicated, in some cases, in lead poisoning. (Note: The community health nurse must assess family for the use of these "medicines" and initiate appropriate follow-up).
Fatigue	Asthma-like symptoms treated with western health care practices, including oxygen and medications.
Mal de ojo	A sudden and unexplained illness including vomiting, fever, crying, and restlessness in a usually well child (most vulnerable) or adult. Brought on by an admiring or covetous look from a person with an "evil eye." It can be prevented if the person with the "evil eye" touches the child when admiring him or her if the child wears a special charm. Treated by a spiritualistic sweeping of the body with eggs, lemons, and bay leaves accompanied by prayer.
Pasmo	Paralysis-like symptoms in the face and limbs treated by massage.
Susto	Anorexia, insomnia, weakness, hallucinations, and various painful sensations brought on by traumatic situations such as witnessing a death. Treatment includes relaxation, herb tea, and prayer.

Adapted from The National Coalition of Hispanic Health and Human Services Organization, 1988; and Spector, 2000.

which is a condition of depression in women (similar to a midlife crisis in American culture) is treated by having the patient lie on the floor while her body is stroked by the curandero (native healer) until the depression passes. Latino culture includes beliefs that witchcraft, or "brujeria," and evil eye, or "mal de ojo," are supernatural causes of illness that cannot be treated by "Anglo" medicine. "Empacho," a stomach ache in children that occurs after a traumatic event, is treated by the curandero with herbal mixtures made into teas. After tender, loving care and a bowel movement, the child is "healed" (Table 4–3). Like Asians, Latinos believe in "hot" and "cold" categories of foods that influence their diet during illness. Many Latinos tend to be oriented to the present and are not as concerned about keeping time schedules or preparing for the future.

Disadvantaged Populations

The final cultural community selected for this discussion is made up of groups of people who are economically, physically, or emotionally disadvantaged. Each of these groups also can be said to have their own subcultures or microcultures. The poor, the homeless, migrant workers who are eco-

nomically disadvantaged, the developmentally delayed, the deaf, the blind, or persons with physical disabilities often form their own communities, with certain distinct beliefs and practices characterizing their culture.

ECONOMICALLY DISADVANTAGED POPULATIONS

Low-income populations are microcultures in most industrialized countries. Over 1 billion people—nearly a sixth of humanity—will enter the 21st century doomed to poverty because they are unable to read, write, or master other skills necessary to hold a job. The economically disadvantaged population can easily be misunderstood by health professionals (see Chapter 32). Although they may share the same values as the dominant culture, the poor are unable to act on these values and exist in separate microcultures that are diverse and unique. People who are economically disadvantaged come from many ethnic and racial backgrounds and bring the values, beliefs, and customs of their backgrounds with them. Because of this diversity, some have challenged the notion of a culture of poverty, warning of the dangers of stereotyping (Carney, 1992; Martin & Henry, 1989; Pesznecker, 1984). As in any culture, individual variations exist because people belong to overlapping groups, even within a specified culture. Community health nurses need to avoid stereotyping the poor, since this may lead to inaccurate assessments and interventions. What, then, characterizes the poor? Poverty is a state of being economically disadvantaged or, because of extremely limited resources, being unable to obtain adequate food, shelter, clothing, employment, or health care (Montgomery et al., 1996; Northam, 1996). However, the microculture of those in poverty is more than economic. Culture, as was previously discussed, comprises the ideas, values, and behaviors shared by a group that provide a design for living. When a person or group of persons is poor, regardless of the circumstances leading to that poverty, those individuals learn a set of behaviors and practices enabling them to cope with life. These behaviors and practices make up the microculture of the poor.

Three attributes, in particular, characterize the poor. One is that people experiencing poverty live mostly in the present (Strauss, 1967). Much of the teaching of health practitioners emphasizes prevention and thus is future oriented. Taking vitamins, eating well-balanced meals, or getting a routine mammogram all involve a future orientation, a view conflicting with the priorities of most people in poverty. Economically disadvantaged persons may have an orientation to the present because frequently they must meet immediate needs at the expense of long-term gains.

A second attribute is that the lives of many in poverty "are uncertain, dominated by recurring crises" (Strauss, 1967, p. 10). Our larger society espouses a value of ordered, controlled, and well-planned lives. We advocate crisis prevention. For the poor, including migrant farm workers and urban homeless people, the demands of daily living with limited resources require adaptation on a day-to-day and even moment-by-moment basis. The poor experience a barrage of stressors, such as inability to find employment, housing, respectful treatment, or freedom from violence, that limit their ability to cope (Pesznecker, 1984). In many instances, positive health may be valued by this group but is unattainable; thus, they learn to live with illness and crisis.

A third attribute for many of the economically disadvantaged is the lack of a stable environment. Certain groups—the homeless, migrant workers, and transient populations, in particular—have no permanent housing; their lives are characterized by a high rate of mobility. Migrant farm laborers work the southern states in the winter and then move north in the summer months. Their mobility makes it difficult to provide continuous or comprehensive health services, which, in turn, accounts for "a higher rate of respiratory, infectious, and digestive diseases than the general population" (Watkins et al., 1990, p. 568). The migrant farm worker population in the United States, an estimated 3 million, includes whites, American blacks, Hispanics, Haitians, and a small percentage of other minorities, although most migrant workers are from Mexico (Watkins et al., 1990). Migrant groups may retain some of their ethnic heritage but add their own cultural characteristics (see Chapter 33).

Many of the poor have learned to accept their life conditions

and to make the most of them. Despite limited resources and often limited education, some have positive health practices, although most have "compromised physical or psychosocial health. . . . Lack of resources and options for coping lead to poor nutritional and other health habits that become extremely difficult to change" (Carney, 1992, p. 74). Some religious groups choose poverty as a way of life, and others, although poor economically, have learned to accept and live happily with limited material resources. Differences in lifestyle, dress, and behavior easily lead the community health nurse to make assumptions about this group that may not be correct. For instance, the poor have been characterized as having low self-esteem (Robertson, 1969). Although this sometimes may be true, it is not fair or accurate to make such a generalization. Rather, these groups need caring professionals who understand and appreciate their values and needs and who offer health assistance within the context of their unique microcultures.

PHYSICALLY DISABLED OR DEVELOPMENTALLY DELAYED POPULATIONS

Persons with varying disabilities often form their own communities for employment, recreation, and mutual support. In turn, these communities develop their own microcultures. These include the deaf community (Holm, 1991), the physically disabled community, the community of developmentally delayed and mentally retarded citizens, disabled veterans, and the blind. A problem created by well-meaning parents, teachers, and health professionals is to try to "fix" these people to be as "normal" as possible. Although this might seem reasonable in some respects, the implication is that they are deficient or inferior. Physically disabled people find this approach deeply debilitating and oppressive. It is a form of ethnocentrism. In the deaf community, the attempt to normalize, which is the integration model, is challenged by some deaf adults, parents of deaf children, and health care providers. "Many believe that a bilingual and bicultural model should be substituted for the integration model. This involves a profound shift in thinking. Deafness would be celebrated as a distinct, unique culture rather than treated as a problem to be fixed. A bicultural model views deafness as qualitatively different, but not worse and not broken" (Conflict and Change Center, 1992).

In 1994, Disabilities Services at the University of Minnesota proposed replacing the medical model with an interactional model (Table 4–4), which implicitly supports the bicultural view.

TRANSCULTURAL COMMUNITY HEALTH NURSING PRINCIPLES

Culture profoundly influences thinking and behavior and has an enormous impact on the effectiveness of health care. Just as physical and psychological factors determine

TABLE 4-4. Cultural Views of People With Disabilities

Medical Model	Interaction Model
Disability is a deficiency or abnormality.	Disability is a difference.
Being disabled is negative.	Being disabled, in itself, is neutral.
Disability resides in the individual.	Disability derives from interaction between the individual and society.
The remedy for disability–related problems is a cure or normalization of the individual.	The remedy for disability–related problems is a change in the interaction between the individual and society.
The agent of remedy is the professional.	The agent of remedy can be the individual, an advocate, or anyone who affects the arrangements between the individual and society.

From *Workshop on meaningful access for people with disabilities.* University of Minnesota Disabilities Services, Minneapolis, May 18, 1994.

clients' needs and attitudes toward health and illness, so, too, does culture. Kark emphasized that "culture is perhaps the most relevant social determinant of community health" (1974, p. 149). Culture determines how people rear their children, react to pain, cope with stress, deal with death, respond to health practitioners, and value the past, present, and future. Culture also influences diet and eating practices. In fact, partly because of culturally derived preferences, dietary practices are very difficult to change (Nakamura, 1999).

Despite its importance, the client's culture often is mis-understood or ignored in the delivery of health care (Leininger, 1995). Nurses must avoid ethnocentric attitudes and must attempt to understand and bridge cultural differences when working with others. Nurses must develop knowledge and skill in serving multicultural clients and must put their responses to experiences within the context of their lives; otherwise, their understanding and interpretation of their experience will be limited (Meleis, 1997).

Overcoming ethnocentrism requires a concerted effort on the nurse's part to see the world through the eyes of clients. It means being willing "to examine one's own culture care-

CLINICAL CORNER   Maria Juarez

Maria Juarez, a 53-year-old Mexican-American widow, was referred to a community health nursing agency by a clinic. Her married daughter reported that Mrs. Juarez was having severe and prolonged vaginal bleeding and needed medical attention. The daughter had made several appointments for her mother at the clinic, but Mrs. Juarez had refused at the last minute to keep any of them.

After two broken home visit appointments, the community health nurse made a drop-in call and found Mrs. Juarez at home. The nurse was greeted courteously and invited to have a seat. After introductions, the nurse explained that she and the others were only trying to help. Mrs. Juarez had caused a lot of un-necessary concern to everyone by not cooperating, she scolded in a friendly tone. Mrs. Juarez quickly apologized and explained that she had felt fine on the days of her broken appointments and saw no need "to bother" anyone. Questioned about her vaginal bleeding, Mrs. Juarez was evasive. "It's nothing," she said. "It comes and goes like always, only maybe a little more." She listened politely, nodding in agreement as the nurse explained the need for her to see a physician. Her promise to come to the clinic the next day, how-ever, was not kept. The staff labeled Mrs. Juarez unre-liable and uncooperative.

Mrs. Juarez had been brought up in traditional Mexican-American culture that taught her to be sub-missive and interested primarily in the welfare of her husband and children. She had learned long ago to ignore her own needs and found it difficult to identify any personal wants. Her major concern was to avoid causing trouble for others. To have a medical prob-lem, then, was a difficult adjustment. The pain and bleeding had caused her great apprehension. Many Mexican Americans have a particular dread of sick-ness and especially hospitalization. Furthermore, Mrs. Juarez's culture had taught her the value of mod-esty. "Female problems" were not discussed openly. This cultural orientation meant that the sickness threatened her modesty and created intense embar-rassment. Conforming to Mexican-American cultural values, she had first turned to her family for support. Often, only under dire circumstances do members of this cultural group seek help from others; to do so means sacrificing pride and dignity. Mrs. Juarez agreed to go to the clinic because refusal would have been disrespectful, but her fear of physicians and her reluctance to discuss such a sensitive problem kept her from going. Mrs. Juarez was being asked to take action that violated several deeply felt cultural values. Her behavior was far from unreliable and uncoopera-tive. With no opportunity to discuss and resolve the conflicts, she had no other choice.

fully and become aware that alternative viewpoints are possible" (Eliason, 1993, p. 226). It means attempting to understand the meaning of other people's culture for them, and it means appreciating their culture as important and useful to them. Ignoring consideration of clients' different cultural origins often has negative results, as illustrated by the Clinical Corner about Maria Juarez.

Culture is a universal experience. Each person is part of some group, and that group helps to shape the values, beliefs, and behaviors that make up their culture. In addition, every cultural group is different from all others. Even within fairly homogeneous cultural groups, there are subcultures and microcultures with their own distinctive characteristics. Further differences, based on such factors as socioeconomic status, social class, age, or degree of acculturation, can be found within microcultures. These latter differences have been called intraethnic variations (Friedman, 1990), which only underscore the range of culturally diverse clients served by community health nurses.

Given such diversity, community health nurses face a considerable challenge in providing service to cross-cultural groups. This kind of practice, known as **transcultural nursing,** means culturally sensitive nursing service to people of an ethnic or racial background different from the nurse's. Community health nurses in transcultural practice with client groups can be guided by several principles: (1) develop cultural self-awareness, (2) cultivate cultural sensitivity, (3) assess client group's culture, (4) show respect and patience while learning about other cultures, and (5) examine culturally derived health practices.

Develop Cultural Self-Awareness

The first transcultural nursing principle focuses on the nurse's own culture. Self-awareness is crucial for the nurse working with people from other cultures (Leininger, 1995). "A first step in developing cultural sensitivity is to examine one's own culture carefully and become aware that alternative viewpoints are possible" (Eliason, 1993, p. 226). Nurses must remember that their culture often is sharply different from the culture of their clients. **Cultural self-awareness** means recognition of one's own values, beliefs, and practices that make up one's culture. It also means becoming sensitive to the impact of one's culturally based responses. The community health nurse who assisted Mrs. Juarez probably thought that she was being friendly, efficient, and helpful. In terms of her own culture, this nurse's behavior was intended to reassure clients and meet their needs. Unaware of the negative consequences of her behavior, the nurse caused damage rather than met needs.

To gain skill in understanding their own culturally based behavior, nurses can complete a cultural self-assessment by analyzing the following points:
- Influences from own ethnic and racial background
- Own typical verbal and nonverbal communication patterns
- Own cultural values and norms
- Own religious beliefs and practices
- Own health beliefs and practices

Start with a detailed list of values, beliefs, and practices relative to each point. Next, enlist one or more close friends to call attention to selected behaviors to bring these to a more conscious level. Videotaping practice interviews with colleagues and actual interviews with selected clients creates further awareness of the nurse's culturally based unconscious responses. Finally, ask selected clients to critique nursing actions in contrast with client culture. Feedback from clients' perspectives can bring many of the nurse's own cultural responses to light.

Because culture is mostly tacit, as discussed earlier in this chapter, it takes conscious effort and hard work to bring the nurse's own culture to the surface. By doing so, however, the nurse will be rewarded first with a more effective understanding of self, and second with an enhanced ability to provide culturally relevant service to clients.

Cultivate Cultural Sensitivity

The second transcultural nursing principle seeks to expand the nurse's awareness of the significance of culture on behavior. Nurses' beliefs and ways of doing things frequently conflict with those of their clients. A first step toward bridging cultural barriers is recognition of those differences and the development of cultural sensitivity. **Cultural sensitivity** requires recognizing that culturally based values, beliefs, and practices influence people's health and lifestyles and need to be considered in plans for service (Gerrish, 1998; Spradley, 1988). Mrs. Juarez's values and health practices sharply contrasted with those of the clinic's staff. Failure to recognize these differences led to a breakdown in communication and ineffective care. Once differences in culture are recognized, it is important to accept and appreciate them. A nurse's ways are valid for the nurse; clients' ways work for them. The nurse visiting the Kim family avoided the dangerous ethnocentric trap of assuming that her way was best, and she consequently developed a fruitful relationship with her clients.

As a part of developing cultural sensitivity, nurses need to try to understand clients' points of view. They need to stand in their shoes, to try to see the world through their eyes. By listening, observing, and gradually learning other cultures, the nurse must add a further step of choosing to avoid ethnocentrism. Otherwise, the nurse's view of a different culture will remain distorted and perhaps prejudiced. The ability to show interest, concern, and compassion enabled Sandra Josten to win the trust and respect of the Native American women. It told the Kims that their nurse cared about them. These nurses attempted to understand the feelings and ideas of their clients, thus establishing a trusting relationship and opening the door to the possibility of the clients adopting healthier behaviors.

Assess Client Group's Culture

A third transcultural nursing principle emphasizes the need to learn clients' cultures. All clients' actions, like our own, are based on underlying culturally learned beliefs and ideas. Mrs. Kim did not like milk because her culture had taught her that it was distasteful. Also, many Asians are lactose intolerant. The Native American women's response to waiting or keeping someone else waiting was influenced by their value of patience. There usually is some culturally based reason that causes clients to engage in (or avoid) certain actions. Instead of making assumptions or judging clients' behavior, the nurse first must learn about the culture that guides that behavior (Lester, 1998). During a cultural assessment, the nurse obtains health-related information about a designated cultural group concerning their values, beliefs, and practices (see Research: Bridge to Practice). One study showed that client behavior was interpreted differently by professionals of a different culture than by professionals of the clients' culture (Tripp-Reimer, 1982). Learning clients' culture first is critical to effective nursing practice. The Giger and Davidhizar transcultural assessment model (1995) considers six interrelated factors for assessing differences between people in cultural groups: communication, space, time, social organization, environmental control, and biological variations (Bechtel et al., 1998; Davidhizar et al., 1998) (Fig. 4–2). Understanding these phenomena is a first step toward appreciating the diversity that exists among people from different cultural backgrounds. Interviewing members of a subcultural group can provide valuable data to enhance understanding.

To fully understand a group's culture, it should be studied in depth, as Bernal maintains:

> **Although a general knowledge base and skills are applicable transculturally, immersion in a given culture is necessary to understand fully the patterns that shape the behavior of individuals within that group. Experience with one group can be helpful in understanding the concept of diversity, but each group must be understood within its own ecologic niche and for its own historical and cultural reality (1993, p. 231).**

Practically speaking, however, it is not possible to study in depth all of the cultural groups that the nurse encounters. Instead, the nurse can conduct a cultural assessment by questioning key informants, observing the cultural group, and reading additional information in the literature. The data can be grouped into six categories:

1. *Ethnic or racial background:* Where did the client group originate and how does that influence their status and identity?
2. *Language and communication patterns:* What is the preferred language spoken and what are their culturally based communication patterns?
3. *Cultural values and norms:* What are their values, beliefs, and standards regarding such things as roles, education, family functions, child-rearing, work

---

RESEARCH Bridge to Practice

Hanson, M.J. (1997). The theory of planned behavior applied to cigarette smoking in African-American, Puerto Rican, and non-Hispanic white teenage females. *Nursing Research, 46*(3), 155–162.

Cigarette-smoking intention in three groups of teenage females is explored to evaluate the adequacy of Ajzen's theory of planned behavior in predicting behavior. Ajzen's theory is designed to predict behavior and enhance understanding of its psychological determinants, providing a framework within which to study cigarette smoking. According to the theory, intention to perform or to not perform a behavior is the immediate determinant of the behavior, with intention being a direct function of three independent variables: attitude, subjective norm, and perceived behavioral control. Consequently, a person's intention to smoke cigarettes is a function of attitude toward smoking, perception of what significant others would think about smoking, and perception about self-control over the behavior of smoking.

The sample consisted of 430 study subjects closely divided into three groups of English-speaking African-American, Puerto Rican, and non-Hispanic white 13- to 19-year-old female teens. Smokers and nonsmokers were about equally represented. The instrument used was the Fishbein/Ajzen-Hanson questionnaire, constructed in accordance with the Theory of Planned Behavior.

Findings support the theory for smoking intention among female African-American teens but not for their counterparts. The results suggest that for female African-American teens, attitude toward smoking, perception of what significant others would think about their smoking, and perception about self-control over smoking all directly influence intention to smoke. Cultural values and beliefs may partially account for the ethnic differences in subjective norm as a predictor of smoking intention and thus may be partly related, at least regarding lack of parental influence, to the decline in the number of traditional families among whites in the United States. African-Americans have strong kinship bonds with extended family, which may partially account for the direct effect of subjective norm on smoking intention in this study.

Further study is recommended to increase the number of questionnaire items to improve reliability and in future studies. Specific information about teenagers' cultural beliefs and values should be gathered. Research demonstrates that significantly better results are obtained when health-promotion messages are tailored to the population (Skinner et al., 1994), with this study providing an initial step in the identification of culturally sensitive predictors of smoking intention among female teens. Additional studies are needed to identify specific beliefs that distinguish between smokers and nonsmokers to use in the development of population-specific smoking prevention programs.

---

and leisure, aging, death and dying, and rites of passage?
4. *Biocultural factors:* Are there physical or genetic traits unique to this cultural group that predispose them to certain conditions or illnesses?
5. *Religious beliefs and practices:* What are the group's religious beliefs and how do they influence life events, roles, health, and illness?

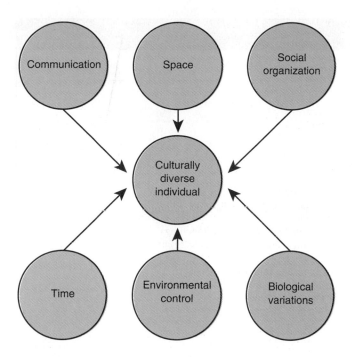

FIGURE 4–2. The Giger and Davidhizar transcultural assessment model (abridged). Shows the culturally diverse individual through communication, space, social organization, time, environmental control, and biological variations. (Adapted from Dowd, S.B., Giger, J.N., & Davidhizar, R. [1998]. Use of Giger and Davidhizar's transcultural assessment model by health professionals. *International Nursing Review, 45* [4], 119–122, 128.)

6. *Health beliefs and practices:* What are the group's beliefs and practices regarding prevention, causes, and treatment of illnesses?

The cultural assessment guide, presented in Table 4–5, gives suggestions for more detailed data collection.

Other cultural assessment guides also are available (Bloch, 1983; Brownlee, 1978; Herberg, 1989; Leininger, 1995; Orque, 1983; Tripp-Reimer, 1985). Tripp-Reimer, Brink, & Saunders (1984) suggests that a thorough cultural assessment may be too time-consuming and costly. Instead, the two-phase assessment process is proposed, as outlined in Table 4–6. Categories to explore in the assessment include values, beliefs, customs, and social structure components. Two methods that have proven highly effective for in-depth study of cultural groups are ethnographic interviewing and participant observation (Spradley, 1979, 1980).

Show Respect and Patience While Learning About Other Cultures

The fourth transcultural nursing principle emphasizes key behaviors for the nurse to practice during the cultural learning process. Respect is the first behavior, and it is shown in many ways. When Sandra Josten involved the Native Amer-

ican women in decisions and gave them choices, she was showing respect. When the nurse gave positive recognition to the importance of the Kim's culture, she was showing respect. Attentive listening is a way to show respect and to learn about their culture (Eliason, 1993). Within the United States, people of minority groups particularly need respect. At times, for groups with limited English skills and a community health nurse who is not bilingual, the use of an interpreter can assist with communication and becomes a necessity (Display 4–5).

A **minority group** is part of a population that differs from the majority and often receives differential and unequal treatment. Their ways contrast with those of the dominant culture. It is difficult for them to retain pride in their lifestyles, or in themselves, when the majority culture suggests that they are inferior. The message may be only implied or even unintentional. Such was the case for Mrs. Juarez as described in the earlier Clinical Corner. The clinic's routine and the manner of the staff were not intended to show disrespect. They did, nevertheless, and Mrs. Juarez was intimidated and unable to receive the help that she needed. Everyone needs respect to enhance pride, dignity, and self-esteem; it is an important contributor to good mental health (Bechtel et al., 1998). Showing respect also is an important means for breaking down barriers in cross-cultural communication. For community health nurses, culturally relevant care means practicing cultural relativism. **Cultural relativism** is recognizing and respecting alternative viewpoints and understanding values, beliefs, and practices within their cultural context.

Besides respect, patience is essential. It takes time to build trust and effect cultural change. It can be difficult to establish the nurse–client relationship when it involves two different cultures. Trust must be won, and winning it may take weeks, months, or years. Time must be allowed for both the nurse and clients to learn how to communicate with one another, to test one another's trustworthiness, and to learn about one another. Change in behavior (learned aspects of the culture) occurs gradually. Some aspects of both the nurse's and the client's cultures can, and probably will, change. The Kims' nurse, Paula Morrow, for example, modified some of her usual practices and adapted them to the Kims' culture and needs. They, in turn, began to assume some American practices and values. However, the process took several months. Time, respect, and patience help to break down cultural barriers.

Examine Culturally Derived Health Practices

The final transcultural nursing principle involves scrutiny of the client group's cultural practices as they affect the group's health status. Once the community health nurse has assessed the culture of the client group, further determinations must be made. Cultural practices affecting the health of the client group need to be examined. Are these behaviors preserving

TABLE 4–5. Cultural Assessment Guide

Category	Sample Data
Ethnic/racial background	Countries of origin Mostly native-born or U.S. born? Reasons for emigrating if applicable Racial/ethnic identity Experience with racism or racial discrimination?
Language and communication patterns	Languages of origin Languages spoken in the home Preferred language for communication How verbal communication patterns affected by age, sex, other? Preferences for use of interpreters Nonverbal communication patterns (eg, eye contact, touching)
Cultural values and norms	Group beliefs and standards for male and female roles and functions Standards for modesty and sexuality Family/extended family structures and functions Values re: work, leisure, success, time Values re: education and occupation Norms for child-rearing and socialization Norms for social networks and supports Values re: aging and treatment of elders Values re: authority Norms for dress and appearance
Biocultural factors	Group genetic predisposition to health conditions (eg, hypertension, anemia) Socioculturally associated illnesses (eg, AIDS, alcoholism) Group attitudes toward body parts and functions Group vulnerability or resistance to health threats? Folk illnesses common to group? Group physical/genetic differences (eg, bone mass, height, weight, longevity)
Religious beliefs and practices	Religious beliefs affecting roles, childbearing and child-rearing, health and illness? Recognized religious healers? Religious beliefs and practices for promoting health, preventing illness, or treatment of illness. Beliefs and rituals re: conception and birth Beliefs and rituals re: death, dying, grief
Health beliefs and practices	Beliefs re: causes of illness Beliefs re: treatment of illness Beliefs re: use of healers (traditional and western) Health promotion and illness prevention practices Folk medicine practices Beliefs re: mental health and illness Dietary, herbal, and other folk cures Food beliefs, preparation, consumption Experience with western medicine

TABLE 4–6. Two-Phased Cultural Assessment Process

PHASE I—DATA COLLECTION

Stage 1	Assess values, beliefs, and customs (eg, ethnic affiliations, religion, decision-making patterns).
Stage 2	Collect problem-specific cultural data (eg, cultural beliefs and practices related to diet and nutrition). Make nursing diagnoses.
Stage 3	Determine cultural factors influencing nursing intervention (eg, child-rearing beliefs and practices that might affect nurse teaching toilet training or child discipline).

PHASE II—DATA ORGANIZATION

Step 1	Compare cultural data with
	    Standards of client's own culture (eg, client's diet compared with cultural norms)
	    Standards of the nurse's culture
	    Standards of the health facility providing service.

Step 2	Determine incongruities in above standards.
Step 3	Seek to modify one or more systems (client's, nurse's, or the facility's) to achieve maximum congruity.

DISPLAY 4–5. **Interpreter Guidelines**

1. Unless the community health nurse is thoroughly effective and fluent in the client's language, an interpreter should be used.
2. Meet with interpreters on a regular basis, since they provide both a window and a mirror when dealing with other clients.
3. Confidentiality must be maintained by the interpreter, who divulges nothing without the full approval of the client and community health nurse.
4. Evaluate the interpreter's style, approach to clients, and ability to develop a relationship of trust and respect. Try to match the interpreter to the client.
5. Be patient. Careful interpretation often requires that the interpreter use long, explanatory phrases.
6. Interpreters must interpret everything that is said by all of the people in the interaction but should inform the community health nurse if the content might be perceived as offensive, insensitive, or harmful to the dignity and well-being of the client.
7. When appropriate, encourage interpreters to explain cultural differences to the client and to yourself.
8. Interpretation conveys the content and spirit of what is said, with nothing omitted or added.
9. Volunteer interpreters receive no fee. Employed interpreters receive their fee or salary from the hiring agency. They should not accept money or favors from clients or the community health nurse. A sincere "thank you" is most appropriate (Kaufert & Putsch, 1997; Putsch, 1985).

and enhancing the group's health or are they harmful to their health? Some traditional practices, such as customary diet, birth rituals, and certain folk remedies, may promote both physical and psychological health. These can be considered healthful. Other practices may be neither harmful nor particularly health promoting but are useful in preserving the culture, security, and sense of identity of a particular ethnic group. Then, some traditional practices may be directly harmful to health. Examples include using herbal poultices to treat an infected wound or "burning" the abdomen to compensate for heat loss associated with diarrhea.

The community health nurse must remember that cultural assessment and aggregate health assessment need to go hand in hand. If the group is experiencing a high incidence of low birth weight babies, pregnancy complications, skin infections, mental illness, or other evidence of health problems, these can be clues to prompt an examination of cultural health practices. Those that are clearly damaging to health can be discussed with group leaders and healers. It is here that knowing their cultural norms for authority and decision-

making can be helpful. Often, a cultural practice can be continued or modified and combined with Western medicine so that respect for the culture is maintained while full treatment efficacy is accomplished.

SUMMARY

Community health clients belong to a variety of cultural groups. A culture is a design for living and provides a set of norms and values that offer stability and security for members of a society and plays a major role in motivating behaviors. The increase in and great variety of cultural groups reinforce the need for community health nurses to understand and appreciate cultural diversity. Ethnocentrism is the bias that a person's own culture is best and others are wrong or inferior. It can create serious barriers to effective nursing care. Understanding cultural diversity and being sensitive to the values and behaviors of cultural groups often is the key to effective community health intervention.

Culture has five characteristics: it is learned from others; it is an integrated system of customs and traits; it is shared; it is tacit; and it is dynamic. Every culture preserves its integrity by deleting nonfunctional practices and acquiring new components that better serve the group. To gain acceptance, nurses must strive to introduce improved health practices that are presented in a manner consistent with clients' cultural values.

Five transcultural nursing principles, drawn from an understanding of the concept of culture, can guide community health nursing practice:
1. Develop cultural self-awareness.
2. Cultivate cultural sensitivity.
3. Assess client group's culture.
4. Show respect and patience while learning other cultures.
5. Examine culturally derived health practices.

ACTIVITIES TO PROMOTE CRITICAL THINKING

1. Based on your own cultural background, how would you feel and what behaviors would you exhibit if you were:
   a. A client sitting in a clinic waiting room in a foreign country whose language you did not know?
   b. Part of a nutrition class being told to eat foods you had never heard of before?
   c. Visited in your home by a nurse who told you to discipline your child in a way that contradicted everything you had been reared to believe about parenting?

2. Describe three tacit cultural rules that govern your own behavior. How might these affect your interaction with clients from another culture?

3. What does the term ethnocentrism mean to you? Have you ever experienced someone else being ethnocentric in their attitude toward you? If so, describe that experience. Using Bennett's stages of cross-cultural sensitivity, explore where your own attitudes are on the continuum toward several of the cultural groups with which you regularly come in contact or from which you know people well.

4. Imagine that you are assigned to work with a Mexican-American migrant population. What are the steps that you would take to gather the appropriate information to provide culturally relevant nursing service? What sources might provide that information?

5. A Hmong father, who severely beat his 12-year-old son with a belt, leaving cuts and bruises, is charged with child abuse. "If I can't discipline my son, how can he be a good kid?" said the father (Bonner, 1994, p. 1). What nursing responses would show respect for this cultural group's norms and values and yet be constructive in resolving the cultural conflict?

6. On the Internet, find web sites that elaborate on transcultural nursing and cross-cultural health care concerns. Print materials of interest and develop a resource file for your professional use.

7. Interprofessional communication techniques among diverse health care disciplines is imperative to effective caregiving. How comfortable are you with knowing the linguistic style, practice, and research backgrounds of social workers, pharmacists, physical therapists, educators, psychologists, and others? Seek out a colleague from a different interprofessional discipline and discuss developing a shared language (Milligan et al., 1999) (see Clinical Corner).

REFERENCES

Bechtel, G.A., Davidhizar, R., & Tiller, C.M. (1998). Patterns of mental health care among Mexican Americans. *Journal of Psychosocial Nursing, 36*(11), 20–27.

Bell, R. (1994). Prominence of women in Navajo healing beliefs and values. *Nursing and Health Care, 15*(5), 232–240.

Bennett, L. (1962). *Before the Mayflower: A history of the black American, 1619–1962.* Chicago: Johnson.

Bennett, M. (1991). Toward a developmental model of intercultural sensitivity. In M. Paige (Ed.), *Education for the intercultural experience.* Yarmouth, ME: Intercultural Press.

Bernal, H. (1993). A model for delivering culture-relevant care in the community. *Public Health Nursing, 10*(4), 228–232.

CLINICAL CORNER | **The Importance of Cultural Sensitivity**

In Australia, well-intentioned government officials, including representatives of the health ministry, identified problems related to substandard housing among a particular aggregate of aboriginal people. To assist this community, the officials spent a great deal of time, energy, and finances planning and building homes for the Aborigines. The homes were small but modern and offered many of the conveniences that officials believed would improve the quality of life for the community.

The Aborigines were appreciative of the group's efforts and moved into their new homes. Before long, however, officials realized that one by one the community was moving back to its "substandard" housing. When queried about their lack of appreciation for the improved lifestyle, the group informed the officials that their life line was their watering hole and that the houses were not only uncomfortable to them but were too far from their watering hole.

Soon, all of the aboriginal families had returned to living on the land, and the homes were part of a veritable ghost town in the middle of nowhere.

Question

1. What does the term *globalization not gobbleization* mean to you?

2. Was the aboriginal community truly "poor," as the officials seemed to think?

3. Discuss your perception of the following issues:

   Cultural imposition

   Cultural poverty

   Dignity and spirit

4. If you were assigned to the international health team that was to return to the community to try again to improve their quality of life, what steps would you take to ensure that previous mistakes are not repeated?

Bloch, B. (1983). Bloch's assessment guide for ethnic/culture variations. In M. Orque & B. Bloch (Eds.), *Ethnic nursing care*. St. Louis: C.V. Mosby.

Bonner, B. (1994). Hmong parents feeling pressure to spare the rod. *St. Paul Pioneer Press, 146*(54), 1A, 5A.

Brownlee, A.T. (1978). *Community, culture, and care*. St. Louis: C.V. Mosby.

Carney, P. (1992). The concept of poverty. *Public Health Nursing, 9*(2), 74–80.

Conflict and Change Center. (1992). Conflict and change in the deaf and hearing cultures. *Conflict/change process* (spring; Vols. 1–3). Minneapolis: University of Minnesota,

Davidhizar, R., Dowd, S.B., & Giger, J.N. (1998). Educating the culturally diverse healthcare student. *Nurse Educator, 23*(2), 38–42.

Dehn, M. (1997). Cactus juice, copper bracelets, and garlic: Self-care issues facing community health nurses. In B. Spradley & J. Allender (Eds.), *Readings in community health nursing* (5th ed.). Philadelphia: Lippincott-Raven Publishers.

Dowd, S.B., Giger, J.N., & Davidhizar, R. (1998). Use of Giger and Davidhizar's transcultural assessment model by health professionals. *International Nursing Review, 45*(4), 119–122, 128.

Eliason, M.J. (1993). Ethics and transcultural nursing care. *Nursing Outlook, 41*(5), 225–228.

Fielo, S.C. & Degazon, C.E. (1997). When cultures collide: Decision making in a multicultural environment *Nursing and Health Care Perspectives, 18*(5), 238–244.

Foster, G.M. (1962). *Traditional cultures and the impact of technological change*. New York: Harper.

Friedman, M. (1990). Transcultural family nursing: Application to Latino and black families. *Journal of Pediatric Nursing, 5*(3), 214–222.

Gerrish, K. (1998). Preparing nurses to care for minority ethnic communities. *International Nurses Review, 45*(4), 115–118, 127.

Hall, E.T. (1959). *The silent language*. Garden City, NY: Doubleday.

Hansen, J.C. (1996). Grandparents remembered: Grandfather Chin. *Generations, 20*(1), 75–76.

Hanson, M.J. (1997). The theory of planned behavior applied to cigarette smoking in African-American, Puerto Rican, and non-Hispanic white teenage females. *Nursing Research, 46*(3), 155–162.

Herberg, P. (1989). Theoretical foundations of transcultural nursing. In J.S. Boyle & M.N. Andrews (Eds.), *Transcultural concepts in nursing care* (pp. 1–60). Glenview, IL: Scott, Foresman/Little, Brown College Division.

Holland, L. & Courtney, R. (1998). Increasing cultural competence with the Latino community. *Journal of Community Health Nursing, 15*(1), 45–53.

Holm, C. (1991). Deafness: Common misunderstandings. In B. Spradley (Ed.), *Readings in community health nursing* (4th ed.) (pp. 544–549). Philadelphia: J.B. Lippincott.

Kark, S.L. (1974). *Epidemiology and community medicine*. New York: Appleton-Century-Crofts.

Kaufert, J.M. & Putsch, R.W. (1997). Communication through interpreters in healthcare: Ethical dilemmas arising from differences in class, culture, language, and power. *The Journal of Clinical Ethics, 8*(1), 71–87.

Leininger, M. (1991a). *Culture care diversity and universality: A theory of nursing*. New York: National League for Nursing Press.

Leininger, M. (1991b). Transcultural care principles, human rights, and ethical considerations. *Journal of Transcultural Nursing, 3*, 21–23.

Leininger, M. (1995). *Transcultural nursing: Concepts, theories, research and practice* (2nd ed.). New York: McGraw Hill.

Lester, N. (1998). Cultural competence: A nursing dialogue. *American Journal of Nursing, 98*(8), 26–33.

Lin-Fu, J.S. (1991). Population characteristics and health care needs of Asian Pacific Americans. In B. Spradley (Ed.), *Readings in Community Health Nursing* (4th ed.). Philadelphia: J.B. Lippincott.

Magar, V. (1990). Health care needs of Central American refugees. *Nursing Outlook, 38*(5), 239–242.

Martin, M.E. & Henry, M. (1989). Cultural relativity and poverty. *Public Health Nursing, 6*(1), 28–34.

Mead, M. (1960). Cultural contexts of nursing problems. In F.C. MacGregor (Ed.), *Social science in nursing*. New York: Wiley.

Meleis, A.I. (1997). Immigrant transitions and health care: An action plan. *Nursing Outlook, 45*(1), 42.

Milligan, R.A., Gilroy, J., Katz, K.S., Rodan, M.F., & Subramanian, K.N. (1999). Developing a shared language: Interdisciplinary communication among diverse health care professionals. *Holistic Nursing Practice, 13*(2), 47–53.

Montgomery, L.E., Kiely, J.L., & Pappas, G. (1996). The effects of poverty, race, and family structure on U.S. children's health: Data from the NHIS, 1978 through 1980 and 1989 through 1991. *American Journal of Public Health, 86*(10), 1401–1405.

Muecke, M.A. (1983). Caring for Southeast Asian refugee patients in the United States. *American Journal of Public Health, 73*(4), 431–438.

Murdock, G. (1972). The science of culture. In M. Freilich (Ed.), *The meaning of culture: A reader in cultural anthropology* (pp. 252–266). Lexington, MA: Xerox College Publishing.

Nakumura, R.M. (1999). *Health in America: A multicultural perspective*. Boston: Allyn and Bacon.

Northam, S. (1996). Access to health promotion, protection, and disease prevention among impoverished individuals. *Public Health Nursing, 13*(5), 353–364.

Orque, M.S. (1983). Orque's ethnic/cultural system: A framework for ethnic nursing care. In M.S. Orque, B. Bloch, & L.S. Montroy (Eds.), *Ethnic nursing care*. St. Louis: C.V. Mosby.

Pesznecker, B.L. (1984). The poor: A population at risk multidimensional model of poverty: Practice implications. *Public Health Nursing, 1*(4), 237–249.

Porter, C. & Villarruel, A. (1993). Nursing research with African American and Hispanic people: Guidelines for action. *Nursing Outlook, 41*(2), 59–67.

Putsch, R.W. III. (1985). Cross-cultural communication: The special case of interpreters in health care. *Journal of the American Medical Association, 254*(23), 3344–3348.

Robertson, H.R. (1969). Removing barriers to health care. *Nursing Outlook, 17*, 43–46.

Seideman, R., Williams, R., Burns, P., Jacobson, S., Weatherby, F., & Primeaux, M. (1994). Culture sensitivity in assessing urban Native American parenting. *Public Health Nursing, 11*(2), 98–103.

Skinner, C.S., Strecher, V.J., & Hospers, H. (1994). Physicians' recommendations for mammography: Do tailored messages make a difference? *American Journal of Public Health, 84*(1), 43–49.

Spector, R.E. (2000). *Cultural diversity in health and illness* (5th ed.) Stamford, CT: Appleton & Lange.

Spradley, J.P. (1979). *The ethnographic interview.* New York: Holt.

Spradley, J.P. (1980). *Participant observation.* New York: Holt.

Spradley, J.P. (1988). *Your owe yourself a drunk: An ethnography of urban nomads.* Lanham, MD: University Press of America.

Spradley, J.P. & McCurdy, D.W. (2000). *Conformity and conflict: Readings in cultural anthropology* (10th ed.) Boston: Allyn and Bacon.

Stehr-Green, J.K. & Schantz, P.M. (1986). Trichinosis in Southeast Asian refugees in the United States. *American Journal of Public Health, 76*(10), 1238–1239.

Strauss, A.L. (1967). Medical ghettos. *Trans-Action, 4*(62), 7–15.

Taylor, R. (1998). Check your cultural competence. *Nursing Management, 29*(8), 30–32.

The National Coalition of Hispanic Health and Human Services Organization. (1988). *Delivering preventive health care to Hispanics: A manual for providers.* Washington, DC: The National Coalition of Hispanic Health and Human Services Organization.

Tripp-Reimer, T. (1982). Barriers to health care: Variations in interpretation of Appalachian client behavior by Appalachian and non-Appalachian health professionals. *Western Journal of Nursing Research, 4*(2), 179–191.

Tripp-Reimer, T. (1985). Cultural assessment. In J. Bellack & P. Bamford (Eds.), *Nursing assessment.* North Scituate, MA: Duxbury.

Tripp-Reimer, T., Brink, P.J., & Saunders, J.M. (1984). Cultural assessment: Content and process. *Nursing Outlook, 32*(2), 78–82.

U.S. Bureau of the Census. (1998a). *Current population reports* (P20-507). Washington, DC: U.S. Government Printing Office.

U.S. Bureau of the Census. (1998b). *Current population reports* (P20-508). Washington, DC: U.S. Government Printing Office.

U.S. Bureau of the Census. (1998c). *Current population reports* (P20-512). Washington, DC: U.S. Government Printing Office.

U.S. Department of Commerce. (1998). *Statistical abstract of the United States, 1998* (118th ed.). Washington, DC: Government Printing Office.

Watkins, E., Larson, K., Harlan, C., & Young, S., (1990). A model program for providing health services for migrant farmworker mothers and children. *Public Health Reports, 105*(6), 567–575.

West, E.A. (1993). The cultural bridge model. *Nursing Outlook, 41*(5), 229–234.

SELECTED READINGS

Allen, L.B., Glicken, A.D., Beach, R.K., & Naylor, K.E. (1998). Adolescent health care experience of gay, lesbian, and bisexual young adults. *Journal of Adolescent Health, 23*(4), 212–220.

Andrews, M.M. & Boyle, J.S. (1999). *Transcultural concepts in nursing care* (3rd ed.) Philadelphia: Lippincott Williams & Wilkins.

Applewhite, S. (1995). Curanderismo: Demystifying the health beliefs and practices of elderly Mexican Americans. *National Association of Social Workers, 20*, 247–253.

Balcazar, H., Peterson, G.W., & Krull, J.L. (1997). Acculturation and family cohesiveness in Mexican American pregnant women: Social and health implications. *Family Community Health, 20*(3), 16–31.

Buehler, J. (1993). Nursing in rural native American communities. *Nursing Clinics of North America, 28*(1), 211–217.

Choudhry, U.K. (1997). Traditional practices of women from India: Pregnancy, childbirth, and newborn care. *Journal of Obstetric, Gynecologic, and Neonatal Nursing, 26*(5), 533–539.

Culley, L.A. (1995). A critique of multiculturalism in health care: The challenge for nurse education. *Journal of Advanced Nursing, 23*(2), 564–570.

Davis, L.A. & Winkleby, M.A. (1993). Sociodemographic and health-related risk factors among African-American, Caucasian, and Hispanic homeless men: A comparative study. *Journal of Social Distress and the Homeless, 2*, 83–101.

Davis, R. (1997). Community caring: An ethnographic study within an organizational culture. *Public Health Nursing, 14*, 92–100.

De Santis, L. & Thomas, J. (1992). Health education and the immigrant Haitian mother: Cultural insights for community health nurses. *Public Health Nursing, 9*(2), 87–96.

Delgado, M. & Barton, K. (1998). Murals in Latino communities: Social indicators of community strengths. *Social Work, 43*(4), 346–356.

Eliason, M. & Macy, N. (1992). A classroom activity to introduce cultural diversity. *Nursing Education, 17*, 32–36.

Fox, P.G., Cowell, J.M., & Montgomery, A.C. (1994). The effects of violence on health and adjustment of Southeast Asian refugee children: An integrative review. *Public Health Nursing, 11*(3), 195–201.

Gerrish, K., Husband, C., & Mackenzie, J. (1996). *Nursing for a multi-ethnic society.* Buckingham: Open University Press.

Grossman, D. (1994). Enhancing your "cultural competence." *American Journal of Nursing, 94*(7), 58–62.

Grossman, D. (1996). Cultural dimensions in home health nursing. *American Journal of Nursing, 96*(7), 33–36.

Hall, S.L., Giger, J.N., & Davidhizar, R.E. (1996). Cultural beliefs, values, and healing practices: Impact on the perinatal period. *Journal of Nursing Science, 1*(3–4), 99–104.

Holmes, C.A. & Warelow, P.J. (1997). Culture, needs and nursing: A critical theory approach. *Journal of Advanced Nursing, 25*, 463–470.

Kim, Y.Y. (1992). Intercultural communicative competence: A systems theoretic view. In W.B. Gudykunst & Y.Y. Kim (Eds.), *Readings on communication with strangers.* New York: McGraw-Hill.

Larson, E. (1995). New rules for the game: Interdisciplinary education for health professionals. *Nursing Outlook, 43*, 180–185.

Lea, A. (1994). Nursing in today's multicultural society: A transcultural perspective. *Journal of Advanced Nursing, 20*, 307–313.

Lyon, J.L., et al. (1988). Mormon health. *Health Values, 12*(3), 37–44.

Nolt, S. (1992). *A history of the Amish*. Intercourse, PA: Good Books.

Stevens, G.L. (1998). Experience the culture. *Journal of Nursing Education, 37*(1), 30–33.

Stewart, M. (1998). Nurses need to strengthen cultural competence for the next century to ensure quality patient care. *American Nurse, 30*(1), 26–27.

Xiaoming, L., Howard, D., Stanton, B., Reachuba, L., & Cross, S. (1998). Distress symptoms among urban African American children and adolescents. *Archives of Pediatric and Adolescent Medicine, 152,* 569–577.

Yi, J.K. (1996). Factors affecting cervical cancer screening behavior among Cambodian women in Houston, Tex. *Family Community Health, 18*(4), 49–57.

Values and Ethics in Community Health Nursing

KEY TERMS

- Autonomy
- Beneficence
- Distributive justice
- Egalitarian justice
- Equity
- Ethical decision-making
- Ethical dilemma
- Ethics
- Fidelity
- Instrumental values
- Justice
- Moral
- Moral evaluations
- Nonmaleficence
- Respect
- Restorative justice
- Self-determination
- Self-interest
- Terminal values
- Value
- Value systems
- Values clarification
- Veracity
- Well-being

LEARNING OBJECTIVES

Upon mastery of this chapter, you should be able to:

- Describe the nature of values and value systems and their influence on community health.
- Identify personal and professional values that you bring to decision-making with and for community health clients.
- Articulate the impact of key values on professional decision-making.
- Discuss the application of ethical principles to community health nursing decision-making.
- Use a decision-making process with and for community health clients that incorporates values and ethical principles.

In the United States, community health nurses face an expanding number of ethical dilemmas every day. Imagine, for example, that you are providing health care to a population of migrant vineyard workers whose housing lacks toilets, heating, and equipment for cooking and refrigerating food. You report the situation to your supervisor, but you are told to ignore the conditions because the wineries that employ the workers contribute heavily to a much-publicized clinic for all of the region's children. What would you do? Or what if you were working in a homeless shelter and were told to evict someone who would not agree to take a tuberculin test? Would your decision change if the resident were elderly or the mother of a newborn?

Within the United States, many marginalized people are failed by the public health care system or go without any health care at all. At the same time, affluent individuals enjoy a wide variety of health care options, including preventive screenings and classes. Community health nurses often are confronted by this disparity when making ethical decisions about client care.

In addition to these dilemmas within U.S. borders, progress in the United States often is linked to exploitation of people in less-developed countries and contributes to widening disparities in health, wealth, and human rights. Failure to respond to such global challenges only leads to greater poverty and deprivation, continuing conflict, escalating migration, and the spread of infectious disease, all adding to our ethical dilemmas (Benatar, 1998) (see The Global Community).

Not only disparity but also advances in technology contribute to ethical dilemmas. Some of these include computerized record-keeping systems that make client information readily

THE GLOBAL COMMUNITY

The Globalization of Public Health: An Ethical Mandate

Communicable diseases and other health care concerns know no national boundaries. Contaminated exported feedstuff transmits bovine spongiform encephalopathy ("mad cow disease") to cattle herds in many European countries; the weakness of national policies and actions for health affect residents in the United States who consume winter fruits and vegetables, grown and inspected under questionable conditions in South America in the midst of a political uprising; the sneezing and coughing passenger on an international flight may have infected a family member with some unknown disease, which then is passed to unsuspecting contacts. There is a need for global awareness, analysis, and action of public health authorities to eliminate, interrupt, or contain the potential risks to international public health in the global community.

Nations cannot remain isolated. According to Yach and Bettcher (1998, p. 738–739), "There is a need for all health professionals and the general public to receive information regularly about the health consequences of globalization in order to promote awareness of the transnational dimensions of health. Efficient information and surveillance systems are a top priority."

In this new millennium, the world is increasingly confronted with problems that could affect future generations. The globalization of the dangers and challenges of war, terrorism, and an international marketplace calls for addressing international policy issues. It is ethically imperative that policy development moves beyond its myopic view and provincialism.

accessible, raising issues of confidentiality, client's rights, and informed consent. Technology also forces nurses to confront the issues of assisted suicide and euthanasia. Organ, tissue, and limb transplants and the question of who is to receive them are further ethical questions.

Underlying every issue and influencing every ethical and professional decision are values. Ethics and values are inextricably intertwined in professional decision-making, since values are the criteria by which decisions are made. This chapter explores (1) the nature and function of values and value systems, (2) the role of values and value systems in ethical decision-making, (3) the central values related to health care choices and their potential conflicts, and (4) the implications of values and ethics for community health nursing decision-making and practice.

VALUES

What are values? A **value** is something that is perceived as desirable or "the way things ought to be" (Ellis & Hartley, 1998; Prilleltensky, 1997). A value motivates people to be-

have in certain ways that are personally or socially preferable. As seen in Chapter 4, a group's culture often is defined by its members' common or shared values.

Standards for Behavior

In general, values function as standards that guide actions and behavior in daily situations. Once internalized by an individual, a value such as honesty becomes a criterion for that individual's personal conduct. Values may function as criteria for developing and maintaining attitudes toward objects and situations or for justifying a person's own actions and attitudes. Values also may be the standard by which people pass moral judgment on themselves and others.

Values have a long-term function in giving expression to human needs. The strong motivational component of values help people to adjust to society, defend egos against threat, and test reality (Priester, 1992). In addition, values are used as standards to guide presentation of the self to others, to ascertain personal morality and competency, and to persuade and influence others by indicating which beliefs, attitudes, and actions of others are worth trying to reinforce or change. As a practitioner, values act as a compass to direct the nurse when working with clients (Gorin & Arnold, 1998).

Qualities of Values

The nature of values can be described according to five qualities: endurance, hierarchical arrangement, prescriptive-proscriptive belief, reference, and preference.

ENDURANCE
Values remain relatively stable over time and persist to provide continuity to personal and social existence. Enduring religious beliefs, for example, offer stability to many people. This is not to say that values are completely stable over time; values do change throughout a person's life. Yet social existence in the community requires standards within the individual as well as an agreement on standards among groups of individuals. As Kluckhohn (1951, p. 400) once pointed out, without values, "the functioning of the social system could not continue to achieve group goals; individuals . . . could not feel within themselves a requisite measure of order and unified purpose." A group's culture, as discussed in the previous chapter, provides such a set of enduring values. Thus, by adding an element of collective purpose in social life, values most often guarantee endurance and stability in social existence.

HIERARCHICAL SYSTEM
Isolated values usually are organized into a hierarchical system in which certain values have more weight or importance than others. For instance, in a team sport such as baseball, values regarding individual performance, batting and run-

ning records, speed, and throwing and catching all fall into a hierarchy, with the values of team and winning being at the top. As an individual confronts social situations throughout life, isolated values learned in early childhood come into competition with other values, requiring a weighing of one value against another. Concern for others' welfare, for instance, competes with self-interest. Through experience and maturation, the individual integrates values learned in different contexts into systems in which each value is ordered relative to other values.

PRESCRIPTIVE-PROSCRIPTIVE BELIEFS

Rokeach (1973) describes values as a subcategory of beliefs. He argues that some beliefs are descriptive or capable of being true or false (eg, the chair on which I am sitting will hold me up). Other beliefs are evaluative, involving judgments of good and bad (eg, that was an excellent lecture). Still other beliefs are prescriptive-proscriptive, determining whether an action is desirable or undesirable (eg, that music is too loud, or those baseball fans shouldn't yell when the pitcher is winding up). Values, he says, are prescriptive-proscriptive beliefs. They are concerned with desirable behavior or what ought to be. Parents' values about child behavior, for example, determine how they choose to discipline their children. Values have cognitive, affective, and behavioral components. According to Rokeach, to have a value, it is important to (1) know the correct way to behave or the correct end state for which to strive (cognitive component); (2) feel emotional about it: be affectively for or against it (affective component); and (3) take action based on it (behavioral component).

REFERENCE

Values also have a reference quality. That is, they may refer to end states of existence called **terminal values,** such as spiritual salvation, peace of mind, or world peace, or they may refer to modes of conduct called **instrumental values,** such as confidentiality, keeping promises, and honesty. The latter can have a moral focus or a nonmoral focus, and these values may conflict. For example, a nurse may experience a conflict between two moral values such as whether to act honestly (tell a client about a fatal diagnosis) or to act re-

spectfully (honor the family's request not to tell the client). Similarly, the nurse can experience conflict between two nonmoral values such as whether to plan logically (design a traditional group intervention for mental health clients) or to plan creatively (design an innovative field experience). The nurse also experiences conflict between a nonmoral value and a moral value, such as whether to act efficiently or to act fairly when establishing priorities for funding among community health programs.

Adults generally possess only a few—perhaps no more than 20—terminal values, such as peace of mind or achievement. These are influenced by complex physiologic and social factors. The needs of security, love, self-esteem, and self-actualization, proposed by Maslow (1969), are believed to be the greatest influences on terminal values. Although a person may have only a few terminal values, the same person may possess as many as 50 to 75 instrumental values. Any single instrumental value or several combined also may help to determine terminal values. For example, instrumental values of acceptance, taking it easy, living one day at a time, or not being concerned about the future can shape the terminal value of peace of mind, or instrumental values of hard work, driving oneself to compete, or not letting anyone get in the way can influence the terminal value of achievement. Figure 5–1 illustrates the influence of instrumental values and human needs on the development of terminal values.

PREFERENCE

A value shows preference for one mode of behavior over another, such as exercise over inactivity, or it may show a preference for one end state over another, such as trimness over obesity. The preferred end state, or mode of behavior, is located higher in the personal value hierarchy.

Value Systems

Value systems generally are considered organizations of beliefs that are of relative importance in guiding individual behavior (Prilleltensky, 1997; Rokeach, 1973). Instead of being guided by single or isolated values, however, behavior at

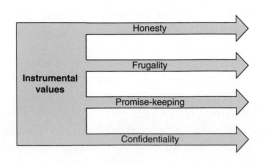

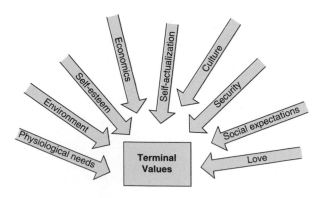

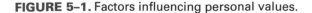

FIGURE 5–1. Factors influencing personal values.

any point in time (or over a period of time) is influenced by multiple or changing clusters of values. Thus, it is important to understand how values are integrated into a person's total belief system, how values assume a place in a hierarchy of values, and how this hierarchical system changes over time.

HIERARCHICAL SYSTEM OF VALUES

Learned values are integrated into an organized system of values, and each value has an ordered priority with respect to other values (Rokeach, 1973). For example, a person may place a higher value on physical comfort than on exercising. This system of ordered priority is stable enough to reflect the continuity of someone's personality and behavior within culture and society, yet it is sufficiently flexible to allow a re-ordering of value priorities in response to changes in the environment or social setting, or changes based on personal experiences. Behavioral change would be regarded as the visible response to a reordering of values within an individual's hierarchical value system.

CONFLICT BETWEEN VALUES IN A SYSTEM

When an individual encounters a social situation, several values within the person's value system are activated rather than just a single value. All of the activated values are not compatible with one another. Thus, conflict between values occurs. This conflict between values is a part of the decision-making process, and resolving these value conflicts is crucial to making good decisions. Community health nurses face conflicting values when they seek to promote the well-being of certain individuals, a result that may come at the expense of the public good. Even within a single community agency, nurses may find that they prioritize client service or programming values differently.

Some values seem to consistently triumph over others and seem to be stronger directives for individual behavior, such as the value placed on high achievement in the United States. It is this persistence on the part of some values, such as individualism versus community, that makes universal coverage and other issues so controversial in health care reform (Stewart, 1997). Other values lose their positions of importance in a value hierarchy. It is this changing arrangement of values in a hierarchical system that determines, in part, how conflicts are resolved and how decisions are made. Thus, people's value systems function as a learned organization of principles and rules that help them to choose between alternative courses of action to reach decisions.

Values Clarification

One way to understand the influence and priority of values in your own behavior as well as that of community health clients is to use various values-clarification techniques in decision-making. **Values clarification** is a process that helps to identify the personal and professional values that guide your actions by prompting you to examine what you believe

about the worth, truth, or beauty of any object, thought, or behavior and where this belief ranks compared with your other values (Catalano, 2000; Davis & Aroskar, 1997; Hamilton, 1996). Since individuals are largely unaware of the motives underlying their choices, values clarification is important for understanding and shaping the kind of decisions people make. Only by understanding your values and their priority can you ascertain whether your choices are the result of rational thinking or of external influences, such as cultural or social conditioning. Values clarification by itself does not yield a set of rules for future decision-making and does not indicate the rightness or wrongness of alternative actions. It does, however, help to guarantee that any course of action chosen by people is consistent and in accordance with their beliefs and values.

PROCESS OF VALUING

Before values clarification can take place, it must be understood how the process of valuing occurs in individuals. Uustal (1977) lists the following seven steps:

1. Choose the value freely and individually.
2. Choose the value from among alternatives.
3. Carefully consider the consequences of the choice.
4. Cherish or prize the value.
5. Publicly affirm the value.
6. Incorporate the value into behavior so that it becomes a standard.
7. Consciously use the value in decision-making.

These steps provide specific actions for the discovery and identification of people's values. They also assist the decision-making process by explicating the process of valuing itself. For example, some people may choose to value honesty in a presidential candidate. They choose this over other values, such as knowledge of foreign affairs or public-speaking ability, because, considering the consequences, they want a leader who will deliver on promises made, who will be the person represented to the public during campaigning. They prize this value of honesty, affirm it publicly, and consciously use it as a standard when deciding whom to vote into office or reject based on the candidate's record of honesty.

VALUES-CLARIFICATION STRATEGIES

Uustal (1978) offers several strategies of values clarification that are ultimately useful to the decision-making process in community health nursing practice. Strategy 1 is a way for nurses to come to know themselves and their values better (Fig. 5–2). Strategy 2 assists in discovering value clusters and the priority of values within personal value systems (Fig. 5–3). Strategy 3 can be used to examine personal responses to selected issues in nursing practice. Each response helps to establish priorities of values by asking the nurse to choose among the alternatives presented or to indicate degree of agreement or disagreement (Fig. 5–4). Other values-clarification strategies are included in the critical thinking activities at the end of this chapter to assist in understanding personal ordering of values and to help when considering

---

Name Tag

Take a piece of paper and write your name in the middle of it. In each of the four corners, write your responses to these four questions:

1. What two things would you like your colleagues to say about you?
2. What single most important thing do you do (or would you like to do) to make your nurse-client relationships positive ones?
3. What do you do on a daily basis that indicates you value your health?
4. What are the three values you believe in most strongly?

In the space around your name, write at least six adjectives that you feel best describe who you are.

Take a closer look at your responses to the questions and to the ways in which you described yourself. What values are reflected in your answers?

FIGURE 5–2. Values clarification strategy 1.

directions for change. These strategies also help the nurse to assist community health clients to become clearer about their own values.

All of these strategies can be used to analyze and understand how values are meaningful to people and ultimately influence their choices and behavior. Clarification of a person's values is the first step in the decision-making process and affects the ability of people to make ethical decisions. Values

---

Patterns

Which of the following words describe you? Draw a circle around the seven words that best describe you as an individual. Underline the seven words that most accurately describe you as a professional person. (You may circle and underline the same word.)

ambitious	reserved	assertive	opinionated
concerned	generous		independent
easily hurt	outgoing	reliable	indifferent
capable	self-controlled		fun-loving
suspicious	solitary	likable	dependent
intellectual	argumentative	dynamic	unpredictable
compromising	thoughtful	affectionate	obedient
logical	imaginative		self-disciplined
moody	easily led	helpful	slow to relate

Reflect on the following questions:

1. What values are reflected in the patterns you have chosen?
2. What is the relationship between these patterns and your personal values?
3. What patterns indicate inconsistencies in attitudes or behavior?
4. What patterns do you think a nurse should cultivate?

FIGURE 5–3. Values clarification strategy 2.

Forced Choice Ranking

How do you order the following alternatives by priority? (There is no correct set of priorities.) What values emerge in response to each question?

1. With whom on a nursing team would you become most angry? The nurse who
   _____ never completes assignments.
   _____ rarely helps other team members.
   _____ projects his or her feelings on clients.

2. If you had a serious health problem, you would rather
   _____ not be told.
   _____ be told directly.
   _____ find out by accident.

3. You are made happiest in your work when you use
   _____ your technical skills in caring for adults with complex needs.
   _____ your ability to compile data and arrive at a nursing diagnosis.
   _____ your ability to communicate easily and skillfully with clients.

4. It would be most difficult for you to
   _____ listen to and counsel a dying person.
   _____ advise a pregnant adolescent.
   _____ handle a situation of obvious child abuse.

FIGURE 5–4. Values clarification strategy 3.

clarification also promotes understanding and respect for values held by others, such as community health clients and other health care providers. As pointed out by Uustal (1977, p. 10), "Nurses cannot hope to give optimal, sensitive care to any patient without first understanding their own opinions, attitudes, and values." This values-clarification process provides a backdrop for next exploring the role of values in ethical decision-making.

ETHICS

Values are central to any consideration of ethics or ethical decision-making. Yet it is not obvious at first what counts as an ethical problem in health care or in the practice of community health nursing. Most nurses easily recognize the moral crisis in some kinds of decisions, for example, whether to let seriously deformed newborn infants die, whether to terminate pregnancies resulting from rape, or whether to provide universal health care coverage. However, there are other, less obvious moral dilemmas that are faced in the routine practice of community health nursing that often are not considered to be ethical in nature. What is "ethics" and what is "ethical"? Merriam-Webster defines **ethics** as "a set of moral principles or values; a theory or system of moral values" (1999). Ethics, Catalano explains, "are declarations of what is right or wrong, and of what ought to be" (2000, p. 113). **Ethical decision-making,** then, means making a choice that is consistent with a moral code or that can be justified from an ethical perspective. Of necessity, the decision-maker must exercise moral judgment. Remember that the term **moral** refers to conforming to a standard that is right and good. Aroskar points out that all nurses, "as moral agents, make decisions that have direct and indirect consequences for the welfare of themselves and others" (1995, p. 135). The next section examines how a nurse makes these moral decisions.

Identifying Ethical Situations

Ethics involves making evaluative judgments. To be ethically responsible in the practice of nursing, it is important to develop the ability to recognize evaluative judgments as they are made and implemented in nursing practice. Nurses must be able to distinguish between evaluative and nonevaluative judgments. Evaluative statements involve judgments of value, rights, duties, and responsibilities. Examples are, "parents should never strike their children," or "it is the duty of every citizen to vote." Among the words to watch for are verbs such as *want, desire, refer, should,* or *ought* and nouns such as *benefit, harm, duty, responsibility, right,* or *obligation.*

Sometimes, the evaluations are expressed in terms that are not direct expressions of evaluations but clearly are functioning as value judgments. For example, the American Nurses Association (ANA) *Code for Nurses With Interpretive Statements* states that "the nurse provides services . . . unrestricted by considerations of social or economic status, personal attributes, or the nature of health problems" (1985, p. 5). In this statement, the ANA could be describing the facts about the way all nurses behave. However, it is not true that all nurses behave in this manner. Rather, this statement prescribes behavior that nurses ought to follow: providing services without discrimination is an ethical ideal.

Another important step is to distinguish between moral and nonmoral evaluations (Thompson & Thompson, 1992; Veatch, 1997). **Moral evaluations** refer to judgments that conform to standards of what is right and good. Moral evaluations assess human actions, institutions, or character traits rather than inanimate objects such as paintings or architectural structures. They are prescriptive-proscriptive beliefs having certain characteristics that separate them from other evaluations such as aesthetic judgments, personal preferences, or matters of taste. Moral evaluations also have distinctive characteristics:

1. The evaluations are ultimate. They have a preemptive quality, meaning that other values or human ends cannot, as a rule, override them (Beauchamp & Childress, 1994).
2. They possess universality or reflect a standpoint that applies to everyone. They are evaluations that everyone in principle ought to be able to make and understand, even if some individuals, in fact, do not (Veatch, 1997).
3. Moral evaluations avoid giving a special place to a per-

son's own welfare. They have a focus that keeps others in view, or at least considers one's own welfare on a par with that of others (Beauchamp & Childress, 1994).

Resolving Moral Conflicts and Ethical Dilemmas

When judgments involve moral values, conflicts are inevitable. In clinical practice, the nurse may be faced with moral conflicts such as the choice between preserving the welfare of one set of clients over that of others. For example, the nurse may have to choose whether to keep a promise of confidentiality to persons who are HIV positive when these individuals continue to have unprotected sex with unknowing partners. Nurses may have to choose between protecting the interests of colleagues or the interests of the employing institution. They may have to decide whether to serve future clients by striking for better conditions or to serve present clients by refusing to strike. Each decision involves a potential conflict between moral values and is called an **ethical dilemma.** An ethical dilemma occurs when morals conflict with one another, causing the nurse to face a choice with equally unsatisfying alternatives (Davis & Aroskar, 1997). It can create a decision-making problem, even in ordinary nursing situations.

Decision-Making Frameworks

To resolve ethical dilemmas or the conflict between moral values in community health nursing practice, and to provide morally accountable nursing service, several frameworks for ethical decision-making have been proposed. Among these frameworks, three key steps are considered as fundamental to choosing alternative courses of action that reflect moral reasoning: (1) separate questions of fact from questions of value, (2) identify both clients' and nurse's value systems, and (3) consider ethical principles and concepts.

The identification of clients' values and those of other persons involved in conflict situations is an important part of ethical decision-making. For example, what are Mr. Bell's values? What are the values of neighbors who are concerned but feel that they can no longer care for him? What are the nurse's values? What are the values of the nurse's employing agency? An ethical decision-making framework that includes the identification and clarification of values impinging on the making of ethical decisions is outlined here:

1. Review the situation.
   a. What health problems exist?
   b. What decisions need to be made?
   c. Separate ethical components of the decisions from those decisions that can be made solely on a scientific knowledge base.
   d. Identify all individuals or groups affected by the decision.

CLINICAL CORNER **Mr. Bell**

Community health nurses encounter value differences every day, and value differences, in turn, create ethical problems. Consider, for example, the dilemma faced by one nurse in Seattle on her first home visit to an elderly man, Mr. Bell. Referred by concerned neighbors, this 82-year-old gentleman was homebound and living alone with severe arthritis under steadily deteriorating conditions. Overgrown shrubs and vines covered the yard and house, making access impossible except through the back door. A wood-burning stove in the kitchen was the sole source of heat, and that room, plus a corner of the dining room, were Mr. Bell's living quarters. The remainder of the once-lovely three-bedroom home, including the bathroom, was layered with dust, unused. His bed was a cot in the dining room; his toilet, a two-pound coffee can placed under the cot. Unbathed, unshaven, and existing on food and firewood brought by neighbors, Mr. Bell seemed to be living in deplorable conditions. Yet he prized his independence so highly that he adamantly refused to leave.

The conflict of values between Mr. Bell's choice to live independently and the nurse's value of having him in a safer living situation raises several ethical questions. When do health practitioners or family members have the right or duty to override an individual's preferences? When do neighbors' rights (Mr. Bell's home was an eyesore and his care was a source of anxiety for his neighbors) supersede one homeowner's rights? Should the nurse be responsible when family members can help but won't take action? Mr. Bell had one son living in a neighboring state.

In this case, the nurse entering Mr. Bell's home applied her values of respect for the individual and his right to autonomy even at the risk of public safety. Not until he fell and broke a hip did he reluctantly agree to be moved into a nursing home.

---

2. Decide what further information is needed before a decision can be made.
3. Identify ethical issues. Discuss historical, philosophical, and religious bases for these issues.
4. Identify your own values and beliefs. Identify professional responsibilities dictated by the ANA's *Code for Nurses With Interpretive Statements*.
5. Identify values and beliefs of other people involved in the situation.
6. Identify any value conflicts.
7. Decide who should make the decision. Determine the nurse's role in making the decision.
8. Identify the range of possible decisions or actions. Determine implications for all people involved. Identify how suggested actions conform to the ANA's code for nurses.
9. Decide on a course of action and follow through.
10. Evaluate the results of the actions or decisions and what has been learned for use in reviewing and resolving similar future situations (Thompson & Thompson, 1992).

Other frameworks can be used. The framework for ethical decision-making in Display 5–1 helps to organize thoughts and acts as a guide through the decision-making process. The steps help to determine a course of action, with heavy responsibility at the evaluation level: here the outcomes need to be judged and decisions repeated or rejected in future situations. Figure 5–5 summarizes several views in the field on ethical decision-making. This framework advocates keeping multiple values in tension before resolution of conflict and action on the part of the nurse. It suggests that value conflict is not capable of resolution until all possible alternative actions have been explored. Final resolution of the ethical conflict occurs through conscious choice of action even though some values would be overridden by other stronger, presumably moral values. The triumphant values would be those values located higher in the decision-maker's hierarchy of values.

DISPLAY 5–1. A Framework for Ethical Decision-Making

1. *Clarify the ethical dilemma:* Whose problem is it? Who should make the decision? Who is affected by the decision? What ethical principles are related to the problem?
2. *Gather additional data:* Have as much information about the situation as possible. Be up to date on any legal cases related to the ethical question.
3. *Identify options:* Brainstorm with others to identify as many alternatives as possible. The more options identified, the more likely it is that an acceptable solution will be found.
4. *Make a decision:* Choose from the options identified and determine the most acceptable option, the one more feasible than others.
5. *Act:* Carry out the decision. It may be necessary to collaborate with others to implement the decision and identify options.
6. *Evaluate:* After acting on a decision, evaluate its impact. Was the best course of action chosen? Would an alternative have been better? Why? What went right and what went wrong? Why?

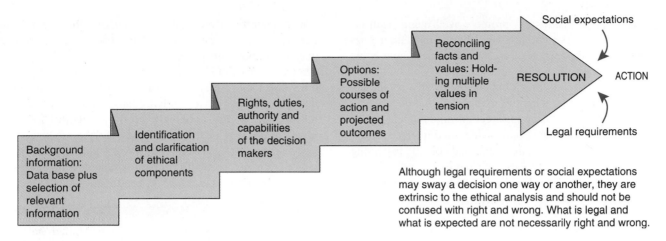

Figure 5–5. An ethical decision-making framework. Although legal requirements or social expectations may sway a decision one way or another, they are extrinsic to the ethical analysis and should not be confused with right and wrong. What is legal and what is expected are not necessarily right and wrong.

Basic Values That Guide Decision-Making

When applying a decision-making framework, certain values influence community health nursing decisions. Three basic human values are considered key to guiding decision-making in the provider–client relationship and can be used with the framework of Thompson and Thompson (1992): self-determination, well-being, and equity (Davis and Aroskar, 1997; President's Commission for the Study of Ethical Problems in Medicine and Biomedical and Behavioral Research [President's Commission], 1982).

SELF-DETERMINATION

The value of **self-determination** or individual autonomy is a person's exercise of the capacity to shape and pursue personal plans for life. Self-determination is instrumentally valued because self-judgment about a person's goals and choices is conducive to an individual's sense of well-being. Thus, respecting self-determination is based on the belief that better outcomes will result when self-determination is respected. The outcomes that could be maximized by respecting self-determination include enhanced self-concept, enhanced health-promoting behaviors, and enhanced quality of care. Self-determination is a major value in the United States but does not receive the same emphasis in all societies or ethnic groups.

In health care contexts, the desire for self-determination has been of such high ethical importance in United States' society that it overrides practitioner determinations in many situations. An early survey undertaken by the President's Commission (1982) showed that 72% of those surveyed said they would prefer to make decisions jointly with their physicians after treatment alternatives had been explained. Physician responses in the same survey, however, indicated that most physicians (88%) believed that patients wanted doctors to make decisions for them. The wide difference between patient expectations regarding self-determination and physi-

cian beliefs indicates that self-determination on the part of patients was at high risk in most health care contexts. Although the situation has improved, many physicians and other health providers fail to recognize the high value attributed to self-determination by many consumers or the differences in views of self-determination among ethnic groups.

Mohr (1996) sees this conflict between provider and consumer as broader. When self-determination deteriorates into self-interest, it poses a major road block to equitable health care. **Self-interest** is the fulfillment of one's own desires without regard for the greater good. Consumers mostly have to fend for themselves when they encounter the world of for-profit health care, just as they do in other commercial markets, where "buyer beware" is the standard (Mohr, 1996).

Self-determination and taking personal responsibility for health care decisions should be nourished when providing health care. This includes informing clients of options and the reasoning behind all recommendations (Davis & Aroskar, 1997; President's Commission, 1982). Yet self-determination and personal autonomy, at times, is impermissible or even impossible. For example, society must impose restrictions on acceptable client choices, such as child abuse and other abusive behaviors, or situations in which clients are not competent to exercise self-determination, as is true for certain levels of mental illness or dementia. There are two situations in which self-determination should be restricted: (1) when some objectives of individuals are contrary to the public interest or the interests of others in society, and (2) when a person's decision-making is so defective or mistaken that the decision fails to promote the person's own values or goals. In these situations, self-determination is justifiably overridden on the basis of the promotion of one's own well-being or the well-being of others, another important value in health care decision-making.

WELL-BEING

Well-being is a state of positive health. Although all therapeutic interventions by health care professionals are intended to improve clients' health and promote well-being, well-intended interventions sometimes fall short if they are in conflict with clients' preferences and needs. Determining what constitutes health for people and how their well-being can be promoted often requires a knowledge of clients' subjective preferences. It is generally recognized that clients may be inclined to pursue different directions in treatment procedures based on individual goals, values, and interests. Community health nurses, who are committed not only to helping clients but also to respecting their wishes and avoiding harming them, must understand each client group's needs and develop reasonable alternatives for service from which clients may choose (see Clinical Corner). In addition, when individuals are not capable of making a choice, the nurse or other surrogate decision-maker is obliged to make health care decisions that promote the value of well-being. This may mean that the alternatives presented by the nurse for choice are only the alternatives that will promote well-being. With shared decision-making, the nurse not only seeks to understand clients' needs and develop reasonable alternatives to meet those needs, but also to present the alternatives in a way that enables clients to choose those they prefer. Well-being and self-determination are, therefore, two values that are intricately related when providing community health nursing service.

EQUITY

The third value important to decision-making in health care contexts is the value of **equity,** which means being treated equally or fairly. The principle of equity implies that it is unjust (or inequitable) to treat people the same if they are, in significant respects, unalike. In other words, different people have different needs in health care, but all must be served equally and adequately. Equity generally means that all individuals should have the same access to health care according to benefit or needs (see Levels of Prevention).

The major problem with this definition of equity, of course, is that it assumes that an adequate level of health care can be economically available to all citizens. In times of limited technical, human, and financial resources, however, it may be impossible to fully respect the value of equity. Choices must be made and resources allotted while the value obligations of professional practice create conflicts of values that seem impossible to resolve. Many of these conflicts are reflected in current health care reform efforts that focus on access of services, quality of services, and the way to control rising costs. However, the following represent the most pressing aggregate health problems related to inequities in the distribution of and access to health and illness care facing our nation:

Too many women go without preventive care. The overall rate of infant mortality in the United States is worse than that of 22 other countries in the world. The rate for people of color—African Americans, Hispanics, and Native Americans—is twice that of European Americans (Singh & Yu, 1995). Forty percent of the pregnancies in white and Hispanic females are unintended, whereas 70% of the pregnancies in African-American females are unintended. Poverty is strongly related to difficulty in accessing family planning services.

Immunization rates for some diseases are at dangerously low levels. For example, only 43% of children between the ages of 19 months and 35 months were immunized for varicella (chickenpox) in 1998 (U.S. Dept. of Health and Human Services, 2000).

The uninsured are likely to go without physician care. Differences in access to expensive, discretionary procedures emerge according to health insurance status, race, and other sociodemographic factors of the client. The poor are only two thirds as likely to obtain the needed services.

Evidence of excess mortality rates for fetuses and infants continues among members of certain races. African-Americans experience a rate of 13.4 per 1000, whereas the rates are 4.6 for Asians and 6.4 for

---

CLINICAL CORNER   A Family Living in Poverty

Contrasting value systems may be seen in many community health practice settings. Andrea Varga, a community health nurse, experienced such a contrast on her first home visit to a family living in poverty. Referred by a school nurse for recurring problems with head lice and staphylococcal infections, the family was living in the worst conditions that the nurse had ever seen. Papers, moldy food, soiled clothing, and empty beer cans covered the floor. Andrea recoiled in dismay. The children, home from school, were clustered around the television. Their mother, a divorced, single parent, unkempt and obese, sat smoking a cigarette with a can of beer in her hand. Although she worked as a waitress part time, she had been unable to earn enough money to support herself and the children, so the family was now temporarily receiving state aid. The mother's main pleasure in life was watching soap operas on television. The nurse interpreted the situation through the framework of her own value system in which health and cleanliness were priorities. Yet the mother, who might have shared those values in the past, appeared to prize freedom and pleasurable diversion, perhaps as a way to cope with her situation. In this instance, it is possible that environmental influences reordered the family's value-system priorities. Rather than imposing her own values, Andrea chose to determine the priorities of the family, assessed their needs, and began where they were.

LEVELS OF PREVENTION

DISTRIBUTIVE JUSTICE FOR BATTERED WOMEN AND CHILDREN

GOAL

To change the proposed state law that would eliminate funding of shelters for battered women and children to a law preserving resources for this population.

PRIMARY PREVENTION

Early advocacy through active lobbying against the bill and garnering community support in favor of the revised law.

SECONDARY PREVENTION

Advocate for amendments to the proposed law to preserve limited funding for shelters.

TERTIARY PREVENTION

After the proposed law has passed and funding is eliminated, seek private resources to fund shelters (such as a private foundation or a women's coalition) and propose a new bill to match private funding for shelters at the next legislative session.

white infants during the perinatal period (U.S. Dept. of Health and Human Services, 2000).

Social Security, without supplements, limits access. The elderly find themselves paying higher out-of-pocket costs and higher insurance premiums, often with forced choices. Prescription and drug coverage and provisions for long-term care may not be available for most, and basic entitlements continue to be reduced.

Environmental hazards threaten global health. Global trade, travel, and changing social and cultural patterns make the population vulnerable to diseases endemic to other parts of the world as well as to diseases previously unknown. Pollution of air, water, and soil to support industry contributes to pathogen mutations and threatens public health (Chafey, 1996).

To promote the achievement of equity, self-determination, and clients' well-being, certain conclusions drawn from the literature can enhance community health nursing's practice (Chafey, 1996; Catalano, 2000; President's Commission, 1982):

1. Society has an ethical obligation to ensure equitable access to health care for all. This obligation rests on the special importance of health care and is derived from its role in relieving suffering, preventing premature death, restoring functioning, increasing opportunity, providing information about an individual's condition, and giving evidence of mutual empathy and compassion.

2. The societal obligation is balanced by individual obligations. Individuals ought to pay a fair share of the cost of their own health care and take reasonable steps to provide for such care when they can do so without excessive burdens.

3. Equitable access to health care requires that all citizens can secure an adequate level of care without excessive burdens. Equitable access also means that the burdens borne by individuals in obtaining adequate care ought not to be excessive or to fall disproportionately on particular individuals. Communities need to be empowered to address distribution problems.

4. When equity occurs through the operation of private forces, there is no need for government involvement. However, the ultimate responsibility for ensuring that society's obligation is met—through a combination of public and private sector arrangements—rests with the federal government.

5. The cost of achieving equitable access to health care ought to be shared fairly. The cost of securing health care for those unable to pay ought to be spread equitably at the national level and should not fall more heavily on the shoulders of particular practitioners, institutions, or residents of different localities.

6. Efforts to contain rising health care costs are important but should not focus on limiting the attainment of equitable access for the least-served portion of the public. Measures designed to contain health care costs that exacerbate existing inequities or impede the achievement of equity are unacceptable from a moral standpoint. Aggregates in the community should be involved in planning and problem solving to increase the distribution of resources where the resources are most needed.

Ethical Decision-Making in Community Health Nursing

The key values described in this chapter of self-determination, well-being, and equity influence nursing practice in many ways. The value of self-determination has implications for how community health nurses:

1. Respect the choices of clients
2. Protect privacy
3. Provide for informed consent
4. Protect diminished capacity for self-determination

The value of well-being has implications for how community health nurses:

1. Reduce or prevent harm and provide benefits to client populations
2. Measure the effectiveness of nursing services
3. Balance costs of services against real client benefits

The value of equity has implications for community health nursing in terms of its priorities for (1) broadly distributing health goods, which are macroallocation issues, and (2) deciding which populations will obtain available health goods and services, which are microallocation issues.

Decisions based on one value mean that this value often will conflict with other values. For example, deciding primarily on the basis of client well-being may conflict with deciding on the basis of self-determination or equity. How community health nurses balance these values may even conflict with their own personal values or the values of the nursing profession. In these situations, values-clarification techniques used with an ethical decision-making process may assist in making decisions that promote the greatest well-being for clients without substantially reducing their self-determination or ignoring equity.

ETHICAL PRINCIPLES

Seven fundamental ethical principles provide guidance in making decisions regarding clients' care: respect, autonomy, beneficence, nonmaleficence, justice, veracity, and fidelity (Aroskar, 1995; Clement, 1996).

Respect

The principle of **respect** refers to treating people as unique, equal, and responsible moral agents. This principle emphasizes people's importance as members of the community and of the health services team. To apply this principle in decision-making is to acknowledge community clients as valued participants in shaping their own and the community's health outcomes. It includes treating them as equals on the health team and holding them and their views in high regard (Chafey, 1996).

Autonomy

The principle of **autonomy** means freedom of choice and the exercise of people's rights. Individualism and self-determination are dominant values underlying this principle. As nurses apply this principle in community health, they promote individuals' and groups' rights to and involvement in decision-making. This is true, however, only as long as those decisions enhance these people's well-being and do not harm the well-being of others (Catalano, 2000). When applying this principle, nurses should make certain that clients are fully informed and that the decisions are deliberate, with careful consideration of the consequences.

Beneficence

The ethical principle of **beneficence** means doing good or benefiting others. It is the promotion of good or taking action to ensure positive outcomes on behalf of clients. In community health, the nurse applies the principle of beneficence by making decisions that actively promote community clients' best interests and well-being. Examples are developing a senior's health program that ensures equal access to all in the community who need it or supporting programs to encourage preschool immunizations.

Nonmaleficence

The principle of **nonmaleficence** means avoiding or preventing harm to others as a consequence of a person's own choices and actions. This involves taking steps to avoid negative consequences. Community health nurses can apply this ethical principle in decision-making by actions such as encouraging physicians to prescribe drugs with the fewest side effects, promoting legislation to protect the environment from pollutants emitted from gasoline even if it raises prices, and lobbying for lower speed limits or gun control to save lives.

Justice

The principle of **justice** refers to treating people fairly. It means the fair distribution of both benefits and costs among society's members. Decisions about equal access to health care, equitable distribution of services to rural as well as urban populations, not limiting amount or quality of service because of income level, and fair distribution of resources all draw on the principle of justice.

Within this principle are three different views on allocation, or what constitutes the meaning of "fair" distribution. One, **distributive justice,** says that benefits should be given first to the disadvantaged or those who need them most (see Levels of Prevention). Decisions based on this view particularly help the needy, although it may mean withholding good from others who also are deserving but less in need. The second view, **egalitarian justice,** promotes decisions based on equal distribution of benefits to everyone, regardless of need. The third, **restorative justice,** says that benefits should go primarily to those who have been wronged by prior injustice, such as victims of crime or racial discrimination. The principle of justice seeks to promote equity, a value that was discussed in the previous section.

Veracity

The principle of **veracity** refers to telling the truth. Community clients deserve to be given accurate information in a timely manner. To withhold information or not tell the truth can be self-serving to the nurse or other health care provider and hurtful as well as disrespectful to clients. Truth-telling treats clients as equals, expands the opportunity for greater client involvement, and provides needed information for decisions (Catalano, 2000).

Fidelity

The final ethical principle of **fidelity** means keeping promises. People deserve to count on commitments being met. This principle involves the issues of trust and trustworthiness. Nurses who follow through on what they have said earn their clients' respect and trust. In turn, this influences the quality of the nurse's relationship with clients, who then are more likely share information, leading to improved decisions. Conversely, when a promise such as a commitment to institute child care during health classes is not kept, community members may lose faith and interest in participation.

Ethical Standards and Guidelines

As the number and complexity of ethical decisions in community health increase, so, too, does the need for ethical standards and guidelines to help nurses make the best choices possible. The ANA's *Code for Nurses With Interpretive Statements* (1985) provides a helpful guide. Some health care organizations and community agencies, using the ANA code or a similar document, have developed their own specific standards and guidelines.

More health care organizations are using ethics committees or ethics rounds to deal with ethical aspects of client services (Mitzen, 1998). These committees are common in the acute care setting and focus on such issues as caregiving dilemmas that may involve practitioner negligence or poor client outcomes and the related health care decisions. However, these committees also function in a variety of community health care settings. In long-term care and home care settings, such a committee may consider conflicts in client care issues that involve family members. In public health agencies, clients with complicated communicable disease diagnoses and health care provider concerns are discussed as they relate to policy, protocols, and the health and safety of the broader population.

SUMMARY

Values and ethical principles have significance for our global community as well as our local community. They strongly influence community health nursing practice and ethical decision-making. Values are lasting beliefs that are important to individuals, groups, and cultures. A value system organizes these beliefs into a hierarchy of relative importance that motivates and guides human behavior. Values function as standards for behavior, as criteria for attitudes, as standards for moral judgments, and give expression to human needs. The nature of values can be understood by examining their qualities of endurance, their hierarchical arrangement, as prescriptive-proscriptive beliefs and by examining them in terms of reference and preference.

The nurse often is faced with decisions that affect client's values and involve conflicting moral values and ethical dilemmas. Understanding what personal values are and how they affect behavior assists the nurse in making ethical evaluations and addressing ethical conflicts in practice. Various strategies can guide the nurse in making these decisions, such as values clarification, which clarifies what values are important, and several frameworks for ethical decision-making. Two frameworks described in this chapter include the identification and clarification of values impinging on the making of ethical decisions.

Three key human values influence client health and nurse decision-making: the right to make decisions regarding a person's health (self-determination), the right to health and well-being, and the right to equal access and quality of health care. At times, these values are affected by another's or a system's value of self-interest. Seven fundamental principles guide community health nurses in making ethical decisions: respect, autonomy, beneficence, nonmaleficence, justice, veracity, and fidelity.

ACTIVITIES TO PROMOTE CRITICAL THINKING

1. Describe where you stand on the following issues. For each statement, decide whether you strongly agree, agree, disagree, strongly disagree, or are undecided.
   a. Clients have the right to participate in all decisions related to their health care.
   b. Nurses need a system designed to credit self-study.
   c. Continuing education should not be mandatory to maintain licensure.
   d. Clients always should be told the truth.
   e. Standards of nursing practice should be enforced by state examining boards.
   f. Nurses should be required to take relicensure examinations every 5 years.
   g. Clients should be allowed to read their health record on request.
   h. Abortion on demand should be an option available to every woman.
   i. Critically ill newborns should be allowed to die.
   j. Laws should guarantee desired health care for each person in this country.
   k. Organ donorship should be automatic unless a waiver to refuse has been signed.
2. In a grid similar to the one below, write a statement of belief in the space provided and examine it in relation to the seven steps of the process of valuing. Areas of confusion and conflict in nursing practice that should be examined are peer review, accountability, confidentiality, euthanasia, licensure, clients' rights, organ donation, abortion, informed consent, and terminating treatment.

   To the right of your statements, check the appropriate boxes indicating when your beliefs reflect one or more of the seven steps in the valuing process. Is your belief a value according to the valuing process?
3. Rank in order the following 12 potential nursing actions, using 1 to indicate the most important choice in a client–community health nurse relationship and 12 to indicate the least important choice.

Statement	Freely chosen	Alternatives	Consequences	Cherished	Affirmed	Incorporated	Employed
	1	2	3	4	5	6	7

Touching clients

Empathetically listening to clients

Disclosing yourself to clients

Becoming emotionally involved with clients

Teaching clients

Being honest in answering clients' questions

Seeing that clients conform to professionals' advice

Helping to decrease clients' anxiety

Making sure that clients are involved in decision-making

Following legal mandates regarding health practices

Remaining "professional" with clients

(Add an alternative of your own)

Examine your ordering of these options. What values can be identified based on your responses in this exercise? How do these values emerge in your behavior?

4. Request to attend two or three sessions of an ethics committee meeting of a community health agency. Observe and make notes on (a) what values are evident in the discussion, (b) what ethical principles are used, (c) what decision-making framework is used, and (d) what would you have liked to contribute if you had been a member of the committee.

5. Search the World Wide Web on the Internet for your state's or national legislative activities on bills that might affect the health and well-being of clients. How do you feel about the pieces of legislation? What could a community health nurse do regarding the impending legislation? What could you do right now?

REFERENCES

American Nurses Association. (1985). *Code for nurses with interpretive statements.* Kansas City, MO: Author.

Aroskar, M.A. (1995). Envisioning nursing as a moral community. *Nursing Outlook, 43*(3), 134–138.

Beauchamp, T.L. & Childress, J.F. (1994). *Principles of biomedical ethics* (4th ed.). New York: Oxford.

Benatar, S.R. (1998). Global disparities in health and human rights: A critical commentary. *American Journal of Public Health, 88*(2), 295–300.

Catalano, J.T. (2000). *Nursing now! Today's issues, tomorrow's trends.* (2nd ed.) Philadelphia: F.A. Davis.

Chafey, K. (1996). "Caring" is not enough: Ethical paradigms for community-based care. *Nursing and Health Care: Perspectives on Community, 17*(1), 11–15.

Clement, G. (1996). *Care, autonomy, and justice: Feminism and the ethic of care.* Boulder, CO: Westview Press.

Davis, A. & Aroskar, M.A. (1997). *Ethical dilemmas and nursing practice* (3rd ed.). Norwalk, CT: Appleton & Lange.

Ellis, J.R., & Hartley, C.L. (1998). *Nursing in today's world: Challenges, issues, and trends* (6th ed.). Philadelphia: Lippincott-Raven.

Gorin, S.S. & Arnold, J. (1998). *Health promotion handbook.* St. Louis: Mosby.

Hamilton, P.M. (1996). *Realities of contemporary nursing* (2nd ed.). Menlo Park, CA: Addison–Wesley.

Institute of Medicine. (1993). *Access to health care in America.* Washington, DC: National Academy Press.

Kluckhohn, C. (1951). Values and value-orientations in the theory of action: An exploration in definition and classification. In T. Parsons & E.A. Shils (Eds.), *Toward a general theory of action* (pp. 388–433). Cambridge, MA: Harvard University Press.

Maslow, A. (1969). *Toward a psychology of being* (2nd ed.). New York: Van Nostrand.

Merriam-Webster. (1999). *Webster's dictionary.* Springfield, MA: Merriam-Webster, Inc.

Mitzen, P. (1998). Organizational ethics in a nonprofit agency: Changing practice, enduring values. *Generations, 22*(3), 102–104.

Mohr, W.K. (1996). Ethics, nursing, and health care in the age of "re-form." *Nursing and Health Care: Perspectives on Community, 17*(1), 16–21.

President's Commission for the Study of Ethical Problems in Medicine and Biomedical and Behavioral Research. (1982). *Making health care decisions* (Vol. 1 report). Washington, DC: U.S. Government Printing Office.

President's Commission for the Study of Ethical Problems in Medicine and Biomedical and Behavioral Research. (1983). *Summing up.* Washington, DC: U.S. Government Printing Office.

Prilleltensky, I. (1997). Values, assumptions, and practices: Assessing the moral implications of psychological discourse and action. *American Psychologist, 52*(5), 517–535.

Rokeach, M. (1973). *The nature of human values.* New York: Free Press.

Singh, G.K. & Yu, S.M. (1995). Infant mortality in the United States: Trends, differentials and projections, 1950 through 2010. *American Journal of Public Health, 85*(10), 957–964.

Stewart, M. (1997). Managed care law blocks quality care to indigent patients. *American Nurse, 29*(6), 12.

Thompson, J.E. & Thompson, H.O. (1992, May–June). *Bioethical decision making for nurses.* Lanham, MD: University Press of America.

U.S. Department of Health and Human Services (2000). *Healthy people 2010* (conference edition, in two volumes). Washington, DC: Author.

Uustal, D.B. (1977). The use of values clarification in nursing practice. *Journal of Continuing Education in Nursing, 8,* 8–13

Uustal, D.B. (1978). Values clarification in nursing. *American Journal of Nursing, 78,* 2058–2063.

Veatch, R.M. (Ed) (1997). *Medical ethics* (2nd ed.). Sudbury, MA: Jones & Bartlett Publishers.

Yach, D. & Bettcher, D. (1998). The globalization of public health: II. The convergence of self-interest and altruism. *American Journal of Public Health, 88*(5), 738–741.

SELECTED READINGS

Aroskar, M.A. (1993). Ethical issues: Politics, power, and policy. In D.J. Mason, S.W. Talbott, & J.K. Leavitt (Eds.), *Policy and politics for nurses.* Philadelphia: W.B. Saunders.

Arras, J.D. (1995). *Bringing the hospital home: Ethical and social implications of high-tech home care*. Baltimore: Johns Hopkins University Press.

Beauchamp, D.E. (1985). Community: The neglected tradition of public health. *Hastings Center Report, 15,* 28–36.

Beauchamp, D.E. (1976). Public health as social justice. *Inquiry, 13,* 3–14.

Benjamin, M. & Curtis, J. (1992). *Ethics in nursing* (3rd ed.). New York: Oxford.

Benatar, S.R. (1994). Africa and the world. *South African Medical Journal, 84,* 723–726.

Bubeck, D. (1995). *Care, justice and gender*. Oxford, England: Oxford University Press.

Chally, P.S. (1997). Nursing ethics. In K.K. Chitty (Ed.), *Professional nursing: Concepts and challenges* (pp. 363–384). Philadelphia: W.B. Saunders.

Chally, P.S. & Loriz, L. (1998). Ethics in the trenches: Decision making in practice. *American Journal of Nursing, 98*(6), 17–20.

Chapman, A. (Ed.) (1994). *Health care reform: A human rights approach*. Washington, DC: Georgetown University Press.

Haddad, A.M. (1996). Ethical considerations in homecare of the oncology patient. *Seminars in Oncology Nursing, 12*(3), 226–230.

Hall, K. (1996). *Nursing ethics and law*. Philadelphia: W.B. Saunders.

Howard, R.W. (1995). Human rights and the search for community. *Journal of Peace Research, 32,* 1–8.

Jecker, N.S., Jonsen, A.R., & Pearlman, R.A. (1997). *Bioethics: Introduction to the history, methods, and practice*. Sudbury, MA: Jones & Bartlett Publishers.

Johnstone, M.-J. (1994). *Bioethics: A nursing perspective* (2nd ed.). Philadelphia: W.B. Saunders.

Kane, R.A. & Levin, C.A. (1998). Who's safe? Who's sorry? The duty to protect the safety of clients in home- and community-based care. *Generations, 22*(3), 76–81.

Last, J. (1995). Redefining the unacceptable. *Lancet, 346,* 1642–1643.

Moody, H.R. (1996). *Ethics in an aging society*. Baltimore: Johns Hopkins University Press.

Sevenhuijsen, S. (1998). *Citizenship and the ethics of care*. New York: Routledge.

Smart, N. (1995). World views: *Cross-cultural explorations of human beliefs* (2nd ed.). Englewood Cliffs, NJ: Prentice Hall.

Smith, K.V. (1996). Ethical decision-making in nursing: Implications for continuing education. *Journal of Continuing Education in Nursing, 27*(1), 42–45.

Susser, M. (1993). Public health as a human right: An epidemiologist's perspective on the public health. *American Journal of Public Health, 83*(3), 418–426.

Teeple, G. (1995). *Globalization and the decline of social reform*. Atlantic Highlands, NJ: Humanities Press.

Tronto, J.C. (1998). An ethic of care. *Generations, 22*(3), 15–20.

Waymack, M. (1998). Old ethical frameworks: What works, what doesn't? *Generations, 22*(3), 11–14.

Structure and Function of Community Health Services

LEARNING OBJECTIVES

Upon mastery of this chapter, you should be able to:

▪ Trace historic events and philosophy leading to today's health services delivery.
▪ Outline the current organizational structure of the public health care system.
▪ Examine the three core functions of public health as they apply to health services delivery.
▪ Differentiate between the functions of public versus private sector health care agencies.
▪ Explain the influence of selected legislative acts in the United States on shaping current health services policy and practice.
▪ Examine the public health services provided by selected international health organizations.
▪ Explore how the structure and functions of community health services affect community health nursing practice.

Nurses preparing for population-based practice need to be familiar with how the health care delivery system is organized and operates because it is through this system that community health services are delivered and community health nurses function (see Chapter 3). This system forms an organizing framework for the design and implementation of programs aimed at improving the health of communities and vulnerable groups. It is within this system or framework that community health nurses work. Furthermore, through the vehicle of this system, community health nurses have the opportunity to shape the future of health services and develop innovative and more effective means of improving community health.

Service delivery systems directed at restoring or promoting the public's health have evolved over centuries. The structure, function, and financing of health care systems have changed dramatically during that time. These changes have come about in response to evolving societal needs and demands, scientific advancements, the development of more effective methods of service delivery, new technology, and varying approaches to resource acquisition and allocation (Barton, 1999). Considerable progress has been made toward a healthier global society. At the same time, many problems remain, particularly those of controlling health care costs, equitable distribution and effectiveness of health services, and assuring the quality of and access to those services (Pan American Health Organization, 1998; U.S. Department of Health and Human Services, 2000).

This chapter examines the current structure and functions of community health services in the United States and reviews historical and legislative events that have influenced the planning for and the delivery of those services.

HISTORICAL INFLUENCES ON HEALTH CARE

Health care has changed dramatically from previous centuries. Yet personal and community hygiene and health care seem to have been practiced from the beginning of time. Many primitive tribes engaged in sanitary practices such as burial of excreta, removal of the dead, and isolation of members with certain illnesses. In addition, treatment of the sick included use of a variety of therapeutic agents administered by a "healer." Whether these activities were superstitious, derived from survival needs, or primarily tied to religious beliefs is unknown. Nonetheless, records show that in Egypt and the Middle East, as early as 3000 BC, people were building drainage systems, using toilets and systems for water flushing, and practicing personal cleanliness (Scutchfield & Keck, 1997). The **Hebrew hygienic code,** described in the Bible in Leviticus circa 1500 BC, probably was the first written code in the world and was the prototype for personal and community sanitation. It emphasized bodily cleanliness, protection against the spread of contagious diseases, isolation of lepers, disinfection of dwellings after illness, sanitation of campsites, disposal of excreta and refuse, protection of water and food supplies, and maternity hygiene (Scutchfield and Keck, 1997). Even more advanced were the Athenians, circa 1000 to 400 BC, who emphasized personal hygiene, diet, and exercise in addition to a sanitary environment, albeit for the benefit of the wealthy. Their successors, the Romans, added more community health measures such as laws regulating environmental sanitation and nuisances and construction of paved streets, aqueducts, and a subsurface drainage system.

The Middle Ages (from about 500 to 1500 AD) marked a distinct change in health beliefs and practices in Europe based on the philosophy that to pamper the body was evil. Neglected personal hygiene, improper diets, and accumulation of refuse and body wastes soon led to widespread epidemics and pandemics of disease, including cholera, plague, and leprosy (Hecker, 1839). Increased trade between Europe and Asia, military conquests, and Christian crusades to the Middle East only furthered the spread of disease. Bubonic plague, known as the Black Death, in the mid-1300s was the most devastating of pandemics, reportedly killing over 60 million people—half of the population of the known world (Hecker, 1839). In response to this, in 1348, Venice banned entry of infected ships and travelers—a form of quarantine. **Quarantine** is a period of enforced isolation of persons exposed to a communicable disease during the incubation period to prevent spread of the disease, should infection occur. The first known official quarantine measure was instituted in 1377 at the port of Ragusa (now Dubrovnik in Croatia, formerly Yugoslavia) where travelers from plague areas were required to wait 2 months and be free of disease before entry. Marseilles, in 1383, passed the first quarantine law (Scutchfield and Keck, 1997). During this regressive period in history, health care was scarce, private, and reserved for the wealthy few, whereas public health problems were rampant but only minimally and ineffectively addressed.

By the end of the Middle Ages, more enlightened Europeans began to challenge the prevailing beliefs and conditions. They no longer believed that disease was a punishment for sin. However, traces of stigma regarding such conditions as leprosy and tuberculosis still can be found, and sexually transmitted diseases and AIDS still are regarded by some as punishment for immoral conduct. During the late 18th century, new efforts at reform were influenced by a growing emphasis on human dignity, human rights, and the search for scientific truth. These efforts continued through the 19th and 20th centuries.

Despite such signs of improvement, during the 17th and 18th centuries serious problems persisted and new ones developed. Industrialization, masses of people moving to cities, and low regard for human life all contributed to deplorable living and working conditions. Hundreds of pauper children died in England's abusive but socially approved workhouses and apprentice slavery system. Most of Europe continued in unspeakable misery and filth. Householders dumped their refuse from windows or doors into the streets. Stinking rivers and water supplies were seriously contaminated. Numerous diseases, including cholera, typhus, typhoid, smallpox, and tuberculosis, took a tremendous toll on human life.

Around the turn of the 19th century, England's leaders became increasingly concerned about social and sanitary reform. **Sanitation** referred to the promotion of hygiene and prevention of disease by maintaining health-enhancing (sanitary) conditions. The first sanitary legislation, passed in 1837, established vaccination stations in London. One of the most notable reformers, Edwin Chadwick, published his *Report on an Inquiry Into the Sanitary Conditions of the Laboring Population of Great Britain* in 1842 (Richardson, 1887). Chadwick, the father of modern public health, believed that disease and poverty were related and could be changed. His efforts resulted in passage of the English Public Health Act and establishment of a General Board of Health for England in 1848 (Lewis, 1952). Conditions improved and scientific study advanced in England and, concurrently, in France, Germany, Scandinavia, and other European countries. England, however, set the pace for application of research, particularly with reference to public health measures, through steadily improved legislation. British laws subsequently became the pattern for American sanitary ordinances.

TABLE 6–1. Changes in Health Status and Health Care Services

Turn of the 20th Century	Turn of the 21st Century
MORBIDITY AND MORTALITY	
High communicable disease morbidity and mortality	High chronic disease morbidity and mortality
Little prevention	Old and new sexually transmitted diseases
Infrequent cure	Resurgence of tuberculosis
Life span of 47 y	Life span of 76 y
High infant mortality	Significant infant mortality
High maternal mortality	High teenage pregnancy
Alcohol abuse	Multiple substance abuse
Many undiagnosed and untreated conditions	New strains of multidrug-resistant diseases, long-term chronicity, and disability
ACCESS TO HEALTH CARE	
Access primarily for those who could pay a fee	Access for those with health insurance
No health insurance	Insurance with copayments shifting to managed care
Public health clinics for poor and underserved	Free health clinics for medically indigent
Limited treatments	Multitude of treatments
HEALTH CARE DELIVERY SYSTEM	
Extended hospitalizations	Short-term, acute care hospitalizations
Discharge on recovery	Recovery occurs at home or transitional setting
Extended maternal and newborn hospitalization	Short-stay maternal and newborn care
Many home deliveries	Few home deliveries
Home care not-for-profit agencies	Home care not-for-profit and proprietary agencies
PHN begun in health departments	Shifting PHN role in health
Health department personal care services for poor and underserved	Health department personal care services shifting to managed care systems

PHN, public health nursing.
(Adapted from Erickson, G.P. [1996]. To pauperize or empower: Public health nursing at the turn of the 20th and 21st centuries. *Public Health Nursing, 13*[3], 163–169.)

HEALTH CARE SYSTEM DEVELOPMENT IN THE UNITED STATES

Today's relatively organized health care system was long in developing. Most health-related services in the United States were initially reactive, responding to the pressure of immediate needs and uncoordinated from one locality to another. Over time, events and insights contributed to a gradually improving system of programs and services, along with recognition that the health of individuals was affected by the health of the wider community (Table 6–1).

Precursors to a Health Care System

Early health care in the American colonies consisted of private practice with occasional (but infrequent) governmental action for the public good. Action usually was in the form of isolated local responses to specific dangers or nuisances, such as the 1647 regulation to prevent pollution of Boston Harbor or the 1701 Massachusetts law requiring ship quarantine and isolation of smallpox patients. New York City in the late 1700s formed a public health committee to monitor, among other public concerns, water quality, sewer construction, marsh drainage, and burial of the dead.

The U.S. Constitution, adopted in 1789, made no direct reference to public health, nor was the federal government active in health matters. It was the responsibility of each sovereign state to manage its own health affairs. The first federal intervention for health problems was the Marine Hospital Service Act of 1798. It subsidized medical and hospital care for disabled seamen. During the early years, a scourge of epidemics, especially smallpox, cholera, typhoid, and typhus, caused deaths throughout the colonies and decimated the Native American population (Woodward, 1932). Slave trade further threatened the lives of colonists by introducing diseases such as yaws (an infectious nonvenereal disease caused by a spirochete), yellow fever, and malaria (Marr, 1982). Quarantine efforts under local control proved ineffective. In 1837, Congress finally instituted the national port quarantine system, which was regulated and enforced by the Marine Hospital Service. Epidemics were quickly brought under control, causing society to recognize the benefits of uniform central government policy. Improvements in public health and sanitation generally throughout the states, however, were held back by delayed progress in coping with other competing needs, such as police and fire protection (Table 6–2).

TABLE 6–2. **Societal Events and Situations Affecting Health Care Needs**	
Turn of the 20th Century	**Turn of the 21st Century**
SOCIETAL AND POPULATION SHIFTS	
Industrial society focusing on production	Postindustrial, service and information oriented
Rural to urban	Urban to suburban
Limited violence	Rampant violence
Wide gaps between rich and poor	Widening gaps between rich and poor
Growing philanthropy	Declining support for charitable health care
Intense immigration from eastern Europe	Moderate immigration—Mexico and Asia
ENVIRONMENT	
Overcrowded, unsanitary housing	Unkept low-income public housing
Unsafe workplaces, lack of worker safeguards	Environmental hazards in some workplaces
Child labor	Homelessness
Poor public sanitation	Good public sanitation
Multiple health risks	Increasing environmental and behavioral risks
SKILL CHANGES AND EMPLOYMENT	
Farm to factory	Factory to service and information
Low wages	Improving wages, limited benefits
Not enough jobs	Downsizing, layoffs, corporate streamlining
PEOPLE LIVNG IN POVERTY	
Women and children	Women, children, the aged
Immigrants—European	Immigrants—Hispanic and Asian
Migration—south to north	Seasonal migration of farm workers

The Shattuck Report

The **Shattuck Report,** a landmark document, made a tremendous impact on sanitary progress. Lemuel Shattuck, a layman and legislator, chaired a legislative committee that studied health and sanitary problems in the commonwealth of Massachusetts. In 1850, he produced the "Report of the Sanitary Commission of Massachusetts" (Shattuck et al., 1850). It described public health concepts and methods that form the base for current public health practice. Among his recommendations, Shattuck advocated the establishment of state and local boards of health, environmental sanitation, collection, use of vital statistics, systematic study of diseases, control of food and drugs, urban planning, establishment of nurses' training schools (there were none before this time), and preventive medicine. Unfortunately, almost 25 years passed before the recommendations were appreciated and implemented. A similar report by John C. Griscom conducted about the same time concluded that illness, premature death, and poverty were directly related. He also recommended sanitary reform.

Official Health Agencies

The beginnings of an organized health care system in the United States came in the form of **official health agencies,** later called public health agencies. These were publicly funded and operated by state or local government with a goal of providing population-based health services. Development occurred initially at the local level. Many cities established local boards of health in the late 1700s and early to mid-1800s. Among the earliest were Baltimore, Maryland (1798), Charleston, South Carolina (1815), and Philadelphia (1818). As their efforts expanded from handling public "nuisances" to dealing with epidemics and complex public health problems, local health boards recognized that employment of full-time staff was needed, and thus health departments were formed. The first full-time county health departments were established in 1911 in North Carolina and Washington State. Louisiana formed the nation's first state board of health in 1855, followed by Massachusetts in 1869. A few years later, Massachusetts created the first state department of health. Congress formed a National Board of Health to combat yellow fever in 1878. However, because of poor organization, it existed for only 10 years. Again at the national level, the Marine Hospital Service, now with a broader function, became the Public Health and Marine Hospital Service in 1902. Congress gave it a more clearly defined organizational structure and specific functions for its director, the surgeon general. In 1912, it was renamed the United States Public Health Service.

Rapidly expanding through World War I and the Great Depression, the Public Health Service (PHS) strengthened its research activity through the National Institutes of Health (NIH, founded in 1912), added demonstration projects, and initiated greater cooperation with the states. Responding to increasingly complex needs, the NIH added programs significant to public health such as the Children's Bureau (1912), the National Leprosarium at Carville, Louisiana (1917), examination of arriving aliens (1917), the Division of Venereal Diseases (1918), the Food and Drug Administration (1927), and the Narcotics Division (1929), which later became the Division of Mental Hygiene. Title VI of the 1935 Social Security Act promoted stronger federal support of state and local public health services, including health manpower training.

As health, welfare, and educational services proliferated, the need for consolidation prompted the creation of the Federal Security Agency in 1939. In 1953, it was enlarged and renamed the Department of Health, Education and Welfare (DHEW), established under President Eisenhower. In 1979, education was made a separate cabinet-level department, and the DHEW was renamed the Department of Health and Human Services (DHHS). Other significant events include the establishment during World War II of the Communicable Disease Center in Atlanta, currently the National Centers for Disease Control and Prevention (CDC), and the development after World War II of the National Office of Vital Statistics, now called the National Center for Health Statistics (NCHS).

Voluntary Health Agencies

The private sector responded first to America's health problems and continues to complement and supplement the government's role in providing health services. By the late 1800s, **voluntary health agencies** (later called private agencies) began to emerge. They were privately funded and operated to address specific health needs. The first of these was the Anti-Tuberculosis Society of Philadelphia formed in 1892 to educate the public and the government about tuberculosis, then causing 10% of all deaths. Other agencies followed. The National Society to Prevent Blindness was formed in 1908, the Mental Health Association in 1909, the American Cancer Society in 1913, and in 1921 the National Easter Seal Society for Crippled Children and Adults and the Planned Parenthood Federation of America. Also in the late 1800s, organized charities such as the Red Cross, previously denounced for promoting dependent poverty, began to be recognized for their contributions to health and welfare. Philanthropy, too, became respected with the establishment of the Rockefeller Foundation (1913), followed by the Carnegie-Mellon, Kellogg, and Robert Wood Johnson Foundations.

Health-Related Professional Associations

Many health-related professional associations have influenced the quality and type of community health services delivery. Among these, the National Organization for Public Health Nursing from 1912 to 1952 significantly influenced early preparation for and quality of public health nursing services (Fitzpatrick, 1975). The American Public Health Association (APHA), founded in 1872, maintains a prominent role in the dissemination of public health information, influence on health policy, and advocacy for the nation's health.

Other nursing and community health organizations that have promoted quality efforts in community health include the Association of State and Territorial Directors of Nursing, the Association of State and Territorial Health Officers, the National League for Nursing (NLN), the American Nurses Association (ANA), and the Association for Community Health Nursing Educators (ACHNE).

HEALTH ORGANIZATIONS IN THE UNITED STATES

The historical record demonstrates that people attempted to address community health needs for centuries. Responsibility shifted between private groups and governing institutions. Each arm, public and private, offered a unique perspective, different skills, and different resources. Lack of coordination between them, however, coupled with no method for comprehensive planning and delivery of health services, left huge gaps in some areas and duplication in others. Only within the last century have the two arms gradually begun to work together to create a loosely structured "system" of health care. Barton speaks of the growing interdependence of the public and private sectors (1999). How does that system work today? What are its strengths and weaknesses? To answer these questions, its structure must first be examined. Why look at structure? Because it becomes the operational base for assessment, diagnosis, planning, implementation, and evaluation of services and because it provides a framework for intersystem and intrasystem communication and coordination.

Health services occur at four levels: local, state, national, and international. Like ever-widening concentric circles, these levels encompass broader populations. The organization of health services at each level can be classified under one of two types: public or private.

Public Sector Health Services

Government health agencies, the tax-supported arm of the public health effort, perform a vital function in community health practice. They are the official public health agencies whose areas of jurisdiction and types of service are dictated by law. They coordinate and administer activities that often can be carried out only by group or community-wide action: for example, proper sewage disposal, the provision of sanitary water systems, or regulation of toxic wastes. Many community health activities require an authoritative legal backing to ensure enforcement (another useful function of public health agencies) of control in areas such as environmental pollution, highway safety practices, and proper handling of food. Official or public health agencies provide important record-keeping services including the collection and monitoring of vital statistics. They also conduct research, provide consultation, and sometimes financially support other community health efforts.

CORE PUBLIC HEALTH FUNCTIONS

Public health services encompass a wide variety of activities, but all can be grouped under one of three **core public health functions.** They are assessment, policy development, and assurance (Conley & Dahl, 1993). As discussed in Chapter 3, public health nursing practices as a partner with other public health professionals within these core functions.

Assessment refers to measuring and monitoring the health status and needs of a designated community or population. As a core function, it is a continuous process of collecting data and disseminating information about health, diseases, injuries, air and water quality, food safety, and available resources. "The assessment function identifies trends in morbidity, mortality and causative factors; available health resources and their application; unmet needs; and community perceptions about health issues" (Plumb, 1994, p. 14).

Policy development is the formation of a guide for action that determines present and future decisions affecting the public's health. As a core public health function, good public policy development builds on data from the assessment function and incorporates community values and citizen input. It provides leadership and administration for the development of sound health policy and planning.

Assurance is the process of translating established policies into services. This function ensures that population-based services are provided, whether by public health agencies or private sources. It also monitors the quality of and access to those services. The specific functions under assurance are listed in Table 6–3.

The roles of public health agencies vary by level, with each level carrying out the core functions in different ways

to form a partnership in protecting the public's health (Williams & Torrens, 1999). International health agencies focus on issues of global concern, setting policy, developing standards, and monitoring health conditions and programs. At the national level, government health agencies engage in similar functions aimed at regional or nationwide concerns. The federal level provides funds (ie, through the Medicaid program) and develops policy (ie, air pollution policy) but depends on the states to implement them. Agencies at the federal level also develop facilities and programs for special groups such as Native Americans, migrant workers, inmates of federal prisons, and military personnel and veterans whose health care is not the direct responsibility of any one state or locality. State government health agencies function fairly autonomously while working within federal guidelines. They assess, develop, and monitor statewide health needs and services. At the local level, one may find a city government health agency, a county agency, or a combination of both to assess, plan, and serve the health needs of that locality.

Unlike private organizations that tend to have a specific focus, government health agencies exist to accomplish a broad goal of protecting and promoting the health of the total population under their jurisdiction. Such a task requires a wide range of services and the combined talents of many types of professional disciplines. Among them are nurses, physicians, health educators, sanitarians, epidemiologists, statisticians, engineers, administrators, accountants, computer programmers, planners, sociologists, nutritionists, laboratory technicians, chemists, physicists, veterinarians, dentists, pharmacists, demographers, and meteorologists. Furthermore, public health agencies must function not only on an interdisciplinary basis but on an interorganizational one as well. Other government services, education for example, can meet their goals fairly autonomously. Public health, on the other hand, cannot accomplish its important objectives without the collaboration

---

TABLE 6–3. Core Public Health Functions

CORE PUBLIC HEALTH FUNCTIONS: POPULATION-WIDE SERVICES

Assessment	Health status monitoring and disease surveillance
Policy development	Leadership, policy, planning, and administration
Assurance	Investigation and control of diseases and injuries
	Protection of environment, workplaces, housing, food, and water
	Laboratory services to support disease control and environmental protection
	Health education and information
	Community mobilization for health-related issues
	Targeted outreach and linkage to personal services
	Health services quality assurance and accountability
	Training and education of public health professionals

CORE PUBLIC HEALTH FUNCTIONS: PERSONAL SERVICES AND HOME VISITS FOR PEOPLE AT RISK

Primary care for unserved and underserved people
Treatment services for targeted conditions—eg, AIDS, alcohol and other drug abuse, mental illness
Clinical preventive services—eg, immunization, sexually transmitted diseases, family planning, Women, Infants, and Children
Payments for personal services delivered by others

(From U.S. Public Health Service, 1993.)

of many agencies and organizations, both public and private (Barton, 1999; Williams & Torrens, 1999). A case in point is the working together of many organizations with public health to manage the AIDS epidemic, including educational institutions, welfare agencies, mental health programs, home care services, Medicaid, and private groups.

Thus, many different government agencies contribute to the health of a community. Most obvious are the local and state health departments, which provide a variety of direct and indirect health services, including community health nursing. Other tax-supported agencies that sponsor health care or health-related services include welfare departments, departments of public works, public schools and hospitals, police departments, county agricultural services, and local housing authorities.

LOCAL PUBLIC HEALTH AGENCIES

At the grassroots level, government health agencies vary considerably in structure and function from one locality to the next. This partly results from variations in local needs and size of the community. For example, a rural community served by a county or state health department may have widely differing needs and services than a densely populated urban community. Differing health care standards and regulations, as well as the type and stipulations of funding sources, also contribute to variations in the structure and function of health agencies. Nonetheless, each local governmental health agency shares some commonly held responsibilities, functions, and structural features.

The primary responsibilities of the local health department are (1) to assess its population's health status and needs, (2) to determine how well those needs are being met, and (3) to take action toward satisfying unmet needs (Scutchfield & Keck, 1997). Specifically, local government health agencies should fulfill the core functions as follows:

Assess and monitor local health needs and the resources for addressing them.

Develop policy and provide leadership in advocating equitable distribution of resources and services, both public and private.

Ensure availability, accessibility, and quality of health services for all members of the community.

Keep the community informed on how to access public health services.

The local health agency is a critical level of health services' provision because of its closeness to the ultimate recipients: health care consumers.

The structure of the local health department varies in complexity with the setting. Rural and small urban agencies need only a simple organization, whereas large metropolitan agencies require more complex organizational structures to support the greater diversity and quantity of work. A local board of health generally holds the legal responsibility for the health of its citizens. Health board members may be appointed by the mayor if the board of health serves a city, or by a board of supervisors if the board of health serves a

county, or they may be publicly elected. In turn, the board of health appoints a health officer, usually a physician with public health training, who employs the remaining staff of the health department, including public health nurses, environmental health workers, health educators, and office personnel. Others, like nutritionists, statisticians, epidemiologists, social workers, physical therapists, veterinarians, or public health dentists, may be added as needs and resources dictate.

Revenue to support local health department expenditures comes from a variety of sources. State and county general appropriations make up the largest share of the local health department's budget, with additional funds provided through special levies and programs such as school health, Headstart, air pollution, toxic substance control, primary care, immunizations, fees, and private foundation grants. Federal funds provide another source of revenue targeted at specific efforts like AIDS research and services, family planning, child health, environmental protection, and hypertension and nutrition programs. Fees, reimbursements and additional miscellaneous sources, such as state laboratory revenues and food supply supplements, make up the remaining portion of the budget. Figure 6–1 depicts the organization of one local health department serving a population of approximately 300,000.

STATE PUBLIC HEALTH AGENCIES

State-level government health agencies, too, vary in structure and how they carry out the core functions. Each state, as a sovereign government, establishes its own state health department, which in turn determines its goals, actions, and administrative structure. The state health department is responsible for providing leadership in and monitoring of comprehensive public health needs and services in the state. It establishes statewide health policy standards, assists local communities, allocates funds, promotes state-level health planning, conducts and evaluates state-level health programs, promotes cooperation with voluntary (private) health agencies, and collaborates with the federal government for health planning and policy development (Scutchfield & Keck, 1997). Of the various levels of government health agencies, the states recently have played the most pivotal role in health policy formation.

General functions of state health departments include the following (Scutchfield & Keck, 1997):

1. Statewide health planning
2. Intergovernmental and other agency relations
3. Intrastate agency relations
4. Certain statewide policy determination
5. Standard setting
6. Health regulatory functions

Specifically, the Institute of Medicine (1988) described the role of state government related to health. Summarized, it includes the following:

Collect data statewide to assess health needs.

Ensure an adequate statutory base for state health activities.

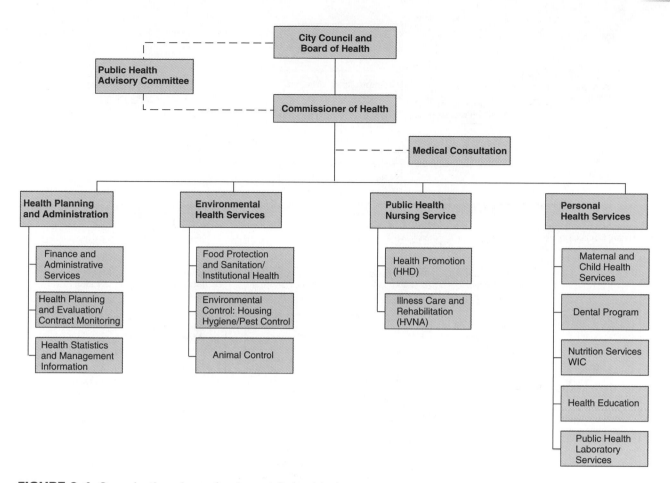

FIGURE 6–1. Organization chart of a city public health department.

Establish statewide health objectives (holding localities accountable where power for implementation has been delegated).

Ensure statewide development and maintenance of essential personal, educational, and environmental health services.

Solve problems that threaten the health of the state.

Support local health services (when needed to achieve adequate service levels) through subsidies, technical and administrative assistance, or direct action.

State public health agencies face a challenge in addressing the health-related issues confronting them. Health insurance, long-term care, organ transplants and donations, AIDS, care of the **medically indigent** (those unable to pay for and totally lacking in medical services), malpractice, and certificates of need for new health services are among the problems faced by most states. Clearly, state health departments must collaborate closely with other agencies, such as social services, education, public works, the legislature, and the housing bureau, to effectively solve such problems. Thus, the solution of state health problems and delivery of health services requires the functioning of an interdependent network of organizations, many of which are not health agencies per se.

Budgetary sources for operating a state health department include state-generated funds, federal grants and contracts, and fees and reimbursements. A large source of federal monies to the states comes through the Department of Agriculture, which has supported the Women, Infants, and Children (WIC) Program, a supplemental nutrition program.

Each of the 50 state health departments in the United States has developed its own unique structure. Some are strongly centralized organizations, and others are decentralized. All are overseen by a director of public health, but titles vary. Under the director are several divisions or bureaus. Those most commonly found in state health department organizational structures are environmental health, disease prevention and control, community health services, maternal and child health, health systems and technical services, laboratory services, and state center for health statistics. Figure 6–2 shows an organizational chart of a state health department.

NATIONAL PUBLIC HEALTH AGENCIES

The national level of public health organization consists of many government agencies. They can be clustered into four groups. First and most directly focused on health is the **Public Health Service.** It is an umbrella organization concerned with the broad health interests of the country and is directed by the Assistant Secretary for Health. The PHS is made up of six functional branches: the CDC, the Food and Drug Administration, the NIH, the Substance Abuse and Mental

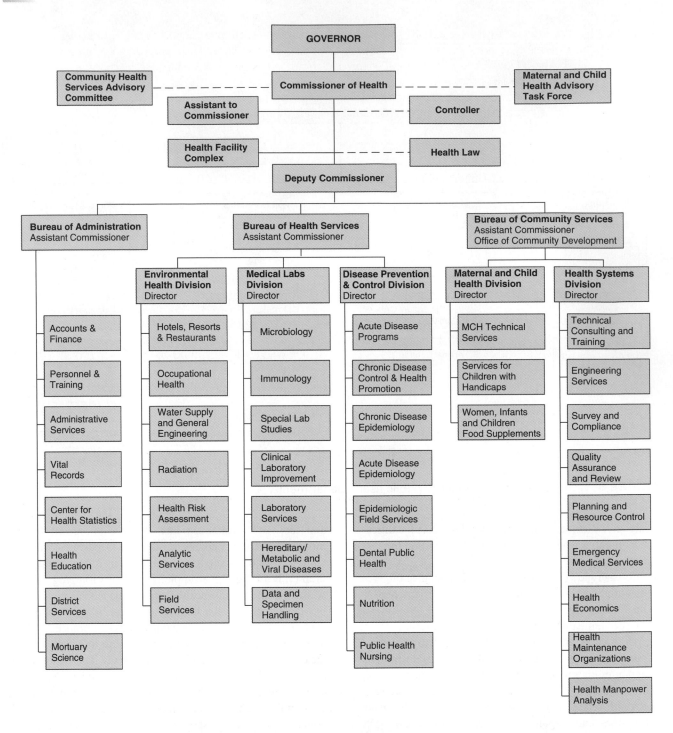

FIGURE 6–2. Organization chart of a state public health department.

Health Services Administration, the Health Resources and Services Administration, and the Agency for Toxic Substances and Disease Registry. One of its major functions through these six branches is the administration of grants and contracts with other government agencies, private organizations, and individuals. In some instances, as with the Indian Health Service, the PHS provides hospital, clinical, and other types of health services for Native Americans on reservations and for Eskimos. Through the CDC and the NIH, it provides epidemiologic surveillance and numerous research programs. Through the Food and Drug Administration, the PHS monitors the safety and usefulness of various food and drug products as well as cosmetics, toys, and flammable fabrics.

Through its staff offices, the PHS offers other services. It has responsibility for the formation, planning, and evaluation of health policy; health promotion; health services management; health research and statistics; intergovernmental affairs; legislation; population affairs; and international health.

It provides financial assistance to the states through grants-in-aid—monies raised by Congress through taxes for specific purposes. It also offers consultation through a National Advisory Health Council and special advisory committees made up of lay experts. The PHS maintains 10 regional offices to make its services more readily available to the states. These offices are located in New York, Boston, Philadelphia, Atlanta, Chicago, Kansas City, Dallas, Denver, Seattle, and San Francisco. Figure 6–3 portrays the PHS organizational structure. Table 6–4 depicts total public health funding through various programs and agencies proposed in fiscal years 1999 and 2000.

At the federal level, the primary agencies concerned with health are organized under the **Department of Health and Human Services (DHHS)**. The PHS is one of five major units in this department. The other four are the Office of Human Development Services, the Health Care Financing Administration, the Family Support Administration, and the Social Security Administration. Figure 6-4 depicts this department's organization. Within the DHHS, clusters of federal agencies deal with the needs of special population groups such as the elderly (Administration on Aging), farm-

ers (Agricultural Extension Service), Native Americans (Bureau of Indian Affairs), and the military (Veterans Administration). Another cluster addresses special programs or problems. Examples are the Bureau of Labor Standards, the Office of Education, the Bureau of Mines, the Department of Agriculture, and the Bureau of Labor Statistics. A final cluster of federal agencies focuses on international health concerns of interest to the nation. Two important ones are the Office of International Health, part of the PHS, and the U.S. Agency for International Development (USAID), under the Department of State.

Private Sector Health Services

The nongovernmental and voluntary arm of the health care delivery system includes many types of services. Private nonprofit health, which includes most hospitals, and welfare agencies make up one large group. Privately owned (proprietary) for-profit agencies are another. Private professional health care practice, composed largely of physicians in solo

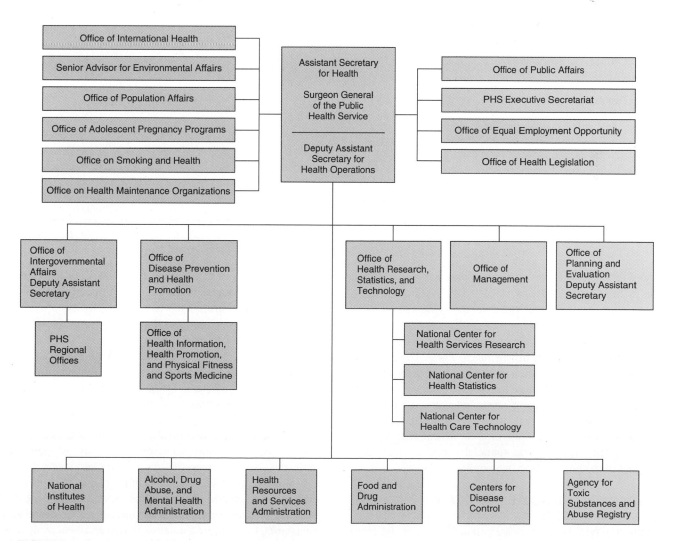

FIGURE 6–3. The United States Public Health Service.

TABLE 6-4. Public Health Funding: Budget Proposal 1999–2000*

Program/Agency	Fiscal Year 1999	Fiscal Year 2000
Agency for Health Care Policy and Research	182	218
Agency for Toxic Substances and Disease Registry	76	64
Centers for Disease Control and Prevention		
Selected programs		
Prevention block grant	150	120
Childhood immunization (Section 317)	421	526
HIV prevention	657	666
STD prevention	124	131
Chronic/environmental disease prevention	474	493
Tobacco	74	101
Infectious diseases	258	301
NIOSH	200	212
National Center for Health Statistics	95	110
Elimination racial/ethnic disparities	10	35
CDC total:	2915	3116
Environmental Protection Agency	7600	7200
Food and Drug Administration programs		
Example program: Tobacco	34	68
FDA total:	1134	1350
Health Resources and Services Administration		
Selected programs		
Health professions	302	212
Community/migrant health centers	920	940
Maternal and child health block grant	700	695
Ryan White AIDS programs	1411	1511
Family planning	215	240
HRSA total:	4130	4172
Indian Health Service	2652	2822
National Institutes of Health	15,709	16,018
Occupational Safety and Health Administration	354	389
Substance Abuse and Mental Health Services Administration	2488	2627

CDC, Centers for Disease Control and Prevention; FDA, Food and Drug Administration; HRSA, Health Resources and Services Administration; NIOSH, National Institute for Occupational Safety and Health.
*All numbers are in millions of dollars and are rounded to the nearest million.
(From the American Public Health Association [1999, March]. President's proposal gives public health short shrift. *The Nation's Health, 1,* 6.)

practice (about two fifths) and group practice (three fifths), forms a third group (DeLew et al., 1992). These are the non–tax supported, nongovernmental dimension of community health care.

Private health services are complementary and supplementary to government health agencies. They often meet the needs of special groups, such as those with cancer or heart disease; they offer an avenue for private enterprise or philanthropy; they are freer than government agencies to develop innovations in health care; and they have been spurred to development, in part, by impatience or dissatisfaction with government programs. Their financial support comes from voluntary contributions, bequests, or fees.

FOR-PROFIT AND NOT-FOR-PROFIT HEALTH AGENCIES

Proprietary health services are privately owned and managed. They may be nonprofit or for-profit. Many hospitals and nursing homes offer nonprofit services but must generate sufficient revenues to keep ahead of operating costs. Often, one or more special services offered by a hospital generate enough income to cover the drain from more expensive programs or uncompensated care. As more hospitals have merged or been integrated into larger health conglomerates, the practice often has been to establish a separate, for-profit corporation that generates revenues so that the basic organization can retain its nonprofit, tax-exempt status.

Examples of for-profit health services include a wide range of private practices by physicians, nurses, social workers, psychologists, and laboratory and x-ray technologists. With the greater demand for home care services since the 1980s, the number of new, for-profit services, such as home care agencies, nursing personnel pools, and durable medical equipment supply companies, has increased. Medicare's annual costs for home care services per enrollee went from $4.00 in 1969 to $258.00 in 1994. When all personal health

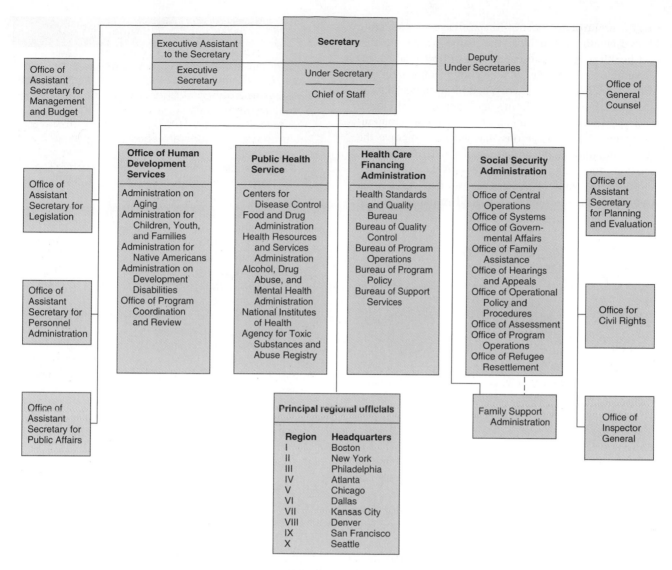

FIGURE 6–4. The United States Department of Health and Human Services.

expenditures are considered (hospital care, physician services, and home health), it costs Medicare $4484 per year per enrollee; private health insurance companies (including those covering dental needs, which Medicare does not cover), $1453; and an undetermined amount comes out of the client's pocket each year for basic health care services (Levit et al., 1996). In response to these escalating home care costs to Medicare, the Balanced Budget Act of 1997 was passed, which was intended to "increase efficiency, reduce fraud, and curtail growth in the home care industry while saving Medicare an estimated $1.6 billion during the first year" (Flaherty, 1998, p. 6). Instead, it reduced Medicare reimbursement by 31% to the for-profit home care agencies, causing 10% of them to close nationwide, placing some clients in jeopardy. The more restrictive reimbursement system in place from 1998 to 1999 was intended to be an interim system, but changing it has been postponed indefinitely because of the potential year 2000 computer problems at the Health Care Financing Administration (Flaherty, 1998).

Not-for-profit private health agencies are organizations established and administered by private citizens for a specific health-related purpose. Often, this purpose is seen as a special need either not addressed or served inadequately by government. An example is visiting nurse associations, which were formed to provide care for the sick in their homes. The contribution of the private, not-for-profit health agency then becomes complementary to public health services.

Three types of private, not-for-profit health agencies have specialized interests. Some, such as the American Cancer Society and the American Diabetes Association, are concerned with specific diseases. Others, such as the National Society for Autistic Children, Planned Parenthood Federation of America, and the National Council on Aging, focus on the needs of special populations. A third group, including agencies such as the American Heart Association and the National Kidney Foundation, is concerned with diseases of specific organs. All of these agencies are funded through private contributions.

Another group of private, not-for-profit agencies affecting health and health care includes the many foundations that support health programs, research, and professional education. Examples include the W.K. Kellogg Foundation, the Pew Charitable Trust, the Robert Wood Johnson Foundation, and the Bush Foundation. Some agencies, like the United Way, exist to fund other voluntary efforts. Another group includes professional associations that work to improve the public's health through the promotion of standards, research, information, and programs. Examples are the APHA, the NLN, the ANA, and the American Medical Association (AMA). These organizations are funded primarily through membership dues, bequests, and contributions.

FUNCTIONS OF PRIVATE-SECTOR HEALTH AGENCIES

The general functions of private-sector health agencies are as follows:

1. Detecting unserved needs or exploring better methods for meeting needs already addressed
2. Piloting or subsidizing demonstration projects
3. Promoting public knowledge
4. Assisting official agencies with innovative programs not otherwise possible
5. Evaluating official programs and assuming a public advocacy role
6. Promoting health legislation
7. Planning and coordinating to promote collaboration among voluntary services and between voluntary and official agencies
8. Developing well-balanced community health programs that seek to make services relevant and comprehensive

Future functions of both private and public sectors most likely will remain much the same. However, the structure of the organizations within both sectors is changing dramatically and will continue to do so as managed care organizations blur the lines between private and public sectors. The movement toward national managed care and its effect on health care delivery is discussed in Chapter 7.

The blurring of the private and public health care sectors has opened the doors to emerging creative health care services. An example of public and private cooperation in the delivery of health care is described in Display 6–1.

INTERNATIONAL HEALTH ORGANIZATIONS

The health of countries around the world cannot be ignored. Besides important humanitarian and moral concerns, there are pragmatic reasons for addressing health issues at the international level. Today, health—along with politics and economics—has become a global issue. Health care among 65% to

---

DISPLAY 6–1. Community Partnerships

Community partnerships are emerging between cities, communities, and other groups, such as businesses, governmental agencies, academic institutions, and voluntary organizations, to meet the health and related needs of citizens. Both government and foundations are encouraging these as an answer to unmet needs.

The Kentucky Partnership for Farm Family Health and Safety began with funds from the Kellogg Foundation but now is a nonprofit, independent, community-based organization. Farm wives have been identified and trained in health education and health-related services and serve as the health "officers" for farm and rural families. This type of community-based organization is being replicated in various counties in Kentucky and in other states to meet the needs of rural farm families.

Organizations such as these highlight the weaknesses and gaps in the U.S. system. They also provide direction for the future of primary care in the United States while assisting all involved to understand the value of interprofessional collaboration. This type of partnering in an organization is becoming more common as they link the private and public sectors and create many new and exciting roles for the professional nurse in the community.

80% of the world's population, or about 3 billion people, continues to be based on traditional medicine. At the same time, the ever-changing global electronic information technologies are revolutionizing health practices with distance education, training, and telemedicine, allowing the transmission of health information to create a more level field for the delivery of health services in all countries (Alleyne, 1998). The nations of the world are dependent on another for goods and services, and, as in any set of interdependent systems, a problem in one nation has repercussions on others. The Director-General of the World Health Organization (WHO) states that "all countries, their governments, their civil societies, and their individuals . . . can be partners who are willing to share and exchange the life-enhancing information and technology that is already at the fingertips of the rich but as yet beyond the reach of the poor"; such is the political vision of WHO (WHO, 1998, p. 6). Furthermore, the constitution of the WHO considers that the health of all people is fundamental to the attainment of peace and security (WHO, 1998). It may not seem possible that the health of a resident of a country 9000 miles away can affect a student from the United States. However, when taking a transnational flight for a school holiday, for example, to Mazatlan, Mexico, Jamaica in the Caribbean, or Bermuda in the Atlantic, the student will be seated among groups of tourists and business people from many nations of the world. There is close scrutiny of airline passengers for passports, visas, customs regulations, weapons, and drugs, but does anyone know whether a passenger from a developing country—who is sitting next to the student for a 6-, 8-, or 10-hour flight—has an airborne communicable disease that is resistant to known antibiotics? (See The Global Community I.)

International cooperation in health dates back to early concerns for epidemics. In 1851, representatives from 12 countries met in Paris for the First International Sanitary Conference. They later established a more permanent organization, the Office Internationale d'Hygiene Publique in 1907. Epidemics on the American continent also prompted representatives from 21 American republics to meet for the First International Sanitary Conference in Mexico City in 1902. In that same year, they formed the International Sanitary Bureau, later renamed the Pan American Health Organization (PAHO). After World War I, the League of Nations in 1921 formed a health organization, which merged with the Office Internationale d'Hygiene Publique (Weindling, 1995).

World Health Organization

The **World Health Organization,** an agency of the United Nations, was developed to direct and coordinate the promotion of health worldwide. It was formed after World War II in 1948 and assumed the functions of the League of Nation's Health Organization. The PAHO remained separate but became WHO's regional office for the Americas. WHO began its existence with 61 member nations, one of which was the United States. By 1998, it had expanded its membership to 191 nations and two associate members (WHO, 1998).

The mission of WHO is to serve as the one directing and coordinating authority on international health. From its inception, WHO has influenced international thinking with its classic definition of health as "a state of complete physical, mental, and social well-being and not merely the absence of disease or infirmity" (WHO, 1998). WHO's primary function is to help countries improve their health status and services by assisting them to help themselves and each other. To accomplish this, it provides member countries with technical services, information from epidemiology and statistics, advisory and consulting services, and demonstration teams.

In the last 20 years, WHO had a realistic expectation that by the year 2000, no individual citizen in any country should have a level of health below an acceptable minimum, and that the global community would later adopt a new strategy to take people further toward the goal of health for all in the future (WHO, 1998). The target date of the year 2000 was intended as a challenge to the member nations. Although the goal has not been met entirely, the WHO continues to emphasize sustaining primary health care, environmental health, control of infectious and diarrheal diseases, maternal and child health care, nutrition, injury prevention, and occupational health (WHO, 1998). These emphases point to a change in focus from primarily reactive programs, like stopping epidemics and instituting quarantines, to adding a more positive stance of promoting the health status of the world community (Display 6–2).

THE GLOBAL COMMUNITY I

There is good news in the developing world (the developing world consists of 90 countries that were seen as presenting the most difficult development challenges in the 1960s and reviewed based on developmental statistics over the last 30 years). Broad changes over the last 30 years have benefited these nations and the world as a whole. "Conditions in the developing world have improved more in the second half of the 20th century than in the previous 500 years" (U.S Agency for International Development, 1998, p. 6).

1968 the Developing World	1998 the Developing World
53% of the people were illiterate	Literacy has risen by almost 50%
62% of these illiterate people were women	Girls and women have significantly closed the gap in gender disparity in education
The average woman had six children	The average woman now has three children
More than one in eight of those children did not live to see their first birthday	Infant mortality had been halved
Nearly 12 million infants died each year, mostly from preventable diseases	5 million fewer children die every year
40% of the people had malnutrition	17% of the people have malnutrition
75% of the people did not have access to clean water or sanitation	The percentage of population with access to clean water has tripled, and access to sanitation has doubled
Life expectancy was just over 50 years	Life expectancy rose more than 10 years
80% of the countries were not democracies	71 more nations have become free or partly free
Annual per capita income was about $700	Annual per capita income rose more than 60%
More than half of the people lived on less than a dollar a day	The percentage of people living in absolute poverty has been cut almost in half

In addition to its headquarters in Geneva, Switzerland, the WHO has six regional offices. The office for the Americas, the PAHO, is located in Washington, DC. The other regional offices are in Copenhagen for Europe, Alexandria for the eastern Mediterranean, Brazzaville for Africa, New Delhi for southeast Asia, and Manila for the western Pacific. Its funding comes from member countries and from the United Nations. It holds an annual World Health

---

DISPLAY 6-2. The 21st Century Goals of the International Community

By 2005
End gender discrimination in education.
Implement strategies that will reverse current losses of environmental resources by 2015.
Build capacity for democratic and accountable governing, protection of human rights, and respect for the rule of law.

By 2015
Cut extreme poverty in half.
Secure universal primary education for all.
Reduce infant mortality rates by two thirds.
Cut the number of mothers who die giving birth by 75%.
Make family planning services available to all who want them.

(U.S. Agency for International Development, 1998.)

Assembly to discuss international health policies and programs.

The WHO publishes several periodicals of interest to the global community, which are available through subscription for a fee and in partial text through WHO's web sites:

Bulletin of the World Health Organization—bimonthly
International Digest of Health Legislation—quarterly
Weekly Epidemiological Record—weekly
WHO Drug Information—quarterly
World Health—bimonthly
World Health Forum—quarterly
World Health Statistics Quarterly—quarterly

Pan American Health Organization

The **Pan American Health Organization** serves as the central coordinating organization for public health in the Western Hemisphere. Founded in 1902, it is the oldest continuously functioning international health organization in the world. Its budget comes from assessments contributed by the American Republics member countries, augmented by funds from WHO, the United Nations, and a variety of other sources, including private donations.

As WHO's regional office for the Americas, PAHO disseminates epidemiologic information, provides technical assistance, finances fellowships, and promotes cooperative research and professional education. An annual conference convened by PAHO provides an opportunity for delegates from all the member nations to discuss issues of concern and plan strategies for addressing health needs. Periodicals published by PAHO include *Perspectives in Health,* published biannually, and *Bulletin of the Pan American Health Organization,* published quarterly.

United Nations International Children's Emergency Fund

Organized in 1946, the United Nations Children's Fund, now the **United Nations International Children's Emergency Fund (UNICEF),** was established initially as a temporary emergency program to assist children of war-torn countries. That focus has broadened, and it has become a permanent agency. It now promotes child and maternal health and welfare globally through a variety of programs and activities. Some include provision of food and supplies to underdeveloped countries, immunization programs in cooperation with WHO, disease control, prevention demonstrations, and, in particular, promotion of family planning in developing countries. Its International Children's Center, opened in the 1940s, has made a significant international impact with its teaching, research, publications, and cooperation on projects related to the health and welfare of children.

Other International Health Organizations

Many other organizations deal with health concerns at the international level. The United Nations Educational, Scientific, and Cultural Organization (UNESCO) offers assistance on international health matters. The Southeast Asia Treaty Organization and the North Atlantic Treaty Organization both have health components. The World Bank addresses health problems through funding and technical assistance. The Food and Agricultural Organization works to improve world food supplies.

In addition to these international organizations, most developed countries have agencies that provide assistance, some in major proportions, to underdeveloped countries. The United States has many agencies, both within the federal government and the private sector, that provide other countries with health-related assistance. Government examples include the U.S. Agency for International Development, Office of International Health in DHHS, the CDC, the Fogarty International Center in the NIH, and the Peace Corps. Examples of private agencies include Project HOPE, International Planned Parenthood Federation, CARE (the Cooperative for Assistance and Relief Everywhere), International Women's Health Coalition, and private foundations and missionary groups.

A description of a fascinating public health agency in Australia is provided in The Global Community II. For a more comprehensive view of world health and international health concerns, see Chapter 21.

SIGNIFICANT LEGISLATION

During the 20th century in the United States, an ever-widening sense of responsibility for health in the public sector led to passage of an increasing amount of health-related legislation. Some acts are of particular significance to the financing and delivery of community health services.

THE GLOBAL COMMUNITY II

The Royal Flying Doctor Service: The Outback, Alice Springs, Australia

The story of the Royal Flying Doctor Service (RFDS) began with one man's frustration. John Flynn was a young Presbyterian minister working in the remote Outback and felt helpless and dismayed that so many people died or suffered because they were too far from medical help. He was a man of vision and saw the possibilities of two new industries that were in their infancy in the 1920s: radio and aviation. Together with Alf Traeger, who devised a transmitter for use in remote areas with no power supply to bring communications to the Outback (an area almost the size of the United States of America and larger than all of Europe), and Hudson Fysh, a young aviator (who later founded Quantas Airlines), they set up the fledgling Flying Doctor Service, which had its first mercy flight in 1928.

The service now is world famous and serves people living in remote communities in some of the harshest conditions on earth. The Central Station, located in the heart of Australia in Alice Springs, provides nearly 30,000 patient contacts a year, including field clinics and remote medical consultations. This station's 10 aircraft make nearly 10,000 flights, about half of which are evacuation flights. Over 150 nurses work for the RFDS. They practice in remote field clinics and are team members with physicians on rescue flights. The flights rarely land at an official airport; most likely, it is the airstrip of a sheep station (a large ranch the size of some small states), with the ill or injured person brought by four-wheel drive vehicle to the airplane. The distances are too great and too remote for the rescue team to get directly to the victim in most cases. If the rescue is for people involved in an automobile crash, the pilot will use the road as a landing strip.

This is a different type of population-based health care that encompasses predominantly public health nursing along with emergency flight nursing and obstetrics. The caregivers (doctors, nurses, Aboriginal health workers, and allied health professionals) refer to the *Central Australian Rural Practitioners Association* (CARPA) *Standard Treatment Manual* for caregiving (CARPA, 1997). Since 98% of the RFDS's clients are Aboriginal, the treatment manual includes protocols that best represent practice for the common presenting problems in remote areas among native people, while highlighting the role of native healers. The manual provides due consideration for the cultural aspects of therapy and recognition of the need to facilitate self-management when possible, since the clients may be hundreds of kilometers from a town large enough to support health care services and the RFDS' remote field clinic may meet at the end of landing strip on a large sheep station only once a month.

The daily operating costs of the RFDS are covered by a combination of federal, state and territory government grants, as well as donations from corporations and the public. They serve anyone in need. A tourist may be visiting the Australian Outback and become injured while hiking up Ayres' Rock (Uluru); the RFDS would assist that person in the same way that they would respond to an Aboriginal woman who needs help during a complicated delivery but who is living 600 km from the nearest health care practitioner.

Because the work environment is so stressful, a 24-hour, confidential Bush Crisis Line has been established. The personal support telephone network assists remote-area health professionals and their families in dealing with normal responses to difficult situations and helps them to maintain the well-being of themselves and their families by effectively managing cumulative and traumatic stress.

(CARPA, 1997; Royal Flying Doctor Service, 1999)

The Shepard-Towner Act of 1921

The Shepard-Towner Act of 1921 provided federal grant-in-aid funds to the states for administration of programs to promote the health and welfare of mothers and infants. The act expired in 1929, but it set a pattern for maternal and child health programs that later was revived and strengthened through the successful and far-reaching efforts of the Children's Bureau, housed in the Department of Labor. Through the leadership of this bureau, many programs were instituted that enhanced children's health. Among them were services targeting prematurity, perinatal mortality, nutrition, mental retardation, audiology, rheumatic fever, cerebral palsy, epilepsy, dentistry, juvenile delinquency, and the problems of migrant workers' children (Elliot, 1962). The Children's Bureau maintained its impact through several administrative changes (moved to the Federal Security Agency in 1946 and to the DHEW in 1953, becoming the Office of Child Development) but was phased out in 1972. For several years, federal advocacy for maternal and child health per se was considerably weakened.

The Social Security Act of 1935

The Social Security Act of 1935 had tremendous consequences for public health. In addition to its revolutionary welfare insurance and assistance programs, which particularly benefited high-risk mothers and children, Title VI of the act financially assisted states and localities in providing public health services. These funds were and still are allocated on the basis of population, public health problems, economic need, and need for training public health personnel. Many of the grants had to be matched by the states or localities. This served to increase their knowledge of and commitment to health programs. The act strengthened local health departments and health programs in most states (Scutchfield & Keck, 1997; Williams & Torrens, 1999).

The Hill-Burton Act (Hospital Survey and Construction Act) of 1946

The Hill-Burton Act of 1946 was an important breakthrough in nationwide health facilities planning. It marked the first real effort to link health planning with population need on a comprehensive basis. The act provided federal funds to states for hospital construction. Allocation of funds, however, was contingent on the states forming planning councils to survey and document needs for new facilities and other capital expansion. The Hill-Harris Amendments in 1954 shifted the emphasis from purely construction to broader health planning based on needs assessment (Hyman, 1982).

The Maternal and Child Health and Mental Retardation Planning Amendments of 1963

The Maternal and Child Health and Mental Retardation Planning Amendments of 1963 opened the door for improved services to selected mothers and children. Recognizing the nation's high perinatal mortality rate and the accompanying problems of premature births, handicapping conditions, and mental retardation, Congress, through this law, authorized project grants to fund projects offering comprehensive care to high-risk, low-income mothers and children. It also provided grants to states to design comprehensive programs addressing mental retardation.

The Heart Disease, Cancer, and Stroke Amendments of 1965 (PL. 89-239)

The Heart Disease, Cancer, and Stroke Amendments of 1965 are noteworthy for their establishment of regional medical programs, one of the first real efforts at comprehensive health planning. Fifty-six regions in the United States were designated, each charged with the responsibility to evaluate the overall health needs of its region and cooperate with other regions for program development. Although the amendments initially were categoric (limited to heart disease, cancer, and stroke), amendments in 1970 expanded the focus. The act was important for two additional reasons: it encouraged local participation in health planning, previously done at federal and state levels; and it funded program operations and planning.

The Social Security Act Amendments of 1965 (PL. 89-97)

The Social Security Act Amendments of 1965 addressed a concern for some type of national health insurance. Title XVIII, Medicare, provided federally funded health insurance for the elderly (65 years and older) and disabled. Title XIX, Medicaid, is a joint federal-state welfare assistance program serving the blind, certain families with dependent children, the disabled, and eligible elderly. These two pieces of legislation (Medicare and Medicaid) have enabled many of the poor, disabled, and elderly to receive quality health care, which otherwise would not be available to them (Scutchfield & Keck, 1997; Williams & Torrens, 1999). More information on Medicare and Medicaid can be found in Chapter 7.

The Comprehensive Health Planning and Public Health Service Amendments Act (Partnership for Health Act) of 1966 (PL. 89-749)

The Comprehensive Health Planning and Public Health Service Amendments Act (Partnership for Health Act) of 1966 promoted further advances in comprehensive health planning. It established comprehensive health planning agencies and coordinated the many categoric health and research efforts into an integrated system. It emphasized comprehensive

health planning and cost containment at local, state, and regional levels. Its goals were improved efficiency and effectiveness of health care. Many problems, including unclear expectations, uncertain funding, and limited authority, prevented full accomplishment of these goals.

The Health Manpower Act of 1968 (PL. 90-490)

The Health Manpower Act of 1968 increased the supply of health personnel by providing federal money to educational institutions for construction, training, special projects, student loans, and scholarships. The act replaced several previous acts with similar goals but whose efforts were fragmentary in addressing the problem. Among them were the Nurse Training Act (1966) and the Allied Health Professions Personnel Training Act (1966). In 1976, Congress passed the Health Professions Education Assistance Act (PL. 94-484) to effect a better balance between the country's health needs and the supply of available health professionals. One of its major emphases was to address the problem of physician maldistribution between underserved (rural) and overserved (urban) areas through educational incentive programs.

The Occupational Safety and Health Act of 1970 (PL. 91-956)

The Occupational Safety and Health Act of 1970 provides protection to workers against personal injury or illness resulting from hazardous working conditions. This and other acts affecting the working population, such as workers' compensation, toxic substance control, access to employee exposure and medical records, and "right-to-know" legislation, are discussed in Chapter 29.

The Professional Standards Review Organization Amendment to the Social Security Act of 1972 (PL. 92-603)

The Professional Standards Review Organization Amendment to the Social Security Act of 1972 had two goals: cost containment and improved quality of care. Professional Standards Review Organization (PSRO) legislation created autonomous organizations, external to hospitals and ambulatory care agencies, to monitor and review objectively the quality of care delivered to Medicare and Medicaid patients. The PSRO review boards, composed mostly of physicians, examined such things as need for care, length of stay, and quality of care against predetermined standards developed locally. Failure to meet standards could mean denial of federal funding. The PSRO concept has created considerable controversy, partly because the two mandated goals, cost containment and quality of care, are potentially incompatible. The federal government's primary emphasis on costs frequently clashed with local concerns for quality. Also, the lack of criteria or standards for review and the governing performed primarily by physicians has made it hard to evaluate the program's success. Some studies, however, indicate a substantial cost saving in Medicare expenditures (Hyman, 1982).

The Health Maintenance Organization Act of 1973 (PL. 93-222)

The Health Maintenance Organization Act of 1973 adds federal support to the concept of prepayment for medical care. Congress authorized funding for feasibility studies, planning, grants, and loans to stimulate growth among qualifying health maintenance organizations (HMOs). In addition, this act requires a business employing 25 people or more to offer a HMO health insurance option, if such an option is available locally.

The National Health Planning and Resource Development Act of 1974 (PL. 93-641)

The National Health Planning and Resource Development Act of 1974 was a major breakthrough in comprehensive health planning. Replacing the Partnership for Health Act, it combined Hill-Burton, comprehensive health planning agencies, and regional medical programs into a single, new program. It fostered not only comprehensive health planning, but regulation and evaluation, and promoted collaborative efforts among regional, state, and federal governments. An important contribution of this act was its emphasis on consumer involvement in health planning. The act was divided into two titles. Title XV, National Health Planning and Development, established national health priorities and assisted the development of area-wide and state planning through health systems agencies and state health planning and development agencies. Title XVI, Health Resources Development, coordinated health facilities planning with health planning, replacing Hill-Burton (Hyman, 1982).

The National Center for Health Statistics (PL. 93-353)

The NCHS, established in 1974, arose from the earlier National Office of Vital Statistics and became part of the CDC under the PHS in 1987. The NCHS operates 11 data collection systems that provide vital information for public health planning and service delivery. Display 6–3 lists these data collection systems.

The Omnibus Budget Reconciliation Act of 1981 (PL. 97-35)

The Omnibus Budget Reconciliation Act (OBRA) of 1981 had a profound effect on public health. In this act, Congress halted the progress made in most of the public health laws of the previous 45 years, substantially reducing their funding authorization. To shift more power to the states and cut the budget, the Reagan administration consolidated categoric grants into four block grants. The first block grant targeted general preventive health services; the second addressed alcohol, drug abuse, and mental health; the third focused on maternal and child health; and the fourth addressed primary care, which covered federal support for community health centers. Although block grants provide some advantages, these came with limiting restrictions on the amount and use of the funds. The result was a significant reduction in funding for state and local health programs. Under OBRA, new legislation was introduced in 1987 to increase quality control in nursing homes and home care.

DISPLAY 6–3. The National Center for Health Statistics Data Collection Systems

1. Basic vital statistics are collected by each state on such things as births, deaths, marriages, pregnancy terminations, and divorces. The Center publishes monthly and annual reports on these data.
2. Vital statistics follow-back surveys are conducted periodically to obtain further information on previously gathered data.
3. National Survey of Family Growth studies such things as fertility, family planning practices, family formation and dissolution, and matters affecting maternal and child health.
4. National Health Interview Survey is a continuous nationwide survey of illness and disability—their amount, distribution, and affects—in the United States. The results are published in Series 10 of Vital Health Statistics.
5. National Medical Care Utilization and Expenditure Survey was conducted once in 1980 to describe medical services' use and expenditures.
6. National Ambulatory Medical Survey occasionally gathers data from physicians on ambulatory services by specialty and target population.
7. National Health and Nutrition Examination Survey provides physical, physiologic, and biochemical data related to nutrition of national population samples.
8. National Hospital Discharge Survey provides annual data on such things as length of stay, diagnosis, procedures performed, and patient use patterns.
9. National Nursing Home Survey collects data from nursing home residents and staff regarding need, level of care, costs, and use patterns.
10. National Master of Facility Inventory identifies and classifies (according to type of beds) all facilities that offer 24-hour care, including hospitals, nursing homes, and residential care facilities.
11. National Health Professions Inventories and Surveys draw from state data systems to describe the distribution and education of health personnel. Statistics on mental health are collected through the National Institute of Mental Health.

(National Center for Health Statistics: (1981). Data systems of the National Center for Health Statistics, Series 1[16] (DHHS Publication No [PHS] 82-1318, Hyattsville, MD. U.S. Department of Health and Human Services.)

The Social Security Amendments of 1983 (PL. 98-21)

The Social Security Amendments of 1983 became law in response to accelerating health care costs. The act represented a major reform in health care financing from retrospective to prospective payment. It introduced a billing classification system of 467 diagnosis-related groups, which provide Medicare payment to hospitals based on a fixed rate set in advance (Scutchfield & Keck, 1997; Williams & Torrens, 1999). The fixed payment could not be increased if hospital costs for care exceeded that amount. Conversely, if costs were less than the paid amount, the hospital could keep the difference. Thus, a positive incentive was introduced to reduce hospital costs while offering a negative incentive for early patient discharge.

The Consolidated Omnibus Budget Reconciliation Act of 1985

The Consolidated Omnibus Budget Reconciliation Act (COBRA) of 1985 required employers to provide extended (up to 36 months) group-rate insurance coverage for laid-off workers and their dependents. This proved to be expensive for employers. The act also expanded Medicaid services and permitted states to offer hospice services to the terminally ill Medicaid recipient.

Omnibus Budget Reconciliation Act Expansion of 1986

Omnibus Budget Reconciliation Act Expansion of 1986 promoted a prospective payment system for hospital outpatient service. In 1989, a further OBRA expansion regulated fee schedules for physicians encouraging less "high-tech" use. Under OBRA, the Agency for Health Care Policy and Research also was established in 1989 to study the effectiveness of health care services.

The Medicare Catastrophic Coverage Act of 1988 (PL. 100-360)

The Medicare Catastrophic Coverage Act of 1988 (MCCA) expanded Medicare benefits significantly. Coverage was extended to include a portion of outpatient prescription drug costs and greater posthospital extended care facility and home health benefits. Also, MCCA set limits on beneficiary liability and provided increased inpatient hospital benefits.

The Family Support Act of 1988

The Family Support Act of 1988 reformed the federal welfare system to emphasize work and child support. It established child support programs, work opportunities, and basic skill and training programs. It included a requirement that recipients seek employment and that states establish an education, training, and work program.

The Health Objectives Planning Act of 1990 (PL. 101-582)

The Health Objectives Planning Act of 1990 was significant for its support of the report by the Institute of Medicine, *Healthy People 2000,* with funding to improve the health status of the nation. Funding for health promotion and disease prevention was added in the 1991 legislative session.

Preventive Health Amendments of 1992

The Preventive Health Amendments of 1992 placed a focus by the federal government on preventive health and primary prevention initiatives. It changed the name of the Centers for Disease Control to the Centers for Disease Control and Prevention. It enhanced services to Migrant Health Centers, especially in maternal and child health and community education. It promoted international exchange programs for public health officials from the around the world who are interested in working in another country.

Personal Responsibility and Work Opportunity Reconciliation Act of 1996

The Personal Responsibility and Work Opportunity Reconciliation Act of 1996 is commonly known as the "Welfare Reform Bill." It amended the Social Security Act to reform the federal welfare system imposing a 5-year lifetime limit on welfare benefits. It also changed Aid to Families With Dependent Children to Temporary Assistance to Needy Families. Finally, it restricted benefits to legal immigrants.

IMPLICATIONS FOR COMMUNITY HEALTH NURSING

The structure and functions of the health care delivery system, as well as particular legislation, have had a significant impact on community health nursing. Community health nurses have had to learn to adapt to a constantly changing system. They have developed innovative modes of service delivery, such as community-based nursing centers for health education, counseling, and screening of low income populations. They have learned to practice in a variety of settings extending beyond homes, work sites, schools, churches, clinics, and voluntary agencies. They have acquired skills in teamwork, leadership, and political activism. They have recognized the importance of outcomes research to document the value of nursing interventions with at-risk populations.

Community health nurses incorporate the three core public health functions as they provide care to aggregates in the community (ANA, 2000). The following activities for each core function demonstrate this:

ASSESSMENT
Assess the health needs of aggregates
Collect data on health and safety hazards in the community
Determine unmet community health needs
Identify available health resources
POLICY DEVELOPMENT
Incorporate community values and input in agency policy formation
Formulate plans and policies that address community health needs
Advocate for the health of the public and promote interprofessional collaboration

ASSURANCE

Translate intent of agency policies into needed services

Assure access to services by community members

Implement and provide services through programs

At the national, state, and local level, community health nursing has important ties to both private and public health agencies. Community health nurses may be employed by either type of organization. When serving in the public sector, they often provide consultation, serve on boards, volunteer their services, or collaborate with private sector health organizations to ensure quality and access of care to the broader community. Examples include joint efforts to promote certain types of health legislation or collaboration to produce and disseminate health education materials targeting specific populations. Sometimes, community health nursing services operate within one organization that combines public and private sector organization and funding. An example is the Metropolitan Visiting Nurse Association of Minneapolis, Minnesota, which has been a combined public-private agency supported by taxes and voluntary funds.

Community health nurses also have many opportunities to serve in international health. Some work with WHO, PAHO, or other agencies to assist in direct-care projects such as famine relief, immunization efforts, or nutritional screening and education programs. Other nurses serve as health planners, assist with policy development, conduct collaborative needs-assessment projects and research efforts, or engage in program development.

SUMMARY

Many factors and events have influenced the current structure, function, and financing of community health services. Understanding these gives the community health nurse a stronger base for planning for the health of community populations.

Historically, health care has progressed unevenly, marked by numerous influences. Primitive practices of early centuries were replaced with more advanced sanitary measures by the Greeks and Romans. The Middle Ages saw a serious health decline in Europe, with raging epidemics leading to extensive 19th-century reform efforts in England and later in the United States.

Organized health care in the United States developed slowly. Public health problems, such as need for isolation of communicable disease and control of environmental pollution, prompted the gradual development of official interventions. For example, quarantines to control the spread of communicable disease were imposed in the late 1700s. Sanitary reform was pursued more vigorously during the 1800s. Local, then state, health departments were formed starting in the late 1700s. By the early 1900s, the federal government had assumed a more active role in public health with a proliferation of health, education, and welfare services.

For years, efforts to address community health needs have been made by private individuals and public agencies. These two arms of service have not been coordinated in the past and only gradually, during this century, have begun to work together to form an emerging health care system.

The public arm of health services includes all government, tax-supported health agencies and occurs at four levels: local, state, national, and international. Each level deals with the health needs of the population encompassed by its boundaries. Each level has a different structure and set of functions. Public health services include three core public health functions: assessment, policy development, and assurance.

Private health services are the unofficial arm of the community health system. They include voluntary nonprofit agencies as well as privately owned (proprietary) and for-profit agencies. Their financial support comes from voluntary contributions, bequests, or fees. Private health organizations often supplement and complement the work of official agencies.

The delivery and financing of community health services has been significantly affected by various legislative acts. These acts have prompted such innovations as health insurance and assistance for the poor, the elderly, and the disabled; money to train health personnel and conduct health research; standards for health planning and delivery; health protection for workers on the job; and the financing of health services.

ACTIVITIES TO PROMOTE CRITICAL THINKING

1. Interview someone at your local health department. How do the services offered compare with those listed in this chapter? What is the role of community health nursing? How does the role of the community health nurse incorporate the core public health functions?

2. Make an on-site visit to your state health department. Compare its functions with the core public health functions described in this chapter. Identify areas where improvement may be needed.

3. Conduct an interview on site with someone at a private health agency, voluntary agency, or community-based organization. Compare their functions with those listed in this chapter for private health agencies. Describe how this agency works collaboratively with public health agencies and other community organizations. What is the role of the nurse in this agency?

4. Look up various international health agencies on the Internet and explore web sites that discuss current international health care issues. What topics are of concern currently? Are new epidemics or emerging strains of a virus being highlighted? What could a

community health nurse in your local community do with this information?

5. Form two teams with your classmates and debate the pros and cons of a strong federal role in health care provision as opposed to decentralized (state and local) control.

6. Interview two consumers about their perception of problems and strengths of our health care system. Select people representing distinctly different age groups and life situations, such as a 25-year-old mother of three children and a 75-year-old widower.

REFERENCES

Alleyne, G.A.O. (1998). First word. Intersection 2000: Past roads meet future highways. *Perspectives in Health, 3*(1).

American Nurses Association. (2000). *Public health nursing: A partner for healthy populations.* Washington, DC: American Nurses Publishing.

The American Public Health Association. (1999). President's proposal gives public health short shrift. *The Nation's Health, 1,* 6.

Barton, P.L. (1999). *Understanding the U.S. health service system.* Chicago: AUPHA Press.

Central Australian Rural Practitioners Association (CARPA). (1997). *Central Australian Rural Practitioners Association standard treatment manual* (3rd ed.). Alice Springs: Central Australian Rural Practitioners Association.

Conley, E. & Dahl, J. (1993). *Public health nursing within core public health functions: A progress report from the public health nursing directors of Washington.* Olympia: Washington State Department of Health.

DeLew, N., Greenberg, G., & Kinchen, K. (1992). A layman's guide to the U.S. health care system. *Health Care Financing Review, 14*(1), 151–169.

Elliot, M. (1962). The Children's Bureau: Fifty years of public responsibility for action in behalf of children. *American Journal of Public Health, 52,* 576.

Erickson, G.P. (1996) To pauperize or empower: Public health nursing at the turn of the 20th and 21st centuries. *Public Health Nursing, 13*(3), 163–169.

Fitzpatrick, M.L. (1975). *The National Organization for Public Health Nursing 1912–1952: Development of a practice field.* New York: National League for Nursing.

Flaherty, M. (1998). Close to closure: Home care agencies feel the budget squeeze. *Nurseweek, 11*(19), 1, 6.

Hecker, J.F.C. (1839). *The epidemics of the Middle Ages.* London: Trubner and Company.

Hyman, H. (1982). *Health planning: A systematic approach* (2nd ed.). Rockville, MD: Aspen Systems.

Levit, K.R., Lazenby, H.C., Sivarajan, L., et al. (1996). National health expenditures, 1994. *Health Financing Review, 17*(3), 205–242.

Lewis, R.A. (1952). *Edwin Chadwick and the public health movement, 1832–1854.* New York: Longman's.

Marr, J. (1982, winter). Merchants of death: The role of the slave trade in the transmission of disease from Africa to the Americas. *Pharos,* 31.

Pan American Health Organization. (1998). *Health situation in the Americas: Basic indicators 1998* (Health Situation Analysis Program, Division of Health and Human Development). Washington, DC: Pan American Health Organization.

Pickett, G. & Hanlon, J. (1990). *Public health: Administration and practice* (9th ed.). St. Louis: Times Mirror/Mosby.

Plumb, D. (1994, September). The roles and responsibilities of state and local public health agencies [position paper]. *The Nation's Health, 24*(8), 13–15.

Richardson, B.W. (1887). *The health of nations: Vol. 2. A review of the works of Edwin Chadwick.* London: Longmans, Green.

Royal Flying Doctor Service. (1999). Alice Springs, Australia: Central Station.

Scutchfield, F.D. & Keck, C.W. (1997). *Principles of public health practice.* Albany, NY: Delmar Publishers.

Shaffer, F. (1988). DRGs: A new era for health care. *Nursing Clinics of North America, 23*(3), 453–463.

Shattuck, L., et al. (1850). *Report of the Sanitary Commission of Massachusetts.* Cambridge, MA: Harvard University Press (originally published by Dutton & Wentworth in 1850).

Turnock, B.J. 1997). *Public health: What it is and how it works.* Gaithersburg, MD: Aspen Publishers.

U.S. Agency for International Development. (1998). *Making a world of difference: Celebrating 30 years of development progress.* Washington, DC: Author.

U.S. Department of Health and Human Services. (2000). *Healthy people 2010* (conference edition in two volumes). Washington, DC: U.S. Government Printing Office.

U.S. Public Health Service. (1993). *The Core Functions Project: Health care reform and public health. A paper on population-based core functions.* Washington, DC: U.S. Public Health Service, Office of Disease Prevention and Health Promotion.

Weindling, P. (Ed.) (1995). *International health organizations and movements, 1918–1939.* Cambridge: Cambridge University Press.

Williams, S.J. & Torrens, P.R. (1999). *Introduction to health services* (5th ed.). Albany, NY: Delmar Publishers.

Woodward, S.B. (1932). The story of smallpox in Massachusetts. *New England Journal of Medicine, 206,* 1181.

World Health Organization. (1998). *World health report 1998: Life in the 21st century. A vision for all.* Geneva: Author.

INTERNET RESOURCES

Care: www.care.org

World Health Organization: http://www.who.org

Pan American Health Organization: http://www.paho.org

Department of Health and Human Services, Health Resources and Services Administration: http://www.hrsa.dhhs.gov

Central Australian Rural Practitioners Association: carpastm@taunet.net.au

U.S. Agency for International Development: http://www.info.usaid.gov

SELECTED READINGS

American Public Health Association. (1994). Cairo summit spells hope for women's health. *The Nation's Health,* 23.

Berkowitz, B. (1995). Health system reform: A blueprint for the future of public health. *Journal of Public Health Management Practice, 1,* 1–6.

Berkowitz, B. (1995). Improving our health by improving our system: Transitions in public health. *Family Community Health, 18*(3), 37–44.

Brown, E.R. (1997). Leadership to meet the challenges to the public's health. *American Journal of Public Health, 87*(4), 554–557.

Bulger, R.J. (1998). Treating individuals while tending to populations. *Western Journal of Medicine, 168*(1), 54–59.

Conley, E. (1995). Public health nursing within core pubic health functions: "Back to the future." *Journal of Public Health Management and Practice, 1*(3), 1–8.

Dahlgren, G. & Whitehead, M. (1992). *Policies and strategies to promote equity in health.* Copenhagen: World Health Organization, Regional Office for Europe.

Danzinger, S. & Gottschalk, P. (Eds.) (1993). *Uneven tides: Rising inequality in America.* New York: Russell Sage Foundation.

Fairbanks, J. & Wiese, W.H. (1997). *The public health primer.* Thousand Oaks, CA: Sage Publications, Inc.

Fielding, J. & Halfon, N. (1994). Where is the health in health system reform? *Journal of the American Medical Association, 272,* 1292–1296.

Fronstin, P. (1997). *Trends in health insurance coverage* (Issue Brief No. 185; pp. 1–19). Washington, DC: Employee Benefits Research Institute.

Greenberg, G. & Kinchen, K. (1992). A layman's guide to the U.S. health care system. *Health Care Financing Review, 14*(1), 151–169.

Halverson, P.K., Kaluzny, A.D., & McLaughlin, C.P. (1997). *Managed care and public health.* Gaithersburg, MD: Aspen.

Hash, M. (1988). *Nursing practice in the 21st century: Structuring and financing of community health services. Community nursing organizations* (*CNOs*) (American Nursing Foundation No. CH-18; pp. 36–40). Kansas City, MO: American Nurses Association.

Himali, U. (1995). Managed care: Does the promise meet the potential? *The American Nurse, 27*(4), 1, 14–16.

Institute of Medicine. (1988). *The future of public health.* Washington, DC: National Academy Press.

Knight, W. (1998). *Managed care: What it is and how it works.* Gaithersburg, MD: Aspen.

Kovner, A.R. & Jonas, S. (1999). *Jonas and Kovner's health care delivery in the United States.* New York: Springer Publishing Company.

Krieger, N., Chen, J.T., & Ebel, G. (1997). Can we monitor socioeconomic inequalities in health? A survey of U.S. Health Department's data collection and reporting practices. *Public Health Reports, 112,* 481–491.

Pollack, A.M. & Rice, D.P. (1997). Monitoring health care in the United States: A challenging task. *Public Health Reports, 112,* 108–113.

Rosen, G. (1958). *A history of public health.* New York: MD Publications.

Shalala, D.E. (1993). Nursing and society: The unfinished agenda for the 21st century. *Nursing and Health Care, 14*(6), 289–291.

Swinson, A. (1965). *The history of public health.* Exeter, England: A. Wheaton & Co.

U.S. Agency for International Development. (1996). *Saving lives today and tomorrow: A decade report on USAID's child survival program.* Arlington, VA: Center for International Health Information.

Wilkinson, R.G. (1996). *Unhealthy societies: The afflictions of inequality.* London: Routledge.

Economics of Health Care

KEY TERMS

- Capitation rates
- Competition
- Cost sharing
- Diagnosis-related groups
- Gross national product
- Health care economics
- Health maintenance organization
- Macroeconomic theory
- Managed care
- Managed competition
- Medicaid
- Medicare
- Microeconomic theory
- National health insurance
- Preferred provider organization
- Prospective payment
- Rationing
- Regulation
- Retrospective payment
- Single-payer system
- Third-party payments
- Universal coverage

LEARNING OBJECTIVES

Upon mastery of this chapter, you should be able to:

- Define the concept of health care economics.
- Describe three sources of health care financing.
- Compare and contrast retrospective and prospective health care payment systems.
- Analyze the issues and trends influencing health care economics and community health services delivery.
- Explain the causes and effects of health care rationing.
- List the pros and cons of managed competition as opposed to a single-payer system.
- Explain the philosophical implications of health care financing patterns on community health nursing's mission and values.

Nurses concerned with the delivery of needed community health services also must understand how those services are financed. In an era when health care resources are limited and provider organizations are competing for scarce dollars, it is essential for nurses to be knowledgeable about the issues related to health care financing and about ways to obtain funding to address identified health needs in the community.

Behind the financing of health care lies the science of **health care economics.** The field of economics, as a whole, is a science that describes and analyzes the production, distribution, and consumption of goods and services. It also is concerned with a variety of related problems such as finance, labor, and taxation. It studies and seeks to promote the best use of scarce resources for the greatest good of society. The science of health care economics describes and analyzes the production, distribution, and consumption of health care goods and services to maximize the administration of scarce resources to benefit the most people. The goal of health economics—similar in some ways to that of public health—is to promote the greatest good for the greatest number using available resources and knowledge.

This chapter summarizes the changing picture of health care economics and its financial incentives and disincentives for enhancing the public's health. More extensive treatment of these subjects is found in the Selected Readings section.

ECONOMIC THEORIES AND CONCEPTS

Health economics can be better understood by examining the two basic theories underlying the science of economics. The first is microeconomics, and the second is macroeconomics. In addition, concepts of health care payment are discussed.

Microeconomics

Microeconomic theory is concerned with supply and demand. Economists using microeconomic theory study the supply of goods and services as these relate to consumer income allocation and distribution. They further study how this allocation and distribution affects consumer demand for these goods and services. Supply and demand influence each other and, in turn, affect prices. An increase in or oversupply of certain products leads to less overall consumption (decreased demand) and lowered prices. The opposite also is true. Limited availability of desired products means that supply does not meet demand, and prices increase. Microeconomic theory is useful for understanding price determination, resource allocation, consumer income, and spending distribution at the level of individuals and organizations.

Macroeconomics

Macroeconomic theory is concerned with the broad variables that affect the status of the total economy. Economists using macroeconomics study factors influencing employment, income, prices, and economic growth rates. Their focus is on the larger view of economic stability and growth. Macroeconomic theory is useful for providing a global or aggregate perspective of the variables affecting the total economic picture.

The economics of health care encompasses both microeconomics and macroeconomics, examining an intricate and complex set of interacting variables. It is concerned with supply and demand: Is the supply of available resources sufficient to meet the demand for use by consumers? It examines costs and benefits, cost effectiveness, and cost efficiency: Are the resources expended achieving the desired outcomes? It studies the allocation of scarce resources for health care: Where should resources, such as funding for health programs and services for at-risk populations, be applied when there are insufficient resources to address all of the needs?

Health economics is a major field of study in and of itself. Health economists draw on economic theory to study and develop an understanding of the factors influencing the financing and delivery of health services. Macroeconomic theory has been useful in providing a large-scale perspective on health care financing that has resulted in various proposals for national health plans, health care rationing, competition, and managed care. These concepts are described later in the chapter. Microeconomic theory may prove more useful if health care competition increases, since the success of the supply-and-demand concept depends on a competitive market. The pros and cons of competition also are examined later in this chapter. Issues such as cost containment, competition between providers, accessibility of services, quality, and need for accountability continue to be targets of major concern for the 21st century.

Payment Concepts in Health Care

Reimbursement for health care services generally has been accomplished through one of two approaches: retrospective or prospective payment. Conceptually, these approaches are opposite one another. It is helpful to understand their differences and their meaning for the financing and delivery of health services, past and present.

RETROSPECTIVE PAYMENT

A traditional form of reimbursement for any kind of service, including health care, is **retrospective payment,** which means to reimburse for a service after it has been rendered. A fee may be established in advance. However, payment of that fee occurs after the fact, or retrospectively. This is known as the fee-for-service (FFS) approach.

In health care, limited accountability in the use of retrospective payment has created several problems. With third-party payers serving as intermediaries, neither consumers nor providers of health services were accountable for containing costs. Patients and providers alike often insisted on expensive or unnecessary tests and treatments. Because reimbursement was made retrospectively by the insuring agency, there was no incentive to keep a lid on this spending. Third-party reimbursement increased, along with rising physician fees, to create an inflationary spiral of escalating costs. Abuse of the FFS system made it more difficult to develop retrospective payment for other health care providers, including nurses.

A further problem associated with the FFS concept was its tendency to encourage sickness care rather than wellness services. Physicians and other providers were rewarded financially for treating illness. There were few incentives for prevention or health promotion in an industry that reaped its revenues from keeping hospital beds full and caring for the sick and injured. Although retrospective payment worked well in other industries, from a cost containment as well as a public health perspective, it was problematic in health care.

PROSPECTIVE PAYMENT

Prospective reimbursement, although not a new concept, was implemented for inpatient Medicare services in 1984 in response to the health care system's desperate need for cost containment. It has since influenced the Medicaid program as well as private health insurers. The prospective payment form of reimbursement has essentially eliminated the retrospective payment system (Hanchak et al., 1996). **Prospective payment** is a payment method based on rates derived from predictions of annual service costs that are set in advance of service delivery. Providers receive payment for services according to these fixed rates set in advance (Harrington & Estes, 1997). Payments may be in the form of premiums paid before receipt of service or in response to fixed rate (not cost) charges. To correct unlimited reimbursement patterns and counteract disincentives to contain costs, prospective payment involves four steps (Dowling, 1979):

1. An external authority is empowered (by statute, market power, or voluntary compliance by providers) to set provider charges, third-party payment rates, or both.
2. Rates are set in advance of the prospective year during which they will apply and are considered fixed for the year (except for major, uncontrollable occurrences).
3. Patients, third-party payers, or both pay the prospective rates rather than the costs incurred by providers during the year (or charges adjusted to cover these costs).
4. Providers are at risk for losses or surpluses.

The concept of prepayment, or consumers paying in advance of health care, has existed for many years. As far back as 1933, prepaid medical groups were advocated to reduce costs and make services more accessible (Hyman, 1982). This pattern of prepayment for comprehensive services has since continued in a variety of forms. Examples of early plans were the Health Insurance Program of Greater New York City and the Kaiser Plan. The success of these two plans helped to influence the growth of the health maintenance organization (HMO), a type of managed care discussed later in this chapter.

Prospective payment, then, imposes constraints on spending and gives incentives for cutting costs. The Federal government therefore enacted a prospective payment plan (Social Security Amendments Act) in 1983. The plan, called **diagnosis-related groups** (DRGs), is a billing classification system based on 23 major diagnostic categories and 467 DRGs that provides fixed Medicare reimbursement to hospitals. This system was enacted to curb Medicare spending in hospitals and to extend the program's solvency period. This regulatory approach changed Medicare hospital reimbursement "from a cost-based retrospective system, in which a hospital was paid its costs, to a fixed-price prospective payment system to create incentives for hospitals to be efficient in the delivery of services" (DeLew et al., 1992, p. 162).

Indeed, the prospective payment system (PPS) has reduced Medicare's rate of increase in inpatient hospital spending and increased hospital productivity (Levit et al., 1996). It also reduced hospital stays and unnecessary admissions and created a boom in home health care (D'Angelo & D'Angelo, 1999). A spinoff, however, was fierce competition among providers and mounting concern over quality of care—in hospitals, ambulatory settings, and home care.

The PPS concept also has proven useful from a public health perspective. Prepaid services create incentives for providers to keep their enrollees healthy, thus reducing provider costs. A potential, indirect benefit from fixed rates and reduced costs is that more of the health care dollar is available for spending on prevention programs.

Further understanding of health economics and its impact on community health and community health nursing can be obtained by examining methods of health care financing, issues and trends influencing health care economics, and the effects of financing patterns on community health practice.

SOURCES OF HEALTH CARE FINANCING: PUBLIC AND PRIVATE

Financing of health care significantly affects community health and community health nursing practice. It influences the type and quality of services offered as well as the way those services are used. Sources of payment may be clustered into three categories: third-party payments, direct consumer payment, and private or philanthropic support.

Third-Party Payments

Third-party payments are monetary reimbursements made to providers of health care by someone other than the consumer who received the care. The organizations that administer these funds are called third-party payers because they are a third party, or external, to the consumer-provider relationship. Included in this category are four types of payment sources: private insurance companies, independent health plans, government health programs, and claims payment agents (Harrington & Estes, 1997).

PRIVATE INSURANCE COMPANIES

Private insurance companies market and underwrite policies aimed at decreasing consumer risk of economic loss because of a need to use health services. In 1994, private health insurance paid $266.8 billion in benefits while taking in $313.3 billion in premiums. Although these numbers seem large, they represent decelerating growth by private health insurance resulting from a shift by employees to lower cost managed-care plans offered through the workplace (Foster Higgins Survey and Research Services, 1994). No private insurer directly delivers health services although some, such as John Hancock, have subsidiary proprietary home health agencies.

There are three types of private insurers. First are commercial stock companies that sell health insurance, generally as a sideline. They are private stockholder-owned corporations, such as Aetna, Travelers, and Connecticut General, that sell insurance nationally. Mutual companies, a second type that operates in the national marketplace, are owned by their policyholders. Examples are Mutual of Omaha, Prudential, and Metropolitan Life. The third type, nonprofit insurance plans, include companies such as Blue Cross, Blue Shield, and Delta Dental. These operate under special state-enabling laws that give them an exclusive franchise to the whole state (or a part of it) and to a specific type of insurance. For example, Blue Cross, in most instances, sells only hospital coverage; Blue Shield, only medical insurance; and Delta Dental, only dental insurance. Because they are non-profit, they are tax-exempt and at the same time subject to tighter state regulation than the commercial health insurance companies. Combined, the nonprofit and commercial carriers have sold most of the private health insurance in the United States recently (Lee & Estes, 1997).

INDEPENDENT HEALTH PLANS

Independent or self-insured health plans underwrite the remaining private health insurance in the United States. These plans have been offered through several hundred smaller organizations such as businesses, unions, consumer cooperatives, and medical groups. The HMOs and various companies' self-insured plans also are included in this category. They may sell only health insurance, or in some cases, they also may provide health services; they focus on a localized population. As a group, they generate a large amount of premium revenues but only a small percentage of the amount generated by the nonprofit and commercial health insurance companies. In the late 1980s, the United States had over 1000 for-profit, commercial health insurers and 85 Blue Cross and Blue Shield plans. The managed care movement since has become one of the most common and rapidly expanding forms of health insurance (Wolf & Gorman, 1996).

GOVERNMENT HEALTH PROGRAMS

Government health programs make up the largest source of third-party reimbursement in the United States. The government's four major health insurance programs are Medicare, Medicaid, the Federal Employees Health Benefits Plan, and the Civilian Health and Medical Program of the Uniformed Services. Combined, government funding is responsible for a lower portion of health care financing in the United States than in other countries in the world: just over 43.5% compared with 98% for Norway, 86% for the United Kingdom, 75% for Canada, and 72% for Australia (U.S. Department of Commerce, 1998). Of the government's health insurance programs, Medicare and Medicaid constitute the largest.

Medicare

Medicare, known as Title XVIII of the Social Security Act Amendments of 1965, provides mandatory federal health insurance for adults aged 65 and older and certain disabled persons. It is the largest health insurer in the United States, covering about 16% of the population. Of Medicare's almost 39 million beneficiaries, 12% (4.5 million people in 1996) are younger than 65 years of age and are disabled, whereas another 9% are aged 85 years and older (The Henry J. Kaiser Family Foundation [Kaiser Family Foundation], 1998a). The Medicare population is projected to

grow to 44.5 million by 2008 and to over 63 million by 2027 (Figs. 7–1 and 7–2).

Medicare is administered by the Health Care Financing Administration (HCFA) of the U.S. Department of Health and Human Services. Part A of Medicare, the hospital insurance program, covers inpatient hospitals, limited-skilled nursing facilities, and home health and hospice services to participants eligible for Social Security. It is financed through trust funds derived from employment payroll taxes. Part B, the supplementary and voluntary medical insurance program, primarily covers physician services but also covers home health care for beneficiaries not covered under part A. It is funded through enrollee monthly premiums (about 25%) and a tax-supported federal subsidy (about 75%).

Until recently, Medicare had been managed in the same manner for over 30 years. In August 1997, President Clinton signed the Balanced Budget Act (P.L. 105–33), which took effect in 1998. This act provided Medicare beneficiaries with markedly different options. In addition, the National Bipartisan Commission on the Future of Medicare was established by Congress in 1997 to consider options to preserve the fiscal integrity of the program while sustaining health coverage for an aging baby boom generation. One of the plans being considered by this committee is an increase in the eligibility age for Medicare from 65 to 67 over a 24-year span. This could save $620 billion over 30 years and would affect the entire baby boom generation. Decisions on this plan have not been made. Financing Medicare benefits into the future while maintaining or improving coverage for elderly and disabled beneficiaries remains the major challenge facing the program (Firshein, 1999; Kaiser Family Foundation, 1998a).

Among the most significant alterations brought about by the Balanced Budget Act are those to the fast-growing managed-care side of Medicare, which in 1998 covered about 15% of enrollees. To control Medicare costs while expanding the range of available health care options, beneficiaries are offered a new

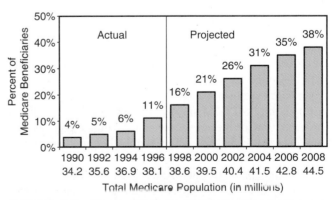

SOURCE: Health Care Financing Administration, *Medicare managed care contract report summary*, December 1990, 1992, 1994, 1996; Congressional Budget Office, *The economic and budget outlook: fiscal years 1999–2008*, January, 1998.

FIGURE 7–1. Enrollment in Medicare HMOs and other Medicare+Choice plans, 1990–2008.

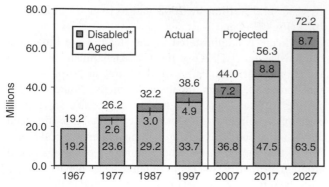

*Includes beneficiaries whose eligibility is based solely on end-stage renal disease (96,000 in 1997).
SOURCE: Health Care Financing Administration, Office of the Actuary, April 1998.

FIGURE 7–2. Number of Medicare beneficiaries, fiscal year 1967–2027.

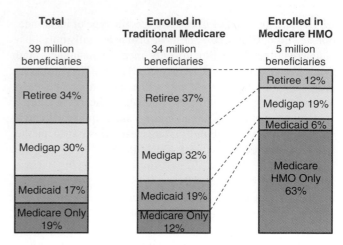

Note: Retiree includes those with retiree health and Medigap; Medigap also includes "other."
SOURCE: Eppig, F. & Chulis, G. (Fall 1997). Trends in medicare supplementary insurance, 1992-96, *Health Care Financing Review, 19* (1), 201–206.

FIGURE 7–3. Medicare beneficiaries by supplemental coverage, 1996.

program called Medicare+Choice. This program seeks to accelerate the migration of patients away from Medicare's traditional and more expensive FFS program into various managed care options. Enrollees opting to remain in traditional Medicare will continue to be covered by the traditional FFS program, which gives patients unlimited choice of doctors, hospitals, and other providers. Those moving to the Medicare+Choice will have a limited choice of providers but, in return, will be offered options such as joining coordinated care plans, including HMOs, preferred provider organizations (PPOs), provider-sonsored organizations, private FFS plans, and on a limited basis, medical savings account plans. With this new law, Medicare has changed from a FFS, when-you-are-sick program to a preventive and wellness program (U.S. Department of Health and Human Services, 1997).

Although Medicare attempts to meet a need among the elderly in the United States, it has significant gaps. Medicare has high deductibles, no cap on out-of-pocket expenditures, and no outpatient prescription drug coverage. As a result, it covers less than half of the elderly's total health spending and is less generous than health plans typically offered by large employers. In 1997, beneficiaries spent an average of 21% of their household income for health services and premiums. To cover cost sharing and supplement Medicare's benefit package, two thirds of all Medicare beneficiaries have additional insurance divided evenly between Medigap policies and retiree health benefits (Kaiser Family Foundation, 1998a) (Fig. 7–3).

Medicare funding, drawn primarily from working people's taxes to benefit the elderly, will need to find new revenue sources in the future. As the population of elderly increases, fewer workers will be available to support the program. In 1960, there were five workers for each Medicare beneficiary. Projections for the year 2040 have said that there will be just 1.9 workers for each beneficiary (DeLew et al., 1992).

Medicaid

Medicaid, known as Title XIX of the Social Security Act Amendments of 1965, provides medical assistance for individuals and families with low incomes and resources. It is jointly funded between federal and state governments to assist the states in the provision of adequate medical care to eligible needy persons. The states have some discretion in determining which groups their Medicaid programs will cover and the financial criteria for Medicaid eligibility. To be eligible for federal funds, however, states are required to provide Medicaid coverage for most individuals who receive federally assisted income maintenance payments, as well as for related groups not receiving cash payments. The following are examples of the mandatory Medicaid eligibility groups (U.S. Department of Health and Human Services, 1998):

Recipients of Aid to Families With Dependent Children (AFDC)

Supplemental Security Income recipients

Infants born to Medicaid-eligible pregnant women

Children younger than age 6 and pregnant women who meet the state's AFDC financial requirements or whose family income is at or below 133% of the federal poverty level

Recipients of adoption assistance and foster care under title IV-E of the Social Security Act

Certain Medicare beneficiaries (qualified disabled workers and certain poor Medicare recipients)

Special protected groups who lose cash assistance because of the cash programs' rules

Coverage includes preventive, acute, and long-term care services. Potential Medicaid recipients must apply for coverage and prove their eligibility in terms of category and limited income.

In 1996, 41.3 million low-income Americans were enrolled in Medicaid at a cost of $155 billion (Kaiser Family Foundation, 1998c). As with Medicare, Medicaid programs moved to a managed care concept, following mandates within the Balanced Budget Act of 1997. The move has not been without its problems for those receiving Medicaid. Medicaid beneficiaries are economically disadvantaged, frequently reside in medically underserved areas, and often have more complex health and social needs than do Americans with higher incomes. Early evidence on the implementation of Medicaid managed care shows some improvement in access to a regular provider but more difficulties in obtaining care and dissatisfaction with care compared with those in Medicaid FFS (Kaiser Family Foundation, 1998c). Nevertheless, Medicaid's use of managed care has grown dramatically; Medicaid recipients enrolled in a broad array of managed care arrangements increased from 10% in 1991 to 37% in 1996 and are projected to continue to increase (U.S. Dept. of Health and Human Services, 1998). The future success of Medicaid managed care depends on the adequacy of the **capitation rates** (a fixed amount of money paid per person by the health plan to the provider for covered services) and the ability of state and federal government to monitor access and quality. Quality performance standards are evolving, and ensuring access and quality of care in a managed care environment will require fiscally solvent plans, established provider networks, education of providers and beneficiaries about managed care, and awareness of the unique needs of the Medicaid population (Kaiser Family Foundation, 1998c).

Other Government Programs

A federal health insurance program known as the Consolidated Omnibus Budget Reconciliation Act developed in 1985—this one designated to be self-financing—protects the unemployed who have lost their benefits. Another workers' compensation program is state administered and requires employers to pay health care costs of workers who sustain illness or injury associated with their jobs. In addition to third-party reimbursement, the government offers some direct health services to selected populations, including Native Americans, military personnel, veterans, merchant marines, and federal employees.

CLAIMS PAYMENT AGENTS

Claims payment agents administer the claims payment process of government third-party payments. That is, the government contracts with private agents to handle the claims payment process. More than 80% of the government's third-party payments have been handled by these private contractors, who sometimes are known as fiscal intermediaries (when processing Medicare hospital claims), carriers (when dealing with insurance under Medicare), or fiscal agents (as applied to Medicaid programs). As an example, Blue Cross, in addition to being a private insurance company, also is a claims payment agent for Medicare.

Direct Consumer Reimbursement

A second major source of health care financing comes from direct fees paid by consumers. This refers to individual out-of-pocket payments made for several different reasons. One is payments made by individuals who have no insurance coverage so that fees must be paid directly for health and medical services. Another is for limited coverage and exclusions (services for which the consumer must bear the entire expense). For example, many individuals carry only major medical insurance and must pay directly for physician office visits, prescriptions, eye glasses, and dental care. In other instances, the insurance contract may include a deductible amount that must be paid by the insuree before reimbursement begins (eg, the first day of hospital care under Medicare must be paid by the patient, which was $768 per benefit period in 1999). The contract may be established on a copayment basis, which determines a percentage to be paid by the insurer and the rest by the individual. Or, the individual may pay the remainder of a health service bill after the insurer has paid a previously agreed-on fixed amount, such as a fixed coverage for labor and delivery. Direct consumer payment has accounted for approximately one third of total personal health care expenditures in the United States.

Private Support

Private or philanthropic support, a third source, contributes both directly and indirectly to health care financing. Many private agencies fund programs, underwrite research, and provide benefits for people who otherwise would go without services. In addition, volunteerism, the efforts of numerous individuals and organizations who donate their time and services, provides tremendous cost savings to health care institutions. It also enables many individuals to receive services, such as home-delivered meals or transportation to health care facilities, at no charge. Philanthropic financing of health care has significantly decreased in the last two decades. However, continued private support is essential, particularly when federal and state monies for health and social programs have been severely restricted (Williams & Torrens, 1999).

TRENDS AND ISSUES INFLUENCING HEALTH CARE ECONOMICS

Cost Control

Control of rapidly rising costs has been one of the largest driving forces behind health care reform in the 1980s and 1990s. Despite a variety of cost-control strategies tried by public and private-sector payers, health care costs have continued to rise. Health expenditures in 1980 accounted for 9.1% of the **gross national product** (GNP), which is the total value of all goods and services produced in the United States economy in 1 year. Health expenditures rose to 12.6% of the GNP by 1990, to 14.1% in 1994, and then modified somewhat to 14% in 1997 (U.S. Department of Commerce, 1998). In 1999, HCFA estimated that health expenditures would rise to $2.1 trillion by the year 2007, but with managed care, the impact of HMOs, and the general concern about health care costs held by all members of the health care community, this prediction has not held true (Federwisch, 1999). "The United States spends more on health care services than does any other nation—on average, more than twice as much per person as the other OECD countries [Organization for Economic Cooperation and Development made up of 15 nations including the U.S.]" (DeLaw et al., 1992, p. 151). Of the United States' total health care spending in 1996, hospital care accounted for about 47%; physician services, 14%; nursing home care, 10%; home health care, 4%; public health activities, 7.5%; and administration, 3%. The missing percentages are for items not listed separately (U.S. Department of Commerce, 1998). Figure 7–4 portrays the nation's health dollar—its source and its destination in 1994.

Health care costs in the United States remain high; however, they have decelerated from the escalating costs experienced during the 1970s and 1980s, when they were spiraling out of control. A major factor contributing to the high health care costs of those two decades was that health care providers were rewarded for focusing on the tertiary level of preventative care—the highest level of health care services and the most expensive—rather than focusing on the less-expensive primary and secondary health care practices.

Since the early 1990s, out-of-pocket health care expenditures for clients have dropped (Levit et al., 1996). Areas that did see increases include nursing home care, medications, and dental care costs. However, the overall trend is hopeful. The more moderate rise in the cost of health care has resulted from the reduction and elimination of the FFS payment system and its replacment by the primary prevention–focused PPS.

A focus on primary prevention demands a paradigm shift in thinking about the practice and delivery of health care. It is one that fits more closely with the mission of public health. It expects that citizens are involved in their health care, are knowledgeable about their health status, manage self-care practices, and modify lifestyle behaviors to promote wellness. This creates a rich environment for community health nursing to work in collaboration with primary care practitioners and other health care professionals to keep the cost of health care under control while providing quality care focusing on primary prevention.

Cost sharing is a cost-containment strategy in which consumers pay a portion of health care costs. Insurance deductibles of $100 to $500 per person per year are typical, as are coinsurance rates of 20% per service. Cost sharing has

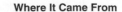
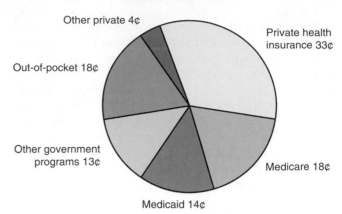

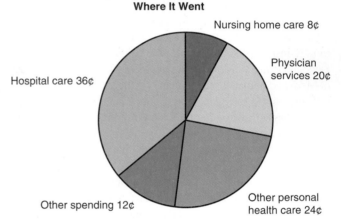

Note: Other private includes industrial in-plant health services, nonpatient revenues, and privately financed construction. Other personal health care includes dental, other professional services, home health care, drugs, and other nondurable medical products, vision products and other durable medical products, and other miscellaneous health care services.
Other spending covers program administration and the net cost of private health insurance, government public health, and research and construction.

FIGURE 7–4. The nation's health dollar—where it came from and where it went in 1994. (*Health Care Financing Review* [1996], *17*(3), 217.)

successfully reduced utilization of health services without having negative health effects. Utilization review techniques have further enhanced utilization and cost control. However, the usefulness of cost sharing, when considering coverage for low-income and some elderly persons, appears to have limited value (Sultz & Young, 1999).

Global Cost Control

Internationally, health care expenditures also are of concern. Health care costs consumed a greater percentage of the Unites States' GNP in most of the OECD countries from 1980 to 1997. Health care expenditures remained the same over those 17 years in Turkey and Sweden and decreased in Denmark. Public health expenditures rose 60% in the United States during those years, while in other countries, the increase was more modest, and in four countries—Denmark, Ireland, Italy, and Sweden—it decreased. It seems likely that the health of citizens in the countries who have been spending less on health care over the last 20 years or who have spent a smaller share of their GNP might be poorer (U.S. Department of Commerce, 1998); however, this is not necessarily true. The United States ranks below 16 other countries, including Italy and Sweden, in life expectancy (Display 7–1). Using health care dollars wisely, promoting health through primary prevention, and combining other factors such as heredity, diet, exercise, attitude, and a moderate pace of life all contribute to longevity.

Access to Health Services: The Uninsured and Underinsured

A growing segment of the U.S. population has limited or no access to health care because they are without coverage for health services. The consequences of not getting needed medical care are not trivial and can result in unnecessary hospitalization and serious health problems. Over 41 million Americans were uninsured in 1998—nearly 18% of the total nonelderly population (Kaiser Family Foundation, 1998b). This is an increase from 14% in 1991. Who are the uninsured? They are predominantly workers and their families, many of whom have low incomes. Display 7–2 highlights some of the dramatic figures among the uninsured population.

DISPLAY 7–2. Who Are the Uninsured?

- Eight of 10 of the uninsured are full-time workers or their dependents.
- Only 10% of the uninsured are in families with no connections to the work force.
- Over half of the uninsured (54%) have low incomes, making less than 200% of the federal poverty level.
- The poor comprise a fifth of the uninsured population.
- The near-poor run the highest risk of being uninsured because they may not qualify for Medicaid and often cannot afford health insurance.
- Twenty-seven percent of the near-poor are uninsured.
- Partly because of Medicaid's eligibility categories, low income, young men are more likely to be uninsured than women—nearly half (46%) are uninsured compared with 27% of low-income, young women.
- Although most (56%) of the uninsured are white, Hispanics (22%) and African Americans (17%) are over represented among the uninsured population.

The Henry J. Kaiser Family Foundation. [1998b, July]. *Uninsured facts: The uninsured and their access to health care.* Washington, DC: Author.)

DISPLAY 7–1. Life Expectancy in Selected Countries

Country	1998	Projected for 2000
United States	76.1	76.3
Australia	79.9	80.4
Austria	77.3	77.6
Belgium	77.4	77.7
Canada	79.2	79.6
France	78.5	78.8
Germany	77.0	77.3
Greece	78.3	78.6
Hong Kong	78.8	79.0
Italy	78.4	78.6
Japan	80.0	80.2
Netherlands	78.0	78.3
Spain	77.6	77.9
Sweden	79.2	79.4
Switzerland	78.9	79.1
Taiwan	76.8	78.2
United Kingdom	77.2	77.5

The poor and the elderly are among the most vulnerable to access problems. Although the PPS has cost-saving benefits, it also has negative effects. The PPS has shortened hospital length of stays, on average by 24%. But researchers from RAND–University of California, Los Angeles found "that under PPS elderly patients were 43 percent more likely to be discharged in an unstable condition than before" and that the risk of dying for these patients was much higher than before (Warden, 1993). Measures were taken to reduce risks to discharged patients with a broadening array of home care services expanding since the 1980s (see Chapter 37). To control costs in the health care setting, the Balanced Budget Act also affected home care services. It is projected to reduce federal government spending on the program by $116.4 billion between fiscal years 1998 and 2002 and by making numerous changes to the way programs operate (Harris, 1998). This is another example of reducing costs at the more expensive tertiary level of prevention. As a result, real people with disease processes in progress are affected.

Medicare+Choice, created in 1997, was intended to increase beneficiary participation in HMOs and other private plans.

Because beneficiaries enrolled in HMOs are on average healthier than those in the traditional

Medicare program, according to many studies, the Medicare HMO program has resulted in increased Medicare spending, rather than achieving expected savings. The new law requires that beginning January 1, 2000, the Health Care Financing Administration (HCFA) adjusts payments to plans for the health status of enrollees to more accurately reflect the health needs of enrollees and prevent financial losses to the program (Kaiser Family Foundation, 1998a).

The Medicaid program, too, depends on managed care to deliver services to the 41.3 million Americans enrolled in Medicaid in 1996. In 1997, all states (except Alaska and Wyoming) were pursuing some managed care initiatives (Fig. 7–5). Because Medicaid operates under tight budget constraints, this has resulted in provider payment rates that often are substantially below market rates, contributing to access problems. Capitation rates need to be sufficient to ensure that plans are able to care for Medicaid enrollees. The future success of Medicaid managed care depends on the adequacy of the capitation rates and the ability of state and federal government to monitor access and quality (Kaiser Family Foundation, 1998c).

In the private sector, numerous firms do not offer health insurance to their employees; nearly 80% of the uninsured are employees of these firms or are their dependents (Kaiser Family Foundation, 1998b). Self-employed individuals also find it difficult to pay the higher costs of insurance premiums without the benefit of group rates. Consequently, many of the self-employed can access health services only by making expensive out-of-pocket payments.

Managed Care

The term **managed care** became popular in the late 1980s and early 1990s. It refers to systems that coordinate medical care for specific groups to promote provider efficiency and control costs. Although the term is relatively new, the concept has been practiced for many years through a variety of models of alternative health care delivery. It is a cost control strategy used in both public and private sectors of health care. Care is "managed" by regulating the use of services and levels of provider payment. This approach includes the use of HMOs and PPOs. In contrast to FFS models, these operate on a prospective payment basis and control costs by managing utilization and provider payments. The managed care model encourages the provision of services within fixed budgets, thus avoiding cost escalation. However, if a system rewards increased FFS billings, managed care can provide only a partial solution to controlling utilization. These are issues that different managed care organizations (MCOs) are trying to eliminate.

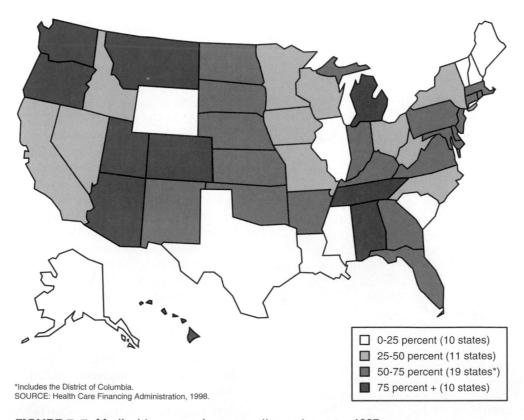

*Includes the District of Columbia.
SOURCE: Health Care Financing Administration, 1998.

☐ 0-25 percent (10 states)
▨ 25-50 percent (11 states)
▨ 50-75 percent (19 states*)
■ 75 percent + (10 states)

FIGURE 7–5. Medicaid-managed care enrollment by state, 1997.

HEALTH MAINTENANCE ORGANIZATIONS

A **health maintenance organization** (HMO) is a system in which participants prepay a fixed monthly premium to receive comprehensive health services delivered by a defined network of providers to plan participants. The HMOs are the oldest model of coordinated or managed care. Several HMOs have existed for decades, but many have developed recently. Enrollees benefit from lower costs, less cost sharing, and minimal billing paperwork.

From 1930 to 1965, the HMO movement, supported initially by the private sector, gradually gained federal backing. Group plans were a part of Medicare and Medicaid bills and the Partnership for Health Act. The HMO Act of 1973 demonstrated stronger federal support. Amendments to this act in 1976 lifted restrictions and further encouraged HMO growth. Currently, there are numerous HMOs with much internal diversity in the industry. However, HMOs continue to claim unique properties (Harrington & Estes, 1997):

There is a contract between the HMO and the beneficiaries (or their representative), the enrolled population.

They absorb prospective risk.

A regular (usually monthly) premium to cover specified (typically comprehensive) benefits is paid by each enrollee to the HMO; few additional charges are levied because the payment mechanism is not FFS.

They have an integrated delivery system with provider incentives for efficiency. The HMO contracts with professional providers to deliver the services due the enrollees; the basis for reimbursing those providers varies among HMOs.

Official encouragement, government subsidies, and the pressures for cost control spurred the growth of HMOs. Some HMOs follow the traditional model that employs the health professionals, such as physicians and nurses, builds their own hospital and clinic facilities, and serves only their own enrollees. Other HMOs provide some services while contracting for the rest. Variations of the HMO model include solo practice physicians (some also continuing FFS medicine) who affiliate with hospitals. Americans enrolled in HMOs—whether through government programs like Medicare, employer-based programs, or private insurers—number more than 130 million people (American Public Health Association [APHA], 1998a). The HMOs have been viewed as a positive alternative delivery system because of their potential for conserving costs resulting from their emphasis on prevention, health promotion, and ambulatory care, with a concomitant reduction in hospital and medical care utilization. However, some have questioned whether the cost savings might result partly from favorable selection of enrollees. Quality concerns also have been raised about the danger of underserving enrollees to stay within payment limits (Sultz & Young, 1999; APHA, 1998a). A Harris poll conducted in 1990 showed that only 7% of those surveyed were "very interested" in joining an HMO, and 63% were "hardly interested" or "not at all interested" (Merline, 1993). Nevertheless, since the expanding years of HMOs in the early 1990s, many have chosen a managed care plan, and by 1997, over 130 million people were enrolled in an HMO (APHA, 1998a).

> The American Public Health Association has significant concerns about the ongoing changes in the organization and financing of medical care and health services and the impact of these changes on public health. While managed care arrangements hold the promise of providing affordable, quality health care for our nation, reports of financial considerations taking precedence over patients' health deserve attention. Specific issues of concern include denials of necessary care, underfunding of public health and prevention services, lack of accountability, loss of choice of health care provider, inadequate access to care (especially specialists), lack of comparable and consumer-friendly information and data about health plans, and abuses in marketing (APHA, 1998a).

These concerns did not go unattended. The Health Insurance Portability and Accountability Act of 1996 and the Newborns' and Mothers' Health Protection Act of 1996 were passed by the 104th Congress of the United States and were signed into law by the President. Both significant pieces of legislation addressed health care concerns among the nation's citizens and official organizations such as the APHA. The Health Insurance Portability and Accountability Act assured people that they would not lose health care coverage if they changed jobs. In addition, for a while in the United States, insurance for labor and delivery hospitalization covered only 24 hours or less after the delivery. Infants and mothers were being sent home in unstable postdelivery conditions. Newborns would go home when younger than 1 day, in some cases so soon after birth that body temperature was not stabilized and the ability to suck and take the breast or formula was not established. The Newborns' and Mothers' Health Protection Act eliminated such "drive-by deliveries," ensuring that mothers and newborns would have the right to remain in the acute care setting for at least 48 hours, covered by their insurance plan. Furthermore, in 1998, the 105th Congress considered the Patients' Bill of Rights, modeled after recommendations from the Advisory Commission on Consumer Protection and Quality, which stipulated that managed care plans (APHA, 1998a):

Provide emergency services

Are legally liable for medical malpractice

May not use "gag" clauses in provider contracts

Offer sufficient access to specialists, including direct access to specialists for ongoing treatment and obstetricians-gynecologists for women

Offer an external, accessible, independent appeals process for service denials

May not retaliate against "whistle blowers"

May not offer financial incentives to providers to discourage service utilization by patients

Incorporate quality assurance programs

Reimburse for approved clinical trials

APHA policy supports all of these reforms as they address, at the federal level, some of the problems occurring in the HMO plans during the years of significant growth.

PREFERRED PROVIDER ORGANIZATIONS

A **preferred provider organization** is another model of managed or coordinated care that developed earlier than the HMO. A PPO is a network of physicians, hospitals, and other health-related services that contracts with a third-party payer organization to provide comprehensive health services to subscribers on a fixed FFS basis. Because of contractual fixed costs, employing organizations who subscribe can offer medical services to their employees at discounted rates. In PPOs, consumer choice exists. Enrollees have a choice among providers within the plan and contracted providers out of the plan. The PPOs practice utilization review and use formal standards for selecting providers.

Despite achieving large discounts (approximately 10% to 20%), some nationwide PPOs (Blue Cross and Blue Shield) pay at rates substantially above Medicare levels, attracting a bevy of providers (Verrilli & Zuckerman, 1996). Enrollment in PPOs grew from about 10 plans in 1981 to over 700 plans in 1994. The number of people enrolled in PPOs also increased from an estimated 10.4% of individuals with private insurance in 1988 to 43% in 1993 (Employee Benefit Research Institute, 1995). These numbers leveled off as the decade came to a close. Early use of PPOs appeared to promote cost savings, but the long-range cost effectiveness of this model has yet to be proved, especially with the expansion of HMOs.

Other variations on managed care models continue to appear. One is the point-of-service network, which combines HMO cost containment with PPO freedom to choose providers. Enrollees may use their HMO's physicians or may select outside physicians by paying a higher coinsurance charge (Sultz & Young, 1999). Issues of cost, quality, extent of coverage, and freedom to choose providers remain dominant in discussions of the managed care concept.

Health Care Rationing

The concept of **rationing** in health care refers to limiting the provision of adequate health services to save costs, but in so doing jeopardizing the well-being of some groups of people. Rationing implies that resources are limited and therefore must be used sparingly. Its effect is to restrict people's choices and deny access to beneficial services. Although some consumer choice is involved, mostly it is the providers and insurers of health services who are unilaterally making rationing decisions to contain costs. When rationing occurs, there always is the danger of compromising what is acceptable to consumers and the quality of services that they receive.

Rationing in health care has been practiced for many years. With limited resources for health services delivery, government programs have had to establish strict eligibility levels and monitor the use of these resources sparingly to ensure their most equitable distribution. Private insurers, to maintain organizational viability and some kind of profit margin, have engaged in rationing to exclude enrollees at greatest risk of health problems (Sultz & Young, 1999). Advances in knowledge and technical capabilities through research and technology compounds rationing decisions. When several individuals need an organ transplant and only one organ is available, what criteria should be used to select the recipient? Now that it is known that certain lifestyle behaviors, such as smoking or driving without restraints, create health risks, should people who engage in these activities pay a higher price for health care or should they be excluded from certain services? Should a younger person needing specialized surgery take priority over an elderly person needing similar care? There are no easy answers. Providers and insurers have struggled with these difficult policy issues for years. In today's health economics, the problems are even more complex.

Competition and Regulation

Competition and regulation in health economics often have been viewed as antagonistic and incompatible concepts. **Competition** means a contest between rival health care organizations for resources and clients. **Regulation** refers to mandated procedures and practices affecting health services delivery that are enforced by law. In a society where freedom of choice and individualism have long been valued, competition provides opportunities for entrepreneurism, free enterprise, and scientific advancement. Yet to promote the public good, oversee equitable distribution of health services, and foster community-wide participation, regulation also serves an important role. Health care incorporates four major kinds of regulation: (1) laws, (2) regulations, (3) programs, and (4) policies (Brown, 1992). Laws that regulate health care include any legislation that governs financing or delivery of health services, such as legislation regulating Medicare reimbursement to hospitals. Regulations "clarify and guide implementation" (Brown, 1992, p. 20); they are issued under the authority of law and are part of most federal health care programs. Examples include regulations governing project grants such as HMO development, formula grants such as Hill-Burton, and entitlements such as Medicare and Medicaid. Regulatory programs are created from free-standing legislative enactments and are designed to accomplish specific goals such as accreditation and licensing rules for hospitals, public health agencies, and other health service providers. Regulatory policies have a broader focus and involve "decisions that shape the health care system by constraining the flow of resources into it and setting limits on key players' freedom of action" (Brown, 1992, p. 21). Examples of regulatory policies are found by reviewing state or federal budget proposals for funding programs such as health manpower training, research, and technology development.

From the 1950s through the 1970s, the federal government assumed a strong role in the regulation of health services. First, federal subsidy of health care costs increased, and there was greater federal control of state programs. Health services became regionalized and more comprehensive. Federal appropriations supported operational as well as capital and planning costs. There was greater federal support for health research and the training of health professionals. Group medical practice multiplied as a cost-saving measure. Over 60% of the population was covered by some form of prepaid health insurance, largely because of the effects of Medicare and Medicaid. There was an increase in inter-agency health planning cooperation and im-

proved health program evaluation. Neighborhood health centers, community mental health centers, and other programs developed to improve health care access for everyone. Although costs were rising, it was a period of relative economic stability that emphasized quality of care. During this period, the federal government assumed a major role, regulating the planning, use, and reimbursement of health care services.

In the early 1980s, the passage of the Omnibus Budget Reconciliation Act caused dramatic changes affecting health care. The federal government, having failed to contain rising health care costs, shifted responsibility for the public's health and welfare back to state and local governments. Large amounts of federal funding for health research, health manpower training, and public health programs were withdrawn. Continued escalation of health care costs prompted a concentrated effort among public and private providers alike to find cost-containment measures. From all this grew the competition-versus-regulation debate (see Bridging Financial Gaps).

Competition, its proponents say, offers wider consumer choice and positive incentives for cost containment and en-

Bridging Financial Gaps

Chronically Ill Equally Satisfied With Medicare HMOs as Traditional Care: Older Americans Report, October 9, 1998, pp. 325–326, Sachs Group, *info@sachs.com*

The Sachs Group (a health care market research company) studied 16,200 seniors in 33 market areas for overall satisfaction with Medicare HMO plans. The results dispelled several common myths or perceptions associated with selection, enrollment, satisfaction, and care of the chronically ill. The findings are particularly significant because chronically ill seniors are heavy users of health care services. Key findings include:

- Medicare HMO members receive more preventive care than seniors in Medicare only, and more HMO members used physician services than their counterparts in other plans.
- Chronically ill seniors are nearly as likely to enroll in Medicare HMOs as their counterparts in Medicare supplemental and Medicare only plans.
- The results challenge the perception that managed care may not be appropriate health coverage for seniors with chronic conditions.
- In five areas—member services, physician access, medical quality, cost, and plan benefits—chronically ill HMO members surveyed were equally satisfied as chronically ill Medicare supplemental plan members.
- Among seniors with chronic illnesses, 92% in Medicare HMOs were satisfied with costs vs. 86% for Medicare only and 83% for Medicare supplemental members.
- In the area of medical management, such as policies regarding specialty referrals, chronically ill Medicare

supplemental plan members were most satisfied (95%), followed by chronically ill Medicare only members (90%) and chronically ill Medicare HMO members (86%).
- Medicare HMO members utilize primary care physician and urgent care services more often, but emergency and home health services less often, than members of other Medicare plan types.
- For six out of eight preventive services and screenings examined, Medicare HMO members received equal or more care than Medicare supplemental and Medicare only members. These six services include cholesterol screenings, colorectal cancer tests, prostate exams, mammograms, pap smears, and routine physicals.
- More than 50% have been enrolled in their plans for more than 5 years, and chronically ill seniors choose health plans for the same reasons as healthy seniors. Top selection drivers were hospital location, physician location, physician location, and prescription drug benefits.

To further improve satisfaction and decrease disenrollment of chronically ill seniors, Medicare HMOs can take several approaches: engage members by encouraging them to participate in services and offerings, particularly those of a preventive nature; empower members to take an active role in managing their health; adjust the policy to better meet members' prescription needs, and streamline the referral processes and educate members and physicians to improve satisfaction with medical management. HMOs' emphasis on outpatient and preventive care may contribute to improved health and, ultimately, increased retention of the chronically ill.

hanced efficiency (Sultz & Young, 1999); that is, consumers are free to select among various health plans on the basis of cost, quality, and range of services. Competing providers must develop efficient production and distribution methods to stay in business, and consumers, because of the required cost sharing that is part of the competition model, are more likely to use only necessary services. Examples of competition are increasingly evident as more health plans, including HMOs and PPOs, vie with insurance companies for subscribers. Many hospitals, too, compete aggressively for patients. For example, some hospitals now promote their services with advertisements depicting the new mother and father having a candlelight dinner in the hospital with their newborn infant in the bassinet beside them, or the surgical center promoting the "hotel guest" concept with dramatically appointed rooms and meals and lodging for a guest.

Although it appears that competition offers the best service for the least cost, regulation advocates, for almost 20 years, argued that there are at least four problems associated with the competition model: (1) consumers often do not make proper health care choices because of limited knowledge of health services; (2) competition may discriminate against enrolling certain consumers, especially high-risk, high-cost patients, thus excluding those who may need services the most; (3) the competition model may not encourage enough teaching and research—expensive elements of our present system; and (4) quality may be sacrificed to keep down costs (Cascio, 1998; Sultz & Young, 1999). Regulation advocates conclude that standardization and controls are needed to guarantee quality and equal access. Leaders in the field have concluded that both competition and regulation are needed (APHA, 1998b; Burris, 1997). With foresight, McNerney said, "It is rapidly becoming apparent that what we need is a proper balance between competition and regulation with more effective links . . . [and] regulation [should be] used as a force to keep the market honest" (1980, p. 1091).

MANAGED COMPETITION

The idea of managed competition was born from the controversy over competition versus regulation and was driven by the need for health care reform. **Managed competition,** it was hoped, would combine market competition to achieve cost savings with government regulation to achieve expanded coverage (Merline, 1993). This idea, whose origin is credited to economist Alain C. Enthoven of Stanford University, has played a major part in debates on health care reform. It seeks to address the two fundamental issues driving reform: cost containment and universal access to health care.

Managed competition was seen as a market-based solution that placed accountability for resolving the health care crisis with the insurance industry. Under this concept, sponsors in the form of collective purchasing agents represent consumers clustered into large groups. The sponsors negotiate with insurers or health plans to offer subscribers an array of choices based on costs and quality among various health plans. Insurers must accept all applicants without excluding those at poorer risk and at the same time must control costs (Mucklo, 1993).

Under managed competition, consumers would choose between competing health insurance plans in the form of "super-HMOs" that are for-profit and privately owned. These plans must "compete for managed care contracts from large employers and group purchasers known as 'health insurance purchasing cooperatives'" (HIPCs) (Young, 1993, p. 945). The proposed HIPCs would be mostly geographically based (region or state), quasigovernmental organizations that would consolidate purchasing power in the health care market. The HIPCs would contract only with insurers whose plans both meet federal guidelines and include a mandated package of basic benefits (Merline, 1993), hence, the "managed" or regulated segment. Insurance companies also would have to prepare regular reports on the quality of their services to give consumers a basis for making an informed comparison among plans. Other common features of managed competition proposals included regulation that prevents screening out high-risk enrollees, penalties for companies that try to achieve better risk pools, community ratings to prevent companies from setting rates by risk pool, and guaranteed coverage for all who apply (Congressional Budget Office, 1993).

Proponents of managed competition cite many advantages. Managed competition would encourage insurance companies to compete on price and quality of services to attract enrollees. It would also offer consumers tax incentive to purchase the lowest cost plans that meet minimum benefits requirements. Managed competition, although market driven, would be highly regulated to ensure quality and access. Besides HIPCs, some managed care proposals include the formation of two additional government bodies: "a National Health Board to set the minimum benefits package, and an Outcomes Management Standards Board to set standards for the health plans' reporting on the quality of their care" (Merline, 1993, p. 2). Thus, managed competition, as a reform concept, would have the potential for reducing expenditures and improving access to health care coverage.

There are problems, however, with managed competition. It remains untested anywhere in the world, and many believe that it will fail to achieve the needed cuts in the growth of health care spending. Similar models, such as HMOs and the Federal Employee Health Benefits Program, have failed to slow health care inflation (Kronick et al., 1993). Nearly 25% of U.S. health care spending has gone to billing and bureaucracy because of the heavy administrative burden imposed by multiple private insurers; this is compared with only 11% of Canadian health care spending. Private insurance overhead in the United States averages 13% of premiums, whereas for Medicare and Medicaid administration it is less than 3%, and for Canada's single-payer system it is less than 1%. Some critics believe that managed competition's regulations will result in additional administrative layers, increasing overhead and driving health care costs even higher (Young, 1993).

Some argue that managed care networks, which enhance managed competition and enable health insurance plans to control cost and quality, also would limit consumers' choices in selecting their own providers and hospitals. Consumers would have to pay out of pocket if they choose services outside of the network. Cost-saving incentives built into managed competition networks still have the potential for reduced quality of services and denial of care to enrollees.

Another major criticism of managed competition is its potential failure to provide equitable and universal coverage. Proposals differ about whether employers are required to provide health insurance coverage for their employees. One study done by the Employee Benefits Research Institute in 1993 shows that large employers would benefit financially under managed competition, whereas small businesses would find the cost burden heavy, and many individuals, such as the self-employed, would remain uninsured (Mucklo, 1993). Questions remain concerning the tax treatment of health insurance premiums, how sponsors should be organized, and what standard benefits should be offered. A basic benefits package, critics argue, must address special concerns affecting such groups as women and the elderly, including coverage for long-term care, home care, mental health, abortions, and prescriptions. Competition among providers would be inefficient in rural areas with fewer providers, such as county nursing agencies and isolated small-town hospitals scattered over great distances.

Although the private insurance industry and many physicians endorse the managed competition concept, a growing number of groups in the United States strongly oppose it. Among the organizations opposing managed competition and supporting some kind of single-payer plan are the American Nurses Association, the National League for Nursing, the National Women's Health Network, the APHA, Physicians for a National Health Program, the American Association for Retired Persons, and the Older Women's League. Dissatisfaction with managed competition as a reform solution has spurred a host of different proposals, all addressing cost savings and access issues.

UNIVERSAL COVERAGE AND A SINGLE-PAYER SYSTEM

A different approach to health care reform emphasizes universal health insurance coverage through a stronger role played by government. This so-called **single-payer system** would replace the nearly 1500 health insurance companies in the United States with a single, public-sector insurer that would entitle all citizens to **universal coverage.** Efforts to accomplish this approach have been evident for many years.

Growing concern over the cost and accessibility of health services in the 1960s and again in the mid-1970s led to a renewed focus on **national health insurance** (NHI) as a solution, whereby health insurance coverage would be provided for all citizens through a single-payer system. Since 1912, NHI has been debated while its proponents have sought comprehensive health care protection for the aged and needy, in particular. Numerous attempts to pass some form of NHI have resulted in piecemeal legislation that added various benefits for Social Security recipients. The Kerr-Mills Bill (1960) set a precedent of public financing for elderly persons who were "medically needy" but not on public assistance. Medicare (1965) was the first compulsory NHI program in the United States. By 1997, it reached 39 million people—only 13% of the population (APHA, 1998a).

In the 1970s, the debate over NHI revived in full force. Many proposed NHI bills were considered by Congress. The seeming consensus over the need for government to ensure access to needed health services for the total population was misleading. Divergent interests and conflicting philosophies led to heated debate with four issues emerging as core areas of controversy. First was the public-private mix. What should be the amount and nature of private health insurance involvement in the public program? Second was the cost-sharing issue. To what extent should consumers share in the cost of the coverage? Third, what should be the amount and nature of cost and quality controls built into the program? And fourth, should a NHI program be used as a vehicle for reform of the health care provision system? Resolution depended, in part, on reconciling the major roles of large private health insurers, hospitals, and the medical profession along with the nation's inherent aversion to direct government intervention.

In the 1980s, study of NHI as an important concept continued. In 1977, Somers and Somers recommended that NHI in its ideal form should include the following, and the intents remain current:

1. Universal coverage regardless of income
2. Equitable financing using multiple sources but channeled through one mechanism
3. Comprehensive and balanced benefit structure
4. Incentives for efficient and effective use of resources and discouragement of health care price inflation
5. Controlled competition in the underwriting and administration of the program
6. Appropriate and feasible consumer options
7. Administrative simplicity
8. Flexibility
9. Acceptability to providers and consumers

These recommendations continue to be viable and have permeated discussions on health care reform in the 1990s and into the 21st century.

Some proponents of universal coverage point to Canada's health care system as a model to emulate. Under the Canada Health Act, each provincial government is responsible for providing health care to all citizens. Each province must develop a plan that meets the following criteria (Young, 1993):

1. Provides universal coverage that does not interfere with reasonable access
2. Makes benefits transferable between provinces
3. Provides insurance for all medically necessary services
4. Is publicly administered and nonprofit

Canadian health services are primarily tax supported through provincial financing and national government subsidies. The system has been successful, but Canada has faced threats to that success in the form of a high national debt, a soaring budget deficit, rising health care costs, and an aging population, which "account(s) for about 50% of all health care dollars spent" (Barnhill, 1992, p. 44). Still, the principle of spreading the financial risk for health care over the entire population has worked in many countries, including Canada. Furthermore, polls indicate that most Americans "would prefer government-financed national health insurance" (Young, 1993, p. 946). Canada has taken some measures to keep its health care costs under control. Total health expenditures as a percentage of their GNP rose to 9.7% in 1995 but fell to the 1990 level of 9.3% by 1997 (U.S. Department of Commerce, 1998).

As a strategy for health care reform, proponents say a major advantage of the single-payer approach is that accountability for cost saving, quality, and access lie with a single payer, most likely the government. This contrasts with accountability resting in multiple, competing insurers under managed competition. Other advantages include its more comprehensive approach to reform, its limiting the role of private insurance, and eliminating the tie between health insurance and employment. Furthermore, a single-payer approach would significantly reduce administrative expenditures by eliminating the overhead costs of multiple private insurers. Supporters of a single-payer system, including the nursing and public health professions who are concerned for at-risk populations, believe that it offers the best approach for getting rid of inequities in the system, providing universal access, and reducing soaring costs.

Those supporting universal health care and a single-payer system stress guidelines to be incorporated into reform proposals. The Older Women's League summarizes them as follows:

"• Universal access not tied to employment;
• Comprehensive benefits including preventive, diagnostic, mental health and treatment services;
• Long-term care available at home and in institutions;
• Choice of providers;
• Cost controls;

• and public funding through a progressively financed plan and public administration" (1993, p. 1)

Health Care Reform

Consumers and professionals agree that health care reform is needed in the United States. The disagreement lies in the form that it should take. At issue is a fundamental conflict in values between advocates of the managed competition model and advocates of the universal coverage, or single-payer plan. On the one hand are those who strongly value the competition model, which ensures a free market, individualism, and the right to choose the type of health care desired.

On the other hand, proponents of universal coverage argue that more comprehensive benefits are needed to include the unemployed or physically or economically disadvantaged who cannot afford health care. Furthermore, they argue that universal coverage emphasizes prevention and primary health care as key factors in reducing long-range health care costs and, more importantly, in ensuring improved levels of health for the public. Nursing's Agenda for Health Care Reform supports this emphasis by promoting nurses as primary providers of health care, a role enthusiastically endorsed by Donna Shalala, who became U.S. Secretary of Health and Human Services in 1993, in a keynote address to the National League for Nursing's 20th Biennial Convention in 1991 (Shalala, 1993).

Designers of health reform have faced a difficult challenge in reconciling these conflicting views. As a result, elements of both models were used to shape an improved system. Reform proposals included an incremental plan that allowed for a flexible transition and opportunities for states to experiment with both approaches.

Sultz and Young (1999) point out the importance of separating the task of financing (how insurance funds are collected) from disbursement (how providers receive payment). Financing might be tried through an income-based premium that would go into a publicly administered health insurance fund. Method of collection and administration are undecided. Japan and Germany have used a payroll-collection method for years to successfully finance their health care. Supplemental financing (to adjust for low-income or no-income households) might come from an extra tax on the affluent or a tax on products that are known to contribute directly to health care costs, such as alcohol and tobacco. Disbursement of health insurance funds could occur in at least two ways. First, a strictly federal program could enroll all Americans who are not privately insured and disburse funds through a program like Medicare. A second option could be to disburse capitated funds from the federal government to states for payment to providers. In some cases, state funds could supplement federal disbursement. Forms of either the single-payer or managed competition models could be tried to accomplish disbursement, allowing states to adjust for local preferences and existing delivery systems (Sultz & Young, 1999).

Another aspect of health care reform that has been considered is a global budget. This means that a single, nationwide health budget, whose funding might come from the income-based premiums (mentioned earlier) plus supplemental sources, would help to control certain aspects of national health spending. The amount of money in this budget would help to determine the size of disbursements to federal programs, like Medicare, and to the states. States still could choose to spend more on health care out of their own resources.

A standard set of benefits, set by law and enjoyed by the entire population, regardless of age, health, income, and employment status, is an important health care reform element. Many countries have successfully implemented such a package under a plan called a "statutory" model. Various versions of this model have worked well in Austria, France, Belgium, Japan, Germany, the Netherlands, and Switzerland. In this model, health insurance falls under the rubric of social security and is funded through government-mandated payroll premiums or taxes. Payment is made to private-sector health insurers, called "sickness funds" in some countries. Individuals select among nationwide plans and choose their doctor and hospital. Reimbursement for services is made directly to providers by insurers. This model eliminates the need for separate programs such as Medicaid and Medicare. It also provides uniform and comprehensive benefits (Randal, 1993).

Other issues to be addressed in health reform include making the FFS system more accountable, eliminating adverse risk selection, and providing informed choices to consumers. Whereas reform is underway, there continues to be a need for advocates of universal access and cost containment to influence the process. Furthermore, health reform proposals must be encouraged to focus on the central question: Do they fund the promotion of health and prevention of illness or simply pay for the diagnosis and treatment of those who are already ill? World Bank evaluations show that public health interventions repeatedly have been found to be more cost effective than medical services, yet health reform proposals have paid minimal attention to this critical issue (Freeman & Robbins, 1994). Community health nurses can play an influential role in emphasizing the importance of incorporating health promotion services into future health reform efforts through political involvement and policy development. An example of such policy development is the international effort to control population expansion (see The Global Community).

The need for health care reform, however, is not new. Perkins examined the work of the 1927 to 1932 Committee on the Costs of Medical Care. Over 70 years ago, the committee defined *costs* as the major problem and *business models of organization* as the major solution (Perkins, 1998).

THE GLOBAL COMMUNITY

Global Health Economics

Health economics on a global scale is directly tied to an alarming rate of world population expansion. World population growth was relatively slow in earlier centuries, taking hundreds of thousands of years to reach 10 million by about 8000 BC and 100 million about the time of Christ. By 1950, it was 2.5 billion, and it more than doubled to 5.5 billion by 1993. The urgency of the situation prompted representatives of the national academies of science throughout the world to convene a "science summit" on world population in New Delhi, India, in October 1993. Participants developed a joint statement calling for the governments of all countries "to adopt an integrated policy on population and sustainable development on a global scale" (Mehra, 1994, p. 7). The Statement reflected "continued concern about the intertwined problems of rapid population growth, wasteful resource consumption, environmental degradation and poverty" (Mehra, 1994, p. 7). The scientists argued that worldwide social, economic, and environmental problems could not be successfully addressed without a stable world population and urged a goal of zero population growth by the end of the next generation. They recommended equality for women, free choice on family size, access to family planning and contraceptive options, and elimination of unsafe sexual practices. They concluded that the responsibility lies with both the public and private sectors of the international community (Mehra, 1994).

EFFECTS OF HEALTH ECONOMICS ON COMMUNITY HEALTH PRACTICE

Health economics has significantly affected community health and community health practice by advancing (1) disincentives for efficient use of resources, (2) incentives for illness care, and (3) conflict with public health values.

Disincentives for Efficient Use of Resources

All of the system structures that directly or indirectly promote cost escalation and prevent cost containment contribute to disincentives for efficient use of resources. For example, retrospective financial reimbursement, with its lack of setting limits, encourages spending on nonessential tests and treatments and drives up costs. Tax-deductible employer contributions for health care coverage and nontaxable employee health benefits encourage unnecessary use of services and drive up costs. Lack of cost sharing by consumers and no financial risk for decisions made by providers create further disincentives to keep costs down.

Community health has been affected in several ways.

Abuse of resources in some parts of the system means a depletion in other areas. Community and public health programs recently have experienced diminished federal and state allocations and severe budget cuts affecting even basic community health services. Competition from the private sector in home care and other community services, such as health education programs, has forced traditional public health agencies to reexamine their programs and seek new avenues for service and new revenue sources. Costs indirectly affect even appropriate use of nursing personnel in community health. Failing to recognize the differences in skills of community health nurses and less-prepared personnel, proliferating agencies in community health often have hired persons underqualified to give the needed high-caliber and comprehensive care. Finally, the advent of prospective payment and limits on the length of stay have encouraged early hospital discharge, resulting in more acutely ill people needing home care services. The immediate effect has been an increase in the demand for highly skilled and more expensive home care services, which requires changes in provision patterns of community health care. The long-range effects of this phenomenon on family stress and caregiver health, on community health care reimbursement, and on the nature and structure of community health services, including the role of the community health nurse, have yet to be determined.

Incentives for Illness Care

The traditional American health care system inadvertently tends to promote illness because health care providers have primarily been rewarded for treating problems, not for preventing them. Hospitals have had more income when their beds stayed full of sick or injured people. The bulk of most reimbursable health services has centered around treating illness or disability in hospitals, nursing homes, and ambulatory care facilities using physicians or skilled nursing care in the home—situations in which the individual must play the role of patient. Health promotional nursing activities such as comprehensive prenatal, maternal, and infant care; health education; childhood immunizations; and home services to enable the elderly to live independently have not been covered by most insurers.

A system that financially supports illness care affects community health practice in several ways. The number and severity of health problems in a community increase when individuals postpone care because they cannot afford visits to the doctor or clinic. It has been more difficult to encourage community clients to assume responsibility for their own health and to engage in self-care and prevention. Furthermore, such illness-oriented incentives create a basic societal valuing of illness care that, conversely, devalues wellness care. Health promotion and disease prevention efforts become second-ranked priorities in competition for scarce resources. In communities where a greater proportion of community health practice is spent on treatment of disorders and rehabilitation, resources are limited for prevention and health promotion. Prepayment methods and the growth of managed care have been positive moves in the direction of a more wellness-oriented financial incentive structure. A HMO has the incentive to offer preventive and health-promoting services such as early detection and treatment of symptoms, regular physical examinations, and health teaching. Health care reform proposals show promise of greater recognition of the cost-saving value of prevention efforts.

Managed care has evolved and can be described as having three stages: event-driven cost avoidance, value improvement, and health improvement (Goldsmith et al., 1995). Initially, MCOs focused on event-drive cost avoidance. Strategies included decreasing inpatient days, decreasing specialty physician use, using physician extenders, and implementing provider discounting. This then evolved into a second stage in which the principal objective was to control resource intensity and improve the delivery process. Strategies used to meet this objective included capitation of specialists, controls on units of service, patient-focused redesign, clinical pathways, and total quality management.

> **The emphasis, however, is now shifting to a focus on community- based health status improvement that goes beyond just measuring utilization of care or mortality outcomes. This focus calls for new strategies, such as community health assessments, identification of high-risk individuals, targeted interventions, case management, and management of illness episodes across the continuum (Weiss, 1997, p. 28).**

Weiss believes that community health assessments will become standard quality tools for MCOs. Community assessments establish the baseline health status of a community and measure changes in the health of the community over time. Community health assessments must include source information that is both primary (health status assessment surveys, focus groups, and satisfaction surveys) and secondary (data collected by public health agencies and state agencies, such as birth rates, mortality rates, and incidence of communicable diseases in the community).

Improving the health status of a community mandates that the MCO—the organization providing health care services through managed care, such as a HMO, or PPO—be actively involved in accurately assessing the community's health status and the major issues facing the community. This would involve "informing health care consumers of how to care for themselves and empowering them to do so, and developing a community action plan that fosters collaboration among organizations and focuses on preventive service strategies" (Weiss, 1997, p. 29). Are these not the proposals that public health has been making for over a century? Perhaps the incentive to keep costs down will be the motivation needed to work with clients at the primary prevention level of care. Although public health proponents have advocated preventive care as the best care for the individual, family, and community as long as the goal of community health is reached, the motivating factor becomes insignificant. If the community health approach is embraced by MCOs, the conflict with public health can be minimized and perhaps eliminated.

Managed Care and Public Health Values

Competition in health care is a reality with which community health practice must cope. Although competition offers several benefits, it poses some dilemmas for community health that may be difficult to resolve. Values underlying the competition model can be in direct conflict with several basic public health values. Competition for the healthier and younger enrollee, for example, encourages MCOs to develop market strategies that entice the client to choose one over another—a win-lose situation for the MCO: one MCO wins while another loses. Public health, however, operates on the basis of collaboration and cooperation. Competition among MCOs serves a selected market partly determined by those able to purchase products or services.

Public health is committed to serving all persons in need, regardless of ability to pay (Young, 1993). Traditionally, the competition model MCOs has focused on individuals and has been oriented to the present; public health is concerned with aggregates and is future oriented, emphasizing prevention. Competition established relatively fixed limits for service, whereas public health must remain flexible if it is to respond to the health needs of the entire population. These dramatic differences between MCOs and public health are beginning to blur and out of necessity will continue to be less adversarial and more collegial. By shifting their focus to community health as a systems outcome, MCOs can create several positive changes, including a safe environment, wholesome nutrition, healthy lifestyle, adequate education, sufficient income, meaningful spirituality, challenging work, recreation, and functional families (Weiss, 1997).

If enrollees in health insurance programs, from Medicare, Medicaid, or other MCOs, become empowered to assume responsibility for their own self-care and well-being, a cooperative and collaborative relationship can be achieved between MCOs and public health. Healthy competition may remain between MCOs for enrollees, but this level of competition will help to decrease costs and improve quality of care, as has occurred with telephone services and utility companies. Consumers can select their service providers, choosing the one that best fits their needs. Competition always has improved services and lowered costs in other markets, such as among retailers, and should do the same in the health care industry.

There are philosophical differences plus constraints, such as civil service restrictions and political influences, under which most public health agencies must operate, which makes it difficult for them to compete. Likewise, MCOs have stockholders, boards of directors, employees, and state and federal regulations that they must satisfy. Public health agencies must remain committed to providing the health promotion and disease prevention services that are their public trust. This may become the commitment of MCOs as they see the cost savings and health benefits of disease prevention. Yet some aspects of competition seem necessary if both forms of health care delivery are to stay in business. Exclusion from health care competition, freedom from unreasonable constraints, and dependable financial support are needed to maintain the organizational viability of many public health agencies. Competition also may stimulate new and innovative community health services and the introduction of new roles and revenue sources for traditional public health agencies. The evolution of the reform of health care implementation may see public and private health care developing partnerships, with MCOs contracting with public health agencies for certain services, and MCOs more effectively expanding the reach of public health agencies into the suburbs or rural areas. Reform will need to continue to address issues affecting delivery of public health services.

SUMMARY

Health care economics studies the production, distribution, and consumption of health care goods and services to maximize the use of scarce resources to benefit the most people. This science underlies the financing of the health care system. It is influenced by microeconomics as well as macroeconomics.

Health care is funded through public and private sources, which fall into three categories: third-party payers, direct consumer payment, and private support. Health care services have been reimbursed either retrospectively, typical of FFS plans, or prospectively, typical of most HMOs.

Several issues and trends have influenced community health care financing and delivery and are important to understanding health care economics and helping to improve community health. They include cost control, financial access, managed care, health care rationing, competition and regulation, managed competition, universal coverage and a single-payer system, and health care reform.

The changing nature of health care financing has adversely affected community health and its practice in three important ways: (1) retrospective payment without limiting costs, tax-deductible employer contributions for health care coverage and nontaxable employee health benefits, plus a lack of consumer involvement in cost sharing all have created disincentives for efficient use of resources; (2) because the health care system traditionally has reimbursed only for treatment of the ill or disabled with no reward for health promotion and prevention efforts, it has promoted incentives to focus only on illness care; and (3) the competition model, which has long driven up health care costs and eliminated many from being able to afford health care services, has generated a conflict with the basic public health values of health promotion and disease prevention for all persons. Health care reform efforts in the 1990s focused on reversing these patterns by combining positive elements of competition, free enterprise, and regulation to allow all individuals access to adequate health care and to bring MCOs more in line with the goals of public health.

ACTIVITIES TO PROMOTE CRITICAL THINKING

1. Compare and contrast the goal of public health with the goal of health care economics.
2. Interview a community nursing administrator to determine the impact that managed care has had on community health and the delivery of community health nursing services.
3. Discuss the pros and cons of prospective payment versus retrospective reimbursement. How has each influenced community health and health care?
4. Form two teams with your classmates and debate the advantages and disadvantages of managed competition as opposed to universal coverage and a single-payer system.
5. On the Internet or in the library, locate recent articles on health care reform, managed care, and the public health response. What are the current thoughts on health care reform and managed care? What are the effects on public health services and the agencies?
6. Access www.apha.com on the Internet and read the most recent position statements or legislature affecting public health. What are some of the concerns? What can you do about the issues as a student?

REFERENCES

American Public Health Association. (1998a). *Managed care reform: Fact sheet*. Washington, DC: Author.

American Public Health Association. (1998b). *Regulatory reform: Fact sheet*. Washington, DC: Author.

Brown, L.D. (1992, winter). Political evolution of Federal health care regulation. *Health Affairs*, 17–37.

Burris, S. (1997). The invisibility of public health: Population-level measures in a politics of market individualism. *American Journal of Public Health, 87*(10), 1607–1610.

Cascio, W.F. (1998). Learning from outcomes: Financial experiences of 300 firms that have downsized. In M. Gowling, J. Kraft, & J.C. Quick (Eds.), *The new organizational reality: Downsizing, restructuring and revitalization*. Washington, DC: American Psychological Association.

Congressional Budget Office. (1993, May). *Managed competition and its potential to reduce health spending*. Washington, DC: The Congress of the United States.

D'Angelo, F.G. & D'Angelo, A.M. (1999). Financial, legal, and ethical issues when providing health care for elderly clients at home. In S. Zang & J.A. Allender (Eds.), *Home care of the elderly* (pp. 17–33). Philadelphia: Lippincott Williams & Wilkins.

DeLew, N., Greenberg, G., & Kinchen, K. (1992). A layman's guide to the U.S. Health care system. *Health Care Financing Review, 14*(1), 151–169.

Dowling, W.L. (1979). Prospective rate setting: Concept and practice. *Topics in Health Care Financing, 3*(2), 35–42.

Employee Benefit Research Institute. (1995). *Sources of health insurance and characteristics of the uninsured: Analysis of the March 1994 current population survey* (Issue Brief No. 158). Washington, DC: Author.

Federwisch, A. (1999). Runaway costs: How can we rein in healthcare expenses? *NurseWeek, 12*(4), 1, 10.

Firshein, J. (1999). Medicare panel weights higher eligibility age. *AARP Bulletin, 40*(2), 6, 17.

Foster Higgins Survey and Research Services. (1994). *National survey of employer-sponsored health plans, 1994: Report*. New York: Author.

Freeman, P. & Robbins, A. (1994). National health care reform minus public health: A formula for failure. *Journal of Public Health Policy, 15*(3), 261–282.

Goldsmith, J., Goran, M.D., & Nackel, J.G. (1995, September–October). Managed care comes of age. *Healthcare Forum Journal*, 14–24.

Hanchak, N.A., Schlackman, N., & Harmon-Weiss, S. (1996). U.S. Healthcare's quality-based compensation model. *Health Care Financing Review, 17*(3), 143–159.

Harrington, C. & Estes, C.L. (1997). *Health policy and nursing: Crisis and reform in the U.S. health care delivery system* (2nd ed.). Boston: Jones & Bartlett.

Harris, M.D. (1998). The impact of the Balanced Budget Act of 1997 on home healthcare agencies and nurses. *Home Healthcare Nurse, 16*(7), 435–437.

The Henry J. Kaiser Family Foundation. (1998a, July). *The Medicare program: Medicare at a glance*. Washington, DC: Author.

The Henry J. Kaiser Family Foundation. (1998b, July). *Uninsured facts: The uninsured and their access to health care*. Washington, DC: Author.

The Henry J. Kaiser Family Foundation. (1998c, June). *Medicaid facts: Medicaid and managed care*. Washington, DC: Author.

Hyman, H. (1982). *Health planning: A systematic approach* (2nd ed.). Rockville, MD: Aspen.

Kronick, R., Goodman, D., Wennberg, J., & Wagner, E. (1993).

The marketplace in health care reform: The demographic limitations of managed competition. *The New England Journal of Medicine, 328*(2), 148–152.

Lee, P.R. & Estes, C.L. (1997). *The nation's health* (5th ed.). Boston: Jones & Bartlett.

Levit, K.R., Lazenby, H.C., Sivarajan, L., et al. (1996). National health expenditures, 1994 (HCFA Publication No. 03383). *Health Care Financing Review, 17*(3), 205–242.

Longest, B.B., Jr. (1994). *Health policy making in the United States.* Ann Arbor, MI: AUPHA Press.

McNerney, W.J. (1980). Control of health care costs in the 1980s. *The New England Journal of Medicine, 303,* 1088–1095.

Mehra, L. (1994). Science academies call for action on population. *World Health, 47*(3), 7.

Merline, J. (1993, April 5). What is "managed competition"? *Investor's Business Daily,* 1–3.

Mucklo, M. (1993, April 15). Health care reform: Managed competition and beyond. *Medical Benefits, 10*(7), 1–2.

Older Women's League (1993). Speak up on universal health care. *The OWL Observer, 13*(1), 1.

Perkins, B.B. (1998). Economic organization of medicine and the committee on the costs of medical care. *American Journal of Public Health, 88*(11), 1721–1726.

Randal, J. (1993, May). Wrong prescription: Why managed competition is no cure. *The Progressive,* 22–25.

Shalala, D.E. (1993). Nursing and society: The unfinished agenda for the 21st century. *Nursing and Health Care, 14*(6), 289–291.

Somers, A.R. & Somers, H. (1977). *Health and health care: Policies in perspective.* Germantown, MD: Aspen.

U.S. Department of Commerce. (1998). *Statistical abstract of the United States, 1998* (118th ed.). Washington, DC: U.S. Government Printing Office.

U.S. Department of Health and Human Services. (1996). *HCFA statistics.* Washington, DC: Author.

U.S. Department of Health and Human Services. (1997, November 29). *Medicare home health: Differences in service use by HMO and fee-for- service providers. Government Accounting Office report.* Washington, DC: Author.

U.S. Department of Health and Human Services. (1998, March). *Medicaid statistics* (HCFA Publication No. 10129). Baltimore, MD: Center for Medicaid and State Operations.

Verrilli, D.K. & Zuckerman, S. (1996). Preferred provider organizations and physician fees (HCFA Publication No. 03383). *Health Care Financing Review, 17*(3), 205–242.

Warden, C. (1993, July 2). Is health-care rationing next? It might control costs but patients will suffer. *Investor's Business Daily,* 1–3.

Weiss, M. (1997). The quality evolution in managed care organizations. *Journal of Nursing Care Quality, 11*(4), 27–31.

Williams, S.J., & Torrens, P.R. (1999). *Introduction to health services* (5th ed.). Albany, NY: Delmar Publications.

Wolf, L.F. & Gorman, J.K. (1996). New directions and developments in managed care financing (HCFA Pub. No. 03383). *Health Care Financing Review, 17*(3), 1–5.

Young, Q. (1993). Health care reform: A new public health movement. *American Journal of Public Health, 83*(7), 945–947.

INTERNET RESOURCES

Kaiser Family Foundation: www.kff.org
Medicare: www.medicare.gov
Health Care Financing Administration (HCFA): www.hcfa.gov
Joint Commission on Accreditation of Healthcare Organizations (JCAHO): www.jcaho.org
National Committee for Quality Assurance (NCQA): www.ncqa.org

SELECTED READINGS

Ansell, D, Schiff, G., Dick, S., Cwiak, C., & Wright, K. (1998). Voting with their feet: Public hospitals, health reform, and patient choices. *American Journal of Public Health, 88*(3), 439–441.

Bodenheimer, T.S. & Grumbach, K. (1995). *Understanding health policy: A clinical approach.* Norwalk, CT: Appleton & Lange.

Coile, R.C. (1998). *Millennium management: Better, faster, cheaper strategies for managiang 21st century healthcare organizations.* Chicago: Health Administration Press.

Congressional Budget Office. (1993, May). *Managed competition and its potential to reduce health spending.* Washington, DC: The Congress of the United States.

Enthoven, A. & Kronick, R. (1989). A consumer-choice health plan for the 1990s. *The New England Journal of Medicine,* January 5, 29–37; January 12, 94–101.

Halverson, P.K., Kaluzny, A.D., & McLaughlin, C.P. (1997). *Managed care and public health.* Gaithersburg, MD: Aspen.

Jones, L.D. (1997). Building the information infrastructure required for managed care. *Image: Journal of Nursing Scholarship, 29*(4), 377–382.

Knight, W. (1998). *Managed care: What it is and how it works.* Gaithersburg, MD: Aspen.

Krahn, M., et al. (1998). Costs and cost-effectiveness of a universal, school-based hepatitis B vaccination program. *American Journal of Public Health, 88*(11), 1638–1644.

Lundeen, S.P. (1997). Community nursing centers: Issues for managed care. *Nursing Management, 28*(3), 35–37.

Mechanic, D. (1996) Changing medical organization and the erosion of trust. *Milbank Quarterly, 74,* 171–189.

Mechanic, D. (1998). Topics for our times: Managed care and public health opportunities. *American Journal of Public Health, 88*(6), 874–875.

On-Lok, Inc. (1995). *PACE fact book: Information about the Program of All-Inclusive Care for the Elderly.* San Francisco: On Lok, Inc.

Porter-O'Grady, T. (1994). Building partnerships in health care: Creating whole systems change. *Nursing and Health Care, 15*(1), 34–38.

Primas, P., Mileham, T., Toronto, C., & McCoy, B. (1994). Breaking the cycle of disadvantage: A nursing system of health care. *Nursing and Health Care, 15*(1), 10–17.

Rassell, M.E. (1995). Cost sharing in health insurance: A reexamination. *New England Journal of Medicine, 332,* 1138–1143.

Resnick, C. & Tighe, E.G. (1997). The role of multidisciplinary community clinics in managed care systems. *Social Work, 42*(1), 91–98.

Rovner, J. (1997). Medicare's new alphabet soup. *AARP Bulletin, 38*(10), 4–6.

Schnurer, E.B. (1998). A health-care plan most of us could buy: It's right under Congress' nose. *The Washington Monthly, 30*(4), 20–25.

The Twentieth Century Fund Press. (1995). *Medicare reform: A twentieth century fund guide to the issues.* New York: Author.

Uchitelle, L. & Kleinfield, N.R. (1996, March 3). On the battlefields of business: Millions of casualties. *New York Times,* 14–16.

Vladeck, B.C. & King, K.M. (1995). Medicare at 30: Preparing for the future. *Journal of the American Medical Association, 274,* 259–262.

Wiener, J.M. (1996). Managed care and long-term care: The integration of financing and services. *Generations, 20*(2), 47–52.

Zwerdling, M. (1994). The health care delivery system in the year 2000: Nursing care for the societal client. *Nursing and Health Care, 15*(8), 422–424.

Communication, Collaboration, and Contracting

KEY TERMS

- Active listening
- Brainstorming
- Channel
- Collaboration
- Communication
- Contracting
- Critical pathway
- Decoding
- Delphi technique
- Electronic meetings
- Empathy
- Encoding
- Feedback loop
- Formal contracting
- Informal contracting
- Message
- Nominal group technique
- Nonverbal messages
- Nursing informatics
- Paraphrasing
- Receiver
- Sender
- Verbal messages

LEARNING OBJECTIVES

Upon mastery of this chapter, you should be able to:

- Identify the seven basic parts of the communication process.
- Describe four barriers to effective communication in community health nursing and how to deal with them.
- Explain three sets of skills necessary for effective communication in community health nursing.
- Discuss four techniques for enhancing group decision-making.
- Describe five characteristics of collaboration in community health.
- Compare the three phases common to the collaboration process.
- Identify four features of contracting in community health nursing.
- Discuss the value of contracting to both clients and community health nurses.
- Design an aggregate level contract useful in community health nursing.

Communication, collaboration, and contracting are primary tools for community health nurses. They form the basis for effective relationships that contribute both to the prevention of illness and to the protection and promotion of aggregate health. To use them skillfully in community health practice, it is important to understand the meaning and value of these concepts. For the nurse accustomed to communicating one-on-one with clients, communication with aggregates and a host of professionals requires new skills. The computer, with its Internet and e-mail capabilities, adds another dimension to communication and brings the world into the home and work settings. Unlike ordinary social relationships, collaborative relationships are based on a team approach with shared responsibilities and mutual participation in establishing and carrying out goals. Clients and health care professionals enter into a working agreement, or contract, tailored to address specific client needs. The concept of contracting can further assist the collaborative process. This chapter examines these tools and discusses their integration into community health nursing practice.

COMMUNICATION IN COMMUNITY HEALTH NURSING

Groups cannot exist without communication, nor can nurses practice without communication. These facts often are taken for granted, since most people spend close to 70% of their waking hours communicating: speaking, listening, reading, or writing. Yet the quality of people's communication has far-reaching effects. Lack of effective communication can lead to misunderstanding, poor performance, interpersonal conflict, ineffective programs, weak public policy, and many other undesirable outcomes (Marshall & Housman, 1999). To communicate, people must "construct shared realities—create shared meanings" (Shockley-Zalabak, 1994, p. 2). In other words, they must engage in an exchange that is both understood and meaningful. **Communication** means to transfer meaning and enhance understanding. "A sentence is situated in a world of reality, the external world of objects and events, the internal world of one's intentions and experiences, and the social world of norms and shared values" (Hiraki, 1998, p. 115).

Communication is the lifeblood of effective community health nursing practice. It provides a two-way flow of information that nourishes professional-client and professional-professional relationships. It also establishes the base of information on which health planning decisions are made and programs developed. For communication to take place, clients and professionals send and receive messages. As participants in the communication process, community health nurses play both roles: sender and receiver. The nurse working with a group of abused women must learn to "read" the messages these women send. Similarly, as a member of a health planning team, the nurse must be able to elicit ideas as well as contribute to the planning process by speaking and acting in ways that communicate effectively.

Communication serves several functions in community health nursing. It provides information for decision-making at all levels of community health. From the choice of goals for a small group to health policy affecting a population at risk, decisions are enhanced through effective communication. It functions as a motivator by clarifying information so that consensus is reached and the people involved can move forward with commitment to shared goals. Effective communication facilitates expression of feelings and promotes closer working relationships. It also controls behavior by providing clear expectations and boundaries for group-member actions.

The Communication Process

Communication occurs as a sequence of events or a process. The process is made up of seven basic parts that need to work together to result in the transference and understanding of meaning. They are as follows: (1) the message, (2) a sender, (3) a receiver, (4) encoding, (5) a channel, (6) decoding, and (7) a feedback loop.

The first part of the communication process is a **message,** which is an expression of the purpose of communication. Without the message, there can be no communication. The next two parts are a sender and a receiver. The **sender** is the person (or persons) conveying a message, and the **receiver** is the person (or persons) to whom the message is directed and who is its actual recipient. The fourth step is the act of

encoding, which refers to the sender's conversion of the message into symbolic form. This involves how the sender translates the message to the receiver. It can be accomplished through verbal or nonverbal means. For example, a nurse teaching breathing techniques to a prenatal class may explain verbally while also demonstrating the correct procedures. The degree of the sender's success in encoding is influenced by the sender's communication skills, knowledge about the topic of the message, attitudes related to the message and the receiver, and the beliefs and values held by the sender. The fifth part involves a **channel,** or the medium through which the sender conveys the message. The channel may be a written, spoken, or nonverbal expression. Examples include a letter stating a request, a report providing information, a written health plan, a verbal message for clarification, or a facial expression indicating confusion. Communication channels may be formal, such as a written grant proposal, or informal, like a face-to-face verbal statement or an e-mail message.

Once the sender has conveyed a message through a channel, the receiver must translate the message into an understandable form, called **decoding,** which is the sixth part of the communication process. The receiver's ability to decode the message is influenced by knowledge of the topic, skills in reading and listening, attitudes, and sociocultural values. The seventh and final part is a **feedback loop,** which refers to the receiver, indicating that the message has been understood (decoded) in the way that the sender intended (encoded). It requires feedback from the receiver to the sender, serving as a check on the success of the transference of meaning. Figure 8–1 portrays the seven steps of the communication process.

Communication Barriers

Community health nurses should be aware of the barriers that block effective communication. This section discusses four that pose particular problems: selective perception, language barriers, filtering, and emotions (Robbins, 1998).

SELECTIVE PERCEPTION
Receivers in the communication process interpret a message through their own perceptions, which are influenced by their own experience, interests, values, motivations, and expectations. They project this perceptual screen onto the communication process as they decode a message. They might distort or misinterpret meaning from the sender's original intent. For example, the nurse may propose a class session on nutrition to a group of elderly persons who may translate that message to mean a focus on dieting, which is not the intended meaning. Nurses can overcome this barrier by using the feedback loop to ask clients or others involved to restate their understanding of the message, such as asking the elderly clients in the example just given what the term *nutrition* means to them. This provides an opportunity for clarification and correction of misunderstandings, which is an essential step in the communication process.

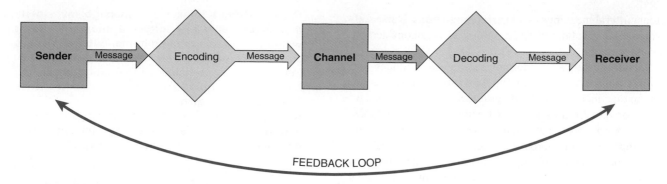

FIGURE 8–1. The communication process (feedback loop).

LANGUAGE BARRIERS

People interpret the meaning of words differently, depending on many variables such as age, education, cultural background, and primary spoken language. An adolescent understands the terms "cool," "tight," and "dude" to mean that something is fashionable or desirable, whereas an 80-year-old woman might not understand the current slang terms. In community health, nurses work with a wide range of clients and professionals whose disparate ages, education, and cultural backgrounds lead to different speech patterns. The use of scientific terminology or jargon by some health professionals can be confusing, as in the case of the Hmong refugee woman who was asked if her son had experienced enuresis. Using unfamiliar terms can become barriers to communication. Client differences must be taken into consideration during the communication process.

FILTERING INFORMATION

A third barrier to communication is filtering, which means manipulation of information by the sender to influence the receiver's response. To gain favor with receivers, senders sometimes say what they believe receivers want to hear rather than the whole truth (Robbins, 1998). Clients sometimes use filtering during a needs assessment process, giving only partial or distorted information because they think this is what health professionals want to hear. Another intent of filtering is to slant information. Prepared minutes from a meeting or a department's quarterly report can emphasize some points and omit or deemphasize others, giving (sometimes unintentionally) false impressions that influence decision-making.

EMOTIONAL INFLUENCE

How a person feels at the time a message is sent or received influences its meaning. Senders can distort messages and receivers can interpret messages incorrectly when emotions cloud their perception. Emotions can interfere with rational and objective reasoning, thus blocking communication. Nurses need to be aware of their own emotions as they send messages. They also need to ascertain the emotional status of clients or health professionals with whom they are communicating to avoid misunderstandings.

Core Communication Skills

Overcoming the barriers to effective communication just described requires the development of sound communication skills. Community health nurses need to cultivate three sets of communication skills: sending skills, receiving skills, and interpersonal skills.

SENDING SKILLS

Sending skills enable nurses to transmit messages effectively. Through these skills, nurses convey information to clients and other persons. Two important considerations influence clarity and effectiveness of message sending. First, the extent of the nurse's self-awareness affects the communication. Does the nurse feel anxious, angry, tired, impatient, or concerned? Does the nurse find certain individuals irritating or offensive? What motives and interests prompt the communication? Second, the nurse's awareness of the receivers influences the sending of messages. What do clients or the professionals with whom the nurse is interacting want or need? Is the message suited to their cultural backgrounds and level of understanding? Does the message have significance for them? How are receivers responding as the nurse sends the message?

Two main channels are used to send messages: nonverbal and verbal. **Nonverbal messages** are those conveyed without words and constitute nearly two thirds of the messages transmitted in normal communication (Brill, 1973). People send messages nonverbally in many ways. Personal appearance, dress, posture, facial expression, and physical distance between sender and receiver all communicate messages. These nonverbal statements may enhance or discredit what someone says verbally (Robbins, 1998). Body language often speaks louder than words. Facial expressions convey acceptance or rejection, interest or boredom, anger or patience, fear or confidence. Gestures and bodily movements such as clenched hands, crossed arms, tapping a finger, hands on hips, or a turned shoulder all communicate messages. Eye contact or lack of it carries additional meaning. Tone of voice and use of silence also send nonverbal messages. Accepting food in certain situations may communicate acceptance and the desire to be friendly. Nonverbal messages may have different cultural meanings or social interpretations. Nurse self-awareness and validation of meaning can save considerable misunderstanding.

Verbal messages are communicated ideas, attitudes, and feelings transmitted by speaking or writing. Nurses cannot assume that the intent of their words always is understood by clients or other professionals. Effective sending skills depend on asking for feedback to make certain that receivers have understood the verbal message's intent. Communication is more effective if speakers avoid using jargon that is unfamiliar to clients. Like all occupations, nursing has its own vocabulary or jargon that may not be understood by clients, perhaps making them feel ignorant or inferior. For example, the terms "critical pathways" or "case management approach" might have little meaning to a community group. Nurses must make special effort to avoid using jargon that is part of nursing's everyday speech. The basic rules for effective sending can be summarized in this manner:

1. Keep the message honest and uncomplicated.
2. Use as few words as possible to state it.
3. Ask for reactions (feedback) to make certain that it is understood.

RECEIVING SKILLS

Receiving skills are as important to communication as sending skills and involve not only listening to what people say, but also observing their behavior. They enable nurses to receive accurate and complete messages. If members of a seniors' exercise class agree to certain exercises but do not participate in them, they are sending a message. What message is their behavior sending? Were the proposed exercises too difficult? Did they misunderstand the nurse's instructions on how to perform the exercise? Are they resisting in other areas of the program? Effective receiving skills require attention to nonverbal as well as verbal messages and seeking feedback to understand their meaning.

An essential skill needed for receiving messages is **active listening** or reflective listening, the skill of assuming responsibility for and understanding the feelings and thoughts in a sender's message. Instead of expecting clients or others to help the nurse understand, the nurse should actively work to discover what clients mean. Understanding the message from the sender's perspective demands careful attention. It arises from a genuine interest in what the speaker has to say. Active listeners demonstrate their interest, perhaps by sitting forward, sustaining eye contact, nodding the head, and asking occasional questions for clarification (Northouse & Northouse, 1997). At times, **paraphrasing,** or stating back to the sender what was heard by the receiver, is helpful in clarifying the sender's meaning. This helps the nurse to avoid daydreaming or pretending to be listening, both of which block communication. Also, the content and feeling of the sender's message is overwhelming at times, and the nurse becomes preoccupied with formulating a response rather than actively listening. In these situations, paraphrasing can help the nurse to stay focused. An example of the skill of paraphrasing is as follows:

Client: "I don't think I can manage my elderly mother at home any longer. I know she never wanted to go to a nursing home, but with my job and the kids, caring for her is becoming impossible. My husband is so helpful, I feel guilty burdening him. But I'll be going against my mother's wishes if I place her somewhere."

Nurse: "You feel frustrated caring for your mother and your family while maintaining a job and you're not sure what is the best action to take?"

Nurses also can listen actively by asking reflective questions that restate what clients or others have said to clarify the received meaning. Reflective questions have a twofold purpose: to show a sincere attempt to understand the senders' messages, and to make clear that the messages and the people who send them are important to the nurse. An example of a reflective question follows:

Class members state, "Quitting smoking is impossible." The nurse asks, "Do you feel you can't quit smoking?"

Active listening helps to communicate acceptance and increase trust, especially when the listener refrains from making any negative judgments of the message or the way it is delivered. A critical response to the message by the listener cuts off communication. Active listening enables nurses to encourage clients to deliberate carefully and to exercise problem-solving skills; it avoids the pitfall of telling receivers what to do.

INTERPERSONAL SKILLS

Effective communication in community health nursing also requires interpersonal skills. Three types of interpersonal skills build on sending and receiving skills but go beyond the mere exchange of messages. They are showing respect, empathizing, and developing trust.

Showing Respect

Showing respect means conveying the attitude that clients and others have importance, dignity, and worth. Community health nurses can express respect by treating ideas and comments as valuable and worthy of attention. Nurses can demonstrate an interest in wanting to understand the situation from the other person's point of view. Nurses show respect by the manner in which they address people, for instance, by using the courtesy titles of "Mr." or "Mrs." until it is determined how the client wants to be addressed. On a more subtle level, the tone of voice either can show respect or make people feel inferior and insignificant. Clients, community members, and other professionals need to feel respected if they are to enter fully into the mutual exchange necessary for effective communication (Display 8–1).

Empathizing

Empathizing is another important interpersonal skill. **Empathy** is the ability to communicate understanding and vicariously experience the feelings and thoughts of others (Balzer-

Most poorly educated populations, those with the lowest literacy levels, have the highest mortality and morbidity rates. Yet it has been well documented that most "health information materials cannot be read or comprehended by low-literacy adults" (Plimpton & Root, 1994, p. 83). Communication with these high-risk groups needs to be simplified and include easy-to-read materials. At the same time, there is the danger of communication being so simple that the reader feels insulted. Low literacy does not necessarily mean low intelligence. How does the nurse find the right balance?

The goal of communication is to achieve understanding. If clients are to understand health communication—whether the messages are spoken or written—they must be given ample opportunity to provide feedback. Pamphlets and other written health information should be reviewed by their intended audiences before final printing and distribution. Proposed users should comment on readability and acceptability of both text and graphics. With spoken communication, nurses should regularly solicit feedback to make certain that messages are understood.

Riley, 1996). Nurses show empathy by reflecting another person's feelings and expressing that message in the receiver's language. The same terms and, if possible, the same tone of voice as the other person's should be used. For example, the nurse should assume a serious manner if the speaker seems serious. Empathy conveys the message, "This is the way it seems to me. Is that correct?" The nurse should keep validating the speaker's true feelings to be certain that the message is being interpreted correctly. Empathy focuses attention on receivers and their feelings and reduces clients' anxiety and defensiveness. It shows that the nurse shares their concerns and makes them feel that their contributions are valued (Balzer-Riley, 1996).

Developing Trust

Developing trust is necessary for effective communication. Clients and others will not express their true feelings if they do not fully trust the nurse. Many times, clients say what they think the nurse wants to hear. They may agree to a plan of action simply because they do not want to displease the nurse, or they may hide true feelings because they think that the nurse is eager for a decision. Agreeing with others, especially people who are in powerful positions and from different cultures, is the polite and respectful thing to do in some cultures. The nurse unaware of this may interpret the client's agreeing as understanding, and a "teachable moment" is gone.

Nurses develop trust in the communication process by showing that they truly accept others, that they believe in

them as people. Trust generates trust; as the nurse shows confidence in clients and the other professionals with whom the nurse is communicating, they will respond in kind. Treating people as fully participating partners in the communication process means demonstrating that they are trustworthy and responsible. Trust also is developed through an open, honest, and patient approach with others. Candid discussion in a flexible time frame encourages people to share their real feelings and to move at their own pace. As trust develops, communication becomes more free flowing and productive.

Factors Influencing Communication

Effective communication, both sending and receiving, is strongly influenced by three factors: previous experiences, culture, and relationships.

Previous experiences of both sender and receiver influence their perceptions and the meanings they attach to messages. For example, adolescents who are having difficulty with parents' authority may hear the nurse's suggestion to "learn more about sexually transmitted diseases" as a command or effort to exert control. Requests for clarification help to verify that messages are being received as intended.

The respective cultures of sender and receiver influence understanding and acceptance of messages. A nervous laugh, appropriate as an outlet in one culture, may appear rude and disrespectful to someone from another culture. Silence, which in Native American cultures indicates patience and thoughtfulness, may be interpreted as weakness or indifference to someone not familiar with their cultural practices. With many clients, the nurse has to communicate cross-culturally, which requires patience and constant effort to ensure accurate and inoffensive messages (Airhihenbuwa, 1995; Kreps & Kunimoto, 1994).

Because much of community health nursing involves groups, the relationships among group members can significantly influence communication effectiveness. When many people are involved, group communication patterns can be complex, and interaction requires skill on the nurse's part to elicit feedback from all members and to generate a common understanding among the group.

Group Decision-Making

An important aspect of communicating with groups in community health is group decision-making. Community health nurses are regularly involved in this activity. "Nurses working in the community often face different decision-making challenges from those encountered by their hospital colleagues" (Bryans & McIntosh, 1996, p. 24). Thus, nurses need to understand how groups function as they make decisions and to learn techniques for facilitating group decision-making (Orme & Maggs, 1993).

GROUP FUNCTIONS IN DECISION-MAKING

Groups, regardless of size, perform many functions. Four functions are of particular relevance to group decision-making:

1. Group members share information. In community health nursing, groups often include clients, health professionals, and community members who share their experience and expertise to arrive at solutions and decisions.
2. Groups present diverse views, which enriches the number and types of alternatives in the problem-solving process.
3. Groups influence their members' thinking by broadening their perspectives and presenting new ways of thinking about the issues. This influencing function can improve the quality of the group decision-making.
4. Groups progress toward consensus or resolution by discussing a set of alternatives and arriving at solutions. Time pressures and desire for completion help to move this process along.

TECHNIQUES FOR ENHANCING GROUP DECISION-MAKING

As a member of many decision-making groups in the community, the community health nurse can facilitate the process through certain techniques. Robbins (1998) describes four useful strategies: brainstorming, nominal group technique, delphi technique, and electronic meetings.

Brainstorming

Brainstorming is an idea-generating process that encourages group members to freely offer suggestions. When brainstorming, members sit around a table (if group size permits) and take turns presenting ideas. They are encouraged to be creative and unusual; thus, no idea is too bizarre. Furthermore, no criticism or discussion is allowed until all ideas have been exhausted and recorded. This technique is helpful for generating creative possibilities and is the most useful in the early stages of decision-making.

Nominal Group Technique

Nominal group technique is a group decision-making method in which ideas are pooled and discussed face to face after members initially think and write down their ideas independently. In this approach, members meet together but spend time silently writing down their ideas first. Afterward, members take turns presenting one idea at a time to the group without discussion until all ideas have been recorded. Discussion then follows for clarifying and judging. Next, members independently and silently rank-order the ideas and read these rankings to the group. This allows the decisions to be narrowed down to the one with the highest aggregate ranking.

Delphi Technique

Delphi technique is a method of arriving at group consensus through a systematic pooling of individuals' judgments by using a written questionnaire and suggestions. Members do not need to be physically present to participate. It follows a series of steps:

1. Identify problem or topic and design questionnaire to elicit responses from members.
2. Members respond independently and anonymously and return questionnaire.
3. Compile responses centrally, then send results and a new questionnaire to members.
4. Members offer new responses or solutions, based on earlier results, and return these.
5. Repeat steps 3 and 4 as needed until consensus is reached.

This process is useful for polling experts who may be geographically distant from one another. It also provides a way to reach a decision without group members unduly influencing each other. Its disadvantages are that it is time-consuming and can be expensive.

Electronic Meetings

Electronic meetings provide a fourth group decision-making method. This method, currently used more in business settings, applies nominal group technique combined with computer technology. Group members sit around a large table furnished with a computer terminal for each person. As issues are presented, members use their computers to key in their responses, which are anonymously displayed on a large projection screen. Group decisions also are displayed for group viewing. This method promotes greater honesty and speed; in fact, experts claim that electronic meetings are 55% faster than face-to-face meetings (Robbins, 1998).

In community health, availability of such technology may be limited in many settings. Nonetheless, computer-assisted decision-making is becoming increasingly useful and available. Computers are used in conjunction with other group decision-making techniques for recording ideas and research findings, tabulating rankings, and conducting simulations.

NURSING INFORMATICS

Nursing informatics is a term for the collective technologic sciences currently available to nurses in the health care delivery system for the delivery of nursing care. One of the most useful definitions of nursing informatics comes from Graves and Corcoran:

> **A combination of computer science, information science, and nursing science designed to assist in the management and processing of nursing data, information, and knowledge to support the practice of nursing and the delivery of nursing care (1989, p. 227).**

The computer is changing all aspects of health care in addition to the documentation process for health care professionals (Thede, 1998). This is seen most vividly in acute care settings, especially surgical and intensive care settings. Physicians and other practitioners use the computer to research diseases, treatment methodologies, and the most current therapies used among colleagues. Consultation regarding complex client health problems is enhanced by computers with two-way visual capabilities. Gebbie (1999), in an editorial in the *American Journal of Public Health,* suggests a core curriculum for all employed public health professionals to include nine topics, with informatics being one of them. Turley (1996) suggests that because informatics is developing as a discipline, a model for nursing informatics can provide a framework for interdisciplinary study and research, thus enhancing decision-making.

In many community health settings, the computer has been used to compile client health records; for Medicare, Medicaid, and other insurance billing; and for community health nursing assignments. More and more, community health nurses will be accessing computerized nursing information systems that assist with quality measurement and improvement (see Chapter 12), home visiting documentation according to protocol computer tools, documentation of all client contact, time management, and work schedules (McCloskey & Maas, 1998). The technique of documenting everything on paper in handwriting is being replaced. Client "charts" are becoming client disks and are accessed by passwords with laptop computer technology that can be brought into the home. For all students early in the educational process, required courses include typing and computer technology so that students can efficiently use the "writing and documenting" format of the 21st century.

COLLABORATION IN COMMUNITY HEALTH NURSING

Collaboration for community health nurses means a purposeful interaction between nurses, clients, other professionals, and community members based on shared values, mutual participation, and joint effort (Hooper-Briar & Lawson, 1996). This definition highlights two basic features of collaboration: it has a goal, and it involves several parties assisting one another to achieve that goal. The overriding purpose or goal of collaboration in community health practice is to benefit the public's health. To that end, many players must work together. There are key strategies for establishing partnerships and collaboration with interprofessional team members:

- Think "outside of the box" when looking for partners or collaborators.
- The partners have to be part of the planning.
- Plans are *guides* toward a goal—stay flexible.
- When adding new partners, be prepared to re-plan.
- Maintain different levels of collaboration (different team members have more resources, come in later to the project, or leave the project earlier).
- Use consensus-building techniques that are creative and visual.
- Establish a shared vision, then share the plans and the leadership (Allender et al., 1997).

Addressing the needs of aggregates requires a variety of team players. Community health nursing practice draws on the expertise and assistance of numerous individuals. The list includes health planners and policy makers, epidemiologists, biostatisticans, community citizens, demographers, environmentalists, educators, politicians, housing experts, safety professionals, and industrial hygienists in addition to physicians, social workers, psychologists, physical therapists, and most of the other professionals involved in health services. Depending on the need to be addressed, community health nurses may work with many of these people on a single project. Furthermore, perhaps the most important team players are community clients—those populations and groups who are the targets of community health services. Clients' perspectives and expressions of need provide important information for the planning and delivery of services. Their participation, either collectively or through representatives, ensures more comprehensive and accurate information as well as commitment to fully using the health programs designed for their benefit. Stevens and Hall emphasize the importance of gaining the community's perspective and add, "To facilitate dialogue with communities, we must form alliances and build coalitions with community groups" (1992, p. 6).

Characteristics of Collaboration

To explore the meaning of collaboration in the context of community health nursing, this section examines five characteristics that distinguish collaboration from other types of interaction: shared goals, mutual participation, maximized resources, clear responsibilities, and set boundaries.

SHARED GOALS

First, collaboration in community health nursing is goal directed. The nurse, clients, and others involved in the collaborative effort recognize specific reasons for entering into the relationship. For example, a lumber company with 150 employees seeks to develop a wellness program. The community health nurse, company employee representatives, a safety expert, an industrial hygienist, a health educator, an exercise therapist, a nutritionist, and a psychologist might work together to develop specific physical and mental health goals. The team enters into the collaborative relationship with broad needs or purposes to be met and specific objectives to accomplish.

MUTUAL PARTICIPATION

Second, in community health nursing, collaboration involves mutual participation; all team members contribute (Baldwin, 1996). Collaboration involves a reciprocal exchange in which individual team players discuss their intended involvement and contribution. The lumber company representatives may outline assessed areas of need such as back strengthening exercises to facilitate lifting and reduce strain.

The professionals, including the nurse involved in the collaboration, will offer their own specific ideas and expertise to design the wellness program.

MAXIMIZED USE OF RESOURCES

A third characteristic of collaboration is that it maximizes the use of community resources. That is, the collaborative effort is designed to draw on the expertise of those most knowledgeable and in the best positions to influence a favorable outcome. If the lumber company team has identified a need for health education materials, the nurse and other members of the collaborating team may explore health education resources through the local health department and within their own profession.

CLEAR RESPONSIBILITIES

Fourth, the collaborating team members assume clearly defined responsibilities. Like a football team, each member in the collaborative effort plays a specific role with related tasks. The nurse may play a case management or group leadership role, whereas others assume roles appropriate to their areas of expertise. Effective collaboration clearly designates what each member will do to accomplish the identified goals. The nurse, for example, might coordinate the planning effort for the lumber company wellness program and work with the health educator to develop classes on various topics. The psychologist might advise on a chemical dependency program, and the industrial hygienist would provide assistance with safety measures. Each member of the team develops an understanding of individual responsibilities based on realistic and honest expectations. This understanding comes through effective communication. The collaborating group explores necessary resources, assesses their capabilities, and determines their willingness to assume tasks.

SET BOUNDARIES

Fifth, collaboration in community health practice has set boundaries, with a beginning and an end that fall within the goals of the communication (Bisch, 1998). An important part of defining collaboration is determining the conditions under which it occurs and when it will be terminated. The temporal boundaries sometimes are determined by progress toward the goal, sometimes by the number of team member contacts, and often by setting a time limit. The collaborating group might target 6 months as a completion date for the lumber company wellness program and establish a time line with designated activities to reach the goal. Once the purpose for the collaboration has been accomplished, the group as a formal entity can be terminated.

Fostering Client Participation

This chapter has stressed that communication and collaboration are based on mutual participation. The extent of clients' involvement in that participation varies, however, depending on their readiness and ability to participate. The client's level of wellness at the time of initial professional–client encounter directly influences participation. Some people are not physically or emotionally well enough to assume an active role in the relationship. Women recently discharged from the hospital after a mastectomy, for example, have many physical and emotional adjustments with which to cope. Their families, too, must expend additional energies to provide needed support and to cope with the temporary loss of the woman's usual role in the family. They may find it difficult to engage actively in identifying their needs and goals at the start of the collaborative process. The nurse may have to take stronger initial leadership; however, the goals of collaboration are not abandoned. Gradually, as the client's wellness level improves, the nurse can encourage more active participation.

Sometimes a client's previous experiences with health personnel limit participation in collaboration. Clients from poverty-stricken areas, from different cultural backgrounds, or with little education may need extensive encouragement to participate actively (Kreps & Kunimoto, 1994). Also, clients who were not previously encouraged to participate in decision-making by physicians, nurses, or other professionals may follow the pattern of a passive role in collaboration. Unless the nurse persists in efforts to reduce the dependence of clients, the relationship can fall short of the therapeutic goals (Ignatavicius & Hausman, 1995).

The nurse's own view of collaboration also influences the degree of client participation. Nurses accustomed to relating to clients in an adult-to-child manner restrict client involvement. If nurses see their position as more informed and the clients' position as one of complete ignorance and need, a paternalistic relationship may develop. All clients have resources on which to build, and the community health nurse helps clients to discover them and use them to enhance collaboration and attain health goals.

Clients who initiate or seek service frequently are best able to assume an active participant role, such as abused women seeking protection or elderly widowed persons seeking support. They have already demonstrated a sense of responsibility for their health by identifying a need and asking for assistance. They also are experts regarding their situation. This intimate knowledge of the problem makes the client an expert partner and a colleague in problem-solving. As McCloskey & Maas state, "In a collaborative relationship, colleagues work together as partners with trust and respect for each other's skills" (1998, p. 160). The nurse still must work carefully to build mutual participation and respond with concern and caring to foster continued interest and participation by clients.

Structure of Collaborative Relationships

Effective collaboration occurs within a particular structure and sequence. During this process, the work of identifying and meeting the client's needs takes place. Because the relationship is bound by time, the structure involves several phases: (1) a beginning phase when the team relationship is just being established; (2) a middle, working phase; and (3) a termination phase when the relationship ends.

The first phase is a period of establishing and defining the team relationship. All of the team members, including clients, are getting to know each other; they seek to establish communication patterns and develop trust. From these bases, they identify the clients' needs and determine the goals toward which they will work.

The middle phase occurs when team members start working together to accomplish desired goals. Their work may include assessment and planning as well as implementation and evaluation. The cycle of the nursing process is repeated as needed during this working phase until goals are satisfactorily accomplished.

The termination phase occurs when the need for team members to work together has ended. When team members have grown close in the relationship, termination can be difficult. Termination should never be abrupt or without participation. It often requires careful advance preparation to make certain that all parties understand when and why it is taking place. Termination helps to ensure a clear-cut end to the collaborative relationship. For example, a nurse, physician, social worker, psychologist, and nutritionist collaborated with a refugee group for nearly a year. As the group's multiple needs declined, the professionals began to taper off their assistance. Two months before ending the relationship, termination of the group was discussed. At first, client group members were frightened at the loss of group support, but slowly they took ownership and control, and with their newly acquired skills they assumed more responsibility for their health needs (Bragg, 1997).

CONTRACTING IN COMMUNITY HEALTH NURSING

Contracting means negotiating a working agreement between two or more parties in which they come to a shared understanding and mutually consent to the purposes and terms of the transaction. Some kinds of contracts are familiar, such as when a buyer signs a contract agreeing to pay a certain amount for a car over a certain period of time. Paying tuition for an education still involves a form of contracting: although no formal document is signed, students agree with an educational institution on a purpose (to obtain a degree) with the terms of the contract being regular tuition payments and regular learning opportunities over a specified period of time.

In contrast to legal contracts, which are written and legally binding, contracts in a collaborative relationship or a nurse–client alliance (Wills, 1996) are flexible and changing and are based on mutual understanding and trust. Sloan and Schommer (1997) describe the community nursing contract as a working agreement that may be renegotiated continuously between clients and health professionals. The flexibility built into contracting makes it a valuable tool for community health nurses.

The same format is followed with clients receiving home health care services. The contract that develops from this partnership between client and home health care nurse often is referred to as a **critical pathway** or "written plans for patient care with a timetable" (England, 1996, p. 18). This type of contract represents a more formal form of contracting: it is typically a fiscally driven and agency-required tool designed to document standards and quality of care while reducing costs (see Chapters 12 and 37).

Characteristics of Contracting

The concept of contracting as used in the collaborative relationship incorporates four distinctive characteristics: partnership and mutuality, commitment, format, and negotiation.

PARTNERSHIP AND MUTUALITY

All aspects of contracting involve shared participation and agreement between team members; they become partners in the relationship. There is also a mutuality to the nurse–client relationship: if we were to document nurse–client collaboration on a continuum, paternalism would be at one extreme and autonomy at the other. "Mutuality is the mid-point or balance of these two extreme positions" (Henson, 1997, p. 77). For example, a parenting group of 15 couples requested community health nursing involvement. The group entered into a mutual partnership with the nurse and came to an agreement on what they needed and what the nurse could provide. Together they developed goals, outlined methods to meet those goals, explored resources to help achieve them, defined the time limits for the contract, and outlined their separate responsibilities. The contract involved reciprocal negotiation and shared evaluation. A partnership with mutuality means that all parties are responsible for setting up and carrying out the terms of the agreement within a dynamic balance (Henson, 1997).

COMMITMENT

Second, every contract implies a commitment. The involved parties make a decision that binds them to fulfilling the purpose of the contract. In community health collaboration, contracting does not mean making a binding agreement in the legal sense; rather, it is a pledge of trust and dedication. Accompanying that sense of dedication is a strong motivation to see the contract through to completion. All parties feel responsible for keeping promises; all want to achieve the intended outcomes. When the nurse and the parenting group identified their separate tasks, they committed themselves: "Yes, we will do thus and so."

FORMAT

Format, the third distinctive feature of contracting, involves outlining the specific terms of the relationship. Clients and professionals gain a clear idea of the purpose of the relationship, of their respective responsibilities, and of the specific limits within which they will work. The format of contracting provides the framework for collaboration. Once the terms of the contract have been spelled out, there is no question about what has to be done, who is to do it, or within what time frame it is to be accomplished. This format helps to avoid the difficulty of terminating long-term relationships and shifts health care responsibilities from the professionals to the individual or group. At times, having something in writing helps the client "legitimize" the nurse–client interaction. The goals and specific objectives are visualized and can be referred to and followed by all parties.

NEGOTIATION

Finally, contracting always involves negotiation. The nurse and other team members propose to accept certain responsibilities and then ask if clients agree. The nurse might ask, "What do you feel you can do to achieve this goal?" A period of give-and-take then occurs in which ideas are discussed and conclusions and consensus are reached. Team members may find over time that terms or goals on which they had agreed need modification. For example, perhaps clients have assumed more responsibility than they can realistically handle at that point in time and need to redefine their specific responsibilities. Perhaps the nurse feels a need to involve another professional in the collaborative process. Kreps and Kunimoto (1994) emphasize the importance of effective interpersonal communication between clients and professionals to keep contracts updated. Negotiation during contracting allows for changes that facilitate the ultimate achievement of goals. It provides built-in flexibility and encourages ongoing communication among all team members. Negotiation gives contracting a dynamic quality (Henson, 1997).

Value of Contracting

The value of contracting has been demonstrated in many settings and disciplines. Contracts have been used for many years in psychiatric and other nursing settings to promote client self-respect, problem-solving skills, autonomy, and motivation (Johnson, 1992; England, 1996). Other disciplines, such as social work, have long used contracting as a tool in the helping relationship to enhance realistic planning and emphasize partnership (Sauer, 1973). Educational contracts between students and instructors have proven valuable for facilitating learning (Corrigan and Udas, 1996). In the Levels of Prevention display, the three levels of prevention (see Chapters 1 and 3) are used to provide a framework of care for elderly clients in a contract format.

Community health nursing also has used the concept of contracting for many years. Without always labeling it as contracting, community health nurses have used these techniques with clients who, for example, want to lose weight. In

LEVELS OF PREVENTION

GOAL
Population of elderly will experience healthful living to the full extent of their ability.

PRIMARY PREVENTION
OBJECTIVE

Group of healthy elderly will interact with the community health nurse on a monthly basis during the senior center health clinic with the goal of maintaining or raising their level of well-being and ability to function.

METHOD

1. Assess group members' current health status.
2. Identify specific activities that will improve healthy elderly persons' current health status and functional ability.
3. Provide "homework" for elders to work on between meetings with the community health nurse.
4. Implement and evaluate identified activities.

SECONDARY PREVENTION

1. Identify factors contributing to resolution of elderly group's existing health limitations and functional status.
2. With the elders, select appropriate activities to achieve individual and group goals designed to resolve health limitations and improve functional status.
3. Implement and evaluate identified activities.

TERTIARY PREVENTION

1. Identify factors that prevent recurrence of health problems or that restore the elderly to a healthful level of functioning within their limitations.
2. With the elders, select appropriate activities to prevent recurrence of health problems or to restore the elders to a healthful level of functioning within their limitations.
3. Implement and evaluate identified activities.

this case, the contract involved mutually agreeing to certain exercise and eating patterns for clients and teaching and support responsibilities for the nurse. Often, they have set a time limit, such as 6 months, within which to achieve the intended weight loss. In each case, a partnership developed, with agreement about the purpose of the relationship and the conditions under which it would be carried out. Nurses and clients were, in effect, contracting.

As more nurses seek to promote client autonomy and self-care, the wide applicability of contracting to nursing practice is being increasingly recognized (Bohny, 1997; Balzer-Riley, 1996; Wandel et al., 1991). Community health nurses have provided care for infants on total parenteral nutrition (Cady et al., 1991) and have worked with outpatients receiving chemotherapy (Hiromoto et al., 1991) and with prenatal groups, postpartum mothers, and home health clients (Smith, 1994; Lorig et al., 1993; Humphrey & Milone-Nuzzo, 1991).

The advantages of contracting in community health nursing are summarized as follows:

1. It involves clients in promoting their own health.
2. It motivates clients to perform necessary tasks.
3. It focuses on clients' unique needs, regardless of aggregate size.
4. It increases the possibility of achieving health goals identified by collaborating team members.
5. It enhances all team members' problem-solving skills.
6. It fosters client participation in the decision-making process.
7. It promotes clients' autonomy and self-esteem as they learn self-care.
8. It makes nursing service more efficient and cost-effective.

Potential Problems with Contracting

Emphasis on contracting as a method rather than a concept can create problems. If a client has experienced contracts only in a business setting, it is possible to carry the stereotype of a cold, formal arrangement into the nursing practice setting. Some nurses fear that asking clients to negotiate a contract will place clients under stress, impede the development of trust, and negatively influence the relationship (Lindell, 1986). Others have found that some clients may prefer to have the nurse make decisions for them and are not ready to enter into any kind of negotiation. These problems in contracting can be overcome by nurses understanding the true concept of contracting.

Process of Contracting

Contracting applies basic principles of adult education: self-direction, mutual negotiation, and mutual evaluation (Gustafson, 1977). It need not be a formal, written, or complex negotiation. Sloan and Schommer (1991) demonstrate that contracting can be formal or informal, written or verbal, simple or detailed, and signed or unsigned by clients and nurse. It should be adapted to the particular client's abilities to assess, plan, implement, and evaluate, which may vary greatly from situation to situation. Like all nursing tools, contracting enhances client health only if adapted to each particular set of client needs and abilities.

Contracting follows a sequence of steps. As a working agreement, it depends on knowing what clients want, agreeing on goals, identifying methods to achieve these goals, knowing the resources that collaborating members bring to the relationship, using appropriate outside resources, setting limits, deciding on responsibilities, and providing for periodic reviews. Each of these tasks requires discussion among members of the contractual group. The tasks are incorporated into the contracting process described in eight phases by Sloan and Schommer (1997):

1. *Exploration of needs:* Assessment of clients' health and needs by clients, nurse, and other relevant persons
2. *Establishment of goals:* Discussion and agreement between contracting members on goals and objectives

3. *Exploration of resources:* Defining what each member has to offer and can expect from the others; identifying appropriate resources and agencies
4. *Development of a plan:* Identifying methods, activities, and a time line for achieving the stated goals
5. *Division of responsibilities:* Negotiating the activities for which each member will be responsible
6. *Agreement on time frame:* Setting limits for the contract in terms of length of time or number of meetings
7. *Evaluation:* Periodic and final assessment of progress toward goals occurring at agreed-on intervals
8. *Renegotiation or termination:* Agreement to modify, renegotiate, or terminate the contract

As community health nurses use this process to negotiate a contract, they must adapt it to each situation. The sequence of phases may change, and some steps may overlap. Nevertheless, the basic elements remain important considerations for successful contracting (Fig. 8–2).

Levels of Contracting

Community health nurses use contracts at levels ranging from formal to informal. The degree of formality depends on the demands of the situation. To fund a community health

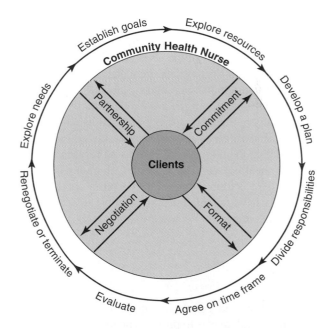

FIGURE 8–2. The concept and process of contracting. Contracting is based on four distinctive features shown here as spokes that support a wheel. These features form the basis for a reciprocal relationship between clients, nurse, and other persons. This relationship is not static; it is a dynamic process that moves through phases, represented here as the outer rim of the wheel. The process moves forward, focused on meeting clients' needs, and enables the collaborating group to facilitate ultimate achievement of clients' goals.

program for preventing child abuse, for example, a formal contract in the form of a written grant proposal may be needed; or to conduct a wide-scale needs assessment of a homeless population, the services of an epidemiologist and statistician may require a formal contract to clarify roles and expectations. **Formal contracting** involves all parties negotiating a written contract by mutual agreement, signing the agreement, and sometimes having it witnessed or notarized. This level of contract has been used with mental health or substance-abusing clients, where the seriousness of the working agreement and the need to actively involve clients are important aspects of therapy.

Some situations best lend themselves to a modified and less formal use of contracting in which the nursing plan becomes the written contract. For example, a school nurse forms a support group for pregnant adolescents. The nurse uses modified contracting by discussing with the girls the purpose of the group and the number of sessions needed and by obtaining their agreement to attend all sessions.

Informal contracting involves some form of verbal agreement about relatively clear-cut purposes and tasks. A client group may agree to prioritize their list of needs, the nurse may agree to conduct health teaching sessions, the social worker may agree to obtain informational materials, and so on. Sometimes, nurses use contracting informally without realizing it. They conclude a session with clients by agreeing with them about the purpose and time of the next meeting. Conscious use of contracting, however, is a more effective way to provide structure for the relationship and foster client involvement, regardless of the level at which it is applied.

The level of contracting also may change during the development of communication and collaboration. Clients often need education about their options. Initially, they may have difficulty in identifying needs and making choices. The professional team can work to promote clients' self-confidence and help them to assume increasing responsibility for their own health (see The Global Community display). Through these efforts, contracting becomes a consciously recognized part of the relationship. Clients can become fully participating partners.

THE GLOBAL COMMUNITY

International Collaboration and Contracting

One example of collaboration and contracting is from the World Health Organization (WHO) south-east Asian region, where many of the 10 countries still are plagued with high maternal mortality (Bisch, 1998). An alarming 40% of estimated maternal deaths worldwide occur in this region alone. Trained personnel, competent to carry out the services safely and effectively, were needed so that when programs were started, they would be involved among groups of health care workers extended over professional and nonprofessional boundaries. Working together, community health nurses were responsible for "linking care delivery across multiple settings and coordinating the work of those who are delivering the care to ensure that peoples' needs are met," (Bisch, 1998, p. 52). Partnerships were established that were "based on a shared vision, commitment to common goals, mutual trust, respect for the different contributions of others, shared responsibilities and shared ownership of the process and outcomes," (Bisch, 1998, p. 53). Contracting is inherent in the role of the private sector, industry, universities, professional bodies, nongovernmental organizations, and communities that worked together as partners to deal with maternal mortality in this region.

Other international organizations have engaged in a form of health contracting for many years. Agencies like The American Refugee Committee and the Peace Corps have established agreements with authorities in third-world countries to develop health programs and provide services to prevent health problems and promote the health of at-risk populations. Sanitation programs, mass immunization efforts, flood and famine relief, and treatment and prevention of such diseases as tuberculosis, HIV disease, and cholera are examples. The concept of contracting applies equally at the international level. Needs must be explored, goals established, resources explored, a plan developed, responsibilities assigned, a time frame agreed on, progress and outcomes evaluated, and interventions renegotiated or terminated. As a part of the collaborative team, community health nurses can play an important role in international contracting.

SUMMARY

Communication and collaboration are important tools for community health nurses to promote aggregate health. Communication involves the transfer and understanding of meaning between individuals. The communication process comprises seven parts: a message, a sender, a receiver, encoding, a channel, decoding, and a feedback loop. Barriers to effective communication include selective perception, language barriers, clients filtering out parts of the message, and emotional influence. Core skills essential to effective communication in community health nursing include sending skills, which allow the nurse to transmit messages effectively; re-

ceiving skills, which allow the nurse to receive accurate and complete messages; and interpersonal skills, which allow the nurse to interact and respond to the messages from clients. These skills include special techniques of active listening, the ability to show respect regardless of the message (whether positive or negative), the ability to empathize with clients' thoughts and feelings, and the ability to develop trust. Many factors can influence the quality of communication, such as negative previous experience, cultural influence, and relationships among the people involved. The community health nurse must consider all of these factors when trying to foster good communication.

In community health, nurses frequently need to promote communication in groups and in group decision-making. Decisions made by groups have many advantages, including the members sharing their experience and expertise, diversity of opinions, potential for broadening members' perspectives, and a focus on arriving at consensus solutions. There are several methods of enhancing group decision-making, including brainstorming, nominal group technique, delphi technique, and electronic meetings. Nursing informatics, or all of the computer-generated tools created to enhance communication, is changing the form of communicating in community health nursing, as it has in the acute care setting.

Collaboration is a purposeful interaction between nurse, clients, community members, and other professionals based on mutual participation and joint effort. It is characterized by shared goals, mutual participation, maximized use of resources, clear responsibilities, and set boundaries. Clients play an important role in the collaborative relationship.

Contracting also is a helpful tool in promoting clients' participation, independence, and motivation. It is used at all levels in community health nursing to promote partnership in the collaborative process, to encourage commitment to health goals, and to ensure a format and a means for negotiation among the collaborating group. Contracts can be formal or informal, written or verbal, simple or complex. The nurse must know the needs and abilities of clients and must tailor the type of contracting to best suit the client's particular situation.

ACTIVITIES TO PROMOTE CRITICAL THINKING

1. Discuss how you would handle the communication barrier of selective perception with a group of clients.
2. Practice active listening with a colleague and analyze the factors that interfered with your total concentration. Identify three actions to take to improve your active listening and apply them during the next week, keeping a log of your progress.
3. Use nominal group technique with a group of classmates to arrive at a rank-ordering of barriers to cross-cultural communication. What did you learn about arriving at a quality decision in the process?
4. Organize a group of classmates to represent a group of clients, professionals, and community members who are collaborating to address the needs of an inner city homeless population. Analyze how well you integrated the five characteristics of collaboration into your activity.
5. Explain the concept of contracting as it applies to aggregates. Discuss its four distinctive characteristics and the advantages that contracting offers to the community health nurse.

6. Develop a hypothetical contract with a group of elderly widows who need support and outlets for their loneliness. What other community members and professionals might be helpful as part of a collaborative team to address the widows' needs?
7. Become a good listener. This exercise asks you to list your closest friends, relatives, school, and work associates. Rank them on a scale of 1 to 10, 1 meaning always fascinating and 10 the most boring. If you find that you've labeled most as boring, you probably have one of two problems: (1) you're socializing or working with the wrong people, or (2) you're a poor listener. The likelihood is the latter. To improve listening skills, compliment people and encourage them; this will increase the chance that they will continue conversing with you, a skill valuable in both your personal and professional life.
8. Experiment in communication. This can be used with your peers or as part of a group teaching project on communication with elementary or high school students:
Purpose
   To demonstrate the differences between one-way and two-way communication and to demonstrate the advantages of the latter.
Setting
   Can be conducted in the classroom with any size group. Each person will need paper and pencil.
Procedure
   Have the group members select one person who everyone believes can communicate clearly and effectively. Have this person be out of sight of the "receivers" but clearly heard and have the "sender" describe to the group a diagram that they are to draw. Using Diagram 1 (p. 150), the sender explains the diagram so the receivers are able to recreate it exactly. Each receiver is to follow the sender's directions without having any communication with the sender or other group members. Time the exercise. When the receivers are finished, rank accuracy of the receiver's drawings by placing them on a Likert scale, as follows:

1 Least accurate--x----x----------x--Most accurate 10

   Ask receivers how they felt and how the sender probably felt. Ask the sender how she or he felt. Next, begin the two-way communication demonstration by allowing the sender to remain in sight of the group as Diagram 2 is explained to be drawn. Allow the receivers to ask questions. The sender may reply but may not use gestures. Record the time and rank for accuracy. Discuss how the receivers felt and how the sender probably felt. Ask the sender how she or he felt this time.

Analysis

1. Two-way communication takes longer.
2. Two-way communication results in greater accuracy among the drawings.
3. In one-way communication, the sender often feels relatively confident; the receiver, uncertain or frustrated.
4. In two-way communication, the sender may feel frustrated or angry; the receiver relatively confident.

Compare your findings with these.

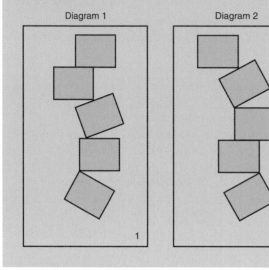

Diagram 1   Diagram 2

REFERENCES

Airhihenbuwa, C.O. (1995). *Health and culture.* Thousand Oaks, CA: Sage.

Allender, J.A., Carey, K.T., Castanon, J.G., Garcia, B., Gonzalez, B., Hedge, G., Herrell, A., Kiyuna, R., Rector, C., & Henderson-Sparks, J. (1997, April). *Interprofessional training project: California State University, Fresno. Serving children and families.* Monmouth, OR: Teaching Research Division.

Baldwin, D.C. (1996). Some historical notes on interdisciplinary and interprofessional education and practice in health care in the USA. *Journal of Interprofessional Care, 10*(2), 173–187.

Balzer-Riley, J. (1996). *Communications in nursing: Communicating assertively and responsibly in nursing. A guidebook* (3rd ed.). St. Louis: Mosby.

Bisch, S.A. (1998). Sharing in practice: New partnerships for health. *International Nurses Review, 45*(2), 51–54, 60.

Bohny, B. (1997). A time for self-care: Role of the home healthcare nurse. *Home Healthcare Nurse, 15*(4), 281–286.

Bragg, M.E. (1997). An empowerment approach to community health education. In B.W. Spradley & J.A. Allender (Eds.), *Readings in community health nursing* (5th ed.). Philadelphia: Lippincott-Raven, 504–510.

Brill, N.I. (1973). *Working with people: The helping process.* Philadelphia: J.B. Lippincott.

Bryans, A. & McIntosh, J. (1996). Decision-making in community nursing: An analysis of the stages of decision-making as they relate to community nursing assessment practice. *Journal of Advanced Nursing, 24,* 24–30.

Cady, C., et al. (1991). Using a learning contract to successfully discharge an infant on home total parenteral nutrition. *Pediatric Nursing, 17*(1), 67–71, 74.

Corrigan, D. & Udas, K. (1996). Creating collaborative, child- and family-centered education, health, and human services systems. In J. Sikula, T. Buttrey, & E. Guyton (Eds.), *The handbook of research on teacher education* (2nd ed., pp. 893–921). New York: Simon and Schuster Macmillan.

England, M. (1996). Content domain for caregiver planning identified by adult offspring caregivers. *Image: Journal of Nursing Scholarship, 28*(1), 17–22.

Gebbie, K.M. (1999). The public health workforce: Key to public health infrastructure. *American Journal of Public Health, 89*(5), 660–661.

Graves, J. & Corcoran, D. (1989). The study of nursing informatics. *Image: Journal of Nursing Scholarship, 21*(3), 227–231.

Gustafson, M.B. (1977). Let's broaden our horizons about the use of contracts. *International Nursing Review, 24*(1), 18–19.

Henson, R.H. (1997). Analysis of the concept of mutuality. *Image: Journal of Nursing Scholarship, 29*(1), 77–81.

Hiraki, A. (1998). Corporate language and nursing practice. *Nursing Outlook, 46*(3), 115–119.

Hiromoto, B.M., et al. (1991). Contract learning for self-care activities: A protocol study among chemotherapy outpatients. *Cancer Nursing, 14*(3), 148–154.

Hooper-Briar, K. & Lawson. H. (Eds.) (1996). *Expanding partnerships for vulnerable children, youth and families.* Washington, DC: Council on Social Work Education.

Humphrey, C.J. & Milone-Nuzzo, P. (1991). *Home care nursing: An orientation to practice.* Norwalk, CT: Appleton & Lange.

Ignatavicius, D.G. & Hausman, K.A. (1995). *Clinical pathways for collaborative practice.* Philadelphia: W.B. Saunders.

Johnson, L. (1992). Interactive planning: A model for self-empowerment. *Nursing Administration Quarterly, 16*(3), 47–57.

Kreps, G.L. & Kunimoto, E.N. (1994). *Effective communication in multicultural health care settings.* Thousand Oaks, CA: Sage.

Lindell, A.R. (1986). Clinical contractual agreements: Liability or blessing? *Journal of Professional Nursing, 2*(3), 138.

Lorig, K.R., Mazonson, P.D., & Holman, H.R. (1993). Evidence suggesting that health education for self-management in patients with chronic arthritis has sustained health benefits while reducing health care costs. *Arthritis Rheumatology, 36,* 439–446.

Marshall, S.G. & Houseman, C.A. (1999). *Communicating in nursing.* Philadelphia: Lippincott Williams & Wilkins.

McCloskey, J.C. & Maas, M. (1998). Interdisciplinary team: The nursing perspective is essential. *Nursing Outlook, 46*(4), 157–163.

Northouse, P.G. & Northouse, L.L. (1997). *Health communication: Strategies for health professionals* (3rd ed.). Norwalk, CT: Appleton & Lange.

Orme, L. & Maggs, C. (1993). Decision-making in clinical practice: How do expert nurses, midwifes and health visitors make decisions? *Nurse Education Today, 13,* 270–276.

Plimpton, S. & Root, J. (1994). Materials and strategies that work in low literacy health communication. *Public Health Reports, 109*(1), 86–92.

Robbins, S.P. (1998). *Organizational behavior* (8th ed.). Upper Saddle River, NJ: Prentice-Hall.

Sauer, J.K. (1973, summer). The process of contracting in the helping relationship. *Minnesota Welfare*, 12–14, 23.

Shockley-Zalabak, P. (1994). *Understanding organizational communication*. New York: Longman.

Sloan, M. & Schommer, B.T. (1997). The process of contracting in community nursing. In B.W. Spradley & J.A. Allender (Eds.), *Readings in community health nursing* (5th ed.). Philadelphia: Lippincott-Raven.

Smith, E.C. (1994). A model of caregiving effectiveness for technologically dependent adults residing at home. *Advances in Nursing Science, 17*(2), 27–40.

Stevens, P.E. & Hall, J.M. (1992). Applying critical theories to nursing in communities. *Public Health Nursing, 9*(1), 2–9.

Thede, L.Q. (1998). *Computers in nursing: Bridges to the future.* Philadelphia: Lippincott Williams & Wilkins.

Turley, J.P. (1996). Toward a model for nursing informatics. *Image: Journal of Nursing Scholarship, 28*(4), 309–313.

Wandel, J.C., et al. (1991). Case report: The care of patients with behavioral problems [including commentary by P. Mian and D. Danis]. *Journal of Professional Nursing, 7*(2), 126–135.

Wills, E.M. (1996). Nurse-client alliance: A pattern of home health caring. *Home Healthcare Nurse, 14*(6), 455–459.

INTERNET RESOURCES

American Medical Informatics Association (AMIA):

http://www.amia.org.

AMIA Nursing Informatics Working Group:

http://www.gl.umbc.edu/~abbott/nursinfo.html

British Computer Society Nursing Specialist Group:

http://www.man.ac.uk/bcsnsg

Canada's Health Informatics Association:
http://www.coachorg.com

Midwest Alliance for Nursing Informatics:
http://www.maninet.org

Virtually Informatics Nursing:

http://milkman.cac.psu.edu/~dxm12/vin.html

Health Informatics Society of Australia (Vic.), Inc.:

http://www.hisavic.aus.net

National League for Nursing's Council for Nursing Informatics (CNI):

http://www.nln.org/info-councils-executive.htm#cni

Whole Nurse Informatics Page:

http://www.wholenurse.com/informatics.htm

SELECTED READINGS

Butterfoss, F.D., et al. (1993). Community coalitions for prevention and health promotion. *Health Education Research, 8*(3), 315–30.

DeLellis, A.J., Henry, J., & Decker, L.E. (1998). Collaboration between schools of nursing and local education agencies to provide health care services to pre-kindergarten through twelfth grade students: Elements of cooperative agreements. *Public Health Nursing, 15*(2), 104–108.

Douglas, G., Robbins, W., & Sullivan-Paal, C. (1994). Beyond rhetoric: Building and achieving community consensus in planning and developing an innovative public health nurse-midwifery education program. *Public Health Nursing, 11*(3), 181–187.

DuBrin, A.J. (1997). *Human relations interpersonal, job-oriented skills* (6th ed.). Upper Saddle River. NJ: Prentice-Hall.

Edwards, J.B., Stanton, P.E., & Bishop, W.S. (1997). Interdisciplinarity: The story of a journey. *Nursing and Health Care Perspectives, 18*(3), 116–117.

Farley, S. (1993). The community as partner in primary health care. *Nursing and Health Care, 14*(5), 244–249.

Hanna, K.M. (1993), Effect of nurse-client transaction on female adolescents' oral contraceptive adherence. *Image: Journal of Nursing Scholarship, 25*(4), 285–290.

Hooper-Briar, K. & Lawson, H. (1994). *Serving children, youth and families through interprofessional collaboration and service integration: A framework for action.* Oxford, OH: The Institute for Educational Renewal at Miami University and The Danforth Foundation.

Kalisch, B. (1973). What is empathy? *American Journal of Nursing, 73*, 1548–1552.

Katzenbach, J.R. & Smith, D.K. (1993). *The wisdom of teams: Creating the high performance organization.* Boston: Harvard Business School Press.

Knapp, M. (1995). How shall we study comprehensive, collaborative services for children and families? *Educational Researcher, 24*, 5–16.

Kristjanson, L. & Chalmers, K. (1990). Nurse-client interactions in community-based practice: Creating common ground. *Public Health Nursing, 7*(4), 215–223.

Leviton, L.C., Needleman, C.E., & Shapiro, M.A. (1997). *Confronting public health risks: A decision maker's guide.* Thousand Oaks, CA: Sage.

McCloskey, J.C. (1995) The nurse executive: The discipline hearts of a multidisciplinary team. *Journal of Professional Nursing, 11*, 202.

McDonald, C.J. (1997) The barriers to electronic medical record systems and how to overcome them. *Journal of the American Medical Information Association, 4*, 213–221.

Nicoll, L.H. (1998). *Nurses' guide to the Internet.* Philadelphia: Lippincott-Raven.

Noone, C., Cavanaugh, J., & McKillip, C. (1995). Computerized documentation in home health. *Journal of Nursing Administration, 25*(1), 67–69.

Polivka, B.J. (1995). A conceptual model for community interagency collaboration. *Image: Journal of Nursing Scholarship, 27*(2), 110–115.

Wilson, A. (1998). Education is the key to understanding outcomes. *Home Healthcare Nurse, 16*(11), 785.

Wright, J., Henry, S., Holzemer, W., & Falknor, P. (1993). Evaluation of community-based nurse case management activities for symptomatic HIV/AIDS clients: California pilot care and waiver projects for HIV/AIDS. *Journal of Association of Nurses in AIDS Care, 4*(2), 37–47.

Health Promotion Through Education

KEY TERMS

- Accommodation (Piaget)
- Adaptation (Piaget)
- Affective domain
- Anticipatory guidance
- Assimilation (Piaget)
- Cognitive domain
- Gestalt-field
- Learning
- Operationalize
- Psychomotor domain
- Teaching

LEARNING OBJECTIVES

Upon mastery of this chapter, you should be able to:

- Identify how the nurse collaborates with other professionals using *Healthy People 2010* as a guide for educational and community-based programs.
- Describe the community health nurse's role as educator in promoting health and preventing or postponing morbidity.
- Identify educational activities for the nurse to use that are appropriate for each of the three domains of learning.
- Select learning theories that are applicable to an individual, family, or aggregate client.
- Identify health teaching models for use when planning health education activities.
- Select teaching methods and materials that facilitate learning for clients at different developmental levels.
- Develop teaching plans focusing on primary, secondary, and tertiary levels of prevention for clients of all ages.
- Identify teaching strategies for the community health nurse to use when encountering clients with special learning needs.
- Locate appropriate multimedia resources to enhance client learning.

Think of a time when you were so influenced by a teacher that you stopped an unhealthy habit, altered a long-held belief, or embarked on a new endeavor. What precisely was it that motivated the change? Was it simply the content of the teaching, or was it how the teacher presented the content? What is good teaching, and why is it important to community health nursing?

Teaching has been a critical part of the community health nurse's role since the origins of the profession and frequently is the primary role or function. Community health nurses develop partnerships with clients to achieve behavior changes that promote, maintain, or restore health. This partnership focuses on self-care—the ability to effectively advocate and manage a person's own health. The rationale for health teaching is to equip people with the knowledge, attitudes, and practices that will allow them to live the fullest possible life for the greatest length of time. The goals of *Healthy People 2010* emphasize not only health status and longevity but also the quality of our lives; they state that even the later years should be full of vigor (U.S. Department of Health and Human Services, 2000). Table 9–1 provides a list of *Healthy People 2010 objectives* for educational, community-based programs.

When the community health nurse identifies a need that is best met through health edu-

Objective	2010 Goals	Baseline
High school completion	Increase the high school completion rate to at least 90%.	85%
School health education	Increase to at least 70% the proportion of middle/junior high and senior high schools that require 1 school year of health education.	28%
Undergraduate health risk behavior information	Increase to at least 25% the proportion of undergraduate students attending postsecondary institutions who receive information from their college or university on all six priority health risk behavior areas—behaviors that cause unintentional and intentional injuries, tobacco use, alcohol and other drug use, sexual behavior, dietary patterns that cause disease, and inadequate physical activity.	6%
School nurse-to-student ratio	Increase to at least 50% the proportion of the middle/junior and senior high schools that have a nurse-to-student ratio of at least 1:750.	28%
Work site health-promotion programs	Increase to 100% the proportion of work sites (with more than 50% employees) that offer a comprehensive health-promotion program to their employees.	95%
Participation in employer-sponsored health-promotion activities	Increase to at least 50% the proportion of all employees (over age 18) who participate in employer-sponsored health-promotion activities.	28%
Patient satisfaction with health care provider communication	This objective is developmental: increase the proportion of patients who report that they are satisfied with the patient education they receive from their health care organization.	—
Community-based health promotion	This objective is developmental: increase the proportion of tribal and local health service areas or jurisdictions that have established a community health promotion program that addresses multiple *Healthy People 2010* focus areas.	—
Culturally appropriate community health-promotion programs	Increase the proportion of local health departments to at least 50% that have established culturally appropriate and linguistically competent community health-promotion and disease-prevention programs for racial and ethnic minority populations.	13–27%
Elderly participation in community health promotion	Increase to at least 90% the proportion of people age 65 and older who have participated during the preceding year in at least one organized health-promotion program.	12%

(U.S. Department of Health and Human Services. [2000, January]. *Healthy People 2010* [conference edition in two volumes]. Washington, DC: Author.)

TABLE 9–1. Healthy People 2010 Objectives for Educational and Community-Based Programs

cation, the nurse is faced with a series of questions: How can I teach effectively? What content should I cover? What method of presentation will communicate most effectively? What resources can I use as teaching tools? How do I know when the client has grasped the information or mastered the skills? How do I help clients with special learning needs? In other words, what makes teaching effective, how are teaching skills acquired, and how is mastery measured? This chapter addresses these questions and discusses teaching as a basic intervention tool in community health nursing practice.

Teaching is a specialized communication process in which desired behavior changes are achieved. The goal of all teaching is learning. Learning is thought to mean gaining knowledge, comprehension, or mastery. These are nebulous terms, and a more acceptable definition suggests that **learning** is a process of assimilating new information that promotes a permanent change in behavior. All people have been presented with information that was not interesting, relevant to their needs, or comprehensible. In such situations, learning was difficult, if not impossible. The nurse as a teacher seeks to transmit information in such a way that the client demonstrates a relatively permanent change in behavior. Af-

ter learning, clients are capable of doing something that they could not do before learning took place (Hergenhahn & Olson, 1997). Effective teaching is a cause; learning becomes the effect. To teach effectively, especially in the community where teaching is the focus of care, nurses need to understand the various domains of learning and related learning theories.

THE DOMAINS OF LEARNING

Learning occurs in several realms or domains: cognitive, affective, and psychomotor. Understanding the differences among the domains and the related role of the nurse provides the background necessary to teach effectively.

Cognitive Domain

The **cognitive domain** of learning involves the mind and thinking processes. When the meaning and relationship of a series of facts is grasped, cognitive learning is experienced.

The cognitive domain deals with the recall or recognition of knowledge and the development of intellectual abilities and skills (Bloom, 1956). There are six major levels in the cognitive domain (Gronlund, 1970): knowledge, comprehension, application, analysis, synthesis, and evaluation. To **operationalize** these levels (ie, put these ideas or concepts into words that can be used), verbs are used. As the goal of the learning or behavioral objective changes, so do the verbs, indicating the learning to be accomplished within that particular level of the cognitive domain. Notice that the objectives at the beginning of each chapter in this text follow this format, using a variety of verbs to indicate the expected level of learning. A representative sample of behavioral objectives focusing on nutrition and appropriate cognitive-level verbs is included in the discussion of each level.

KNOWLEDGE

Knowledge, the lowest level of learning, involves recall. If students remember material previously learned, they have acquired knowledge. This level may be used with clients who are unable to understand underlying reasons or rationales, such as people who have had strokes or young children. Stroke clients may need to remember that medication should be taken daily, that regular exercise restores function, and that drinking alcohol should be avoided, although they may not grasp the reasons behind these measures. Five-year-olds may need to identify healthful foods rather than understand why they are nutritious.

A knowledge-level behavioral objective might be: The client can *recall* the names of six fruits to eat as nutritious snacks. Other knowledge-level verbs include define, repeat, list, and name.

COMPREHENSION

The second level of cognitive learning, comprehension, combines remembering with understanding. Teaching aims at instilling at least a minimum understanding. Nurses want clients to grasp the meaning and to recognize the importance of suggested health behaviors.

An example of a comprehension-level behavioral objective might be: The pregnant client will *describe* a well-balanced diet during pregnancy. Other appropriate verbs at the comprehension level include discuss, explain, identify, tell, and report.

APPLICATION

Application is the third level of cognitive learning in which the learner is able to not only understand material but also apply it to new situations. Application approaches the possibility of self-care when clients use their knowledge for improvement of their own health. The test of application is a transfer of understanding into practice. Thus, to encourage application, the nurse can design teaching plans that show clients how to put knowledge into practice. For example, a program using this approach to prevent relapse in women who quit smoking during pregnancy resulted in decreased use of tobacco products among the women in the study for

up to 6 months postpartum (McBride et al., 1999). In the home setting, a nurse may suggest that a diabetic client write down glucometer readings to show the nurse at the next visit. A school nurse could ask adolescents in a weight-loss group to keep a diet record for a week, draw up a diet plan, and share this plan with the group at the next meeting. In contrast, the construction worker who understands on-the-job hazards but seldom wears a protective hat in the work area has yet to transfer knowledge and comprehension into practice.

An example of an application-level behavioral objective might be: The client will *practice* eating well-balanced meals at least two times a day. Other verbs at this level include apply, use, demonstrate, and illustrate.

ANALYSIS

The fourth level of cognitive learning is analysis: at this level, the learner breaks down material into parts, distinguishes between elements, and understands the relationships among the parts. This level of learning becomes a preliminary step toward problem-solving. The learner carefully scrutinizes all of the variables or elements and their relationships to each other to explain the situation. A family that studies its own communication patterns to identify sources of conflict is using analysis. A mother analyzes when she seeks to determine the cause of an infant's crying. After viewing the total situation, she breaks it down into variables such as hunger, pain, overstimulation, loneliness, type of crying, and intensity of crying. She examines these parts and draws conclusions about their relationships. In health teaching, community health nurses foster clients' analytic skills by (1) demonstrating how to isolate the parts in a situation, and (2) encouraging them to consider the relationship of the parts and draw conclusions from their thinking.

An analysis-level behavioral objective for senior citizens trying to learn more about low-fat foods might be: The seniors should be able to *compare* the fat content in a variety of packaged foods. Other verbs at the analysis level include differentiate, contrast, debate, question, and examine.

SYNTHESIS

Synthesis, the fifth level of cognitive learning, is the ability not only to break down and understand the elements of a situation, but also to form elements into a new whole. Synthesis combines all of the earlier levels of cognitive learning to culminate in the production of a unique plan or solution. Clients who achieve learning at this level not only analyze their problems but also find solutions for them. For example, a nurse may assist mental health clients in a therapy group to examine their frequent depression and then to generate their own plan for alleviating it. A young couple who want to toilet train their 2-year-old child learns the physiologic and psychological dimensions of toilet training, analyzes their own situation, and then develops strategies (their own plan) for training the child. Nurses facilitate synthesis by assisting and encouraging clients to develop their own solutions with specific plans. When a problem is identified, the client should be asked, "What are

TABLE 9–2. Cognitive Learning: Case Study in Controlling Diabetes

Level	Illustrative Client Behavior	Illustrative Nurse Behavior
Knowledge (recalls, knows)	States that insulin, if taken, will control own diabetes	Provides information
Comprehension (understands)	Describes insulin action and purpose	Explains information
Application (uses learning)	Adjusts insulin dosage daily to maintain proper blood sugar level	Suggests how to use learning
Analysis (examines, explains)	Discusses relationships between insulin, diet, activity, and diabetic control	Demonstrates and encourages analysis
Synthesis (integrates with other learning, generates new ideas)	Develops a plan, incorporating above learning, for controlling own diabetes	Promotes client formulation of own plan
Evaluation (judges according to a standard)	Compares degree of diabetic control (outcomes) with desired control (objectives)	Facilitates evaluation

some possible causes? Do you see anything that has been over-looked about the problem?" If the client asks for a solution, the nurse should encourage synthesis by asking, "What are some possible solutions to this problem that you might carry out?"

An example of a synthesis-level behavioral objective for a client on a sodium-restricted diet might be: The client will be able to *prepare* an enjoyable meal using low-sodium foods. Other verbs at this level include compose, design, formulate, create, and organize.

EVALUATION

The highest level of cognitive learning is evaluation: at this level, the learner judges the usefulness of new material compared with a stated purpose or specific criteria (Gronlund, 1970). Clients can learn to judge their own health behavior by comparing it with standards established by others—such as complete abstinence from smoking, maintenance of normal weight, or exercising three times a week—or clients may establish their own criteria. For example, a parent support group might design activities to enhance parent-child communication, then judge their performance by using their desired outcomes as evaluation criteria. When nurses aim for this level of client learning, they have made self-care a concrete objective. Evaluation, because it goes beyond attempts at problem-solving, enables the client to judge the adequacy of solutions, to critique lifestyle and health-related behavior, and to anticipate needed improvements.

An example of a behavioral objective at the evaluation level might be: The clients in a nutrition class will be able to *measure* the cholesterol content in one portion of the low-cholesterol dish they brought to share. Other verbs at this level include judge, rate, choose, and estimate.

HOW TO MEASURE COGNITIVE LEARNING

Cognitive learning at any of the levels described can be measured easily in terms of learner behaviors. Nurses know, for instance, that clients have achieved teaching objectives for the application of knowledge when their behavior demonstrates actual use of the information taught. Client roles in cognitive learning range from relatively passive (at the knowledge level) to active (at the evaluation level). Con-versely, as clients become more active, the nurse's role becomes less directive. Notice that not all clients need to be brought through all levels of cognitive learning, nor does every client need to reach the evaluation level for each aspect of care. For some clients and situations, comprehension is an adequate and effective level; for others, the nurse should focus on the application level as the level of achievement. Table 9–2 illustrates client and nurse behaviors for each cognitive level.

Affective Domain

The **affective domain** in which learning occurs involves emotion, feeling, or affect. This kind of learning deals with changes in interest, attitudes, and values (Bloom, 1956). Here, nurses face the task of trying to influence what clients value and feel. Nurses want them to develop an ability to accept ideas that promote healthier behavior patterns even though those ideas may conflict with their own values.

Attitudes and values are learned (Bigge, 1982). They develop gradually, as the way an individual feels and responds is molded by family, peers, experiences, and societal influences. These feelings and responses are the result of imitation and conditioning. In this way, clients acquire their health-related beliefs and practices. Because attitudes and values become part of the person, they are difficult to change unless the nurse is aware of how they develop.

Affective learning occurs on several levels as learners respond with varying degrees of involvement and commitment. At the first level, learners are simply receptive; they are willing to listen, show awareness, and be attentive. The nurse aims at acquiring and focusing learners' attention (Gronlund, 1970). This limited goal may be all that clients are ready for at the early stages of the nurse-client relationship.

At the second level, learners become active participants by responding to the information in some way. Examples are a willingness to read educational material, to participate in discussion, to complete assignments such as keeping a diet record, or to voluntarily seek out more information.

At the third level, learners attach value to the information.

TABLE 9–3. Affective Learning: Case Study in Family Planning

Level	Illustrative Client Behavior	Illustrative Nurse Behavior
Receptive (listens, pays attention)	Attentive to family planning instruction	Directs client's attention
Responsive (participates, reacts)	Discusses pros and cons of various methods	Encourages client involvement
Valuing (accepts, appreciates commits)	Selects a method for use	Respects client's right to decide
Internal consistency (organizes values to fit together)	Understands and accepts responsibility for planning for desired number of children	Brings client into contact with role models
Adoption (incorporates new values into lifestyle)	Consistently practices birth control	Positively reinforces healthy behaviors

Valuing ranges from simple acceptance through appreciation to commitment. For example, a nurse taught members of a therapy group several principles concerning group effectiveness. An explanation of the importance of a democratic group process and ways to improve group skills was given. Members showed acceptance when they acknowledged the importance of these ideas. They showed appreciation of the ideas by starting to practice them. Commitment came when they assumed responsibility for having their group function well.

The final level of affective learning occurs when learners internalize an idea or value. The value system now controls learner behavior. Consistent practice is a crucial test at this level. Clients who know and respect the value of exercise but only occasionally play tennis or go for a walk have not internalized the value. Even several weeks of enthusiastic jogging are not evidence of an internalized value. If the jogging continues for 6 months, a year, or longer, learning may have been internalized.

Affective learning often is difficult to measure. This elusiveness may influence community health nurses to concentrate their efforts on cognitive learning goals instead. Yet client attitudes and values have a major effect on the outcome of cognitive learning—desired behavioral changes. Therefore, both cognitive and affective domains must remain linked in teaching; otherwise, results quickly fade.

Attitudes and values can change in the same way that they were first learned, that is, through imitation and conditioning (Hergenhahn & Olson, 1997; Redman, 1996). Role models, particularly those from the client's peer group who practice the desired health behaviors, can be a strong influence. Support groups like mastectomy clubs or chemical dependency support groups can have a powerful role-model effect. Frequently, the nurse may be viewed as a role model by clients; thus, nurses should be careful to demonstrate healthy behaviors.

Attitudes often change when the nurse provides clients with a satisfying experience during the learning process. The nurse who recognizes clients' participation in a group, praises them for completing assignments, or commends them for sticking to diet plans will have more success than the nurse who only criticizes failures. Another point to remember is that clients can develop a close relationship with the nurse during the teaching-learning process. When this oc-

curs, some limited sharing of the nurse's experiences in managing personal health issues may be appropriate to let clients know that the nurse, too, is human. This can be an effective addition to teaching strategies if it feels comfortable and is used wisely. Table 9–3 shows client and nurse behaviors for each level of affective learning.

To influence affective learning requires patience. Values and attitudes seldom change overnight. Remember that other forces continue to reinforce former values. For example, a middle-aged housewife may want to pursue a career for self-fulfillment, but she might not do so because she has children in high school and feels that their needs come first. A young man can verbalize to the nurse the importance of safe sex but is uncomfortable discussing the subject with his partner, jeopardizing his compliance with the nurse's instruction.

Psychomotor Domain

The **psychomotor domain** includes visible, demonstrable performance skills that require some kind of neuromuscular coordination. Clients in the community need to learn skills such as infant bathing, temperature taking, breast or testicular self-examination, prenatal breathing exercises, range-of-motion exercises, catheter irrigation, walking with crutches, and how to change dressings.

For psychomotor learning to take place, three conditions must be met: (1) learners must be capable of the skill, (2) learners must have a sensory image of how to perform the skill, and (3) learners must practice the skill.

The nurse must be certain the client is physically, intellectually, and emotionally capable of performing the skill. An elderly diabetic man with tremulous hands and fading vision should not be expected to give his own insulin injections; it could frustrate and harm him. An accessible person more physically capable should be enlisted and taught the skill. Clients' intellectual and emotional capabilities also influence their capacity to learn motor skills. It may be inappropriate to expect persons of limited intelligence to learn complex skills. The degree of complexity should match the learners' level of functioning. However, educational level should not be equated with intelligence. Many clients may have had limited formal schooling but are able to learn com-

TABLE 9–4. Nurse Behaviors in Psychomotor Learning		
The Nurse	**Provides Sensory Image**	**Encourages Practice**
Determines capability: Assesses client's physical, intellectual, and emotional ability	Demonstrates and explains	Uses guidance and positive reinforcement

plex skills for themselves or as a caregiver after thorough instruction. Developmental stage is another point to consider in determining whether it is appropriate to teach a particular skill. For example, most children can put on some article of clothing at 2 years of age but are not ready to learn to fasten buttons until well past their third birthday.

Learners also must have a sensory image of how to perform the skill through sight, hearing, touch, and sometimes taste or smell. This sensory image is gained by demonstration. To teach clients motor skills effectively, the nurse has to provide them with an adequate sensory image. The nurse must demonstrate and explain slowly, one point at a time, and sometimes repeatedly, until clients understand the proper sequence or combination of actions necessary to carry out the skill.

The third necessary condition for psychomotor learning is practice. After acquiring a sensory image, clients can start to perform the skill. Mastery comes over time as clients repeat the task until it is smooth, coordinated, and unhesitating. During this process, the nurse should be available to provide guidance and encouragement. In the early stages of practice, the nurse may need to use hands-on guidance to give clients a sense of how the performance should feel. When clients give a return demonstration, the nurse can make suggestions, give encouragement, and thereby maximize the learning. For example, a nurse demonstrates passive range-of-motion exercises on a client's wife to show her how the exercises should feel (giving her a sensory image). Then the wife learns to do them for her husband. During practice, feedback from the nurse enables the wife to know if the skill is being performed correctly.

The psychomotor domain, like the cognitive and affective domains, ranges from simple to complex levels of functioning. It is necessary to exercise judgment in assessing clients' ability to perform a skill. Even clients with limited ability often can move to higher levels once they have mastered simple skills. Nurse behaviors that influence psychomotor learning are shown in Table 9–4.

LEARNING THEORIES

A *learning theory* is a systematic and integrated look into the nature of the process whereby people relate to their surroundings in such ways as to enhance their ability to use both themselves and their surroundings more effectively. Nurses have and use a particular theory of learning, whether consciously or unconsciously, and that theory, in turn, dictates their way of teaching. It is useful to discover what that learning theory is and how it affects the nurse's role as health educator.

Some of the learning theories developed by educational psychologists in the 20th century remain influential. They are grouped into four categories: behavioral, cognitive, social, and humanistic. Recently, the adult learning theory of Malcolm Knowles (1980, 1984, 1989) has influenced client teaching. A brief examination of these categories and the specific theories of each follows.

Behavioral Learning Theories

Behavioral theory (also known as stimulus-response or conditioning theory) approaches the study of learning by focusing on behaviors that can be observed, measured, and changed. Developed early in the 20th century, behavioral theory work primarily is associated with three famous names: Ivan Pavlov (1957), Edward Thorndike (1932, 1969), and B.F. Skinner (1974, 1987). Essentially, to a behavioralist, learning is a behavioral change—a response to certain stimuli. Thus, the behaviorialistic teacher seeks to significantly change learners' behaviors through a series of selected stimuli.

The stimulus-response "bond" theory proposes that with conditioning, certain causes (stimuli) evoke certain effects (responses). The teacher promotes acquisition of the desired stimulus-response connections so that transfer of learning can occur in another situation having the same stimulus-response elements. Pavlov's early work with stimulus-response and involuntary reflex actions is the best-known application of this theory. Pavlov conditioned a dog to anticipate food by ringing a bell at feeding time. Initially, the dog would salivate as the food was brought to the cage. However, after time, the dog would salivate at hearing the bell, before seeing or smelling the food.

Two other behavioral theories are conditioning with no reinforcement (Thorndike) and conditioning through reinforcement (Skinner). No-reinforcement theorists focus on the learner's innate reflexive drives to accomplish the desired response after conditioning, such as when the nurse repeatedly emphasizes to a group of pregnant women that their prenatal classes promote a positive delivery experience and healthy newborns. In contrast, the reinforcement theorists

TABLE 9–5. Piaget's Five Phases of Cognitive Development

Age	Stage	Behavior
Birth to 2 y	Sensorimotor stage	The child moves focus from self to the environment (rituals are important).
2–4 y	Preconceptual stage	Language development is rapid and everything is related to "me."
4–7 y	Intuitive thought stage	Egocentric thinking diminishes, and words are used to express thoughts.
7–11 y	Concrete operations stage	Child can solve concrete problems and recognize others' viewpoints.
11–15 y	Formal operations stage	Child uses rational thinking and can develop ideas from general principles (deductive reasoning) and apply them to future situations.

use successive, systematic changes in the learner's environment to enhance the probability of desired responses. For example, a school nurse might give rewards (balloons, coloring books, crayons) to children who attend each class on safety.

Cognitive Learning Theories

Jean Piaget is the most widely known cognitive theorist. His theory of cognitive development has contributed to the theories of Kohlberg (moral development) and Fowler (development of faith). Piaget (1966, 1970) believed that cognitive development is an orderly, sequential, and interactive process in which a variety of new experiences must exist before intellectual abilities can develop. His work with children led him to develop five phases of cognitive development, from birth to 15 years of age (Table 9–5).

Each stage signifies a transformation from the previous one, and a child must move through each stage sequentially. The three abilities of **assimilation** (reacting to new situations by using skills already possessed), **accommodation** (being sufficiently mature so that previously unsolved problems can now be solved), and **adaptation** (the ability to cope with the demands of the environment) are used to make the transformation. Nurses must understand their audience's learning stage to ascertain how to approach teaching for that developmental stage. The nurse can see how the use of puppets with 3-year-olds may be a beneficial addition to a presentation on safety, whereas a group of young teens with diabetes can respond to the consequences of taking or not taking their insulin.

The **Gestalt-field** family of cognitive theories assumes that people are neither good nor bad—they simply interact with their environment, and their learning is related to perception (Wertheimer, 1959, 1980). Thus, this theory defines learning as a "reorganization of the learner's perceptual or psychological world" (Bigge, 1982, p. 57).

The first Gestalt-field theory, called *insight theory,* regards learning as a process in which the learner develops new insights or changes old ones. Learners sense their way intuitively and intelligently through problems. However, the "insight" is useful only if the learner understands its significance. For example, Lana dropped out of high school after the birth of her daughter and realizes, after attending a career planning class offered by a community health nurse, that she

has limited job skills and if she had learned how to use a computer, she could get a better job. This learner understands the significance of her insight. The second theory, *goal-insight,* is similar to the insight theory but goes beyond intuitive hunches to tested insights. Teachers subscribing to this theory promote insightful learning but assist learners in developing higher-quality insights. For example, Lana takes a beginning and then an advanced computer class and is offered a higher-paying job. The community health nurse discusses Lana's successes with her, asks if she ever thought about going to college, and mentions the added benefits of college-level course work. Lana reflects on this for a while and begins to think about completing the requirements to go to junior college because she could be promoted to supervisor if she had an associate degree. In the third theory, *cognitive-field theory,* the learner is seen as purposive and problem-centered. Teachers seek to help learners gain new insights and restructure their lives accordingly. For example, Lana confers with the community health nurse about her choices and has changed her thinking about herself so much that she is planning to get an apartment in a neighborhood that is better for her child and may continue taking classes " for the fun of it" after she completes her degree in a few months.

Social Learning Theories

The aim of social learning theory is to explain behavior and facilitate learning. An important social theorist, Bandura (1977, 1986) points out that apparent but not real relationships often are dysfunctional, producing undesirable or inappropriate behavior. He describes three ways that dysfunctional beliefs develop:

In coincidental association, outcomes typically are preceded by numerous events, and the client selects the wrong events as a predictor of an outcome. For example, Jolene Smyth had a negative experience with a man who wore a hearing aid. Afterward, all of her experiences with men who wore hearing aids were negative. She reached the conclusion that all men who wear hearing aids are undesirable. This client's beliefs became a self-fulfilling prophecy.

In inappropriate generalization, one negative experience provokes negative feelings for future experiences.

For example, Sue Nortly had a purse snatched by a teenager and generalizes that all teenagers are bad. Three-year-old Ryan Link accidentally drank some spoiled milk. He now generalizes that milk tastes bad and refuses to drink it.

In perceived self-inefficacy, "Persons who judge themselves as lacking coping capabilities, whether the self-appraisal is objectively warranted or not, will perceive all kinds of dangers in situations and exaggerate their potential harmfulness" (Bandura, 1986, p. 220). For example, an older client, Bill Hall, tells the community health nurse about two missing social security checks, but he refuses to take a bus to the post office. He states that he does not know what to say to the postal clerk and has read about senior citizens getting mugged on buses. He refused to follow up on his lost income.

Social learning theory focuses on the learners. They are benefitted by role models, building self-confidence, persuasion, and personal mastery. Self-efficacy can lead to the desired behaviors and outcomes. Jolene may begin to separate her negative experiences with men from their hearing disabilities after attending a class on building self-esteem suggested by the nurse. Through some positive experiences with teenagers organized by the nurse, Sue may learn that not all teenagers are bad. The nurse can suggest to Ryan's mother that he may be persuaded to drink chocolate milk. She then can slowly reintroduce plain milk. Bill might find the courage and self-confidence to solve future problems after his nurse introduces him to another gentleman in the apartment complex who feels confident in the neighborhood.

Humanistic Learning Theories

Humanistic theories assume that there is a natural tendency for people to learn and that learning flourishes in an encouraging environment. Two of the best-known humanists are Abraham Maslow and Carl Rogers. Abraham Maslow developed the classic hierarchy of human needs in the 1940s. It suggests that a person's first needs are physiologic (eg, air, food, water). Once these are met, people work to fulfill safety and security needs. Third is the need for love and a sense of belonging, then come self-esteem needs (positive feelings of self-worth). Only when these needs are met do people work toward self-actualization or becoming all that we can be (Maslow, 1970).

In community health nursing, the clients' needs must be considered when planning health education programs. For example, it would be difficult for a group of young mothers to concentrate on learning about proper infant nutrition if they are worried about their babies crying in the next room. Their need to care for their children (need of love and belonging) would be greater than the need to learn about future health considerations (self-esteem, self-actualization). Likewise, it is impossible for learning to take place if the room is so warm that the participants are falling asleep (physiologic needs are not being met).

Carl Rogers developed the client-centered counseling approach that has long been important in psychotherapy. He believed the role of therapist should be nondirective and accepting and proposed approaching clients in a warm, positive, and empathetic manner to get in touch with the their feelings and thoughts. Rogers soon applied his beliefs to education, suggesting that the learning environment be learner centered (1969, 1989). The outcome of a learner-centered educational environment is that the students become more self-directed and guide their own learning. Rogers believed that the learner is the person most capable of deciding how to find the solutions to problems. The client identifies the problem and, given time and space, can find a way through the problem to a solution. The nurse acts as a facilitator in this learning process. As an example, a 55-year-old man wants to quit smoking after a prolonged upper respiratory infection, aggravated by his habit, and has come to a stop-smoking class conducted by a nurse in the county health department.

Knowles' Adult Learning Theory

In the last 20 to 30 years, a variety of techniques have been developed to help adults learn. One of the main discoveries is that adults as learners are different from children. They do not learn differently but are different kinds of learners. Knowles suggests that there are four characteristics of adult learners, and these characteristics have implications for adult learning (1984). Display 9–1 describes the characteristics of adult learners and implications for nurses working with adults.

HEALTH TEACHING MODELS

Theories on learning provide a general understanding of how people learn. In addition, various health teaching models specifically focus on explaining individual health experiences, behaviors, and actions. These models fit with the learning theories to give nurses a more accurate picture of the client and the clients' learning needs. Five useful ones are described here: the Cloutterbuck Minimum Data Matrix (CMDM), the Health Belief Model (HBM), the Health Promotion Model (HPM), and the PRECEDE and PROCEED models.

The Cloutterbuck Minimum Data Matrix

The CMDM generates a comprehensive base of client information. This information is prerequisite to the in-depth level of critical analysis and synthesis needed to produce quality health care outcomes in the 21st century. It assumes an interdisciplinary perspective and educates the nurse to recog-

DISPLAY 9–1. Characteristics and Implications for Knowles' Adult Learning Theory

Characteristics	Learning Implications
Self-concept	Openness and respect between teacher and learner.
Adult learners are self-directed.	The learner plans and carries out own learning activities.
	Learner evaluates own progress toward self-chosen goals.
Experience	Teaching methods focus on experiential activities.
Adults have a lifetime of experience and define self in terms of this experience.	Discovering how to learn from experience is key to self-actualization.
	Mistakes are opportunities for learning.
Readiness to learn	Experiential learning opportunities focus on requirements for occupational and social roles.
Learning is focused on social and occupational roles.	Learning peaks when there is a need to know.
	Adults can best assess own readiness to learn and teachable moments.
Adults have a problem-centered time perspective.	Teaching needs to be problem-centered rather than theoretically oriented.
	Teacher needs to teach what the learners need to learn.
	Learners need to apply and try out learning quickly.

nize and incorporate client diversity into care. In teaching, it assists the nurse in conceptualizing clients beyond the institutional, individual, and biomedical perspectives (Cloutterbuck & Cherry, 1998). The model helps the nurse to discern the life circumstances or chain of events that have jeopardized a client's health (Fig. 9–1).

The model "is comprised of a set of empirical variables known to influence consumer health status, behavior, and outcomes" (Cloutterbuck & Cherry, 1998, p. 386). For example, in the personal variables dimension, there are items such as age, ethnicity, level of education, and self-care practices. These variables are distributed across three dimensions: personal, situational, and structural. Information generated by the CMDM creates a more comprehensive profile than information gathered in the traditional biomedical health care system. This information, such as client health beliefs and practices and a broad range of personal factors, can be instrumental in helping the nurse design and implement health education programs to promote positive changes in clients' health. Although community health nurses have a long tradition of considering the client holistically, this ma-

trix helps the nurse visualize the complexity of factors influencing clients' health. It helps to identify and challenge assumptions, recognize the importance of context, imagine and explore alternatives, and use reflective skepticism. When the nurse approaches individuals, families, and groups prepared with complete information, all of the caregiving—especially the appropriateness and effectiveness of the teaching—will be enhanced.

Health Belief and Health Promotion Models

This section describes two closely associated health models. The Health Belief Model (HBM), which was developed by social psychologists and brought to the attention of health care professionals by Rosenstock (1966), has undergone much empirical testing. The HBM is useful for explaining the behaviors and actions taken by people to prevent illness and injury. It advances that readiness to act on behalf of a person's own health is predicated on the following:

Perceived susceptibility to the condition in question
Perceived seriousness of the condition in question
Perceived benefits to taking action
Barriers to taking action
Cues to action, such as knowledge that someone else has the condition or attention from the media
Self-efficacy—the ability to take action to achieve the desired outcome (Strecher & Rosenstock, 1997)

Pender's Health Promotion Model (HPM) (1987) modifies the HBM and focuses on *predicting* behaviors that influence health promotion. In addition, Pender's model includes the variable of interpersonal influence of others, including family and health professionals. Pender's model includes perceptual factors and a description of how those factors are operationalized (Table 9–6).

The PRECEDE and PROCEED Models

First publicized by Green and Kreuter (1991), the PRECEDE model was developed for educational diagnosis. The acronym PRECEDE stands for Predisposing, Reinforcing, and Enabling Causes in Educational Diagnosis and Evaluation. It includes seven levels in formulating educational diagnoses (Table 9–7).

The community health nurse's role of teacher focuses heavily on assessment and identification of strengths and weaknesses at each level. From the information gathered, the nurse can develop a diagnostic statement describing the learning needs of clients.

The PROCEED model had been associated with the PRECEDE model as the community health nurse *proceeds* to plan, implement, and evaluate health education programs. This acronym stands for Policy, Regulatory, and Organizational Constructs for Educational and Environmental Development. The four steps in this model include implementa-

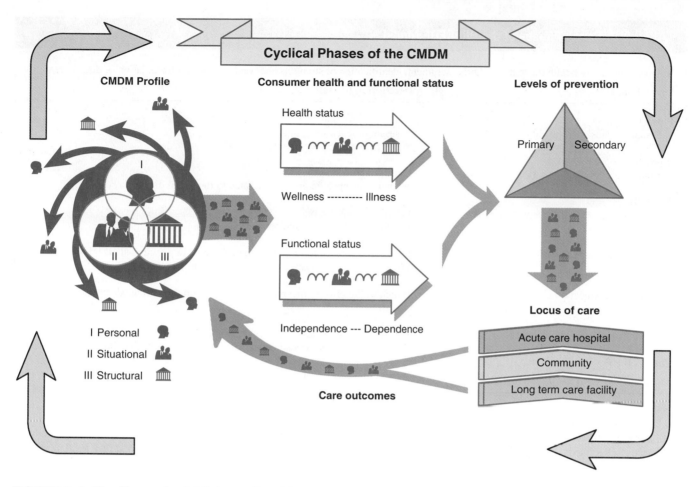

FIGURE 9–1. The Cloutterbuck Minimum Data Matrix as a tool to promote health education.

TABLE 9–6. Principles of Pender's Health Promotion Model

Perceptual Factors	Description
Health importance	Perceived value of health to life and daily functioning
Perceived control of health	Perceived ability to control health: internally, externally, and by chance
Perceived self-efficacy	Perceived ability to take action that achieves the desired outcome
Personal health definition	What health means to the client
Perceived health status	How individual views own health
Perceived benefits of behaviors that promote health	View of positive outcomes occurring from health-promoting behaviors
Perceived barriers to behaviors that promote health	View of things hindering health-promoting behaviors

Modifying Factors	Description
Demographics	Age, sex, race, location
Biologic	Weight, fat distribution, height
Interpersonal	Interactions with family, health care providers
Situational	Societal factors making health-promoting activities available
Behavioral	Established skills and knowledge
Cues to action	Internal (feelings of self) and external cues (media)

TABLE 9–7. Seven Phases of the PRECEDE Model

Role of community health nurse as teacher: assessment, identification of strengths and weaknesses, and formulation of diagnoses.

Level (Phases)	Description (Questions)
Phase I Social diagnosis	Assessing the learner's quality of life. What are the group's general concerns?
Phase II Epidemiologic diagnosis	Identifying health problems. What are the specific problems related to the social diagnosis?
Phase III Behavioral and environmental diagnosis	Identifying risk factors. What are the health related behaviors?
Phase IV Educational diagnosis	Identifying predisposing, reinforcing, and enabling factors at each level. What are the predisposing, enabling, and reinforcing factors?
Phase V Analysis of educational diagnosis	Which of the priority factors will be focused on during the educational plan?
Phase VI Administrative and policy-making diagnosis	Assessing administrative and organizational resources. What specific objectives and resources are needed for the health education plan?
Phase VII Evaluation	What are the results of the educational plan?

tion, process, impact, and outcome evaluation of the teaching process (Richards, 1997). The nurse builds on the assessment and diagnosis formulated from the PRECEDE model. The steps are similar to the nursing process and, because of this familiarity, have become useful tools for nurses teaching in the community.

TEACHING AT THREE LEVELS OF PREVENTION

Nurses should develop teaching programs that coincide with the level of prevention needed by the client. The three levels (defined in Chapter 1) of primary, secondary, and tertiary prevention are reinforced in Table 9–8.

Ideally, the nurse focuses teaching at the primary level. If nurses were able to reach more people at this level, it would help to diminish the years of morbidity and limit subsequent infirmity. Many people experience disabilities that might have been prevented if primary prevention behaviors had been incorporated into their daily activities. The primary level of prevention is not possible in all cases, however, so a significant share of the nurse's time is spent teaching at the secondary or tertiary level. An example of this is an 88-year-old woman with a fractured hip who has returned home after 3 weeks of physical therapy at a skilled nursing facility. The nurse assesses the client's environment, gait, functional limitations, safety, and adherence to medication and initiates needed referrals. The teaching focuses on rehabilitation and

prevention of a secondary problem that may affect the healing process and the client's health and safety in general (see Levels of Prevention).

EFFECTIVE TEACHING

Teaching is an art. It can be performed with such skill and grace that the client becomes a part of a well-orchestrated event with learning as the natural outcome. Instead of relying on prescribed teaching methods, the skillful nurse can make judgments based largely on client qualities, situations, and needs that guide the experience to fruition. Thus, the desired changes emerge in the course of the interaction rather than at a level conceived before the teaching (Eisner, 1985). Before the community health nurse can reach this level of artistry, there is much to learn about being an effective teacher.

Teaching-Learning Principles

Teaching lies at one end of a continuum. At the other end is learning. Without learning, teaching becomes useless in the same way that communication does not occur unless a message is both sent and received (Lorig, 1995). Both the teacher and the learner have responsibilities on that continuum. Learners must take responsibility for their own learning (Bastable, 1997). Teachers obstruct that process if they assume complete responsibility for bringing about changed behavior. Clients

TABLE 9–8. Teaching at Three Levels of Prevention

Level	Focus	Examples
Primary prevention	Health teaching	Health education: a nurse teaches a class on sensible weight control for teenagers
	Specific protection	Immunizations: a nurse teaches the importance of pneumonia and flu vaccines for seniors, followed by an immunization clinic
Secondary prevention	Early diagnosis	Screening and case-finding: a nurse takes blood pressures on all family members at each home visit and teaches them the importance of maintaining a healthy blood pressure reading
	Prompt treatment	Treatment: a nurse teaches clients how to navigate through the complexities of the health care delivery system for clients to receive prompt treatment
Tertiary prevention	Maintenance	Maintenance: a nurse observes clients with TB taking their oral medication (DOT therapy) where they live on a daily basis, and incorporates teaching about the importance of diet, rest, and exercise to prevent a secondary health problem
	Rehabilitation	Restore function: a nurse teaches a stroke survivor about home safety, alternative housing options, physical therapy, and retraining opportunities

can be directed toward health knowledge, but will not learn unless they have the desire to learn. Teaching, then, becomes a matter of facilitating both the desire and the best conditions for satisfying it. Teaching in community health nursing means to influence, motivate, and act as a catalyst in the learning process. Nurses bring information and learner together and stimulate a reaction that leads to a change (Redman, 1996). Nurses facilitate learning when they make it as easy as possible for clients to change. To do this, the nurse needs to understand the basic principles underlying the art and science of the teaching-learning process and the use of appropriate materials to influence learning (Table 9–9).

CLIENT READINESS

Clients' readiness to learn influences teaching effectiveness (Babcock & Miller, 1994). Two facets of client readiness have been identified. Emotional readiness, a state of receptivity to learning, and experimental readiness, the learner's knowledge and understanding, both must be assessed by the nurse. For instance, one community health nurse found that a young primipara was not ready for prenatal teaching on fetal growth and development. She had strong fears, the nurse discovered, that "losing her figure" would make her sexually unattractive to her husband. Until these anxieties had subsided, the teaching would remain ineffective. Clients' needs, interests, motivation, stress, and concerns determine their readiness for learning.

Another factor that influences readiness is educational background. If a group of women who never completed grade school meet to learn how to care for a sick person in the home, material should be presented simply, factually, and in terms that they understand. To discuss complex concepts of health, illness, and scientific research would be above their level of readiness. However, increasingly complex concepts can be introduced as the nurse works with the women and assesses their readiness to assimilate advanced concepts.

Maturational level also affects readiness. An adolescent mother who still is working on normal developmental tasks of her age group, such as seeking independence or selecting a career path, may not be ready to learn parenting skills. Readiness of the client determines the amount of material presented in each teaching session. The pace or speed with which information is presented must be manageable. A moderate amount of anxiety often increases client receptivity to learning; however, high or low levels of anxiety can have the opposite effect.

CLIENT PERCEPTIONS

Clients' perceptions also affect their learning, serving as a screening device through which all new information must pass (Rankin & Stallings, 1996). Individual perceptions help people interpret and attach meaning to things. A wide range of variables affects human perception. These variables include values, past experiences, culture, religion, personality, developmental stage, educational and economic level, surrounding social forces, and the physical environment. One client may view the experience of parenting as a positive, growth-producing relationship; another may see it as a conflict-ridden, unhappy experience to avoid. Each kind of perception has a different consequence for teaching and learning. In another example, the nurse working with adolescents to educate them about the dangers of substance abuse should understand that adolescents seeking independence need to feel that they have options and choices and do not want to be told what to do.

Frequently, clients use selective perception. They screen out some statements and pay attention to those that fit their values or personal desires. For example, a nurse is teaching a client the various risk factors in coronary disease; the individual screens out the need to quit smoking and lose weight, paying attention only to factors that would not require a drastic change in lifestyle. Nurses must know their clients, un-

LEVELS OF PREVENTION

TEACHING AUTO SAFETY USING THREE LEVELS OF PREVENTION

GOAL
To prevent auto crashes

PRIMARY PREVENTION
Use passive restraints, air bags
Driver education programs
Public education: drinking and driving, fatigue, mechanical failures, emergency actions
Driving safe speeds for road, weather, and traffic conditions
Regular checks of vehicle for safety, equipment, lights, brakes
Suspension of license when appropriate
Retesting drivers for knowledge of laws and auto handling, vision tests at intervals and as driver ages

GOAL
To provide immediate and adequate response at the scene of auto crashes

SECONDARY PREVENTION
Cellular phones, early reporting of crashes by passing motorists
Emergency medical services for treatment at the scene
Professional specialties in emergency medical services
Public education in first-aid
Cross-training of ambulance drivers, police, and fire fighters as paramedics in all communities
Develop and upgrade trauma centers and reporting systems
Teach necessary care to family members

GOAL
To provide appropriate rehabilitative services to injured passengers and/or pedestrians

TERTIARY PREVENTION
Develop or use existing rehabilitation programs with physical therapy, occupational therapy, speech therapy
Educate industry on the employment of disabled individuals (Americans With Disabilities Act)
Develop community services for disabled, job retraining programs
Financial assistance during rehabilitation and job training
Aid to totally disabled and partial aid to those unable to support self totally but still able to work part time

derstand their backgrounds and values, and learn about their perceptions before health teaching can influence their behavior.

EDUCATIONAL ENVIRONMENT

The setting in which the educational endeavor takes place has a significant impact on learning (Breckon et al., 1998). Students probably have had the experience of sitting in a cold room and trying to concentrate during a lecture or of being distracted by noise, heat, or uncomfortable seating. Physical conditions such as ventilation, lighting, decor, room temperature, view of the speaker, and whispering need to be controlled to provide the environment most conducive to learning.

Equally important for learning is an atmosphere of mutual respect and trust. The nurse needs to convey this attitude both verbally and nonverbally. The way the nurse addresses clients, shows courtesies, and gives recognition makes a considerable difference in establishing clients' respect and trust. Both nurse and clients need to be mutually helpful and considerate of one another's needs and interests. All participants in the educational experience should feel free to express ideas, know that their views will be heard, and feel accepted despite differences of opinion and perspective. According to Knowles, this requires that the nurse refrain from seeming judgmental or inducing competitiveness among learners. Knowles adds that the teachers share their own feelings and knowledge "as a colearner in the spirit of inquiry" (1980, p. 58).

CLIENT PARTICIPATION

The degree of participation in the educational process directly influences the amount of learning (Weimer, 1996). One nurse discovered this principle while working with a group of clients nearing retirement. After talking to them about the changes that they would face and receiving little response, the nurse shifted to a different method of teaching. Pamphlets on social security benefits were distributed, and everyone was asked to read them during the week and come the next week with questions generated by the pamphlets. This strategy prompted the group to slowly begin to participate in their own learning.

When the nurse works with clients in a learning context, one of the first questions to discuss is, what does the client want to learn? As Carl Rogers (1969, p. 159) states:

> **Learning is facilitated when the student participates responsibly in the learning process. When he chooses his own directions, helps to discover his own learning resources, formulates his own problems, decides his own course of action, lives with consequences of each of these choices, then significant learning is maximized.**

The amount of learning is directly proportional to the learners' involvement. A group of senior citizens attended a class on nutrition and aging, yet made few changes in eating patterns. It was not until the members became actively involved in the class, encouraged by the nurse to present problems and solutions for food purchasing and preparation on limited budgets, that any significant behavioral changes occurred.

Contracting, in which the client participates in the process as a partner to determine goals, content, and time for learning, can contribute to client learning. Contracting in the context of teaching can develop a sense of accountability in clients for their own learning. Contracting is discussed in Chapter 8.

SUBJECT'S RELEVANCE TO CLIENT

Subject matter that is relevant to the client is learned more readily and retained longer than information that is not mean-

TABLE 9–9. Seven Principles for Maximizing the Teaching-Learning Process

Teaching Principles	Learning Principles
1. Adapt teaching to clients' level of readiness.	1. The learning process makes use of clients' experience and is geared to their level of understanding.
2. Determine clients' perceptions about the subject matter before and during teaching.	2. Clients are given the opportunity to provide frequent feedback on their understanding of the material taught.
3. Create an environment that is conducive to learning.	3. The environment for learning is physically comfortable; offers an atmosphere of mutual helpfulness, trust, respect, and acceptance; and allows for free expression of ideas.
4. Involve clients throughout the learning process.	4. Clients actively participate. They assess needs, establish goals, and evaluate their learning progress.
5. Make subject matter relevant to clients' interest and use.	5. Clients feel motivated to interest and learn.
6. Ensure client satisfaction during the teaching-learning process.	6. Clients sense progress toward their goals.
7. Provide opportunities for clients to apply material taught.	7. Clients integrate the learning through application.

(Adapted from Knowles, M. [1980]. *The modern practice of adult education: Androgogy versus pedagogy* [2nd ed.]. Chicago: Follett.)

ingful (Lorig, 1995). Learners gain the most from subject matter immediately useful to their own purposes. This is particularly true of adult learners who have more life experiences that can be related to learning and who tend to see the immediate relevance of the material taught (Knowles, 1980).

Consider two middle-management men taking a physical fitness course offered by their employer. One, the father of a Boy Scout, has agreed to co-lead his son's troop on a 2-week backpacking trip in the mountains. He wants to get in shape. The second man is taking the course because it is required by the company. Its only relevance to his own purposes is that it prevents incurring his boss's disfavor. There is little question about which man will learn and retain the most. The course has considerable relevance and meaning to the first man and little to the second.

Relevance also influences the speed of learning. Diabetics who must give themselves daily injections of insulin to live learn that skill quickly. When clients see considerable relevance in the learning, they accomplish it with speed. According to Rogers (1969), 65% to 85% of the time allotted for learning various subjects could be deleted if learners perceived the material to be related to their own purposes. This is seen in the short period of time that it takes for families to learn the skills needed to provide home care for a family member in need (Baltazar et al., 1999).

When subject matter is relevant to the learner, there also is greater retention of knowledge. On seeing the usefulness of the material, the learner develops a strong motivation to acquire it and use it and is less likely to forget it. Even in instances when a previously learned motor skill has not been used for years, it often is quickly recaptured when it is needed.

CLIENT SATISFACTION

Clients must derive satisfaction from learning to maintain motivation and increase self-direction (Redman, 1996). Learners need to feel a sense of steady progress in the learn-

ing process. Obstacles, frustrations, and failures along the way discourage and impede learning. Many stroke clients with potential for rehabilitation give up trying to regain speech or move paralyzed limbs because they become too frustrated, discouraged, and dissatisfied. On the other hand, clients who experience satisfaction and progress in their speech and muscle retraining maintain their motivation and work on exercises without prompting (Diamantopulos, 1999). Nurses can promote client satisfaction through support and encouragement.

Realistic goals contribute to learner satisfaction. Objectives should be set within the learner's ability, thereby avoiding the frustration resulting from a task that is too difficult and the loss of interest resulting from one that is too easy. Setting objectives requires agreement on goals, periodic reviews, and revision of goals if they become too easy or too difficult. Nurses further promote clients' learning satisfaction by designing tasks with rewards. One nurse led a class for obese adolescents, and together they set the goal of a weekly 2-lb weight loss. The school nurse helped the group to design a plan that included counting calories, reducing fat in their diets, increasing physical activity, and a buddy system to bring about a behavior change. As members in the group achieved monthly goals, they were encouraged to reward themselves with a pair of earrings, new nail polish, or a special outing as a group. These students found this learning experience satisfying because goals were attainable and their progress was rewarded. Instead of competing with one another, the group set out to help each member achieve the goal. As a result, most kept the weight off after the class had finished.

CLIENT APPLICATION

Learning is reinforced through application (Hergenhahn & Olson, 1997). Learners need as many opportunities as possible to apply the learning in daily life. If such opportunities arise during the teaching-learning process, clients can try out new knowledge and skills under supervision. Learners are given an opportunity to begin integrating the learning into their daily lives at a time when the teacher is there to help reinforce that pattern. Take a prenatal class as an example. The learning only begins with explanations of proper diet, exercise, breathing techniques, hygiene, and avoidance of alcohol and tobacco. More learning occurs as the group members discuss these issues and apply them intellectually, exploring ways to practice them at home. Additional reinforcement comes by demonstrating how to do these activities. Sample diets, demonstrations of exercises, posters, pamphlets, or models may be used. The group can begin application in the classroom by making diet plans, exercising, role-playing parenting behavior, or engaging in group problem-solving. The members then can be encouraged to apply these activities on a daily basis at home and to share their results at future sessions.

Frequent use of newly acquired information fosters transfer of learning to other situations. The major goal of prevention and health promotion depends on such a transfer. For instance, mothers who learn and practice a well-balanced diet, free of non-nutritious snacks, can be encouraged to offer more nourishing foods to other family members. A family that practices asepsis and good handwashing techniques when caring for a postsurgical wound can learn to transfer this same principle to prevention of infection in daily living.

Teaching Process

The process of teaching in community health nursing follows steps similar to those of the nursing process:

1. *Interaction:* Establish basic communication patterns between clients and nurse.
2. *Assessment and diagnosis:* Determine clients' present status and identify clients' need for teaching (keeping in mind that clients should determine their own needs).
3. *Setting goals and objectives:* Analyze needed changes and prepare objectives that describe the desired learning outcomes.
4. *Planning:* Design a plan for the learning experience that meets the mutually developed objectives; include the content to be covered, sequence of topics, best conditions for learning (place, kind of environment), methods, and materials (eg, visual aids, exercises). A written plan is best; it may be part of the written nursing care plan.
5. *Teaching:* Implement the learning experience by carrying out the planned activities.
6. *Evaluation:* Determine whether learning objectives were met and if not, why not. Evaluation measures progress toward goals, effectiveness of chosen teaching methods, or future learning needs.

INTERACTION
Reciprocal communication must take place between the nurse and client. It is essential in the helping relationship and requisite to effective use of the nursing process. Community

health nurses need to develop good questioning techniques and listening skills to determine clients' learning needs and levels of readiness (see Chapter 8).

ASSESSMENT AND DIAGNOSIS
Identifying clients' learning needs presents a challenge to the nurse. Too often, teaching occurs based on the nurse's assumption of what the learner needs to know. In client education, nurses have a responsibility to tailor teaching to clients' real and perceived needs. Knowles (1980, 1984, 1989) describes educational needs as gaps between what people know and what they need to know to function effectively. He relates that the potential learners, the sponsoring organization, and the community all help to determine the needs to be addressed in the teaching-learning situation.

Assessing educational needs may be accomplished in several ways. The nurse can use surveys, interviews, open forums, or task forces that include representative clients as members. The principle to remember is that clients should be involved in identifying what they want to learn. When a "need" to learn something, such as the importance of immunizing children, is identified by the nurse rather than by clients, the nurse may need to "sell" clients on the importance of the topic. Nurses need to use approaches that assist clients toward their own awareness of the need.

SETTING GOALS AND OBJECTIVES
Once a need has been clearly identified, the nurse and clients can establish mutually agreed-on goals and objectives. Goals are broad statements of intent, and objectives are more specific descriptions of intended outcome (Mager, 1975). Sometimes in a teaching situation, an objective may be broken down into short-term and long-term goals. For example, the nurse may have identified a group's desire to stop smoking. The need and teaching goals might be stated thus:

Need: A group of smokers wish to stop their addiction to nicotine.

Short-term goal: All members of the group will stop smoking within 1 month.

Long-term goal: Ninety percent of group members will remain tobacco-free for 6 months.

Objectives should be stated in measurable behavioral terms, using a grammatical structure that contains a subject, verb, condition/criteria, and a time frame. That is, each objective should include a single idea that describes an outcome that can be measured within a certain timeframe. To accomplish the short- and long-term goals of smoking cessation, educational objectives are developed from the levels of cognitive learning covered earlier in this chapter. Each behavioral objective is stated in measurable terms and includes a verb that coincides with one of the six levels within the cognitive domain (Display 9–2). Objectives might appear like this:

At the end of the program all clients should be able to:

1. *List* three reasons why smoking is unhealthy.
2. *Identify* at least two factors that influenced their smoking habit.

DISPLAY 9–2. Verbs for Stating Cognitive Outcomes

Knowledge	Comprehension	Application	Analysis	Synthesis	Evaluation
Define	Translate	Interpret	Analyze	Compose	Judge
Repeat	Restate	Apply	Distinguish	Plan	Appraise
Record	Describe	Employ	Appraise	Propose	Evaluate
List	Discuss	Use	Calculate	Design	Rate
Recall	Recognize	Practice	Experiment	Formulate	Value
Name	Explain	Operate	Differentiate	Arrange	Revise
Relate	Express	Schedule	Test	Assemble	Score
Underline	Identify	Sketch	Compare	Collect	Select
	Locate	Shop	Contrast	Construct	Choose
	Report	Practice	Criticize	Create	Assess
	Review	Demonstrate	Diagram	Set up	Estimate
	Tell		Inspect	Organize	Measure
			Debate	Manage	
			Inventory	Prepare	
			Question		
			Relate		
			Categorize		
			Examine		

3. *Apply* a series of action steps leading to smoking cessation within 1 month.
4. *Examine* the steps as they contribute to living tobacco-free in the first 3 months.
5. *Design* a way to live a fulfilled, tobacco-free life.
6. *Evaluate* successful strategies to remain tobacco-free for 6 months.

Each of these objectives (1) refers to a subject, (2) can be readily measured because each describes a specific outcome, condition, criterion, or expected behavior, (3) uses a verb for stating cognitive outcomes, and (4) includes a specific time frame. Well-written objectives meet these four criteria and enhance evaluating the success of the educational effort.

PLANNING

Teaching preparation can be done formally or informally. Generally, it is best to have a written plan when teaching groups. This plan should include the following: (1) subject, (2) intended audience, (3) dates, time, and place, (4) short- and long-term goal statements, (5) teaching-learning methods, (6) activities and assignments, (7) course outline of topics, and (8) evaluation method and criteria.

TEACHING

The class, seminar, or workshop should be conducted according to the plan described earlier. Even with one-on-one teaching, these eight steps should be planned in advance, since each client has a different cultural background, education, intellectual level, and learning need. Using a variety of teaching methods addresses unique needs of the learners and makes the teaching interesting. Include and combine such methods as lectures, discussions, role playing, demonstrations, and videos (see Teaching Methods and Materials later in this chapter).

If necessary, make assignments such as readings, presentations, keeping journals, practice experiences, or return demonstrations designed to reinforce and synthesize the learning. The teaching methods used and activities selected are important parts of the teaching plan. The teacher will find that a well-designed plan enhances the smoothness and effectiveness of the teaching situation; problems in teaching often can be related back to a poorly developed plan.

EVALUATION

The final step of evaluation is a critical one in the teaching-learning process. According to Tyler, "evaluation is the process for determining the degree to which changes in behavior are actually taking place" (1949, p. 106). At this point, the nurse determines whether the goals and objectives for the educational experience have been met, and if not, why not. Clear, measurable objectives facilitate evaluation. For example, to measure the third objective in the stop-smoking program previously noted, "Apply a series of action steps that will lead to smoking cessation within 1 month," the nurse may ask group members to share the steps that they will use and then have a group discussion about the ideas shared. To measure the sixth objective, "Evaluate successful strategies to remain tobacco-free for 6 months" would require follow-up contacts and relying on self-reporting. Sussman and colleagues (1993) found, on evaluation, that a combined intervention of teaching youth necessary refusal skills, or saying "no," and an awareness of social misperceptions was the most effective way to reduce tobacco use in a school-based prevention project with teenagers. Each intervention alone was not effective. A well-developed evaluation component revealed this important finding. Adatsi (1999) reports that a smoking-cessation program in Duluth, Minnesota, followed 195 clients for 1 year after participation in a program and found that 49% had remained tobacco-free for 1 year. The American Lung Association estimates that only 20% to 30% of smokers typically remain abstinent 1 year after quitting. They attributed the success to gearing intervention to the client's stage of readiness to quit based on a model that describes four stages through which smokers move as they attempt to change their smoking habit. In addition, the participants got the support of planned and periodic contact from program staff over the 12 months, which included evaluation of strategies that worked for the participant's individual stage and those that did not.

If objectives have not been met or have been met only partially, this too requires attention. The nurse should explore this outcome with the clients to determine what hindered their success and what action might be helpful. Partially met objectives give the nurse a place to begin with the group at follow-up sessions and should not be considered a failure.

Teaching Methods and Materials

Teaching occurs on many levels and incorporates various types of activities. It can be formal or informal, planned or unplanned. Formal presentations, such as lectures with groups, generally are planned and fairly structured. Some teaching is less formal but still is planned and relatively structured, as in group discussions in which questions stimulate exploration of ideas and guide thinking. Informal levels of teaching, such as counseling or **anticipatory guidance** (the client is assisted in preparing for a future role or developmental stage), require the teacher to be prepared, but there is no defined plan of presentation. All nurses use one or a combination of methods and a variety of materials to facilitate the teaching-learning process. However, nurses need to expand their repertoire of teaching methods and to avoid relying on one or two methods. Generating a variety of teaching methods stimulates creative thinking. Nurses use knowledge from physiology, pathology, sociology, and psychology in their practice, and when teaching, nurses can benefit from using concepts, principles, and teaching methods from education, especially adult education. This chapter closes by discussing four commonly used teaching methods (lecture, discussion, demonstration, and role playing), teaching materials for enhancing learning, and how to effectively teach the client with special learning needs (see Research: Bridge to Practice).

LECTURE

The community health nurse sometimes presents information to a large group, such as a local parent-teacher association, a women's club, or a county board of commissioners. Under such circumstances the lecture method, a formal kind of presentation, may be the most efficient way to communicate general health information. However, lecturers tend to create a passive learning environment for the audience unless strategies are devised to involve the learners. Many individ-

RESEARCH Bridge to Practice

Lerman, L.M., Young, H.M., Powell-Cope, G., Georgiadou, F., & Benoliel, J.Q. (1994). Effects of education and support on breast self-examination in older women. *Nursing Research, 43*(3), 158–163.

This study was designed to determine the effects of education and structured support on breast self-examination (BSE), frequency, proficiency, and perceived control in women older than 50 years of age who were subscribers of a health maintenance organization. One year of follow-up at 6- and 12-month intervals was planned. The women received one-on-one instruction and supervised practice of BSE. They also were randomly assigned to a control group of no support, peer support group, or selected partner support group. The BSE performance was measured by self-report of frequency and proficiency in addition to an expert rating of demonstrated behavior. Research assistants conducted interviews in the participants' homes on three occasions: initially, at 6 months, and at 12 months.

Results indicate no significant differences across the three support groups on any variables on all three occasions using a variety of tests, including analysis of variance, chi-square, the Wilcoxon Z test, and the Kruskal-Wallis test. There were significant, positive findings with BSE frequency, proficiency, and perceived skill. Frequency increased to 98% at the 6-month interval and 63% at 12 months. Self-report proficiency doubled at 6 months and continued to increase by 1 year, as did perceived skill.

The results led the researchers to conclude that the motivation of the women to change their behavior and the strong teaching program given to all women contributed most to the changes in behavior. The strong internal motivation and intense teaching may have reduced the need for external motivation in the form of a support partner initially. Perhaps the support partner would have helped the waning internal motivation at a later time during the follow-up period.

uals are visual rather than auditory learners. To capture their attention, slides, overhead projections, computer-generated slide presentations, or videotapes can supplement the lecture. Allowing time for questions and discussion after a lecture also actively involves the learners. This method is best used with adults, but even they have a limited attention span, and a break at least midway through a presentation of 1 hour or longer will be appreciated. Distributing printed material that highlights and summarizes the content shared, or supplements it, also reinforces important points.

DISCUSSION

Two-way communication is an important feature of the learning process. Learners need an opportunity to raise questions, make comments, reason out loud, and receive feedback to develop understanding. When discussion is used in conjunction with other teaching methods such as demonstration, lecture, and role playing, it improves their effectiveness. In group teaching, discussion enables clients to learn from one another as well as from the nurse. The nurse must exercise leadership in controlling and guiding the discussion so that learning opportunities are maximized and objectives are met. Discussions that are organized around specific questions or topics are more fruitful.

DEMONSTRATION

The demonstration method often is used for teaching psychomotor skills and is best accompanied by explanation and discussion, with time set aside for return demonstration by the client or caregiver. It gives clients a clear sensory image of how to perform the skill. Because a demonstration should be within easy visual and auditory range of learners, it is best to demonstrate in front of small groups or one to one. Use the same kind of equipment that clients will use to show exactly how the skill should be performed, and provide learners with ample opportunity to practice until the skill is perfected.

This is an ideal method to use in the client's home as well as in groups. The materials and supplies that the client will use when unaided by the nurse should be used in the demonstration. This might be the time when the nurse uses improvising skills. Helping families figure out ways to accomplish goals with materials found at home often becomes the hallmark of an experienced community health nurse. The new mother learns how to bathe her baby safely in the kitchen sink. The nurse assists several low-income parents in using household items to make inexpensive toys (mobiles from coat hangers, string, and pictures from a magazine or bean bags using dry beans and scraps of fabric). The husband learns how to change dressings over his wife's central line site using sterile technique while conserving supplies purchased on their fixed income. Each activity takes a different type of psychomotor skill and ingenuity on the part of the nurse (Fig. 9–2).

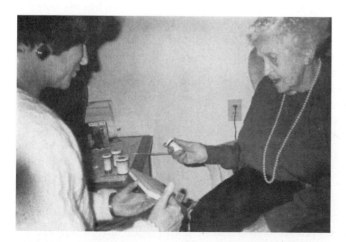

FIGURE 9–2. Teaching methods and tools vary with clients' learning needs. On this home visit, the nurse uses a weekly medication container to help an elderly woman with limited vision devise a plan for taking her medications.

ROLE PLAYING

At times, having clients assume and act out roles maximizes learning. A parenting group, for example, found it helpful to place themselves in the role of their children; their feelings about various ways to respond became more apparent. Reversing roles can effectively teach spouses in conflict about better ways to communicate. To prevent role playing from becoming a game with little learning, plan the proposed drama with clear objectives in mind. What behavioral outcomes should be achieved? Define the context, the "stage," clearly so that everyone shares in the situation. Then define each role ahead of time, making sure that participants understand their performance roles. Emphasize that no wrong or right performance exists, and that participants should behave the way people behave in everyday life. Avoid having people play themselves; it can embarrass them and make it difficult for them to achieve objectivity. After the drama has concluded, elicit discussion with carefully prepared questions. This technique can be used with staff, coworkers, young children, teenagers, and adults. However, this technique can be a risk-taking experience for people, and they may be reluctant to participate. The nurse needs to use judgment, to begin with volunteers, and to avoid pushing this technique on unwilling or nonreceptive people. Build up to full participation.

TEACHING MATERIALS

Many different kinds of teaching materials are available to the nurse. They often are used in combination and are useful during the teaching process. Visual images—pictures, slides, posters, chalkboards, flannel boards, videotapes, bulletin boards, flash cards, pamphlets, flyers, charts, and gestures—can enhance most learning. Some tools, such as tapes and compact discs, provide an auditory stimulus. Americans readily learn from television; it appeals to sight and sound and grabs attention. Education through television can be more effective and efficient than traditional teaching methods (Schoenbeck, 1992). There are many programs on educational television channels and network channels that can be recommended by the nurse. Other tools, such as anatomic models and improvised or purchased equipment, allow clients both visual and tactile learning. Still others, such as interactive computer games or instruction, actively involve learners.

The choice of teaching materials varies with clients' interests, abilities, and the resources available. Teaching often occurs in casual conversations, spontaneously in situations in which clients raise unexpected questions, or when a crisis arises. In these instances, nurses draw on their background of knowledge and exercise professional judgment in their selection of content, methods, and materials.

Several different types of printed educational support materials are available, such as pamphlets, brochures, booklets, flyers, and informational sheets. Each should be evaluated for its appropriateness and effectiveness with particular individuals, families, or groups. Many come from state and local official sources. Nurses can create their own handouts by using a computer, customizing them to the needs of individual clients (Gabello, 1997). The Internet has vast health resources that can be combined with the desktop publishing capabilities of the nurse's computer to create one-of-a-kind material for clients. Other materials come from nonprofit national agencies such as the American Diabetes Association, the March of Dimes, the American Association for Retired Persons, and the American Heart Association. Materials from these sources can be acquired in mass quantity for free or at a nominal cost to the nurse or agency. Major manufacturers of infant formulas, foods, diapers, and toys are good sources for literature on growth and development, safety, and caring for infants and children. Pharmaceutical companies develop educational material for the public along with the manufacturers of in-home supplies and equipment. Usually, these are excellent sources of information for families or groups; however, the nurse needs to assess the material for appropriateness. Also beware that the commercial message in the literature does not outweigh the educational impact, making it misleading or confusing to the client.

Factors to be considered with all educational literature include the material's content, complexity, and reading level. There are several ways to assess the readability of the printed word. One that is easy to use is the Fog Index. It is a rough way of determining the years of schooling needed to understand printed material. It works by analyzing words and sentence length. The higher the Fog Index, the more difficult the reading level. A Fog Index of 6 is a sixth-grade reading level, and 11 is the junior year in high school. The steps include the following:

1. Take a sample of approximately 100 words. Count the number of sentences. When semicolons and commas are used instead of periods, count each clause as a separate sentence.
2. Divide the number of sentences into the exact number of words, which gives the words per sentence.
3. Count the words with three or more syllables, excluding those that became three syllables because of "es" or "ed" at the end. Also, do not count names.
4. Add the number of words with three or more syllables to the average number of words per sentence.
5. Multiply the total by .04.
6. Use the resulting whole number (without rounding) as the Fog Index. The number is the years of schooling needed to understand the writing sample.

Culturally appropriate health education materials must be acquired or developed for the predominant cultural and linguistic minority populations taught by the nurse. "Developing printed materials is an important first step, but the development of videos and public service announcements in these languages is also necessary" (Williamson et al., 1997, p. 20).

Finally, nurses teach by example. Actions speak louder than words. If a nurse teaches the importance of washing hands to reduce disease transmission and then begins a dressing change without hand washing, the message of observed actions carries more impact than the words. Nurses who exhibit healthy practices use themselves as tools and serve as role models as well as health teachers.

CLIENTS WITH SPECIAL LEARNING NEEDS

At times, the nurse experiences a challenging teaching situation with an individual, family, or group. These challenges may involve clients with cultural or language differences, hearing impairments, developmental delays, memory losses, visual perception distortions, problems with fine or gross motor skills, distracting personality characteristics, or demonstrations of stress or emotions. Regardless of the situation, the nurse will feel most comfortable and confident if prepared to deal with these situations before experiencing them.

Before beginning to teach a client, family, or aggregate, thorough preparation is important for successful learning. This includes finding out whether it is possible to teach in English or whether other modifications are needed as the teaching plan is being developed (MacDonald, 1998). Nurses should never assume anything, including the primary language spoken by clients, their visual or hearing ability, or capacity to understand. When teaching unfamiliar groups, a center manager, a caretaker, or program director can give information regarding the interests and abilities of the members. These human resources are invaluable in planning any teaching when English may be a second language or when other barriers exist that may impede success if they are not known by the nurse. The phases of the nursing process continue to guide the nurse as a teacher.

Another difficulty that can arise is unexpected behavior from a client that disrupts the group process. The client may monopolize the discussion, answer questions asked of others, burst out with personal experiences that have no relevance to the topic, become irate at the comments of others, or sit silently and never speak. This can be unnerving to even the most experienced nurse. Any behavior that has the potential to distract the other learners needs to be diffused by the nurse. This is accomplished by caringly giving the recognition sought by the person while also setting limits. More information on client behavior and appropriate communication techniques can be found in Chapters 8 and 23.

SUMMARY

Much of community health nursing practice involves teaching. More than simply giving health information to clients, the purpose of teaching is to change client behavior to healthier practices. When these practices are internalized and implemented regularly, years of morbidity and premature mortality can be avoided, contributing to the quality and length of the human life span. *Healthy People 2010* focuses on teaching to improve the quality of life.

Understanding the nature of learning contributes to the effectiveness of teaching in community health. Learning occurs in three domains: cognitive, affective, and psychomotor. The cognitive domain refers to learning that takes place intellectually. It ranges in levels of learner functioning from simple recall to complex evaluation. As learners move up the scale of cognitive learning, they become more self-directed; the nurse then assumes a more facilitative role.

Affective learning involves the changing of attitudes and values. Learners may experience several levels of affective involvement from simple listening to adopting the new value. Again, as the client increases involvement, the nurse becomes less directive.

Psychomotor learning involves the acquisition of motor skills. Clients who learn psychomotor skills must meet three conditions: they must be capable of the skill; they must develop a sensory image of the skill; and they must practice the skill.

Learning theories can be grouped into four broad categories: (1) behaviorist theories, which view learning as a behavioral change through stimulus-response or conditioning; (2) cognitive learning theories, which seek to influence learners' understanding of problems and situations through promoting their insights; (3) social learning theories, which explain dysfunctional behavior and facilitate learning; and (4) humanistic theories, which assume that people have a natural tendency to learn and that learning flourishes in an encouraging environment. Knowles' adult learning theory provides a framework to understand adult characteristics and appropriate teaching interventions.

Health teaching models work together with the learning theories to give nurses a more accurate picture of the client and the client's learning needs. Five models were explored. The CMDM is designed as a teaching mechanism to create a comprehensive base of client information that enhances all care, including client teaching. The HBM is useful in explaining the behaviors that are triggered by people in an interest in preventing diseases, and the HPM modifies the HBM and focuses on predicting behaviors that influence health promotion. The PRECEDE model, an acronym standing for Predisposing, Reinforcing, and Enabling Causes in Educational Diagnosis and Evaluation, is designed to address educational diagnosis focusing heavily on assessment and identification of strengths and weaknesses. The fifth model, PROCEED, is an acronym for Policy, Regulatory, and Organizational Constructs for Educational and Environmental Development. The steps in this model include implementation, process, and impact and outcome evaluation of the teaching process, building on the assessment and diagnosis formulated from the PRECEDE model.

Teaching in community health nursing is the facilitation of learning that leads to behavioral change in the client. Ideally, this is done at the primary level of prevention. However, much of the nurse's work is done at the secondary and tertiary level. The nurse uses several teaching-learning principles to facilitate the learning process, such as clients' readiness for learning, clients' perceptions, learners' physical and emotional comfort within an educational setting, degree of client participation, relevant subject matter, allowing clients to derive satisfaction from learning, and reinforcing learning through application.

The teaching process in community health nursing is similar to the nursing process, including steps of interaction, assessment and diagnosis, goal setting, planning, teaching, and evaluation. The teaching may be formal or informal, planned or unplanned, and methods may range from structured lecture presentations to demonstration and role playing. Selection of teaching materials depends on how well they suit learners and helps to meet the desired objectives. Sources of teaching materials that are free or inexpensive can enhance the nurses' teaching but need to be evaluated for effectiveness. The nurse needs to know how to help learners with special needs, those with physical or mental disabilities, those from a different culture or who speak a different language, and those who monopolize the discussion, become emotional, or even are hostile. The nurse must be prepared for each situation to effectively teach the individual, family, or group.

ACTIVITIES TO PROMOTE CRITICAL THINKING

1. What learning theories discussed in this chapter most closely reflect your own position? How can they be applied in your practice?
2. A children's day-care center is located in your service area. What populations in this setting could be potential recipients of health teaching? How would you assess each group's learning needs?
3. Your city governmental officials often make decisions that appear to reflect a lack of knowledge regarding health and health care. How might you "educate" them using the concepts and principles described in this chapter?
4. Discuss the differences between cognitive, affective, and psychomotor learning. Why do cognitive and affective learning need to be linked in health teaching?
5. Develop a flyer or program for an educational presentation for clients using behavioral objectives that match the learning level desired.
6. Select one of the health teaching models. Use the steps in the model to plan an educational program for a group of teenagers at the local high school. How did the use of the model enhance your teaching?
7. Explore the possible use of role models as teaching tools for community health nursing practice. What examples exist in your community? What new ones might you develop?

8. You are teaching an aggregate of middle-aged women about menopause. One woman monopolizes the class by telling stories and talking negatively about her husband. The other women are getting upset with her. How do you resolve the situation?

9. Using the Internet, locate web sites of companies, public service agencies, and voluntary health agencies that offer free or low-cost educational material. Either request useful material to be used with clients now or bookmark a selection of sites for you to refer to later as needed, developing a resource file.

REFERENCES

Adatsi, G. (1999). Health going up in smoke: How can you prevent it? *American Journal of Nursing, 99*(3), 63–67.

Babcock, D.E. & Miller, M.A. (1994). *Client education: Theory and practice.* St. Louis: Mosby.

Baltazar, V., Ibe, O.B., & Allender, J.A. (1999). Maintaining optimum nutrition among elderly clients at home. In S. Zang & J.A. Allender (pp. 98–121), *Home care of the elderly.* Philadelphia: Lippincott Williams & Wilkins.

Bandura, A. (1977). *Social learning theory.* Englewood Cliffs, NJ: Prentice-Hall.

Bandura, A. (1986). *Social foundations of thought and action: A social cognitive theory.* Englewood Cliffs, NJ: Prentice-Hall.

Bastable, S.B. (1997). *Nurse as educator: Principles of teaching and learning.* Boston: Jones and Bartlett Publishers.

Bigge, M.L. (1982). *Learning theories for teachers* (4th ed.). New York: Harper.

Bloom, B. (Ed.). (1956). *Taxonomy of educational objectives: The classification of educational goals. Handbook I: Cognitive domain.* New York: Longman.

Breckon, D.J., Lancaster, B., & Harvey, J.S. (1998). *Community health education: Settings, roles, and skills for the 21st century* (4th ed.). Gaithersburg, MD: Aspen.

Cloutterbuck, J.C. & Cherry, B.S. (1998). The Cloutterbuck minimum data matrix: A teaching mechanism for the new millennium. *Journal of Nursing Education, 37*(9), 385–393.

Diamantopulos, D. (1999). Caring for the elderly client with neurological deficits. In S. Zang & J.A. Allender (pp. 388–411), *Home care of the elderly.* Philadelphia: Lippincott Williams & Wilkins.

Eisner, E.W. (1985). *The educational imagination* (2nd ed.). New York: Macmillan.

Gabello, W.J. (1997, February 15) How computers enrich patient education. *Patient Care,* 88–113.

Green, L.W., & Kreuter, M.W. (1991). *Health promotion planning: An educational and environmental approach* (2nd ed.). Mountain View, CA: Mayfield.

Gronlund, N.E. (1970). *Stating behavioral objectives for classroom instruction.* New York: Macmillan.

Hergenhahn, B.R. & Olson, M. (1997). *An introduction to theories of learning* (5th ed.). Upper Saddle River, NJ: Prentice-Hall.

Knowles, M. (1980). *The modern practice of adult education: Androgogy versus pedagogy* (2nd ed.). Chicago: Follett.

Knowles, M. (1984). *The adult learner: A neglected species* (3rd ed.). Houston: Gulf Publishing.

Knowles, M. (1989). *The making of an adult educator: An autobiographical journey.* San Francisco: Jossey-Bass.

Lerman, L.M., Young, H.M., Powell-Cope, G., Georgiadou, F., & Benoliel, J.Q. (1994). Effects of education and support on breast self-examination in older women. *Nursing Research, 43*(3), 158–163.

Lorig, K. (1995). *Patient education: A practical approach* (2nd ed.) Newbury Park, CA: Sage.

Mager, R.F. (1975). *Preparing instructional objectives* (2nd ed.). Belmont, CA: Pitman Learning.

Maslow, A.H. (1970). *Motivation and personality* (2nd ed.). New York: Harper and Row.

McBride, C.M., Curry, S.J., Lando, H.A., et al. (1999). Prevention of relapse in women who quit smoking during pregnancy. *American Journal of Public Health, 89*(5), 706–711.

Pavlov, I.P. (1957). *Experimental psychology and other essays.* New York: Philosophical Library.

Pender, N.J. (1987). *Health promotion in nursing practice* (2nd ed). Los Altos, CA: Appleton & Lange.

Piaget, J. (1966). *The origin of intelligence in children.* New York: Norton.

Piaget, J. (1970). Piaget's theory. In P.H. Mussen (Ed.), *Charmichael's manual of child psychology: Vol. 1.* New York: Wiley.

Rankin, S.H. & Stallings, K.D. (1996). *Patient education: Issues, principles, and guidelines* (3rd ed.). Philadelphia: Lippincott-Raven.

Redman, B.K. (1996). *The practice of patient education* (8th ed.). St. Louis: Mosby.

Richards, E. (1997). Motivation, compliance, and health behaviors of the learner. In S.B. Bastable (Ed.), *Nurse as educator: Principles of teaching and learning* (pp. 124–144). Boston: Jones & Bartlett.

Rogers, C. (1969). *Freedom to learn.* Columbus, OH: Merrill Publishing Co.

Rogers, C. (1989). *Freedom to learn for the eighties.* Columbus, OH: Merrill Publishing Co.

Rosenstock, I.M. (1966). Why people use health services. *Milbank Memorial Fund Quarterly, 44,* 94–127.

Schoenbeck, S.B. (1992). Teaching the nurse to teach with health information videos. *Journal of Nursing Staff Development, 8*(2), 66–71.

Skinner, B.F. (1974) *About behaviorism.* New York: Knopf.

Skinner, B.F. (1987). *Upon further reflection.* Englewood Cliffs, NJ: Prentice-Hall.

Strecher, U.J. & Rosenstock, I.M. (1997). The health belief model. In K. Glanz, F.M. Lewis, & B.K. Rimer (Eds.), *Health behavior and health education: Theory, research and practice* (2nd ed., pp. 41–59). San Francisco: Jossey-Bass.

Sussman, S., Dent, C.W., Stacy, A.W., et al. (1993). Project towards no tobacco use: 1-year behavior outcomes. *American Journal of Public Health, 83*(9), 1245–1250.

Thorndike, E.L. (1932). *The fundamentals of learning.* New York: Teachers College Press.

Thorndike, E.L. (1969). *Educational psychology.* New York: Arno Press.

Tyler, R.W. (1949). *Basic principles of curriculum and instruction.* Chicago: University of Chicago Press.

U.S. Department of Health and Human Services. (1998). *Healthy people 2010 objectives: Draft for public comment.* Washington, DC: Office of Public Health and Science.

Wertheimer, M. (1959 [1945]). In M. Wertheimer (Ed.), *Productive thinking.* New York: Harper & Row.

Wertheimer, M. (1980). Gestalt theory of learning. In G.M. Gazda & R.H. Corsini (Eds.), *Theories of learning: A comparative approach.* Ithasca, IL: Peacock.

Williamson, E., Steccih, J.M., Allen, B.B., & Coppens, N.M. (1997). The development of culturally appropriate health education materials. *Journal of Nursing Staff Development, 13*(1), 19–23.

SELECTED READINGS

Bortz, W.M., II (1991). *We live too short and die too long.* New York: Bantam Books.

Bortz, W.M. II (1996). *Dare to be 100.* New York: Simon & Schuster.

Camp, C.J., Judge, K.S., Bye, C.A., et al. (1997). An intergenerational program for persons with dementia using Montessori methods. *The Gerontologist, 37*(5), 688–692.

Doak, C.C., Doak, L.G., & Root, J.H. (1996). *Teaching patients with low literacy skills.* Philadelphia: Lippincott-Raven.

Engs, R.C. (1998). Using magic for AIDS prevention: Some teaching techniques. *Journal of Health Education, 29*(1), 43–45.

Freire, P. & Shor, I.(1987) *A pedagogy for liberation: Dialogues on transforming education.* Basingstoke, Hampshire: MacMillan Education.

Graham, B.A. & Gleit, C.J. (1998). Teaching in selected settings. In M.D. Boyd, B.A. Graham, C.J. Gleit, & N.I. Whitman (Eds.), *Teaching in nursing practice: A professional model* (3rd ed., pp. 41–63). Stamford, CT: Appleton & Lange.

Greiner, P.A. & Valiga, T.M. (1998). Creative educational strategies or health promotion. *Holistic Nursing Practice, 12*(2), 73–83.

Knowles, M. (1975). *Self-directed learning: A guide for learners and teachers.* New York: Associated Press.

Lewin, K. (1951). *Field theory in social science.* New York: Harper Publishing Co.

London, F. (1995). Teach your patients faster better. *Nursing 95, 68,* 70.

Margargal, P. (1997). Show and do, not tell and give: Teaching techniques for thee community client. *DNA Reporter, 22*(4), 20.

O'Donnell, L.N., San Doval, A., Duran, R. & O'Donnell, C. (1995). Video-based sexually transmitted disease patient education: Its impact on condom acquisition. *American Journal of Public Health, 85*(6), 817–822.

Owen, N., Bauman, A., Booth, M., et al. (1995). Serial mass media campaigns to promote physical activity: Reinforcing or redundant? *American Journal of Public Health, 85*(2), 244–248.

Polomeno, V. (1997). High-risk pregnancy: Teaching activities and strategies. *International Journal of Childbirth Education, 12*(3), 14–17.

Regan-Smith, M.G. (1997). How teachers can promote meaningful learning. *Journal of Cancer Education, 12*(3), 149–151.

Rydholm, L. (1997). Patient-focused care in parish nursing. *Holistic Nursing Practice, 20,* 47–60.

Sachdeva, A.K. (1996). Use of effective feedback to facilitate adult learning. *Journal of Cancer Education, 11*(2), 106–118.

Sechrist, W. (1997). Teaching idea. How can I choose a sexual partner who doesn't have HIV? *Journal of Health Education, 28*(5), 311–313.

Schonfeld, D.J., O'Hare, L.L., Perrin, E.C., Quackenbush, M., Showalter, D.R., & Cicchetti, D.V. (1995). A randomized, controlled trial of a school-based, multifaceted AIDS education program in the elementary grades: The impact on comprehension, knowledge, and fears. *Pediatrics, 95*(4), 450–486.

Sheridan-Leos, N. (1995). Women's Health Lotería: A new cervical cancer education tool for Hispanic females. *ONF, 22*(4), 697–700.

Spilberg, M.L. (1997). Breast mapping provides alternative method to perform BSES. *Alternative Therapies in Clinical Practice, 4*(6), 211–214.

Vaillancourt, M.V., et al. (1997). From formal to friendly: Creating materials that work with adolescents. *Journal of School Health, 67*(7), 294–295.

Wallerstein, N. & Bernstein, E. (1994). Introduction to community empowerment, participatory education, and health. *Health Education Quarterly, 21,* 141–148.

Weimer, M. (1996). *Improving your classroom teaching.* Newbury Park, CA: Sage Publications.

Whitman, N.I. (1998). Assessment of the learner. In M.D. Boyd, B.A. Graham, C.J. Gleit, & N.I. Whitman (Eds.), *Teaching in nursing practice: A professional model* (3rd ed., pp. 157–180). Stamford, CT: Appleton & Lange.

The Community Health Nurse as Leader, Change Agent, and Case Manager

KEY TERMS

- Autocratic leadership style
- Autonomous leadership style
- Case management
- Change
- Empirical-rational change strategy
- Empowerment
- Evolutionary change
- Force field analysis
- Leadership
- Normative-reeducative change strategy
- Participative leadership style
- Planned change
- Power
- Power bases
- Power-coercive change strategy
- Power sources
- Revolutionary change
- Stages of change
- Transactional leadership style
- Transformational leadership style

LEARNING OBJECTIVES

Upon mastery of this chapter, you should be able to:

- Describe three characteristics of leadership.
- Summarize five leadership theories.
- Compare and contrast five leadership styles.
- Describe five leadership functions.
- Differentiate between four power bases and four power sources.
- Discuss the concept of empowerment and its significance for community health nursing.
- Explain the three stages of change.
- Discuss the eight steps in planned change.
- Identify three planned change strategies.
- Summarize six principles for effecting change in community health.
- Describe the case-management role of the community health nurse.

Influencing people to change to healthier beliefs and practices lies at the heart of all community health nursing. With clients at every level, from families and groups to large aggregates, the ability to influence change requires knowledge and skill in the practice of leadership, the acquisition and use of power, the management of change, and skillful case management.

How do nurses carry out their roles as both leaders and change agents at the aggregate level? Many examples can be cited. A community health nurse becomes a member of the Governor's Commission on the Handicapped. In addition to recognizing the entire state as a community and the handicapped as a special population, the nurse assists the commission to formulate new policies for meeting the needs of the handicapped. Another nurse, as a member of a metropolitan health planning board, works to improve health care for a group of Hmong immigrants from Southeast Asia. In a rural community of farms and small towns, the county health department nurse organizes a grassroots task force concerned about the increasing injuries from farm machinery. The task force decides to survey farm families to determine the causes and develop preventive measures. All three of these nurses are involved in leadership and change at the aggregate level. They are working to change people's beliefs regarding health and healthful activities and to involve them in creating organized responses to community problems.

Community health nurses also lead people to change at the organizational level. For example, a staff nurse in a public-health nursing agency who feels overburdened by paperwork, is burned out, and lacks clear goals for daily tasks observes that other staff members seem to be feeling the same. At a staff meeting, the nurse brings up the problem of job stress and suggests that everyone read an article on the subject to discuss at the next staff meeting. The first discussion is successful, and a regular staff-development meeting evolves with rotating leadership. Over a few months' time, the staff begins to feel more focused in their work and more capable of coping with job stress. Consequently, their morale improves. This is an example of how a nurse can lead informally to bring about organizational change. The result not only left individuals feeling better able to cope with their jobs, but also improved the health of the organization and the quality of its services.

Many nurses do not see themselves as leaders, nor do they wish to become leaders. These nurses often assume that leadership entails a formal position with heavy administrative responsibilities. Although this sometimes is the case, leadership also takes place informally in nursing practice. Being an expert practitioner, case manager, and role model for peers are important leadership roles. In other words, nurses can be leaders in the profession and within their organization by the nature of their nursing skills and should remember that professional accountability includes this leadership role.

Many nurse theorists advocate that all nurses should exercise leadership and accept responsibility for continually revitalizing professional nursing practice, broadening nursing's sphere of influence, and improving health services (Swansburg & Swansburg, 1999). Habel (1999) declares, "The world is in the midst of a major transformation as civilization moves from the industrial era into the communication age and beyond. The changes affecting the world and the healthcare industry will provide unique opportunities for nurses who develop their leadership potential" (p. 10). For community health nurses, the opportunities for leadership are staggering. Among them are the need to influence health reform, promote healthy public policies, and design more effective health services (O'Neil, 1998). Other authors stress that community health nurses must prepare themselves to move into leadership positions (Michaels, 1997; Salmon, 1993).

Becoming an effective leader, change agent, and case manager requires specialized knowledge and skills. This chapter examines the theoretical and applied aspects of leadership, power, and change. It describes how leadership, empowerment, and effecting change are inextricably linked, and how community health nurses incorporate them into practice.

WHAT IS LEADERSHIP?

Leadership has been studied for decades, and many theorists in the social sciences and business domains have contributed to its definition. One noteworthy definition identifies **leadership** as an interpersonal process in which one person influences the activities of another person or group of persons toward accomplishment of a goal (Robbins, 1993). Therefore, leadership simply is the use of personal characteristics or qualities to influence others (Bleich, 1999). Leadership involves creating a vision and guiding and directing people's beliefs and behavior toward fulfilling that vision. It accomplishes goals with and through people (Hersey & Blanchard, 1993). To lead requires interacting with other people to influence them to achieve a goal.

Three major characteristics of leadership are implied in these descriptions: it involves a purpose or goal, it is interactive with people, and it influences people.

Leadership Is Purposeful

Leadership always has a goal (Bleich, 1999; Robbins, 1993). No act of leadership exists without a reason. A mayor seeks low-cost housing for the poor; a community health nurse wants to see teenaged parents develop parenting skills; a minister desires transportation that is accessible to the physically handicapped. In each instance, the leader has a purpose and involves others in accomplishing that purpose. A leader works to achieve goals by making them clear, attainable, specific, and agreeable to the follower constituency.

Leadership Is Interpersonal

Leadership always involves a social exchange, a relationship between the two parties of leader and followers (Bleich, 1999). These parties mutually agree on roles and share information in a variety of patterns: a community agency's director of nursing sets policy and standards for client services; a nurse chairing a community task force makes informal suggestions to members. In both cases, the leader and followers must maintain a relationship that fosters ongoing communication and facilitates the movement-toward-a-goal process.

Leadership Is Influential

Leadership is influential, that is, it motivates others to change their behaviors and achieve a goal (Habel, 1999). Leaders are creative problem solvers who use their imagination to visualize new connections between ordinary events to continually analyze the efficiency of the status quo and to ask "what if" questions (Kerfoot, 1998). For example, in a suburb of a large city, a nurse received reports that several children had encountered rats while playing, and two children had been bitten. A casual survey revealed alleys with piles of garbage and trash that attracted rats. The nurse, as a leader, wanted to influence or motivate members of the community to eliminate this public health problem. To achieve this goal, the nurse needed to influence local citizens. The nurse began by inviting the parents of children who had encountered rats to call their neighbors together. At that meeting, the nurse facilitated the discussion and offered suggestions; the group decided to form a task force and hold a cleanup day with proper disposal of refuse and adequate containers. As a leader, this nurse offered guidance and direction, thus influencing the ideas and activities of this group of followers. In this situation, the nurse analyzed the efficiency of the status quo and asked the "what if" questions. In summary, then, leadership in community health means to influence people toward development of an optimally healthy lifestyle and environment. Any purposeful effort to influence behavior is an example of leadership; thus, every community health nurse can act as a leader (Michaels, 1997).

LEADERSHIP THEORIES

Some nurses effectively influence change in community health. Others do not. What explains the difference? What accounts for effective leadership? Six theoretical approaches provide insight into the nature of leadership: trait theory, behavioral theory, contingency theory, leadership style theories, transformational theory, and charismatic theory.

Trait Theory

"The 'great man,' or 'trait' theory, was derived from the Greek philosopher Aristotle's belief that only a few people are born with the traits necessary to be great leaders" (Habel, 1999, p. 11). During the Industrial Revolution, researchers theorized that certain individuals exhibited specific personality qualities—or traits—that made them leaders, including intelligence, enthusiasm, self-confidence, charisma, and decisiveness (Table 10–1). They concluded at first that leaders were born with these characteristics but later determined that, for some, these traits were acquired. However, trait theorists were unable to identify specific qualities possessed by *all* leaders. For example, Geier (1967) reviewed 20 different research investigations that had isolated 80 different traits of leaders, but only five traits were common to four or more of the studies. Recent research has identified six traits that distinguish leaders from nonleaders: (1) desire to lead, (2) ambition and energy, (3) intelligence, (4) self-confidence, (5) honesty and integrity, and (6) job-relevant knowledge (Kirkpatrick & Locke, 1991).

The trait theory has had only limited success in enlarging our understanding of leadership. Its flaws include a failure to examine the needs of followers. Additionally, it did not clarify the relative importance of various traits as different traits take on greater or lesser importance, depending on the leadership situation (Robbins, 1993; Yukl, 1997). Finally, it did not reveal whether traits are already present or acquired as a result of leadership.

TABLE 10–1. Leadership Qualities Enhancing Effectiveness		
Intelligence	Personality	Abilities
Knowledge	Adaptability	Social participation
Decisiveness	Creativity	Interpersonal skills
Speaks fluently	Cooperativeness	Ability to enlist
Judgment	Self-confidence	cooperation
ability	Emotional stability	Tact and diplomacy
	Independent	Popularity and
	thinking	prestige
	Personal integrity	

(Adapted from Bass & Stogdill, 1990; Gibson et al., 1999; and Swansburg, 1996.)

Behavioral Theory

Dissatisfied with the limitations of the trait approach, researchers began in the 1940s to focus on the behavior of leaders during interaction with followers. Behavioral theory proposed that leaders' behavior, rather than leaders' personality traits, were the chief determinants of who would become leaders and how effective they would be. This approach held out the hope that leadership ability could be developed.

As stated earlier, leadership involves accomplishing goals with and through people. Consequently, behavioral theorists determined that leaders must be concerned with production to achieve goals and with relationships to show concern for people. These two dimensions, concern for people and concern for productivity or tasks, became the focus of many studies (Blake & Mouton, 1964; Hersey & Blanchard, 1993; Robbins, 1993). Research showed that leaders who exhibited high concern for tasks while neglecting concern for people tended to be less effective (Fig. 10–1). Similarly, leaders demonstrating high concern for people with little emphasis on tasks did not yield desired results. Research reveals that leaders who showed high concern for people and a high concern for production (see Fig. 10–1, upper right quadrant) were the most effective. The behavioral research findings, however, could not demonstrate a leadership style that was effective in all situations.

Contingency Theory

Contingency theory describes leadership in terms of the leader's ability to adapt to the situation. It became the focus of research starting about the mid-1960s, when researchers recognized that predicting leadership success was more complex than had been envisioned previously. One type of leadership used in one organization was not always successful in another organization. Leadership success was contingent on the situation that dictated which style of leadership should be used.

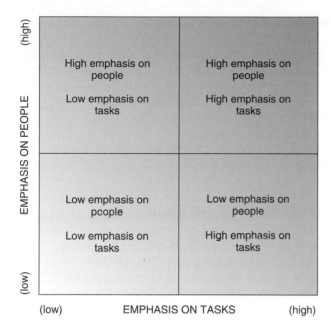

FIGURE 10–1. Leadership behavior grid. (Adapted from Blake and Morton, 1964 and Hersey and Blanchard, 1993.)

As researchers began to examine situational factors that influenced leadership effectiveness, several contingency models emerged. Fiedler's model indicates three measures of the kind of power and influence that the group gives to its leader: the relationship between the leader and the group members, the group's task structure, and the positional power of the leader (Fiedler, 1969). Because every situation is unique, leadership is a dynamic process of adapting the leader's style to the demands of the situation. Hersey and Blanchard (1993) refer to this process as "adaptive leader behavior" and say that leadership style should be adapted to followers' level of maturity, immaturity, or their ability and willingness to assume responsibility. Its implications for community health nursing are summarized as follows: the more nurses adapt their style of leadership behavior to meet the particular situation and the needs of clients or followers, the more effective they will be in reaching health-related goals (Fiedler, 1969; Swansburg & Swansburg, 1999).

Attribution Theory

Attribution theory says that leadership is made up of a set of characteristics ascribed or attributed to leaders by other people. For example, Mother Theresa was considered exceptionally inspiring and humane, characteristics that were attributed to her because of people's perceptions of her style and accomplishments. People also judge whether the leader's behavior is a personal attribute (internally caused) or is dictated by the situation (externally caused) (Robbins, 1993). This theoretical approach combines aspects of trait,

behavioral, and contingency theories to explain leadership style and effectiveness.

Charismatic Theory

Charismatic theory says that leadership occurs because of a magnetic and inspirational personality and behavior. The charismatic leader inspires others by getting an emotional commitment from them and arousing strong feelings of loyalty and enthusiasm (Habel, 1999). Charismatic theory is similar to attribution theory in that followers attribute extraordinary leadership ability to someone who exhibits exceptional appeal and persuasive ability. An example is Martin Luther King, Jr. Habel (1999) describes charismatic leaders as follows:

1. Emerge during a crisis
2. Advocate a vision that differs from the status quo
3. Accurately assess the situation
4. Communicate self-confidence
5. Use personal power
6. Make self-sacrifices
7. Use unconventional strategies

According to Marriner-Tomey (1996), followers of charismatic leaders:

1. Trust in the leader's beliefs
2. Have similar beliefs
3. Exhibit affection for, obedience to, and unquestioning acceptance of the leader
4. Believe that they can contribute to the mission advocated by the leader

Research shows a high correlation between charismatic leadership and followers' high performance and satisfaction. Furthermore, additional research demonstrates that individuals can learn "charismatic" behaviors (Marriner-Tomey, 1996; Robbins, 1993). Thus, this type of leadership is not limited solely to those who are born with these qualities.

LEADERSHIP STYLES

Early research by Kurt Lewin in the 1930s examined three general styles of leadership related to forces within the leader, within the group members, and within the situation: (1) autocratic, (2) participative (democratic), and (3) autonomous (formerly called laissez-faire) (Hersey & Blanchard, 1993; Swansburg & Swansburg, 1999). Recently, theorists have distinguished between a transactional style of leadership and a transformational style.

Autocratic Leadership Style

Autocratic leadership style is an authoritarian style in which leaders use their power (usually the power of their position) to influence their followers. The autocratic leader makes decisions alone and gives orders, expecting others to obey without question. This style generally is evident in the military. Suggestions from followers are not, as a rule, invited or accepted. The leader is dominant, and followers have little power or freedom of choice. This type of leader is more interested in task accomplishment than with concern for followers. In an extreme crisis, an autocratic style can enhance results and even survival. Sometimes, a nurse finds that members of a group expect to be led in an autocratic style. They may see the nurse as the qualified expert among them. However, autocratic leadership has a tendency to promote hostility, aggression, or apathy, which decreases initiative. Autocratic leadership must be used with caution, and many current organizational structures do not lend themselves to its practice (Robbins, 1993; Swansburg & Swansburg, 1999).

Participative Leadership Style

Participative leadership style is a democratic style in which leaders involve followers in the decision-making process (Swansburg & Swansburg, 1999). These leaders are people oriented and focus on relationships and teamwork. This form of leadership has become increasingly popular because it promotes followers' self-esteem and increases motivation and productivity. Leaders using this style encourage all members of the group to have a voice and participate in consensus decision-making. Some participative leaders encourage followers to exercise more freedom and power than others. Generally, however, this leadership style allows followers considerable freedom to make choices (Terry, 1993).

Autonomous Leadership Style

Autonomous leadership style is facilitative and encourages group members to select and carry out their own activities and to function independently. The leader's role is to set general parameters and to facilitate followers' progress. This style is used in certain industries where creative design of new products, such as computer applications or medical technologies, is being encouraged. It is effective in a group whose members have both the motivation and competence to achieve the goals. Although someone is formally the leader, this style uses little or no direct influence; rather, the leader exercises indirect influence by establishing an overall purpose and encouraging follower creativity and innovation. In some situations, where more guidance and direction is needed, this laissez-faire approach results in low productivity and follower frustration (Swansburg & Swansburg, 1999).

Building on these leadership styles, Hersey and Blanchard (1993) developed a continuum of leader behavior (Fig. 10–2) that describes style in relation to concern for people versus concern for production. Research shows that autocratic leaders are concerned about goals and are more task oriented, whereas participative leaders are more concerned about people and emphasize relationships.

Transformational Versus Transactional Leadership Styles

In **transactional leadership,** leader and followers engage in a reciprocal transaction. During this transaction, the roles and tasks of the followers are clarified and assigned as the

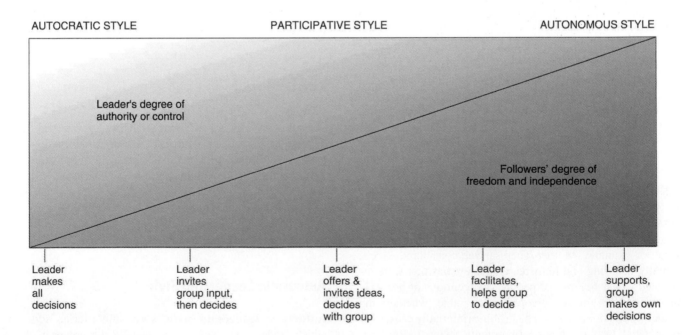

FIGURE 10–2. Leadership styles continuum. (Adapted from Hersey and Blanchard, 1993.)

group works to accomplish the goal. Most of the early leadership theories describe transactional leadership.

In the last decade, the literature has increasingly emphasized a type of leadership that is more charismatic (Bass, 1990; Cottingham, 1990; Terry, 1993). **Transformational leadership** is leadership that inspires followers to high levels of commitment and effort to achieve group goals (Robbins, 1993). Transformational leaders gain the respect and trust of their followers; instill in them a sense of pride and mission; communicate high expectations; promote intelligent, rational problem-solving; and give followers individualized consideration (Bass, 1990). It is leadership that creates purposes for institutions (Cottingham, 1990).

Closely related to transformational leadership is the reflective leadership view, an ethical perspective proposed by Robert Terry (1993), director of the Hubert H. Humphrey Institute of Public Affairs Education for Reflective Leadership Program at the University of Minnesota. He emphasizes that true leadership must be transformative rather than transactional to effect positive change. He states that a leader is an ethically motivated person who sees the possibilities for improvement in a situation and works in concert with followers to effect the change. Transformational leaders effectively use the following strategies (Cottingham, 1990):

1. Get to know the followers
2. Help the followers to learn and develop
3. Give generous feedback
4. Give responsibility and status
5. Give rewards to the followers
6. Communicate information

Nurses are being challenged to engage in transformational leadership (Beecroft, 1993; Porter-O'Grady, 1992); however, nurses need to determine the most appropriate leadership style by assessing the unique qualities of each situation, their followers' needs and degree of independence, and their own personalities and abilities.

LEADERSHIP FUNCTIONS

What are the functions of leadership in community health nursing? Michaels (1997) describes community nursing leaders as professionals who embrace challenges; synthesize, process and promote healing; analyze; and cure. Leaders challenge the process and inspire shared visions, enabling others to perform to their ultimate ability. Leaders know how to ask the right questions, how to develop problem-solving networks to find solutions to these questions, and how to marshal human energy and commitment to create the solutions. Specifically, five essential functions are required for effective leadership at any level: (1) the creative function, (2) the initiating function, (3) the risk-taking function, (4) the integrative function, and (5) the instrumental function. These functions do not occur in any particular order; rather, they operate simultaneously throughout the leadership process.

Creative Function

Leaders must be creative and must envision new and better ways to solve problems. This first step involves creative thinking about problems, which includes developing methods and activities for carrying out their solutions. This function requires knowledge to stimulate sensory perceptions, curiosity, openness, sensitivity to problems, and flexibility (Swansburg, 1996). For instance, a group of nursing students participated in a community leadership experience in an alternative high school for 400 adolescent parents of 200 children. After a community assessment, the students planned a health fair focusing on issues identified as needed by the mothers and their children. But after they began working on their health fair plan, their creativity sparked dozens of new ideas, and the services at the health fair expanded from providing screening and health information to formalizing a baseline of health data on all of the teenagers and "making plans to enlist future nursing students to participate in, and provide leadership for, the implementation of targeted health programs" (Mellon & Nelson, 1998, p. 122).

The creative leadership function includes generating ideas and developing designs for action. It also involves risk-taking and inventive problem-solving when buffering resisting forces. Finally, it includes empowering others to use their own creativity to accomplish goals (Hagberg, 1994; Swansburg, 1996).

Initiating Function

A leader introduces change and sets its process in motion. For a nurse, the initiating function includes convincing clients or followers of the need for change, starting the problem-solving process, and launching the activities needed to carry out the plan. Like all of the other leadership functions, it requires decision-making skills. For example, after seeing an increased number of adolescent pregnancies in the high school, a school nurse convinces the board of education of the need for a sex education program initiated at the junior high school level. The nurse also works to establish a prenatal counseling group and initiates a series of parenting seminars tailored to the teenaged parents in the high school. The initiating function begins the process toward goal accomplishment. It is the stimulus that starts clients or followers on their way to meet personal or agency goals.

Risk-Taking Function

Every leader is faced with uncertainty, and to proceed under uncertain conditions is to be a risk-taker. Leaders cannot guarantee outcomes. Most nurses working with families or groups in the community frequently encounter unpredictable variables. Examples include the uncertainty about whether new government policies will alter programs and funding or whether a proposed program will be well received by clients and will bring about the needed change. The leadership process requires careful planning based on all available data and the creation of scenarios to predict all possible obstacles and outcomes. It requires preparation of alternative courses of action, should earlier plans fail. Nevertheless, some variables cannot be predicted beyond a certain point, and leaders must be willing to take risks and expose themselves to possible failure and embarrassment. Taking risks also means that they may expose clients or followers to potential negative outcomes. Effective leaders, however, take calculated risks; they weigh the potential consequences, pro and con, of each action before proceeding. Their concern is to minimize perceived barriers and harmful consequences and maximize positive outcomes for followers.

Integrative Function

The integrative aspect of the leadership role focuses on strengthening collective ties and uniting clients or followers through a strong sense of purpose. The leader reminds the followers of their goals, encourages pride in their group identity, stabilizes intragroup relations, and mediates interpersonal conflict (Kouzes & Posner, 1995). Community health nurses working with families, groups, and aggregates frequently find members at odds or cross-purposes with one another. Individuals in any group setting tend to have their own hidden agendas and separate needs. One job of the nurse leader is to keep the client group on target by clarifying and reinforcing the goals that they have mutually identified. The integrative function requires good interpersonal skills for establishing positive relationships with, as well as between, followers. This function supports the aim of promoting member commitment and cooperation.

Instrumental Function

Leaders also must keep followers moving in the right direction; this is the purpose of the instrumental or facilitative function. Inspired by vision and goals, the leader serves as an enabler to move followers to act (Hersey & Blanchard, 1993; Kouzes & Posner, 1995). For nurse leaders, this function involves good communication. They must keep in constant touch with clients or followers to make certain that goals and activities are understood and agreed on, and to encourage both negative and positive feedback. Leaders further stimulate followers to progress toward achievement of goals by reinforcing desired behaviors and by setting the pace themselves. The latter is particularly important for gaining followers' respect and sustained commitment. To set the pace means that nurse leaders must demonstrate competence, practice what they preach, and demonstrate their belief in the followers and in what the followers are being asked to accomplish.

POWER AND LEADERSHIP

Power is the ability to influence or control other people's behavior to accomplish a specific purpose. Leadership and power are closely related, since leaders use power in the process of achieving goals. The concept of power has both positive and negative connotations. Positive synonyms for power are strength, energy, force, and might. Although the power to influence people for good is a goal in community health, power also may be abused. Authority, control, domination, coercion, and manipulation are negative terms often associated with power.

Although power often is viewed as being exercised by the leader, many see power as a social relationship of mutual dependency (Robbins, 1993). A leader has only as much power over the followers as the followers grant to the leader. The leader is dependent on the followers. At the same time, the greater the followers' dependency on the leader, the greater is the power that the leader has over the followers.

If a college student is financially dependent on parents, the parents have a certain economic power over the student. But the amount of power held by the parents also depends on how much the student earns independently and spends. People make choices. Followers can choose how dependent on the leader they wish to be, as well as the amount of power that they wish to exercise for themselves. Leaders also can choose the amount of power that they exert and the degree of their dependency on their followers. Thus, the amount of power a person has over others is determined by two things: (1) the amount that a person chooses to take, and (2) the amount that others are willing to give.

Power Bases and Power Sources

Where does power originate? What gives people the ability to influence others? In 1959, French and Raven identified five bases of power: (1) coercive power, which uses force to gain compliance; (2) reward power, which provides something of value in exchange for compliance; (3) expert power, which exerts influence by using special knowledge or skills; (4) legitimate power, which is derived from the person's position or title; and (5) referent power, which comes from other people's admiration and emulation of the power holder. These five categories proved useful but did not clearly distinguish between bases of power and sources of power (Willey, 1990).

POWER BASES
Power bases refer to knowledge or skills possessed by the power holder that enable the power holder to exert influence over others. As a power holder, a person's power bases are the things controlled by the person. Power bases come from four types of power: information power, persuasive power, reward power, and coercive power.

Information Power

Information power refers to a person's access to or possession of valued information. It often has been said that knowledge is power. When individuals control unique information needed for such things as decision-making, they are in positions of power. The Internet gives information power, which is an empowering experience. Being knowledgeable about computers and how to retrieve global data can empower nurses and clients alike.

Persuasive Power

Persuasive power is the ability to influence people to adopt changed beliefs and actions through convincing discussion. The discussion may take such forms as argumentation, entreaty, or expostulation. A political leader who arouses a crowd to rally around a certain cause and a clergyman passionately raising money for the poor are both using persuasive power.

Reward Power

Reward power is the ability to influence people by granting rewards that they view as valuable. People comply with a request if they believe that a positive benefit will result from their compliance. They are thus voluntarily granting power to the person giving the reward. When a child is offered candy for good behavior or an employee a raise in salary if performance improves, the individuals offering the benefits have reward power.

Coercive Power

Coercive power refers to forced compliance based on fear. People comply with orders if they believe that not doing so would result in penalty, pain, or death. A mother threatening her children with loss of their allowance to get them to complete their homework has coercive power. A robber holding a gun to the head of a jewelry store owner has coercive power.

POWER SOURCES

Power sources refer to qualities or situations from which the power holder gains a power base (Robbins, 1993). Although individuals may hold one or more of the types of power just described in their power base, the question still remains: "Where does that power originate?" Robbins describes four sources of power: a person's position, personal qualities, expertise, and opportunities.

Position or Legitimate Power

Position or legitimate power means the ability to influence or control people as a result of a formal position. A formal position of authority, such as a corporation's chief executive officer, a classroom teacher, or head of a nursing department, gives the person power over those who are lower in the structural hierarchy. Position power enables a person to use various power bases. For example, a college professor exercises persuasive and reward power, a police officer uses coercive power, and a secretary applies information power.

Personal or Referent Power

Personal or referent power is the ability to influence others because of the person's personality. Trait theory and charismatic theory demonstrate that personal characteristics or personality style are a source of power. An individual who is charming, articulate, or physically dominating usually influences others through personal power.

Expert Power

Expert power refers to the ability to influence people based on specialized knowledge or skills. Expertise in some specialized area enables one to use one or more of the power bases. For example, a computer expert's knowledge is the source for information power as well as persuasive power when making computer-related decisions. Nurses, physicians, environmentalists, epidemiologists, and tax accountants have expert power.

Opportunity Power

Opportunity power is the ability to influence people by taking advantage of a special or timely situation. Rosa Parks seized an opportune moment in history to create awareness and change concerning civil rights. (Although her significant contributions to civil rights bravely began almost 50 years ago, when she refused to give up her seat on a bus in 1955 to a white passenger, she received the nation's highest civilian honor, a Congressional Gold Medal, in 1999 for her subsequent civil rights work.) In a crisis (eg, at the scene of a car accident), someone who does not necessarily have a position of power often emerges to take charge and tell people what to do. That person is using opportunity power. Being in the right place at the right time and using that opportunity to influence people is drawing on opportunity power.

Empowerment for Change in Community Health

Community health nurses need to develop their sources of power. Nurses can move into positions of influence in the health system as professional practitioners, managers, teachers, researchers, and consultants. They can use these positions to exercise information power, persuasion power, reward power, or coercive power to effect change. Nurses also can capitalize on their personal characteristics as a power source. Self-knowledge becomes critical in cultivating this power source. Nurses need to know their own strengths, limitations, and proclivities to find and sharpen the traits that will enhance their ability to influence people. Developing expertise is another source of nurse empowerment. In community health, nurses who expand their knowledge and competence in such areas as group dynamics, health policy and politics, computer technology, epidemiologic research, occupational health, school health, environmental health, health planning, or community assessment can use this expertise to build their power base of knowledge, persuasion, reward, and coercion. Nurses also need to take better advantage of opportunities in their personal and professional lives where they can influence decisions because of their rich power bases (Kerfoot, 1998). Sometimes, nurses shy away from chances to serve on influential committees in the community, testify before the legislature on important health issues, attend community meetings where issues are being aired, or provide input for planning decisions. These are only a few of the opportunities when community health nurses can gain power and influence change. Nursing's input into health reform discussions is a prime example of gaining nursing power and influence.

Empowerment is a process of developing knowledge and skills that increase a person's mastery over life-changing decisions (Kreisberg, 1992). To empower means to enable. As community health nurses learn to empower themselves, they can then empower others. Empowerment is therapeutic physically, mentally, and spiritually for the nurse, the agency, and the community (Swanson, 1996). To empower people in the community requires helping them to develop competence to take charge of their lives and find ways to meet their own needs (Zerwekh, 1992). It means helping them to develop knowledge and skills so that they can participate in their social and political worlds (Krichbaum, 1993). Nurses can assist community clients to develop the four power sources for themselves: using their position, capitalizing on personal characteristics, developing expertise, and taking advantage of opportunities. The elderly population, for example, could be encouraged to take advantage of a local election (opportunity power) to lobby for crime prevention. Adolescents could participate in school educational projects to gain knowledge (expert power) about family values and sexuality. Such programs have proved effective in preventing teenage pregnancy (American Hospital Association, 1994).

Vulnerable groups in the community, such as the homeless or abused women and children, often perceive themselves to be powerless. To promote client choice and self-determination requires empowering strategies that foster clients' self-esteem. To promote client self-esteem, nurses can provide consistent affirmations, set clear expectations, encourage increasing responsibility, model empowering behavior, facilitate client choices, and promote a sense of meaning and hope (Zerwekh, 1992). When people are unable to act in a positively autonomous manner (eg, abusive parents or the mentally ill), the nurse may need to use persuasive or coercive power bases to protect them and the people affected by their actions.

Empowerment of self and others is germane to effective leadership for community health nurses (Eng et al., 1992; Michaels, 1997). The use of power can and should be a positive force for protecting and promoting aggregate health.

THE NATURE OF CHANGE

To be a leader is to effect change in people's behaviors (McPherson, 1991). When nurses suggest that families adopt healthier communication patterns, they are asking them to change. Teaching parenting skills to teenagers is introducing a change. Promoting a community's self-determination in choosing a safer environment requires that the individuals involved must change. Because community health nursing's responsibility is to accomplish health goals and thus promote change, nurses cannot lead without introducing change into people's lives. Therefore, it becomes imperative for community health nurses to understand the nature of change, how people respond to it, and how to effect change for improved community health.

Definitions and Types of Change

Change is "any planned or unplanned alteration of the status quo in an organism, situation, or process" (Lippitt, 1973, p. 37). This definition explains that change may occur either by design or by default. Over the years, various theorists have contributed to understanding the nature of change. From a systems perspective, change means that things are out of balance or the system's equilibrium is upset (Spradley, 1980; Swansburg & Swansburg, 1999). For instance, when a community is devastated by a flood, its normal functioning is thrown off balance. Adjustments are required; new patterns of behavior become necessary. Other theorists explain change as the process of adopting an innovation (Spradley & McCurdy, 1994). Something different, such as an organization-wide smoke-free policy, is introduced; change occurs when the innovation is accepted, tried, and integrated into daily practice. Some have explained change in terms of its effect on behavior—that change requires adjustment in thinking and behavior and that people's responses to change vary according to their perceptions of it. Change threatens the security that people feel when following established and familiar patterns (Callan, 1993). It generally requires adopting new roles. Change is disruptive.

The way people respond to change depends partly on the type of change. The change process can be described as sudden or drastic (revolutionary) or gradual over time (evolutionary).

Evolutionary change is change that is gradual and requires adjustment on an incremental basis. It modifies rather than replaces a current way of operating. Some examples of evolutionary change include becoming parents, gradually cutting back on the number of cigarettes smoked each day, and losing weight by eliminating desserts and snacks. Because it is gradual, this kind of change does not require radical shifts in goals or values. "People resist discarding their own ideas. Accepting another's idea reduces their self-esteem" (Swansburg, 1996, p. 298). Gradual change may "ease the pain" that change brings to some individuals. This type of change sometimes may be viewed as reform.

Revolutionary change, in contrast, is a more rapid, drastic, and threatening type of change that may completely upset the balance of a system. It involves different goals and perhaps radically new patterns of behavior (Swansburg, 1996). Sudden unemployment, stopping smoking overnight, losing the town's football team in a plane accident, suddenly removing children from abusive parents, or suddenly replacing human workers with computers are examples of revolutionary changes. In each instance, the people affected have little or no advance warning and little or no time to prepare. High levels of emotional, mental, and sometimes physical energy and rapid behavior change are required to adapt to revolutionary change. If the demands are too great, some may experience defense mechanisms such as incapacitation, resistance, or denial of the new situation. (See Chapter 20 for a detailed discussion of coping with stress and defense mechanisms.)

The impact of a proposed change on a system clearly depends on the degree of the change's evolutionary or revolutionary qualities, a factor to be considered in planning for change. Some situations lend themselves better to one kind of change than the other. A community in need of improved facilities for the handicapped, such as ramps and wider doors, can introduce this change on an evolutionary, incremental basis, whereas a community involved in an unsafe, intolerable, or life-threatening situation, such as a flood or serious influenza epidemic, may require revolutionary change.

Stages of Change

The phrase **stages of change** refers to the three sequential steps leading to change that include unfreezing (when desire for change develops), changing (when people accept and try out new ideas), and refreezing (when the change is integrated and stabilized in practice). These stages were first described by Kurt Lewin and have become a cornerstone for understanding the change process (Lippitt et al., 1958; Noone, 1987).

UNFREEZING

The first stage, unfreezing, occurs when a developing need for change causes disequilibrium in the system. A system in disequilibrium is more vulnerable to change. People are motivated to change either intrinsically or by some external force. People have a sense of dissatisfaction; they feel a void that they would like to fill. The unfreezing stage involves initiating the change.

Unfreezing may occur spontaneously. A family requests help in solving a problem with alcoholism; a group seeks assistance in adjusting to retirement; a community desires a solution to noise pollution. However, the nurse as change agent may need to initiate the unfreezing stage by attempting to motivate clients, through education or other strategies, to see the need for change.

CHANGING

The second stage of the change process, changing, occurs when people examine, accept, and try the innovation. For instance, this is the period when participants in a prenatal class are learning exercises or when the elderly in a senior citizens' center are discussing and trying ways to make their apart-

ments safe from accidents. During the changing stage, people experience a series of attitude transformations, ranging from early questioning of the innovation's worth to full acceptance and commitment to accomplishing the change. The change agent's role during this stage is to help clients see the value of the change, encourage them to try it out, and assist them in adopting it (Cobb-McMahon et al., 1984).

REFREEZING

The third and final stage in the change process, refreezing, occurs when change is established as an accepted and permanent part of the system. The rest of the system has adapted to it. Because it is no longer viewed as disruptive, threatening, or new, people no longer feel resistant to it. As the change is integrated, the system becomes refrozen and stabilized. It is evident that refreezing has occurred when weight loss clients, for example, are routinely following their diets and losing weight, or when senior citizens are using grab bars in their bathrooms and have removed scatter rugs from their homes, or when a community has erected stop signs and established crosswalks at dangerous intersections.

Refreezing involves integrating or internalizing the change into the system and then maintaining it. Because a change has been accepted and tried does not guarantee that it will last (Spradley, 1980). Often, there is a tendency for old patterns and habits to return; consequently, the change agent must take special measures to ensure maintenance of the new behavior. A later section discusses ways to stabilize change.

PLANNED CHANGE

Planned change is a purposeful, designed effort to effect improvement in a system with the assistance of a change agent (Spradley, 1980). Planned change is crucial to the development of successful community health nursing programs. The following characteristics of planned change are key to its success:

The change is purposeful and intentional: There are specific reasons or goals prompting the change. These goals give the change effort a unifying focus and a specific target. Unplanned change occurs haphazardly, and its outcomes are unpredictable.

The change is by design, not by default: Thorough, systematic planning provides structure for the change process and a map to follow toward a planned destination.

Planned change in community health aims at improvement: That is, it seeks to better the current situation, to promote a higher level of efficiency, safety, or health enhancement. Planned change, however, aims to facilitate growth and positive improvements. Plans to provide shelter and health care for a homeless population, for example, are designed to improve this group's well-being.

Planned change is accomplished through an influencing agent: The change agent is a catalyst in developing and carrying out the design; the change agent's role is a leadership role.

Planned Change Process

The planned change process involves a systematic sequence of activities that follows the nursing process. Following its eight basic steps leads to the successful management of change: (1) recognize symptoms, (2) diagnose need, (3) analyze alternative solutions, (4) select a change, (5) plan the change, (6) implement the change, (7) evaluate the change, and (8) stabilize the change (Spradley, 1980). Figure 10–3 shows how forces acting on a system create a need for change using the planned change model.

STEP 1: RECOGNIZE (ASSESS) SYMPTOMS
The first step in managing change is to recognize and assess the symptoms that indicate a need for change. In this step, it is necessary to gather and examine the presenting evidence, not diagnose or jump ahead to treatment. For instance, assume that a group of clients shows interest in receiving help

with parenting skills. The nurse cannot assume that these clients feel inadequate in the parent role, nor can the nurse assume that they lack information about parenting or are having difficulty with their children. The nurse must assess the specific needs to discover that some of the parents have trouble talking to their teenagers, others wonder if their children's behavior is normal, a few question how strictly they should set limits, and still others are not certain about how to handle punishment. These symptoms are pieces of evidence that will assist diagnosis in the next step. This first step is an assessment phase. Before moving on, however, change agents need to ask themselves what are their motives for pursuing this change. Inappropriate motives of the change agent, such as wanting to feel needed, can cloud judgment and interfere with effective management of change.

STEP 2: DIAGNOSE NEED
Diagnosis means to analyze the symptoms and reach a conclusion about what needs changing. First, describe the situation as it is now (the real) and compare it with the way it should be (the ideal). For example, loud arguing and conflict may be normal and functional behavior for an adolescent support group. There is no discrepancy between the real and the ideal and, therefore, no need for change within the group.

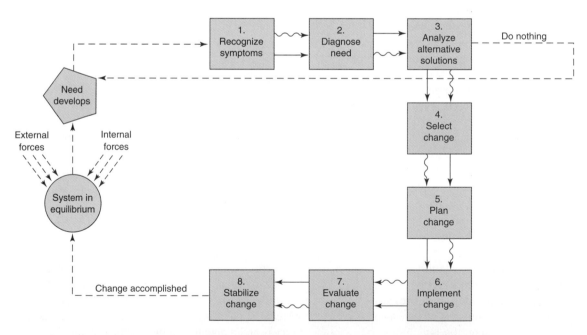

FIGURE 10–3. Planned change model. The planned change process begins when one recognizes a need. When the change agent fails to respond to a need for change, the need continues and may escalate. Client system (those involved and affected by the change) and change agent must work together throughout the entire planned change process. Their respective roles vary depending on the situation and the players' abilities, but no planned change is truly effective without utilization of this collaborative relationship. The client system (*wavy arrow*), which may be an entire community, will fluctuate in its involvement with the change process. The change agent (*straight arrow*), as a good leader, analyzes the situation thoroughly, plans carefully, and sets a steady course for effecting the change.

If, however, there is a discrepancy between the real and the ideal, then a need exists and a change effort is justified (Hersey & Blanchard, 1993). For example, the community health nurse, in talking with a group of parents, hears the following comment, "I'm not sure how much freedom to allow Karen. She came in late twice last week and I'm not sure how to punish her." Clearly, the nurse notices a discrepancy between this family's present and ideal situations; hence, there is a need.

The next step is to determine the nature and cause of the need. Gathering data by questioning clients, checking the literature, or seeking consultation is important for making a more accurate diagnosis. The parents should be questioned in more detail about the difficulties that they are having with their children. Asking questions such as: How do they feel about being parents? What are the most difficult aspects of parenting for them? Have they read any books or used any other resources to help them in their parenting activities? To whom do they talk about parenting problems? When they have a problem handling the raising of their children, how do they usually solve it? Secondary data should be obtained by checking the literature to determine the most effective approaches to solving parenting problems or by consulting an expert on family life to get ideas about what this group of parents might need. The parents also should be asked directly what information they desire or need. Conclusions should be drawn about the specific changes needed for these parents. Unless the diagnosis is made accurately, the entire change effort may address the wrong problem. Also, the client system should help to diagnose. Ask the parents what it is that they want and need.

The findings should be formulated into a single, diagnostic statement that also includes the cause. After data collection, the nurse discovers that the parents are insecure in their parenting roles, partially because of lack of knowledge about how to carry out parental responsibilities, but primarily because they lack a supportive reference group. Most of them live some distance from relatives or no longer maintain close ties with relatives. The diagnosis for these parents is insecurity in the parenting role because of a lack of support and knowledge.

STEP 3: ANALYZE ALTERNATIVE SOLUTIONS

Once the diagnosis and its cause are determined, it is time to identify solutions or alternative directions to follow. Brainstorming is helpful here, and the client system should be involved as much as possible in the process. Reviewing the literature is helpful at this point to suggest solutions tried by others. Make a list of all reasonable, broad alternatives and then analyze them thoroughly to determine the advantages, disadvantages, possible consequences, and risks involved in each. For the parents, general alternatives might be considered such as family counseling, a support group, or education in family life. Each of these alternatives has some advantages and disadvantages toward meeting the parents' need for confidence in their roles.

Next, each alternative should be analyzed. For example, the counseling solution could provide insight and awareness into family behavior. It would give family members opportunities to express feelings and gain understanding of how other members feel. However, it would not provide a frame of reference that they could use to compare their own parenting behaviors with other acceptable ones, nor would it provide adult peer support for the parents. The consequences of this alternative most likely would be to promote parents' self-understanding and better family communication. Risks would include the possibility that children, especially teenagers, might not be willing to participate and that parents might not gain self-confidence in their roles. Each alternative should be examined to determine its usefulness and feasibility, again using literature and other resources, such as consultants, to learn the best ways to meet the parents' need for change.

STEP 4: SELECT A CHANGE

After having carefully analyzed all alternatives, the best solution must be selected. The parents favor the idea that the best solution seems to be a parenting support group. The risks involved in the choice of change should be reexamined, such as whether this action might be too costly in time, money, or potential for failure. Ways to reduce these risks might be explored.

To know what the change is aiming to accomplish, a clearly stated goal should be formulated. For this parenting group, the mutually agreed-on goal is to provide a supportive, reinforcing climate while increasing members' parenting skills.

STEP 5: PLAN THE CHANGE

Step 5 is at the heart of planned change because at this stage, the change agent and client system together prepare the design, the blueprint that guides the change action. In steps 1 through 4, data are gathered, a diagnosis is made, resources are assessed, and a goal is established—all preparatory actions for planning the change. The plan tells the change agent and client system how to meet that goal. Preferably, they develop the plan together.

Talk with the parents about ways to meet their goal, considering such possibilities as weekly discussion groups on selected topics, monthly meetings with an informed speaker, or reading books and articles on parenting with regular sessions to discuss their application. After analysis and discussion, the group decides to meet one evening a month, rotating the location between members' homes. Group sessions will include a variety of approaches: a speaker will be invited every 4 months, a book or article discussion will be held quarterly, and the remaining meetings will be spent on topics of the group's choice. All sessions will provide opportunities for parents to discuss their concerns or problems. The nurse and the group design this plan around a set of objectives.

The most important activity in planning is to have clear, specific objectives. These should be measurable and, preferably, stated as outcomes. For example, the following objective is measurable and describes an outcome: "By the end of the second session, each parent in the group will have participated in the discussion at least once." It is helpful to prepare a list of activities to help accomplish each objective and to develop a time plan. It also is important to assess the potential costs in terms of time, money, materials, and the number of people needed and to determine the resources available. Design the evaluation plan and start a list of ways to stabilize (refreeze) the change.

During planning, it is useful to perform a **force field analysis** (Hersey & Blanchard, 1993), a technique developed by Kurt Lewin (1947) for examining all positive (driving) forces and negative (restraining) forces influencing a change situation. Force field theory says that there are driving forces, which favor change, and restraining forces, which decrease or discourage change. Examples of driving forces include clients' desire to be healthier, more productive, or have a safe environment. Examples of restraining forces include apathy, fear of something new, low self-esteem, or hostility. When the strength of the driving forces is equal to the strength of the restraining forces, equilibrium exists. To introduce a change and move the client system to a higher level of health, that balance must be altered. To do so, the change agent either increases the driving forces, decreases the restraining forces, or both. The change agent uses force field analysis to study both sets of forces and to develop strategies to influence the forces in favor of the change (see Fig. 10–3).

The procedure for conducting a force field analysis follows a few simple steps. The change agent may perform the analysis alone but preferably consults with clients and a change-planning resource group such as community health colleagues. The steps for conducting force field analysis are as follows:

1. Brainstorm to produce a list of all driving and restraining forces. (For the parenting group, one driving force is the parents' desire to be more successful parents; a restraining force might be lack of group agreement on discussion topics.)
2. Estimate the strength of each force.
3. Plot the forces on a chart such as the one shown in Figure 10–4.
4. Note the most important forces, then research and analyze them.
5. List and document possible responses or actions that might strengthen each important driving force or weaken each important restraining force.

Finally, as a consideration in planning the change and in analyzing the driving and restraining forces, study the social network and interaction of the system involved in the change. The change agent needs to be aware of formal and informal leaders, cliques within larger groups, influential persons, and all other social network influences on the change process. For instance, one nurse attempting to improve the infant-feeding practices of a group of young southeast Asian mothers failed to consider the strong cultural influence of the infants' grandmothers living nearby. The older women had strong opinions based on long-held cultural traditions about what infants were to eat and how they were to be fed. To ignore their influence could cause the proposed change to fail; involving the grandmothers could be a way of turning their influence into a driving force for the change.

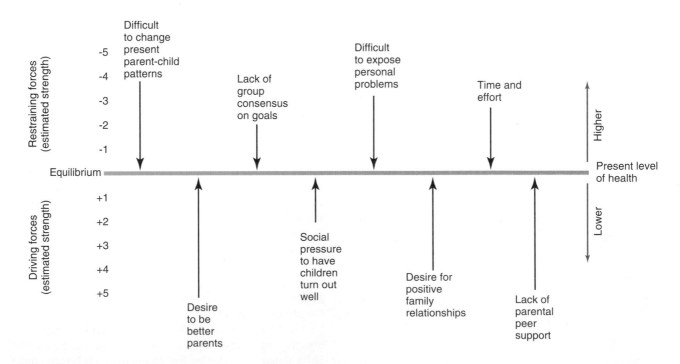

FIGURE 10–4. Analysis of restraining and driving forces.

STEP 6: IMPLEMENT THE CHANGE

The implementation step involves enacting the change plan. Because the objectives and activities have been clearly defined in previous steps, the change agent and client system know what needs to be done and how to begin the process. For example, the parenting group and their nurse–change agent begin group discussions meeting every Tuesday evening at a local school.

At the start of implementation, be certain that all persons concerned clearly understand and are prepared for the change. When working with an aggregate, for example, the nurse may do most of the planning with a few key members. The nurse must be sure that each member who will be affected by the proposed change understands (1) what to expect, (2) the meaning of the change, and (3) what will be required of them in adapting to it. An unprepared client system, especially in a large group or organization, may bring disaster (Kanter, 1983; Swansburg, 1996). No matter how well a change effort is planned, people who are unprepared for it may resist it strongly and render it useless.

When implementing change that will affect a large group of people, such as introduction of a mass screening or immunization program, it is helpful to do a pilot study. The pilot study is done to test the change on a small scale to iron out problems and revise the change before implementing it in the larger system. One advantage of a pilot study is that it demonstrates the change to the client system on a small scale, which is less threatening, so that clients are more receptive. It gives people time to adjust their thinking and to discover that the change will not disrupt their lives too much or require drastic adaptations.

STEP 7: EVALUATE THE CHANGE

The success of step 7 depends on how well the change is planned. Well-written objectives with specific criteria for their measurement will make the evaluation step simpler. However, evaluation does not end with saying whether the objectives were met. Each objective requires analysis: (1) Was it met? (2) What evidence (documentation) shows that it was met? (3) Was it accomplished using the best means possible, or would another method have been better? The objective for the parenting group stated that each member should enter into the discussion by the end of the second session. Although this objective could be easily evaluated by the nurse leader, the objective could have been improved by more a specific description of how this participation would occur. A better method to achieve this objective would have been to suggest that more active group members could solicit ideas from those who did not have an opportunity to speak. This would facilitate more group participation rather than the nurse leader calling on nontalkers to speak. Finally, considering the evaluation, the change agent makes needed modifications in the change before stabilization.

STEP 8: STABILIZE THE CHANGE

The final step in the planned change process requires taking measures to reinforce and maintain the change (see Fig. 10–3). A well-developed change plan includes a design for stabilization. The change agent actively encourages continued use of the innovation by establishing two-way communication; thus, future resistance can be overcome, and the client's full commitment to the change can be maintained (Noone, 1987). Stabilization occurs by soliciting reactions from the client system. Do the clients perceive any potential problems? Do they have doubts? Reinforcing the desired behavior and following up on the change as long as necessary will help to ensure its permanence. Alcoholics Anonymous, for example, stabilizes the change to nondrinking by providing a regular support group that reinforces the nondrinking pattern. The group rewards compliance with praise and replaces drinking with other satisfying experiences, such as social acceptance, to keep the alcoholic from returning to the old behavior. In the example of the parenting group, the nurse stabilizes changed behaviors by focusing on the group's increased confidence in their parenting roles and emphasizing the increased success with coping with their children. The group decides to reward successes by giving a "Parent of the Month" plaque to the member who demonstrates the most growth in parenting skills and agrees to nominate one member as "Parent of the Year" in the community newspaper contest. When stabilization occurs and the system achieves a new equilibrium (see Fig. 10–3), the change agent–client system relationship can be terminated for this specific change effort.

Applying Planned Change to Larger Aggregates

We have viewed the planned change process primarily in the context of introducing change to smaller aggregates. Community health nurses also use these eight steps when managing change at the organization, population group, community, and larger aggregate levels. For example, a nurse may suspect that there is a widespread lack of confidence among young parents. This hypothesis could be tested through a survey using a mailed questionnaire to determine parenting needs among the entire community's population of young parents. If symptoms are present (step 1), the nurse, in collaboration with health department personnel or other appropriate professionals, could analyze the symptoms and reach a diagnosis (step 2), perhaps that many young parents in the community are lacking in confidence and knowledge of parenting skills. Several approaches to meeting this need could be considered, such as instituting a parenting center in the community with satellite clinics; organizing churches, clubs, or both to sponsor parenting support groups; or working through the community college system to hold workshops and classes on parenting skills (step 3). The most feasible and useful alternative could be selected (step 4), and a parenting program for the community planned (step 5) and implemented (step 6). The nurse, with parents and other professionals involved, then would evaluate the outcomes (step 7) and make necessary adjustments in the parenting program be-fore finally stabilizing it (step 8), making certain that this change, undertaken to meet a population group need, re-mained an established and effectively functioning service (see The Global Community).

THE GLOBAL COMMUNITY

Leadership and Effecting Change Globally

We live in a global community. The problems and affairs of one country can no longer be viewed in isolation; rather, they influence trade, economic conditions, health, and welfare on an international level. Wars, terrorism, famine, floods, earth-quakes, population overcrowding, limited food supply, eco-nomic disasters, and epidemics of communicable diseases are among the many events that have a global impact. Public health leadership is needed to address these problems, and this leadership must be population and prevention focused. Nurses can take leadership to help solve some of these major issues:

1. World population is increasing by 100 million per year (Beaglehole & Bonita, 1997). The distribution of this growth is predominantly in the poorest developing countries.
2. Premature mortality (between ages 15 and 60 years) "varies about tenfold among countries: from more than 50% in parts of sub-Saharan African to about 5% in Switzerland and Japan" (Beaglehole & Bonita, 1997, p. 24–25).
3. In 1990, it was estimated that 9.2% of the world's population was older than 65 years. By 2025, the world's elderly population may be around 1.2 billion, or 14% of the population, with most of the increase occurring in poor countries (Department of International Economic and Social Affairs, 1995). This adds to the need for health services to address chronic disabilities (World Health Organization [WHO], 1994).
4. Environmental health problems and disease distribution follow similar global patterns.
5. One disease of worldwide concern is AIDS. About 17 million adults and 1.5 million children have been infected with HIV (WHO, 1996). By the year 2000, 40 million people are expected to be infected with HIV, and the total death toll from AIDS is expected to exceed 8 million by the year 2000 (Beaglehole & Bonita, 1997).

Community health nurses face an unparalled opportunity to provide leadership and influence change internationally. Many nurses already serve in influential positions with national and international organizations assisting developing countries such as the World Health Organization, the Pan American Health Organization, and the Peace Corps. However, more community health nurse leaders are needed to effect improve-ment in global health.

Planned Change Strategies

The literature describes three general change strategies (Bennis et al., 1985; Haffer, 1986). In a given situation, the change agent may use one or a combination of these strate-gies to effect a change: (1) empirical-rational, (2) normative-reeducative, and (3) power-coercive (Lundeen, 1992).

EMPIRICAL-RATIONAL CHANGE STRATEGIES

Empirical-rational change strategies are strategies used to effect change based on the assumption that people are ratio-nal, and when presented with empirical information will adopt new practices that appear to be in their best interest. To use this approach, which is common in community health, new information is offered to people. For instance, most fam-ily planning programs use empirical-rational strategies. Clients are given basic information on reproductive anatomy and physiology, and they are told about the benefits of con-traception with an explanation of a variety of family planning methods. Health workers hope that once clients have this in-formation, they will adopt some method of family planning. Some clients respond well to this approach, whereas others do not. The difference lies in client ability and interest in self-help. The nurse–change agent uses empirical-rational strate-gies with clients who can assume a relatively high degree of responsibility for their own health. In some respects, this set of strategies parallels the participative leadership style (see Fig. 10–2), which fosters maximum client autonomy.

NORMATIVE-REEDUCATIVE CHANGE STRATEGIES

Normative-reeducative change strategies are strategies used to influence change that not only present new informa-tion but directly influence people's attitudes and behaviors through persuasion (Flynn, 1992). It is a sociocultural reed-ucation. This approach assumes that people's attitudes and practices are determined by sociocultural norms and that they need more than presentation of information to change behavior (Chin & Benne, 1985). This approach strengthens client self-understanding, self-control, and commitment to new patterns through direct urging and influence. For exam-ple, a health education program that aims to increase safety practices in an industrial setting not only provides safety information such as posters and warning signs but also uses persuasive tactics such as individual rewards for safe practices, division recognition for minimum number of acci-dents, or discipline for noncompliance. Nurses use normative-reeducative strategies with clients who have a measure of self-care skill but at the same time need external assistance to effect lasting behavioral change. This type of client is found in teaching, counseling, and therapy situations.

POWER-COERCIVE CHANGE STRATEGIES

Power-coercive change strategies use coercion based on fear to effect change. Change agents may derive power from the law (such as health regulations or administrative policies), from position (such as political, social, or managerial positions), from a group (such as a social, work, or professional group), or from personal power (such as personal charisma, competence, or respect of followers). They use this power to coerce change; the result is forced compliance on the part of the client system. Some situations, particularly those that are life-threatening, may require power-coercive strategies. In community health practice, power-coercive strategies may be used with people who cannot help themselves or in situations that threaten individuals' safety or the public's health. An example is the stringent enforcement of infection control policies regarding the treatment of contaminated objects, such as all used needles and the safe disposal of infectious wastes. In another example, if officials find a restaurant in violation of health codes, they will either force compliance with the code or close the restaurant. Occasionally, clients cannot exercise responsibility because of temporary or permanent physical or psychological incapacitation, such as the mentally ill, abusive parents, or developmentally disabled persons. In such cases, the nurse may need to use the power of the law (eg, with abusive parents) to effect changes that are in clients' best interests. Although power-coercive strategies are appropriate in some situations, they should be used with caution because they can rob people of opportunities to grow in autonomy and capacity for self-care.

Planned change strategies may be combined; for instance, a normative-reeducative approach might have a power-coercive backup. This combination is evident in programs that educate and persuade groups of people to be immunized against an impending epidemic or to keep their garbage contained to avoid insect and rodent infestation. Behind this normative-reeducative strategy is an implied coercive threat of official disapproval, or worse, of noncompliance.

The effectiveness of a change strategy, then, varies with each situation and particularly with the degree of client capacity for self-care. As in the approach to leadership styles and use of power discussed earlier in the chapter, the nurse–change agent adapts strategies to fit each change situation.

Principles for Effecting Positive Change

Community health nurses introduce change every day that they practice. Every effort to solve a problem, prevent another from occurring, meet a potential community need, or promote people's optimal health requires changes. To make these changes truly successful so that desired outcomes are reached, they must be managed well. The following six principles provide guidelines for effecting positive change: (1) principle of participation, (2) principle of resistance to change, (3) principle of proper timing, (4) principle of interdependence, (5) principle of flexibility, and (6) principle of self-understanding.

PRINCIPLE OF PARTICIPATION

Persons affected by a proposed change should participate as much as possible in every step of the planned change process (Marriner-Tomey, 1996). This involvement is important for several reasons. Collaboration with those who have a vested interest in the change can produce a wealth of ideas and insights that can greatly improve the change plan. Furthermore, such participation can help remove obstacles and reduce resistance. Participation ensures a greater likelihood that the change will be accepted and maintained (Kanter, 1983; Flynn, 1992). One nurse, for instance, when planning with a school's parent-teacher association for a drug education program, involved students as well as teachers and parents. As a result, she secured all their support and cooperation, gained many helpful suggestions that she herself had not considered, and discovered that students were more responsive to the program because the change plan was specifically tailored to their needs.

PRINCIPLE OF RESISTANCE TO CHANGE

Because all systems instinctively preserve the status quo, the change agent can expect people to resist change (Swansburg, 1996). The homeostatic mechanism operating in any system seeks to maintain equilibrium; change poses a threat to that stability and security. Furthermore, all systems experience inertia; that is, they resist beginning movement. People do not undertake a change until they are convinced of its worth. Resistance may also come from a conflict over goals and methods or from misunderstanding about what the change will mean and require. Involving people in the planned change process, discussed in the previous section, is one way to overcome resistance. Another way is establishing and maintaining open lines of communication in order to make ideas clearly understood and to resolve disagreements quickly (Lundeen, 1992). Prepare people thoroughly for the change, provide support and patience during the change process, and encourage response and expression of feelings.

PRINCIPLE OF PROPER TIMING

Sometimes a change, even a well-designed and much needed one, should be postponed because the present is not the right time to introduce it. For example, perhaps the client system is experiencing too many other changes to handle the stress of this one. Other projects or activities in which the client system is currently engaged may compete for energy and other resources, depleting the energy and resources needed to make the proposed change successful. For example, in November, some middle-aged women, eager to start a book club that focused on discussion of preparing for menopause, had to postpone the project because the holidays were approaching. Shopping, entertaining, and vacations made it impossible to give the kind of time and energy needed to make the book club effective.

Proper timing is as important to a planned change as well-timed seed planting is to a good harvest. The change idea must be appropriate, the change recipient prepared, the climate right, and the resources available before the change can be fostered to grow into full maturity and usefulness (Cobb-McMahon et al., 1984; Flynn, 1992).

PRINCIPLE OF INTERDEPENDENCE

Every system has many subsystems that are intricately related to and interdependent upon one another. A change in one part of a system affects its other parts, and a change in one system may affect other systems (Chin, 1980). For example, a county community nursing agency made a change in its use of home health aides. Because many homebound clients needed more care than the agency staff could provide, the agency contracted with a private home-care service for extra home health aides. These paraprofessionals worked in the homes of agency clients, supplementing the care given by agency staff. The private company preferred to supervise its own aides, whereas the county agency had a policy of using community health nurses to supervise aides. The county agency was legally responsible and professionally accountable for the quality of care given to clients. The private company wanted to retain control of its workers. The matter was resolved by contracting with a different private service that would accept the county agency's supervision. The change, however, had affected the roles of nurses and aides within the system as well as the relationships between the two systems.

This principle of interdependence reminds the nurse that change does not take place in a vacuum. When workers learn new health and safety practices associated with their jobs, their relationships with one another, and their bosses, their overall productivity in the organization may easily be affected. One must anticipate and prepare for the impact of the proposed change on the clients involved, other persons, departments, organizations, or even geographic areas.

PRINCIPLE OF FLEXIBILITY

Unexpected events can occur in every situation. This fifth principle emphasizes two points. First, the nurse needs to be able to adapt to unexpected events and make the most of them. Perseverance and flexibility are the marks of a creative change manager (Swansburg, 1996). One community health nurse had tried unsuccessfully to contact a young mother who was reportedly abusing her 2-year-old son. After several phone calls and visits to an empty house, she finally found the mother and son at home with a neighbor who insisted on staying for the entire visit. At first the nurse was irritated by the neighbor's presence and viewed it as interfering with her goal of getting to know the mother and child. Then she realized that this situation offered an opportunity to learn more about the situation through the neighbor's input and viewed it as an opportunity to influence another client as well. She asked if the neighbor had children and began to include them both in the discussion and explained what she had to offer in terms of health teaching and support. This nurse was flexible in her approach to this situation.

The second point to remember about flexibility is that a good change planner anticipates possible blocks or problems by preparing strategies and alternative plans. During step 3 of the planned change process, it is helpful to rank the alternative solutions considered. Then, if the first choice does not work out for some reason, an alternative is ready to be put into action. Flexibility involves a willingness to consider a variety of options and suggestions from many sources (Swansburg, 1996).

PRINCIPLE OF SELF-UNDERSTANDING

Self-understanding is essential for an effective change agent (Hersey & Blanchard, 1993). A leader and change agent should be able to clearly define his or her role and learn how others define it. It is important to understand one's values and motives in relation to each change that one might ask people to make. Nurses as well should understand their personality traits and typical leadership styles to capitalize on or alter them in order to be more effective leaders and change agents. Understanding oneself is crucial to learning to make use of one's best qualities and skills to effect change.

CASE MANAGEMENT IN COMMUNITY HEALTH NURSING

One of the most important leadership roles of a community health nurse is that of case manager. **Case management** refers to a strategy of face-to-face relationships across a variety of health care services and their representatives and over a period of time for managing the risk associated with vulnerable groups (Michaels, 1997). For community health nurses, this has been the method of caregiving for almost 100 years (Knollmueller, 1989). However, it was introduced in the acute care setting, with enthusiasm, in the 1990s as a "delivery innovation" and a panacea for harnessing escalating costs and insurance premium increases (Lynn & Kelley, 1997; Roughan, 1997).

Regardless of the setting or wellness level of the client population, case management takes interdisciplinary collaboration, the working together of professionals across health, education, and welfare domains, moving clients toward specific measurable outcomes. The nurse works with clients using all agencies and services available to reach predetermined goals.

The settings in which community health nurses work frequently incorporate the case-management role as part of third-party reimbursement partnerships. For instance, a school nurse may conduct annual physical examinations, including hearing and vision screening, height and weights, and a head-to-toe assessment, on high-risk students receiving Medicaid or for those on the Children's Health Insurance Program (CHIP) (see Bridging Financial Gaps).

The nurse plans follow-up when assessment data determine there is the potential for or an existing health problem. This may take the form of nutrition classes for a group of children and their parents or referring a child to an ophthalmologist for

Bridging Financial Gaps

Leavitt, J.K. (1998). The Children's Health Insurance Program: Send in the nurses! *Nursing Outlook, 46*(4), 185.

Beginning in 1998, every state in the union engaged in decisions about a new public health program called the Children's Health Insurance Program (CHIP). This is the largest public program of health insurance since the enactment of Medicare and Medicaid in 1964. However, few nurses have been part of creating the plans for this program. Where are these experts? Not only are nurses not involved, but the American Nurses Association and the American Academy of Nursing have offered little information or encouragement for involvement. Some nursing leaders are working with legislators on CHIP through state nursing associations because of established working relationships, but the impact is not what it could be if more nurses were involved.

As part of the Balanced Budget Act of 1997, CHIP was enacted to extend health benefits to children who have no insurance. The children who will benefit most are those whose family income falls just above the Medicaid eligibility limits. Coded as Ti-

tle XXI of the Social Security Act, CHIP is a federal grant-in-aid to states, enabling them to provide health insurance for 11 million low-income children with a budget of over $40 billion over 10 years. Levels of benefits, amount of cost sharing, coverage choices, outreach, and participating providers must be decided by each state. Nurses have a major stake in each of the processes. Unless they are at the table during decision-making, they are less likely to be reimbursed for nursing care. Those currently making the decisions are insurance companies and pediatricians.

What should nurse leaders do? (1) Become informed about CHIP in your state. (2) Act as an information source for the public and nursing colleagues. (3) Ask your state nurses association to become actively involved in policy deliberations if they are not already involved. (4) Join with others—coalitions and advocates—who are working with policy-makers. (5) Contact state representatives and offer to advise them about policy options and research information. (6) If you cannot be involved, find a colleague who can.

---

strabismus. Additionally, the nurse collaborates with others working in the best interest of the child, such as the school dietitian, physical education and classroom teachers, family physician, or other helping professionals already working with the families of children with nutrition problems. For the child with strabismus, the nurse coordinates follow-up with the classroom teacher, medical specialist, family, and hospital staff if correction of the problem entails surgery.

Populations at risk in the community benefit from the intensive relationship that promotes coordination of care through the case-management delivery system. The most effective case manager benefits from utilizing leadership skills, including creativity and flexibility, developing her or his power base, tapping the appropriate power sources, and participating as an effective change agent. High-risk populations depend on the case-management skills of the nurse.

COMMUNITY HEALTH NURSES' LEADERSHIP ROLES

Community health nurses exercise the functions of leadership in ever-widening spheres of influence, as shown in Figure 10–5. The central aim of this leadership role is to positively influence community health. The first area of focus is to improve the immediate environment, which includes physical, psychological, social, and spiritual factors, by influencing consumer health-related behavior. Community health nurses exercise leadership when they influence the quality of nursing practice of their coworkers through, for instance, providing opportunities for professional growth and development and peer review and consultation. They may also influence the service provi-

sion vehicle, the agency or organization through which care is offered, by accepting a formal leadership position or by serving on committees and taking an active part in quality management and improvement. For example, listed below are some areas of influence associated with various positions in a large community health nursing agency:

Director: Influences organizational policy and decision-making

Associate director: Influences management of specific aspects of the organization

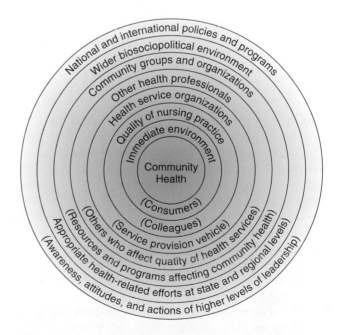

FIGURE 10–5. Areas of potential leadership influence within community health nursing practice.

Supervisor: Influences structure and process of providing services

Case manager: Influences coordination of assessment and referral activities

Team leader: Influences day-to-day quality of nursing practice

Staff nurse: Influences client health, behavior, and environment

In other settings for community health nursing practice, such as rural or occupational environments, there may be only one nurse present to provide leadership that encompasses many, if not all, of these activities. Beyond the agency itself, the leadership role of each nurse extends to influencing those community attitudes, programs, and environmental factors that affect community health. Each nurse must assess the situation and determine the kind and extent of leadership needed.

Community health nurses may influence other professionals involved in the health system through ongoing communication to promote awareness of health needs and facilitate development of appropriate services. Nurses may influence groups and organizations, such as clubs, churches, or the legislature, by keeping them informed about health problems and suggesting ways they can improve community health levels. Extending their leadership influence even wider, community health nurses may focus on the wider biosociopolitical environment of the city, county, state, or region (Salmon, 1993). For example, a nurse may support anti-smoking programs or may campaign for proper disposal of toxic waste. Finally, community health nursing leadership may extend to influencing national and international policies and programs that affect health, such as those of the World Health Organization. Participating in citizens' lobbies, serving on national committees, or contacting senators and representatives at the national and international levels are some of the many possible actions nurses could take. The number of spheres in which the community health nurse exercises a leadership role varies, depending on health needs, the work situation, the nurse's abilities, and available time.

Conditions for Effective Nursing Leadership

The ultimate test of nurse leadership is in the outcomes. Are goals met? What did the leader accomplish? Reaching a successful outcome involves certain factors. Adherence to these factors will contribute to positive results, but violation of one or more of them will create negative results. They form the conditions necessary for leadership to be effective.

1. Team members, followers, or clients must have the background knowledge of what is being suggested, advised, or directed in order to make compliance possible.
2. Team members, followers, or clients must be able to carry out the suggestion. They must have access to the needed resources or have their abilities developed as needed (Swansburg, 1996).

3. The required action must be consistent with the personal values and interests of team members, followers, or clients.
4. The required action must be consistent with the collective purposes, values, and norms of the team members, followers, or clients—that is, be in tune with group or agency goals (Swansburg, 1996).

Central and most important to effective leadership is a relationship of trust, respect, and mutual exchange between leader and followers. It is through this transformational relationship that community health nurses can satisfy the conditions for effective leadership and accomplish positive health outcomes.

Effectiveness of Followers

A great deal of attention has been focused on leadership. Yet for every leader there must be followers. There is evidence that the success of leadership depends on the effectiveness of followers (Hollander & Offermann, 1990). Simple observation demonstrates that some followers do a good job of supporting leader goals, while others may be indifferent or incompetent. What role do followers play in successful leadership outcomes? It is becoming evident that ineffective followers may be more of a handicap to accomplishing goals than ineffective leaders (Robbins, 1993).

Four qualities are characteristic of effective followers:

1. *Commitment:* They are committed to the vision, goals, and purpose of the leadership effort, in addition to concern for their own goals. They are physically and psychologically dedicated to their work.
2. *Self-management:* Effective followers manage their own lives well, working independently and not needing close supervision. They are disciplined and can think and solve problems for themselves.
3. *Integrity:* Effective followers are honest and trustworthy. Their ideas, judgment, and ability to follow through can be trusted. They have high moral and ethical standards, acknowledge their mistakes, and give credit where it is appropriate.
4. *Competence:* Effective followers learn to master the skills necessary for accomplishing leadership goals. They seek to expand their competence and have higher standards for their own performance than the job requires (Kelley, 1988).

As a community health nurse you can seek to enhance these qualities in yourself when you perform a follower role as well as encourage these traits in clients.

SUMMARY

Community health nurses, at every level of practice, must be leaders and change agents in order to influence people to adopt healthier behaviors. Formally or informally, they act as leaders to change people's health beliefs and practices and promote organized responses to community health problems. For example, they may provide leadership in initiating programs to meet the needs of at-risk populations, such as the homeless, or may lead groups, such as the elderly, toward self-empowerment.

Leadership includes three important characteristics: it is purposeful, it is interpersonal—involving interaction with others—and it is influential in that the change agent influences others toward accomplishing a goal. Several theories assist in understanding leadership. Their differing emphases include personality traits, leader behaviors, adapting leadership to the situation, differing leadership styles, attributed qualities, and charisma. Leadership styles may be autocratic, participative, or autonomous. In additon, some leadership is transactional, focused more on roles, tasks, and accomplishing goals, whereas other leadership is transformational, emphasizing inspiring motivation and commitment in followers.

Leadership influence depends on the use of power. This power is based on the ability to use information, be persuasive, grant rewards, and enforce compliance. The sources of these abilities or power bases come from the leader's position of authority or influence, the leader's personality, the leader's expertise, and effective use of opportunities. Nurses need to empower themselves and others to effect change in community health.

The purpose of leadership is to effect change, which alters the equilibrium in a system; it may occur gradually, with time for people involved to adjust, or it may occur in a drastic fashion, such as in a crisis or natural disaster. Change occurs in three stages: unfreezing when the system is ready for change, changing when the innovation is implemented, and refreezing when the change is stabilized.

Planned change is a purposeful, designed effort to effect improvement in a system with the help of a change agent. It involves a process of eight steps, similar to the nursing process, which nurses can use to create change. These steps include the following: assessing symptoms, diagnosing need, analyzing alternative solutions, selecting a change, planning the change, implementing the change, evaluating the change, and stabilizing the change. During planned change, the nurse can use one or a combination of three major strategies: a rational approach of providing information to influence people to change, an educative approach of combining new information with persuasion to effect change, and a coercive approach of enforcing compliance. Several important principles serve as guidelines for community health nurses to effect change. They include involving all persons affected by the change, introducing change in a timely fashion, considering the impact of the change on other systems, being flexible, and understanding oneself and one's own qualities, which can be groomed to provide the most effective leadership.

Case management is an important leadership function in an agency employing community health nurses. In this role, the nurse coordinates client care, collaborating with other professionals to meet client needs. Although this role is familiar to the public health sector, it is an innovative caregiving method in other health care settings.

Finally, effective leadership incorporates the functions of creative problem-solving, initiating ideas and events, taking risks, uniting people around a purpose, and facilitating movement toward the goal. Community health nurses use these leadership functions in the context of ever-widening spheres of potential influence. They inspire and motivate people to believe in themselves, develop high self-esteem, and empower themselves to solve problems and effect change.

ACTIVITIES TO PROMOTE CRITICAL THINKING

1. As a staff community health nurse with case-management responsibilities, you have been asked to chair an ad hoc committee in your health department made up of interdisciplinary colleagues and community members. The committee's task is to plan a health fair for the local community.
   a. As chairperson of the committee, discuss how you would exercise each of the five leadership functions as you chair the planning committee.
   b. Identify and analyze your own sources of power and bases of power. Which of these power bases and sources would you use to influence committee members and community citizens?
   c. Describe your leadership style and determine whether it is appropriate for this situation and group.
   d. Outline the specific planned change steps that your committee needs to ensure a successful health fair with outcomes that promote improved levels of community health.
   e. Select one specific objective of your health fair (eg, cholesterol screening of an at-risk aggregate with reduced cholesterol levels in a year). Does the proposed objective require an evolutionary or revolutionary change in citizens' health-related behaviors? Justify your choice of the type of change.
   f. Explain the strategies that you would use to effect the change.
   g. Six principles for effecting positive change are presented in this chapter. Briefly discuss how you would use each one as you and your committee develop the health fair.
   h. How would your role of case manager in this agency assist you in your work on this committee?
   i. As the committee leader, you suggest that someone use the Internet to search for resources to help the committee enhance the materials available at the health fair. What appropriate health fair materials can you find on the Internet?

2. Characteristics of leadership exercise: The purpose of this exercise is to identify the characteristics of an effective leader. This exercise has six steps, which can be done with a large group of peers or with students in grades 7 to 12 as part of a teaching project.

   a. Give each group member 10 minutes to individually list the characteristics of an effective leader, stated in single words, phrases, or short sentences. Identify the most important characteristic by making a check next to it.

   b. Divide the group into equal subgroups of 8 to 10 members, each of which is to select two observers from among its members.

   c. Instruct the observers separately to look for persons who exhibit some of the leadership characteristics that are being identified in their groups.

   d. Instruct each group to share among themselves within a 20-minute period the lists of characteristics previously prepared by individual members and to collectively agree on the priority order of the characteristics.

   e. For the next 10 minutes, have each group discuss the process by which they worked, with contributions by the observers. Were there effective leaders in the subgroups? What characteristics did they display?

   f. During a final 10-minute period, discuss with the whole group the styles of behavior that seemed particularly helpful in sharing views on leadership characteristics. Discuss learning outcomes of the exercise.

REFERENCES

American Hospital Association. (1994, Sept. 5). Fostering a culture of innovation. *American Hospital Association News,* 6.

Bass, B.M. (1990, December). Transformational leadership: Beyond initiation and consideration. *Journal of Management,* 693–703.

Bass, B.M. & Stogdill, R.M. (1990). *Bass and Stogdill's Handbook of leadership: Theory, research, and managerial applications* (3rd ed.). New York: Free Press.

Beaglehole, R. & Bonita, R. (1997). *Public health at the crossroads: Achievements and prospects.* Cambridge, UK: Cambridge University Press.

Beecroft, P.C. (1993). Where are the transformational leaders? *Clinical Nurse Specialist, 7*(4), 163.

Bennis, W.G., Benne, K.D., & Chin, R. (1985). *The planning of change* (4th ed.). New York: Holt.

Blake, R.R. & Mouton, J.S. (1964). *The managerial grid.* Houston: Gulf.

Bleich, M.R. (1999). Managing and leading. In P. Yoder-Wise (Ed.), *Learning and managing in nursing* (2nd ed., pp. 3–20). St. Louis: Mosby.

Callan, V.J. (March, 1993). Individual and organizational strategies for coping with organizational change. *Work & Stress,* 63–75.

Chin, R. (1980). The utility of system models and developmental models for practitioners. In J. Riehl & S. Roy (Eds.), *Conceptual models for nursing practice* (2nd ed.). New York: Appleton-Century-Crofts.

Chin, R. & Benne, D. (1985). General strategies for effecting changes in human systems. In W.G. Bennis, K.D. Benne, & R. Chin (Eds.), *The planning of change* (4th ed.). New York: Holt.

Cobb-McMahon, B., Williams, D., & Davis, J. (1984). Changing health behavior of community health clients. *Journal of Community Health Nursing, 1*(1), 27–31.

Cottingham, C. (1990). Transformational leadership: A strategy for nursing. In E. Hein, & M.J. Nicholson (Eds.), *Contemporary leadership behavior* (3rd ed., pp. 71–75). Glenview, IL: Scott, Foresman/Little, Brown Higher Education.

Department of International Economic and Social Affairs. (1995). *Periodical on aging, 1*(1). New York: United Nations.

Eng, E., et al. (1992). Community empowerment: The critical base for primary health care [review]. *Family and Community Health, 15*(1), 1–12.

Farley, S. (1996). Leadership. In R.C. Swansburg (Ed.), *Management and leadership for nurse managers* (2nd ed., pp. 422–441). Boston: Jones & Bartlett.

Fiedler, F.E. (1969). Style or circumstance: The leadership enigma. *Notes & Quotes, 358,* 3.

Flynn, B.C. (1992). Healthy cities: A model of community change. *Family and Community Health, 15*(1), 13–23.

French, J., Jr. & Raven, B. (1959). The bases of social power. In D. Cartwright (Ed.), *Studies in social power.* Ann Arbor: University of Michigan, Institute for Social Research.

Geier, J.G. (1967, December). A trait approach to the study of leadership in small groups. *Journal of Communication,* 316–323.

Gibson, J., Ivancevich, J., & Donnelly, J. (1999). *Organizations: Behavior, structure, processes* (10th ed.). Hightstown, NJ: McGraw-Hill.

Habel, M. (1999). Wanted: Nurse leaders for the new millennium. *NurseWeek, 12*(9), 10–11.

Haffer, A. (1986). Facilitating change: Choosing the appropriate strategy. *Journal of Nursing Administration, 16*(4), 18–22.

Hagberg, J.O. (1994). *Real power.* Salem, WI: Sheffield Publications.

Hersey, P. & Blanchard, K. (1993). *Management of organizational behavior: Utilizing human resources* (6th ed.). Englewood Cliffs, NJ: Prentice-Hall.

Hollander, E.P. & Offermann, L.R. (1990, February). Power and leadership in organizations. *American Psychologist,* 179–189.

Kanter, R.M. (1983). *The change masters.* New York: Simon & Schuster.

Kelley, R.E. (1988, November–December). In praise of followers. *Harvard Business Review,* 142–148.

Kerfoot, K. (1998). Management is taught, leadership is learned. *Pediatric Nursing, 24*(3), 273–274.

Kirkpatrick, S.A. & Locke, E.A. (1991, May). Leadership: Do traits matter? *Academy of Management Executive,* 48–60.

Knollmueller, R. (1989). Case management: What's in a name? *Nursing Management, 20*(10), 38–42.

Kouzes, J. & Posner, B. (1995). *The leadership challenge: How to get extraordinary things done in organizations*. San Francisco: Jossey-Bass.

Kreisberg, S. (1992). *Transforming power, domination, empowerment and education*. New York: State University of New York Press.

Leavitt, J.K. (1998). The Children's Health Insurance Program: Send in the nurses! *Nursing Outlook, 46*(4), 185.

Lewin, K. (1947). Frontiers in group dynamics: Concept, method, and reality in social science: social equilibria and social change. *Human Relations, 1, 5*.

Lippitt, G.L. (1973). *Visualizing change: Model building and the change process*. La Jolla, CA: University Associates.

Lippitt, R., Watson, J., & Westley, B. (1958). *The dynamics of planned change*. New York: Harcourt.

Lundeen, S.P. (1992). Leadership strategies for organizational change: Applications in community nursing centers. *Nursing Administration Quarterly, 17*(1), 60–68.

Lynn, M.R. & Kelley, B. (1997). Effects of case management on the nursing context: Perceived quality of care, work satisfaction, and control over practice. *Image: Journal of Nursing Scholarship, 29*(3), 237–241.

Marriner-Tomey, A. (1996). *Guide to nursing management and leadership* (5th ed.). St. Louis: Mosby.

McPherson, W. (1991). Leadership is about change. *Nursing Standard. 5*(36), 51.

Mellon, S. & Nelson, P. (1998). Leadership experiences in the community for nursing students: Redesigning education for the 21st century. *Nursing and Health Care Perspectives, 19*(3), 120–123.

Michaels, C. (1997). Leading beyond traditional boundaries: A community nursing perspective. *Nursing Administration Quarterly. 22*(1), 30–37.

Noone, J. (1987). Planned change: Putting theory into practice—utilizing Lippitt's theory. *Clinical Nurse Specialist 1*(1), 25–29.

O'Neil, E. (1998). The leadership challenges in health care. *Front and Center, 2*(3), 2.

Porter-O'Grady, T. (1992). Transformational leadership in an age of chaos. *Nursing Administration Quarterly, 17*(1), 17–24.

Robbins, S.P. (1993). *Organizational behavior* (6th ed.). Englewood Cliffs, NJ: Prentice-Hall.

Roughan, J. (1997). Case management: From outside to inside the care process. *The Journal of Care Management, 3*(6), 37–38, 41.

Salmon, M. (1993). An open letter to public health nurses [Editorial]. *Public Health Nursing, 10*(4), 211–212.

Spradley, B. (1980). Managing change creatively. *Journal of Nursing Administration, 10*(5), 32–37.

Spradley, J. & McCurdy, D. (1994). *Conformity and conflict: Readings in cultural anthropology* (8th ed.). New York: Harper Collins.

Swansburg, R.C. (1996). *Management and leadership for nurse managers* (2nd ed.) Sudbury, MA: Jones & Bartlett.

Swansburg, R.C. & Swansburg, R.J. (1999). *Introductory management and leadership for nurses* (2nd ed.). Sudbury, MA: Jones & Bartlett.

Terry, R. (1993). *Authentic leadership: Courage in action*. San Francisco: Jossey-Bass.

Willey, E.L. (1990). Acquiring and using power effectively. In E. Hein & M.J. Nicholson (Eds.), *Contemporary leadership behavior* (3rd ed., pp. 189–193). Glenview, IL: Scott, Foresman/Little, Brown Higher Education.

World Health Organization (1994). Population and health. *World Health, 47*(3), 3–31.

World Health Organization (1996, July 5). *Weekly Epidemiological Record, 27*.

Yukl, G.A. (1997). *Leadership in organizations* (4th ed.). Englewood Cliffs, NJ: Prentice Hall.

Zerwekh, J.V. (1992). The practice of empowerment and coercion by expert public health nurses. *Image: Journal of Nursing Scholarship, 24*(2), 101–105.

SELECTED READINGS

Allen, D.W. (1998). How nurses become leaders: Perceptions and beliefs about leadership development. *Journal of Nursing Administration, 28*(9), 15–19.

Andrews, M. (1993). Importance of nursing leadership in implementing change. *British Journal of Nursing, 2*(8), 437–439.

Daly, G.M. & Mitchell, R.D. (1996). Case management in the community setting. *Nursing Clinics of North America, 31*(3), 527–534.

Dietzen, J. (1997). Decision support systems: Technology enhancing case management. *The Journal of Care Managmenet, 3*(6), 12, 14–15.

Ellefsen, B. (1998). Influence and leadership in community-based nursing in Norway. *Public Health Nursing, 15*(5), 348–354.

Halper, J. (1998). The nurse case manager in multiple sclerosis. *The Journal of Care Management, 4*(19), 12–24.

Harris, M.D. (1998). Home healthcare nurses as leaders. *Home Healthcare Nurse, 16*(8), 540–546.

Highsmith, C. (1998). Case management strategies for "difficult" clients. *The Journal of Care Management, 4*(1), 26–28, 31.

Lamb, G.S. (1995). Case management. *Annual Review of Nursing Research, 13,* 117–136.

Lamb, G.S. & Stempel, J.E. (1994). Nurse case management from the client's view: Growing as insider-expert. *Nursing Outlook, 42,* 7–13.

Misener, T.R., et al. (1997). National Delphi study to determine competencies for nursing leadership in public health. *Image: Journal of Nursing Scholarship, 29*(1), 47–51.

Novik, L.F., Woltring, C.S., & Fox, D.M. (1997). *Public health leaders tell their stories*. Gaithersburg, MD: Aspen.

Porter-O'Grady, T. (1996). The seven basic rules for successful redesign. *Journal of Nursing Administration, 26*(1), 46–53.

Porter-O'Grady, T. & Wilson, C.K. (1995). *The leadership revolution in health care*. Gaithersburg, MD: Aspen.

UNICEF. (1995). *The state of the world's children, 1995*. New York: Oxford.

Research in Community Health Nursing

KEY TERMS

- Conceptual model
- Control group
- Descriptive statistics
- Experimental design
- Experimental group
- Generalizability
- Inferential statistics
- Instrument
- Meta-analysis
- Nonexperimental design
- Qualitative research
- Quantitative research
- Quasi-experiment
- Randomization
- Reliability
- Research
- True experiment
- Validity

LEARNING OBJECTIVES

Upon mastery of this chapter, you should be able to:

- Explain the difference between quantitative research and qualitative research.
- Describe the eight steps of the research process.
- Differentiate between experimental and nonexperimental research design.
- Analyze the potential impact of research on community health nursing practice.
- Evaluate the application of a community-based research study.
- Identify the community health nurse's role in conducting research and using research findings.

Students new to community health nursing often ask, "Can anything I do really make a difference in the lives of my clients?" They are often shocked and discouraged by the crushing poverty they see, the overwhelming sense of helplessness of some of their clients, and the continual recurrence of substance abuse, domestic violence, job failures, and criminal activity. They may ask, "Why should I bother to make home visits to pregnant teens? Why should I offer health-education classes at the local homeless shelter? Will it really matter?"

Recent community health nursing research validates that nursing care *does* matter and that you really *can* make a difference. For example, David Olds and his colleagues (1997) conducted a 15-year longitudinal study and found that regular visits by public health nurses to poor, unmarried women and their first-born children resulted in dramatic differences when compared with similar mothers and children in a control group. Many of the women in the study were under the age of 19, and nurses made an average of 9 prenatal visits and 23 child-related visits (up to age 2). There were statistically significant differences on the following outcomes:

- Fewer subsequent pregnancies and live births
- Greater spacing between first and second births
- Fewer incidences of reported child abuse and neglect
- Fewer months on public assistance and food stamps
- Fewer arrests and convictions
- Less reported impairment by alcohol or other drug use

The effects of the intervention continued for up to 15 years after the birth of the first child. This is powerful evidence for the effectiveness of regular public health nursing visits to this vulnerable client group. Such evidence is only gleaned through conducting formal nursing research.

Research is defined as the systematic collection and analysis of data related to a particular problem or phenomenon. Research that is properly conducted and analyzed has the potential to yield valuable information that can affect the health of large groups of people. Indeed, it often serves as the basis for changing health care policies and programs. In the current national atmosphere of managed care and steadily rising health care costs, the importance of valid research on how health care dollars can be spent to benefit the greatest number of people cannot be overemphasized.

This chapter examines research as it relates to community health nursing. It discusses the differences between quantitative and qualitative research and then describes the eight steps in the research process. A community-based research study is analyzed, and the nurse's role with respect to research in community health is discussed.

QUANTITATIVE AND QUALITATIVE RESEARCH

Scientific inquiry through research is generally pursued by means of two different approaches: Quantitative research and qualitative research. **Quantitative research** concerns data that can be quantified or measured objectively. An example is a study that measured cardiovascular reactivity and central adiposity in older African Americans (Waldstein, Burns, Toth & Poehlman, 1999). Researchers measured waist circumference, mental-stress–induced systolic and diastolic blood pressure and heart rate responses, along with body composition, metabolic factors such as fasting insulin, high-density and low-density lipoprotein cholesterol levels (HDL, LDL), and health practices in a small group of male and female subjects. They found that those subjects with higher waist circumference had significantly greater stress-induced systolic and diastolic blood pressure and heart rate reactivity, as well as greater fasting insulin levels, lower HDL cholesterol levels, and greater body mass index compared with subjects with lower waist circumference.

Quantitative research is helpful in identifying a problem or a relationship between two or more variables, such as cardiovascular reactivity and central adiposity. In so doing, quantitative studies tend to examine isolated parts of problems or phenomena and thus do not generally pay attention to the larger context or overall health of individuals. Thus, quantitative research involves a reductionistic tendency (focusing on the parts rather than the whole) and, if used exclusively, can limit nursing knowledge because many of the important aspects of client services such as quality of life, grieving, and spirituality cannot be measured objectively.

A more subjective or qualitative approach is needed to study areas that need a broader focus or that do not lend themselves to objective measurement. **Qualitative research** emphasizes subjectivity and the meaning of experiences to individuals. An example of this type of research is a study

that examined the expectations of subjects seeking presymptomatic gene testing for Huntington's disease (Williams, Schutte, Evers & Forcucci, 1999). Semistructured interviews were conducted with a small group of asymptomatic adult subjects with a family history of Huntington's disease who were requesting gene identification at a genetic counseling program. Researchers found common expectations that included anticipating relief from uncertainty, making plans for their future life decisions and health care, wanting to know the fate of their children, anticipating the forfeiture of family support, needing relief from self-monitoring, looking into the unknown, and making plans for disclosure.

Qualitative research methods can be as rigorous and systematic as quantitative research methods, although the design and purpose of the approaches differ. The choice of one approach over the other is largely determined by the nature of the phenomenon to be examined.

It is not uncommon to find research studies in which both approaches are used. A study on the sleep patterns of sheltered battered women (Humphreys, Lee, Neylan & Marmar, 1999) used both quantitative methods (ie, self-report questionnaires; an actigraph, which senses movement; sleep diaries) and a qualitative approach (ie, open-ended interview questions). Results revealed that most subjects had disturbed sleep patterns and daytime fatigue, and common patterns were identified (eg, difficulty falling asleep, waking early in the morning, waking often during the night).

Another method of analyzing research in community health uses a statistical procedure, known as **meta-analysis,** that allows researchers to evaluate the results of many similar quantitative research studies in an attempt to integrate the findings. By combining results of many similar studies, meta-analysis affords greater statistical power and can give the researcher a more complete overall perspective, especially when research on a certain issue may seem inconclusive (Gordis, 1996). An example of this type of research is the meta-analysis of randomized controlled trials to determine if dietary interventions change diet and cardiovascular risk factors (Brunner et al., 1997). Seventeen randomized controlled trials of dietary behavior interventions were analyzed and found to be modestly effective in changing diet and reducing cardiovascular risk, and this status was maintained for 9 to 18 months. The researchers concluded that dietary advice and population-based public health measures to improve diets may be the most cost-effective way to decrease cardiovascular risk.

STEPS IN THE RESEARCH PROCESS

All effective research follows a series of predetermined, highly specific steps. Each step builds on the previous one and provides the foundation for the eventual discussion of findings. Alone or in collaboration with others, investigators use the following eight steps to complete a research project:

1. Identify an area of interest.
2. Formulate a research question/statement.
3. Review the literature.
4. Select a conceptual model.
5. Choose a research design.
6. Collect and analyze data.
7. Interpret results.
8. Communicate findings.

Although the process remains the same for any nurse conducting research, the area of interest may vary depending on specialty.

Identify an Area of Interest

Identifying the problem or area of interest is frequently one of the most difficult tasks in the research process. Be certain that the problem or interest is not too broad, that you have the resources and opportunity to study it, and that it has relevance to community health nursing practice.

The problem needs specificity (ie, it must be specific enough to direct the formulation of a research question). For example, concern about quality of services for the mentally ill is too broad a problem; instead, you could focus on availability of health services for the homeless mentally ill in your community.

The problem must also be feasible. Feasibility concerns whether the area of interest can be examined given available resources. For example, a state-wide study of the needs of pregnant adolescents might not be practical if time or funding is limited, but studying the same group in a given school district could be feasible.

The meaning of the project and its relevance to nursing must also be considered, such as exploring the implications for nursing practice in the study of pregnant adolescents. Areas for study often evolve from personal interests, clinical experience, or philosophical beliefs. The nurse's specialty influences the selection of a problem for study and also the particular perspective used. The community health nurse functions within a context that emphasizes disease prevention, wellness, and the active involvement of clients in the service they receive. Clients' physical and social environments, as well as their biopsychosocial and spiritual domains, are of major concern. Community health nurses think in terms of the broader community; therefore, their research efforts are developed with the needs of the community or specific populations in mind.

Problems recently identified and studied within community health nursing include questioning the quality of maternal caregiving (Byrd, 1999), positing if child abuse predicts adolescent pregnancy (Fiscella, Kitzman, Cole, Sidora & Olds, 1998), evaluating the effectiveness of prenatal and infancy home visitation by nurses (Olds et al., 1999), predicting participants at prostate cancer screenings at worksites (Weinrich, Greiner, Reis-Starr, Yoon & Weinrich, 1998), and determining the impact of ethnicity, family income, and parent education on children's health and use of health services (Flores, Bauchner,

Feinstein & Nguyen, 1999). Each of these problem areas provides direction for the formulation of related research questions.

Formulate a Research Question/Statement

The research question or statement reflects the kind of information desired and provides a foundation for the remainder of the project. How the question or statement is phrased suggests the research design for the project. For example, the question, "What are nurses' attitudes toward patients diagnosed with HIV?" determines that the design will be a simple, nonexperimental, exploratory one. In contrast, the question, "What is the effect of an educational program on nurses' attitudes toward individuals diagnosed with HIV?" suggests an experiment that will evaluate an intervention designed to influence nurses' attitudes.

Well-formulated research questions identify (1) the population of interest, (2) the variable or variables to be measured, and (3) the interventions (if being used). It is extremely important when formulating research questions that specific terms be used to clearly represent the variables being studied. For example, if stress is identified as the variable measured in the research question, then it is important to note how the researcher is defining stress. The researcher must focus only on the "stress" experienced by clients, for instance, and must be careful not to measure other related variables such as anxiety or depression. Consistency of terms used is crucial to the success of a project, so investigators must formulate the research question carefully.

Good examples of research questions addressed recently by community health nurses include the following:

What is the impact of Medicaid managed care [variable] on community clinics in Sacramento County [population of interest]? (Korenbrot, Miller & Greene, 1999)

What clinician follow-up [variables] is provided to children screened for lead poisoning [population of interest]? (Markowitz, Rosen & Clemente, 1999)

Will a low-intensity educational approach to weight gain prevention [intervention] for adults [population of interest] increase weighing frequency and healthful dieting practices and reduce weight gain [variables]? (Jeffery & French, 1999)

What are the roles of geographic area, socioeconomic status, household type, and availability of medical care [variables] to premature mortality in the United States [population of interest]? (Mansfield, Wilson, Kobrinski & Mitchell, 1999)

Review the Literature

There are two phases to a review of the literature. The first phase consists of a cursory examination of available publications related to the area of interest. Although several nursing research journals publish studies reflecting all areas of nursing practice, most specialty areas have journals dedicated to specific interests. *Public Health Nursing, Family and Community Health, Journal of Community Health Nursing, Journal of School Health,* and *Journal of School Nursing* are some of the journals that publish the results of research of interest to community health nurses. In this phase, the investigator develops a somewhat superficial but sufficient knowledge about the area of interest to make a decision about the value of pursuing a given topic. If considerable research has already been conducted in the area, the investigator may decide to ask a different question or to pursue another area of interest.

The second phase of the literature review involves an in-depth, critically evaluated search of all publications relevant to the topic of interest. The goal of this phase is to narrow the focus and increase depth of knowledge. Journal articles describing research conducted on the topic of interest provide the most important kind of information, followed by clinical opinion articles (information on the topic described by experts in the field) and books. Journal articles provide more up-to-date information than books, and systematic investigations provide a foundation for other studies.

Criteria for compiling a good review of the literature include (1) articles that closely relate to the topic of interest (relevancy); (2) current articles that provide up-to-date and recent information (usually within the past 5 years; those written before the 5-year period are included based on their importance to the area of interest); and (3) inclusion of primary and secondary sources. A *primary source* is a publication that appears in its original form. A *secondary source* is an article in which one author writes about another author's work. Primary sources are preferred over secondary sources because the information can be reviewed in its original form and affords the investigator a more accurate and first-hand account of the study from which personal conclusions can be drawn. For example, English (1998) describes the extent and consequences of child abuse, citing many other studies, including one by Ernst, Angst, and Foldenyi (1993) that concluded that some children internalize their maltreatment by experiencing depression, substance abuse, sleep disturbances or eating disorders, whereas others externalize reactions to abuse by shoplifting, attempting suicide, or being physically aggressive. The English article is important and useful for understanding child abuse and its consequences, but it becomes a secondary source for knowing about the results of the earlier longitudinal epidemiologic study on sexual abuse in childhood. Direct reading of the Ernst, Angst and Foldenyi article would provide a primary source for information gained specifically from that research.

A major component of a review of literature is the investigator's critical evaluation of information collected. The conceptual base and research methods of studies must be critically assessed regarding the appropriateness of the methods used and the conclusions drawn, as well as how carefully the research was conducted. Examining the primary literature source assists this process. For nurses unskilled in this type of assessment, consultation with an experienced researcher can be helpful.

After a careful and comprehensive review of the litera-

ture, the investigator writes a clear description of the information related to the area of interest. Conflicting findings are included, and each study/article is referenced. This review provides the basis for the proposed study.

Select a Conceptual Model

In relation to research, a **conceptual model** is a framework made up of ideas for explaining and studying a phenomenon of interest. A conceptual model conveys a particular perception of the world; it organizes one's thinking and provides structure and direction for research activities.

All fields of study, whether they be nursing, psychology, sociology, or physics, specify the major concerns and boundaries for their activities. Nursing is concerned with the interaction between humans and the environment in relation to health (Burns & Groves, 1999). Nursing conceptual models such as Orem's (1985) self-care model or King's (1989) open systems model reflect the boundaries and major concerns of nursing as a profession. Although nurse investigators frequently and successfully use conceptual models developed within other fields, the advantage of using nursing models is that they provide an understanding of the world in terms of nursing's major concerns.

The investigator can become familiar with various conceptual models by reviewing the literature in the area of interest as well as by reading any of the many texts available on conceptual models. A thorough understanding of the major concepts of a potential model and their relationships is necessary before attempting to use a model as a framework for a study. For example, Bear, Brunnell and Covelli (1997), in establishing a nurse-managed senior health clinic, used Cox's Interactional Model for Client Health Behavior as a framework for delivery of care and as a basis in the design of evaluation methods for the clinic (Cox, 1986; Cox, Sullivan & Roghmann, 1984). Use of this model ensured a nursing focus for delivery of primary care to seniors and provided a conceptual basis for ongoing and evaluative research (Fig. 11–1). The tools used to document client data and nurse practitioner contact and services were based on the concepts identified in this model. A client satisfaction tool was used to measure the seniors' happiness with the health information, affective support, and professional technical competencies provided or demonstrated by the nurse practitioner. A later study by Bear and Bowers (1998) demonstrated that the client satisfaction tool they developed, based on Cox's model, was a valid and reliable instrument.

Choose a Research Design

The design of a research project represents the overall plan for carrying out the study. This overall plan guides the conduct of the study and, depending on its effectiveness, can influence investigators' confidence in their results. A major consideration in selecting a particular design is to try to con-

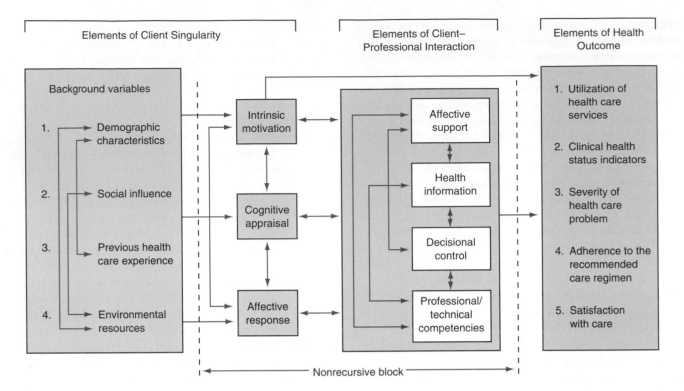

Elements of Client Singularity

Elements of Client–Professional Interaction

Elements of Health Outcome

Background variables

1. Demographic characteristics

2. Social influence

3. Previous health care experience

4. Environmental resources

Intrinsic motivation

Cognitive appraisal

Affective response

Affective support

Health information

Decisional control

Professional/technical competencies

1. Utilization of health care services

2. Clinical health status indicators

3. Severity of health care problem

4. Adherence to the recommended care regimen

5. Satisfaction with care

Nonrecursive block

Client singularity—unique characteristics of each client
Client–professional interaction—competencies demonstrated by a provider that are affected by client singularity and can influence health outcomes—"fit" of responses to client
Health outcome—client health behavior/health status

FIGURE 11–1. Cox's interaction model of client health behavior. (Adapted from Cox, C. L. [1982]. An interaction model of client health behavior: A theoretical prescription for nursing. *Advances in Nursing Science,* 5[1],47.)

trol as much as possible those factors that are not included in the study but can influence the results. For example, Douglas, Mallonee and Istre (1999) wanted to discover the percentage of homes with functioning smoke alarms. They initially conducted a telephone survey, a commonly used method of survey research in community health, and found that 71% of households reported functioning smoke alarms. Concerned that this might be an inflated number, they conducted an on-site survey to confirm the results. After face-to-face interviews, they found that only 66% of householders reported having functioning alarms. However, when researchers actually tested the smoke alarms in those homes, only 49% were fully functioning. By having researchers actually test the smoke alarms, this design controlled for inflated results of the more convenient and economic telephone survey. As a community health nurse, you will need to determine the most efficient and cost-conscious methods of obtaining necessary data.

Complete descriptions of various research designs and specific methodologies are available in basic nursing research texts. For the purposes of this chapter, a few important considerations underlying design selection are described. First, within quantitative approaches, there are two major categories of research design: experimental and nonexperimental (or descriptive).

Experimental design requires that the investigators institute an intervention and then measure its consequences. Investigators hypothesize that a change will occur as a result of their intervention, and then they attempt to test whether their hypothesis was accurate.

Experimental design requires investigators to randomly assign subjects to an **experimental group** (those receiving the intervention) and a **control group** (those not receiving the intervention). This process, called **randomization,** is the systematic selection of research subjects so that each one has an equal probability of selection. For example, Krieger, Collier, Song and Martin (1999) conducted a randomized controlled trial to assess the effectiveness of amplified tracking and follow-up services provided by community health workers in promoting medical follow-up for people found to have high blood pressure at community outreach clinics. Subjects were assigned to one of two groups: amplified (intervention group) or usual referral protocol (control group). The goal was for the subjects to complete a medical follow-up visit within 90 days of referral. The amplified intervention group had more follow-up visits (65.1% compared with 46.7% for the control group).

Another important distinction made within the experimental category of research is between true experiments and quasi-experiments. **True experiments** are characterized by instituting an intervention or change, assigning subjects to groups in a specific manner (randomization), and comparing the group of subjects who experience the manipulation to the control group. **Quasi-experiments** lack one of these elements, such as the randomization of subjects. Community health nurses conduct quasi-experiments more often than true experiments because it is often difficult (sometimes impossible) to randomize subjects.

A quasi-experimental study was conducted by Chen (1999) to evaluate the effectiveness of health-promotion counseling by home care nurses in Taiwan. Family caregivers were assigned (but not randomly) to either the treatment or control groups. After receiving health promotion information during their routine home care visits, treatment subjects showed significant improvement on the health promotion scale that was used as a pre-test and post-test. Those receiving routine home care visits without health promotion counseling did not show significant differences in their pre- and post-test scores. The researcher concluded that counseling during the home care visits promoted adoption of a healthier lifestyle for those subjects who participated in the intervention.

Nonexperimental designs (also called *descriptive designs*) are used in research to describe and explain phenomena or examine relationships among phenomena. Examples of this approach could include examining the relationship between sex and smoking behaviors among adolescents, describing the emotional needs of families of clients with Alzheimer's disease, or determining the attitudes of parents in a given community toward sex education in the schools. In each of these instances, the focus of the research would be on the relationships observed or the description of what exists.

These nonexperimental designs are often the precursors of experiments. For example, DeSantis, Thomas and Sinnett (1999) examined attitudes and values regarding sexuality in a small group of Haitian immigrant parents and their adolescent children. Interviews with the subjects revealed that there were considerable differences between parents and adolescents regarding the topics of sex education, contraception, and expectations about premarital sexual intercourse. Both adolescents and parents lacked accurate information about contraception, yet both believed that the main responsibility for education about sexuality and contraception remained with parents. The researchers determined that there was a need for culturally appropriate sexuality and reproductive health education. Once this intervention is developed, further research can evaluate its appropriateness and, ultimately, its effectiveness. Other lines of clinically based research can also be designed. The choice of research design influences the generalizability of the results, and the attention given to the details of the study affects the value of the knowledge derived.

Collect and Analyze Data

The value of the data collected in any research project largely depends on the care taken when measuring the concepts of concern or variables. The specific tool, often a questionnaire or interview guide, used to measure the variables in a study is called an **instrument.** The accuracy of the instrument used and the appropriateness of the choice of instruments can clearly influence the results.

VALIDITY AND RELIABILITY

To evaluate instrument accuracy, two tests are used: Validity and reliability. **Validity** is the assurance that an instrument measures the variables it is supposed to measure. If a written questionnaire is the instrument being used in the study, questions included on the questionnaire would be evaluated to make certain they are appropriate to that subject (content validity) and whether the variable of interest is actually being measured (construct validity).

For example, Christensen, Moran and Wiebe (1999) noted that not all people think rationally about health; thus, they developed a 20-item questionnaire, called the Irrational Health Belief Scale (IHBS) to measure irrational health beliefs. An example of a question on the IHBS is: "Your doctor recommends a new medication for an ongoing health problem and indicates that about 10% of patients experience unpleasant side effects from the medicine. You think to yourself, 'If anyone is going to have side effects, it's going to be me.'" After an extensive search of the literature, they modeled their questionnaire after a previously published one and tested it on 392 undergraduate psychology students. The subjects also completed other instruments that measured similar constructs, as well as their general health practices. The correlation with those other scales formed the basis of the IHBS's construct validity. A second validation study, with 107 insulin-dependent diabetic subjects, used the same instruments and the IHBS, along with a measurement of adherence to a specific medical regimen. Both studies demonstrated that irrational health beliefs are associated with health-related behavior for both healthy and diabetic populations.

Reliability is how consistently an instrument measures a given research variable within a particular population. Test-retest reliability ensures that similar results are obtained by the same instrument in the same population on two separate testings. If similar results are obtained on two separate occasions, the test can be considered reliable. A questionnaire is internally consistent to the extent that all of its subparts measure the same characteristic. In the study by Christensen and coworkers, test-retest reliability was done by administering the questionnaire twice (with an 18-month interval between testings) to the first group of subjects. Their responses were similar enough each time to indicate a high stability of the questionnaire. Statistical tests and measurements are often used to analyze subjects' responses to questionnaires in order to evaluate internal consistency.

Unfortunately, within the area of community health nursing research, instruments appropriate to the measurement of nursing concepts are often not available. Researchers may use questionnaires that have been designed and tested by other investigators, or they may begin the tedious task of developing their own. Both approaches to measuring the variables of interest are acceptable; however, using available instruments of known reliability and validity saves considerable time.

METHODS OF COLLECTING DATA

A variety of methods can be used to collect data. They include self-report (subjects report their own experience verbally or in written form), observation (investigators observe subjects and document their observations), physiologic assessment (measures of physical evidence such as blood pressure, impaired mobility, and so forth), and document analysis (review and analysis of written materials such as health records). For example, using the four methods mentioned above, investigators examining the stress level of the caregiver when a family member chooses to die at home might:

1. Design or use an existing written questionnaire or interview schedule (self-report)
2. Outline a schema (such as a list of potential stress-induced behaviors) for observing caregivers as they function in the home (observation)
3. Measure various physiologic indicators of stress such as hypertension, insomnia, poor diet (physiologic assessment)
4. Ask caregivers to keep a diary of their activities and feelings for 2 weeks, then analyze the diaries for evidence of stress (document analysis)

In most instances, the nature of the data to be collected dictates the best method of collection. One or more methods may be appropriate, given the topic of concern. In the example above, a combination of the first three would probably be appropriate, or the diary could be substituted for the questionnaire.

METHODS OF ANALYZING DATA

Once collected, data must be analyzed so a meaningful interpretation can be made. Statistical procedures reduce great amounts of information to smaller chunks that can be easily interpreted. When deciding on an appropriate statistical procedure, it is helpful to consider the two major categories of statistical analysis: descriptive and inferential statistics.

Descriptive statistics describe in quantitative or mathematical terms the data collected. Commonly used descriptive statistics include calculating the average number or mean of a particular set of occurrences or calculating standard deviations (how much each score on the average deviates from the mean) and percentages. For example, an investigator analyzing data collected from 50 chronic pain clients might find their mean pain score to be 4.96 (scale used 0 = no pain, 10 = worst pain) with a standard deviation of 0.83. These descriptive statistics suggest that clients are grouped around the middle of the pain scale and differ very little in the amount of pain they experience. The investigator may also report that over 95% of the female clients experience pain between 4 and 6 on the 10-point pain scale. These descriptive statistics can be reported graphically (using graphs or charts) or in written form as shown in Table 11–1.

Inferential statistics involve making inferences about

TABLE 11–1. **Pain**		
Value	Frequency	Percent (%)
3.00	1	2.0
4.00	11	22.0
5.00	30	60.0
6.00	6	12.0
7.00	1	2.0
8.00	1	2.0
MEAN 4.96	STANDARD DEVIATION 0.83	

features of a population based on observations of a sample. For example, the Gallup Poll, which surveys a sample of the population to determine what opinion they hold on a particular topic (eg, favorite presidential candidate), uses inferential statistics to estimate the proportion of the total population that favors that candidate. The potential for **generalizability,** the ability to apply the research results to other similar populations, has great value to health professionals. It allows researchers to test their hypotheses on smaller groups before instituting widespread changes in methods, programs, and even national health policies.

Inferential statistics are also used to test hypotheses in research, and provide information about the likelihood that an observed difference between two or more groups, for instance, could have happened just by chance or may be due to some intervention or manipulation. These statistical procedures enable one to determine the extent to which changes or differences between sets of data are attributable to chance fluctuations and to estimate the confidence with which one can make generalizations about the data (Brockopp & Hastings-Tolsma, 1994). For example, in the previously cited study by Kreiger and colleagues (1999) that assigned subjects with high blood pressure to an intervention group (amplified tracking and follow-up services) and a control group (usual referral protocol), the differences between the two groups in the number of subjects who presented for follow-up could be tested using inferential statistics. That would give researchers a better sense of whether the differences between those numbers were due to their intervention or to experimental error or chance. There are many inferential statistical techniques, and they vary considerably in their complexity; however, the goal of each technique is the same.

It is often appropriate to use both descriptive and inferential statistics to analyze the data from a study. For example, in a study designed to examine the effects of prenatal education on the health status of pregnant women, investigators might, using inferential statistics, find a significant difference in health status between the group who experienced the educational program (experimental group) and the group who did not (control group). The investigators might also use descriptive statistics to report the percentage of women from the experimental group who attended all classes and the means and standard deviations for the women's health status scores (see The Global Community).

Interpret Results

The explanation of the findings of a study flows from the previously formulated research plan. Findings need to make sense in relation to the identified conceptual framework, research question, literature review, and methodology. When findings support the directions developed in the research plan, their interpretation is relatively straightforward. For example, a group of community health nurse investigators might design a study to determine the effect of parenting classes on the self-esteem of single welfare mothers between the ages of 21 and 35. They could use Coopersmith's (1967) ideas on self-esteem as their conceptual model, hypothesize that self-esteem will improve as a result of the classes, and design an experiment to test their idea. If self-esteem does, in fact, increase, their finding flows logically from their framework.

If the findings do not support the hypothesis of the study, investigators question various aspects of the research in order to develop an explanation. In this instance, a number of questions could be posed. Coopersmith posited that self-esteem would relate to feelings of success in a given endeavor. Can that position be inaccurate? Could the parenting classes have been ineffective? Perhaps they did not enhance feelings of success. Were there problems with the methodology used—were there too few subjects or intervening occurrences that affected the results? All of these questions and more could be considered in an attempt to explain the results.

If the study is descriptive in nature (ie, one that was designed to describe particular characteristics of a population), the direction of the findings is not a concern. A detailed, accurate report of the results and their implications is appropriate. Given either an experimental or descriptive design, the importance of accuracy cannot be overemphasized. Leaps of faith when reporting the results of a study are not appropriate unless labeled as such. One could not conclude, for example, from the study on the parenting classes that these classes develop expert parenting skills, given that parenting skills were not assessed.

A valuable contribution can be made to the advancement of nursing knowledge when investigators use their results to make suggestions for future research. The investigators' knowledge of a particular area and their experience in conducting a specific study give them an excellent background for identifying future research possibilities.

Communicate Findings

The findings of nursing research projects need to be shared with other nurses regardless of the study's outcome. Findings contrary to the researcher's expectation are a valuable contribution to other researchers and consumers of research. Negative as well as positive findings can make a valuable contribution to nursing knowledge and influence nursing practice.

The research report should include the key elements of the research process. The research problem, methodology used, results of the study, and the investigators' conclusions and

---

THE GLOBAL COMMUNITY

Tuberculosis (TB) is a worldwide concern. Drug-resistant organisms have spurred more closely supervised methods of treatment. Directly observed therapy (DOT) is used in the United States and around the world to ensure patient compliance with medication regimens. In a study from South Africa, researchers determined that twice-weekly DOT for HIV and non-HIV TB patients was effective in curing most adherent patients, despite their HIV status or previous treatment history (Davies Connolly, Sturm, McAdam & Wilkinson, 1999).

A group of Italian researchers wanted to determine whether DOT was cost-effective in countries that have a low prevalence of tuberculosis (Migliori et al., 1999). They conducted an economic analysis of two possible scenarios: The first scenario followed current policy (generally longer inpatient stays), and the second was a hypothetical policy oriented toward outpatient care. Both scenarios included DOT for care outside the hospital, and both were compared according to cost per case treated successfully. Loss of productivity and other indirect costs were also included in the analyses. Economic profiles of enrolled patients were collected, and treatment lasted for a mean of 6.6 months. The second scenario (outpatient care) was determined to be the most cost-effective, although representing only a minor change in policy, and it reflected a large amount of savings (estimated to be over US $50 million per year). Although non-DOT was the least costly follow-up to administer, DOT reflected only a "modest economic burden," and it appeared to be the most practical in terms of other indirect costs (eg, loss of productivity).

Georgia Tate, a supervising public health nurse in a rural, agricultural area of California, has noted that medication compliance for TB clients in her county has been poor, and, until DOT was instituted several years ago, it had become a very serious public health concern because of medication-resistant strains of tuberculosis. Her county health department serves a relatively sparsely populated, geographically large area (5000 square miles). A high percentage of the population were born outside the United States, and, because of the large farms in the area, about 15% to 20% of the population are migrant farm workers, largely from Mexico. A fairly recent influx of Russian and Middle Eastern immigrants has further strained the health system, and compliance with tuberculin skin testing and immunization laws has been difficult to track. Tate has read about the effectiveness of DOT in other countries and other areas of the United States, and she believes it has been worthwhile in her rural county, but she must constantly prove the cost-effectiveness of her TB program, including DOT, to her county health department budget officer.

1. What information could you gather to assist Georgia Tate in researching the effectiveness of DOT to prove her case to her budget officer? What references might be most promising? What types of local data could you collect and how would you analyze the data?
2. How can studies like the ones from South Africa and Italy be useful to community health nurses in the United States? Why is a global perspective useful?
3. Think of several research questions that you could pose regarding tuberculosis and treatment interventions such as DOT. What type of research design would be most appropriate to each question? How would you collect and analyze data? Think of methods you could employ to share the results of your research.

recommendations are presented. Whether investigators are presenting their findings verbally or writing for publication, they need to discuss the implications of their findings for nursing practice.

IMPACT OF RESEARCH ON COMMUNITY HEALTH AND NURSING PRACTICE

Research has the potential to have a significant impact on community health nursing in three ways: (1) on public policy and the community's health, (2) on the effectiveness of community health nursing practice, and (3) on the status and influence of nursing as a profession. Community health nurses have been involved in research addressing all three of these dimensions.

Public Policy and Community Health

Research with policy implications for addressing the health needs of aggregates has been conducted on numerous topics. Many studies done by nurses and others examine issues related to prevention, lifestyle change, quality of life, and health needs of specific at-risk populations (see References at the end of this chapter). The results of these studies can influence public policy, the quality of services, and, in turn, the public's health.

For example, in a study done by Keyserling and associates (1999), nurses at 17 health departments screened 781 subjects and enrolled 468 of them in their Food for Heart Program to provide nutritional counseling for those rural residents at high risk for heart disease. The majority of those enrolled were overweight, and 60% had two or more risk factors for coronary heart disease. Although the results showed that subjects had relatively modest high-fat meat and snack food consumption, there was an excessive consumption of sweets along with a clearly inadequate intake of fruits and vegetables and a modest consumption of complex carbohydrates. Their mean cholesterol was 257 mg/dL. Clearly, this study has implications for health policy and nursing practice. Because the number and proportion of the overweight adults in this country have continued to rise and are expected to increase, the significance, both in terms of quality of life for those at risk of coronary heart disease and cost savings to the health care system, cannot be overemphasized. Actions to be taken should include regular nutritional counseling in addition to blood pressure and cholesterol screenings for high-risk populations.

Community Health Nursing Practice

A primary purpose for conducting community health research is to gain new knowledge that will improve health services and promote the public's health. Consequently, most nursing research has implications for nursing practice. Many studies focus on a specific health need or at-risk population and then suggest nursing actions to be taken based on study findings. An example is Tarkka, Paunonen, and Laippala's (1999) examination of the social support provided by public health nurses and first-time mothers coping with child care. When their infants were 3 months old, 271 first-time mothers completed a questionnaire to assess the degree to which they were coping with child care. The mother's competence and her coping provided the strongest correlation. However, both mother and child characteristics (eg, health, depression, attachment, relationship with spouse) predicted first-time mother's coping with child care, as did social support from both public health nurses and the mother's own social networks. The results from this study provide useful information for nurses in targeting the unmet needs of this population.

Some nursing research specifically targets the improvement of nursing practice. For example, Capps, Pinger, Russell, and Wood (1999) conducted a statewide assessment of the general knowledge and professional practices of local health department nurses with regard to Lyme disease (LD). Nurses (n = 226) from 80 health departments in Indiana took a self-administered questionnaire about Lyme disease. Areas where nurses had weaker knowledge included symptoms of LD, case definition, and reporting criteria. However, nurses demonstrated the most knowledge in the area of personal protection against LD. Conclusions of this study noted that better dissemination of LD information among public health nurses, as well as the general public, was needed, along with extended surveillance activities.

Nursing's Professional Status and Influence

The third way in which research has a significant impact on community health nursing is its potential to enhance nursing's status and influence. As community health nursing research sheds light on critical health needs of at-risk populations, exposes deficiencies in the health care system, demonstrates more efficient and cost-effective methods for delivering services, and documents the effectiveness of nursing interventions, the profession will gain a stronger voice and have a greater impact on health policy and programs.

Flynn (1998) summarized trends affecting community health nursing practice and outlined examples of effective community-based research and practice, forming the conclusion that quality services are provided that can control costs. The advantages of community health nursing include a focus on health promotion and disease prevention; provision of services across the lifespan where people live, work, and learn; development of community capacity building for health; and working with partnerships, coalitions, and policy makers to promote a healthier environment. In a review of the literature covering considerable research, Deal (1994) underscores these points and describes the effectiveness of services provided by community health nurses. In addition to home-based interventions, community health nurses have been effective in developing community partnerships in maternal and child health; developing cost-effective, community-based follow-up preventive services; promoting health in day care centers; developing programs for vulnerable populations; promoting multidisciplinary approaches to working with high-risk youth; and assisting in development of effective health policies. Both Flynn's and Deal's reviews provide strong documentation for the effectiveness of community health nursing interventions. This kind of information must be made visible and used to influence legislators, planners, administrators, and other decision makers in health care. As this occurs, nursing's status and influence will increase.

THE COMMUNITY HEALTH NURSE'S ROLE IN RESEARCH

Community health nurses have two important responsibilities with respect to research in community health: (1) to apply research findings and (2) to conduct nursing research. First, because research results provide essential information for improving health policy and the delivery of health services, community health nurses need to be knowledgeable consumers of research. That is, they need to be able to critically examine research reports and apply study findings to improve the public's health.

Rankin and Esteves (1998) describe the steps you can take to thoroughly assess a research study. You begin by looking carefully at several things:
1. The title
2. The abstract
3. The journal in which the article is found
4. Author information

Abstracts afford you an opportunity to quickly preview the article. The quality of the journal (eg, history, circulation, caliber of editorial board) is another consideration. Authors' educational and affiliative credentials can give clues to their credibility and could reveal any financial interest they might have in relation to their research outcomes. For instance, authors whose research studies are funded by drug companies may have a conflict of interest, and the results of those studies could be questioned. You can examine the currentness of references and the extensiveness of the authors' literature review. When reading the article, you should keep in mind the steps in the research process and note how carefully the authors followed each one. Questions you may want to ask include:

Did the author clearly state the research question?
Was the literature review complete and current?
Was there an appropriate conceptual framework?
How was the sample selected?
Did the methodology follow logically from the research question and the conceptual framework?
Were the instruments described in sufficient detail, and were they valid and reliable?

Did they clearly identify the method of data collection and data analysis?

You then should carefully review the findings and discussion sections of the research article and determine what implications this study might have for your practice. Talk with your colleagues and peers about the implications of the study and ways you might either replicate it or extend that line of research.

Community health nurses have many opportunities to apply the results of other investigators' research, but a necessary prerequisite is to be informed about research findings. As an essential part of their role, community health nurses must read the journals in public health and community health nursing. Subscribing to some of these journals enables nurses to make regular review of research an ongoing part of their professional practice. Nursing agencies and employment sites in community health can encourage nurses to become more knowledgeable about research findings by subscribing to journals and circulating them among staff, by holding seminars to discuss recent research results, and by promoting nurses' application of research findings in their practice.

Second, although the amount and quality of community health nursing research are expanding, many more community health nurses need to conduct research themselves. An increasing number of nurses have developed skill in research through advanced preparation and conduct investigations related to aggregate health needs. Other community health nurses work collaboratively with trained investigators on a variety of research projects affecting community health. Whether these projects are initiated by the nurse or whether the nurse is involved as a team member, it is an opportunity to influence the types of research questions that are addressed and the way in which the research is carried out, ultimately affecting the community's health.

SUMMARY

Involvement in community health nursing research can be an exciting opportunity to contribute to the body of nursing knowledge and influence changes in nursing practice and in community health programs and policies. Research findings also enable community health nurses to promote health and prevent illness among at-risk populations.

Research is defined as the systematic collection and analysis of data related to a particular problem or phenomenon.

Quantitative research concerns data that can be measured objectively. It is helpful in identifying a problem or a relationship between two or more variables; however, because it requires the researcher to focus on the parts, if used exclusively it can limit nursing knowledge.

Qualitative research emphasizes subjectivity and the meaning of experiences to individuals.

The research process includes eight steps:
1. Identify an area of interest.
2. Specify a research question or statement.

3. Review the literature.
4. Select a conceptual model.
5. Choose a research design.
6. Collect and analyze data.
7. Interpret the results.
8. Communicate the findings.

Although the process is the same regardless of nursing specialty, community health nurses have a unique opportunity to expand nursing knowledge in relation to community health issues and the health needs of aggregates.

Research has a significant impact on community health and nursing practice in three ways. It provides new knowledge that helps to shape health policy, improve service delivery, and promote the public's health. It contributes to nursing knowledge and the improvement of nursing practice. Research also offers the potential to enhance nursing's status and influence through documentation of the effectiveness of nursing interventions and broader recognition of nursing's contributions to health services.

The nurse must become a responsible user of research, keeping abreast of new knowledge and applying it in practice. The nurse must learn to evaluate nursing research articles critically, assessing their validity and applicability to their own practice. Nurses should subscribe to and read nursing research journals and discuss research studies with colleagues and supervisors. More community health nurses must also conduct research studies of their own or in collaboration with other community health professionals. It is this commitment to the use and conduct of research that will move the nursing profession forward and enhance its influence on the health of populations at risk.

ACTIVITIES TO PROMOTE CRITICAL THINKING

1. As a community health nurse working in a large city, you notice a group of small children playing in a vacant, unfenced lot bordered by a busy street. List three research questions you might consider using to study the situation.
2. You want to determine whether a group of sexually active teenagers who are at risk of AIDS would be receptive to an educational program on AIDS. Formulate a research question, describe a conceptual framework you might use in your study, and defend your choice.
3. Select a community health nursing research article from the references and readings listed in this chapter (or choose one of your own) and analyze its potential impact on health policy and on community health nursing practice.
4. You have just completed a study on the effectiveness of a series of birth control classes in

three high schools, and the results show a reduction in the number of pregnancies over last year. Describe three ways in which you could disseminate this information to your nursing colleagues and other community health professionals.
5. You are alarmed to note that the new area to which you have been assigned has high rates of tuberculosis. Using the Internet and your college library databases to research this topic, determine the most effective forms of treatment and discuss the feasibility of implementing some new approaches with your specific target population.

REFERENCES

Alexander, J., & Kroposki, M. (1999). Outcomes for community health nursing practice. *Journal of Nursing Administration, 29*(5), 49–56.

Arlotti, J. P., Cottrell, B. H., Lee, S. H., & Curtin, J. J. (1998). Breastfeeding among low-income women with and without peer support. *Journal of Community Health Nursing, 15*(3), 163–178.

Bachman, J. G., Freedman-Doan, P., O'Malley, P. M., Johnston, L. D., & Segal, D. R. (1999). Changing patterns of drug use among US military recruits before and after enlistment. *American Journal of Public Health, 89*(5), 672–677.

Bear, M., & Bowers, C. (1998). Using a nursing framework to measure client satisfaction at a nurse-managed clinic. *Public Health Nursing, 15*(1), 50–59.

Bear, M., Brunell, M. L., & Covelli, M. (1997). Using a nursing framework to establish a nurse-managed senior health clinic. *Journal of Community Health Nursing, 14*(4), 225–235.

Bechtel, G. A. (1998). Parasitic infections among migrant farm families. *Journal of Community Health Nursing, 15*(1), 1–7.

Brockopp, D., & Hastings-Tolsma, M. (1994). *Fundamentals of nursing research.* Boston: Jones and Bartlett.

Brunner, E., White, I., Thorogood, M., Bristow, A., Curle, D., & Marmot, M. (1997). Can dietary interventions change diet and cardiovascular risk factors? A meta-analysis of randomized controlled trials. *American Journal of Public Health, 87*(9), 1415–1422.

Bunting, S. M., Bevier, D. J., & Baker, S. K. (1999). Poor women living with HIV: Self-identified needs. *Journal of Community Health Nursing, 16*(1), 41–52.

Burns, N., & Groves, S. K. (1999). *Understanding nursing research* (2nd ed.). Philadelphia: W. B. Saunders.

Byrd, M. (1999). Questioning the quality of maternal caregiving during home visiting. *Image: Journal of Nursing Scholarship, 31*(1), 27–32.

Capps, P. A., Pinger, R. R., Russell, K. M., & Wood, M. L. (1999). Community health nurses' knowledge of Lyme disease: Implications for surveillance and community education. *Journal of Community Health Nursing, 16*(1), 1–15.

Chen, M. Y. (1999). The effectiveness of health promotion counseling to family caregivers. *Public Health Nursing, 16*(2), 125–132.

Christensen, A. J., Moran, P. J., & Wiebe, J. S. (1999). Assessment of irrational health beliefs: Relation to health practices and medical regimen adherence. *Health Psychology, 18*(2), 169–176.

Coopersmith, S. (1967). *The antecedents of self-esteem.* San Francisco: Freeman & Company.

Cox, C. L. (1982). An interaction model of client health behavior: A theoretical prescription for nursing. *Advances in Nursing Science, 5*(1), 41–56.

Cox, C. L., Sullivan, J. A., & Roghmann, K. J. (1984). A conceptual explanation of risk-reduction behavior and intervention development. *Nursing Research, 33*(3), 168–173.

Davies, G. R., Connolly, C., Sturn, A. W., McAdam, K. P., & Wilkinson, D. (1999). Twice-weekly, directly observed treatment for HIV-infected and uninfected tuberculosis patients: Cohort study in rural South Africa. *AIDS, 13*(7), 811–817.

Deal, L. W. (1994). The effectiveness of community health nursing interventions: A literature review. *Public Health Nursing, 11*(5), 315–323.

DeSantis, L., Thomas, J. T., & Sinnett, K. (1999). Intergenerational concepts of adolescent sexuality: Implications for community-based reproductive health care with Haitian immigrants. *Public Health Nursing, 16*(2), 102–113.

Douglas, M. R., Mallonee, S., & Istre, G. R. (1999). Estimating the proportion of homes with functioning smoke alarms: A comparison of telephone survey and household survey results. *American Journal of Public Health, 89*(7), 1112–1114.

English, D. (1998, Spring). The extent and consequences of child maltreatment. *The Future of Children, 8*(1), 39–53.

Ernst, C., Angst, J., & Foldenyi, M. (1993). The Zurich study: Sexual abuse in childhood, frequency and relevance for adult morbidity data of a longitudinal epidemiological study. *European Archives of Psychiatry and Clinical Neuroscience, 242*(5), 293–300.

Fiscella, K., Kitzman, H. J., Cole, R. E., Sidora, K. J., & Olds, D. (1998). Does child abuse predict adolescent pregnancy? *Pediatrics, 101*(4), 620–624.

Flores, G., Bauchner, H., Feinstein, A. R., & Nguyen, U. S. (1999). The impact of ethnicity, family income, and parenting education on children's health and use of health services. *American Journal of Public Health, 89*(7), 1066–1071.

Flynn, B. C. (1998). Communicating with the public: Community-based nursing research and practice. *Public Health Nursing, 15*(3), 165–170.

Gordis, L. (1996). *Epidemiology.* Philadelphia: W. B. Saunders.

Herrmann, M. M., Van Cleve, L., & Levisen, L. (1998). Parenting competence, social support, and self-esteem in teen mothers case managed by public health nurses. *Public Health Nursing, 15*(6), 432–439.

Humphreys, J. C., Lee, K. A., Neylan, T. C., & Marmar, C. R. (1999). Sleep patterns of sheltered battered women. *Image: Journal of Nursing Scholarship, 31*(2), 139–143.

Hutin, Y. J., Bell, B. P., Marshall, K. L., Schaben, C. P., Dart, M., Quinlisk, M. P., & Shapiro, C. N. (1999). Identifying target groups for a potential vaccination program during a hepatitis A community-wide outbreak. *American Journal of Public Health, 89*(6), 918–921.

Jeffery, R. W., & French, S. A. (1999). Preventing weight gain in adults: The pound of prevention study. *American Journal of Public Health, 89*(5), 747–751.

Keyserling, T. C., Ammerman, A. S., Atwood, J. R., Hosking, J. D., Krasny, C., Zayed, H., & Worthy, B. H. (1999). A cholesterol intervention program for public health nurses in the rural southeast: Description of the intervention, study design, and baseline results. *Public Health Nursing, 16*(3), 156–167.

King, I. M. (1989). King's general systems framework. In J. Riehl-Sisca (Ed.), *Conceptual models for nursing practice* (3rd ed.; pp. 149–158). Norwalk, CT: Appleton & Lange.

Korenbrot, C. C., Miller, G., & Greene, J. (1999). The impact of Medicaid managed care on community clinics in Sacramento County, California. *American Journal of Public Health, 89*(6), 913–917.

Krieger, J., Collier, C., Song, L., & Martin, D. (1999). Linking community-based blood pressure measurement to clinical care: A randomized controlled trial of outreach and tracking by community health workers. *American Journal of Public Health, 89*(6), 856–861.

Mansfield, C. J., Wilson, J. L., Kobrinski, E. J., & Mitchell, J. (1999). Premature mortality in the United States: The roles of geographic area, socioeconomic status, household type, and availability of medical care. *American Journal of Public Health, 89*(6), 893–898.

Markowitz, M., Rosen, J. F., & Clemente, I. (1999). Clinician follow up of children screened for lead poisoning. *American Journal of Public Health, 89*(7), 1088–1090.

McBride, C. M., Curry, S. J., Lando, H. A., Pirie, P. L., Grothaus, L. C., & Nelson, J. C. (1999). Prevention of relapse in women who quit smoking during pregnancy. *American Journal of Public Health, 89*(5), 706–711.

Migliori, G. B., Ambrosetti, M., Besozzi, G., Farris, B., Nutini, S., Saini, L., Casali, L., Nardini, S., Bugiani, M., Neri, M., & Raviglione, M. C. (1999). Cost-comparison of different management policies for tuberculosis patients in Italy. *Bulletin of the World Health Organization, 77*(6), 467–476.

Oberski, I. M., Carter, D. E., Gray, M., & Ross, J. (1999). The community gerontological nurse: Themes from a needs analysis. *Journal of Advanced Nursing, 29*(2), 454–462.

Olds, D., Eckenrode, J., Henderson, C., Kitzman, H., Powers, J., Cole, R., Sidora, K., Morris, P., Pettitt, L., & Luckey, D. (1997). Long-term effects of home visitation on maternal life course and child abuse and neglect: Fifteen-year follow-up of a randomized trial. *Journal of the American Medical Association, 278*(8), 637–643.

Olds, D., Henderson, C. R., Kitzman, H. J., Eckenrode, J. J., Cole, R. E., & Tatelbaum, R. C. (1999). Prenatal and infancy home visitation by nurses: Recent findings. *The Future of Children, 9*(1), 44–65.

O'Malley, P. M., & Johnston, L. D. (1999). Drinking and driving among US high school seniors, 1984–1997. *American Journal of Public Health, 89*(5), 678–684.

Orem, D. E. (1985). *Nursing: Concepts of practice* (3rd ed.). New York: McGraw-Hill.

Perilla, J. L., Wilson, A. H., Wold, J. L., & Spencer, L. (1998). Listening to migrant voices: Focus groups on health issues in south Georgia. *Journal of Community Health Nursing, 15*(4), 251–263.

Puskar, K. R., Tusaie Mumford, K., Sereika, S., & Lamb, J. (1999). Health concerns and risk behaviors of rural adolescents. *Journal of Community Health Nursing, 16*(2), 109–119.

Rankin, M., & Esteves, M. D. (1998). How to assess a research study. Lippincott-Raven Publishers Continuing Education Online. Available: http://www.ajn.org/continuing/ce/viewarticle.

Rosenstock, I. M. (1966). Why people use health services. *Millbank Memorial Fund Quarterly, 44,* 94–127.

Tarkka, M. T., Paunonen, M., & Laippala, P. (1999). Social support provided by public health nurses and the coping of first-time mothers with child care. *Public Health Nursing, 16*(2), 114–119.

Waldstein, S. R., Burns, H. O., Toth, M. J., & Poehlman, E. T. (1999). Cardiovascular reactivity and central adiposity in older African Americans. *Health Psychology, 18*(3), 221–228.

Weinrich, S. P., Greiner, E., Reis-Starr, C., Yoon, S., & Weinrich, M. (1998). Predictors of participation in prostate cancer screening at worksites. *Journal of Community Health Nursing, 15*(2), 113–129.

Williams, J. K., Schutte, D. L., Evers, C. A., & Forcucci, C. (1999). Adults seeking presymptomatic gene testing for Huntington disease. *Image: Journal of Nursing Scholarship, 31*(2), 109–114.

INTERNET RESOURCES

American Nurses Foundation
www.nursingworld.org/anf/

National Institute of Nursing Research
www.nih.gov/ninr

Sigma Theta Tau International Registry of Nursing Research
www.stti.iupui.edu/library/registry.html

SELECTED READINGS

Chapman, S., Borland, R., Scollo, M., Brownson, R. C., Dominello, A., & Woodward, S. (1999). The impact of smoke-free workplaces on declining cigarette consumption in Australia and the United States. *American Journal of Public Health, 89*(7), 1018–1023.

Cohen, D., Scribner, R., Bedimo, R., & Farley, T. A. (1999). Cost as a barrier to condom use: The evidence for condom subsidies in the United States. *American Journal of Public Health, 89*(4), 567–568.

DiFranza, J. R., & Librett, J. J. (1999). State and federal revenues from tobacco consumed by minors. *American Journal of Public Health, 89*(7), 1106–1108.

Froom, P., Kristal-Boneh, E., Melamed, S., Gofer, D., Benbassat, J., & Ribak, J. (1999). Smoking cessation and body mass index or occupationally active men: The Israeli CORDIS Study. *American Journal of Public Health, 89*(5), 718–722.

Griffin, J. F., Hogan, J. W., Buechner, J. S., & Leddy, T. M. (1999). The effect of a Medicaid managed care program on the adequacy of prenatal care utilization in Rhode Island. *American Journal of Public Health, 89*(4), 497–501.

Haapanen-Niemi, N., Miilunpalo, S., Vuori, I., Pasanen, M., & Oja, P. (1999). The impact of smoking, alcohol consumption, and physical activity on use of hospital services. *American Journal of Public Health, 89*(5), 691–698.

Hellerstedt, W. L., Olson, S. M., Oswald, J. W., & Pirir, P. L. (1999). Evaluation of a community-based program to improve infant immunization rates in rural Minnesota. *American Journal of Preventive Medicine, 16*(3 Suppl), 50–57.

Heymann, S. J., & Earle, A. (1999). The impact of welfare reform on parents' ability to care for their children's health. *American Journal of Public Health, 89*(4), 502–505.

Kaiser, K. L., Miller, L. L., Hays, B. J., & Nelson, F. (1999). Patterns of health resource utilization, costs, and intensity of need for primary care clients receiving public health nursing case management. *Nursing Case Management, 4*(2), 53–62.

Klevens, R. M., Diaz, T., Fleming, P. L., Mays, M. A., & Frey, R. (1999). Trends in AIDS among Hispanics in the United States, 1991–1996. *American Journal of Public Health, 89*(7), 1104–1106.

Leininger, M. M. (Ed.). (1985). *Qualitative research methods in nursing.* Orlando, FL: Grune & Stratton.

Lindsey, E., Sheilds, L., & Stajduhar, K. (1999). Creating effective nursing partnerships: Relating community development and participatory action research. *Journal of Advances in Nursing, 29*(5), 1238–1245.

Mainous, A. G., Hueston, W. J., Love, M. M., & Griffith, C. H. III. (1999). Access to care for the uninsured: Is access to a physician enough? *American Journal of Public Health, 89*(6), 910–912.

Nawaz, H., Adams, M. L., & Katz, D. L. (1999). Weight loss counseling by health care providers. *American Journal of Public Health, 89*(5), 764–757.

Neugebauer, R., Wasserman, G. A., Fisher, P. W., Kline, J., Geller, P. A., & Miller, L. S. (1999). Darryl, a cartoon-based measure of cardinal posttraumatic stress symptoms in school-age children. *American Journal of Public Health, 89*(5), 758–761.

Odhiambo, J. A., Borgdorff, M. W., Kiambih, F. M., Kikbuga, D. K., Kwamanga, D. O., Ng'ang'a, L., Agwanda, R., Kalisvaart, N. A., Misljenovic, O., Nagelkerke, N. J., & Bosman, M. (1999). Tuberculosis and the HIV epidemic: Increasing annual risk of tuberculous infection in Kenya, 1986–1996. *American Journal of Public Health, 89*(7), 1078–1082.

Porter, K. R., Thomas, S. D., & Whitman, S. (1999). The relation of gestation length to short-term heat stress. *American Journal of Public Health, 89*(7), 1090–1092.

Rodriguez, M. A., McLoughlin, E., Bauer, H. M., Paredes, V., & Grumbach, K. (1999). Mandatory reporting of intimate partner violence to police: Views of physicians in California. *American Journal of Public Health, 89*(4), 575–578.

Snider, D. E., & Stroup, D. F. (1997). Defining research when it comes to public health. *Public Health Reports, 112,* 29–112.

Southwick, K. L., Guidry, H. M., Weldon, M. M., Mert, K. J., Berman, S. M., & Levine, W. C. (1999). An epidemic of congenital syphilis in Jefferson County, Texas, 1994–1995: Inadequate prenatal syphilis testing after an outbreak in adults. *American Journal of Public Health, 89*(4), 557–560.

Stein, Z. A. (1999). Silicone breast implants: Epidemiological evidence of sequelae. *American Journal of Public Health, 89*(4), 484–487.

Sullivan, K. (1999). Managed care plan performance since 1980: Another look at 2 literature reviews. *American Journal of Public Health, 89*(7), 1003–1008.

Will, J. C., Denny, C., Serdula, M., & Muneta, B. (1999). Trends in body weight among American Indians: Findings from a telephone survey, 1985 through 1996. *American Journal of Public Health, 89*(3), 487–489.

Yusuf, H. R., Rochat, R. W., Baughman, W. S., Gargiullo, P. M., Perkins, B. A., Brantley, M. D., & Stephens, D. S. (1999). Maternal cigarette smoking and invasive meningococcal disease: A cohort study among young children in metropolitan Atlanta, 1989–1996. *American Journal of Public Health, 89*(5), 712–717.

Quality Measurement and Improvement in Community Health Nursing

KEY TERMS

- Audit
- Benchmarking
- Concurrent review
- Peer review
- Quality assurance
- Quality care
- Quality circles
- Quality improvement
- Quality indicators
- Quality measurement
- Retrospective review
- Risk assessment
- Standards of care
- Total quality management

LEARNING OBJECTIVES

Upon mastery of this chapter, you should be able to:

- Develop a working knowledge of quality improvement and management terms.
- Discuss five factors affecting quality measurement and improvement in community health nursing.
- Compare and contrast six models for measuring and improving the quality of care and their usefulness in community health nursing.
- Identify six techniques used in quality measurement and improvement in community health programs.
- Discuss the role of the nurse within quality measurement and improvement programs in community health nursing agencies.

Think about your most recent experience at your health care provider's office, clinic, or hospital. What were your expectations for the care you would receive and the manner in which that care would be provided? Were these expectations met? Why or why not? How would you approach the task of measuring and improving the quality of the care that you received? Indeed, what is quality care?

Quality is a relative term that describes something with high merit or excellence as compared to an accepted standard or norm. In industry, for example, products are typically measured against a predetermined standard of quality established by field testing. Quality experts test sample products for durability, consistency of performance, and other characteristics, and then recommend improvements in the products to meet consumer expectations. Most companies constantly monitor and control their purchase of supplies, their methods of production, their products' packaging, and their distribution networks to ensure that standards are met and that customers are satisfied.

In health care, the wide variety of situations, roles, settings, and services makes identification and adoption of quality standards somewhat more challenging. But during the past 50 years, serious efforts have been made to set standards for measuring and improving health care services. **Quality care** means that the services provided match the needs of the population, are technically correct, and achieve beneficial results.

The escalating costs of health care in recent years have caused consumers and third-party payers to demand quality care at more reasonable costs. Efforts to control costs have led to changes in the health care delivery system, most notably the emergence of managed care. Health care costs are largely beyond a community health nurse's direct control, but nurses do have control over the delivery of quality care, and they can evaluate the quality of their own nursing care and the outcomes of that care. They can use these evaluations to determine whether clients are receiving the best service possible and how to use limited resources to support the most critical improvements and programs.

This chapter discusses how quality services in the community are measured and improved and the pivotal role of the community health nurse in achieving quality care.

TERMINOLOGY OF QUALITY IMPROVEMENT AND MANAGEMENT

As you progress through this chapter, you will encounter many new terms specific to the focus of quality improvement and management you are reading. However, the terms presented in this section are used more generally in quality measurement and improvement literature and provide you with a foundation to understand the concepts in this chapter. In addition, some terms are no longer in general use and are described to provide you with the historical development of quality management.

Formal quality management in the health care field began in earnest in the early 1970s. Nursing's efforts were in **quality assurance,** developed and used during the 1950s and 1960s, predating those of other health care fields. Quality assurance efforts included initial setting of standards, formal auditing, and **peer review,** in which peer professionals use an organized system to assess the quality of care being delivered (Phaneuf, 1976). It includes methods of ensuring that quality care is being delivered by using the following three-phase process: (1) comparing a health care situation with preestablished criteria believed to represent quality care; (2) identifying care strengths, deficiencies, and opportunities for improvement; and (3) introducing changes in the health care system. (The term *quality assurance* can be misleading and is no longer used. It assumes that if the three-phase process is carried out, quality care is ensured. It certainly may improve care by identifying areas needing to be modified or enhanced, but *ensuring* quality is a more ambitious outcome than the behaviors in the process can accurately deliver.)

Faced with limited resources available and escalating costs of care, health care agencies began in the 1980s to engage in **quality measurement** to be able to identify services and programs that best serve the needs of the community. Studying the impact of intervention and instituting tighter controls on the delivery of specific community health nursing services may not automatically result in satisfied clients or healthier clients; however, such methods can contribute to **quality improvement** of the care delivered by the health care organization.

Quality indicators or quality-focused objectives are used to determine whether a goal has been achieved and to measure client outcomes or process outcomes (eg, all clients receive a home visit within 24 hours of the agency receiving the referral). Quality indicators ensure that quality issues are dealt with routinely within all organizational program evaluations.

Total quality management (TQM) is a comprehensive term referring to the systems and activities used to achieve all aspects of quality care within a given agency. Quality indicators are a part of this broader concept.

FACTORS AFFECTING QUALITY MEASUREMENT AND IMPROVEMENT

A variety of factors promote quality measurement and improvement. These include (1) professional self-regulation of clinical competence, (2) certification and accreditation, (3) legislation and regulation, (4) reimbursement, and (5) consumer demands.

Nursing's Self-Regulation

In the mid-1800s, nurses began to assume responsibility for maintaining standards in the services they provided by requiring minimum levels of education. Nursing education began with a few intuitive, service-minded people who applied practical knowledge in the care of the ill. By the late 19th century, it became formalized, with many hospitals providing 1- to 3-year training programs for nurses. By the 1920s, the education of nurses began to be standardized with mandatory licensure nationwide. Educational opportunities, with programs developed in colleges and universities, improved options. Today, it includes standardized basic and advanced clinical preparation, with many options, including advanced practitioner and doctoral preparation in nursing.

Various accrediting organizations were established in the early 1900s to oversee and stimulate nursing schools to keep up with changes in health care. Two of the most influential organizations are the American Nurses Association (ANA), which began in the 1890s, and the National League for Nursing (NLN), which was formed in 1952 from seven organizations established in the early 1900s (see Chapter 2). The NLN offers voluntary accreditation for nursing programs and works closely with schools to maintain standards of educational programs. The ANA first developed functions, standards, and qualification committees in 1952. In 1973, ANA's Congress for Nursing Practice published a generic Standards of Nursing Practice out of the work of these committees, laying the foundation for professional nursing practice (ANA, 1998; Dean-Barr, 1994). This generic standard served as the root of today's current standards of practice in 10 nursing specialties. In 1983, the ANA developed **standards of care,** which are desired goals that can help plan and evaluate school nursing practice (ANA, 1983). A recent set of standards was developed in 1999 for public health nursing (Display 12–1) and home health nursing (see Chapter 37) (ANA, 1986a, 1999).

In its 1988 Peer Review Guidelines, the ANA proposed that nurses bear primary responsibility and accountability for the quality of nursing care their clients receive (ANA, 1988).

DISPLAY 12–1. ANA Scope and Standards for Public Health Nursing

The public health nurse:
1. Assesses the health status of populations using data, community resources identification, input from the population, and professional judgment.
2. Analyzes collected assessment data and partners with the people to attach meaning to those data and determine opportunities and needs.
3. Participates with other community partners to identify expected outcomes in the populations and their health status.
4. Promotes and supports the development of programs, policies, and services that provide interventions that improve the health status of populations.
5. Assures access to and availability of programs, policies, resources, and services to the population.
6. Evaluates the health status of the population.
7. Systematically evaluates the availability, accessibility, acceptability, quality, and effectiveness of nursing practice for the population.
8. Evaluates his or her own nursing practice in relation to professional practice standards and relevant statutes and regulations.
9. Acquires and maintains current knowledge and competency in public health nursing practice.
10. Establishes collegial partnerships while interacting with health care practitioners and others, and contributes to the professional development of peers, colleagues, and others.
11. Applies ethical standards in advocating for health and social policy and delivery of public health programs to promote and preserve the health of the population.
12. Collaborates with the representatives of the population and other health and human service professionals and organizations in providing for and promoting the health of the population.
13. Uses research findings in practice.
14. Considers safety, effectiveness, and cost in the planning and delivery of public health services when using available resources, to ensure the maximum possible health benefit to the population.

(From American Nurses Association [1999]. *Scope and standards of public health nursing practice.* Washington, DC: Author.)

Each nurse is responsible for interpreting and implementing the standards of nursing practice and must participate with other nurses in the decision-making process for auditing, peer review, and assessing and evaluating the quality of nursing care being delivered. Peer review is an ongoing process of assessing performance against the standards and criteria that indicate quality care in a specific agency. It involves periodic review of caregiving practices by staff nurses who may make shared home visits with their peers or observe peers teaching groups of clients, or implementing the services of programs or projects.

Over the past 35 years, nursing has developed increasingly more formalized nursing care review models and implemented them throughout the profession. The ANA has contributed to formal quality improvement evaluative processes through development of models, quality of care and peer review guidelines, and nursing care standards, including those for community health nursing and home health nursing. In addition, nursing case management and managed care concepts are incorporated in publications produced by the ANA since 1982. Nursing has adapted and applied these models, guidelines, standards, and concepts in many inpatient, ambulatory care, and community nursing settings (ANA, 1999, 1998, 1986b).

The American Nurses Credentialing Center (ANCC) was established in 1989 and assumed responsibility for the ANA certification programs (Bulechek & Maas, 1994). It provides clinical certification for nurses in over 25 clinical specialties. The most common ANCC certifications that community health nurses may find helpful to hold include:
Nurse Generalists
    College health nurse
    Community health nurse
    Home health nurse
    School nurse
    Women's health
Nurse Practitioner (NP)
    Ambulatory nurse practitioner (ANP)
    Family nurse practitioner (FNP)
    Geriatric nurse practitioner (GNP)
    Pediatric nurse practitioner (PNP)
    School nurse practitioner (SNP)
Clinical Nurse Specialist (CNS)
    CNS in community health nursing
    CNS in home health nursing
Nurse Administrator
    Nursing administration
    Nursing administration advanced

Certification examinations and ongoing continuing education units (CEUs) provide additional means for achieving and maintaining a high level of nursing skills. In addition, associations of nurses in specific disciplines influence the standards of care provided by supporting their own certification programs and establishing a forum of support for nurses through regularly scheduled meetings and periodic conferences focusing on advances in that specific discipline.

By 1952, all states, the District of Columbia, and United States' territories had enacted nurse practice acts to ensure that minimum standards of education, practice, and expertise are maintained. In addition to graduating from a state-approved school of nursing and passing a state-recognized examination, nurses are required to accrue an annual or biannual number of CEUs as part of their qualifications for nursing license renewal (Mitchell & Grippando, 1993; Ellis & Hartley, 1998).

Certification and Accreditation of Health Care Organizations

The many responsibilities that hospitals and other health care organizations have to their clients, staffs, boards of directors, and funders complicate their functioning and have the potential to compromise care. As they have developed and diversified, many methods for managing their large staffs, multiple departments, and missions have emerged. Institutional attention to quality-of-care issues first appeared in the 1940s and 1950s. At that time, it became clear that organizations delivering health care services needed to monitor those services in order to meet the goals of the organization and its consumers, and to survive in a competitive environment. External certification and accreditation processes began about the same time (Catalano, 2000). These processes verified an organization's ability to provide adequate service. Voluntary accreditation boards, such as the Joint Commission on Accreditation of Healthcare Organizations (JCAHO), examine all types of health care organizations to help them attend to all facets of their operations, and thus establish appropriate priorities (JCAHO, 1992). For example, they certify all organizations receiving Medicare and/or Medicaid dollars. In reviewing an organization for accreditation, they consider how quality is affected by such factors as staff recruitment, organizational structure, management effectiveness, billing practices, and planning. They also require evidence of effective quality measurement and improvement programs in all agencies that they certify.

Through the 1970s, accrediting bodies focused most of their attention on hospitals. In the 1980s, the attention shifted to include ambulatory or outpatient care, long-term care, and home health care. That shift occurred for many reasons, but the high costs of care and competition for health care dollars were the leading reasons why those agencies sought accreditation (Ellis & Hartley, 1998). Since 1965, the Community Health Accreditation Program, Inc. (CHAP), a subsidiary of the National League for Nursing, has set a standard of excellence through its accreditation services and publications geared to home health care, hospice care, and community health care organizations since 1965 (CHAP, 1993; Koerner, 1997). As an independent evaluating body based on a voluntary commitment to excellence by home and community health care organizations, CHAP is attempting to determine levels of excellence (quality) in home care services. One effort, the In Search for Excellence project, funded by the W. K. Kellogg Foundation, is designed to strengthen the quality of care delivered at home by (1) defining quality outcomes using consumer feedback, (2) developing a system to assess quality using these outcomes, and (3) incorporating the process into CHAP's process of accreditation (CHAP, 1993; Peters, 1992). Project leaders work together with as many people as possible through advisory groups, expert consultants, and consumers to define the important values in home care. The project has combined various beliefs about quality to develop the following definition of quality:

The degree to which consumers progress toward desired outcomes, which they have established with the guidance and support of health care providers. These providers are part of an administratively and financially sound organization that monitors competent staff and an environment encouraging personal excellence (Peters, 1992, p. 24).

Legislation and Regulation

Legislation and regulation of health care services are the functions of individual states. Agencies must be licensed by the state, staffed by trained and licensed people, and prepared to provide the services offered. State licensure or accreditation standards are monitored by regular state inspections and annual surveys. If an agency provides a variety of technically sophisticated services, such as mammography or ultrasound, additional state inspections may occur (Fintor et al., 1998).

Most often, health care organizations apply for and receive federal or state grants to support specific programs or services. These grants are often a major part of the agency budget, and, if these services do not maintain a specified standard of quality, funding will be discontinued. The withdrawal of financial support may cause other services to be discontinued as well, leaving clients with fragmented or discontinuous care.

Financial Reimbursement

As mentioned above, financial reimbursement is often linked to the state through grants. They provide funding for immunization programs, maternal and infant services, and other specific programs. Without this important source of financial support, many agencies would have to limit services. Other sources of funding include Medicare, Medicaid, and private insurers. These federal, state, and privately financed programs for large populations in the United States have very rigid rules and regulations regarding standards of care provided to beneficiaries.

Monitoring of specific aspects of care is often done in response to funders' requirements for periodic progress reports rather than as part of a program of quality management. If monitoring is done only for reimbursement purposes, the total quality of the program is not the agency goal, as it should be. Health care agencies cannot survive without relying on reimbursement sources, but quality management should be a mission of the agency regardless of the source of funding.

Consumer Demands

Which health care provider or health care agency consumers choose to use is often based on presumed or assumed caregiving services and the quality of those services. Health care consumers are provided with many choices when selecting health care services, which contributes to competition in the health care marketplace. This competition is beneficial to consumers. When consumers are knowledgeable receivers of health care services, they can demand quality care as they define it. They make decisions regarding health care services based on such quality domains as:

- Proficiency (capability, expertise, or knowledge of the staff and the manner in which services are provided)
- Judgment (consistency, objectivity, and reasonable interpretation of regulations), responsiveness (timeliness, assistance, and guidance)
- Communication (clarity of verbal and written expression)
- Accommodation (the behavior or interpersonal skills of staff)
- Relevance (significance and pertinence of the encounter with staff) (Andrzejewksi & Lagua, 1997)

The decisions regarding these domains are based on consumers' perception of the care received. This perception is an important piece of the quality measurement and improvement program within an organization.

MODELS FOR QUALITY MANAGEMENT AND IMPROVEMENT

Models of client caregiving are based on structure, process, and outcome: *ideally,* they provide *structure* to guide nurses through the *nursing process* to reach desired *client outcomes.* Each of the following models has all three components, some working more effectively than others, depending on the agency and its philosophy. Six quality management models are presented in this section: the Donabedian model, the Quality Health Outcomes model, the ANA model, the upwardly spiraling feedback loop model, the Omaha classification system, and the Hoesing and Kirk quality management model.

Donabedian Model

Donabedian (1966, 1985) proposed a model for the structure, process, and outcome of quality that is widely used as the framework for more elaborate models.

> **The structure of the care environment, the processes responsible to improve or stabilize the patient's health status, and the resultant outcomes need to be causally linked indicators of quality in order to have an organization-wide appreciation of quality . . . (Sainfort, Ramsey, Ferreira & Mezghani, 1994, p. 75).**

The Donabedian paradigm is recognized as a method of measuring quality as structure, process, and outcome and can be depicted in the following linear model:

Structure →	Process →	Outcomes
Facility resources, personnel mix and skills, philosophy, policies, client mix	Standards, attitudes, nursing care plans, effectiveness, client satisfaction	Client health care goals met, efficiency and effectiveness of services

Quality Health Outcomes Model

Mitchell and colleagues (1998) have taken the time-tested Donabedian model a step further. The quality health outcomes model includes the client in the model and proposes a two-dimensional relationship among components. Interventions always act through the system and the client, thus creating a dynamic model. The uniqueness of this model is the posit that there are "dynamic relationships with indicators that not only act upon, but reciprocally affect the various components" (Mitchell, Ferketich & Jennings, 1998, p. 43). A major criticism of other models is that they do not lend themselves to the population focus of community health nursing. However, this model includes community as a client. Figure 12–1 depicts the structure of this model.

ANA Model

The ANA provides a quality improvement model based on standards of care and quality indicators within the Donabedian framework of structure, process, and outcomes (Dienemann, 1992). Adopted by the ANA in 1975, the model was developed by Lang to depict the multiple components of evaluating client care (ANA, 1975). The ANA model has changed as more information is gathered through research and as the profession of nursing grows; however, it has proved beneficial over time (Bull, 1996). This circular and continuous model suggests ongoing evaluation. Its core includes the agency's philosophy or mission statement, which identifies the values of the agency and reflects its views of clients, nursing, the community, and health. Defining the beliefs of the agency is the first step in improving quality. The three components of structure, process, and outcomes are depicted as pie-shaped wedges around this central core. Specific nursing actions are added to more closely interrelate each section and make the transition to the next section smoother (Fig. 12–2).

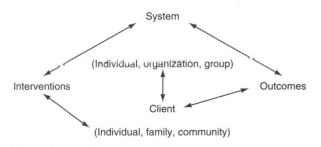

FIGURE 12–1. Quality health outcomes model.

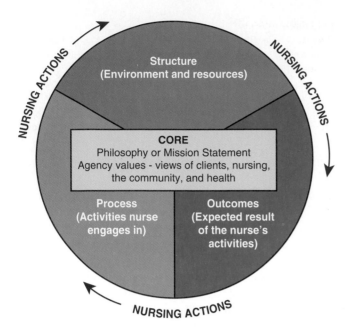

FIGURE 12–2. The ANA quality assurance model.

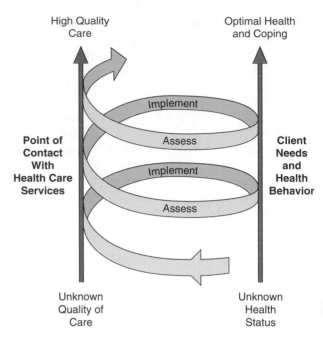

FIGURE 12–3. Upwardly spiraling quality assurance feedback loop.

Although each component is important, agencies rely on positive client outcomes as key indicators of success. Successful outcomes are the purpose of the agency's existence and the key to evaluation by accrediting bodies. Moreover, continued reimbursement by third-party payers, such as private insurance companies, Medicare, and Medicaid, depends on successful outcomes.

Upwardly Spiraling Feedback Loop Model

This model takes the ANA model one step further. It adds a feedback loop that makes the process dynamic and subject to change in response to ongoing feedback, which is used to assess and then implement revisions in care or plans. The model in Figure 12–3 illustrates this idea. The right pole of the model represents the continuum of a client's health needs and personal health behaviors from a client's current status to optimal health and coping. The left pole depicts the contact between clients and the health care system. The spiral's movement from pole to pole demonstrates the quality assessment activities that nurses use to assess their clients, revise nursing care or plans, and implement changes. Any changes are assessed again at a future date as part of the ongoing review process.

This ongoing and repetitive process should result in improvements in the quality of care and the clients' health. The model makes two basic assumptions: first, that specific nursing activities are known to maintain and promote health; second, that positive results are brought about by positive interventions.

This model shows the distance between the two poles of client needs and behaviors and contacts with the health care delivery system. It demonstrates that nurses should step back

from the everyday demands of direct client care and assess that care and the desired outcomes. More specifically, stepping back from the process prompts nurses to do the following:

1. Identify and prioritize the health problems and needs of the populations served.
2. Determine the systems, nursing actions, or outcomes in terms of client behaviors that are facilitated by the nurse.
3. Examine the success or failure of nursing efforts with a specific group.
4. Adjust nursing care, systems, or client goals as needed.
5. Plan for future quality assessments.

Omaha System

This model was developed and refined during four research projects conducted between 1975 and 1992 in the Omaha Visiting Nursing Association. It was designed to increase the effectiveness and efficiency of nursing practice in the agency (Bowles & Naylor, 1996; Martin, Leak & Aden, 1997). It is a comprehensive model and includes:

Patient classification scheme—offers nurses a holistic, standardized method for client assessment and nursing diagnosis and problem identification

Intervention scheme—provides a framework for documenting plans and interventions in the client record

Supervisory shared visit tool—a supervisor's evaluation instrument

Problem rating scale for outcomes—used to document client progress in the record and during case conferences

The Omaha system has measurement approaches that make a useful model for determining the quality of nursing care to individuals and families. Evaluation focuses on process indicators, client outcome measures, and satisfaction with care (Bowles & Naylor, 1996; Martin, Leak & Aden, 1997). By using this multifocal approach, measuring nursing practice becomes comprehensive. However, this model was designed to evaluate care to individuals and families. As a result, evaluating care to populations needs a different set of indicators that must include health trend data, morbidity and mortality statistics, and community system comparisons.

For example, the Omaha System was used with an aggregate when a group of county health department community health nurses conducted an assessment of the community's need for a satellite health clinic in a rural part of the county. The nurses gathered data on population needs, age, health status, and accessibility to health care by surveying clients living in rural zip codes who use the main health department. They also conducted a survey by mail to additional residents not presently using the health department clinic system for immunizations, TB and STD/HIV screening, and well-baby visits to see whether these people had unmet needs. After carefully analyzing the data, they began three 4-hour clinics the first week of each month in an empty storeroom of the community pharmacy.

After funding the clinics for 6 months, the health department evaluated the effectiveness of this nursing service. The number of emergency-room visits for infants in the area was compared with the number of visits before the satellite clinic, and the number of cases of flu and pneumonia among residents over 65 was compared with the same period previous to the rural clinic. Finally, clients were surveyed for satisfaction with nursing care and services, and were asked if there were additional services they needed. Survey outcomes were supportive of continuing the present clinics and adding an additional well-baby clinic, a dental clinic, and a prenatal clinic. Clients liked the convenience; older residents did not have to drive the 35 miles to the main clinic; parents kept up with their children's immunizations closer to the recommended schedule, and they liked the shorter wait; and HIV follow-up included the formation of an HIV/AIDS support group for clients/families in the rural area, meeting a need no one had previously identified. The nurses incorporated clinic responsibilities with home visits in the area on the clinic day and were able to do case finding, improving the overall health of this rural area.

The nurses were evaluated and their charts audited using the traditional tools, and clients received the same periodic surveys. Case conferences continued to be held among the nurses serving the rural area, and, at times, cases were presented among the larger group of nurses. By modifying the comprehensive Omaha Visiting Nursing Association measurement approaches, they met quality measurement needs of a population.

Hoesing and Kirk Quality Management Model

This final model focuses on the "big picture" and provides the clarity needed to manage quality and to monitor and evaluate the results (Hoesing & Kirk, 1990). The model is designed for supervisory and administrative personnel as well as for the individual professional nurse (Fig. 12–4). The model begins with defining the major nursing responsibilities within the agency. "If nurses know what is desired and expected of them, they will also have direction and a knowledge of what it is they are working toward in achieving goals, as well as objective measures to monitor and evaluate results" (Hoesing & Kirk, p. 11).

The key to this quality management model is identifying measurable and verifiable indicators and being able to easily access timely and accurate information about them. Hoesing and Kirk use concepts of standards of care, practice, and finance (Kirk & Hoesing, 1991). Information gathered from monitoring the major responsibility areas is collected, organized, and analyzed. From the data, it can be determined whether the indicator is being met or exceeded and the appropriate action to take. The next steps in the process are to communicate feedback and information, praise the staff, and then go on to develop even higher targets to promote a level of improved quality. For example, within a community health agency, a clinical performance indicator might be that nurses complete client assessments during the first home visit 95% of the time. If that 95% goal or indicator is met, feedback in the form of praise is shared with the staff and a higher target can then be implemented (97.5%). Agencies might use this model to determine whether it would ever be practical to expect 100% compliance with an indicator. For instance, would it ever be possible to expect 100% of the assessments completed on the first home visit? There may be circumstances beyond the nurse's control, such as a crisis may occur in the home at the time of the visit or the client may be aphasic and the caretaker may be unavailable at the time.

An example of a client outcome indicator might be that on a scale of 1 to 10, client satisfaction should be at least 8. If that is not met because the results are 7.2, then these data are shared; some praise may be in order, especially if previous surveys indicated that client satisfaction had been 6. However, discussion may lead to changes in any or all parts of the program to achieve a higher level of client satisfaction. The more that successes, problems, and information are shared with agency staff, the greater the potential for quality improvement.

TECHNIQUES OF QUALITY MEASUREMENT AND IMPROVEMENT

"Quality is not an event, it's a way of life, a way to conduct business, an ongoing quest for excellence" (Kirk & Hoesing, 1990, p. 93). This quote embodies the main principle of quality management. Programs that promote quality should consider quality to be an ongoing process and a standard rather than an afterthought of a specific event. The many terms used

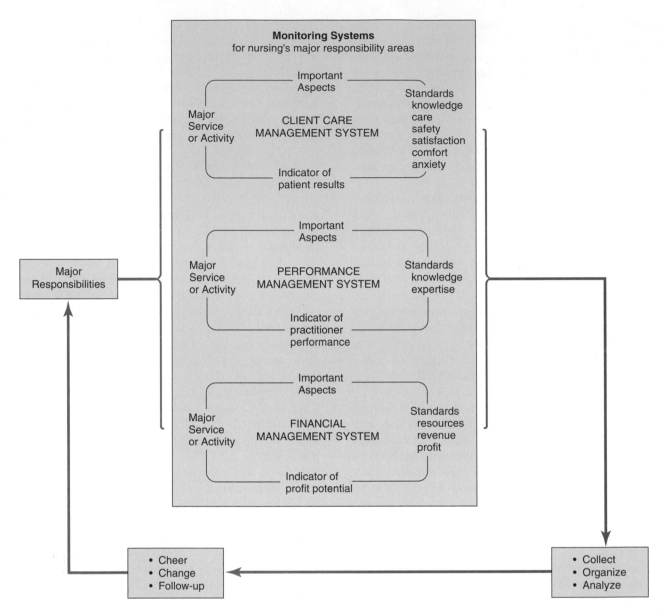

FIGURE 12–4. The Hoesing and Kirk quality management model.

for describing various aspects of quality management may seem confusing, if not overwhelming. To evaluate a quality business, which any health care agency can and should be, several techniques may be used.

Assessing Risk

Risk assessment is a process of identifying factors that lead to negative events. It can be a formal process that uses a tool, such as a questionnaire or a checklist called a *risk assessment inventory* (RAI). It can also proceed informally (eg, a nurse with knowledge about primary health promotion is aware that children are at higher risk for preventable diseases if they are not immunized, and that pregnant women who gain

over 50 lb during pregnancy are at an increased risk for complications).

An RAI is designed to inventory specific factors that put people at a higher risk for certain events. For example, falls among older adults are often viewed as single events. However, their occurrences have been associated with a number of intrinsic (client or host) and extrinsic (environmental) factors (Fortin, Yeaw, Campbell & Jameson, 1998). Intrinsic factors include aspects of the older person's physical and mental health, such as dizziness, weakness, difficulty ambulating, poor vision, confusion, and/or impaired memory or judgment. Medication use, including sedatives or psychotropic drugs, is another intrinsic factor. Extrinsic factors are associated with the environment. They include proper footwear, lighting, glare, slippery and wet surfaces, and obstacles. Just one of the above factors could cause a fall, but most often falls are "multifactorial" (Staab & Hodges, 1996).

Knowing a population's risk factors for certain events helps with planning prevention strategies. Once the potential for risks is determined and assessed, plans can begin with designing goals and objectives for the intervention strategy.

Setting Measurable Goals and Objectives

Planned programs should have specific goals to help identify who the program is supposed to serve, what services are provided, the length of time in which the services are provided, and the resources that are needed. Then, measurable objectives are developed that describe the expected outcomes. Using selected verbs indicates the expected level of achievement, such as clients will be able to demonstrate safe administration of insulin after three home visits, or parents will have their infants' recommended immunizations up to date by 24 months of age. This is done when developing an educational program (see Chapter 9) or an entire health program or service. These statements of measurable goals are then examined during the program evaluation. Without such statements, accurate evaluations cannot be conducted.

In evaluating programs and care, outcomes must be measured against certain standards. Standards are generic guidelines of expected functioning and can focus on the client, the caregiver, or the organization (finances). All care and services must also be measured against these guidelines. The core standards of care, practice, and finance must be integrated and compatible if they are to ensure quality care.

Evaluating Outcomes

The outcomes or results of care (having the right things happen) are the desired effect of the structure (having the right things) and the processes (doing the right things) as described in the models earlier. The more recent focus on client outcomes demands continued analysis of structure and process because it is these two components that produce desirable or undesirable outcomes. With this new focus on outcomes, there has been an impetus to include positive outcome terms such as improved health status, functional ability, perceived quality of life, and client satisfaction (Mitchell et al., 1998). Client satisfaction is measured by how closely a client's expectations of nursing care are to the perception of the nursing care actually received (Andrzejewski & Lagua, 1997; Megivern, Halm, & Jones, 1992). Client satisfaction can be determined by a telephone survey or a mailed questionnaire.

When responses indicate a program is meeting its goals, maintaining set standards, and having positive client outcomes and satisfied clients, that means the program is providing quality care. However, the accuracy of using outcomes as a primary measure of quality care is limited because some clients may have unsatisfactory outcomes de-

spite receiving good care. Factors other than specific health interventions influence outcomes, such as a client's adherence to treatment or the client's ability to respond to care as a result of such situations as a compromised immune system. Nursing staff needs to keep all this in mind when evaluating care (Donabedian, 1969).

Quality indicators of client outcomes are the quantitative measures of a client's response to care. Defining and quantifying client outcomes from these indicators are worthwhile processes that enable the nursing staff to evaluate the results of the care they provide. The goal of care in the community is successful client outcomes. By starting with measurable indicators, successful outcomes can be demonstrated in quantifiable terms. When client care meets the standards set, client satisfaction—another quality indicator—is greater.

Quality indicators are part of the broader quality management program and are used to determine goal achievement. A chart audit is a useful method to measure the frequency of quality indicator occurrence. For example, an agency may have a quality indicator such as all infants less than 6 months of age are weighed on each home visit. Every fifth chart of infants visited in March, June, September, and December during 1 year is audited for documentation of the number of home visits and the number of infant weights recorded. A sampling of charts is sufficient to measure goal achievement and specific quality indicators. It is generally accepted that a sample of 20 randomly selected cases will provide useful information. If the population to be sampled numbers more than 200, some sources recommend that the sample include more than 20 cases.

Quantifying the indicators also can be accomplished through a rate or ratio of events for a defined population and time frame. These indicators can be tailored to express almost any patient outcome (Williams, 1991):

$$\text{outcome indicators} = \frac{\text{number of patient care events}}{\substack{\text{total number of clients or total} \\ \text{number of times at risk for event} \\ \text{during a given period of time}}}$$

$$\substack{\text{occurrence of} \\ \text{UTIs in} \\ \text{clients with} \\ \text{indwelling} \\ \text{urinary} \\ \text{catheters}} = \frac{\substack{\text{number of clients experiencing} \\ \text{urinary tract infections (UTIs)} \\ \text{related to long-term use of} \\ \text{indwelling urinary catheters} \\ \text{from 1/1 to 3/1, 2001}}}{\substack{\text{number of clients with long-term} \\ \text{indwelling urinary catheters} \\ \text{from 1/1 to 3/1, 2001}}}$$

The nursing staff sets a standard for the number of UTIs the agency will tolerate in clients with indwelling urinary catheters (perhaps 5% to 7%, depending on client age, diagnosis, family support, and home environment). This is a quality outcome indicator. It is necessary to have indicators when setting standards in order to measure the success and quality of programs at home or in the community. The same types of indicators are used in acute care settings, using the focus appropriate to that population. If the standards are being met but client outcomes are unacceptable, Nadzam (1991) suggests that the process indicators, such as the catheter care protocol an agency uses, and possible areas of weakness may need further study to identify the cause of the infections. In addition, some state and Medicare regulations mandate that a percentage of records are audited each year.

While striving for excellence and best practices, agencies are using the benchmarking process. **Benchmarking** refers to studying another's processes in order to improve one's own. Internal benchmarking occurs within the organization, between departments or programs. External benchmarking occurs between similar agencies providing like services. For example, a home care agency may have developed a clinical pathway they have found useful with clients with congestive heart failure (CHF); another agency could benefit by using the same clinical pathway. In another example, an agency uses clinical practice guidelines from a specialty organization along with information from a national database; another agency can benefit from this knowledge. This is a way for an agency to identify what is achievable while comparing and contrasting how others provide quality services (McKeon, 1996).

Employing Quality Circles

Nursing staff in the community can use quality circles to improve the quality of care provided to clients. **Quality circles** are a participative management approach in which employees and managers share the responsibility for decision-making and problem solving in client care. The concept of quality circles is based on several well-established motivational and management theories (Herzberg, Mauser & Snyderman, 1968; Maslow, 1954). The quality circles approach has been used in Japan since it was introduced after World War II by Dr. W. Edwards Deming (Swansburg, 1996). Kaoru Ishikawa (1985) is recognized as the motivator for the movement in Japan. More recently, quality circles have been used in American industry as a participative management tool based on W. G. Ouchi's Theory Z (Ouchi, 1981). Quality circles are being used as effective tools in the health care arena (Swansburg, 1996). Although this management technique was at first only used in the acute-care setting, it is now being identified as an excellent tool for those providing care in the home and community. The use of quality circles help home care agencies achieve program goals and multidisciplinary and interdisciplinary collaboration (Schmele, Allen, Butler & Gresham, 1991).

For a quality circle to be an effective problem-solving group, it must incorporate the following:

- Problems are identified and solved by using the energies of nurses working in groups.
- Contributions made by individuals and groups are recognized.
- Continuous mechanisms are in place for further learning, decision-making, and nursing research.
- Processes are instituted for advocacy and negotiation,

power from knowledge, networking through consultation, communication, collaboration, and coordination (O'Brien & McHugh, 1994).

Central to achieving the above purposes is the expectation that the formation of a quality circle ensures unity and a common sense of purpose. Employees are more satisfied in environments that are open and supportive of opportunities for self-determination and creative expression and in which their ideas are valued (Schmele et al., 1991; Swansburg, 1996). The quality circle approach promotes such environments (O'Brien & McHugh, 1994). Staff members share their expertise, experiences, and ideas, and they critique the handling of past situations. This profoundly useful quality improvement tool uses sharing and quality practices to go beyond routine auditing of key nursing activities. The emphasis on group processes facilitates increased understanding among a staff who must consider the quality of care delivered by the department or agency and must work together across a range of skills, management levels, and job assignments to solve problems related to the nursing goals.

Measuring Client Satisfaction

The health care practices that consumers value have been receiving more attention in recent years. The client's perception of quality care has become very important, as health care agencies or programs compete for clients. However, client satisfaction is difficult to define. Many studies using reliable and valid measurement tools indicate that clients identify quality care by such attributes as kindness, pleasantness, the ability to listen and care, flexibility, and proficiency. In addition, the quality of the nurse–client interaction in providing holistic care is frequently mentioned when clients are asked about the quality of care received (Andrzejewski & Lagua, 1997; Green, Hawes, Wood & Woodsong, 1997–1998; Megivern, Halm, & Jones, 1992).

The final step of the nursing process—the evaluation—is often the weakest yet one of the most crucial components. Failure to thoroughly evaluate services and care can result in delivering mediocre nursing care. If the delivery and outcome of care are not evaluated, then care may continue at an unsafe or below minimum standard. No longer will consumers tolerate mediocre care, nor can agencies afford to provide such care. Today's health care consumer demands a high level of quality care from beginning to end. This may begin by the pleasantness and timeliness of the first telephone call and continue with a proficiency and flexibility of services, to the follow-up survey 2 weeks after the termination of service. Questionnaires or telephone surveys can be used to collect feedback from clients. If clients are not satisfied, they may select a different agency, or they may be unreceptive to services by refusing to come to the door or to be at home, which often occurs in public agencies. Lack of follow-up and noncompliance with mutually set goals can often be traced to dissatisfaction with certain aspects of the care received.

In public agencies, many clients do not solicit the services they receive. As a result, adherence with instructions or goals, such as teaching parenting skills to substance abusers, educating pregnant teens, and instructing older adults about their medication, becomes an even more important and challenging issue. Issues of adherence also make it difficult to use questionnaires or surveys to gather information on client satisfaction. Measuring satisfaction, however, may be achieved through qualitative measures, such as statements from clients and family members. Quantitative measures may include such indicators as the number of times clients make themselves available for visits and adhere with caregiving measures. Another factor affecting clients' perceptions of the care they receive is the nurse-to-client ratio. In many public programs, because one-on-one nursing care is not cost-effective, more care is delivered to the aggregate. Using such aggregate approaches as group classes may affect the client's perception of quality service. In addition, only the most motivated and receptive clients may attend group sessions, which means the reticent or disinterested clients do not contribute to an evaluation process.

Auditing

Auditing is another technique for improving quality. An **audit** is an organized effort whereby practicing professionals monitor, assess, and make judgments about the quality and appropriateness of nursing care provided by peers as measured against professional standards of practice. A variety of audit tools can help achieve the best and most comprehensive data. These tools are record reviews, checklists, questionnaires, and surveys. These tools provide the audit committee with quantitative data with which to make decisions about future care as it relates to the agreed-upon standards. Collaborating with the entire staff in the process is essential to increasing incentives for adhering to the standards (Toms, 1992; Twinn, 1997). The information gathered can also support plans for revising the standards as client needs change. In some instances, the audit committee is empowered to implement those changes. Otherwise, the committee should receive follow-up reports on their recommendation from those who have taken the actions. In either case, the results of recommended actions should be reevaluated at a specified future date by the same group (ANA, 1988; JCAHO, 1992). The audit becomes an organized effort practicing professionals can use to monitor, assess, and judge the quality and appropriateness of nursing care provided by peers as measured against professional standards of practice (see The Global Community).

RETROSPECTIVE REVIEW SYSTEM
The most commonly known audit process is the **retrospective review** of client charts. This review is a quality assessment process that examines patterns of care over a specified period of time and includes closed-record audits and a statistical review of trends in services provided. Spe-

THE GLOBAL COMMUNITY

Twinn, S. (1997). Methodological issues in the evaluation of the quality of public health nursing: A case study of the maternal and child health centres in Hong Kong. *Journal of Advanced Nursing, 25,* 753–759.

The demand for the evaluation of health care is occurring at the international as well as the local level. Policy documents from the World Health Organization (WHO), as well as national movements such as the National Health Service and Community Care Act (1990) in the United Kingdom are requiring providers to measure the quality of care.

In Hong Kong, such demands stimulated the development of a collaborative study to evaluate the quality of public health nursing in the maternal and child health centers. The design of the study used both qualitative and quantitative methods of data collection.

The findings revealed three major issues with implications for clinical practice and methodology: the cultural context of care, including client perceptions of care; how health data sources and recording of data were handled; and, finally, the method of data collection, especially the language in the data collection tools.

The findings indicated that the use of "professional language" and the translators with varying degrees of proficiency reduced the validity of the data collected. These findings were especially evident in transcripts from subjects and translators when English was not the first language for either participant. It proved very difficult to get accurate information because questions were not culturally sensitive and the data were filtered through translators with varying degrees of English skills. These issues are important to consider when evaluating care to clients (and using translators) where English is not their first language.

(*Note:* This study clearly denotes the problems nurses can have when attempting to survey clients using tools designed by English-speaking professionals and administering them to culturally, educationally, and linguistically different clients. The use of culturally sensitive and valid tools, along with well-trained translators, will improve the quality of evaluative information.)

cific components of a home visit or care provided are reviewed, such as documented teaching, wound size in millimeters or centimeters, the nurse's signature, or dates of care. However, the assumption that there is a relationship between the quality of documentation and the quality of nursing care is questionable (Edwards, Pickard & Van Berkel, 1991). This type of audit should be viewed as a continuous process of reflective exploration (Campbell & Russo, 1998) rather than an attempt to determine the quality of care. Campbell and Russo advocate the need for exploratory tools as well as evaluative tools. One tool does not give an agency the holistic picture of care provided. An agency that relies on only one tool can get a distorted and incomplete view of the care delivered.

CONCURRENT REVIEW SYSTEM

The Public Health Nursing Services of Baltimore County, Maryland, instituted a **concurrent review** system that uses the chart audit, clients' opinions, and observations of the health center environment (Zlotnick, 1992). This approach combines a retrospective review with assessment of current clients' opinions and observations, while the care is still occurring. The Baltimore system tabulates and consolidates the combined data into a report that is shared with the staff. To understand this audit system, the staff members attend work sessions in which they review one client record using the combined monitoring tools. As a result, staff members gain insight and become invested in the system (Andrzejewski & Lagua, 1997; Zlotnick, 1992).

QUALITY MEASUREMENT AND IMPROVEMENT IN COMMUNITY HEALTH NURSING

Do the people in the health care field know what their customers want, need, and like? Can satisfied consumers of health care services be identified? Often, the answers to these questions are no, leaving health care agencies with little knowledge about how to target their services.

The unique population-focused role of community health carries with it the challenge of sorting out top-priority health care needs from the many competing client needs. There are many areas of community health in which the current system of services does not meet the needs of large segments of the population. Frequently seen are preventable injuries, illnesses, and deaths caused by accidents, chemical abuse, sexually transmitted diseases, domestic violence, violent deaths, and suicide. Deficiencies in health services are also evident in the way care is given to those with existing problems, such as adolescent parents, disabled children, frail elderly, and people entrenched in cycles of poverty and illness.

New and innovative public health programs arise from the realization by public health practitioners that time-honored methods have become ineffective in addressing the problems of those at risk. New strategies need to be found. Such realizations come from scrutinizing public health services. This careful examination requires objective data on services and self-reflection on health care delivered. The process of continually improving and ensuring quality provides a framework for collecting and evaluating these data on an ongoing basis (Harvey, 1991; Peterson, 1991; Swansburg, 1996; Zlotnick, 1992).

Characteristics of Quality Health Care

An agency operates from an agreed-upon definition of quality. That definition is incorporated into an agency's mission statement or philosophy and is the basis on which a quality health care program can be built. In other words, a quality health care program is built on the concepts that the agency and its staff value. Such a program must consider everything that has an impact on the agency and the clients it serves. The following six characteristics are considered essential in the development and maintenance of quality community health programs:

1. It is comprehensive and addresses the interrelated health needs of the entire person or community.
2. It demonstrates organizational competency and operates from within an expertly managed and financially sound organizational system.
3. It demonstrates professional competency and a commitment to an environment that encourages personal excellence among a competent staff.
4. It is accessible and demonstrates that its services are readily available to its clients in a timely manner, despite the financial, cultural, emotional, or geographic barriers that may exist.
5. It is efficient and demonstrates that it consistently makes the best use of available and, at times, limited resources.
6. It is effective and demonstrates its consideration of client priorities and concern with the positive effects of the health status of clients as measured by client outcomes, client satisfaction ratings, and the client's ability to return to the same program when needed.

These six characteristics provide a framework for evaluating the quality of community health care delivery. Consider how these six characteristics might be used to assess a program or services for adolescent mothers. (1) Are we looking at all the health care needs of our typical teen mothers? (2, 3) Is the care being provided and delivered by competent staff who provide excellent care, from an agency that is well managed? (4) Are these young mothers actually functioning at a higher level as a result of our care, and do we connect with these women during their first trimester and find ways to effectively interact with them to meet their needs throughout their pregnancy and postpartum period? (5) Are the services provided consistent with the mother's specific needs, or are they too generalized to make efficient use of available funds? (6) Are the women satisfied with their care and do they return to our agency for continued services after this pregnancy?

Such questions provide the basis for studying each dimension of quality. Each question refers to one of the key dimensions within the agency's mission statement or philosophy (Fig. 12–5).

Pulse Points for Quality

A program of quality has specific pulse points (check points) and outcomes that are determined by the agency's mission statement and are measurable (Peters, 1992). The In Search of Excellence project, funded by the W. K. Kellogg Founda-

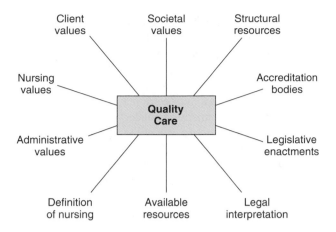

FIGURE 12–5. Factors affecting quality nursing care.

tion to strengthen the home care industry, has identified 11 pulse points for quality. These pulse points are divided into three categories (Peters, 1992):

1. Consumer outcomes
   a. Consumer empowerment
   b. Caregiver relationship
   c. Knowledge and information needs
   d. Family support
   e. Consumer expectations
2. Clinical outcomes
   a. Functional ability
   b. Physiologic functioning
3. Organizational outcomes
   a. Team building
   b. Commitment to quality
   c. Coordination of care
   d. Financial viability

Ideally, a comprehensive community health nursing program will address in some fashion all of the agency services, the processes and resources used to accomplish the services, and client expectations and outcomes. This is done to improve quality and efficiency and are parts of an organized assessment process.

Role of the Nurse in Quality Measurement and Improvement

Although nurses who deliver care directly to clients are not managers as such, improving quality is not only a "management" activity. Community health nurses may not be responsible for a staff or agency budget and functioning, but they are responsible for managing a caseload of clients with needs of varying degrees of urgency. Using the resources available, they must provide priority services that will promote the highest possible level of personal and group functioning and health. Thus, any activities the community health nurse engages in to realize these goals contribute to the quality management program.

Some quality improvement activities for community health nurses include daily prioritizing care needs for a caseload of clients, seeking supervision or skills development for a difficult case, systematizing charting so that needed documentation is efficiently completed (eg, using flow sheets to chart maternal–child health visits), proposing better ways to organize care of chronically ill clients, or establishing new agency procedures. All these actions demonstrate that nurses are evaluating their work and looking for ways to improve care. Staff meetings, quality circle meetings, peer review, and case conferences are common settings for nurses to bring the lessons of their practices to the larger group for examination and potential adoption.

It is the role of nursing administration to develop a formalized quality management program that includes a three-pronged focus, based on a classic approach to quality management: (1) review organizational structure, personnel, and environment; (2) focus on standards of nursing care and methods of delivering nursing care (process); and (3) focus on the outcomes of that care (Donabedian, 1985). These formal evaluations include peer review audits (documented care delivered by peers), client satisfaction assessments, review of agency policies and procedures, analysis of demographic information, and the like (Ellis & Hartley, 1998).

Nurses who are new to formal quality improvement activities in the work setting need to see the value of these efforts and their part in ensuring that quality care is being delivered. Direct service providers are the best judges of care problems and their potential solutions. It is critical, then, that quality assurance reviews and other quality improvement activities focus on issues relevant to staff and client concerns and be structured so they can be accomplished quickly and with minimal effort. When these activities are clear, concise, and well integrated into daily routines, they become less time-consuming. Additionally, staff will clearly see the positive client outcomes as rewards of their contributions to the process. Moreover, when health care providers have the opportunity to systematically examine the care they provide, they will generate useful ideas for improving that care and identify care issues sooner.

Whether small or large, health care agencies are complex organizations with interrelated components. The nursing staff has input into or some control over the quality of care delivered to clients who use the services of the agency. The following is a review of the nurse's role in each of the three areas of structure, process, and outcomes.

STRUCTURE

The organizational structure and financial stability of the agency should allow the mission statement or philosophy to be realized. The agency should be client focused, with sufficient resources to maintain present services and introduce additional services as needed. Public agencies need to operate within budget and also have a well-developed system of acquiring additional funding for new services through grants and contract expansion. Private agencies should operate efficiently enough to realize a profit that encourages the owners and boards of directors to continue to support the services. They should look for additional ways to solicit clients in addition to employing highly motivated and qualified staff.

PROCESS

The agency should maintain standards set by the professional staff that comply with or surpass those recommended by a variety of accrediting bodies mentioned earlier. The staff is encouraged to contribute to evaluation of the standards and revise them as needed. Staff members need to keep themselves current by attending in-services and acquiring additional education appropriate to their job requirements. The staff works collaboratively with others across disciplines to improve the quality of care given in the community by using a variety of participative management tools (audit instruments, quality circles). The agency is supportive of its staff and the needs of individuals. Staff turnover is minimal because employee values are compatible with the goals of the agency. Administration and staff have a compatible working relationship. A system of quality review is in place, and each staff member contributes to this process as a member of a peer review committee or quality improvement or assurance committee. Staff also listens to clients and provides an outlet to evaluate the care received either by questionnaires, surveys, or interviews, and the agency acts on client suggestions and comments.

OUTCOMES

Standards of care are met or surpassed. Client outcomes are consistent with agency goals and quality care. They are measured against set standards. Client satisfaction is monitored, and a system of improving client satisfaction is part of the agency's agenda.

All services an agency provides should be reviewed periodically to determine whether standards are meeting the present needs of the population and whether the nursing staff is implementing these standards. The nursing services used most frequently, such as well-child care, self-care education with chronically ill adults, or various screening programs, are excellent places to begin the review. Generally, these services involve the entire nursing staff and consume a significant amount of nursing care time.

Focusing on commonly served high-risk groups presents an opportunity to optimize care delivery as well as to benefit high-risk clients. Children living in neighborhoods that are known to have high lead toxicity rates from leaded paint in older homes stand to benefit tremendously by a consistently implemented lead screening, treatment, and advocacy program. Without review, such a program may not achieve its goals of decreasing toxic levels of lead in area children.

Incidents of poor client outcome are important areas for further study. Through clinic or home visit records, community nurses can routinely review documentation of deceased or hospitalized clients to assess whether any aspect of the clinic's care or home visit activities might have prevented these occurrences. For instance, a case of a child with re-

peated high serum lead levels who requires hospitalization for chelation might stimulate a clinic's examination of the adequacy of parent education on environmental sources of lead. The clinic could also explore the effectiveness of its advocacy with the area's lead-abatement staff to ensure needed repairs in leaded homes and the removal of families to safe housing while repairs are being made.

As another example, a review of the charts of hospitalized clients who take multiple medications can be conducted to ascertain whether teaching or compliance issues regarding medication contributed to the hospitalization. This may prompt a change in home-visit teaching techniques, an increase in the frequency of visits, or a change in vital-sign parameters for notifying a physician. If problems and deficiencies persist, that could be a clue that the home care nurse needs additional education in this area or that the nurse's caseload is too heavy and therefore exceeds the ability of the nurse to provide minimally expected care. Once the cause is determined, implementation of appropriate changes can commence, after allowing adequate time for the staff to address critical issues. Should additional education be needed, it is the responsibility of the coordinating or in-service nurse to provide or arrange for the needed education.

Given adequate resources, including sufficient time, information, and support, good care is the norm. Occasionally, quality-of-care problems result from an individual provider's performance. Recommendations are made for counseling or other type of intervention by that person's supervisor, and appropriate corrective action should be taken to resolve the problem and preserve the employee's job.

Future Trends

Major changes in quality measurement and improvement have been occurring in recent years.

At present, there are several activities and initiatives that will impact the quality of public health services in the future.

Public health officials representing the Centers for Disease Control and Prevention (CDC), the American Public Health Association (APHA), and state and territorial health offices formed a coalition to develop performance standards for state and local public health systems nationwide (The Nation's Health, 1999). These "partners" believe that performance standards will have a profound impact on the quality of public health delivery systems. The standards will act as critical tools for measuring and refining public health practice, documenting accountability, benchmarking quality improvement in performance, and justifying investment in public health infrastructure (The Nation's Health, 1999). "What gets measured gets done," state the coalition members.

Another community-based group, preferred provider organizations (PPO), is beginning to measure the quality through a long-awaited accreditation process being developed by the National Committee for Quality Assurance (NCQA). This loosely managed delivery system provides health care for 90 million Americans. In 1999, there were no national standards of accreditation for over 1000 PPOs in the United States ("Quality Assurance?," 1999).

The ANA is testing quality indicators for the acute-care setting. In addition, an advisory committee on community-based non-acute care quality indicators has been established. The group is defining and testing the feasibility of an initial set of indicators across health care settings that are nursing sensitive. In other words, the ability to exceed, meet, or fall below expected quality indicators is reflected in the nurse's actions with clients. The group has identified the following areas where there is adequate research of a link to quality care: symptom severity, therapeutic alliance, client satisfaction, protective factors, level of function, risk reduction, and utilization of services.

Medicare has recently developed the Outcome Assessment Information Set (OASIS). This tool will greatly enhance the measurement of quality services to the nation's elders and will create the ability to benchmark with comparable agencies. Similar changes initiated by JCAHO are occurring in home care.

What benefits and costs will potentially be associated with these changes for clients, community health nurses, community health care organizations, and third-party payers? Time will tell what positive, or possibly negative, effects these changes may have. These represent only a few of the quality measurement and improvement activities at the national, state, and local levels of health care delivery in the community. The community health nurse must stay informed of legislative changes affecting how care and services are measured, as well as professional organization standards and agency policies.

the setting of measurable goals and objectives, evaluating outcomes, employing quality circles, measuring client satisfaction, and using retrospective and concurrent review of documentation during the audit process. The current techniques provide new ways to involve staff in participative management opportunities. All services an agency provides should be reviewed periodically to determine whether the current standards are being met. Increasing focus has been placed on quality care indicators, such as client outcomes and client satisfaction, because of the increasing competition among health care providers.

Identifying quality health care characteristics and "pulse points" for quality help the community health care practitioner recognize the quality indicators of best practice. These also give community health nurses direction to their role in quality measurement and improvement. This role is grounded in the structure, process, and outcomes of caregiving and services provided.

Quality measurement and improvement initiatives are a fairly new addition to the health care delivery system, taking hold in the 1970s with nursing in a leadership position. Whether quality measurement and improvement techniques are formally or informally practiced, whenever nurses monitor, assess, and judge the quality and appropriateness of care as measured against professional standards, the interests of clients are being served.

Local agencies, professional organizations, and official agencies at the state and national levels are developing standards, techniques, and tools designed to improve quality, measure care and services, and determine client outcomes. This is likely to continue into the 21st century with a constant view toward positive client outcomes.

SUMMARY

Quality measurement and improvement for community health nursing are vital. Quality measurement and improvement programs seek to ensure that sufficient health care services are provided in a timely manner and that the services being provided are very likely to produce positive effects on the health and perception of health of those being served. Factors affecting the outcome of quality include nursing's self-regulation, certification and accreditation, legislation and regulation, reimbursement, and consumer demands.

The multiple models or frameworks on which quality management systems are based include a classic way of looking at programs through organizational structure, process, and outcomes, and the interrelatedness of each component. However, the six models presented in this chapter are structured in unique ways that enable them to meet the differing needs of community agencies.

Over time, quality management techniques have changed, becoming more inclusive and using participative management systems. Current techniques include risk assessment,

ACTIVITIES TO PROMOTE CRITICAL THINKING

1. Refer to an existing community health nursing program (home health agency, public health nursing service, or an adult health clinic) in your community and evaluate its quality based on the characteristics of a quality community health program.

2. Using one of the six models for quality management discussed in this chapter, create a quality management program in a community family planning agency. Select another model and create a quality management program in a prenatal clinic. How do the different models serve the agencies selected?

3. Select a community program with which you are familiar. Identify one topic for study and develop one or more standards and criteria you can use to measure the actual service provided.

As a school nurse in a large urban high school, your duties have ranged from violence prevention program coordinator and clinic specialist to parent group liaison. The high school is located in the inner city of an East Coast metropolitan area. The demographics of the student population reflect the diversity of the city: 30% of the students are white, 25% are Hispanic, 20% are black, 10% are Southeast Asian, and the remaining 15% represent a wide range of other cultures and ethnicities. There are approximately 3,000 students enrolled in the school.

Until recently, the school's family planning program services have been contracted out to a community-based family planning clinic. The clinic was paid $60,000 per year to provide students with family planning services. Recently, there has been a significant increase in the number of unplanned pregnancies among students at the school. This problem, combined with anticipated budget cutbacks, led the school board to sever its ties with the contracted clinic. With supreme confidence in your abilities, your supervisor has volunteered you for the job of starting up a school-based family planning/STD prevention clinic.

Quality management issues in the past have included:
- School staff does not refer students to the clinic. Rationale is unknown.
- Although the predetermined agreement of $60,000/year is to include all students who may remain anonymous when presenting for care, utilization is reportedly low.
- STD and pregnancy rates have continued to rise in the past 3 years.
- Clients complain of language barriers and culturally insensitive staff members.

Questions
1. What additional information do you need to improve the quality of care given?
2. How will you go about obtaining necessary information?
3. The current budget is $60,000 per year to the contracted agency. The school board has allotted $56,000 for the upcoming fiscal year. Can you provide higher quality care at a lower cost? Brainstorm about your plan; include a budget along with anticipated outcomes.
4. What issues does this scenario elicit regarding:
   Fears and anxiety in this role
   Lack of immediate resources (eg, supervisor)
   Social justice
   Building partnerships within your communities
   Globalization of public health

4. Using the organizational tools (philosophy, mission, procedures, and protocols) of a community agency, participate in a quality circle with peers to improve an identified area of care an agency provides.
5. Using the Internet and selecting various portals, locate recent nursing journal articles focusing on quality measurement and improvement. Are some of the models described in this chapter used? Are there new models in the literature? If there are, how different are they from the ones presented here? Would they be more useful in the community? Why or why not? (See Clinical Corner.)

REFERENCES

American Nurses Association (1999). *Scope and standards of public health nursing practice.* Washington, DC: Author.
———. (1998). *Standards of clinical nursing practice.* Washington, DC: Author.
———. (1988). *Peer review guidelines.* Kansas City, MO: Author.
———. (1986a). *Standards of home health nursing practice.* Kansas City, MO: Author.
———. (1986b). *Community-based nursing services: Innovative models.* Kansas City, MO: Author.
———. (1983). *Standards of school nursing practice.* Kansas City, MO: Author.
———. (1975). *A plan for implementation of the standards of nursing practice.* Kansas City, MO: Author.
Andrzejewski, N., & Lagua, R. T. (1997). Use of a customer satisfaction survey by health care regulators: A tool for total quality management. *Public Health Reports, 112*(3), 206–210.
Bowles, K. H., & Naylor, M. D. (1996). Nursing intervention classification systems. *Image: Journal of Nursing Scholarship, 28*(4), 303–308.
Bulechek, G. M., & Maas, M. L. (1994). Nursing certification: A matter for the professional organization. In J. McCloskey & H. K. Grace (Eds.), *Current issues in nursing* (4th ed., pp. 327–335). St. Louis: Mosby.
Bull, M. J. (1996). Past and present perspectives on quality of care in the United States. In J. A. Schmele (Ed.), *Quality management in nursing and health care* (pp. 141–157). Albany, NY: Delmar.
Campbell, D. T., & Russo, M. J. (1998). *Social experimentation.* Thousand Oaks, CA: Sage.
Catalano, J. T. (2000). *Nursing now! Today's issues, tomorrow's trends* (2nd ed.). Philadelphia: F.A. Davis.
Community Health Accreditation Program, Inc. (CHAP). (1993). *Standards of excellence for community health organizations.* New York: Author.
Dean-Barr, S. L. (1994). Standards and guidelines: How do they

assure quality? In J. McCloskey & H. K. Grace (Eds.), *Current issues in nursing* (4th ed., pp. 316–320). St. Louis: Mosby.

Dienemann, J. (Ed.). (1992). *Continuous quality improvement in nursing.* Kansas City, MO: American Nurses Association.

Donabedian, A. (1985). *Explorations in quality assessment and monitoring* (Vol. 3). Ann Arbor, MI: Health Administration Press.

———. (1969). Medical care appraisal: Quality and utilization. In *Guide to medical care administration.* New York: American Public Health Association.

———. (1966). Evaluating the quality of medical care. *Milbank Memorial Fund Quarterly, 44,* 166–206.

Edwards, N., Pickard, L., & Van Berkel, C. (1991). Community health nursing audit: Issues encountered during the selection and application of an audit instrument. *Public Health Nursing, 8*(1), 3–9.

Ellis, J. R., & Hartley, C. L. (1998). *Nursing in today's world: Challenges, issues, and trends* (6th ed.). Philadelphia: Lippincott.

Fintor, L., et al. (1998). The impact of mammography quality improvement legislation in Michigan: Implications for the National Mammography Quality Standards Act. *American Journal of Public Health, 88*(4), 667–671.

Fortin, J. D., Yeaw, E. M. J., Campbell, S., & Jameson, S. (1998). An analysis of risk assessment tools for falls in the elderly. *Home Healthcare Nurse, 16*(9), 624–629.

Green, A., Hawes, C., Wood, M., & Woodsong, C. (1997–1998). How do family members define quality in assisted living facilities? *Generations, 21*(4), 34–41.

Harvey, G. (1991). An evaluation of approaches to assessing the quality of nursing care using (predetermined) quality assurance tools. *Journal of Advanced Nursing, 16*(3), 277–286.

Herzberg, F., Mauser, B., & Snyderman, B. (1968). *The motivation to work.* New York: John Wiley.

Hoesing, H., & Kirk, R. (1990). Common sense quality management. *Journal of Nursing Administration, 20*(10), 10–15.

Ishikawa, K. (1985). *What is total quality control?* Englewood Cliffs, NJ: Prentice-Hall.

Joint Commission on Accreditation of Healthcare Organizations. (1992). *Ambulatory health care standards manual.* Chicago: Author.

Kirk, R., & Hoesing, H. (1991). *The nurses' guide to common sense quality management.* West Dundee, IL: S-N Publications.

Koerner, S. M. (1997). Quality care in home health nursing. In S. M. Zang & N. C. Bailey (Eds.), *Home care manual: Making the transition* (pp. 537–545). Philadelphia: Lippincott-Raven.

Martin, K., Leak, G., & Aden, C. (1997). The Omaha system. A research-based model for decision making. In B. W. Spradley & J. A. Allender (Eds.), *Readings in community health nursing* (5th ed., pp. 316–324). Philadelphia: Lippincott-Raven.

Maslow, A. (1954). *Motivation and personality.* New York: Harper & Row.

McKeon, T. (1996). Benchmarks and performance indicators: Two tools for evaluating organizational results and continuous quality improvement efforts. *Journal of Nursing Care Quality, 10*(3), 12–17.

Megivern, K., Halm, M. A., & Jones, G. (1992). Measuring patient satisfaction as an outcome of nursing care. *Journal of Nursing Care Quality, 6*(4), 9–24.

Mitchell, P. H., Ferketich, S., & Jennings, B. M. (1998). Quality health care outcomes model. *Image: Journal of Nursing Scholarship, 30*(1), 43–46.

Mitchell, P. R., & Grippando, G. M. (1993). *Nursing perspectives and issues* (5th ed.). Albany, NY: Delmar Publishers.

Nadzam, D. (1991). The agenda for change: Update on indicator development and possible implications for the nursing profession. *Journal of Nursing Quality Assurance, 5*(2), 18–22.

O'Brien, B., & McHugh, M. (1994). Quality circles: One organization's experience. *Journal of Nursing Care Quality, 8*(4), 20–24.

Ouchi, W. G. (1981). *Theory Z.* Reading, MA: Addison Wesley.

Peters, D. A. (1992). A new look for quality in home care. *Journal of Nursing Administration, 22*(11), 21–26.

Peterson, G. (1991). Computer-assisted quality assurance. *ANNA Journal, 16*(3), 288–290.

Phaneuf, M. C. (1976). *The nursing audit and self-regulation in nursing practice.* New York: Appleton-Century-Crofts.

Quality assurance? Accreditation group to evaluate PPOs. (1999). *Nurseweek, 12*(15), 24.

Sainfort, F., Ramsey, J. D., Ferreira, P. L., & Mezghani, L. (1994). A first step in total quality management of nursing facility care: Development of an empirical causal model of structure, process and outcome dimensions. *American Journal of Medical Quality, 9*(2), 74–86.

Schmele, J. A., Allen, M. E., Butler, S., & Gresham, D. (1991). Quality circles in the public health sector: Implementation and effect. *Public Health Nursing, 8*(3), 190–195.

Staab, A. S., & Hodges, L. C. (1996). *Essentials of gerontological nursing: Adaptation to the aging process.* Philadelphia: J. B. Lippincott.

Swansburg, R. C. (1996). *Management and leadership for nurse managers* (2nd ed.). Boston: Jones and Bartlett.

The Nation's Health. (July 1999, Part I). *Coalition unveils standards for public health practice.* Washington, DC: American Public Health Association.

Toms, E. C. (1992). Evaluating the quality of patient care in district nursing. *Journal of Advanced Nursing, 17,* 1489–1495.

Twinn, S. (1997). Methodological issues in the evaluation of the quality of public health nursing: A case study of the maternal and child health centres in Hong Kong. *Journal of Advanced Nursing, 25,* 753–759.

Williams, A. D. (1991). Development and application of clinical indicators for nursing. *Journal of Nursing Care Quality, 6*(1), 1–5.

Zlotnick, C. (1992). A public health quality assurance system. *Public Health Nursing, 9*(2), 133–137.

SELECTED READINGS

Al-Assaf, A. F., & Schmele, J. A. (Eds.). (1993). *The textbook of total quality in healthcare.* New York: National League for Nursing.

Barry, T. L. (1994). Computer support for continuous quality improvement. *Journal of Healthcare Quality, 16*(2), 16–17, 40.

Bull, M. (1994). Patients' and professionals' perceptions of quality in discharge planning. *Journal of Nursing Care Quality, 8*(2), 47–61.

Davis, F. R. (1994). *Total quality management for home care.* Gaithersburg, MD: Aspen.

Gold, M., & Wooldridge, J. (1995). Surveying consumer satisfaction to assess managed care quality: Current practices: New initiatives and approaches in health care quality. *Health Care Financing Review, 16*, 155–159.

Griffiths, P. (1995). Progress in measuring nursing outcomes. *Journal of Advanced Nursing, 21*, 1092–1100.

Hicks, L. L., Stallmeyer, J. M., & Coleman, J. R. (1993). *Role of the nurse in managed care*. Kansas City, MO: American Nurses Association.

Hodges, L. C., Icenhour, M. L., & Tate, S. (1994). Measuring quality: A systematic integrative approach. In J. McCloskey & H. K. Grace (Eds.), *Current issues in nursing* (4th ed., pp. 295–302). St. Louis: Mosby.

Holzemer, W. L. (1994). The impact of nursing care in Latin America and the Caribbean: A focus on outcomes. *Journal of Advanced Nursing, 20*, 5–12.

Iezzoni, L. (1994). *Risk adjustment for measuring health outcomes*. Ann Arbor, MI: Health Administration Press.

Jones, K. R., Jennings, B. M., Mortiz, P., & Moss, M. T. (1997). Policy issues associated with analyzing outcomes of care. *Image: Journal of Nursing Scholarship, 29*(3), 261–267.

Kelly, M. P., Bacon, G. T., & Mitchell, J. A. (1994). Glossary of managed care terms. *Journal of Ambulatory Care Management, 17*(1), 70–76.

Kemp, N., & Richardson, E. (1994). *The nursing process and quality care*. San Diego: Singular Publishing Group.

Lynn, M. R., & Kelley, B. (1997). Effects of case management on the nursing context—Perceived quality of care, work satisfaction, and control over practice. *Image: Journal of Nursing Scholarship, 29*(3), 237–241.

Maas, M. L., Johnson, M., & Moorhead, S. (1996). Classifying nursing-sensitive patient outcomes. *Image: Journal of Nursing Scholarship, 28*(4), 295–301.

Mitchell, P. H., & Shortell, S. M. (1997). Adverse outcomes and variations in organization of care delivery. *Medical Care, 35*(11), NS19–NS32.

Peters, D. A. (1997). Outcomes: The mainstay of a framework for quality care. In B. W. Spradley & J. A. Allender (Eds.), *Readings in community health nursing* (5th ed.). Philadelphia: Lippincott-Raven.

Shaughnessy, P. W., Kramer, A. M., Hittle, D. F., & Steiner, J. F. (1995). Quality of care in teaching nursing homes: Findings and implications. *Health Care Finance Review, 16*(4), 55–83.

Tinetti, M., et al. (1993). Yale factor: Risk factor abatement strategy for fall prevention. *Journal of the American Geriatric Society, 41*(3), 315–320.

Ulrich, B. (1992). *Leadership and management according to Florence Nightingale*. Norwalk, CN: Appleton & Lange.

Warren, B. H. (1994). An outcomes analysis approach to utilization management: Quality assessment of appropriateness of specialty referrals. *American College of Medical Quality, 9*(1), 34—38.

Weiss, M. (1997). The quality evolution in managed care organizations: Shifting the focus to community health. *Journal of Nursing Care Quality, 11*(4), 27–31.

Wildfire, J. B., et al. (1997–1998). The effect of regulation on the quality of care in board and care homes. *Generations, 21*(4), 25–29.

Zinn, J. S., Aaronson, W. E., & Rosko, M. D. (1993). The use of standardized indicators as quality improvement tools: An application in Pennsylvania nursing homes. *American Journal of Medical Quality, 8*, 72–78.

Policy Making and Community Health Advocacy

KEY TERMS

- Community health advocacy
- Distributive health policy
- Health policy
- Lobbying
- Polarization
- Policy
- Policy analysis
- Policy system
- Political action
- Political action committee (PAC)
- Political empowerment
- Politics
- Public policy
- Regulatory health policy
- Special interest group

LEARNING OBJECTIVES

Upon mastery of this chapter, you should be able to:

- Define health policy and explain how it is established.
- Analyze the influence of health policy on community health and nursing practice.
- Explain the role of special interest groups in health care reform and policy making.
- Define political empowerment and describe ways in which community health nurses can become politically empowered.
- Identify the four stages in the policy process and briefly explain what each entails.
- Explain the role of community health nurses in determining a community's health policy needs.
- Identify the ten steps in mobilizing a community for political action.
- Describe the steps involved in how a bill becomes law.
- Explain several methods of communicating with legislators on policy issues.
- List at least four political strategies for community health nursing.

As a nursing student, you probably have a vision of health care that is more accessible, equitable, cost-effective, and quality-oriented than the present system. Unfortunately, as you enter the current health care system, you will soon recognize that vision alone is not enough. For a myriad of reasons, nurses have had a difficult time just making policy makers aware of the value of their input, not to mention their vital role in providing essential health care services. Although most nurses recognize the importance of their role as providers of health care, many do not recognize the importance of their role in influencing or making legislation in relation to their practice or to community health.

Behind all legislation and health care regulation, there are power struggles. Only the naive think that others will be persuaded by the facts alone. There are social and political factions at work, special interest groups, and business and industry—each bringing their power into play. Because the outcomes of these struggles determine the availability and quality of all health and social services, nurses need to develop an operational knowledge of health policy and political process in order to protect individuals, families, communities, and their nursing practice.

Fortunately, nursing's interest and representation in public affairs are growing. Nurses are competing successfully for fellowships in public policy such as the Robert Wood Johnson Health Policy Fellows Program and the Kellogg National Fellowship Program. In 1992, Eddie Bernie Johnson, RN (D., Texas) became the first nurse to be elected to the U.S. House of Representatives. She was one of nine nurses who ran for the 103rd Congress (Mason & Leavitt, 1998).

This chapter examines health policy, the political process involved in determining health policy, and community health nursing's role in the process. The underlying bias is that community health nurses should not only provide input to policy circles through advocacy, but should be leaders who sit at the decision-making tables. The purpose is to emphasize the need for community health nurses to understand their role and power in providing an essential influence and unique perspective in health care.

POLICY MAKING

Policy is an authoritatively stated course of action that guides decision-making. It is how an institution, organization, agency, or government exercises its authority; it is based on that group's goals, and it exists to provide guidelines for operation. Policy can (and should) be written formally, but many policies are unwritten, unclear, or "hidden" to prevent public or legal review. Government policy–whether the government is local, state, or federal–that makes decisions affecting the public is called **public policy** (Dye, 1992).

Policies attempt to express the collective interests and beliefs of the social system or institution that generates them. Public policy usually comes about because policy makers perceive that something is not functioning as it should or the political pressure is so great that a change is mandated. A policy is made because the perceived benefits outweigh the perceived costs, at least to the decision makers (Harrington & Estes, 1997). The "something" needing change can be as large and complex as the health care system or as small and simple as a local agency's title. It should be noted, however, that the latter will not be perceived as small and simple by those with a vested interest in the title. As an example, during the development of the National Institute of Nursing Research (NINR) from the National Center of Nursing Research (NCNR) in 1993, those involved struggled long and hard to secure a title for this institute that accurately reflected its mission.

Policies are enforced by the agency or organization for whom they were created. For example, noncompliance with employment policies in a health care agency, such as not following protocol designed to ensure client safety or not following a specific dress code aimed to identify employees to clients and portray professionalism, may mean termination of services; violation of a government policy, such as illegally selling drugs, may mean paying a fine or imprisonment. Public policy is usually backed by law or regulations.

All public policy is inextricably linked to economics. The growth of our health care system is driven by economic conditions and profit motives as well as competition promoted by the political climate (Harrington & Estes, 1997). Policy problems come about because a policy, to a great extent, determines who gets what in a society or institution. In other words, policy problems occur because resources are being redistributed, resulting in some receiving a greater share and others receiving less.

Health Policy

Health policy is any policy that constitutes the governing framework (structure, process, and outcomes) for providing health services on a local, state, national, or even international level. *Structure* is the number and types of agencies, programs, and services, as well as providers and targeted clients. *Process* is how the agencies, programs, and services are going to be provided, managed, and funded, and how clients are to receive services. *Health policy outcomes* are the actual consequences of a health policy being implemented and are described in terms of effectiveness, efficiency, equity, innovativeness, and empowerment. Figure 13–1 outlines health policy from this perspective.

The passage of health care legislation at the federal and state levels ultimately leads to the implementation of health policy at a local level. For example, the Omnibus Budget Reconciliation Act (OBRA) of 1993 recognized the Vaccines for Children (VFC) program as a critical need. As a result, the President's Childhood Immunization Initiative (CII), a nationwide effort to vaccinate all children in the United States, was implemented in October 1994. This federal health policy provides guidelines and resources by combining the efforts of both public and private health care providers at a local level to vaccinate children, regardless of ability to pay.

Health policy is about health care choices (Mason & Leavitt, 1998) and should reflect a community's values. However, the power to make policy decisions for any community is spread among a number of stakeholders (anyone with a vested interest) who may not live in the community. Because there are so many people with vested interests in the health care system, it is unlikely that anyone can know the real and full impact of a health policy on any one community until after its implementation.

Theoretically, health policy should empower the community for which it is intended, but often conflict can arise over empowerment when one community's empowerment threatens the values of another. For example, there is much conflict and argument over the controversial policies regarding government funding of abortions for low-income women. Some community groups oppose this policy, arguing that it violates the greater policy of preserving life, whereas other groups support it, saying that it protects and promotes the overall health of the community. Such conflict dilutes the empowering ability of a given health policy.

Health policy also empowers the health care provider by deeming the provider's services as essential, subsidizing the provider's education, and directly reimbursing the provider. Because health policy affects a community's health status

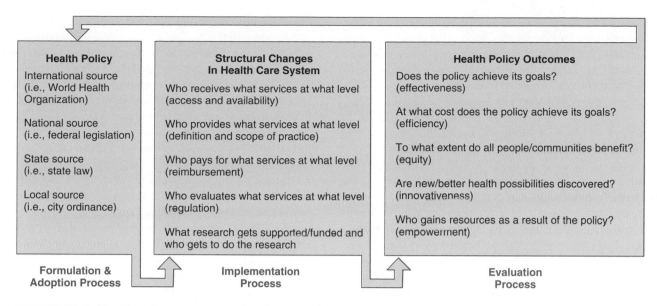

FIGURE 13–1. Health policy as a governing framework.

and determines who will be reimbursed for what by whom, politics are involved at every step of its development, implementation, and evaluation. When health policy fails to provide a workable framework at the community level, the health care needs of communities are not met in a cost-effective manner. For example, in 1996, Congress passed and President Clinton signed a watershed welfare reform bill predicated on a centuries-old notion of "forcing" the poor out of poverty (Brown, 1997). This new law has dramatically eliminated millions of people from receiving federal assistance, but has increased the amount spent on the remaining families and left billions of dollars unspent as the states continue to receive a historically high fixed amount of money based on the numbers of people on old welfare rolls (DeParle, 1999). The percentage unspent is as high as 91% in Wyoming and 76% in Idaho and as low as 6% in Missouri and 4% in Hawaii. The excess federal welfare money has created a "rich new financing stream for anti-poverty efforts" (DeParle, 1999, p. 1), which is baffling some states while inspiring others. For example, New Mexico has been plagued by political infighting between the governor and the state Supreme Court delaying the monies being spent while thousands of jobless New Mexicans have been dropped from the welfare rolls. Nonetheless, New Mexico received $751 million in 1997 and 1998 and by the end of 1998 had $242 million left, or 32% of its total grant. It has plans to spend all the money on "various programs for the poor, such as expanding child-care for low-income workers" (DeParle, 1999, p. 20). These diverse examples are a reminder that the intent of a policy may not be its outcome. The policy intent reflected by this bill was to reduce an expensive government program, but it continues to cost the federal government the same amount of money while denying access to critical safety net programs undermining the health of millions of families in some states.

Health policies can be distributive or regulatory. **Distributive health policy** promotes nongovernmental activities thought to be beneficial to society as a whole. An example of a distributive policy is the Nurse Training Act, Title VIII of the Public Health Service Act established in 1965, which provided federal subsidy for nursing education to address the need for a greater supply of nurses. *Redistributive health policy* changes the allocation of resources from one group to usually a broader or different group. Medicare is an example of redistributive policy in that provisions under Medicare expanded to provide a broader range of benefits and coverage to needy groups, such as the permanently disabled, regardless of age, and for those over age 65.

Regulatory health policy is policy that attempts to control the allocation of resources by directing those agencies or persons who offer resources or provide public services. For example, there are government regulations that set standards for licensure of health care organizations, such as hospitals, and health care providers, such as nurses. Public health often uses regulatory policy to protect the health of the community (Longest, 1998). An example in the United States is the mandatory reporting of certain communicable diseases. On the international level, regulatory health policy is as broad as international communicable disease control, trade, human rights, armed conflict and arms control, and the environment (Fidler, 1999).

Regulatory policy can be further categorized as either competitive or protective. Competitive regulation limits, or structures, the provision of health services by designating who can deliver them. Protective regulation sets conditions under which various private activities can be undertaken. Although professional licensure is most commonly identified by professions as primarily protecting the public, such policy is competitive regulation in terms of its social impact.

Protective regulation is more clearly evident in utilization review organizations (regulatory bodies that critically examine health agency utilization patterns) or certificates of need (the legal requirement for a potential provider agency to demonstrate the need for its services before a license to practice is granted; see Chapter 12).

Health Policy Debate and Interest Groups

Health policy debate revolves around central issues such as the overall cost of health care reform, the amount of control the federal government will exercise over the entire health care system, and the extent to which various individuals and groups, including nurses, will be harmed by reform or perceive they will be harmed by reform. Any policy involving the redistribution of income will be opposed most vigorously by those affected most negatively. For example, early in the nurse practitioner movement, physicians were threatened by the advanced practice status of nurses and how it would influence their client base and income. The effective lobbying and influence of the American Medical Association (AMA), a powerful interest group, contributed to the limits of practice, state by state, for nurse practitioners. However, eleven states now grant nurse practitioners direct third-party reimbursement for their services without a physician as primary care provider (Catalano, 2000).

The most significant obstacles to the passage of effective health care legislation today are special interest groups and partisan politics. A **special interest group** is any group of people sharing a common goal, which is politically active in attempting to influence policy makers to support their goal. Policy solutions are, more often than not, eliminated by the outcry of politically motivated special interest groups. These interest groups come in many forms such as business groups, labor groups, neighborhood groups, minority groups, religious groups, environmental groups, and even nursing specialty groups. The AMA, the tobacco industry, and the National Rifle Association (NRA) constitute three of the most powerful forces in the United States today influencing policy decisions. The impact of these three organizations on health services delivery, on continuing the ill effects of smoking and tobacco use, and on control of gun ownership contributing to high death and injury statistics, is immeasurable. Interest groups employ many tactics to influence policy decisions, including public hearings, campaigns, litigation, protest, public relations, and especially lobbying (Christensen, 1995). **Lobbying** is the process by which an individual or group acts on the behalf of others to influence specific decisions of policy makers, such as legislators. Many special interest groups and organizations employ one or more full-time lobbyists to represent their interests. These individuals work behind the scenes to influence policy makers through informal sessions and written communication in addition to attending hearings and giving public testimony.

The four most powerful special interest groups in health care have been physicians, hospitals, insurance companies, and the drug industry (Lee & Estes, 1997). Physicians recognized the implications and consequences of health policy in relation to their profession decades ago and have become increasingly empowered through most of this century. Medicine's strong social and political influence is the result of many factors, among them a strong professional organization (the AMA), active political lobbying for their interests, and formation of strategic coalitions with respected individuals and scientific groups.

Hospitals have lost some of the power they had earlier in the 20th century as insurance companies have increased in power and influence as a special interest group and increasing numbers of physicians have become associated with health maintenance organizations (HMOs), decreasing their direct influence in hospitals. The most significant impact on the influence of hospitals occurred with the implementation of the prospective payment system in the mid-1980s when hospitals were no longer reimbursed for each day a client was hospitalized but based on a client profile schedule, giving them an incentive to discharge clients quickly. This trend continues today, and clients recuperate at home, not in the hospital.

The influence of insurance companies rose steadily as the influence of the hospital declined, and it remains a formidable force today. It directs the quality and quantity of client care in most instances, and, when including Medicare and Medicaid into the "pool" of insurance companies, the influence is overwhelming.

The drug industry is a fourth special interest group. Billions of dollars are spent annually by drug companies to develop, test, and market new medications. The only way they can recover development costs and make a profit is to ensure their product is sold to millions of clients. Therefore, they must convince primary care providers to prescribe their medications and charge large amounts of money for the product. This cycle of development, marketing, and more development continues in a highly competitive marketplace, and the consumer is an unwitting victim. Elderly clients are the most vulnerable to the spiraling costs of drugs because they are on fixed incomes and live with chronic illnesses requiring long-term polypharmacy. Many may take four, five, or six different medications, with some clients spending more than $1000 a month for their medications.

POLICY, POLITICS, AND COMMUNITY HEALTH NURSING

Health policy provides the conditions for empowering or disempowering certain groups in a variety of ways. Community health nurses must understand that power is an essential and primary concept inherent to all political and policy systems. A power base can be created through collaboration, cooperation, and communication (Catalano, 2000). Nurses have to negotiate and compromise with other interest groups to be politically effective. By forming strong health care coalitions, nurses gain a stronger voice in policy decisions affecting them and their clients (see The Global Community).

THE GLOBAL COMMUNITY

Healthcare Reform in Puerto Rico

Hulme, P.A. & Rios, H (1998). Healthcare reform in Puerto Rico: Managed care in a unique environment. *Journal of Nursing Administration, 28*(2), 44–49.

Puerto Rico is a self-governing U.S. Territory. The 3,500-square-mile island is the smallest and easternmost island of the Greater Antilles. Its 3.7 million people make Puerto Rico one of the most densely populated places on the globe. Puerto Ricans have had U.S. citizenship since 1917, and Spanish and English are official languages.

Nurses are educated in Puerto Rico much the same as in the United States with all levels of entry into nursing and passing a comprehensive examination in Spanish before licensure is granted.

The health of Puerto Ricans has changed dramatically in the last half of the 20th century. Fifty years ago, it had statistics similar to Third World countries, with a life expectancy of 46 years and an infant mortality of 6.8%. Tropical (malaria and intestinal parasites), infectious (TB), and acute illnesses (gastroenteritis) were the leading causes of death. These problems abated with the development of a regional health system, which included environmental health and sanitation departments. Each of the 78 municipalities (similar to counties) had its own primary health center, and, in each of the seven larger regions, a tertiary-care hospital was established where more complex care could be referred. Community health and acute-care nurses were vital to this system. Consequently, by the 1990s, the life expectancy was 74 years and the infant mortality rate was 1.3%. Leading causes of death were chronic and degenerative diseases, but, as in the United States, the ravages of substance abuse, homicide, suicide, and AIDs had begun to take their toll.

Before health care reform, one group of residents paid for health care with private insurance and Medicare, whereas others used the public health care system. The two groups used different facilities, and the systems functioned side by side but were not equal. Those using the insufficiently budgeted public system experienced long waits and overcrowding. All health statistics were worse in the public system, which had seven times fewer physicians working in it.

Health care reform, which began in Puerto Rico in 1994, changed these inequitable public and private systems. Essentially, the public system was privatized, using a managed care approach in which the private insurance companies assumed the financial risk at a predetermined cost per beneficiary. This reform has three goals: (1) improved health care quality and health outcomes, (2) cost control, and (3) equal access to primary physicians. The benefits included immunizations, yearly physicals and screening tests as needed, maternal–child care, primary care for acute and chronic illness, medications, mental health services, dentistry, and special, acute, and emergency care. No one was eliminated from the program because of gender, age, or preexisting condition. Those eligible included people who previously used the public health care system, people on Medicare, all public employees, and people below 200% of the local poverty level. No longer did the department of health provide direct services; instead, it became an overseer of services.

Community health nurses were highly visible in the old system with the severe physician shortage, but the role of nurses under managed care was barely addressed during the legislative process, despite impressive testimony by many nurses. As a consequence of the legislation, nurses lost important roles in the new system. This is of great concern among nursing managers in the United States and Puerto Rico because health outcome goals are likely to be severely affected by the shortsightedness of this decision in the reformed system. Another goal of the program, cost control, may also be compromised because Puerto Rico does not have advanced practice nursing (APN) programs in their schools and the physician power base is strong. In the United States, APNs have proved that they can provide quality primary care while saving money. Puerto Rico could have benefited from including such practitioners in their reform.

Change in this reform is inevitable, and nursing leaders must not let themselves be left out of the planning this time. Schools of nursing need to begin preparing nurses for advanced practice, the nurse practice act in Puerto Rico needs to be reformed, and nurses must lobby, testify, and otherwise make their voices heard.

Politics is inherent in any system where resources are absolutely or relatively scarce and where there are competing interests for those resources. **Politics** is an interactive process of influencing others to make decisions that favor (or at least do not threaten) a person's or group's chosen position and the allocation of scarce resources to support that position (Mason & Leavitt, 1998). For example, nursing's increasing influence on federal research development and funding policies is demonstrated by the NINR being funded for $63,531,000 in 1994, compared with Allied Health's $3,467,000 (Elwood, 1993/1994).

The health care system is governed through complex interactions among different government representatives, health professionals, consumers, third-party payers, and employers who may not agree on one another's roles and jurisdiction in health care. These groups use politics to survive, as well as to pursue their respective health care interests and goals. "There is no single source of governance or health policy, nor is there a single set of shared values or goals among these groups; the health care system is an amalgamation of many different agendas" (Pew Health Professions Commission, 1991, p. 55). Politics in the government is demonstrated by the fact that literally thousands of legislative bills are drafted each year, yet only a few are ever signed into law where they influence citizens. Although the political system within a local community may be less formalized, it has a profound influence on the collective health and well-being of its residents.

In the past, public policy primarily has restricted nurses in three related ways—scope of practice limitations, exclusionary definitions, and limits on eligibility for reimbursement.

Although most community health nursing services constitute primary care by being first contact, continuous, comprehensive, and coordinated (Selker, 1994), most health policy definitions of primary care exclude community health nurses as providers of primary care. As a result, community health nurses are not paid directly for their services, may require physician supervision, and have client responsibilities that continually test their practice limits.

It is a major problem when health policy does not recognize nurses as providing reimbursable health care services or primary care services in any community context. The exclusion of nurses, other than nurse practitioners, in primary care legislation and health policy statements practically eliminates the possibility of community health nurses receiving direct fees for services or even practicing unless under the supervision of a physician. Community health nurses should be one of the major sources of political influence (Hulme & Rios, 1998), although many strong and well-organized forces resist nursing's direct involvement in the politics and policy making of health care.

In spite of health policy restrictions on reimbursement and scope of practice, the demand for community health nursing services is stronger than ever. Community health nursing has grown in part because many areas were abandoned or delegated by physicians, such as home- and community-based ambulatory care and primary care. Finally, the importance and impact of quality community health care is receiving the national and political focus it deserves. In its conclusions, the Pew Health Professions Commission's 1993 report lists 17 competencies for future health care practitioners such as the need to care for the community's health, emphasize primary care, expand access to effective care, practice prevention, involve clients and families in the decision-making process, promote healthy lifestyles, understand the role of the physical environment, accommodate expanded accountability, and participate in a racially and culturally diverse society. Clearly, these are competencies that have long been expected of community health nurses.

Changes in federal health policy may present an opportunity to revisit the issue of giving community health nurses authority consistent with their actual practice. One commonly stated goal of health care reform is to provide more services to more people at a lower cost. Community health nurses are well positioned to do just that.

At the global level, nurses from many different cultures and countries and speaking different languages work in communities to promote the public's health. Protocols developed by the World Health Organization (WHO) are used as health, social, and environmental team members work together. The politics encountered include international as well as regional and those within the WHO (see Chapter 21).

No practicing nurse can escape politics, whether it be in the workplace or in the context of local, state, and federal government. However, there are still many social and professional barriers in place that hinder nurses from becoming a unified, powerful political force. Fragmented communica-

tion patterns isolate individual nurses and prevent them from interacting around issues of health policy beyond their immediate work environment. Also, tight resources limit opportunities and strain nurse relationships in the work environment. In addition, prevailing methods of evaluation and reward in the workplace often undermine attempts to create an environment more conducive to political involvement of nurses beyond their workplace issues. Finally, passivity and apathy are still problems within the profession. We *are* a profession and responsible for ourselves and our practice. Nursing has gained a much stronger political voice in recent years and is learning to build strategic alliances and power bases. Furthermore, it is each nurse's responsibility to continue to value, support, and foster political thinking and behavior that enhances the profession and its future.

Community health nurses need to learn to manage their immediate work environment effectively and be able to participate in the context of a larger political system to support quality health care. They must work to create a supportive health care culture that encourages frequent interaction among the various constituencies. Political involvement is an important means to achieve this goal. They must understand that community health nurses, like all people, may hold significantly different or conflicting opinions about theory, methods, and the direction of health care. These differences should be aired and debated to promote dialogue and creative solutions to health care problems. Community health nurses face an unparalleled opportunity to influence health policy through political involvement (Catalano, 2000).

HEALTH CARE REFORM: IMPLICATIONS FOR COMMUNITY HEALTH

Although the U.S. health care system has made remarkable advances in practice, education, technology, and facilities over the past 50 years, these have come at a very high cost. Furthermore, inflation (double digits in some years) has compounded the problem, so the United States has been spending an extraordinary and disproportionate amount of its national income on health care. In fact, in 1999, 14% of the gross national product (GNP) was spent on health care (Stai, McCormick, Fernandez, Weikel-Magden, & Beyer, 2000).

"Far and away, the most troubling issue in health care is the growing aggregate cost and the seemingly disproportionate share of income that we pay for care when compared to other nations" (Pew Health Professions Commission, 1991, p. 5). According to virtually all measures, health care spending in the United States is the highest in the world (Harrington & Estes, 1997). Recently, annual health care expenses were $1 trillion, representing a rise of 7.4% between 1994 and 1997 alone (Levit et al., 1997).

Four major factors influence rising health care costs: general nationwide inflation in the economy, inflation specific to the health care industry that is over and above the general rate of inflation in the economy, population growth, and changes in the nature and intensity of health care service delivery (Kovner & Jonas, 1999). Furthermore, the American public has expectations of the health care delivery system, nurtured by physicians over the years, that are unrealistic. When resources are finite in a health care system that focuses on secondary and tertiary prevention, the health of people cannot be optimized. However, community health's focus on primary prevention allows the limited resources to be available to those who need them.

There are also problems with accessibility of health care for certain segments of the population. Despite the enormous cost, approximately 44.3 million people lacked health insurance in 1998 (U.S. Department of Health and Human Services, 2000). "Substantial disparities remain in health insurance coverage for certain populations. Among the non-elderly population, approximately 31% of Hispanic persons lacked coverage in 1997, a rate that is double the national average" (U.S. Department of Health and Human Services, 2000, p. 1–9). One in four pregnant women receives no prenatal care, and only 45% and 53% of African-American and Hispanic elders, respectively, received influenza vaccinations (U.S. Department of Health and Human Services, 2000). These figures suggest why the United States ranks among the highest in the industrialized world in infant mortality and 19th in the world in life expectancy (National Center for Health Statistics, 1999). This indicates we are spending more money but getting less for the dollars spent.

President Clinton reenergized the health care debate by making health care reform a major theme of his 1992 presidential campaign and a primary goal of his first term in office. The proposed Clinton plan (the Health Security Act of 1993) was supposed to provide quality health care to everyone, regardless of ability to pay, while curbing the rise of medical costs. This legislation stirred national debate and controversy and ultimately was defeated in 1994. Its defeat demonstrates the complexities of health care reform at the federal level and the influence of partisan politics and special interests of business and labor, the insurance industry, government and education, health care providers, and consumers. The failure of the 103rd Congress to pass the Health Security Act of 1993 gave a signal to the health care industry that attempts to shape the health care system were not likely to come soon from the federal government. In his classic work, Starr (1982, p. 411) stated that health care reform will be elusive "as long as opposing interests remain sufficiently strong to block almost any coherent course of action, conservative or progressive." Indeed, the fiscal need for health care reform may be the only force that can overcome such widespread resistance. The managed care movement that took the United States by storm in the 1990s and continues into the new millennium has made profound changes in health care choices and accessibility for much of the population. These changes are not necessarily perceived as positive by the public. Although it attempts to contain costs while ensuring quality of care, managed care has not solved our problems. We continue to have a health care system that is "costing too much and serving too few" (Bulger, 1997, p. 54).

One group with an enormous stake in health care reform is the disabled community. People with disabilities have significant health care needs, yet are often uninsured or underinsured. This population includes people of all ages, with those over 65 making up a great percentage of the disabled population. The current U.S. system spends enormous sums—mostly out of pocket—on nursing homes and hospitals and much less on outpatient, home health, preventive care, or on personal assistance services where the emphasis should be focused. It is the latter services that the disabled community needs most.

The challenge for U.S. health care reform in this new century is to reduce costs and increase accessibility. What is needed is change from the present uncoordinated system to a consolidated health services delivery system that is accountable for costs, quality, and outcomes. Strategically, enhancing quality health care and reducing health care costs are the primary yardsticks for any health policy. Community health professionals must work to convince the political players that the health of the community is directly tied to quality health services, accessibility, and reasonable costs. As the need to restrain health care spending continues and health care dollars remain tight, "students in the health care professions need to be taught to integrate more fully the principles of community-based comprehensive care" and deliver a more population-based approach to health care (Bulger, 1997, p. 58). Convincing policy makers is key to successful health care reform.

POLITICAL EMPOWERMENT AND PROFESSIONAL ORGANIZATIONS

Because politics is an inherent part of any professional organization's operations, it is through participation in organizations that many nurses develop and refine their political skills. A strong professional organization offers a more collective diversity and realistic forum for political issues and debate and for enhancing a nurse's visibility. Leaders of professional organizations sit on decision-making boards, influence public policy, and define priorities for their communities. Professional organizations become seats of political empowerment. **Political empowerment** is a conscious state in which an individual, group, or organization becomes recognizably influential in determining policy. The nurse who is visible and influential in professional organizations can raise community awareness and mobilize community support.

Professional organizations come under fire by people outside their membership. Some believe professional organizations are nothing more than efforts to carve out turf or claim dominion at the expense of others. Morrison (1993, p. 8) claims that "professional associations . . . have sought to control professional accreditation programs, to establish and maintain rigid scopes of practice that preserve professional monopolies, and to restrict the use of professionals in the work place through control of facility licensure and accreditation schemes."

Regardless of criticisms, professional organizations provide an essential mechanism for nurses to be collectively empowered. One nurse's opinions may not be recognized nor would one nurse have the resources to promote a cause, but several thousand nurses together could. Effective nursing organizations monitor governmental regulations and lobby public officials on a regular basis. They also work together with other organizations to influence how the public views nursing, to set standards for nursing practice, and to participate in interdisciplinary efforts to shape public policy. An example was *Nursing's Agenda for Health Care Reform* (ANA, 1994), which was endorsed by over 60 professional nursing organizations (Display 13–1). This document, presented to legislators and many others, raised national consciousness and gave nursing a strong voice in shaping health reform. It became the policy statement of the nursing profession. However, it is outdated and needs revision to reflect changes since 1994.

Personal politics, as much as any other factor, sharpens conflict among individual nurses and makes communication difficult. The pursuit of personal agendas over the common good results in a piecemeal approach to problems and promotes polarization. **Polarization** is the process by which a group is seriously split into two or more factions over a political issue. Polarization can be so intense that people perceive one another as good or wicked depending on their ideological opinion. One of the primary goals of a professional nursing association is to build a collective voice for nurses. A strong professional association limits polarization by developing the political skills of its members and ensuring that its structure and processes equitably meet the needs of its constituencies. This is the essence of politics—people must listen to one another, learn from other viewpoints, and compromise to ensure the most positive outcomes from their endeavors.

Policy Systems and Policy Analysis

A **policy system** is an entity that receives input from external sources and has legal authority to generate or revise policies governing or managing the constituents it represents. Policy systems, such as city and county governments, are interrelated, complex, and highly political and receive input from many sources such as voters, lobbyists, special interest groups, and the media. Policy systems produce an output by generating policy, which in turn determines feedback for subsequent policy decisions. Their boundaries are defined by their legal authority to make only certain types of policy decisions at a particular level. Ideally, policy systems revise or make policy (output) based on comprehensive, accurate information (input) from a variety of sources, including feedback from all constituencies being affected by the policy.

Policy analysis is the systematic identification of causes or consequences of policy and the factors that influence it (Litman, 1997). Often, nurses confuse policy advocacy with policy analysis. This mistake can be detrimental in community health nursing. Policy advocacy is subjective; policy analysis should be objective. What is most important is that policy analysis should come before policy advocacy.

Community health nurses need a simple policy analysis framework to be effective in any practice arena. Nurses use the framework for determining the intentions and possible capacity of policy systems governing their practice, as well as their community. This framework allows nurses to protect themselves and, most important, to protect clients, whether families or groups.

Nurses can take several approaches when analyzing a policy that affects the health of a community or target population. They can look at the reasons for policy formulation, the groups of people affected by the policy, or the policy's possible long-range consequences. When analyzing policy, nurses need to answer two general questions: (1) who benefits from this policy? and (2) who loses from this policy? Whether the policy should be advocated by the community as a whole depends on the degree to which the policy benefits the community without being detrimental to individuals or the country.

Figure 13–2 provides a simple model for studying health policy. If nurses know something about the forces shaping health policy and the policy process, they are in a better position to influence policy outcomes. The model identifies four major stages in the policy process: formulation, adoption, implementation, and evaluation. Policy formulation involves identifying goals, problems, and potential solutions. Policy adoption involves the authorized selection and specification of means to achieve goals, resolve problems, or both. Implementation follows adoption and occurs when the policy is put to use. Policy evaluation means comparing policy outcomes or effects with the intended or desired effects.

STAGES 1 AND 2: POLICY FORMULATION AND ADOPTION

Health policy formulation is the stage at which a policy is conceptualized and ultimately defined. It is approached in at least two ways. Most commonly, a health problem is identified, such as the increased infant mortality rate associated

---

DISPLAY 13–1. Nursing's Agenda for Health Care Reform

This radical proposal called for "a new paradigm in U.S. health care delivery based upon a community and health model, a patient-focused system of care, patient self-determination with informed consent, a balance of health and illness services, a value on care and caring, and an expanded health care work force with direct consumer accessibility to professional nurses" (Betts, 1996, p. 4).

The proposal called for "a federal standard of a uniform basic benefits package for all U.S. citizens and residents, financed through a public–private partnership, delivering a continuum of services, in convenient, accessible sites by a variety of qualified providers whose activities would balance services for health and illness while improving quality of care, which would be measured and openly reported" (Betts, 1996, p. 4).

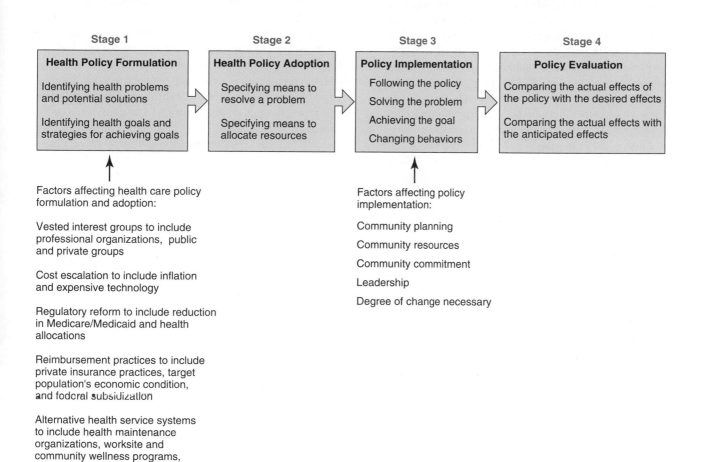

Stage 1	Stage 2	Stage 3	Stage 4
Health Policy Formulation Identifying health problems and potential solutions Identifying health goals and strategies for achieving goals	**Health Policy Adoption** Specifying means to resolve a problem Specifying means to allocate resources	**Policy Implementation** Following the policy Solving the problem Achieving the goal Changing behaviors	**Policy Evaluation** Comparing the actual effects of the policy with the desired effects Comparing the actual effects with the anticipated effects

Factors affecting health care policy formulation and adoption:

Vested interest groups to include professional organizations, public and private groups

Cost escalation to include inflation and expensive technology

Regulatory reform to include reduction in Medicare/Medicaid and health allocations

Reimbursement practices to include private insurance practices, target population's economic condition, and federal subsidization

Alternative health service systems to include health maintenance organizations, worksite and community wellness programs, and managed care

Factors affecting policy implementation:

Community planning

Community resources

Community commitment

Leadership

Degree of change necessary

FIGURE 13–2. Policy analysis model. Policy analysis examines the entire process to determine (1) who benefits from the policy and (2) who loses from the policy.

with teenage pregnancy. Health policy is developed to correct the particular health problem. Another approach to policy formulation emphasizes health planning more than corrective actions, at least initially. This is a goal-oriented approach. Health goals and strategies for achieving the goals are identified. In this more proactive approach, resources may be created as well as allocated for health services. Although both approaches to policy formulation may lead to the solution of a health problem, the goal-oriented approach is less reactive in that it does not require problem identification before the making of health policy.

The social and political conditions that affect policy formulation are limitless, but public need and public demand *should* be the strongest influences (Brown, 1997). Health care providers can stimulate a community to identify its health needs and demand health policies to fulfill its needs. During this process, the community health nurse should recognize that each community is unique, with its own mix of health services and public expectations.

STAGE 3: POLICY IMPLEMENTATION
Implementation of health policy occurs when an individual, group, or community puts the policy into use. It involves overt behavior changes as the policy is put into nursing practice. The degree and extent of compliance with a policy are the most direct measures of the policy's implementation (Harrington & Estes, 1997). *Noncompliance* refers to conscious or unconscious refusal to follow the policy directives. Community health nurses have always been health policy implementers and, recently, evaluators, regardless of whether these roles were consciously chosen.

Implementation of health policy is an essential part of effective, comprehensive client care for many documentable reasons. It should now be apparent that policies come in many forms and may have statutory or nonstatutory origins. Nurses are most cognizant of the latter in the form of procedure manuals and institutional guidelines. Communities are most aware of policies that limit or restructure their activities and growth, such as curfews and zoning regulations.

Once a health policy is written and adopted, its successful implementation depends heavily on the manipulation of many variables. For example, the implementation of day care standards depends, in part, on how they are interpreted and what resources are available to enforce them. The community health nurse as an implementer assesses the capacity of the community to formulate and define strategies that will enhance the community's compliance with the policy. This phase of policy analysis does not focus on the merits or shortcomings of the policy as is done in policy formulation, adoption, and evaluation.

STAGE 4: POLICY EVALUATION

Comparing what a policy does with what it is supposed to do is *evaluation*. Evaluation of a policy should result in continuation of the policy in its original form, revision or modification of the policy, or termination of the policy. Laws and policies are created to express the collective and powerful interests of the political system that generated them (Litman, 1997; Longest, 1998). The need for a particular health policy may be temporary, but a policy is difficult to change once adopted and implemented. Once a policy system is in operation, vested interests evolve as a result and become political influences. These vested interests under the guise of jobs, positions, titles, and wealth are perceptibly jeopardized by any change in the health policy that helped create them. Hence, tradition in the form of old policies tends to prevail.

One form of policy evaluation examines the health outcomes believed to be attributable to the health policy. Indicators such as mortality and morbidity statistics are used. Yet how the outcomes are defined and measured is highly political and more subjective than many recognize. For example, mortality statistics are often treated as objective data, yet how statistics are collected and the formulas used can often render them more subjective. For example, if data regarding driving under the influence of alcohol or drugs are not included in data on deaths from motor vehicle accidents, or if smoking data are left out of data on deaths from lung cancers, policy decisions based on such data may be seriously misdirected.

Perhaps the major premise that should underlie policy evaluation is that the goal of health policy is to design a system whereby health services are equitably distributed and appropriate care is given to the right people at a reasonable cost. This premise leads to the following basic criteria for evaluation:

1. Are the health services appropriate and acceptable to the population?
2. Are the health services accessible (physically and financially)?
3. Are the health services comprehensive?
4. Is there continuity of care?
5. Is the quality of the services adequate?
6. Is the efficiency of the services adequate?
7. Is there an ongoing (formative) evaluation of the services?
8. Is there a final (summative) evaluation of the services?
9. Is appropriate action taken based on the findings of the evaluations?

Regardless of the factors that affect policy evaluation, continual comparison is necessary between what a community believes about and wants in health care and what it is getting. Nurses have a responsibility to increase community awareness of health issues. They help the community make sure that its health needs are met through productive, desirable health policies.

Voices From the Community

The Florence Project—From Cyberspace to City Hall

The Florence Project was born out of a growing group of nurses' interest in raising awareness about unsafe conditions in health care. It started in 1997 as a handful of nurses "venting" on the Internet, via an e-mail list. The small group has grown with a dedicated website getting more than 16,000 hits during a 7-month period. As of May 1998, 400 nurses had registered online as members.

Membership is free, and anyone can enter the chat room. Participants say this opportunity "has given them a sense of community and empowerment" (Ventura, 1998, p. 48). Discussion topics range across health care issues of national, regional, and local concern. Topics include salary, working conditions, and case load issues. The dialogue is informative, and the site also serves as a forum for kinship and activism. Some of the group's grassroots efforts have involved initiating annual May Day rallies around the country to heighten awareness of health care issues among the people in their communities.

In 1998, rallies were planned in nine major U.S. cities in front of state capitols or city halls. Nurses, and in two cities a gubernatorial candidate and a congressman, spoke on health care issues. Promotion by e-mail, word of mouth, flyers, and ads in local papers generated up to 300 attendees. The organizers handed out information on local patient safety and nurse advocacy legislation. One group even offered blood pressure and glucose screening to those in attendance.

The Florence Project is in the process of evolving and continuing to define itself. It is set on becoming a "legitimate" organization with a large grassroots base and is incorporating in Florida to obtain a nonprofit status. Visit the Florence Project at their website and add your thoughts, concerns, and voice from the community (http://www.florenceproject.org).

COMMUNITY HEALTH ADVOCACY

The health of a nation stems from the health of its communities, and nurses have a solid tradition in serving the community's needs (Ventura, 1998; Pew Health Professions Commission, 1993) (see Voices From the Community). Nurses improve the quality of health services through community health advocacy. *Advocacy,* as defined in Chapter 3, refers to the community health nurse's role of pleading the cause of or working on behalf of others. **Community health advocacy** refers to efforts aimed at creating awareness of and generating support for meeting the community's health needs. Both nurses and communities have a common goal—the best possible health services for all. The community health nurse helps communities achieve this goal by being politically active, as well as providing effective health programs (American Public Health Association, 1998). As an advocate, the nurse works directly with community constituencies to support vulnerable groups such as low-income families, children, and the elderly. For example, community health advocacy might mean creating public awareness of the needs of battered women and exerting pressure on policy makers to provide protective legislation, or it might mean demonstrating the effectiveness of early intervention. There is a need for nurses to have good data because they base their practice on evidence derived from well-conducted research.

This recognition of a community's rights in determining its health policies inherently involves conflict. Nurses as community advocates are under pressure to help the population define specific goals, to delegate or implement actions to achieve these goals, and to establish controls to see that a community moves toward these goals. Sometimes, specific health goals prove elusive or they have no validity save that they are agreed upon. One thing is certain—the goals, constraints, and consequences of actions are seldom known precisely at a community level.

Community health advocacy causes change to occur at the community level. The change can be through legislation at local level (traffic laws), state level (revision of nurse practice act), or federal (expansion of Medicaid coverage for a target population). The change can also be regulatory (higher reimbursement for home health care services) or budgetary (federal financing of training for nursing students). To be effective, community health nurses must be an impetus for change at the community level by increasing the community's awareness and supporting the community's decisions regarding health policies.

Determining a Community's Health Policy Needs

Data about a community's problems and needs are often incomplete. This results in ineffective policy decisions and usually occurs because people within a community allow others to determine policy for them instead of with them.

When consultation with important policy implementers such as community leaders or community health nurses is not considered, ineffective health policy is likely to be enacted. Notable efforts to prevent these types of omissions in relation to health care policy have been in the formulation of *Healthy People 2000: National Health Promotion and Disease Prevention Objectives* and in the new *Healthy People 2010* (U.S. Department of Health and Human Services, 1991, 2000). These documents were developed with input from numerous groups and individuals, among whom nursing was well represented. They propose a national strategy for improving the health of the United States over the decade of the 1990s and, in the newer document, the first decade in the new millennium.

It is essential that the community health nurse take an active role in identifying a community's health policy needs. The nurse serves as a facilitator in assessing the community's unique health care needs in relation to its existing health care policies. Legislation and policy must be reviewed from the community's viewpoint, as opposed to an individual's viewpoint. Both public health efforts and community health systems are confronted with conflicting interests when individual rights interfere with aggregate rights. However, the community health nurse's primary mission is to promote and preserve the health of populations or aggregates for the benefit of the entire community (see Research: Bridge to Practice).

To identify the health policy needs of a community requires an ongoing comprehensive assessment of the community, or what some policy analysts call a "community diagnosis." Chapter 18 identifies the dimensions or variables of a community that are important in making a community assessment. Research studies sometimes provide data for policy formulation. A study by Sargent and associates (1999) examined the association between state housing policy and lead poisoning in children in two census tracts in different states. They found that the percentage of children with lead poisoning was three times higher in Providence County, Rhode Island, than in Worcester County, Massachusetts. Although both counties had similar percentages of pre-1950s housing, the researchers concluded that Massachusetts policy, which requires lead paint abatement of children's homes and places liability for lead paint poisoning on property owners, contributed to substantially reduced childhood lead poisoning in that state. Such data can be used to influence policy formation in other parts of the country.

Community Organization for Political Action

Political action refers to actions taken by an individual or group to influence the political decisions of others toward issues or policies beneficial to the welfare of the individual or group. Organizing a particular community for political action involves taking the following steps:

1. In your role as the community health nurse, identify yourself as a potential community organizer. In this

RESEARCH Bridge to Practice

Raube, K. & Merrell, K. 1999. Maternal minimum-stay legislation: Cost and policy implications. *American Journal of Public Health, 89*(6), 922–923.

In the fall of 1996, President Clinton signed the Newborns' and Mother' Health Protection Act requiring insurers to cover hospitalization for a minimum period of time for mothers and newborns after delivery, namely 48 hours after normal vaginal deliveries and 96 hours after cesarean deliveries. Some attribute the swift adoption of federal and state minimum-stay laws, in part, to the absence of compelling data from researchers on the outcome of shorter stays. In the research literature, there is disagreement about the appropriate length of stay for healthy newborns and cost-effectiveness of longer stays.

In this light, the hospital discharge records for over 167,000 women giving birth in Illinois during a 12-month period before the new law were analyzed for client (maternal and infant) outcomes. Readmissions for women who gave birth and received a routine discharge were 1.1% and 2.1% of the newborns during the first 2 weeks of life. Jaundice was the most common cause of newborn readmissions, accounting for more than one third. Using the data from this analysis to determine the percentage of total spending on maternal and infant admissions and readmissions, the net effect of the law ranges from a savings of just 0.1% to a significant cost savings of 20.2%.

Is this policy decision accomplishing what it intended to do—improve client outcomes and save money? The analysis has some important limitations in seeking answers to this question. This study gives no evidence of improved maternal and infant outcomes related to longer hospital care. There is no discussion on promising alternatives such as postdischarge home nursing visits. Public health nursing visits can be made to selected high-risk families on the day of or after discharge for infant and maternal assessment and teaching. Home health care visits can be made to monitor in-home phototherapy to treat newborn physiologic jaundice, once diagnosed by a primary health care provider in an outpatient setting, perhaps eliminating most of the infant readmissions related to jaundice.

This study may highlight that the rush to implement minimum-stay legislation is not accomplishing what it intended to do and is an expensive reaction to outcomes that were not well documented before more cost-effective models of care were tried.

beginning step, nurses must perform a self-assessment in terms of what they have to offer the community.

2. Identify problems, concerns, and issues. This information should come from the community's perspective, not merely that of individuals. Such information may be obtained directly by conducting a survey in the community and indirectly by looking at vital statistics, voting practices, and the lifestyle of the community.

3. Assess the physical community. Physical environment can have a significant influence on a community. Characteristics of the location in which a population lives set the stage for particular health problems and practices. Information about the physical environment can be obtained from a variety of resources, such as doing a windshield survey (see Chapters 16 and 18).

4. Assess community strengths, resources, and interests. This information is an important indicator of the community's health potential and ability to organize for political action. In this step, the nurse identifies community skills and assesses community strengths and limitations.

5. Assess political influences in the community. Each community has its own power base and political structure. Gaining knowledge of community political systems enables the nurse to identify key people and operations that are essential to the successful implementation of health goals. The community health perspective has a political advantage in terms of votes if the community is clearly defined and can be unified on a particular health issue.

6. Evaluate alternative courses of action. Community decision-making is facilitated when the community is well informed. The nurse can play an important role in the decision-making process by helping to identify possible outcomes and alternative courses of action to meet health goals. Each community, as well as each individual, has a different perspective, knowledge level, and ability to make changes. Decision-making will be influenced by the impact the decision can have on the social systems of the community.

7. Redefine objectives, priorities, and the community health nurse's goals. After a careful assessment of the community's needs, the community health nurse must compare the relationship between existing programs and policies as they relate to the defined needs and goals. If an incongruent relationship does exist, plans must be made to redefine and reshape existing and future policy directions.

8. Develop a plan of action. Planning for an entire community requires the nurse to collaborate with other professionals and representatives of the community's social systems. Each member of the planning team is considered an equal resource, and each member's input is vital to the successful implementation of the plan. Target audiences include federal policy officials, state and local policy officials, community groups, the business community, professional groups, major institutions such as hospitals or universities, research organizations, advocacy groups, and the general public.

9. Implement the plan. Implementing the plan first and foremost requires effectively communicating it to those who have a vested interest in such a way they will support it or at least not block it. One must figure out a way of reconciling differences that exist among those who (1) favor taking major action, but in

different ways; (2) favor taking action, but in incremental steps; or (3) only see the necessity of correcting certain problem areas, such as allowing workers to transfer the same health insurance coverage when they change jobs. Implementation of a plan requires several important considerations: involvement by representatives of the population to be affected, proper timing, and preparedness.

When implementing a community action plan, it is critical that the nurse is prepared and understands the common ground that racial and ethnic groups share without losing sight of their differences. Understanding the community's cultural values and media behavior is the first step to bridging cultural gaps. The second step is to choose the right messages. When the Centers for Disease Control and Prevention (CDC) tested public-service announcements about AIDS through focus groups, it found that single-race panels and multicultural panels reacted quite differently. In other words, a multicultural panel's perspective is not complete in itself (Rabin, 1994).

Rabin (1994, p. 57) states,

Messages may or may not be controversial in themselves, but the chance of controversy increases greatly if you don't get permission to relay a message to a particular group. It is critical to win the support, respect, and invitation of community leaders before they can open an effective line of communication with their members.

10. Evaluate the outcome of the planned action. Evaluation of a plan or program requires analyzing the observed outcomes based on the specific goals, objectives, and criteria that were adopted. Evaluation should be a continuous process that guides decision-making for the future.

THE LEGISLATIVE PROCESS AND INFLUENCING LEGISLATION

Theoretically, at the local level, health policies are guidelines for the implementation of health laws. A community's policy system exerts its control in distributing its health resources through its health policies. Sometimes, nurses and clients come to think of policies as statutes and, therefore, as difficult to change as law. In reality, community health policies are often an interpretation of health laws and, at best, serve as a strategy for implementing health laws, whether they be state or federal.

The nurse's role as an indirect care provider includes active involvement in the community's political arena (Ventura, 1998). Nurses particularly have a responsibility to generate new ways of providing health care and to modify or improve existing health care. To influence and initiate changes in the health care system, the nurse needs to know about the legislative process and be directly involved in setting the

health policy agenda for a community. The nurse also needs to know how to influence the passage of legislation or modify existing legislation (Williams, 1983). These skills are essential for all professional nurses because they are major ways that nurses can provide leadership in the improvement of health care.

How a Bill Becomes Law

All state governments and the three branches of the federal government make decisions that affect health care. All nurses have opportunities to provide input on the initiation, formulation, and revision of legislation at the local, state, and federal levels. Proposed drafts of bills originate from many places because the sources of legislative ideas are relatively unlimited. An idea may be forwarded to a legislator by individuals, groups, government agencies, or other interested parties. The process can be initiated when a concerned citizen or group writes or talks to a legislator.

The legislative process is well defined and guided by rules at all levels of government (U.S. House of Representatives, 1981). The process is similar at the state and federal levels, with the exception of some minor peculiarities. Public libraries have copies of a state's legislative process, or you may write to the state's printing office for information.

There is a requirement that certain types of federal bills be started in the House of Representatives, as opposed to the Senate. This may not be true at the state level, depending on the particular state's constitution. Once a senator or representative is found who is willing to author a bill, discussion takes place about what current law needs changing or what needs to be added to existing laws. When authoring a bill, a senator or representative consults with a legislative council. This council consists of legal specialists who assist legislators with the drafting of bills. The drafted bill is returned to its originator in the form of an "author copy." Content is carefully reviewed to ascertain that the bill does, in fact, state what it was intended to state.

A bill can be introduced at any time while the House is in session as long as the sponsoring representative has endorsed the bill and placed the proposal in the House's hopper. The procedure is more formal for the Senate, and any senator can postpone a bill by raising objections to it. All sponsored bills are assigned a legislative number and referred to committee. There are 16 standing committees of the Senate, 22 standing committees of the House of Representatives, and 5 joint committees. Most standing committees have two or more subcommittees.

Formal statements and details pertaining to each bill are published in the *Congressional Record* and printed for distribution. At the federal level, a bill may be considered at any time during the 2-year life of that Congress.

The chairperson of the committee to which a bill has been referred must submit the bill to the appropriate subcommittee assigned to work on it within a specified time period, usually

2 weeks. The exception occurs when the majority of the committee members of the majority party vote to have the bill considered by full committee. Traditionally, many committees and subcommittees have had a policy that any member who insists on a committee hearing on a particular bill should have it. Standing committees must have regular meetings at least once per month while in session, and the chairperson may call additional meetings.

The legislators appointed to a committee conduct the hearing on a bill. At the federal level, a bill may have no hearings or several hearings at one time in different committees. At the federal level, the author of a bill is seldom a member of the committee hearing the bill, whereas at the state level, the bill's author may have connections not available to other legislators or the audience.

The committee chairperson selects individuals to present the first testimony at hearings. Individuals or representatives of groups who have requested to speak about the bill may or may not be called for testimony. Testimony can always be submitted in writing. It is a frustrating political reality that one may go to committee hearings planning to speak or expecting to hear witnesses, only to find that the voting action was determined before the meeting. Astute individuals and groups not only monitor legislation but also tactfully lobby legislators before committee and subcommittee hearings.

After studying a bill and possibly hearing testimony, there are three types of recommendations the committee can make. (1) The committee approves the bill and is ready to forward it (due pass). (2) The committee revises the bill (due pass with amendments). (3) The committee may refer the bill to another committee. If the bill is set aside by any committee, it will eventually die; in so doing, committees can actually veto bills. Bills are usually revised and then forwarded or set aside. If a committee votes to pass a bill, a committee report is written that includes the bill's purpose, scope, and the reasons for the committee's approval. Containing a section-by-section analysis of the bill, the committee's report is one of the most valuable sources of information regarding policy formulation and adoption.

Amendments to state bills and federal bills are handled differently. At the state level, the original bill retains its assigned number throughout the legislative process regardless of amendments. At the federal level, amending occurs in "markup" sessions. A new bill is printed and reintroduced with a new number after each markup session. Obviously, it is more difficult to follow a bill through the federal process. Also, it should be noted that thousands of bills and joint resolutions are introduced each year, yet fewer than 10% are enacted as laws.

After committee action, the bill goes on the calendar and awaits being read before the originating house. The house considers the bill, and, at this point, its author states reasons why the bill is needed and responds to questions. Only legislators of the house may speak at the floor vote. The house may pass the bill or defeat the bill at this third reading. If the author knows in advance that there are not enough votes for the bill's passage, he or she will take action to delay the vote. At this point, considerable compromise, negotiating, trade-offs, and other strategies come into play. Success greatly depends on the author's power base and political maneuvering.

If a bill passes the first house, it is forwarded to the second house. For example, if a bill passes the Senate, it then goes to the House of Representatives. It enters as a new bill with an introduction and first reading. In the second house, the bill will again be assigned to committee. The committee will recommend due pass, due pass as amended, or amend and rerefer. After this committee's actions, the bill has a second reading on the floor of the second house. The third reading results in a floor vote. If there are any changes in the bill by the second house, it is returned to the originating house for concurrence. When significant differences prevent concurrence, the bill is referred to a conference committee consisting of members from both houses.

The conference committee action is a very important step to which the public has no access. This committee determines which version of the bill, or whether a compromise from both versions, will go forward in the conference report. This is a point where a great deal of political trading goes on and major deals are cut. After adoption by both houses, the bill is enrolled and goes to the President.

The President has three options: to sign, hold, or veto the bill. Signing the bill causes it to become law. Holding the bill without signing it may be done for timing or political reasons, but even without signing the bill becomes law after a delay of 10 days if Congress is still in session. Vetoing the bill sends it back to Congress with the President's objections attached. Congress can override this veto by a two-thirds majority vote in both houses, and, if the veto is overridden, the bill becomes law despite the President's objections.

Figure 13–3 outlines the process by which a bill becomes law. The fact remains that statutory law is only the beginning. The legislature enacts statutory law that enables a government agency to administer that law by means of regulation. Law is measured only in court. There are few laws other than criminal law by which one may be cited for noncompliance without going through a report mechanism. The executive branch, as represented by a government agency, administers the law through regulation. In the case of registered nurses, it is the Board of Registered Nursing that administers laws relating to nursing education, licensure, and practice, most often called the Nurse Practice Act. This is also the group accountable for disciplining registered nurses who do not meet the law.

A Political Strategy for Nursing

Community health nursing must be clearly defined as having a necessary and integral role with clear-cut responsibilities in the health care system. The role must be understood and appreciated by the public and legislators. The "selling" or marketing of the role can begin at the community or grassroots

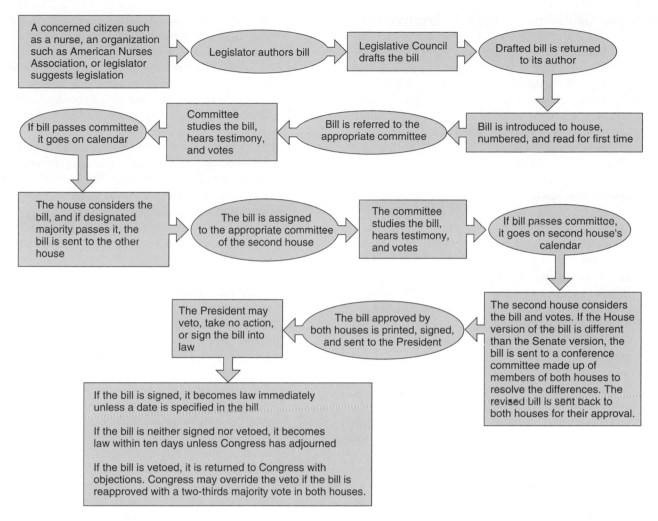

FIGURE 13–3. This flow chart diagrams the legislative process through which a bill becomes a federal law.

level but must also occur at the state and national levels. Ideas of opposition groups or interest groups with conflicting goals must be met with constructive criticism and compromise. During this process of defining and marketing nursing, nurses should present a positive and unified image to the public, the legislators, and opposition groups (Mason & Leavitt, 1998).

Nursing, like all other professions, has internal struggles and disagreements, but these internal disagreements need to be downplayed in the political arena. Nursing needs to present a unified, professional influence. Nursing holds a great deal of power, but that power remains unexerted when we are polarized (Swansburg, 1996). A change in image is overdue. Nurses outnumber all other health care providers and are as well educated as most. They have enhanced the health care system throughout all its struggles. Nurses need to improve their individual and collective self-concept and learn to be personally and politically assertive (Mason & Leavitt, 1998). They must assist each other in achieving the highest possible levels of maturity, education, public service, and professionalism with a focus on growth (Swansburg, 1996).

Nurses must give one another credit for their accomplish-

ments and learn to support and assist one another. Community health as a movement was created by nurses, yet there are many other groups ready to take the credit. Many leaders in nursing have received little recognition from their peers. Nurses need their colleagues' respect and recognition.

A greater financial base for promoting nursing will have to be established. As with any investment, nurses must first invest money in their professional organizations, in supporting the work of nurse lobbyists, and in promoting research and dissemination of information about nursing's contributions, before expecting any returns. Also, it must be recognized there is an inherent risk to be taken by being politically involved before any short-term or, more importantly, long-term gains can be expected. That is, gains for clients and for the profession as a whole have been minimized because, until now, nurses have not taken an active enough role in policy decision-making and they have not unified their political voice. Once the profession as a whole becomes empowered and assumes authority, autonomy, and recognition, individual nurses will be individually empowered to achieve their personal goals.

Individual Guidelines for Political Involvement

Community health nurses need to develop skill and experience to function effectively in the policy/political arena. Three major goals should be accomplished by the nurse as an individual in the political arena: generating support, creating legitimacy, and resolving conflicts. These goals are fulfilled when the community health nurse follows certain guidelines.

GENERATING SUPPORT

1. Present yourself well by promoting a positive and professional image. Dress and act accordingly.
2. Communicate your ideas effectively. Be knowledgeable, prepared, and state your position well. Use clear, concise, and understandable terms.
3. Learn the importance of socialization skills. Legislators attend local social and community functions for constituents. Invite a legislator to attend a social event at which a concern or issue can be discussed in a relaxed manner.
4. Get yourself known. Network both inside and outside the profession.
5. Recognize your skills to initiate, organize, and participate and use the nursing process. Apply these skills to the political process.
6. Know who your representatives are at the local, state, and federal levels and other groups and organizations that share the same legislative goals. Get in touch with them and keep them informed of health issues and their potential impact.
7. Make a concerted effort to influence a legislator to take a particular position on prospective legislation. Offer to write position papers. Become involved in lobbying, writing, and presenting testimony when legislators hold hearings on prospective legislation.
8. Support a candidate's campaign by donating money or by volunteering time and energy. Campaign for candidates who support nursing and community health, provided the rest of their political platform is agreeable. Get involved in campaigns early.
9. Join a **political action committee (PAC),** which is formed by a group or organization to endorse and financially back its candidates and support the group's position on issues.

CREATING LEGITIMACY

1. Keep abreast of current issues in health care and nursing and share information with your colleagues and elected officials.
2. Register to vote and encourage other nurses to do so. Hold a voter registration drive. Be sure to vote and communicate with legislators when a health issue surfaces.
3. Belong to and become involved in professional nursing organizations, such as the American Nurses Association and the National League for Nursing, and outside professional organizations, such as the American Public Health Association and the American Hospital Association.
4. Become involved on committees and boards within your agency and community, such as boards of directors, state boards of registered nursing, health planning boards and committees, city planning boards, and the League of Women Voters.
5. Run for office. Start by running for an office at the local level, or, if you are known in your community, consider state or national office. Nurses need representation from nurses in the governmental system at all levels.
6. Become knowledgeable about the political process. Become familiar with committees handling health care legislation.

RESOLVING CONFLICT

1. Plan your strategies well. Be able and willing to negotiate and compromise with conflicting views or interest groups. However, always keep the goals of nursing as your primary concern over those of other professions.
2. Be proactive rather than reactive on health issues whenever possible. Anticipate health concerns and issues and accumulate resources to be better prepared to negotiate rather than simply reacting to poor policies.
3. Communicate with tact and respect. Each person has a right to his or her own beliefs. Avoid insults and overly aggressive behavior. Balance cooperation, collaboration, strength, and assertiveness. Be positive.
4. Have an open mind in considering issues. Every political position has both pros and cons and should be weighed carefully to avoid a narrow viewpoint. Know opposing viewpoints well and be prepared to provide accurate rebuttal information.

Communicating With Public Officials

One form of political participation is communication with legislators. The purpose of this contact is to sway the public official's view toward or against a specific bill or political position. The nurse can influence a legislator's opinion by means of oral and written communication through telephone calls, personal visits, telegrams, mailgrams, and letters. To be effective as a private citizen or as a member of a group, the nurse needs to know the process and appropriateness of each type of communication.

WRITTEN COMMUNICATION

Legislators and government officials are more likely to be influenced by letters that express personal opinion and provide useful data than by form letters or mass telegrams. Form communications are tallied by an administrative assistant, but personal communication often reaches legislators directly. E-mail may be a legislator's or government official's preferred method of communication. A considerable amount of data convincingly presented is necessary to change a legislator's opinion (Display 13–2).

PERSONAL VISITS

An amazing number of bills are enacted with no input from constituents. Lobbyists exert great influence, as do other legislative colleagues and persons who use their physical proximity to a legislator or the persuasive tactic of trading favors to sway legislators' decisions.

Personal visits by nurses to their legislators can have a profound impact. Many legislators welcome additional expert information and respect the professional commitment involved in making the visit. Because legislators are very busy, with as little as 3 to 5 minutes for an interview, the nurse will make the visit more profitable by sending a one-page briefing sheet or letter before the meeting. Discussion

---

DISPLAY 13–2. Effective Communication With Legislators and Government Officials

Effective communication persuades with facts, logic, and brevity. It requires the nurse to be well prepared. In writing a public official, the following points should be considered:

1. A neat, clear, handwritten letter is acceptable, although a typewritten/computer-generated letter is preferable. Always address the letter appropriately with name and address on the letter and envelope and use appropriate salutations.

U.S President

Name	The President
Address	The White House
	Washington, DC 20500
Salutation	Dear Mr. or Mrs. President:
Closing	Sincerely,

U.S. Senator

Name	The Honorable Jane Doe
Address	United States Senate
	Washington, DC 20510
Salutation	Dear Mr. or Ms. Doe:
Closing	Sincerely,

U.S. Congressperson

Name	The Honorable John Doe
Address	U.S. House of Representatives
	Washington, DC 20515
Salutation	Dear Representative/Congressperson Doe:
Closing	Sincerely,

U.S. Secretary of Health and Human Services

Name	The Honorable Jane Doe
Address	200 Independence Ave, SW
	Washington, DC 20201
Salutation	Dear Ms. Jane Doe:
Closing	Sincerely,

Governor

Name	The Governor
Address	State Capitol
	City, State, ZIP
Salutation	Dear Govenor Doe:
Closing	Sincerely,

Mayor or City Council Member

Name	Mayor (or) Council Member
Address	City Hall
	City, State, ZIP
Salutation	Dear Mayor or Council Member:
Closing	Sincerely,

2. When a bill is in committee, correspond with all members of the committee. The content of the letter may be the same, but each letter should be individually typed or handwritten.

3. Plan the wording of your letter to make points concisely and succinctly. Letters are scanned before they are read. The following is a content outline of what is appropriate to include in the correspondence:
   a. One sentence that clearly states the issue
   b. One sentence that clearly states your individual or group position
   c. A statement that delineates the status of the proposed legislation (eg, where it is in the legislative process and what appears to be its disposition)
   d. A list of the reasons to support or oppose the pending legislation
      (1) Financial
      (2) Groups adversely affected
      (3) Weaknesses of opposing view
      (4) Specific benefits that override weaknesses of your view, benefits of the opposing view, or both
   e. Specific data that support these reasons
      (1) Dollar amounts
      (2) Number of groups affected and their names
      (3) Numbers within those groups
      (4) Delineation of processes, systems, equipment, and loopholes that have adverse or positive effects
   f. A clear, concise statement of the action that you want the legislator to take on the piece of legislation such as to vote for or against the legislation; meet with you or your organization; ask for additional information; convey contents of letter to interested, influential persons; provide you with those persons' names and titles so you can contact them; or other similar action.

with a legislator's staff members can also be worthwhile and may be the only route upen to you. These individuals do the legislator's background research and help to develop the positions and language contained in the bills. Staff members are the gatekeepers and are often more knowledgeable than the legislator about the issues and have more time to discuss them.

Community health nurses, as advocates for a health issue, must know the opposition's arguments and be prepared to counter them. The prepared nurse will communicate far more effectively with the legislator and his or her staff.

ATTENDING HEARINGS AND PROVIDING TESTIMONY

Community health nurses attending a legislative hearing can have considerable impact on a pending bill or proposed regulation. Singly or as an organized group, the nurses' physical presence communicates to legislators that they are concerned, informed, and ready to take action. Again, nurses need to be prepared in advance of the hearing. Resources, such as a government relations committee or the state nurses' association, can provide useful information on the issues surrounding the bill. Other existing communication networks, such as nurses involved in political action committees, can provide additional information.

Once a community health nurse is versed in the particular topic of a bill, he or she may want to provide testimony (Fig. 13–4). Testimony may be given verbally at the time of a hearing, or it may be written in advance. What should be included in one's testimony differs little from what should be included in a letter, with the exception of supportive materials, such as actual research or survey data.

Party politics has significant impact on the conduct of legislative business. At times, votes may reflect party allegiance and platforms rather than the individual legislator's response to the information provided at the hearing or through constituents' letters. Thus, the numbers of any given party in each house can make a considerable difference in passing bills. Organized lobbying groups can exert more pressure on legislators to override party decisions.

If you as a community health nurse support a bill and wish to testify, contact the author of the bill. If you are opposed to a bill and wish to testify, notify the bill's author and the chairperson of the committee in which the bill is being heard. Be sure you are working from or responding to the latest version of a bill (with amendments). Organized groups with registered lobbyists are most familiar with the process and may provide the best entree to the committee hearings as a participant. Remember, votes are counted by the author before a committee meets, and, if the number is not sufficient for a due pass, there are many ways to postpone an official vote.

Running for Public Office or Seeking an Appointment

Perhaps running for public office or seeking an appointment is the best way for your convictions to be expressed and for you to effect change as a community health nurse. Using the steps within the three goals mentioned above of generating support, creating legitimacy, and resolving conflict will place you in the best position to be successful as a candidate for political office or appointment.

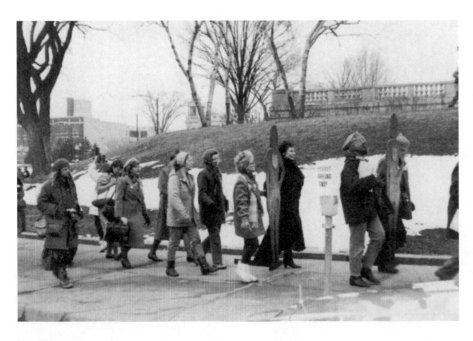

FIGURE 13–4. Community health nurses and friends on their way to testify at a health-related hearing in the state capitol.

The local level is an appropriate beginning for most people just entering the political arena. Become aware of positions coming available to run for and know where your expertise and interest will best be used. Most political positions have terms of office or term limits, where the present person needs to run for the office again or step down. Good beginning positions might be in local educational systems as president of a parent-teachers association or membership on a school board. There are positions on advisory boards, governing boards, or boards of directors for nonprofit organizations, such as the Epilepsy Foundation or the American Cancer Society. Consider a boardmember position for aggregate living centers if your interests are with specific aggregates, health departments, acute-care facilities, and other health- and service-related organizations if your connections are strong in these settings. As you become well known for your work at the local level, consider other political offices, such as a member of a county board of supervisors, city council member, or mayor. You will need to plan your strategy well, organize the necessary funding, and complete the necessary paperwork. Of course, you will need to meet basic eligibility requirements of age, residency, and citizenship. Major political parties provide training for potential candidates.

Once you become known in your community, consider a state or national political office or appointment (American Nurses Association, 1993). Nurses and the community as a whole benefit by representation from nurses in all levels of the government. For community health nurses, the basic skills needed for aggregate nursing can carry over into the policy/politics arena. These skills include the ability to assess aggregate health needs, to communicate and collaborate effectively with others, to educate people regarding health promotion and disease prevention, to conduct and be a consumer of health research, to lead others and effect positive change, and to gain power and wield it effectively. Nurses can speak on issues with a strong voice and influence health and public policy. To do this, they must be prepared to meet the challenge of public service. Again, participating in the steps to meet the three goals mentioned earlier will give nurses that preparation.

The need for nurses prepared to influence the system is even more urgent today as health care policy reaches a crisis in terms of continued rising costs, personnel shortages, and limited access to services—problems not resolved by the managed care movement. Gaining both knowledge and experience in the political arena will build confidence and skill for community health nurses to influence health policy and, ultimately, the public's health.

Nurses must depend on professional and political organizations and current literature for guidance in studying policy and becoming politically active. Many organizations are politically significant to community health nurses; a listing of some at the national level can be found in the Resources at the end of this textbook. The chief objective is to provide directions in which political contacts and knowledge can be developed by the community health nurse.

SUMMARY

The need for health care reform has become critical as the costs of health care continue to rise. The United States spends a disproportionate percentage of the national budget on health care, yet there are still major segments of the population that do not have adequate access to quality health services. Because of these economic concerns, health care reform and policy making have become politically charged issues involving many groups and factions, including not only health care providers and health care professionals but also government, third-party payers, insurance companies, and others with vested interests.

Many people are just beginning to realize that health care is a business. It has always been a business—we are just more aware of it now because of scarcity of resources. Many believe that business interests and efforts to curb rising costs may divert public services away from community health issues, such as preventive and primary care. Community health nurses know community needs and the value of such services and, therefore, need to be a major force in this political arena where health policy decisions are being made. Community health nurses need to become politically aware and active to ensure quality health services—working as community health advocates. They must collaborate with community constituents and with nurses and other professionals to ensure the safety and well-being of groups and populations at risk.

Although nurses' influence has been limited in the past, they must learn how to empower their own profession, themselves, and the communities they work with by becoming politically active and aware. If they are to fulfill their mission of promoting, protecting, and preserving the health of aggregates, they must become policy makers as well as policy implementers. They must learn to use policy systems and the political process so their voice is heard and they have influence in policy decision-making. They must learn to formulate, implement, and evaluate health policies. They must understand the legislative process and how to influence that process. The politically involved nurse should aim to accomplish three primary goals of (1) generating support for his or her views, by communicating ideas effectively and getting to know and influence representatives at local, state, and national levels; (2) creating professional legitimacy such as keeping abreast of current issues in health care and nursing and becoming involved in professional nursing organizations, community boards, and/or committees or running for political office at the local, state or national level; and (3) resolving conflict and being able to effectively negotiate and compromise.

Many resources and opportunities exist to help community health nurses study policy issues and make political contacts. Community health nurses must recognize societal changes and their potential impact on community health. They must also be able to analyze policy and become active in the political process to influence policy decisions that are in the community's best interests.

ACTIVITIES TO PROMOTE CRITICAL THINKING

1. Investigate a major health policy system in your community or state; discover how it works and determine whether community health nurses are represented in this system. Areas to investigate include the boundaries of the system; the authority by which the system generates health policy; how the system receives input (formally and informally); resources the policy system uses and allocates to others; and the system's output over the past few years.

2. Describe a legislative bill related to community health at either the state or federal level and the issues involved in it. Identify who is sponsoring the bill, who is opposing it, and why. Determine who will be affected by the bill, if passed, and in what ways they will be affected. Discuss what you, as a community health nurse, could do to be involved in this bill and then develop a political action plan to support or oppose the bill. Write a letter to your legislator regarding your position.

3. Carefully review your own health care plan and determine whether you believe it is an adequate and equitable plan. Describe the plan and the issues involved in it. Include what health services are covered and who is authorized to provide services and receive direct reimbursement. Also determine who qualifies for the plan and who is excluded and what conditions can disqualify a person or a family once they have the plan. Compare the cost of this plan to one other plan.

4. Attend a meeting of a professional organization, board of directors, government agency, or council when a health policy or health care issue is on the agenda. Analyze the positions of the major interest groups involved and describe to what extent economics comes into the discussion. Describe who controls the discussion and how this is done.

5. Interview a health care administrator in your local area and determine this person's position on health care reform including the rationale for the position. Determine at what level(s) this administrator is politically active and involved in influencing policy.

6. Several websites for government agencies and organizations are shared in this chapter. Contact two or three of them. What resources can you get from these sites? How can you use the information as a community health nurse? Did these sites lead you to other sites? If they did, contact these additional sites and write down the additional website addresses in the margin of the chapter for future reference.

REFERENCES

American Nurses Association. (1994). *Nursing's agenda for health care reform*. Washington, DC: ANA Publications.

———. (1993). *Positioned for power: Obtaining government appointments for nurses*. Washington, DC: ANA Publications.

American Public Health Association. (1998). *APHA advocates' handbook: A guide for effective public health advocacy*. Washington, DC: Author.

Betts, V. T. (1996). Nursing's agenda for health care reform: Policy, politics, and power through professional leadership. (Politics, power, and practice). *Nursing Administration Quarterly, 20,* 1–9.

Brown, E. R. (1997). Leadership to meet the challenges to the public's health. *American Journal of Public Health, 87*(4), 554–557.

Bulger, R. J. (1997). The quest for mercy: The forgotten ingredient in health care reform, Section III—The broadening scope of health care, *Western Journal of Medicine, 167,* 54–72.

Catalano, J. T. (2000). *Nursing now!: Today's issues, tomorrow's trends* (2nd ed.). Philadelphia: F. A. Davis Company.

Christensen, T. (1995). *Local politics*. Belmont, CA: Wadsworth.

DeParle, J. (1999, August 29). Leftover money for welfare baffles, or inspires, states. *The New York Times,* pp. 1, 20–21.

Dye, T. R. (1992). *Understanding public policy*. Englewood Cliffs, NJ: Prentice-Hall.

Elwood, T. (Ed.). (Dec. 1993/Jan. 1994). Clinton health reform bill dropped into congressional hoppers. *Trends: Association of Schools of Allied Health Professions Newsletter, 2.*

Fidler, D. P. (1999). *International law and infectious diseases*. Oxford: Clarendon Press.

Harrington, C., & Estes, C. L. (1997). *Health policy and nursing: Crisis and reform in the U. S. health care delivery system* (2nd ed.). Boston: Jones and Bartlett.

Hulme, P. A., & Rios, H. (1998). Healthcare reform in Puerto Rico: Managed care in a unique environment. *Journal of Nursing Administration, 28*(2), 44–49.

Kovner, A. R., & Jonas, S. (1999). *Jonas and Kovner's health care delivery in the United States*. New York: Springer Publishing Company.

Lee, P. R., & Estes, C. L. (Eds.). (1997). *The nation's health* (5th ed.). Boston: Jones and Bartlett.

Levit, K., et al. (1997). National health expenditures, 1996. *Health Care Financing Review, 19*(1), 161–200.

Litman, T. J. (1997). *Health politics and policy* (3rd ed.). New York: Delmar.

Longest, B. B. (1998). *Health policymaking in the United States* (2nd ed.). Chicago: Health Administration Press.

Mason, D. J., & Leavitt, J. K. (Eds.). (1998). *Policy and politics for nurses: Action and change in the workplace, government, organizations and community* (3rd ed.). Philadelphia: W. B. Saunders.

Morrison, R. D. (1993). *Creating an agenda for change in Virginia: Virginia health care workforce*. A presentation to the twenty-sixth annual meeting, Association of Schools of Allied Health Professions, Galveston, TX, October 28, 1993.

National Center for Health Statistics (1999). *Health, United States 1999*. Washington, DC: U.S. Department of Health and Human Services.

Pew Health Professions Commission. (1993). *Health professions for the future: Schools in service to the nation. A report of the Pew Health Professions Commission.* San Francisco: UCSF Center for the Health Professions.

———. (1991). *Healthy America: Practitioners for 2005. A report of the Pew Health Professions Commission.* Durham, NC: Duke University Medical Center.

Rabin, S. (1994). How to sell across cultures. *American Demographics, 16*(3), 56–57.

Raube, K., & Merrell, K. (1999). Maternal minimum-stay legislation: Cost and policy implications. *American Journal of Public Health, 89*(6), 922–923.

Sargent, J. D., Dalton, M., Demidenko, E, et al. (1999). The association between state housing policy and lead poisoning in children, *American Journal of Public Health, 89*(11), 1690–1695.

Selker, L. G. (1994, March 12–13). *Descriptions of the current and future roles of allied health workers in the direct provision and support of primary care.* White paper presentation at Thomas Jefferson University workshop: The Role of Allied Health in the Delivery of Primary Care. Philadelphia, PA.

Short, P. F., & Banthin, J. S. (1995). New estimates of the underinsured younger than 65 years. *Journal of the American Medical Association, 274,* 1302.

Stai, M., McCormick, C., Fernandez, T., Weikel-Magden, L., & Beyer, M. (2000). Up in smoke: Smoking as an individual and national health risk in the U.S. Stanford University Department of Human Biology web journal: http://sil-8.stanford.edu/webjournal/69/

Starr, P. (1982). *The social transformation of American medicine.* New York: Basic Books.

Swansburg, R. C. (1996). *Management and leadership for nurse managers* (2nd ed.). Boston: Jones and Bartlett.

U.S. Department of Health and Human Services. (2000). *Healthy people 2010* (conference edition in two volumes). Washington, DC: U.S. Government Printing Office.

———. (1991). *Healthy people 2000: National health promotion and disease prevention objectives* (S/N 017-001-00474-0). Washington, DC: U.S. Government Printing Office.

U.S. House of Representatives. (1981). *Our American government: What is it? How does it function? 150 questions and answers* (House Document No. 96-351). Washington, DC: U.S. Government Printing Office.

Ventura, M. J. (1998). Can these nurses make a difference? *RN, 61*(7), 47–49.

Williams, C. A. (1983). Making things happen: Community health nursing and the policy arena. *Nursing Outlook, 31,* 225–228.

INTERNET RESOURCES

Agency for Health Care Research and Quality (AHCRQ)
http://www.ahcrq.gov/info@ahcpr.gov

American Public Health Association (APHA)
http://www.apha.org

The Florence Project
http://www.florenceproject.org

Thomas (U.S. Government Legislative Information)
http://thomas.loc.gov/

SELECTED READINGS

Aday, L. A., Begley, C. E., Lairson, D. R., & Slater, C. H. (1993). *Evaluating the medical care system.* Ann Arbor, MI: Health Administration Press.

American Nurses Association. (1990). *Political and legislative handbook.* Washington, DC: ANA Publications.

Bagwell, M., & Clements, D. (1985). *A political handbook for health professionals.* Boston: Little, Brown.

Burris, S. (1997). The invisibility of public health: Population-level measures in a politics of market individualism. *American Journal of Public Health, 87*(10), 1607–1610.

Chin, P. L. (1993). What can just one nurse do? *Nursing Outlook, 41*(2), 54–55.

Congressional Quarterly. (1991). *How Congress works.* Washington, DC: Author.

Coss, C. (1993). Lillian D. Wald: Progressive activist. *Public Health Nursing, 10*(2), 134–137.

Declercq, E., & Simmes, D. (1997). The politics of "drive-through deliveries": Putting early postpartum discharge on the legislative agenda. *Milbank Quarterly, 75,* 175–202.

deVreis, C. M., & Vanderbilt, M. W. (1993). *The grassroots lobbying handbook* (ANA Pub. No. GR-4). Washington, DC: American Nurses Publishing.

Feldstein, P. J. (1996). *The politics of health legislation: An economic perspective* (2nd ed.). Ann Arbor, MI: Health Administration Press.

———. (1994). *Health policy issues: An economic perspective on health reform.* Ann Arbor, MI: Health Administration Press.

Hall-Long, B. A. (1995). Nursing's past, present, and future political experiences. *Nursing and Health Care, 16*(1), 24–28.

Ham, C. (1997). *Health care reform: Learning from international experience.* Philadelphia: Open University Press.

Helms, L., & Anderson, M. A. (1996). *Nurses as policy analysts and advocates: Avoiding lessons already learned* (series on nursing administration, no. 6). Thousand Oaks, CA: Sage.

Kun, K. E., & Muir, E. (1997). Influence on state legislators. *Public Health Reports, 112*(2), 276–283.

Mackenzie, E. R. (1998). *Healing the social body: A holistic approach to public health policy.* New York: Garland Publishing.

Powell, F. D., & Wessen, A. F. (1998). *Health care systems in transition: An international perspective.* Thousand Oaks, CA: Sage.

Shi, L., & Singh, D. A. (1998). *Delivering health care in America: A systems approach.* Gaithersburg, MD: Aspen.

Thomas, P. A., & Shelton, C. R. (1994). Teaching students to become active in public policy. *Public Health Nursing, 11*(2), 75–79.

Weiss, D. (1995). Challenging our values: Directing health care reform. *Nursing Policy Forum, 1*(1), 22–26.

Weissert, C. S., & Weissert, W. G. (1996). *Governing health: The politics of health policy*. Baltimore: The Johns Hopkins University Press.

Williams, D. M. (1991). Policy at the grassroots: Community-based participation in health care policy. *Journal of Professional Nursing, 7*(5), 271–276.

Williams-Crowe, S., & Aultman, T. (1994). State health agencies and the legislative policy process. *Public Health Reports, 109*(3), 361–367.

Woodworth, J. R., & Gump, W. R. (1994). *Camelot: A role playing simulation for political decision making*. Belmont, CA: Wadsworth.

Epidemiology in Community Health Care

LEARNING OBJECTIVES

Upon mastery of this chapter, you should be able to:
- Explore the historical roots of epidemiology.
- Explain the host, agent, and environment model.
- Describe theories of causality in health and illness.
- Define *immunity* and compare passive, active, cross, and herd immunity.
- Explain how epidemiologists determine populations at risk.
- Identify the four stages of a disease or health condition.
- List the major sources of epidemiologic information.
- Distinguish between incidence and prevalence in health and illness states.
- Use epidemiologic methods to describe an aggregate's health.
- Distinguish between types of epidemiologic studies useful for researching aggregate health.
- Use the seven-step research process when conducting an epidemiologic study.

Epidemiology is the study of the determinants and distribution of health, disease, and injuries in human populations. It is a specialized form of scientific research that can provide health care workers, including community health nurses, with a body of knowledge on which to base their practice and methods for studying new and existing problems. The term is derived from the Greek words *epi* (upon), *demos* (the people), and *logos* (knowledge), thus meaning the knowledge or study of what happens to people. Epidemiologists ask such questions as, What is the occurrence of health and disease in a population? Is there an increase or decrease in a health state over the years? Does one geographic area have a higher frequency of disease than another? What characteristics of people with a particular condition distinguish them from those without the condition? Is one treatment or program more effective than another in changing the health of affected people? Why do some people recover from a disease when others do not? The ultimate goal of epidemiology is to determine the scale and nature of human health problems, identify solutions to prevent disease, and improve the health of the entire population (Beaglehole & Bonita, 1997).

Epidemiology offers community health nurses a specific methodology for assessing the health of aggregates. Furthermore, it provides a frame of reference for investigating and improving clinical practice in any setting. For example, if a community health nursing goal is to lower the incidence of sexually transmitted diseases (STDs) in a given community, such a prevention plan requires information about population groups. How many STD cases have been reported in this community in the past year? What is the expected number of STD cases (the morbidity rate)? What members of the community are at highest risk of contracting STDs? Any program of screening, treatment, or health promotion regarding STDs must be based on this kind of information about population groups in order to be effective. Whether the community health nurse's goals are to improve a population's nutrition, to control the spread of human immunodeficiency virus (HIV), to deal with health problems created by a flood, or to protect and promote the health of battered women, epidemiologic data are essential.

HISTORICAL ROOTS OF EPIDEMIOLOGY

The roots of epidemiology can be traced to Hippocrates, a Greek physician who lived from about 460 to 375 BC and is sometimes referred to as the first epidemiologist. Hippocrates and other members of the Hippocratic School believed that disease not only affects individuals but is a mass phenomenon. This was one of the earliest associations of the occurrence of disease with lifestyle and environmental factors (Beaglehole & Bonita, 1997). However, it was not until the late 19th century that modern epidemiology actually came into existence.

Although they are among history's greatest disasters, epidemic diseases clearly prompted the development of epidemiology as a science. An **epidemic** refers to a disease occurrence that clearly exceeds normal or expected frequency in a community or region. In past centuries, epidemics of cholera, bubonic plague, and smallpox swept through community after community, killing thousands of people, changing the community structure, and altering the lifestyle of masses of people. When an epidemic, such as the plague or acquired immunodeficiency syndrome (AIDS), is worldwide in distribution, it is called a **pandemic.**

Epidemiology became a distinct branch of medical science through its concern with epidemics and pandemics of infectious diseases. In 1348, the Black Death (bubonic plague, pneumonic plague, or referred to as the plague and caused by the bacillus *Yersinia pestis*) swept through continental Europe and England, killing millions of people and lowering the life expectancy to 20 years from 30 to 35 years (Display 14–1). In England alone, approximately one fourth of the population died from the plague. The plague continued in Europe, but with less force, for three centuries and then waned, only to reappear in an epidemic in Hong Kong in 1896. Kitasato, a Japanese bacteriologist, discovered the plague bacillus during this Hong Kong epidemic; within 10 years, epidemiologists had traced its life cycle from rats to their infected fleas that bit humans. Now intervention was possible, and public health officials declared war on rats, seeking to make ships and wharf buildings rat-proof. The first major campaign against rats that took place in California after an outbreak of plague in 1900 was successful. However, wild rodents, especially ground squirrels, remain a natural reservoir of the plague bacillus, as

DISPLAY 14-1. Impact of the Plague

"It was the appearance of the plague in the fourteenth century, and its periodic return throughout the next two centuries, that crystallized the interest in public health that had begun with the isolation of lepers in the thirteenth century. Some cities complied 'books of the dead,' which were comprehensive mortality records used to identify epidemics and follow their course. Mortality rates in the early epidemics were staggering, with up to half of the population dying in cities during the plague pandemic. In response to the first plague pandemic, Northern Italian city-states instituted a series of public health measures designed to protect the health of the elite. For example, the authorities isolated ships suspected of carrying disease; the quarantine lasted for 40 days" (Beaglehole & Bonita, 1997, p. 87).

well as rabbits and domestic cats. Cases still occur occasionally in the western half of the United States with periodic outbreaks in large areas of South America; north-central, eastern, and southern Africa; and central and Southeast Asia (Chin, 1999). The continuing presence of a disease or infectious agent in a given geographic area, such as plague in Vietnam and malaria in the tropics of Brazil and Indonesia, means the disease is **endemic** to that area.

As the threat of the great epidemic diseases declined, epidemiologists began to focus on other infectious diseases such as diphtheria, infant diarrhea, typhoid, tuberculosis, and syphilis. They also studied diseases linked to occupations, such as scurvy among sailors and scrotal cancer among chimney sweeps. In recent years, epidemiologists have turned to the study of major causes of death and disability, such as cancer, cardiovascular disorders, AIDS, violence, mental illness, accidents, arthritis, and congenital defects.

Nursing's epidemiologic roots can be traced back to Florence Nightingale (1820–1910) (Cohen, 1984). Miss Nightingale often obtained advice on issues related to hospital statistics and disease classification from her close friend William Farr, who established the field of medical statistics as chief statistician of England's General Register Office for health and vital statistics. Her detailed records, morbidity (sickness) statistics, and careful description of the health conditions among the military in the Crimean War represent one of the first systematic descriptive studies of the distribution and patterns of disease in a population. She used wedge-shaped graphs, circles, and squares that were shaded and in colors to illustrate preventable deaths of the hospitalized Crimean soldiers as compared with hospitalized soldiers in England at the time. Changes made according to her suggestions brought dramatic proof of the authenticity of her observations and knowledge. Forty out of every 100 British troops (40%) were dying in the Crimea before Miss Nightingale instituted environmental and nutritional changes in the hospital and field.

When her work in the Crimea was finished, the mortality (death) rate was only 2%.

Florence Nightingale's use of statistical data along with her commitment to environmental reform strongly influenced nursing's evolution into a profession whose service addressed public health problems as well as hospital care (Kopf, 1978). As nursing has evolved, community health nurses have been increasingly challenged to intervene at the aggregate level, using epidemiologic approaches to address the needs of high-risk groups and populations.

CONCEPTS BASIC TO EPIDEMIOLOGY

The science of epidemiology draws on certain basic concepts and principles to analyze and understand patterns of occurrence among aggregate health conditions.

Host, Agent, and Environment Model

Through their early study of infectious diseases, epidemiologists began to consider disease states generally in terms of the epidemiologic triad, or the *host, agent, and environment model*. Interactions among these three elements explained infectious and other disease patterns.

HOST

The **host** is a susceptible human or animal who harbors and nourishes a disease-causing agent. Many physical, psychological, and lifestyle factors influence the host's susceptibility and response to an agent. Physical factors include such things as age, sex, race, and genetic influences on the host's vulnerability or resistance. Psychological factors, such as people's outlook and response to stress, can strongly influence host susceptibility. Lifestyle factors also play a major role. Diet, exercise, sleep patterns, healthy or unhealthy habits all contribute to either increased or decreased vulnerability to the disease-causing agent.

The concept of resistance is important for community health nursing practice. People sometimes have an ability to resist pathogens, which is called *inherent resistance*. Typically, these people have inherited or acquired characteristics, such as the various factors mentioned above, which make them less vulnerable. For instance, people who maintain a healthful lifestyle may be exposed to the flu virus but do not contract the disease. Resistance can be promoted through preventive interventions (see Levels of Prevention).

AGENT

An **agent** is a factor that causes or contributes to a health problem or condition. Causative agents can be factors that are present, such as the presence of the bacteria that causes tuberculosis, or factors that are lacking, such as a lack of iron in the body, which causes anemia.

Agents vary considerably and include five types: biologic, chemical, nutrient, physical, and psychological. Biologic agents include bacteria, viruses, fungi, protozoa, worms, and insects. Some biologic agents are infectious, such as influenza virus or HIV. Chemical agents may be in the form of liquids, solids, gases, dusts, or fumes. Examples are poisonous sprays used on garden pests and industrial chemical wastes. The degree of toxicity of the chemical agent influences its impact on health. Nutrient agents include essential dietary components, which, if deficient or taken in excess, can produce illness conditions. For example, a deficiency of niacin can cause pellagra, and too much vitamin A can be toxic. Physical agents include anything mechanical (a chainsaw or an automobile), material (rockslide), atmospheric (ultraviolet radiation); geologic (earthquake), or genetically transmitted that causes injury to humans. The shape, size, and force of physical agents influence the degree of harm to the host. Psychological agents are events producing stress that lead to health problems.

Agents may also be classified as either infectious or noninfectious. Infectious agents cause diseases, such as AIDS or tuberculosis, that are communicable—that is, the disease can be spread from one person to another. Certain characteristics of infectious agents are important for community health nurses to understand. Extent of exposure to the agent, the agent's pathogenicity (disease-causing ability), infectivity (invasive ability), virulence (severity of disease), and the infectious agent's structure and chemical composition all influence its effects on the host. (Chapter 15 examines the subject of communicable disease in greater depth.) Noninfectious agents have similar characteristics in that their relative abilities to harm the host vary with type of agent and intensity, and duration of exposure.

ENVIRONMENT

The **environment** refers to all the external factors surrounding the host that might influence vulnerability or resistance. The physical environment includes factors like geography, climate, weather, safety of buildings, and water and food supply, presence of animals, plants, insects, and microorganisms, which have the capacity to serve as reservoirs (storage sites for disease-causing agents) or vectors (carriers) for transmitting disease. The psychosocial environment refers to social, cultural, economic, and psychological influences and conditions that affect health, such as access to health care, cultural health practices, poverty, and work stressors, which can all contribute to disease or health.

Host, agent, and environment interact with each other to cause a disease or health condition. For example, the agent responsible for Lyme disease is the spirochete *Borrelia burgdorferi;* humans of all ages are susceptible hosts, along with dogs, cattle, and horses. Ticks that feed on wild rodents and deer transfer the spirochete to human hosts after feeding on them for several hours. Environmental factors, such as working or playing in tick-infested areas, influence host vulnerability. The host, agent, and environment model, shown in Figure 14–1, offered the epidemiologists who first studied

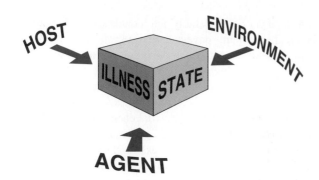

FIGURE 14–1. Epidemiologic triad. Epidemiologists study the causal agent, the susceptible host, and environmental factors that contribute to an illness state (or a wellness state). Intervention may focus on any of these three to prevent the spread of illness or to improve health in a population.

Lyme disease in 1982 a plan for intervention. As soon as the agent was identified, measures could be taken to keep the spirochete from infecting human hosts, such as wearing protective clothing or tick repellent in tick-infested areas and promptly removing surface or attached ticks (Chin, 1999).

Causality

The concept of **causality** refers to the relationship between a cause and its effect. A purpose of epidemiologic study has been to discover causal relationships in order to understand why conditions develop and offer effective prevention and protection. Over the years, as scientific knowledge of health and disease has expanded, epidemiology has changed its view of causality.

ERAS IN THE EVOLUTION OF MODERN EPIDEMIOLOGY

Modern epidemiology can be described as having three distinct eras, each based on causal thinking. They are sanitary statistics, infectious-disease epidemiology, and chronic-disease epidemiology. Eco-epidemiology, a fourth era, is emerging (Susser & Susser, 1996a).

Early causal thinking was dominated by the *miasma theory,* which had its origins in the work of the Hippocratic School and was formally developed in the early 1700s. The miasma theory held that miasma was "composed of malodorous and poisonous particles generated by the decomposition of organic matter" (Beaglehole & Bonita, 1997, p. 87) and was the cause of disease. Prevention based on this theory attempted to eliminate the sources of the miasma or polluted vapors. Despite its faulty reasoning, this type of prevention has had positive consequences in our awareness that decaying organic matter can be a source of infectious diseases. This theory dominated until the first half of the 19th century.

The era of infectious-disease epidemiology was dominated by the *contagion theory* of disease, which had developed by the mid-18th century. Prompted by the development of increasingly sophisticated microscopes, this theory attempted to identify the microorganisms that cause diseases as a first step in prevention. It inspired various theories of immunity and even some initial attempts at vaccination against smallpox. Additionally, once an agent had been identified, measures were taken to contain its spread. Fumigating ships to kill rats, protecting wharf buildings and human habitations against rats, and removing rat food supplies from easy access were all measures taken to protect the public by further preventing the spread of plague bacilli. Following the work of Jacob Henle, Louis Pasteur, and Robert Koch (Dever, 1991), the contagion theory was refined and best known as the germ theory of disease and became predominant in the late 19th century through the first half of the 20th century (Susser & Susser, 1996a).

In the era of infectious disease epidemiology, scientists viewed disease in terms of a simple cause-and-effect relationship. Finding a single cause (plague bacilli) and attacking it (eliminating rats) seemed the solution for preventing many diseases. In the case of bubonic plague, this approach appeared quite effective. However, scientific research eventually revealed that disease causation was much more complex than was first suspected. For example, although most members of a group might be exposed to the plague, many did not contract the disease. With bubonic plague, as with many other infectious diseases, the characteristics of the host can determine the spread of the disease. Not everyone in a population is at risk; it is now known that untreated bubonic plague has a case-fatality rate of only about 50% to 60%. Furthermore, the agent and course of transmission can be quite complex. Although a flea carries the bacilli from rat to human in bubonic plague, many infectious diseases spread directly from one human being to another. Finally, the environment must be considered as part of the cause of disease. Considering the plague again, evidence suggests that it originated in the high steppes of Asia and spread to other parts of the world. However, questions remain as to whether the bacillus spread from rats to ground squirrels or whether it had always been part of the squirrels' ecology.

After World War II, the causative agents of major infectious diseases were identified, methods of prevention recognized, and antibiotics and chemotherapy added to the arsenal to fight communicable diseases. The focus then became to "understand and control the new chronic disease epidemics" (Susser & Susser, 1996a, p. 670). The key figures of R. Doll, A. B. Hill, J. Morris, and T. McKeown completed case-control and cohort studies linking the causative factors of cholesterol levels and smoking with coronary heart disease and tied smoking with lung cancer. The general metaphor of a *black box* (a self-contained unit whose inner processes are hidden from view) is the associated paradigm with this era; it relates exposure to outcome without obligation to interpolate intervening factors or pathogenesis. Just as in earlier

TABLE 14–1. Eras in the Evolution of Modern Epidemiology

Era	Paradigm	Analytic Approach	Prevention Approach
Sanitary statistics (1800–1850)	Miasma: poisoning from foul emanations	Clustering of morbidity and mortality	Drainage, sewage, sanitation
Infectious disease epidemiology (1850–1950)	Germ theory: single agent related to specific disease	Laboratory isolation and culture from disease sites and reproduce lesions	Interrupt transmission (vaccines, isolation, and antibiotics)
Chronic disease epidemiology (1950–2000)	Black box: exposure related to outcome	Risk ratio of exposure to outcome at individual level in populations	Control risk factors by modifying lifestyle (diet), agent (guns), or environment (pollution)
Eco-epidemiology (emerging)	Chinese boxes: relations within and between localized structures organized in a hierarchy of levels	Analysis of determinants and outcomes at different levels of organization using new information systems and biomedical techniques	Apply both information and biomedical technology to find leverage at efficacious levels

Adapted from Susser, M., & Susser, E. (1996). Choosing a future for epidemiology: 1. Eras and paradigms. *American Journal of Public Health, 86* [5], 668–673; and Susser, M., & Susser, E. [1996b]. Choosing a future for epidemiology: II. From black box to Chinese boxes and eco-epidemiology. *American Journal of Public Health, 86* [5], 674–677.)

eras, epidemiologists are faced once more with major mortal diseases of completely unknown origin.

We are entering a new era of eco-epidemiology distinguished by the inclusion of systems at different levels and inclusion of the two factors of transforming global health patterns and technological advances (Susser & Susser, 1996b). This paradigm is called *Chinese boxes*. First, there is a transformation in global health patterns. The HIV epidemic is a good example.

> The causative organism as well as the critical risk factors are known, yet we are failing to control the disease because of our lack of understanding of transmission and illness in the social context. We know which social behaviors need to change, but we know little about how to change them, even when entire societies are at stake (Susser & Susser, 1996a).

This is true for many current chronic diseases. How many nurses smoke? Do you exercise as you know you should? What are we missing to effectively change social behaviors?

The second factor is technology. Developments in technology will drive research primarily in biology and biomedical techniques and in the information system capabilities. For example, possibilities now exist through DNA studies to recognize both viral and genetic components in insulin-dependent diabetes (Solimena & De Camilli, 1995); track HIV, tuberculosis, and other infections from person to person through molecular specificity of the organisms (Alland et al., 1994); and track and mark the first breast cancer gene (Hall et al., 1990). The possibilities of learning through technology have just begun as we enter this fourth epidemiologic era. Table 14–1 summarizes the four eras in the evolution of modern epidemiology.

CHAIN OF CAUSATION

As the scientific community's thinking about disease causation has grown more complex around the tripartite model of host, agent, and environment, epidemiologists have used the idea of a chain of causation (Fig. 14–2). The chain begins by identifying the reservoir (ie, where the causal agent can live and multiply). With plague, that reservoir may be other humans, rats, squirrels, and a few other animals. With malaria, infected humans are the major reservoir for the parasitic agents, although certain nonhuman primates also act as reservoirs (Chin, 1999). Next, the agent must have a portal of exit from the reservoir as well as some mode of transmission. For example, the bite of an *Anopheles* mosquito provides a portal of exit for the parasites, which spend part of their life cycle in the mosquito's body, which thus acts as a mode of transmission. The next link in the chain of causation is the agent itself. Malaria, for instance, actually consists of four distinct diseases caused by four kinds of microscopic protozoa. The next link is the portal of entry. In the case of malaria, the mosquito bite provides a portal of exit as well as a portal of entry into the human host.

The box surrounding this chain of causation in Figure 14–2 represents the environment, which can have a profound influence at almost any point along the chain. Consider the impact of environmental factors in the malaria epidemic of Ceylon in the Indian Ocean off southern India in 1934 to 1935. Historically, malaria occurred frequently in the dry northern area where sparse vegetation allowed pools of water to be exposed to the sun, providing excellent breeding grounds for the *Anopheles* mosquito. In contrast, the more populous southwestern area usually had heavy monsoon rains and was relatively free from malaria. In 1934, however, a severe drought changed this environment drastically;

Environment

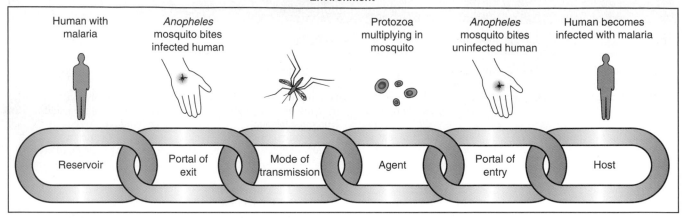

FIGURE 14–2. Chain of causation in infectious disease.

throughout Ceylon, rivers almost dried up, leaving stagnant pools of water for mosquito breeding. Widespread crop failure caused the population to become badly undernourished, which added to the conditions that would foster a malaria epidemic. The epidemic hit in October 1934, affecting 2 to 3 million people and causing 80,000 deaths. The environment must certainly be seen as a major part of this causal chain (Burnet, 1962). A similar tragedy occurred in the African country of Rwanda in July of 1994. Civil war caused a large percentage of the population to flee an unfriendly regime. Hundreds of thousands of people filled refugee camps to overflowing. Conditions of squalor and poor sanitation led to contaminated water and resulted in a large-scale epidemic of cholera, a severe form of bacterial dysentery. Relief workers had limited supplies of intravenous or oral rehydration solutions and could do little to help. Uncounted thousands lost their lives. The unstable political environment, unsanitary conditions, and malnourishment were all part of the causal chain.

MULTIPLE CAUSATION

A more advanced concept of multiple causation has emerged to explain the existence of health and illness states and to provide guiding principles for epidemiologic practice (Dever, 1991). Sometimes discussed as a "web of causation," this model attempts to identify all the possible influences on the health and illness processes (Friedman, 1994). Figure 14–3 shows the web of causation for myocardial infarction; such a health problem cannot be explained in single causal terms, even if that cause represents part of a larger chain. Recognition of multiple causes provides many points of intervention for prevention, health promotion, and treatment. For example, examination of Figure 14–3 suggests interventions such as directly attacking significant coronary atherosclerosis (bypass surgery), reducing the incidence of obesity, helping people stop smoking, developing an exercise program, and making dietary modifications. Figure 14–4 depicts the web of causation for infant mortality. Data from birth and death certificates were used to identify the complex interactions

among multicausal factors that produced a negative health condition leading to infant mortality.

A concept helpful in determining multiple causality is *association*. Events are associated when they appear together more often than they would appear by chance alone. These events may include risk factors or other characteristics affecting disease or health states. Examples are the frequent association of cigarette smoking with lung cancer, obesity with heart disease, or severe prematurity with infant mortality. Thus, study of frequently appearing associated factors suggests possible causality and points for intervention. Contemporary epidemiologists continue to explore new and more comprehensive ways of viewing health and illness. Lifestyle, behavior, environment, and stress of all kinds affect health states.

In the model of host, agent, and environment, one can note a shifting emphasis over time. Early epidemiologists worked to identify and manage the causative agent; the focus of concern was disease states. The emphasis then shifted to the host. Who was susceptible? What characteristics led to susceptibility? Through immunization and health promotion, efforts were made to improve hosts' resistance. Increasingly, however, community health workers have come to realize the limitations imposed on individual control of health. Even those in the best of health cannot withstand toxic agents in the workplace, nuclear wastes in the atmosphere from power plant accidents, or other debilitating conditions created by modern society. More and more, public health professionals are turning to a study of the environment and looking for methods to change environmental conditions that contribute to illness.

Immunity

The concept of **immunity** refers to the host's ability to resist a particular infectious disease-causing agent. This occurs when the body forms antibodies and lymphocytes that react with the foreign antigenic molecules and render them harm-

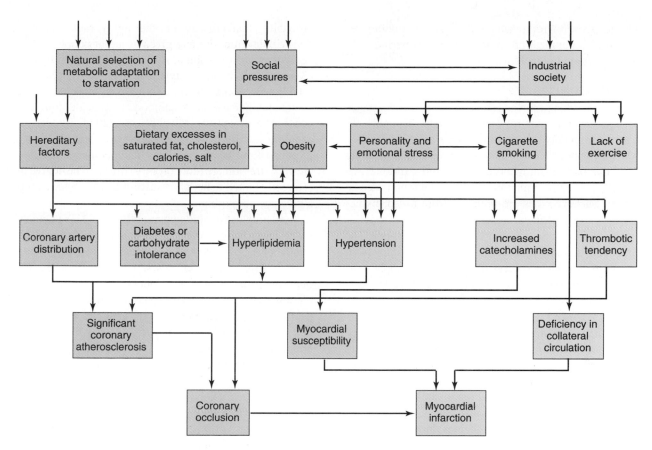

FIGURE 14–3. Web of causation for myocardial infarction. (Adapted from Friedman, G. D. [1987]. *Primer of epidemiology.* New York: McGraw-Hill. Reprinted by permission.)

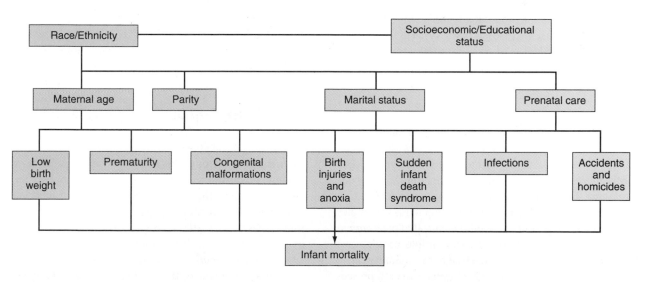

FIGURE 14–4. A web of causation for infant mortality, based on information available from birth and death certificates. (From Anderson, C. T., & McFarlane, J. [2000]. *Community as partner.* [3rd ed.]. Philadelphia: Lippincott Williams & Wilkins.)

less. For community health nursing, this concept has significance in determining which individuals and groups are protected against disease and which may be vulnerable. Four types of immunity are important in community health. They are passive, active, cross, and herd immunity.

PASSIVE IMMUNITY

Passive immunity refers to short-term resistance that is acquired either naturally or artificially. Newborns, through maternal antibody transfer, have natural passive immunity lasting about 6 months. Artificial passive immunity is attained through inoculation with a vaccine that gives temporary resistance. Such immunizations must be repeated periodically to maintain immunity levels.

ACTIVE IMMUNITY

Active immunity is long-term and sometimes lifelong resistance that is acquired either naturally or artificially. Naturally acquired active immunity comes through host infection. That is, a person who contracts a disease often develops long-lasting antibodies that provide immunity against future exposure. Artificially acquired active immunity is attained through vaccine inoculation. Such vaccines are prepared from killed, living-attenuated, or living-virulent organisms administered to artificially produce or increase immunity to a particular disease. The concept of active immunity underlies public health immunization programs that have successfully kept polio, diphtheria, smallpox, and other major diseases under control worldwide.

CROSS IMMUNITY

Cross immunity refers to a situation in which a person's immunity to one agent provides that person with immunity to another related agent. The immunity can be either passive or active. Sometimes, infection with one disease, such as cowpox, gives immunity to a related disease, such as smallpox. The concept of cross immunity has also been useful in the development and administration of vaccines. Inoculation using a vaccine made from one disease organism can provide immunity to a related disease-causing organism. Field trials in Uganda and Papua, New Guinea, and a study in India are exploring the administration of bacille Calmette-Guérin (BCG) vaccine, used to prevent tuberculosis, to people who have been exposed to Hansen's disease (leprosy). This appears to provide them with a degree of cross immunity to the related infectious agent, *Mycobacterium leprae,* and prevents their contracting the disease (Chin, 1999).

HERD IMMUNITY

Herd immunity describes the immunity level present in a population group (Chin, 1999). A population with low herd immunity is one that has few immune members and is consequently more susceptible to the disease. Nonimmune people are more likely to contract the disease and spread it throughout the group, placing the entire population at greater risk. Conversely, high herd immunity means that the immune people in the group outnumber the susceptible people, thus reducing the incidence of disease. High herd immunity (80% or more) provides the population with greater overall protection because nonimmune people are at less risk of disease exposure. Mandatory preschool immunizations and required travel vaccinations are applications of the herd immunity concept.

Risk

To determine the chances that a disease or health problem will occur, epidemiologists are concerned with **risk** or the probability that a disease or other unfavorable health condition will develop. For any given group of people, risk of developing a health problem is directly influenced by their biology, environment, lifestyle, and the system of health care. Situations or factors in these four areas can negatively affect health and increase the likelihood that a health problem will occur. These negative influences are called *risk factors.* For example, low-birth-weight babies (health status) tend to be at greater risk for health problems, and people whose lifestyles are very stressful are more prone to illness. The degree of risk is directly linked to people's susceptibility or vulnerability to a given health problem.

Epidemiologists study populations at risk. A population at risk means a collection of people among whom a health problem has the possibility of developing because certain influencing factors are either present (such as exposure to HIV) or absent (such as lack of childhood immunizations). A population at risk has a greater probability of developing a given health problem than other groups. Epidemiologists measure this difference using relative risk ratio, which statistically compares the disease occurrence in the population at risk with the occurrence of the same disease in people without that risk factor.

$$\text{Relative Risk Ratio} = \frac{\text{Incidence in Exposed Group}}{\text{Incidence in Unexposed Group}}$$

The risk is the same for both groups if the relative risk ratio is 1:1. When the ratio is greater than 1:0, the exposed group is at greater risk. An example is the difference between the incidence of heart disease among smokers (risk factor) as compared with the incidence of heart disease among nonsmokers. Relative risk ratio assists in determining the most effective points for community health intervention with health problems.

Natural History of Disease or Health Condition

Any disease or health condition follows a progression known as its **natural history;** this refers to events preceding its development, during its course, and during its conclusion. This process involves the interaction among host, agent, and environment. The natural progression of a disease occurs in four stages as they affect a population. They are susceptibility, exposure, onset, and culmination (Fig. 14–5).

1. In the *susceptibility stage,* also called the *stage of prepathogenesis,* the disease is not present nor have individuals been exposed. However, host and environment factors could very likely influence people's susceptibility to a causative agent and lead to development of the disease. For example, in 1994 the overcrowded conditions and poor sanitation of Rwandan refugee camps in Africa (described earlier), as well as refugees' stress, fatigue, and malnutrition, made them extremely vulnerable to contracting cholera and other diseases. However, in a later tragedy in Kosovo (1999), the thousands of refugees

Susceptibility	Exposure	Onset	Culmination
Host and environment factors influence population's vulnerability.	Invasion by causative agent; people are asymptomatic.	Disease or condition evident in population.	Disease or condition concludes in renewed health, disability, or death.

| Primary | Secondary | Tertiary |
| Prevention | Prevention | Prevention |

FIGURE 14–5. Natural history stages of a disease or health condition.

fleeing for their lives from Yugoslavian Serbs were housed in refugee border camps with adequate supplies and services, and many found temporary or permanent refuge in other countries, including the United States. They entered a shorter period of stress and fatigue with better nutrition than for those in Rwanda; thus, malnutrition was not as rampant. Because improved conditions in refugee camps eliminated major outbreaks of cholera and other diseases, susceptibility to disease as a group was reduced. Nevertheless, the psychological trauma from the attempts at "ethnic cleansing" of the people in Kosovo remains an existing health problem.

2. The *exposure stage* occurs when individuals have been exposed but are asymptomatic. This stage has also been called *early pathogenesis* because the disease is present in an early form and has begun its work. Vulnerable children who have been exposed to chickenpox (varicella) but do not yet display signs of fever or lesions are an example.

3. During the *onset stage,* signs and symptoms of the disease or condition develop. In the early phase of this period, the signs may only be evident through laboratory tests, such as tubercular lesions on x-ray or premalignant cervical changes evident on Pap smears. Later in this stage, acute symptoms are clearly visible, as in the case of widespread enterocolitis in a salmonellosis (food poisoning) outbreak. Other names for this stage are the *clinical stage* or *early discernible lesions stage* because evidence of the disease or condition is now present.

4. In the *culmination stage,* the disease or health condition is fully advanced and concludes either in a return to health, a residual or chronic form with some disabling limitations, or death. This is also called the *advanced disease stage* because the disease or condition has completed its course. Community health nurses can intervene at any point during these four stages to delay, arrest, or prevent the progress of the disease or condition. Primary, secondary, and tertiary prevention can be applied to the stages (see Levels of Prevention).

Epidemiology of Wellness

The public health science of epidemiology has traditionally studied the occurrence of disease and health problems. Because of their devastating effect on the health of populations, infectious diseases like plague, cholera, and AIDS as well as chronic illnesses like heart disease and cancer and fatal or debilitating injuries all require a continued epidemiologic focus. Nonetheless, the need to examine the epidemiology of wellness grows increasingly urgent.

Epidemiology has moved from concentrating only on illness to examining how host, agent, and environment are involved in wellness at various levels. In response to an escalating need for improved methods for health planning and health policy analysis, epidemiology has developed more holistic models of health. These newer epidemiologic models are organized around four attributes that influence health: (1) the physical, social, and psychological environment, (2) lifestyle with its self-created risks, (3) human biology and genetic influences, and (4) the system of health care organization (Blum, 1981; Dever, 1991). In the United States, establishment of health objectives for the year 2010 (U.S. Department of Health and Human Services, 2000) and greater recognition of the importance and cost-effectiveness of illness prevention and health promotion are driving new efforts at developing policy and research initiatives for public health.

Wellness models that at first focused on individual behavior now include approaches that encompass aggregates. Such a model was used by nurse researchers to study the substance-abuse pandemic (Talashek, Gerace & Starr, 1994). Societal changes, such as the growing elderly population, communication revolution, global economy, environmental threats, technology development, holism and wellness movements, are driving these new approaches.

The natural history stages of disease can apply to one's understanding of any health condition, including wellness states. In stage one, susceptibility, people can become amenable to healthier practices and improved health system organization. In stage two, exposure, a community can learn about these health-promoting behaviors. Stage three, onset, could be a period of trying out the beneficial policies and activities, and stage four, culmination, could be full adoption and a higher level of well-being for the community. This fact has important implications for community health nursing preventive and health promotive practice.

Community health nursing can play a primary role in the investigation and identification of factors that not only prevent illness but also promote health. This means sharpening skills in epidemiologic research to uncover the factors that contribute to a full measure of healthful living. The time for an epidemiology of wellness has come.

Causal Relationships

One of the main challenges to epidemiology is to identify causal relationships in disease and health conditions in

LEVELS OF PREVENTION

PREVENTION DURING NATURAL HISTORY STAGES OF DISEASE

GOAL

Because the events leading to a disease or health condition generally develop over time, there are a number of instances where preventive measures can alter or stop their progress. Community health nurses have a prime opportunity to apply the three levels of prevention—primary, secondary, and tertiary—discussed in Chapter 1—to the natural history progression of a health condition

PRIMARY PREVENTION

Primary prevention, which keeps a health problem from ever occurring, can be applied in both the susceptibility and exposure stages. Susceptible and exposed people are at risk. The number and type of risk factors can be eradicated or reduced through health promotion and protection measures. Health promotion measures might include nutritional counseling, sex education, and smoking cessation. Protective measures might address such areas as improved housing and sanitation, immunizations, and removal of environmental hazards.

Public health efforts using primary prevention have been very successful in reducing disease occurrence with its associated mortality and morbidity. This can be attributed, in particular, to mandatory immunization programs and environmental management.

SECONDARY PREVENTION

Secondary prevention seeks to find and treat existing health problems as early as possible. Secondary prevention measures are used to address the third stage in the natural history of disease, the onset stage, through early detection, diagnosis, and timely treatment. When an illness exists, screening programs can detect such conditions as breast and testicular cancer, hypertension, hearing problems, tuberculosis, and diabetes. Screening tests and early case-finding provide opportunities to diagnose and treat conditions in the early stage of the disease or illness condition's progress. The aim of secondary prevention is to remove the health problem, cure the disease, or at least arrest its progression and prevent associated disability.

TERTIARY PREVENTION

Tertiary prevention seeks to reduce the extent and severity of a health problem in order to minimize disability and restore or preserve function. This level addresses the culmination stage of the natural history of disease process. At this stage, the health condition is advanced; thus, tertiary preventive measures include treatment to arrest further progression of the disease and rehabilitative efforts to limit disability. At the aggregate level, an example of tertiary prevention is providing food, shelter, health services, and training for employment with a homeless population. Another example is group treatment and rehabilitation for adolescent drug users.

Community health nurses apply all three levels of prevention but concentrate their efforts especially on the primary and secondary levels.

populations. As has been suggested in previous sections, the assessment of causality in human health is difficult at best; no single study is adequate to establish causality. Causal inference is based on consistent results obtained from many studies. Frequently, the accumulation of evidence begins with a clinical observation or an educated guess that a certain factor may be causally related to a health problem. A **cross-sectional study** (exploring a health condition's relationship to other variables in a specified population at a certain point in time) can show that the factor and problem coexist. An example is a study of never smokers, former smokers, and current smokers to examine the association of smoking with facial wrinkling (Ernster, Grady, Miike, Black, Selby & Kerlikowske, 1995). Results of the study showed that risk of facial wrinkling was greater in cigarette smokers than in never smokers. A **retrospective study** (looking backward in time to find a causal relationship) allows a fairly quick assessment of whether an association exists. Nonepidemiologic animal studies may suggest a biologic mechanism whereby the factor could cause the disease or condition. At this point, a **prospective study** (looking forward in time to find a causal relationship) is crucial to ensure that the presumed causal factor actually antedates the onset of the health problem. The prospective approach is concerned with current information and provides a direct measure of the variables in question. Finally, if ethically possible, an **experimental study** (in which the investigator controls or changes factors suspected of causing the condition and observes results) is used to confirm the associations obtained from the observational studies. Thus, it often requires many years to accumulate enough evidence to suggest a causal relationship.

Epidemiologically, one can accept that a causal relationship may exist when two major conditions are met: (1) the factor of interest (causal agent) is shown to increase the probability of occurrence of the disease or condition as observed in many studies in different populations, and (2) there is evidence that a reduction in the factor decreases the frequency of the given disease. The synthesis of data begins by selecting as many as possible of all the various types of epidemiologic studies on the problem. After discarding those studies that are not methodologically sound, the studies are reviewed. The better the data meet the following six criteria, the more likely the factor of interest will be one of several causes of the disease:

1. Temporal relationship: Exposure to the suspected factor must precede the onset of disease.
2. Strength of the association: This refers to the ratio of disease rates in those with and without the suspected causal factor. A strong association would be noted when disease rates are much higher in the group with the factor than in the group without it.
3. Dose–response relationship: This relationship is demonstrated if, with increasing levels of exposure to the factor, there is a corresponding increase in occurrence of disease.

4. Consistency: Association is demonstrated in varying types of studies among diverse study groups.
5. Biologic plausibility and coherence of the evidence: The hypothesized cause makes sense based on current biologic knowledge.
6. Lowering of disease risk: Interventions that decrease the exposure or factor result in a lowering of disease risk (relative risk).

The goal of any epidemiologic investigation is to identify causal mechanisms that meet the above criteria and to develop measures for preventing illness and promoting health. The community health nurse may need to gather new data for this type of investigation but should thoroughly examine existing, pertinent data before doing so. This type of information can be obtained by the community health nurse from a variety of sources, discussed in the next section.

SOURCES OF INFORMATION FOR EPIDEMIOLOGIC STUDY

Epidemiologic investigators may draw data from three major sources or a combination of these sources. They are (1) existing data, (2) informal investigations, and (3) scientific studies. The community health nurse will find all three sources useful in efforts to improve the health of aggregates.

Existing Data

A variety of information is available nationally, by states, and by sections, such as counties, regions, or urbanized areas. This information includes vital statistics, census data, and morbidity statistics on certain communicable or infectious diseases. Local health departments often can provide these data on request. Community health nurses seeking information on nearby communities may find local health system agencies helpful. These agencies work to collect health information for groups of counties within states and interact with health planning authorities at the state level. They have access to many types of information and can give advice on specific problems raised by nurses.

VITAL STATISTICS
Vital statistics is a term used for the information gathered from ongoing registration of "vital" events relating to births, deaths, adoptions, divorces, and marriages. Certification of births, deaths, and fetal deaths are the vital statistics most useful in epidemiologic study. The community health nurse can obtain blank copies of a state's birth and death certificates to become familiar with the information contained in each. It will become apparent that much more information is recorded than the fact and cause of death on the death cer-

tificate. Birth certificates also can provide helpful information. For example, the weights of infants and the amount of prenatal care received by their mothers have been used to identify high-risk mothers and infants.

CENSUS DATA
Data from population censuses taken every 10 years in many countries are the main source of population statistics. This information can be a valuable assessment tool for the community health nurse taking part in health planning for aggregates. These population statistics can be analyzed by age, sex, race, ethnic background, type of occupation, income gradient, marital status, or educational level, as well as by other standards, such as housing. Analysis of population statistics can provide the community health nurse with a better understanding of the community and help identify specific areas that may warrant further epidemiologic investigation.

REPORTABLE DISEASES
Each state has developed laws or regulations that require health organizations and practitioners to report to their local health authority cases of certain communicable and infectious diseases that can be spread through the community (Chin, 1999). This reporting enables the health department to take the most appropriate and efficient action. All states require that the diseases subject to international quarantine regulations be reported immediately. These diseases (plague, cholera, yellow fever, and smallpox) are virtually unknown now in developed countries. The World Health Organization announced the global eradication of smallpox in 1980 after more than 10 years of international effort (The World Health Report, 1998). In addition, there are numerous diseases under surveillance by the World Health Organization (eg, louse-borne typhus fever and relapsing fever, paralytic poliomyelitis, malaria, and viral influenza), and these must be reported. The other reportable diseases (varying between 20 and 40 by state) are usually classified according to the speed with which the health department should be notified. Some should be reported by phone or electronic mail, others weekly by regular mail. They vary in potential severity from chickenpox to rabies and include AIDS, encephalitis, meningitis, syphilis, and toxic shock syndrome. Community health nurses should obtain the list of reportable diseases from their local or state health department offices. Following up on occurrences of these diseases is a task frequently assigned to community nursing services.

DISEASE REGISTRIES
In some areas or states, there are disease registries or rosters for conditions with major public health impact. Tuberculosis and rheumatic fever registries were more common in past years when these diseases occurred more frequently. Cancer registries provide useful incidence, prevalence, and survival data and assist the community health nurse in monitoring cancer patterns within a community.

ENVIRONMENTAL MONITORING

State governments, sometimes through health departments and sometimes through other agencies, now monitor health hazards found in the environment. Pesticides, industrial wastes, radioactive or nuclear materials, chemical additives in food, and medicinal drugs have joined the list of pollutants (see Chapter 16 for detailed discussion). Concerned community members and leaders view these as risk factors that affect health at both the community and individual levels. Community health nurses can also obtain data from federal agencies such as the Food and Drug Administration, the Consumer Product Safety Commission, and the Environmental Protection Agency.

NATIONAL CENTER FOR HEALTH STATISTICS HEALTH SURVEYS

On the national level (published data are frequently available also for regions), the National Center for Health Statistics (NCHS) furnishes valuable health prevalence data from surveys of Americans (Scutchfield & Keck, 1997). The Health Interview Survey includes interviews from approximately 40,000 households each year and provides information about the health status and needs of the entire country. The Health Examination Survey reports physical measurements on smaller samples of the population and augments the information provided by interviews. This survey provides prevalence information on injuries, diseases, and disabilities that appear frequently in the population. A third type of NCHS survey is of health records. This survey samples institutional records of hospitals and nursing homes, primarily. This survey provides information on those who are using services from these institutions along with diagnoses and other characteristics. Other NCHS surveys focus on fertility and family planning, follow back studies on vital statistics events, and characteristics of ambulatory patients in physicians' community practices.

Each of these nationally sponsored efforts suggests ways in which community health nurses can examine health problems or concerns affecting their communities. Interviews, physical examinations of samples of community members, and surveillance of institutions, clinics, and private physicians' practices can be carried out locally when needs are identified and funds made available. Other sources may be found in data kept routinely but not centrally on the health problems of workers in local industry or health problems of schoolchildren, a key issue to many community health nurses. Existing epidemiologic data can be used to plan parent education programs, health promotion among students, and almost any other type of service.

Informal Observational Studies

A second information source in epidemiologic study comes through informal observation and description. Almost any client group encountered by the community health nurse can trigger such a study. If, for example, the nurse encounters an abused child at a clinic, screening the clinic's records for possible further instances of child abuse and neglect could lead to more case finding. If several cases of diabetes come to the attention of a nurse serving on a Navajo reservation, a widespread problem might come to light through conducting informal inquiries about the incidence and age of onset of the disease among this Native American population. A nurse working with several elderly widows living alone learned by questioning them that being independent was secondary to staying in their own homes. Interview data revealed that these older widows had learned to accept their aloneness, exercised freedom and delegation in getting things done, practiced safety measures, and took good care of themselves, thus enabling them to continue to live at home (Porter, 1994). Collecting such information, complemented with existing data, could lead to improved understanding and service to the broader population of elderly widows living alone. Informal observational study often raises questions and suggests hypotheses that form the basis for designing larger-scale epidemiologic investigations.

Scientific Studies

The third source of information used in epidemiologic inquiry involves carefully designed scientific studies. Nursing, as a profession, has recognized the need to develop a systematic body of knowledge on which to base nursing practice. Already, systematic research is becoming an accepted part of the community health nurse's role. Findings from epidemiologic studies conducted by or involving nurses are appearing more frequently in the literature. For example, concern about a large number of infant injuries led a nurse and physician research team to study sociodemographic and psychosocial risk factors causing unintentional infant injuries in the home (Harris & Kotch, 1994). They learned that family conflict and maternal unemployment were among predictors for unintentional injury. They also learned that use of social support to alleviate maternal stress resulted in fewer unintentional infant injuries. In another study, conducted in Baltimore, Maryland, researchers examined whether interventions aimed at aggressive and disruptive classroom behavior and poor academic achievement would also reduce the incidence of smoking initiation (Kellam & Anthony, 1998). An epidemiologically based, universal randomized preventive study involved 2,311 boys in two classroom-based interventions or controls. Each intervention was directed at one of the aforementioned two antecedents over first and second grades in 19 urban Baltimore schools. Smoking initiation was reduced in both cohorts for boys at final assessment age of 14 who were assigned to the behavioral intervention. The researchers concluded that targeting early risk antecedents such as aggressive behavior appears to be an important smoking-prevention strategy. Systematic studies such as these, as well as informal studies and existing epidemiologic data, can provide the community health nurse with valuable information that can be used to positively affect aggregate health.

METHODS IN THE EPIDEMIOLOGIC INVESTIGATIVE PROCESS

The goal of epidemiologic investigation is to identify the causal mechanisms of health and illness states and to develop measures for preventing illness and promoting health. Epidemiologists employ an investigative process that involves a sequence of three approaches that build on one another: descriptive, analytic, and experimental studies. All three approaches have relevance for community health nursing.

Descriptive Epidemiology

Descriptive epidemiology includes investigations that seek to observe and describe patterns of health-related conditions that naturally occur in a population. For example, a community health nurse might seek to learn how many children in a school district have been immunized for measles, how many home births occur each year in the county, or how many cases of STDs have occurred in the city in the past month. At this stage in the epidemiologic investigation, one seeks to establish the occurrence of a problem. Data from descriptive studies suggest hypotheses for further testing. Descriptive studies almost always involve some form of broad-based quantification and statistical analysis.

COUNTS

The simplest measure of description is a count. For example, an epidemiologic study of childhood drownings was conducted to provide data for prevention efforts in Harris County, Texas (Warneke & Cooper, 1994). One of the first steps in the research was to make a simple count of the number of child and adolescent (newborn through 19 years) drownings that occurred. The investigators gathered data from death certificates (1983 through 1989) and medical examiner data (1983 through 1990); most of the 196 unintentional drownings occurred in swimming pools, half of which were in apartment complexes and a third of which were in private homes (Fig. 14–6). Obtaining a count of this type always depends on the definition of what one counts. This count, for example, does not represent all drownings occurring in the county, but only those in this age group. As in most kinds of research, availability of data influences the count. Before making use of any statistics, whether from official state offices, the Census Bureau, or a health agency, it is necessary to determine what the information represents.

RATES

Rates are a statistical measure expressing the proportion of people with a given health problem among a population at

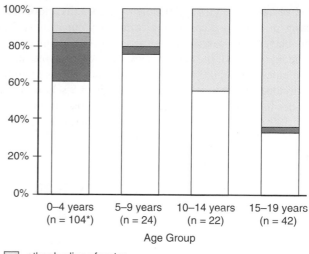

FIGURE 14–6. Percentage distribution for location of submersion, by age group, for unintentional drownings that, according to medical examiner files, occurred in Harris County, Texas, 1983 through 1990, among persons newborn through 19 years. (Warneke & Cooper, 1994, p. 595. Reprinted by permission.)

risk. The total number of people in this group serves as the denominator for various types of rates. To express a count as a proportion, or rate, one must first decide on the population to be studied. If 196 drownings are considered in relation to the total number of children in Harris County, there will be one rate; if they are considered in relation to the total population of children in the state, there will be a different proportion.

In epidemiology, the population represents the universe of people defined as the objects of one's study. Because it is often difficult, if not impossible, to study an entire population, most epidemiologic studies draw a sample to represent that group. For example, in the Baltimore study dealing with behavioral interventions that decrease smoking initiation, the investigators selected a random sample of 2,311 children in 19 classrooms to include as study subjects or controls out of a much larger urban school population (Kellam & Anthony, 1998). Sometimes, it is important to seek a random sample (when everyone in the population has an equal chance of selection for study and choice is made without bias); at other times, a sample of convenience (when study subjects are selected because of their availability) is sufficient. In many small epidemiologic studies, it may be possible to study nearly every person in the population, thus eliminating the need for a sample.

Several proportions have wide use in epidemiology. Those most important for the community health nurse to understand include prevalence rate, period prevalence rate, and incidence rate.

Prevalence refers to all people with a health condition existing in a given population at a given point in time. The prevalence rate describes a situation at one point in time (Friedman, 1994). If a nurse discovers 50 cases of measles in an elementary school, that is a simple count. If that number is divided by the number of students in the school, it describes the prevalence of measles. For instance, if the school has 500 students, the prevalence of measles on that day would be 10% (50 measles/500 population).

$$\text{Prevalence Rate} = \frac{\text{Number of Persons}}{\text{Total Number in Population}}$$

In the study of reported drownings, on the other hand, the investigators had a count for a 7-year period, 1983 to 1990. Rather than portraying only one day, this number covered an extended period of time. Calculating the prevalence rate over a period of time is called a period prevalence rate.

$$\text{Period Prevalence Rate} = \frac{\text{Number of Persons With a Characteristic During a Period of Time}}{\text{Total Number in Population}}$$

Not everyone in a population is at risk for developing a disease, incurring an injury, or having some other health-illness characteristic. The incidence rate recognizes this fact. **Incidence** refers to all new cases of a disease or health condition appearing during a given time. Incidence rate describes a proportion in which the numerator is all new cases appearing during a given time and the denominator is the population at risk during the same period of time. For example, some childhood diseases give lifelong immunity. The children in a school who have had such diseases would be removed from the total number of children at risk in the school population. The incidence rate, after 3 weeks of a measles epidemic in a school, was

$$\frac{200}{1000} \text{ or } \frac{200 \text{ New Cases}}{1000 \text{ Persons at Risk}}$$

during the 3-week time period. The health literature is not always consistent in the use of the term *incidence;* sometimes, this word is used synonymously with *prevalence rates,* and the reader must take this into consideration.

$$\text{Incidence Rate} = \frac{\text{Number of Persons Developing a Disease}}{\text{Total Number at Risk per Unit of Time}}$$

Another rate describing incidence is called an attack rate. An *attack rate* describes the proportion of a group or population that develops a disease among all those exposed to a particular risk. This term is used frequently in investigations of outbreaks of infectious diseases such as influenza. When the attack rate changes, it may suggest an alteration in the population's immune status or that the disease-causing organism is present in a more or less virulent strain.

COMPUTING RATES

To make comparisons between populations, epidemiologists often use a common base population in computing rates. For example, instead of merely saying that the rate of an illness is 13% in one city and 25% in another, the comparison is made per 100,000 people in the population. This population base can vary for different purposes from 100 to 100,000. To describe the **morbidity rate,** which is the relative incidence of disease in a population, one would describe the ratio of the number of sick individuals to a total given population. The **mortality rate** refers to the relative death rate or the sum of deaths in a given population at a given time. Display 14–2 includes formulas for computing rates commonly used in community health.

The goal of descriptive studies is to identify the patterns of occurrence of any health-related condition. They can be retrospective (identify cases and controls, then go back to review existing data) or prospective (identify groups and exposure factors and follow them forward in time). In a descriptive study of child abuse, for example, the investigator would note the age, sex, race or ethnic group, and physical and emotional conditions of the children affected. In addition, data would be collected that described the economic status and occupation of parents, the location and setting of abusive behavior, and the time and season of the year when abuse occurred. In the study on reported drownings in Harris County, Texas (retrospective design), the investigators described the age, sex, and ethnic background of victims and other features such as location and time of drowning. Describing facets of these health conditions provided information for further study as well as suggested avenues for intervention or prevention.

Analytic Epidemiology

A second type of epidemiologic investigation is analytic. **Analytic epidemiology** goes beyond simple description or observation and seeks to identify associations between a particular human disease or health problem and its possible cause(s). Analytic studies tend to be more specific than descriptive studies in their focus. They test hypotheses or seek to answer specific questions and can be retrospective or prospective in design. For example, in a prospective analytic study, several nurses set out to address the question, are paper diapers more effective in controlling fecal contamination than cloth diapers in a day care environment? The nurses studied children and providers in four licensed day care centers in Davidson County, Tennessee (Holaday et al., 1995). A total of 104 children and 25 caregivers participated in the study over a period of 8 weeks. The centers were supplied with cloth and paper diapers, and two centers used cloth diapers for the first 4-week period while the other two used paper, each then switching to the other diaper type for the second 4-week period. The investigators monitored selected rooms twice weekly in each center for the presence of fecal bacteria by sampling of play/sleep area, diaper changing

DISPLAY 14-2. Common Epidemiologic Rates

General Mortality Rates

Crude Morality Rate =

$$\frac{\text{Number of Reported Deaths During 1 Year}}{\text{Estimated Population as of July 1 of Same Year}} \times 100,000$$

Cause-Specific Mortality Rate =

$$\frac{\text{Number of Deaths From a Stated Cause During 1 Year}}{\text{Estimated Population as of July 1 of Same Year}}$$
$$\times 100,000$$

Case Fatality Rate =

$$\frac{\text{Number of Deaths From a Particular Disease}}{\text{Total Number With the Same Disease}} \times 100$$

Proportional Mortality Ratio =

$$\frac{\begin{array}{c}\text{Number of Deaths From a Specific}\\ \text{Cause Within a TIme Period}\end{array}}{\text{Total Deaths in the Same Time Period}} \times 100$$

Age-Specific Mortality Rate =

$$\frac{\begin{array}{c}\text{Number of Persons in a Specific Age}\\ \text{Group Dying During 1 Year}\end{array}}{\begin{array}{c}\text{Estimated Population of the Specific Age}\\ \text{Group as of July 1 of Same Year}\end{array}} \times 100,000$$

Specific Rates for Maternal and Infant Populations

Crude Birth Rate =

$$\frac{\text{Number of Live Births During 1 Year}}{\text{Estimated Population as of July 1 of Same Year}} \times 1,000$$

General Fertility Rate =

$$\frac{\text{Number of Live Births During 1 Year}}{\text{Number of Females Aged 15–44 as of July 1 of Same Year}}$$
$$\times 1,000$$

Maternal Mortality Rate =

$$\frac{\text{Number of Deaths From Puerperal Causes During 1 Year}}{\text{Number of Live Births During Same Year}}$$
$$\times 100,000$$

Infant Mortality Rate =

$$\frac{\text{Number of Deaths Under 1 Year of Age for Given Year}}{\text{Number of Live Births Reported for Same Year}}$$
$$\times 1,000$$

Perinatal Mortality Rate =

$$\frac{\begin{array}{c}\text{Number of Fetal Deaths Plus Infant Deaths}\\ \text{Under 7 Days of Age During 1 Year}\end{array}}{\begin{array}{c}\text{Number of Live Births Plus Fetal Deaths}\\ \text{During Same Year}\end{array}} \times 1,000$$

---

area, and caregivers' and children's hands (Fig. 14–7). No significant differences were found between cloth and paper diapers in the frequency or intensity of fecal contamination. However, the study revealed that sink faucets and caregivers' and children's hands were often contaminated, suggesting the need for further study of handwashing and diapering techniques, use of disinfectant hand creams, and altering the environment by installing automatic, faucet-free handwashing sinks. Like many analytical studies, this one gathered a great deal of descriptive data as well.

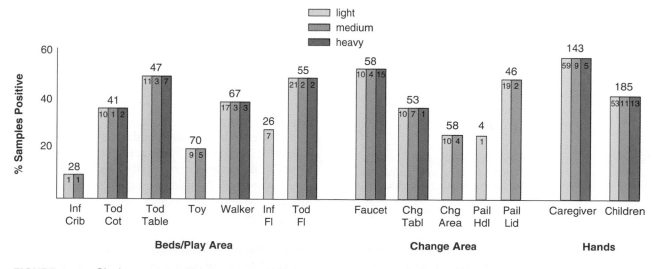

FIGURE 14–7. Cloth vs. paper diaper study. Total fecal cultures by collection site and location: percentage of positive samples from all four centers in both time periods (Holaday, et al, 1995, p. 31). Reprinted by permission. Note: Above each bar is the total number of specimens collected at each site. Within each bar is the number of positive samples that are classified as light, medium, or heavy growth. Inf crib = infant crib; tod cot = toddler cot; tod table = toddler table; inf fl = infant floor; tod fl = toddler floor; chg tabl = diaper change table; chg area = diaper change area; hdl = diaper pail handle; pail lid = diaper pail lid.

Analytic studies fall into three types: prevalence studies, case-control studies, and cohort studies.

PREVALENCE STUDIES

When one examines prevalence, it is helpful to remember that the health condition may be new or may have affected some people for many years. Prevalence studies describe patterns of occurrence, as in the study of reported drownings in Texas and in the study described in Research: Bridge to Practice. They may examine causal factors, but these are always from the same point in time and the same population. Hypothesized causal factors are based on inferences from a single examination and most likely need further testing for validation.

CASE-CONTROL STUDIES

Case-control studies make a comparison between people with a health-illness condition (cases) and those who lack this condition (controls). These studies begin with disease (case) and look back over time for presence or absence of the suspected causal factor in both cases and controls. In the study of early antecedents to prevent smoking initiation, 1,604 students remained in the Baltimore City public schools. Of that number, 700 had participated as study subjects (cases); the 904 other children not experiencing the interventions were the controls. This study then reviewed the history of cases and controls for the presence of aggressive or disruptive behavior among the 1,604 students remaining in the school system. In a case-control study, both groups should share as many characteristics as possible in order to isolate possible causes; randomly selecting first- and second-grade classrooms helps to ensure this. Comparison between

RESEARCH Bridge to Practice

Safety Belt Use After California's Primary Law

Lange, J.E. & Voas, R.B. (1998). Nighttime observations of safety belt use: An evaluation of California's primary law. *American Journal of Public Health, 88*(11), 1718–1720.

In 1993, California was the first state in the country to modify an existing safety belt law from a secondary to a primary enforcement law, meaning that not wearing a safety belt can be the only reason one is stopped by the police. Before this change, if drivers were stopped for another reason, they could also be cited for not wearing a safety belt. This study analyzed what effect this change had on safety belt use among nighttime weekend drivers. Observations were made in two California communities during voluntary roadside surveys conducted every other Friday and Saturday night from 9 PM to 2 AM for 4 years from 1991 to 1995. Over 18,4000 drivers were surveyed. Data collected over the 4 years show that rates of safety belt use rose from 73.0% to 95.6%. High-risk drivers, such as those with a blood alcohol concentration of 0.10 or higher, had rates rise from 53.4% to 92.1%. "Because substantial improvement in safety belt use was seen even in a group of high-risk drivers, the injury reduction benefits of this law may be high" (p. 1718).

one group of children in first grade with another group in their late teens would have invalidated the conclusion in a study on the effects of behavioral interventions.

COHORT STUDIES

A **cohort** is a group of people who share a common experience in a specific time period. Examples are a group of elders or the employees of an industry. In epidemiology, a cohort of people often becomes a focus of study. Cohort studies, rather than measuring the relationship of variables in existing conditions, study the development of a condition over time. A cohort study begins by selecting a group of people who display certain defined characteristics before the onset of the condition being investigated. In studying a disease, the cohort might include individuals initially free of the disease but known to have been exposed to a particular factor. They would be followed over time to evaluate what variables were associated with the development or nondevelopment of the disease. An example is the prospective study of unintentional infant injuries, mentioned earlier (Harris & Kotch, 1994). The subjects, a cohort of 367 mothers, were interviewed 6 to 8 weeks after the newborns' hospital discharge and then again approximately 1 year later. Investigators were able to identify injury predictors (family conflict and maternal unemployment) and also interventions (social support) for reducing the number of injuries.

In actual practice, the various types of studies just discussed are frequently mixed. A case-control study may include description and analysis with a retrospective focus; a cohort study may be conducted prospectively or retrospectively. The study of early antecedents to prevent tobacco smoking (Kellam & Anthony, 1998) was a case-control study, a cohort study, and an experimental study (see below). Flexibility is essential to allow the investigator as much freedom as possible in choosing the most useful methodology.

Experimental Epidemiology

Experimental epidemiology follows and builds on information gathered from descriptive and analytic approaches. It is used to study epidemics, the etiology of human disease, the value of preventive and therapeutic measures, and the evaluation of health services (Timmreck, 1998). In an experimental study, the investigator actually controls or changes the factors suspected of causing the health condition under study and observes what happens to the health state. In human populations, experimental studies should focus on disease prevention or health promotion rather than testing the causes of disease, which is done primarily on animals.

Experimental studies are carried out under carefully controlled conditions. The investigator uses an experimental group and exposes them to some factor thought to cause disease, improve health, prevent disease, or influence health in some way. Simultaneously, the investigator uses a control group that is similar in characteristics to the experimental group but without the exposure factor. An example is a study conducted by several nurses to examine the influence of case management approaches on client use of preventive child health services (Erkel, Morgan, Staples, Assey & Michel, 1994). An experimental group of infants received continuity of care provided by a single public health nurse who integrated case management and preventive services. The control group of infants received the customary pattern of services, which were fragmented and delivered by multiple public health nurses. Findings showed that continuous, integrated public health nursing case management was significantly more effective in achieving client use of preventive child health services and was also one fifth the cost of the control group's fragmented services.

The community health nurse should be alert for opportunities to conduct experimental studies in the course of working with groups. The study need not be elaborate and can provide important data for future nursing practice. For example, a study conducted in Albuquerque, New Mexico, compared 17 schoolboys with violent behavior with a control group of 27 carefully matched students (second through fifth grades) who were not overtly violent at school (Sheline, Skipper & Broadhead, 1994). Data were gathered through questionnaires completed by all students and in-home interviews with parents or guardians. Findings showed that boys from families with absent fathers, divorced parents, or numerous siblings were at higher risk for violent behavior. Lack of parental affection and expression of pride and use of spanking as discipline were parenting practices most strongly associated with violent behavior. The findings suggested the need for programs in parental education and encouragement to show affection and to use other methods of discipline. Similar experimental studies could be done with almost any small group within the community health nurse's practice.

An expanding area of experimental epidemiology involves the use of computers to simulate epidemics. With mathematical models, it is possible to determine the probability of various aspects of disease occurrence. This approach is making an increased contribution to epidemiologists' knowledge of etiology and prevention.

At present, there is a national longitudinal experimental study involving thousands of nurses called the Brigham and Women's Hospital/Harvard Medical School Women's Health Study. It consists of a randomized trial evaluating the balance of benefits and risks of low-dose aspirin and vitamin E in the prevention of cancer and cardiovascular disease. Depending on the random assignment of the nurses, participants are taking 100 mg of aspirin or placebo and 600 IU of vitamin E or placebo. Early in the study, 50 mg of beta carotene or placebo was included in the study, but findings in other studies associated additional beta carotene with a higher risk of lung cancer. It was removed from the study in the mid-1990s. This is a double-blind study (neither the participants or researchers know which subjects are taking the study drugs or placebos). Nurses were selected for this major study because, as an aggregate, they are accessible through RN registry, and it was assumed that nurses, who know the value of research, would have a higher rate of follow-through in taking the test drugs routinely than the general public. Data on the health status of the participants is gathered every 6 months, and the study is presently funded through 2001.

Occasionally, an experiment occurs naturally in which conditions offer the researcher the chance to make important discoveries. John Snow discovered such a "natural experiment" in London in 1854 (Turnock, 1997). In his seminal study of an epidemic of cholera, he observed one group that contracted the disease and another that did not. Closer inspection revealed that the major difference between these groups was their water supply. Eventually, the spread of cholera was traced to the water supply of the group with the high morbidity rate.

A *community trial* is a type of experimental study done at the community level (Timmreck, 1998). In this type of study, geographic communities are assigned to intervention (experimental) or nonintervention (control) groups and compared to determine whether the intervention produces a positive change in the community. Community trials can be extremely expensive and are not undertaken unless there is substantial evidence that the intervention will make a difference at the aggregate level.

The Minnesota Heart Health Program was one such community trial conducted in the Minneapolis/St. Paul area (Mittlemark et al., 1989). This study compared three sets of paired communities in the Upper Midwest. Each pair had one community in the intervention group and one in the nonintervention group. The intervention communities received multiple intervention techniques such as dietary instruction, smoking cessation intervention, and risk factor instruction. Myocardial infarction, stroke, and mortality rates along with other measurements were done at regular intervals to evaluate whether the interventions were improving the health in the communities that received them. Another classic example was the Kingston/Newburgh, New York, study, conducted in the 1950s in which two towns on opposite sides of a river, one whose water system was fluoridated and the other was not, compared dental records and learned that there was an association between fluoridated water and reduced dental caries. One consequence of this study was the development of fluoridated toothpaste.

CONDUCTING EPIDEMIOLOGIC RESEARCH

The community health nurse who engages in an epidemiologic investigation becomes a detective. First, there is a problem to solve, a puzzle to unravel, or a question to answer. Then, one begins to search for basic information, clues that might help answer the question. Information is never self-explanatory, and, like a detective, one must analyze and interpret every additional clue. Slowly, there is a narrowing of possible suspects until the causes of a disease, the consequences of a prevention plan, or the results of treatment are identified. On the basis of this investigation, one can then draw further conclusions and make new applications to improve health services.

As discussed previously, epidemiologic studies are a form of research. The steps outlined below are similar to those discussed in Chapter 11. Epidemiologic research involves seven steps. Both an informal study in the course of nursing practice and the most comprehensive epidemiologic research project can be undertaken with these steps:

1. Identify the problem.
2. Review the literature.
3. Design the study.
4. Collect the data.
5. Analyze the findings.
6. Develop conclusions and applications.
7. Disseminate the findings.

Each of these steps will be considered in the context of a single nursing study examining the untoward effects of in-utero drug exposure for a group of infants and children.

Identify the Problem

Community health nurses are constantly confronted with threats to the health and well-being of the community. Almost daily, questions are raised, puzzles presented, and problems identified. Pregnant women who smoke or use cocaine threaten the health of their unborn children; what can be done to reduce this behavior? Rape is increasing; what can be done to prevent such violence or to bring aid to victims? Children are injured and die from bicycle accidents; why do these occur and how can they be prevented? Many farm workers have been killed or injured in farm equipment accidents; what can be done to prevent them? Any threat to the health of a group offers fertile ground for epidemiologic investigation.

One team of nurse researchers was concerned with the untoward effects of in-utero drug exposure (IUDE) on cognitive development and health problems in infants and children (Butz et al., 1998). Intensive home-based interventions provided by registered nurses proved an effective method to improve cognitive development and reduce health problems in these high-risk infants and children, supporting the view that home visiting should be incorporated into the discharge planning of any IUDE infant.

Review the Literature

All too often, after identifying a problem, health professionals rush to take immediate action without reviewing solutions that have been tried previously. Every epidemiologic investigation should begin with a review of the literature. Even discovering that little research has been done on the problem can be valuable information. Conversely, if many studies have already been conducted on the area, this information can help narrow the study to areas not previously investigated or allow re-

searchers to replicate earlier studies to confirm findings in a different setting. One of the most valuable sources in the literature is the review article, which essentially summarizes all the research that has been conducted on a subject.

A review of the literature often suggests hypotheses from discoveries made in other studies. In the home intervention program for IUDE infants, a review of the literature did provide helpful background information; however, "home intervention studies specifically examining IUDE infants are sparse" (Butz et al., 1998, p. 308). The literature review also revealed that, when interventions were provided, they proved to be an effective method in many other settings with different populations. This assisted the researchers with this study.

Design the Study

The first step in designing a study is to formulate a specific question(s) to answer or perhaps a hypothesis to test. Sometimes, this question or hypothesis may emerge from the review of literature; at other times, it will have to be developed through the researcher's own analysis and hunches. It is a good idea to write out one or more hypotheses to test or questions to answer. The researchers in the IUDE infants study formulated several research questions, which led to a conceptual model for the study that used "a home-based nurse intervention focused on the mother and infant and aimed to reduce infant morbidity" (Butz et al., 1998, p. 308).

The next step is to plan what type or combination of study types will best suit the goals of the research (descriptive, analytic, or experimental) and how the study will be conducted. Will the data be collected retrospectively from existing records, or will new data be collected? Who will conduct interviews? What kinds of data will be needed to measure the outcomes of intervention?

The IUDE infants study was part of a larger, randomized clinical trial, which included 204 mother–infant dyads. This study reported analysis of home visit data for the first 20 enrolled infants and their mothers, and they received a total of 229 home visits.

Collect the Data

Data in the IUDE study were collected from existing records by analyzing the mean length of the home visits, mean scores on the type of educational material provided, the reception of the information by the mother/caregiver, and the quality of the nurse–mother/caregiver relationship. In addition, "clinical follow-up data (immunization status, number of developmental referrals) was collected at 6 months of age and analyzed by frequency distributions" (Butz et al., 1998, p. 310).

It is useful to perform a pilot study that pretests an interview guide or questionnaire. If one wishes to interview women about battering during pregnancy, it might be useful to prepare a guide and interview one or two people, then revise the guide on the basis of one's experience. If developing a questionnaire to assess the nutritional needs of elderly people living alone, it would be helpful to test the survey on some volunteers to determine its clarity and relevance.

In community health nursing, data collection often can occur as part of ongoing practice. Unless the study has been carefully designed, however, one may collect data for months or years, only to discover that important questions have been omitted.

Analyze the Findings

In most epidemiologic studies, data analysis will consist of summarizing the findings, computing rates and ratios, and displaying the findings in tables and graphs. It is at this stage that the data are used to address the original questions or test the original hypothesis. Was the hypothesis supported or not supported by the data? Summarized data can also generate more questions or indicate areas that warrant further investigation. For example, one of the pieces of data accumulated in the IUDE study that was not a main focus of the study was that, on 25 home visits, during 10 of the visits (40%), there was evidence of rats/mice/cockroaches in the home, and, in 4 (16%) of the home visits, there was dust/garbage/clutter/dirt in the home. This leads to additional questions. What housing options are available to these mothers? Who is monitoring the landlord or homeowner responsibilities? Where is the priority of house cleaning among these mothers or other household members? Are there additional services (social, broader based teaching, environmental health referrals, and so forth) nurses provide when making these IUDE home visits?

Develop Conclusions and Applications

Stating conclusions is an outcome of analysis and interpretation. The investigators summarize the results and their meaning for the purpose of making it useful to other health services providers. Many times, the research will have direct practical application for improving health services, continuing or discontinuing services, and conducting future research. It is also important to describe mistakes made and lessons learned about study design and other aspects of the research to assist future investigators.

The researchers' conclusions from the IUDE study were that these 20 mother–infant dyads experienced health (30%) and social (80%) problems, supporting "the suggestion that nurse home visiting programs, if adequately designed and implemented, can expand office and clinic based efforts for high risk infants including IUDE infants" (Butz et al., 1998, p 313).

Disseminate the Findings

Finally, research findings should be shared. Information gained from epidemiologic study must be disseminated throughout the professional community to strengthen the knowledge base for improved practice and to promote future research. The IUDE study was published in *Public Health Nursing* in October of 1998 and describes a portion of the work of David Olds and others over 15 years of a major ongoing study on the outcomes of intensive nurse home visiting among high-risk infants and children (Olds, 1992; Olds, Henderson & Kitzman, 1994; Olds et al., 1997).

SUMMARY

Epidemiology is the study of the distribution and determinants of health, health conditions, and disease in human population groups. It shares with community health nursing the common focus of the health of populations. It is a specialized form of scientific research that can provide public health professionals with a body of knowledge on which to base their practice and methods for studying new and existing problems. To understand epidemiology, one must first understand some basic epidemiologic concepts: the host, agent, and environment model; causality; immunity; the natural history of disease or health conditions; risk; and prevention strategies.

Community health nurses can use three sources of information when conducting epidemiologic investigations: existing epidemiologic data, informal investigations, and carefully designed scientific studies.

Epidemiology employs three investigative approaches: descriptive studies, analytic studies, and experimental studies. Although studies can be either retrospective or prospective, some merely describe existing conditions (descriptive studies), whereas others seek to explain causes (analytic studies). Experimental studies seek to confirm causal relationships identified in descriptive and analytic studies. Analytic studies can be of three types: prevalence, case-control, or cohort. In practice, all these types of studies often become combined in various ways. They also make use of quantitative concepts such as count, prevalence rate, incidence rate, mortality rate, and various types of morbidity (sickness) rates.

Epidemiologic research includes seven steps:
1. Identify the problem, which is usually some threat to the health of a population.
2. Review the literature to determine what other studies have found.
3. Carefully design the study.
4. Collect the data.
5. Analyze the findings.
6. Develop conclusions and applications.
7. Disseminate the findings.

Thinking epidemiologically can significantly enhance community health nursing practice. Epidemiology provides both the body of knowledge—information on the distribution and determinants of health conditions—and methods for investigating health problems and evaluating services.

ACTIVITIES TO PROMOTE CRITICAL THINKING

1. Identify an aggregate-level health problem in your community. Using the host, agent, and environment model, explain who is the host, what is the causative agent(s), and what environmental factors have promoted or delayed the development of the problem.

2. Select an aggregate health (wellness) condition, such as preschoolers' normal growth and development or elders' healthy aging, and list all the causal factors that might contribute to this healthy state. Now, plot these schematically in a diagram (such as Fig. 14–3) to show the web of causation for this condition.

3. Using the same health condition that you selected in the previous exercise, describe the natural history of this condition, outlining its four stages. Identify three preventive nursing interventions, one for each level of prevention, that could apply to this condition.

4. Select an article that reports an epidemiologic study from a recent nursing or public health journal, and record your responses to the following questions:

   a. What prompted the study, and what was its purpose?

   b. Was it descriptive, analytic, or experimental research?

   c. Was the study design retrospective or prospective?

   d. Why did the investigators choose this design?

   e. What existing sources of epidemiologic data did this study use? List all sources specifically, such as *Morbidity and Mortality Weekly Report* or incomes by household in census data.

   f. What were the study findings? Identify the population group that will benefit from this research.

5. Interview one or more practicing public health nurses in your community, and identify an aggregate-level problem that needs epidemiologic investigation. Propose a rough draft study design to research this problem.

6. A major portion of the end of this chapter was devoted to the steps of the epidemiologic process using as an example a portion of the major work of Dr. David Olds. Search the Internet for new data from this ongoing study. It is being replicated by health departments in many other states, and community health nurses may be publishing their data. Look for articles using the key terms Olds Model, home visiting, high-risk infants, and home visit assessment.

REFERENCES

Alland, D., Kalkut, G. E., & Moss, A. R., et al. (1994). Transmission of tuberculosis in New York City: An analysis by DNA fingerprinting and conventional epidemiologic methods. *New England Journal of Medicine, 330,* 1710–1716.

Beaglehole, R., & Bonita, R. (1997). *Public health at the crossroads: Achievements and prospects.* Cambridge, England: Cambridge University Press.

Blum, H. L. (1981). *Planning for health* (2nd ed.). New York: Human Sciences Press.

Burnet, M. (1962). *Natural history of infectious diseases* (3rd ed.). Cambridge, England: Cambridge University Press.

Butz, A. M., et al. (1998). Home intervention for in utero drug-exposed infants. *Public Health Nursing, 15*(5), 307–318.

Chin, J. E. (Ed.). (1999). *Control of communicable diseases manual* (17th ed.). Washington, DC: American Public Health Association.

Cohen, I. (1984). Florence Nightingale. *Scientific American, 250*(3), 128–133.

Dever, G. E. A. (1991). *Community health analysis* (2nd ed.). Gaithersburg, MD: Aspen.

Erkel, E., Morgan, E., Staples, M., Assey, V., & Michel, Y. (1994). Case management and preventive services among infants from low-income families. *Public Health Nursing, 11*(5), 352–360.

Ernster, V., Grady, D., Miike, R., Black, D., Selby, J., & Kerlikowske, K. (1995). Facial wrinkling in men and women, by smoking status. *American Journal of Public Health, 85*(1), 78–82.

Friedman, G. D. (1994). *Primer of epidemiology* (4th ed.). New York: McGraw-Hill.

Hall, J. M., Lee, M. K., Newman, B., et al. (1990). Linkage of early onset familial breast cancer to chromosome 17Q21. *Science, 250,* 1684–1689.

Harris, M. J., & Kotch, J. B. (1994). Unintentional infant injuries: Sociodemographic and psychosocial factors. *Public Health Nursing, 11*(2), 90–97.

Holaday, B., Waugh, G., Moukaddem, V., et al. (1995). Fecal contamination in child day care centers: Cloth vs paper diapers. *American Journal of Public Health, 85*(1), 30–33.

Kellam, S. G., & Anthony, J. C. (1998). Targeting early antecedents to prevent tobacco smoking: Findings from an epidemiologically based randomized field trial. *American Journal of Public Health, 88*(10), 1490–1495.

Kopf, E. W. (1978). Florence Nightingale as statistician. *Research in Nursing and Health, 1*(3), 93–102.

Lange, J. E., & Voas, R. B. (1998). Nighttime observations of safety belt use: An evaluation of California's primary law. *American Journal of Public Health, 88*(11), 1718–1720.

Mittlemark, M., et al. (1989). Prevention of cardiovascular disease: Education strategies of the Minnesota Heart Health Program. *Preventive Medicine, 15,* 1–17.

Olds, D. L. (1992). Home visitation for pregnant women and parents of young children. *American Journal of Diseases of Children, 146*(6), 704–708.

Olds, D. L., et al. (1997). Long-term effects of home visitation on maternal life course and child abuse and neglect: Fifteen-year follow-up of a randomized trial. *Journal of the American Medical Association, 278*(8), 637–643.

Olds, D. L., Henderson, C. R., & Kitzman, H. (1994). Does prenatal and infancy nurse home visitation have enduring effects on qualities of parental caregiving and child health at 25 and 50 months of life? *Pediatrics, 93*(1), 89–98.

Pickett, G., & Hanlon, J. (1990). *Public health: Administration and practice* (9th ed.). St. Louis: Times Mirror/Mosby.

Porter, E. J. (1994). Older widows' experience of living alone at home. *Image: Journal of Nursing Scholarship, 26*(1), 19–24.

Scutchfield, F. D., & Keck, C. W. (1997). *Principles of public health practice*. Albany, NY: Delmar.

Sheline, J. L., Skipper, B. J., & Broadhead, W. E. (1994). Risk factors for violent behavior in elementary school boys: Have you hugged your child today? *American Journal of Public Health, 84*(4), 661–663.

Solimena, M., & De Camilli, P. (1995). Coxsackie viruses and diabetes. *Nature Medicine, 1*(1), 25–26.

Susser, M., & Susser, E. (1996a). Choosing a future for epidemiology: I. Eras and paradigms. *American Journal of Public Health, 86*(5), 668–673.

———. (1996b). Choosing a future for epidemiology: II. From black box to Chinese boxes and eco-epidemiology. *American Journal of Public Health, 86*(5), 674–677.

Talashek, M., Gerace, L., & Starr, K. (1994). The substance abuse pandemic: Determinants to guide interventions. *Public Health Nursing, 11*(2), 131–139.

The World Health Report. (1998). *Report of the director-general.* Geneva, Switzerland: World Health Organization.

Timmreck, T. C. (1998). *Introduction to epidemiology* (2nd ed.). Sudbury, MA: Jones and Bartlett.

Turnock, B. J. (1997). *Public health: What it is and how it works.* Gaithersburg, MD: Aspen.

U.S. Department of Health and Human Services. (1998). *Healthy people 2010 objectives: Draft for public comment.* Washington, DC: U.S. Government Printing Office.

Warneke, C. L., & Cooper, S. P. (1994). Child and adolescent drownings in Harris County, Texas, 1983 through 1990. *American Journal of Public Health, 84*(4), 593–598.

SELECTED READINGS

Blanchard, J. F., et al. (1998). The evolving epidemiology of chlamydial and gonococcal infections in response to control programs in Winnipeg, Canada. *American Journal of Public Health, 88*(10), 1496–1502.

Brown, J. S., & Semradek, J. (1992). Secondary data on health-related subjects: Major sources, uses, and limitations. *Public Health Nursing, 9*(3), 162–171.

Brownson, R. C., Remington, P. L., & Davis, J. R. (Eds.). (1998). *Chronic disease epidemiology and control.* Washington, DC: American Public Health Association.

Cappelleri, J., Eckenrode, J., & Powers, J. (1993). The epidemiology of child abuse: Findings from the second national incidence and prevalence study of child abuse and neglect. *American Journal of Public Health, 83*(11), 1622–1624.

Coughlin, S. S., & Beauchamp, T. L. (Eds.). (1996). *Ethics and epidemiology.* Oxford, England: Oxford University Press.

Curtis, S., & Taket, A. (1996). *Health and societies: Changing perspectives.* London, England: Arnold.

Diez-Roux, A. V. (1998). Bringing context back into epidemiology: Variables and fallacies in multilevel analysis. *American Journal of Public Health, 88*(2), 216–222.

Erickson, G. P. (1992). Epidemiology and biostatistics content in baccalaureate education for community health nursing. *Public Health Nursing, 9*(1), 45–52.

Gorin, S. S., & Arnold, J. (1998). *Health promotion handbook.* St. Louis: Mosby.

Harper, A. C., & Lambert, L. (1993). *The health of populations* (2nd ed.). New York: Springer.

Khoury, M. J. (1997). Genetic epidemiology and the future of disease prevention and public health. *Epidemiologic Reviews, 19,* 175–180.

Lapedes, A. (1998, September 25). Forecasting influenza epidemiology. Available: http://www.acl.lanl.gov/ ~dwf/ predict/influenz.html.

Lee, P. R., & Toomey, K. E. (1994). Epidemiology in public health in the era of health care reform. *Public Health Reports, 109*(1), 1–3.

Lilienfeld, D. E., & Stolley, P. (1994). *Foundations of epidemiology* (3rd ed.). New York: Oxford University Press.

Misener, T. R., Watkins, J. G., & Ossege, J. (1994). Public health nursing research priorities: A collaborative delphi study. *Public Health Nursing, 11*(2), 66–74.

Morton, R. F., Hebel, J. R., & McCarter, R. J. (1996). *A study guide to epidemiology and biostatistics* (4th ed.). Gaithersburg, MD: Aspen.

Ozonoff, D. (1998). The uses and misuses of skepticism: Epidemiology and its critics. *Public Health Reports, 113,* 321–323.

Parascandola, M. (1998). Epidemiology: Second-rate science? *Public Health Reports, 113,* 312–320.

Pearce, N. (1996). Traditional epidemiology, modern epidemiology, and public health. *American Journal of Public Health, 86*(5), 678–683.

Seeff, L. B. (1998, August 31). Epidemiology and natural history of hepatitis C. Available: http://ex/as/;amcemet/pr/jp/heppers/ seef.html.

Toughill, E., Mason, D., Beck, T., & Christopher, M. A. (1993). Health, income, and postretirement employment of older adults. *Public Health Nursing, 10*(2), 100–107.

Unwin, N., Carr, S., & Leeson, J. (1997). *An introductory study guide to public health and epidemiology.* Philadelphia: Open University Press.

Valanis, B. (1998). *Epidemiology in health care* (3rd ed.). Stamford, CT: Appleton & Lange.

Vredevoe, D. L., Brecht, M., Shuler, P., & Woo, M. (1992). Risk factors for disease in a homeless population. *Public Health Nursing, 9*(4), 263–269.

Wallace, R. B. (Ed.). (1998). *Maxcy-Rosenau-Last Public health and preventive medicine* (14th ed.). Stamford, CT: Appleton & Lange.

Weed, D.L. (1998). Beyond black box epidemiology. *American Journal of Public Health, 88*(1), 12–14.

Wilby, M. L. (1998). Improving the health profile: Decreasing risk for cancer through primary prevention. *Holistic Nursing Practice, 12*(2), 52–61.

Willett, W. (1998). *Nutritional epidemiology* (2nd ed.). Washington, DC: American Public Health Association.

Communicable Disease Control

KEY TERMS

- ■ Acquired immunodeficiency syndrome (AIDS)
- ■ Active immunity
- ■ Communicable disease
- ■ Direct transmission
- ■ Fomites
- ■ Herd immunity
- ■ Human immunodeficiency virus (HIV)
- ■ Immunization
- ■ Incubation period
- ■ Indirect transmission
- ■ Infectious
- ■ Isolation
- ■ Passive immunity
- ■ Quarantine
- ■ Reservoir
- ■ Screening
- ■ Surveillance
- ■ Vaccine
- ■ Vector

LEARNING OBJECTIVES

Upon mastery of this chapter, you should be able to:

- ■ Discuss the global and national trends and issues in communicable disease control.
- ■ Describe the three modes of transmission for communicable diseases.
- ■ Explain the strategies used for the three levels of prevention in communicable disease control.
- ■ Explain the significance of immunization as a communicable disease control measure.
- ■ Describe major issues impacting the control and elimination of tuberculosis.
- ■ Differentiate between HIV infection and AIDS.
- ■ Discuss specific ways to prevent sexually transmitted diseases, including HIV/AIDS.
- ■ Identify six globally emerging communicable diseases.
- ■ Describe the nurse's role in communicable disease control.
- ■ Discuss ethical issues affecting communicable disease and infection control.

Communicable diseases pose a major threat to public health and are of significant concern to community health nurses. A **communicable disease** is one that can be transmitted from one person to another. It is caused by an agent that is **infectious** (capable of producing infection) and is transmitted from a source, or **reservoir,** to a susceptible host.

Knowledge of communicable diseases is fundamental to the practice of community health nursing because these diseases typically spread through communities of people. Understanding the basic concepts of communicable disease control, as well as the numerous issues arising in this area, helps a community health nurse work effectively to prevent and control communicable disease in populations and groups. It also helps nurses teach important and effective preventive measures to community members, advocate for those affected, and protect the well-being of uninfected persons (including the nurses themselves).

Several issues and circumstances have emerged during the last quarter century that are important areas of concern to community health nurses.

- • Despite significant declines in mortality, communicable diseases are responsible for persistently high morbidity among various age and population groups.
- • Rates of some communicable diseases, especially tuberculosis (TB) and sexually transmitted diseases, remain disproportionately (in some cases, shockingly) high in selected population groups, a fact often masked when statistics are aggregated.
- • The development of multidrug-resistant strains of bacteria and viruses poses a significant occupational health challenge as well as a practice issue for health workers.

- Lastly, current research reveals that infectious agents may be responsible for a number of the chronic diseases, including some forms of cancer, that have occupied the interest of health care providers in the last few decades.

This chapter provides community health nurses with information to assess the communicable disease burden in a community. It describes ways to plan appropriate prevention interventions, including immunization of children and adults, environmental interventions, community education, screening programs, and case-finding and contact investigation. Ethical issues of communicable disease control are also discussed. A list of communicable disease information sources useful to the nurse is given in the Resources at the back of this book.

BASIC CONCEPTS REGARDING COMMUNICABLE DISEASES

Evolution of Communicable Disease Control

Communicable diseases have challenged health care providers for centuries. They have led to the development of countless nursing and medical preventive measures, from simple procedures such as handwashing, sanitation, and proper ventilation to the research and development of vaccines and antibiotics. Because these preventive measures have greatly reduced the spread of communicable diseases, many people consider communicable diseases to be a threat of the past. Yet this is not so. Communicable diseases, particularly those of epidemic and pandemic proportions such as TB and acquired immunodeficiency syndrome (AIDS), continue to cost millions of lives and billions of dollars to the global human society every year.

As mentioned in Chapter 14, the first documented global threat from a communicable disease began in the 13th century in the form of bubonic plague. It was responsible for killing 25% of the population in some European countries in the years after the Crusades and during the years of exploration and trade by ship in the 1400s to 1600s.

As commerce and industry continued to grow, people migrated from rural areas to towns and cities. However, health and hygiene practices that worked in remote areas did not transfer to the new urban settings. In tenements and overcrowded parts of towns, water for drinking easily became contaminated with human waste; mounting garbage and trash, unable to be composted or buried as was done in farming communities, created a rich habitat for rodents and other animals and insects, encouraging them to breed and act as vectors for many communicable diseases.

It was not until the 1700s and 1800s that the causative organisms for different infectious diseases were first recognized through the assistance of increasingly sophisticated microscopes. With these discoveries came early attempts to create ways to prevent the spread of such organisms, either by decreasing their power or by eliminating them. Milk began to be pasteurized, and efforts to eliminate rats from ships and food storage areas began. These measures began a global effort to eliminate communicable diseases.

One disease, smallpox, is a classic example of a communicable disease control success story. For centuries, smallpox, an infectious disease, killed millions of people and scarred survivors for life. It first responded to a crude vaccine developed, almost accidentally, in the 1800s. The vaccine was studied and perfected and was used globally for decades. A major worldwide eradication campaign began in 1967. The last naturally acquired case of smallpox in the world occurred in October 1977; global eradication was certified 2 years later by the World Health Organization (WHO) and confirmed by the World Health Assembly in May 1980. Since then, no cases of smallpox have been identified in any country (Chin, 1999; World Health Report, 1998). However, the potential threat of biologic warfare using smallpox or other disease organisms raises concerns about how to prepare for the future.

Global Trends

During the last 30 to 40 years, substantial progress has been made in controlling some major infectious diseases around the world, although other diseases have not been managed as well. Some of the major accomplishments include:

- The WHO's Expanded Program on Immunization (EPI) was launched in 1974. As a result, by 1995, over 80% of the world's children had been immunized against *diphtheria, tetanus, whooping cough, poliomyelitis, measles,* and *TB,* compared with fewer than 5% in 1974 (World Health Report, 1998).
- Global eradication of *smallpox* was achieved in 1980.
- The tropical disease *yaws* has virtually disappeared. The first yaws campaign was launched in Haiti in 1950, and, by 1965, 46 million people in 49 countries were successfully treated with penicillin. The disease is no longer a significant problem in most of the world.
- Because of improved sanitation and hygiene in recent decades, outbreaks of *relapsing fever,* transmitted by lice, are rare today.
- In 1988, a campaign for global eradication of *poliomyelitis* by the year 2000 was launched. Reported cases worldwide have declined by over 90% since the campaign began. The poliovirus has disappeared from the Americas, but polio remains in India and is heavily affecting the continent along with areas of Africa and the Eastern Mediterranean (World Health Report, 1998).
- The global threat of *plague* has declined in the last 40 years, largely because of antibiotics and insecticides. However, there is evidence of plague in rodents spreading in parts of the western United States.

- *Leprosy* (Hansen disease), once a major communicable disease, is close to being eliminated. In 1966, there were 10.5 million reported cases worldwide. Through the use of multidrug therapy, the numbers were reduced to 5.4 million in 1985, and in 1999 there were 1.4 cases per 10,000 population. The WHO will no longer consider leprosy a public health problem when there is less than 1 case per 10,000 population.

Some major problem communicable diseases and areas include:

- *Malaria* remains a major threat even with an improved mortality rate in the last 25 years. In 1954, there were 2.5 million deaths annually and 250 million cases worldwide; now, there are 1.5 to 2.7 million deaths and 300 to 500 million cases. Tropical Africa has 90% of the cases, and malaria is endemic in 100 countries. The aim of the current Global Malaria Strategy is to reduce mortality by at least 20% compared with 1995 in at least 75% of affected countries by the year 2000.
- *Cholera* was mainly confined to Asia in the early 20th century through improvements in sanitation elsewhere. However, there has been a series of pandemics affecting much of the world since 1960, becoming more widespread and more frequent in Africa since the 1970s. A new strain, *Vibrio cholerae O139,* was identified in India in 1992. Cholera is endemic in 80 countries and is of concern in all parts of the world. Along with other diarrheal diseases, it ranked as the third leading cause of death worldwide in 1999, mostly among children under age 5 (Gannon, 2000).
- *TB* has made a powerful resurgence in the last 3 decades as many countries let their control programs become complacent. It kills 3 million people a year, with 7.3 million new cases annually. WHO declared TB a global emergency in 1993. One third of the incidence in the last 5 years can be attributed to HIV. Drug-resistant strains of the tuberculosis bacillus have infected up to 50 million people worldwide.
- *Yellow fever* causes about 30,000 deaths each year among 200,000 annual cases. However, since the late 1980s, there has been a dramatic resurgence of the disease in Africa and the Americas. It is endemic in 34 countries in Africa, where immunization programs are weak in the 14 poorest African countries. In 1995, Peru experienced the largest yellow fever outbreak reported from any country in the Americas since 1950.
- *Sleeping sickness* (African trypanosomiasis) cases have doubled in the past few years (World Health Report, 1998).

Our global successes and failures to control communicable diseases are affected by a bevy of factors. First, the geopolitical nature of the area influences who can respond when a communicable disease occurs in a country. Second, the natural and manmade resources of the area influence the health status of the population before a disease strikes and contribute to the population's resistance to the disease and ability to survive once a communicable disease is contracted. Therefore, richer nations have fewer deaths from and incidences of communicable diseases; poorer countries have higher communicable disease incidences and greater numbers of deaths from the disease. Finally, weather and climatic factors can influence health and illness. For example, both droughts and floods can lead to crop failure and subsequent famine. Other such factors include hurricanes, monsoons, earthquakes, tornadoes, floods, and fire.

National Trends

At the turn of the millennium in the United States, we are faced with the emergence of new and newly virulent diseases. The set of revised health objectives in *Healthy People 2010* was written in part to address this challenge in communicable disease control.

NEW, EMERGING, AND RESURGING DISEASES

At the national level, for several decades in the late 20th century, medical research and funding focused on major chronic diseases such as arteriosclerosis and cancer. During those years, we were winning the communicable disease war and, as a nation, became complacent about communicable diseases. Thus, when HIV/AIDS emerged in the early 1980s, we lost valuable time because of our unwillingness or inability to recognize its potential as a major killer among all people. At the same time, we discovered that many of our children were not being immunized against communicable diseases at rates as high as those in poorer nations. Also, we came to see that some diseases, such as *Escherichia coli*–induced diarrhea and TB, were coming back with a vengeance and that our current prevention or treatment regimens were not effective.

We have learned that we will probably always be challenged by communicable diseases. Pathogens that we consider under control because they respond well to current treatment can mutate and produce new, virulent strains; diseases that have been nearly eliminated can emerge again if public health efforts slacken; and diseases eradicated in the United States can revisit us on any one of the hundreds of international flights arriving at our airports each day. As a result, our present concerns focus on three types of communicable disease: new diseases, emerging diseases, and resurging diseases.

Some communicable diseases have been affecting us for centuries or millennia, but a major new disease, HIV/AIDS, which is covered in detail later in this chapter, was first recognized only in 1981. Another new disease, Legionnaires' disease, was first detected in Philadelphia only in 1976. It has occurred sporadically in other countries since then. Both of these diseases are disturbing reminders that new threats to public health are always on the horizon.

Emerging diseases are diseases rarely or never before seen in the United States. These diseases may also be new to public health officials in other countries. Emerging diseases occurring in the United States include the hantavirus, seen in the southwestern United States in 1993; dengue fever, acquired from travel outside the United States among people in Texas in the 1980s; and typhoid, seen in a native Nigerian in New York City in 1994. Typically, diseases uncommon in the United States, such as malaria, plague, Lassa fever, cholera, and yellow fever, accompany people as they travel from one country to another on airlines and cruise ships (Ostroff & Kozarsky, 1998).

Resurging diseases are those communicable diseases that have been endemic in some parts of the world but are now endemic in more countries and are increasing to epidemic proportions in others. Often, the resurgence is due to the emergence of new drug-resistant strains of a familiar organism. TB's resurgence is caused by a bacillus that is multidrug resistant. This is just one of the many diseases becoming drug resistant. The list of diseases that are caused by antimicrobial-resistant organisms includes strains of *Haemophilus influenzae, Neisseria gonorrhoeae, Bordetella pertussis,* and *Streptococcus pneumoniae* (Tenover & Hughes, 1996) (Fig. 15–1). TB is the communicable disease affecting the greatest number of people in the United States with strains of drug-resistant microbes. Hepatitis B, C, and D have resurged and are now seen in increasing numbers because of intravenous drug abuse.

HEALTHY PEOPLE THE PREVENTION AGENDA FOR THE NATION

The new *Healthy People 2010* document groups the nation's health objectives somewhat differently from the previous document, *Healthy People 2000*. Nevertheless, many objectives still focus on infectious diseases and immunizations, aiming to decrease morbidity and mortality from infectious diseases and to increase the number of children and adults immunized. In addition, the document attempts to guide the nation toward health with goals and objectives that include new focus areas, including arthritis, osteoporosis, chronic back conditions, chronic kidney diseases, respiratory diseases, vision and hearing, medical product safety, health communication, and public health infrastructure (U.S. Department of Health and Human Services, 2000).

Healthy People 2010 was formulated with input from over 350 national and 250 state public health, medical, and environmental agencies, in addition to lay advisors from around the country. They began to meet in 1996 to design the structure and content of the document. During its development, the Office of Disease Prevention and Health Promotion accepted electronic comments at its website and in writing, making this truly a document of the people. With so many people involved, achievement of the document's goals is more likely.

Modes of Transmission

As we discussed in Chapter 14, the reservoir of infection can be a person, animal, insect, or inanimate material in which the infectious agent lives and multiplies and which is a source of infection to others. Transmission of a communicable disease can occur by direct or indirect methods.

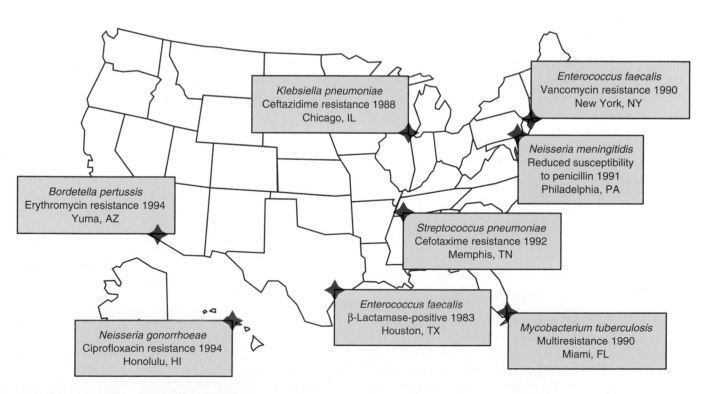

FIGURE 15–1. Map of the United States showing emergence of a number of antimicrobial-resistant organisms.

DIRECT TRANSMISSION

Direct transmission occurs by immediate transfer of infectious agents from a reservoir to a new host. It requires direct contact with the source, through touching, biting, kissing, or sexual intercourse, or by the direct projection of droplet spray onto the conjunctiva or onto the mucous membranes of the eye, nose, or mouth during sneezing, coughing, spitting, singing, or talking. Direct transmission is limited to a distance of a meter (1 yard) or less.

INDIRECT TRANSMISSION

Indirect transmission occurs when the infectious agent is transported within contaminated inanimate materials such as air, water, or food. It is also commonly referred to as *vehicle-borne transmission*. Chapter 16 describes both the government's role and the nurse's role in helping to prevent food and water contamination by infectious agents.

People may be affected by certain communicable diseases merely through carrying on the normal activities of eating food and drinking beverages. Food-borne illnesses frequently reported to the Centers for Disease Control and Prevention (CDC) in the last few years include salmonellosis, a bacterial agent; hepatitis A, a viral agent; and shigellosis, a bacterial agent. The most commonly reported water-borne illness is due to *Giardia lamblia,* an infection-causing protozoan. *Giardia* can also occur as a food contaminant. Most of the disease-causing agents typically found in foods also survive in water to cause disease, although water may provide a less nutritive environment and result in lower concentrations of the agent. Most commonly, exposure to infectious food or water results in symptoms relating to gastrointestinal (GI) function, including diarrhea, nausea, vomiting, stomach cramps, and jaundice. Onset of symptoms may occur within a few hours of exposure or not until days or even weeks later, depending on the organism. This time interval between exposure and onset of symptoms is called the **incubation period.** Note that water-borne pathogens do not only affect the GI tract. The CDC compiles reports as well on skin infections associated with recreational water use.

Bacterial contamination of food resulting in human illness occurs as a result of either infection or intoxication. Infection occurs through ingesting food contaminated with adequate doses of *Salmonella, Shigella, E. coli,* or other pathogens. The cycle begins when the infectious agent multiplies and grows in the food medium. The agent subsequently invades the host after ingestion of the food. Infection then occurs, which is the entry and development or multiplication of an infectious agent in the body usually accompanied by an immune response, such as the production of antibodies with or without clinical manifestation. The infectious organism produces illness by direct irritation of the normal GI mucosa. In contrast, intoxication is caused by the production of toxins as a byproduct of the normal bacterial life cycle. This commonly occurs when cooked food is left standing at room temperature. It is ingestion of the toxin, rather than the microbe itself, that produces the illness.

The distinction between infection and intoxication is relevant for a number of reasons. Toxins may be difficult to isolate and identify, particularly in the absence of the bacteria; thus, some suspected food-borne illnesses go unidentified. Although the bacteria may be killed after heating of foodstuffs before consumption, some bacteria-produced toxins are stable in normal cooking temperatures; thus, the food cannot be rendered safe. A bacteria that establishes itself in the human GI system may require medical treatment to be eradicated. In contrast, people suffering from food intoxication typically require essentially supportive care while in the process of ridding themselves of the toxin.

The most important aspects of food- and water-borne diseases for nurses in community health may be in recognizing that outbreaks of illness affecting large numbers of people continue to occur fairly regularly. This is true despite well-recognized standards for decontamination of water supplies and safe commercial food preparation. Secondly, such outbreaks may not be detectable by usual surveillance means because of individuals' mobility. For example, an outbreak of illness in Minnesota in 1990 was associated with food served on an international airline. Had a large group of the affected travelers not communicated among themselves and with providers, the outbreak may never have been identified. Thirdly, such outbreaks can serve to remind all community health practitioners that there continues to be a need to teach and observe the most basic methods for preventing food and water contamination. Display 15–1 summarizes correct methods for preserving the safety and cleanliness of food.

When transmission occurs through a **vector,** which is a nonhuman carrier such as an animal or insect, it is known as vector-borne transmission. Common vectors include bats,

---

DISPLAY 15–1. Correct Methods for Preserving the Safety and Cleanliness of Food

Before handling food:
- Wash hands and all food preparation surfaces and utensils thoroughly with soap and water.

When preparing food:
- Wash foods that are to be eaten raw and uncooked thoroughly in clean water. This includes foods that are to be peeled that grow on the ground or come in contact with soil.
- Cook all meat products thoroughly.
- Do not allow cooked meats to come in contact with dishes, utensils, or containers used when the foods were raw and uncooked.

When storing leftover foods:
- Cool cooked foods quickly; store under refrigeration in clean, covered containers.

When reheating leftover foods:
- Heat foods thoroughly. Bacteria contaminating food grow and multiply in a temperature range between 39°F and 140°F.

fleas, lice, mosquitoes, raccoons, rats, skunks, squirrels, and ticks. During vector-borne transmission, the infectious agent may be transported mechanically without multiplication or change, or the infectious agent may develop biologically before passage to a susceptible host.

Diseases transmitted through vectors prove challenging in communicable disease control because individuals who become infected typically have no direct personal contact with other infected persons. Rather, isolated cases occur within areas inhabited by the vector. Nevertheless, human history has been significantly affected by vector-borne diseases. Louse-borne typhus and flea-borne plague together were responsible for a majority of devastating epidemics occurring in the last 6 centuries. Currently, mosquito-borne malaria and snail-borne schistosomiasis cause major human suffering to hundreds of millions of people in tropical settings every year. The fact that most of these diseases are endemic to certain areas suggests the need for tight controls for prevention and intervention.

Control strategies directed to vector-borne diseases typically involve complex environmental measures to hinder the vector from reaching the host (see Chapter 16) as well as community education. Such strategies include:

- Reducing the population of insect vectors (eg, by spraying insecticides to kill mosquitoes)
- Treating the natural habitat of the vector to reduce the population density
- Reducing the population of other animal hosts that harbor the vector, as when rats are exterminated to reduce the risk of plague
- Erecting barriers between the susceptible human and the vector, such as use of mosquito nets or screened windows to control malaria or protective clothing and sprays against tick-borne diseases
- Educating the public about preventive and protective measures, including actions to take when attacked by the vector to prevent disease from developing

In the United States, vector-borne illnesses have received renewed attention in recent years with accumulating information about tick-borne Lyme disease, a viral disease transmitted to humans by a tick vector. It results in symptoms of varying severity, including rash, joint pain, progressive weakness, vision changes, and other neuromuscular dysfunctions. Other vector-borne diseases receiving attention in the 1990s include tick-borne fevers, such as Rocky Mountain spotted fever and relapsing fever, and rabies, whose vector usually is a domestic animal, bat, skunk, or raccoon. Occasionally, imported vector-borne tropical diseases, including malaria and dengue fever, are reported. The return of military personnel from southeast Asia through the 1960s and 1970s had a significant effect on the numbers of imported cases of malaria reported in the United States.

AIRBORNE TRANSMISSION

Airborne transmission occurs through droplet nuclei—the small residues that result from evaporation of fluid from droplets emitted by an infected host. They may also be created purposely by atomizing devices or accidentally in microbiology laboratories. Because of their small size and weight, they can remain suspended in the air for long periods of time before they are inhaled into the respiratory system of a host.

Airborne transmission can also occur in dust. Small particles of dust from soil containing fungus spores may cling to clothing, bedding, or floors. Alternatively, the spores may become separated from dry soil by the wind and then be inhaled by the host.

PRIMARY PREVENTION

In the context of communicable disease control, two approaches are useful in achieving primary prevention: (1) education using mass media and targeting health messages to aggregates and (2) immunization.

Education

Health education in primary prevention is directed at both helping at-risk individuals understand their risk status and promoting behaviors that decrease exposure or susceptibility. Chapter 9 deals more extensively with the concepts of learning theory and the variety of health education approaches and materials available to community health nurses today.

USE OF MASS MEDIA FOR HEALTH EDUCATION

All people need to be informed about the risks of communicable diseases. Often, mass media are the most effective way to reach the largest number of people. Additionally, many target groups, such as low-income and racially and ethnically diverse communities at high risk for communicable diseases, are very hard to reach one on one. One way to reach them is through the media. To disseminate public health information to large numbers of people, there are four major roles of the media (Flora & Cassady, 1990).

1. Use the media as a primary change agent; community education programs can successfully increase knowledge about communicable diseases and preventive measures.
2. As a complement to other disease prevention efforts, the media can effectively model preventive behaviors, such as condom use and drug abstinence.
3. As a promoter of communicable disease control programs, the media can help to increase participation of community members in primary prevention services.
4. Disease prevention messages can contribute to creation of a social environment that promotes health (eg, increasing acceptance of regular condom use in the prevention of sexually transmitted disease).

The body of literature on mass communication for promoting health and preventing disease through the voluntary adoption of healthy behaviors is growing rapidly (Maibach & Parrott, 1995).

The urgency to combat AIDS, as well as other life-threatening diseases, provides a strong rationale and impetus for developing effective disease prevention and control messages for dissemination through the media (Fig. 15–2). Messages need to be tailored to the specific characteristics of target audiences and the media channels to which the audiences are exposed. Disadvantaged or stigmatized groups, such as the poor, ethnic minorities, gay men, injection drug users, and prostitutes, are more vulnerable to infectious diseases and need mass media messages targeted to them (Manning, 1995). Those people who watch more television and listen to more radio will respond to health promotion messages using these media more often than groups who do not. A behavior change is essential to control the spread of communicable diseases, and that change depends on successful communication between community health providers and target audiences using the most appropriate media possible (Glanz & Yang, 1996). Participation in media and education efforts depends on groups, such as injection drug users, being aware of available programs and how to access them. Carefully and thoughtfully designed disease prevention messages disseminated through the media are a reliable and effective way of reaching hard-to-reach populations. However, mass media have the potential to undermine traditional customs and beliefs and may serve to sever individuals from their community (Mackenzie, 1998). This reinforces the need to screen selected media with community leaders for effectiveness and appropriateness before use and to plan together educational efforts that meet community needs.

TARGETING MEANINGFUL HEALTH MESSAGES TO AGGREGATES

To effectively deliver a communicable disease prevention message, the message must reach the target (at-risk) population. This requires correctly identifying the characteristics of the target audience, in terms of educational level, salience of the issue, involvement of the target audience with the issue, and access of the target audience to the media channels used (Maibach & Parrott, 1995). Cultural issues affect people's interpretation of messages and must be considered in the presentation of a disease-prevention message to ethnic and racial minority groups (Glanz & Yang, 1996). There are principles for adapting health messages to specific population subgroups (Falvo, 1994; O'Donnell et al., 1995):

1. Develop educational materials from the community perspective, reflecting respect for community values and traditions, relevance to community needs and interests, and participation of the community in the preparation and use of the materials.
2. Ensure that materials are an integral part of a health education program, supported by other components of intervention, not standing alone as the educational program in itself.
3. Materials must be related to the delivery of health services that are available, accessible, and acceptable to the target population.
4. All materials must be pretested and have demonstrated attractiveness, comprehension, acceptability, ownership, and persuasiveness.
5. Materials must be distributed with instructions for their use (ie, how, when, and with whom they are to be used).

Immunization

Control of acute communicable diseases through immunization has been a common practice since the 19th century in the United States. **Immunization** is the process of introducing some form of disease-causing organism into a person's system to cause the development of antibodies that will resist that disease. In theory, this process makes the person immune (able to resist a specific infectious disease-causing agent) to that particular infectious disease. That immunization requirements are acceptable in American society today is evidenced by high levels of immunization in school children and the fact that aggressive enforcement of school im-

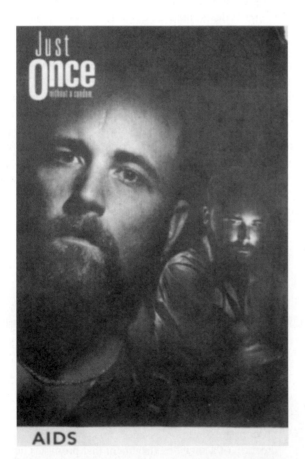

FIGURE 15–2. This poster conveys a powerful message about AIDS.

munization requirements, starting in the late 1970s, has not met with widespread opposition. This is true even during the last decade when common immunizations have been changed, the number of immunizations has increased, and the schedule for administration of vaccines officially changes every January (Selekman, 1998).

The statutes that exist to ensure adequate immunization levels by school entry place the school in the role of controlling agency, whereas public health departments and private health care providers are authorized to administer the required vaccines. An emerging drawback of this mechanism is the fact that many parents delay immunizations until the 5th year (Scutchfield & Keck, 1997). Preschool-aged children represent a major proportion of all cases of immunizable diseases and are the group at highest risk of infection (American Academy of Pediatrics, 1997; Hamlin, Wood, Pereyra & Grabowsky, 1996). Vaccines provide significant cost benefits. For example, for every dollar sent on DTaP, $24 is saved, and $2 is saved for the more recently approved Hib vaccine (U.S. Department of Health and Human Services, 2000).

The national objective, stated in *Healthy People 2000,* is for 90% of American children to be vaccinated by their second birthday with four doses of DPT, three doses of oral polio, and one dose of the combined measles, mumps, and rubella vaccine (U.S. Department of Health and Human Services, 1991). *Healthy People 2010* (U.S. Department of Health and Human Services, 2000) reinforces this by including an objective of reducing or eliminating all indigenous cases of vaccine-preventable disease (Table 15–1).

Although childhood immunization rates historically have been lower in minority populations compared with the white population, rates for minority preschool children have been increasing at a more rapid rate, thereby significantly narrowing the gap (U.S. Department of Health and Human Services, 2000). The National Immunization Survey documents substantial progress toward achieving 1996 Childhood Immunization Initiative coverage goals by racial and ethnic groups. However, efforts to increase vaccination coverage need to be intensified, particularly for children living in poverty (CDC, 1997; U.S. Dept. of Health and Human Services, 2000). Thus, it is critical to discover the social and cultural characteristics affecting health status, attitudes about preventive measures, behaviors in seeking services, acceptability of intervention, and perceptions of health care providers that, in turn, determine parental action in having a child immunized in a regular and timely fashion. This is a unique area of health care delivery, where nurses must rely on parental initiative to obtain a form of care for the well child that may be perceived as producing pain and temporary illness, for no observable benefit.

VACCINE-PREVENTABLE DISEASES

Vaccine-preventable diseases (VPD), such as hepatitis B, *H. influenzae* type b, measles, polio, diphtheria, pertussis, and chickenpox, are diseases that can be prevented through immunization. Immunity may be either passive or active. **Passive immunity** is short-term resistance to a specific disease-caus-

TABLE 15–1. *Healthy People 2010* Vaccine-Preventable Disease (VPD) Objective

Disease	1997	2010 Target
Congenital rubella syndrome	4	0
Diphtheria (people <35 years of age)	4	0
Haemophilus influenzae type b	165	0
Hepatitis B (people <25 years of age)	8,693	0
Measles	135	0
Mumps	612	0
Pertussis (children <7 years of age)	2,633	2,000
Polio (wild-type virus)	0	0
Rubella	161	0
Tetanus (among people <35 years of age)	10	0
Varicella (chickenpox)	4 million*	400,000

*Estimated from the National Health Interview Survey (NNHIS), 1990–1994.

ing organism that may be acquired naturally (as with newborns through maternal antibody transfer) or artificially through inoculation with a vaccine that gives temporary resistance. Such immunizations must be repeated periodically to sustain immunity levels. An example is the influenza vaccination. **Active immunity** is long-term (sometimes lifelong) resistance to a specific disease-causing organism and is also acquired either naturally or artificially. Naturally acquired active immunity occurs when a person contracts a disease, developing long-lasting antibodies that provide immunity against future exposure. Artificially acquired active immunity occurs through inoculation with a vaccine, such as the diphtheria, pertussis, tetanus vaccination series given to children. A **vaccine** is a preparation made either from killed, living attenuated, or living fully virulent organisms and is administered to produce or artificially increase immunity to a particular disease.

Because of the success of immunization strategies, few practicing nurses today have treated clients with tetanus or diphtheria (although some have cared for clients with residual polio disabilities). However, immunizable diseases still exist in force in the developing world today, and outbreaks occur in the United States in groups of unimmunized or susceptible populations. For example, certain people are constitutionally exempt from immunization, others decline immunization for religious or personal reasons, and certain refugee populations can be especially vulnerable. Even with global and national efforts at reducing and eliminating VPD, some national goals have not been met. In fact, statistics for some diseases have gotten worse. Immunization rates of coverage have declined in some areas, with subsequent increases in VPDs such as pertussis. Pertussis increased from 3,450 cases in 1988 to 6,568 cases in 1997 (U.S. Department of Health and Human Services, 1998). The *Healthy People 2010* goal is set at 2,000 cases, and with an intensified VPD effort among the families of highest risk, this goal should be achievable (U.S. Department of Health and Human Services, 2000).

SCHEDULE OF RECOMMENDED IMMUNIZATIONS

An annual schedule for the administration of childhood vaccinations is published based on recommendations by the Advisory Committee on Immunization Practices (ACIP), the American Academy of Pediatrics (AAP), the American Academy of Family Physicians (AAFP), and the CDC (Table 15–2). The CDC also provides schedules for children not receiving their first immunization at birth according to the standard schedule. Current recommendations call for a child to receive ten different vaccines or toxoids (many in combination form and all requiring more than one dose) in six to seven visits to a provider, between birth and school entry, with boosters in the preteen to early teen years (CDC, 2000).

Factors influencing the recommended age at which vaccines are administered include the age-specific risks of the disease, the age-specific risks of complications, the ability of persons of a given age to produce an adequate and lasting immune response, and the potential for interference with the immune response by passively transferred maternal antibodies. In general, vaccines are recommended for the youngest age group at risk whose members are known to develop an acceptable antibody response to vaccination (CDC, 2000). Recommendations for vaccine administration may be revised in light of specific circumstances. For example, in response to a rising incidence of hepatitis B among sexually active individuals, it is now recommended that infants receive hepatitis B vaccine in doses varying depending on whether their mothers have positive or negative responses to the hepatitis B surface antigen (CDC, 2000). In addition, the rotavirus vaccine was eliminated from the 2000 immunization schedule because it caused too many serious illnesses in infants who received it in 1999.

ASSESSING IMMUNIZATION STATUS OF THE COMMUNITY

Determining the immunization status of children in a community can be a time-consuming but worthwhile task. Community health nurses may consider assessing groups of children with some common characteristics such as children served by the Women, Infants and Children program (WIC), served by private medical providers, or attending public schools in various neighborhoods. Because all children attending school in the United States must show proof of immunization upon school entry, review of immunization records at school can provide a means of retrospectively determining the proportion of these children whose immunizations were up to date at age 3 months or age 2 years. The CDC strongly promotes the retrospective school vaccination record survey as a means of estimating current levels and monitoring trends over time in immunization status. If no unusual immunization events occur in the intervening period,

this retrospective record review gives a reasonable estimate of current immunization status of those age groups in the community. In addition, such a record review targeting children who were not up to date on their immunizations before school entry helps identify younger siblings who may also not be up to date.

With increasing numbers of children entering day care services in the preschool years, more states now require immunization for preschool children, often including immunization against influenza, which is not presently required for older age groups. Preschool or day care operators, therefore, now obtain information about immunization status of this younger cohort, a group that has, until now, often escaped surveillance and immunization initiative.

Other community settings where community health nurses may identify underimmunized children include homeless shelters and other public service settings used by families and children, including local religious centers. A family with one underimmunized child may have other underimmunized children of other ages as well as any number of other unmet preventive health care needs, which the community health nurse might help address.

Understanding disease rates and immunization status by race or ethnicity requires population data accurately showing the multicultural composition of the community. Such data can be obtained from census figures and augmented by refugee or immigration records. Noting the racial or ethnic heritage of the underimmunized child may lead to valuable insights about unique barriers for the group that must be addressed to reduce disease rates and increase healthy resilience.

HERD IMMUNITY

Herd immunity is central to understanding immunization as a means of protecting community health. As described in Chapter 14, it is the immunity level present in a particular population of people (Chin, 1999). Low herd immunity occurs when there are few immune persons within a community and the spread of disease is more likely. When more individuals in a community are vaccinated so that a high proportion of the individuals have acquired resistance to the infectious agent, this contributes to high herd immunity. High herd immunity reduces the probability that the few unimmunized persons will come in contact with one another, making spread of the disease unlikely. Outbreaks may occur when immunization falls below 85% (Scutchfield & Keck, 1997) or if unimmunized susceptible persons are grouped together rather than dispersed throughout the immunized community. An example of lack of herd immunity is presented in The Global Community.

BARRIERS TO IMMUNIZATION COVERAGE

Improving immunization coverage requires examination of reasons children are not immunized. Many barriers exist. They include religious, financial, social, and cultural factors, philosophical objections, and provider limitations that form barriers to adequate immunization.

TABLE 15–2. Recommended Childhood Immunization Schedule: United States, January–December 2000

Regular checkups at your pediatrician's office or local health clinic are an important way to keep children healthy.

By making sure that your child gets immunized on time, you can provide the best available defense against many dangerous childhood diseases. Immunizations protect children against: *hepatitis B,* polio, measles, mumps, rubella (German measles), pertussis (whooping cough), diphtheria, tetanus (lockjaw), *Haemophilus influenzae* type b, and *chickenpox.* All of these immunizations need to be given before children are 2 years old in order for them to be protected during their most vulnerable period. Are your child's immunizations up-to-date?

The chart below includes immunization recommendations from the American Academy of Pediatrics. Remember to keep track of your child's immunizations—it's the only way you can be sure your child is up-to-date. Also, check with your pediatrician or health clinic at each visit to find out if your child needs any booster shots or if any new vaccines have been recommended since this schedule was prepared.

If you don't have a pediatrician, call your local health department. Public health clinics usually have supplies of vaccine and may give shots free.

Vaccines[1] are listed under routinely recommended ages. *Bars* indicate range or recommended ages for immunization. Any dose not given at the recommended age should be given as a "catch-up" immunization at any subsequent visit when indicated and feasible. *Ovals* indicate vaccines to be given if previously recommended doses were missed or given earlier than the recommended minimum age.

Age ▶ / Vaccine ▼	Birth	1 mo	2 mos	4 mos	6 mos	12 mos	15 mos	18 mos	24 mos	4–6 yrs	11–12 yrs	14–16 yrs
Hepatitis B[2]	Hep B	Hep B		Hep B							Hep B	
Diphtheria, Tetanus, Pertussis[3]			DTaP	DTaP	DTaP		DTaP[3]			DTaP	Td	
H. influenzae type b[4]			Hib	Hib	Hib	Hib						
Polio[5]			IPV	IPV	IPV[5]					IPV[5]		
Measles, Mumps, Rubella[6]						MMR				MMR[4]	MMR[6]	
Varicella[7]						Var					Var[7]	
Hepatitis A[8]										Hep A[8] in selected areas		

Approved by the Advisory Committee on Immunization Practices (ACIP), the American Academy of Pediatrics (AAP), and the American Academy of Family Physicians (AAFP). On October 22, 1999, the Advisory Committee on Immunization Practices (ACIP) recommended that Rotashield (RRV-TV), the only US-licensed rotavirus vaccine, no longer be used in the United States (*MMWR Morb Mortal Wkly Rep.* Nov 5, 1999;48(43):1007). Parents should be reassured that their children who received rotavirus vaccine before July are not at increased risk for intussusception now.

[1]This schedule indicates the recommended ages for routine administration of currently licensed childhood vaccines as of 11/1/99. Additional vaccines may be licensed and recommended during the year. Licensed combination vaccines may be used whenever any components of the combination are indicated and its other components are not contraindicated. Providers should consult the manufacturers' package inserts for detailed recommendations.

[2]*Infants born to HBsAg-negative mothers* should receive the 1st dose of hepatitis B (Hep B) vaccine by age 2 months. The 2nd dose should be at least 1 month after the 1st dose. The 3rd dose should be administered at least 4 months after the 1st dose and at least 2 months after the 2nd dose, but not before 6 months of age for infants.

Infants born to HBsAg-positive mothers should receive hepatitis B vaccine and 0.5 mL hepatitis B immune globulin (HBIG) within 12 hours of birth at separate sites. The 2nd dose is recommended at 1 to 2 months of age and the 3rd dose at 6 months of age.

Infants born to mothers whose HBsAg status is unknown should receive hepatitis B vaccine within 12 hours of birth. Maternal blood should be drawn at the time of delivery to determine the mother's HBsAg status; if the HBsAg test is positive, the infant should receive HBIG as soon as possible (no later than 1 week of age).

All children and adolescents (through 18 years of age) who have not been immunized against hepatitis B may begin the series during any visit. Special efforts should be made to immunize children who were born in or whose parents were born in areas of the world with moderate or high endemicity of hepatitis B virus infection.

[3]The 4th dose of DTaP (diphtheria and tetanus toxoids and acellular pertussis vaccine) may be administered as early as 12 months of age, provided 6 months have elapsed since the 3rd dose and the child is unlikely to return at age 15 to 18 months. Td (tetanus and diphtheria toxoids) is recommended at 11 to 12 years of age if at least 5 years have elapsed since the last dose of DTP, DTaP, or DT. Subsequent routine Td boosters are recommended every 10 years.

[4]Three *Haemophilus influenzae* type b (Hib) conjugate vaccines are licensed for infant use. If PRP-OMP (PedvaxHIB or ComVax [Merck]) is administered at 2 and 4 months of age, a dose at 6 months is not required. Because clinical studies in infants have demonstrated that using some combination products may induce a lower immune response to the Hib vaccine component, DTaP/Hib combination products should not be used for primary immunization in infants at 2, 4, or 6 months of age unless FDA-approved for these ages.

[5]To eliminate the risk of vaccine-associated paralytic polio (VAPP), an all-IPV schedule is now recommended for routine childhood polio vaccination in the United States. All children should receive four doses of IPV at 2 months, 4 months, 6 to 18 months, and 4 to 6 years. OPV (if available) may be used only for the following special circumstances:

    1. Mass vaccination campaigns to control outbreaks of paralytic polio.

    2. Unvaccinated children who will be traveling in <4 weeks to areas where polio is endemic or epidemic.

    3. Children of parents who do not accept the recommended number of vaccine injections. These children may receive OPV only for the third or fourth dose or both; in this situation, health care professionals should administer OPV only after discussing the risk for VAPP with parents or caregivers.

    4. During the transition to an all-IPV schedule, recommendations for the use of remaining OPV supplies in physicians' offices and clinics have been issued by the American Academy of Pediatrics (see *Pediatrics,* December 1999).

[6]The 2nd dose of measles, mumps, and rubella (MMR) vaccine is recommended routinely at 4 to 6 years of age but may be administered during any visit, provided at least 4 weeks have elapsed since receipt of the 1st dose and that both doses are administered beginning at or after 12 months of age. Those who have not previously received the second dose should complete the schedule by the 11- to 12-year-old-visit.

[7]Varicella (Var) vaccine is recommended at any visit on or after the first birthday for susceptible children, ie, those who lack a reliable history of chickenpox (as judged by a health care professional) and who have not been immunized. Susceptible persons 13 years of age or older should receive 2 doses, given at least 4 weeks apart.

[8]Hepatitis A (Hep A) is shaded to indicate its recommended use in selected states and/or regions; consult your local public health authority. (Also see *MMWR Morb Mortal Wkly Rep.* Oct 01, 1999;48(RR-12); 1–37.) (American Academy of Pediatrics, 2000.)

THE GLOBAL COMMUNITY

Donnelly, J., & Montgomery, D. (1999, March 18). Drug-resistant TB could be "principal epidemic of the next decade." *The Fresno Bee*, pp. A7, A8.

In the fall of 1998, on an 8-hour plane ride from Paris to New York City, a Ukrainian emigre repeatedly coughed. Unknown to the fellow passengers, the man was ill with active tuberculosis. His strain of TB had mutated into an organism able to resist six common antituberculosis drugs.

Two days after arriving in the United States, the man walked into a western Pennsylvania health clinic. The illness was diagnosed, and the airline was called by health investigators. They were able to track down 40 passengers who had sat near the man. Thirteen passengers were found infected with the mutant bacteria.

The heart of the crisis lies in the former Soviet states, particularly in Russia, Belarus, Moldova, and Ukraine. A CDC doctor described the situation as "probably the worst situation for multidrug-resistant TB ever documented in the world." Russia's financial meltdown is playing a direct role in the spread of resistant TB as doctors are unable to treat patients because of a lack of money. When treatment is interrupted, the bacteria grow especially hardy and, in close, unsanitary quarters, such as Russian prisons, easily infect others rapidly.

As the crisis grows in Europe, the chance of outbreaks in the United States grows. With 49 million international travelers coming to the United States each year, it will be impossible to keep TB from foreign sources out. The risk on airplanes, according to the CDC, only occurs on flights lasting 8 hours or more, and then only to those in the vicinity of the infectious person.

The cost of fighting multidrug-resistant TB soars, with a single case costing more than $25,000 because it involves a cocktail of drugs, lengthy hospitalization, and preventive measures for health care providers. In contrast, a 6-month treatment program using common drugs for nonresistant TB costs as little as $50.

This ongoing and potentially increasing problem among international travelers causes concern to public health practitioners and travelers alike. It creates a costly health care crisis that affects people unknowingly during a situation where the victims are unable to prevent their exposure or to protect themselves.

Religious Barriers. The right to religious freedom gives some groups of individuals in the United States the constitutional right to exemption from immunization when they object to vaccination on religious grounds. Children from these families are identified at school entry. Such exemptions must be specifically enacted by law, and although it is not necessary to belong to a specific denomination, courts have required those seeking exemption to demonstrate that such belief against immunization is sincere, and that no clear danger exists due to the particular disease. Problems arise when members of exempted groups are found together in school or community settings, raising the risk of disease spread because of a lower herd immunity.

Financial Barriers. Until recently, finances may have been significant in accounting for immunization delays in families with limited incomes. Such families may have had more immediate priorities than vaccinations for an otherwise well child. In the late 1990s, two major initiatives significantly improved the financing of childhood immunizations. The Vaccines for Children Program and the Child Health Insurance Program cover children on Medicaid, uninsured children, and American Indian and Alaska Native children. In addition, underinsured children who receive immunizations at federally qualified health centers and rural health clinics are covered. These initiatives should eliminate this barrier. Also, the 317 Grant Program and state funds help provide free vaccines for children not covered by the other programs who are served by the public sector, such as those who seek vaccines at health department clinics.

Social Barriers. Educational levels, transportation problems, and access to and overcrowding of facilities pose further barriers to adequate immunization coverage. Formidable quantities of paperwork involved in obtaining informed consent of parents may be intellectually intimidating as well as time consuming. Working parents may find it difficult, if not impossible, to reach an immunization clinic with their child during working hours. Requirements for appointments versus walk-in clinics or for a physical examination before vaccination may present additional deterrents. "Pockets of need" continue to exist in areas of every major city where substantial numbers of underimmunized children live. These areas are of great concern because, particularly in large urban areas with traditionally underserved populations, there is great potential for disease outbreaks (U.S. Department of Health and Human Services, 2000).

Cultural Barriers. Meeting the immunization needs of minority groups may involve cultural barriers related to differing concepts of health care and preventive measures between cultures. Language barriers may intervene to make parents feel confused, overwhelmed, and unable to access services. Depending on how long a family has resided in the United States and the level of active sponsorship, expectations of the health care system for parental action on behalf of the well child may be very unfamiliar.

Philosophical Objections. Many affluent, well-educated, caring parents have philosophical objections to immunization. They fear harm to their children, as has periodically been reported in the media. Parents may object to one or more of the vaccines or prefer to delay or separate the vaccines, thus putting them "behind" in immunizations, according to the AAP schedule. Community health nurses should be aware that caring parents are talking about these issues, reading about them, and trying to make informed decisions about them.

Provider Limitations. Another barrier to immunization coverage is provider limitations. Health care providers may have contact with an eligible child, yet fail to offer the vaccination. This occurs when providers see children for different reasons and do not review their immunization records, missing the opportunity to provide vaccination services at what may be a very convenient time for parents. Sometimes, children come for immunization services and receive some vaccines but not others, although the safety and efficacy of administering multiple vaccines on the same occasion are well established and recommended by the CDC (1994). Providers may erroneously defer administration of a vaccine based on a condition (eg, symptom of illness) that is not a true contraindication to immunization. To address this particular issue, the CDC has developed guidelines for providers showing misconceptions concerning contraindications to vaccination (Table 15–3). Another provider limitation or barrier to timely immunization coverage is that few providers have the initiative and resources to establish a uniform system for recall and notification when the next immunization is due. In the United States, even clients of private providers often are not encouraged or assisted to maintain their own copies of personal written medical records.

PLANNING AND IMPLEMENTING IMMUNIZATION PROGRAMS

Immunization programs targeting specific subgroups can be effective when they include the following: (1) community assessment parameters by race or other cultural groupings in the planning phase; (2) assessment of specific characteristics of the groups such as language, child care practices, preventive health behaviors, extreme poverty, or high illiteracy; and (3) appropriate planning decisions to deal with these potential barriers. Successful outreach efforts are motivated by the desire to reach the target population, even though specific or unusual accommodations must be made. Clinics are scheduled and held at times and places specifically intended to make the service more accessible and convenient to the target group. Materials are designed and presented with the needs and abilities of target parents in mind. Interpreters are present as needed. Display 15–2 outlines the necessary steps and considerations for administering immunization clinics in community settings.

ADULT IMMUNIZATION

Many people erroneously assume that vaccinations are for children only. Well-advertised influenza vaccination campaigns in recent years have helped somewhat to correct this notion. However, media coverage about adverse effects of such vaccination has done little to increase either community or provider enthusiasm about adult vaccination in general. Adults are at increased risk for many VPDs, and approximately 45,000 adult deaths each year are associated with complications from pneumococcal disease and influenza (U.S. Department of Health and Human Services, 2000). As our nation's population ages, increasing numbers of adults will be at risk for these major causes of death and illness.

Adults may require vaccination for a variety of reasons. Occupational exposure to blood, blood products, or other potentially contaminated body fluids provides the basis for Oc-

cupational and Safety Health Administration (OSHA) requirements for hepatitis B vaccine. All persons should receive tetanus vaccine every 10 years unless they have experienced major and/or contaminated wounds. If this is the case, individuals should receive a single booster of a tetanus toxoid on the day of the injury if more than 5 years have elapsed since their last tetanus toxoid dose. In addition to influenza and pneumonia vaccination already mentioned, adult immunizations may also include adult diphtheria/tetanus (DT). Other reasons for adult vaccination include a history of high-risk conditions, such as heart disease, diabetes, and chronic respiratory diseases; international travel; or suspected failure of earlier vaccines to produce lasting immunity. Table 15–4 displays the *Healthy People 2010* objective for influenza and pneumonia vaccines for people over 18 years of age.

A substantial portion of VPDs still occur among adults despite the effectiveness and availability of safe and effective vaccines. At least six reasons contribute to low vaccination levels among adults.

1. Limited comprehensive vaccine delivery systems are available in the public and private sectors.
2. Although statutory requirements exist for vaccination of children, no such requirements exist for all adults.
3. Vaccination schedules are complicated because of the detailed recommendations that may vary by age, occupation, lifestyle, or health condition.
4. Health care providers frequently miss opportunities to vaccinate adults during contacts in offices, outpatient clinics, and hospitals.
5. Comprehensive vaccination programs have not been established in settings where healthy adults congregate (eg, the workplace, senior centers).
6. Clients and providers may fear adverse effects after vaccination.

INTERNATIONAL TRAVELERS, IMMIGRANTS, AND REFUGEES

As Americans interact more and more with their neighbors in other parts of the world, the incidence of Americans with tropical or imported diseases also rises.

> **Virtually any destination can be reached from any other in only 36 hours of travel . . . this is well within the incubation period of most infectious diseases, affording ample opportunity for the unrecognized movement of pathogens from place to place and for rapid global spread of microbial agents (Ostroff & Kozarsky, 1998, p. 231).**

Information necessary for a potential traveler to go to new and exotic places, remain healthy, and return healthy is available from a number of sources. At the very minimum, all international travelers must take steps to be adequately immunized as required by international health practices. These include being immunized with immunoglobulin to prevent hepatitis A, having the necessary chemical prophylaxis on hand (and taking it regularly as instructed) if the traveler is to be in a malarious area, and being knowledgeable about

TABLE 15–3. General and Specific Guide to Contraindications and Precautions to Vaccinations*

True contraindications and precautions	Not contraindications (vaccines may be administered)
General for all vaccines (DTP/DTaP, OPV, IPV, MMR, Hib, Hepatitis B)	

CONTRAINDICATIONS

Anaphylactic reaction to a vaccine contraindicates further doses of that vaccine

Anaphylactic reaction to a vaccine constituent contraindicates the use of vaccines containing that substance

Moderate or severe illnesses with or without a fever

NOT CONTRAINDICATIONS

Mild to moderate local reaction (soreness, redness, swelling) following a dose of an injectable antigen

Mild acute illness with or without low-grade fever

Current antimicrobial therapy

Convalescent phase of illnesses

Prematurity (same dosage and indications as for normal, full-term infants)

Recent exposure to an infectious disease

History of penicillin or other nonspecific allergies or family history of such allergies

---

DTP/DTaP

CONTRAINDICATIONS

Encephalopathy within 7 days of administration of previous dose of DTP

PRECAUTIONS†

Fever of ≥40.5°C (105°F) within 48 h after vaccination with a prior dose of DTP

Collapse or shocklike state (hypotonic-hyporesponsive episode) within 48 h of receiving a prior dose of DTP

Seizures within 3 days of receiving a prior dose of DTP§

Persistent, inconsolable crying lasting ≥3 h within 48 h of receiving a prior dose of DTP

NOT CONTRAINDICATIONS

Temperature of <40.5°C (105°F) following a previous dose of DTP

Family history of convulsions§

Family history of sudden infant death syndrome

Family history of an adverse event following DTP administration

---

OPV¶

CONTRAINDICATIONS

Infection with HIV or a household contact with HIV

Known altered immunodeficiency (hematologic and solid tumors; congenital immunodeficiency; and long-term immunosuppressive therapy)

Immunodeficient household contact

PRECAUTION†

Pregnancy

NOT CONTRAINDICATIONS

Breast-feeding

Current antimicrobial therapy

Diarrhea

IPV

CONTRAINDICATION

Anaphylactic reaction to neomycin or streptomycin

PRECAUTION†

Pregnancy

MMR¶

CONTRAINDICATIONS

Anaphylactic reactions to egg ingestion and to neomycin**

Pregnancy

Known altered immunodeficiency (hematologic and solid tumors; congenital immunodeficiency; and long-term immunosuppressive therapy)

NOT CONTRAINDICATIONS

Tuberculosis or positive PPD skin test

Simultaneous TB skin testing††

Breastfeeding

Pregnancy of mother of recipient

Immunodeficient family member or household contact

(continued)

TABLE 15–3. General and Specific Guide to Contraindications and Precautions to Vaccinations* (Continued)

True contraindications and precautions	Not contraindications (vaccines may be administered)
PRECAUTION† Recent immune globulin administration	Infection with HIV Nonanaphylactic reaction to eggs or neomycin

Hib

CONTRAINDICATION None identified	**NOT A CONTRAINDICATION** History of Hib disease

Hepatitis B

CONTRAINDICATION Anaphylactic reaction to common baker's yeast	**NOT A CONTRAINDICATION** Pregnancy

(From Advisory Committee on Immunization Practices. [1994]. Guide to contraindications and precautions to vaccinations. *Morbidity and Mortality Weekly Report, 43* [RR-1], 24–25.)

*This information is based on the recommendations of the Advisory Committee on Immunization Practices (ACIP) and those of the Committee on Infectious Diseases (Red Book Committee) of the American Academy of Pediatrics (AAP). Sometimes these recommendations vary from those contained in the manufacturer's package inserts. For more detailed information, providers should consult the published recommendations of the ACIP, AAP, and the manufacturer's package inserts.

†The events or conditions listed as precautions, although not contraindications, should be carefully reviewed. The benefits and risks of administering a specific vaccine to an individual under the circumstances should be considered. If the risks are believed to outweigh the benefits, the vaccination should be withheld; if the benefits are believed to outweigh the risks (eg, during an outbreak or foreign travel), the vaccination should be administered. Whether and when to administer DTP to children with proven or suspected underlying neurologic disorders should be decided on an individual basis. It is prudent on theoretical grounds to avoid vaccinating pregnant women. However, if immediate protection against poliomyelitis is needed, OPV is preferred, although IPV may be considered if full vaccination can be completed before the anticipated imminent exposure.

§Acetaminophen given before administering DTP and thereafter every 4 hours for 24 hours should be considered for children with a personal or family history of convulsions in siblings or parents.

¶No data exist to substantiate the theoretical risk of a suboptimal immune response from the administration of OPV and MMR within 30 days of each other.

**Persons with a history of anaphylactic reactions following egg ingestion should be vaccinated only with caution. Protocols have been developed for vaccinating such persons and should be consulted. (*Journal of Pediatrics*, 196–199; 1983; 102. *Journal of Pediatrics*, 1988;113:504–506.)

††Measles vaccination may temporarily suppress tuberculin reactivity. If testing cannot be done the day of MMR vaccination, the test should be postponed for 4 to 6 weeks.

food and water hygiene precautions as well as basic first aid for the care of simple injuries. Yet every year in the 1990s, there were between 1,000 and 1,500 cases of malaria among poorly prepared and careless international travelers from the United States (Ostroff & Kozarsky, 1998). In many major cities of the United States, one finds tropical medicine or travelers' medicine specialists who can assist in being adequately prepared for travel. The CDC offers a travelers' hotline with up-to-date recommendations regarding malaria prophylaxis. Health departments and large libraries usually offer materials on international travel, including those listed in the Resources at the end of this book.

Refugees or international travelers who arrive in the United States are often unfamiliar with its health systems, health precautions, and practices. Refugees and immigrants must follow prescribed guidelines for their acculturation, including extensive health screening mandated by U.S. immigration laws. More than ever before, community health nurses have professional contact with these new Americans, whether close to time of their arrival or later, in schools and immunization clinics or other locations. Visitors from other countries may also require the assistance of community health professionals. For this reason, community health nurses are encouraged to develop and maintain a global perspective on communicable diseases.

SECONDARY PREVENTION

Two approaches to secondary prevention of communicable disease include screening and contact investigation/case-finding.

Screening

The term **screening** is used in community health and disease prevention to describe programs that deliver a testing mechanism to detect disease in groups of asymptomatic, apparently healthy individuals. Familiar examples include the rapid plasma reagin (RPR) test or Venereal Disease Research Laboratory (VDRL) test for syphilis, confirmed by the FTA-ABS, MHA-TP, or TPHA, discussed later in this chapter, the tine or Mantoux tuberculin test for TB; and HIV-1 antibody tests or a sensitive screening test such as the enzyme immunoassay (EIA), confirmed by a supplemental test, such as the Western blot (WB) or an immunofluorescence assay (IFA), discussed later in this chapter (CDC, 1998). Screening is a secondary prevention method because it discovers those who may have already become infected in order to initiate prompt early treatment.

DISPLAY 15–2. Administrative Aspects of Immunization Programs

Study the Target Community

Assess disease incidence and level of immunization coverage.

Identify the target group.

Assess conditions in the community: Is the target group scattered or localized?

Assess level of community involvement and awareness of the problem.

Identify means of communicating with target group: Through the media or through leaders or other.

Consider political and social structure of the community. Identify important leaders.

Identify sites for immunization clinics that are appropriate, accessible, and available.

Plan the Immunization Program

Review budget for immunization services.

Determine goals for clinic performance or outcome measures.

Communicate with target group to notify them of need and promote involvement and participation.

Estimate needs for vaccines and supplies and obtain them. Plan care of vaccines before, during, and after clinic.

Develop team coordination among staff.

Plan clinic logistics: Available supply of needed materials; medical waste disposal; anaphylaxis supplies; records and means of clinic registration; staffing; floor plan for traffic control and efficient management of crowds.

Prepare staff with information regarding objectives for clinic; criteria for who shall not be immunized;

mechanisms for referral of clients with other health needs.

Publicity

Inform target group of date, location, and times of immunization clinic.

Provide information on reasons for and benefits of (and contraindications to) immunization.

Encourage parents to bring existing immunization records to clinic.

Provide contact information for those with questions or inquiries.

Immunization Clinic

Registration system and records (for parent and clinic) ready.

Registrar or assistant(s) ready to assist parents not familiar with language of paperwork.

Parent education: informed consent; reporting of adverse reactions; date next vaccine due.

System for call-back, follow-up.

System for dealing with other health issues and/or adverse events.

Evaluation of Program

Assess numbers of immunizations given in relation to goals.

Assess suitability of approach in identification of target group, selection of sites, means of communication with group, availability of resources, and so forth.

Invite parental as well as community and staff feedback.

Evaluate results in relation to expenditures.

It is important to remember that the screening itself is not diagnostic but rather seeks to identify those persons with positive or suspicious findings who require further medical evaluation and/or treatment. Any community health nurse working with clients in a screening setting must be prepared to clearly and correctly explain to individuals that screening tests are not definitive, and positive findings require subsequent investigation before diagnostic conclusions can be drawn.

Criteria for Screening Tests

There are some important criteria for deciding whether to carry out a screening intervention in a community.

Validity and Reliability. The screening test must be valid and reliable. *Validity* refers to the test's ability to accurately identify those with the disease. *Reliability* refers to the test's ability to give consistent results when administered on different occasions by different technicians.

Test Predictive Value and Yield. The *predictive value* of

TABLE 15–4. 2010 Target for Influenza and Pneumonia Immunization in Adults

Objective: Increase to 90% the rate of immunization coverage among adults 65 years of age or older; 60% for high-risk adults 18 to 64 years of age.

Recommended Immunization	1995	Target 2010
NONINSTITUTIONALIZED ADULTS 65 YEARS OF AGE OR OLDER		
Influenza vaccine	58%	90%
Pneumococcal vaccine	32%	90%
NONINSTITUTIONALIZED HIGH-RISK ADULTS 18 TO 64 YEARS OF AGE		
Influenza vaccine	30%	60%
Pneumococcal vaccine	15%	60%
INSTITUTIONALIZED ADULTS (PERSONS IN LONG-TERM OR NURSING HOMES)		
Influenza vaccine	62%	90%
Pneumococcal vaccine	23%	90%

(U.S. Department of Health and Human Services [2000] *Healthy people 2010* [conference edition in two volumes]. Washington, DC: Author.)

a screening test is important for determining whether the screening intervention is justified. *Yield* refers to the number of positive results found per number tested. The predictive value and the yield of screening tests become important in planning screening programs for communicable disease detection and prevention because they can help planners locate screening efforts in areas or within population groups that are known to be at high risk for the disease. The predictive value of screening tests increases as the prevalence of the disease increases. For example, a screening test for syphilis targeted at the population included in crack-houses in a particular city would have greater predictive value and yield than a screening test for syphilis given to the city population at large.

Epidemiologic criteria for screening interventions for the detection of health problems are as follows:

1. Is the disease an important public health problem?
2. Is there a valid and reliable test?
3. Is there an effective and tolerable treatment that favorably influences the early stages of the disease?
4. Are facilities for diagnosis and treatment after positive screening results available and accessible?
5. Is there a recognizable early asymptomatic or latent stage in the disease?
6. Do clear guidelines for referral and treatment exist?
7. Is the total cost of the screening justifiable compared to the costs of treating the disease if left undiscovered?
8. Is the screening test itself acceptable?
9. Will screening be ongoing?

The ethics or values represented by these statements include a clear and unwavering respect for the dignity and worth of individuals across racial, gender, religious, sexual, tribal, ethnic, and geographic lines (Satcher, 1996). They include a commitment to ensuring that resources are allocated to areas where they will have the most benefit in preventing disease and premature death. They speak to respect for the individual receiving the screening service, that the person should only take on the burden of diagnosis if access to acceptable further intervention exists. Socioeconomically disadvantaged persons are often the most at risk for disease yet the least likely to receive screening services, due to financial barriers including lack of health insurance coverage for preventive care. This type of disparity in health care services needs to be corrected and is an objective of *Healthy People 2010* (U.S. Department of Health and Human Services, 2000).

Contact Investigation/Case-Finding

Another secondary prevention approach is contact investigation and case-finding. In this approach, the community health nurse seeks to discover and notify those who have had contact with a person diagnosed with a communicable disease. The objective in contact tracing and partner notification is specifically to reach contacts of the *index case* (diagnosed person) before the contacts, in turn, become infectious (CDC, 1998). Thus, the rapidity with which contact investigation can be accomplished is a concern.

Healthy People 2010 differentiates between two types of partner notification. *Patient referral* describes those clients who voluntarily advise their partners of the risk of disease and the need for contact with a health provider. *Provider referral* describes the community health workers who contact the individuals exposed to the index case and encourage them to receive appropriate medical care. In both types of notification, clients need information and encouragement as well as assurance of confidentiality.

It is a fact that not all individuals with disease can accurately identify the persons with whom they have had close or intimate contact. This is particularly the case with sexually transmitted diseases associated with drug abuse and the selling of sex for drugs. It is also true in situations involving highly mobile or transient people whose lifestyles preclude establishing relationships that can be traced or followed. These problems lead to the need for alternative approaches in case-finding, including the provision of screening activities in locations where people with similar risky lifestyle behaviors are likely to congregate. It further points to the critical need for tests that provide reliable results very rapidly, because it may not be possible to locate the person 24 hours or 2 weeks later for follow-up.

Contact investigation is most commonly practiced today in sexually transmitted disease and TB control programs. It is also used with some types of food-borne illness outbreak-control efforts. Rapidly evolving diseases and those that produce acute identifiable symptoms are not of concern in contact investigation so much as finding the cases of disease with incipient onset and long periods of infectiousness. The latter allow infected persons to reside and interact extensively in the community in an infectious state without being aware of their illness.

TERTIARY PREVENTION

The approaches to tertiary prevention of communicable disease include isolation and quarantine of the infected person and safe handling and control of infectious wastes.

Isolation and Quarantine

Communicable disease control includes two methods for keeping infected persons and noninfected persons apart to prevent spread of the disease. **Isolation** refers to separation of the infected persons (or animals) from others for the period of communicability to limit the transmission of the infectious agent to susceptible persons. **Quarantine** refers to restrictions placed on healthy contacts of an infectious case for the duration of the incubation period to prevent disease transmission if infection should develop (Chin, 1999).

Transmission by Health Care Workers

The problem of multidrug-resistant organisms has been increasing since the 1960s, when the first strains of methicillin-resistant *Staphylococcus aureus* (MRSA) were identified in the United Kingdom. The prevalence rates vary in location and by size and type of hospital, but resistance rates of 10% to 50% occur in the *S. aureus* isolates cultured and have become one of the most common agents of hospital and community-acquired infections (Dugger, 1997). Clients who are colonized (organisms living in the host with no deleterious effects to the host) or infected (organisms in large enough numbers in a host to cause deleterious effects) with multidrug-resistant strains are discharged into and admitted from the community, reinforcing the problem. This is a special concern for nurses because not only is there potential for the nurse to carry the infectious agent from client to client, but also there is considerable uncertainty about the implications for practice of the nurse who becomes colonized with drug-resistant bacteria in the course of caring for individuals. Although there is no definitive evidence that colonized health workers are implicated in outbreaks of drug-resistant infections, some agencies furlough colonized workers or limit their practice to infected patients. Studies have shown that effective decolonization may take from 3 weeks to a year. Employee health care programs must include infection control policies that address this problem and provide recommendations to the nurse for the prevention not only of infection but also of colonization, and provide agency policies regarding care of the infected or colonized nurse.

Safe Handling and Control of Infectious Wastes

Also important to control of infection in community health is the proper disposition of contaminated wastes. The CDC has developed universal precautions in which it encourages health workers to think of all blood and body fluids, and materials that have come in contact with same, as potentially infectious (Chin, 1999). The universal precautions include:

- Basic handwashing after contact with the client or potentially contaminated articles and before care of other clients
- Appropriate discarding or bagging and labeling of articles contaminated with infectious material before being sent for decontamination and reprocessing
- Appropriate isolation based on the mode of transmission of the specific disease, which includes strict isolation, contact isolation, respiratory isolation, TB isolation (AFB isolation), enteric precautions, and drainage/secretion precautions

The Environmental Protection Agency (EPA) defines infectious waste as "waste capable of producing an infectious disease." The agency notes that for waste to be infectious, it must contain pathogens with sufficient virulence and quantity so that exposure to the waste by a susceptible host could result in an infectious disease. EPA requirements for medical waste disposal are for waste to be segregated into categories of (1) sharps; (2) toxic, hazardous, regulated, or infectious fluids of greater than 20 mL; and (3) other materials. Although incineration has long been recognized as an efficient method of disposing safely of sharps and other contaminated medical waste, fewer incinerators are available now with increasing regulation of emissions, particularly those related to burning chemical wastes.

Four key elements of an infectious waste management program are applicable to community practice. (1) Health professionals must be able to correctly distinguish waste that poses a significant infection hazard from other biomedical waste that poses no greater risk than general municipal waste, and such infectious waste must be clearly defined. (2) The waste management program must have administrative support and authority to institute practice guidelines and provide the containers and other resources needed for safe disposal of infectious wastes. (3) Handling of the infectious wastes must be minimized. Containers should be rigid, leak resistant, impervious to moisture, have sufficient strength to prevent rupture or tearing under normal conditions, and be sealed to prevent leakage. For sharps, containers must also be puncture resistant. (4) There must be an enforcement or evaluation mechanism in place to ensure meeting the goal of reducing potential for exposure to infectious waste in the community.

MAJOR COMMUNICABLE DISEASES IN THE UNITED STATES

There are several communicable diseases that community health nurses encounter in their practice. They are frequently diagnosed and treated in the community. The more common ones, such as TB, HIV/AIDS, gonorrhea, syphilis, chlamydia, genital herpes, viral warts, the hepatitis viruses A, B, C, D, and E, influenza, and pneumonia are discussed here.

Tuberculosis

Tuberculosis (TB), once nearly eradicated, now poses a major threat to the public's health. There is evidence of recent alarming increases in overall rates, sharply disparate rates of TB among minority populations, a fatal association of TB with HIV infection and AIDS, increasing rates of TB among children, and a proliferation of multidrug-resistant strains, presenting a significant threat not only to clients but also to their caregivers.

INCIDENCE AND PREVALENCE

Roughly one third of the world's population is infected with *Mycobacterium tuberculosis*. Thus, 2 billion people in the world have the potential for developing active TB at some point in time (Ginsberg, 1998). In 1997, there were over 7 million new cases of TB, and approximately 3 million people died of it, making TB the leading infectious killer of adults, and this despite the fact that effective antituberculosis treatment has been known since the 1940s (World Health Report, 1998). TB is also the leading cause of death in people infected with the human immunodeficiency virus (HIV) (World Health Organization, 1997).

Exposure to TB does not lead to actual disease in all cases. A long latent period may persist for many years (even for a lifetime) before the infected person develops disease and becomes infectious. The probability of becoming infected depends primarily on the amount of exposure to air contaminated with *M. tuberculosis,* the proximity to the infectious person, and the degree of ventilation. The greatest majority of individuals exposed to infectious cases do not become infected. Of those who do, all but about 5% to 10% will remain disease free, perhaps for a lifetime (Grimes & Grimes, 1997). The remaining 90% harbor the organism, although they are not infectious (capable of spreading infection to others), and represent a persistent pool of potential cases in a population. The likelihood of being among the 10% who develop clinical infectious disease is variable, depending on the initial dose of infection and certain other risk factors. Groups at increased risk include children under age 3, adolescents, young adults, the aged, and the immunosuppressed (Chin, 1999). Unlike some other infectious diseases that spread rapidly in a susceptible community, immunizing or killing large numbers of people, TB can be maintained at endemic levels in populations for generations. Endemic levels are those at which the disease or infectious agent is habitually present in a geographic area, but disease outbreaks are contained to a minimum.

SURVEILLANCE

Variably called *consumption, wasting disease,* and the *white plague,* TB has been one of the greatest scourges since prerecorded historical times. It was the leading cause of death in the United States through the 1930s because no cure was available. A diagnosis of TB was a slow death sentence, and the best chance of recovery was rest, sunshine, and plenty of food. Consequently, sanatoriums—rest homes where patients followed a prescribed routine every day—were built and were occupied for months until recovery or death (CDC, 1995a) (Fig. 15–3).

Surveillance of a disease refers to the continuous scrutiny of all aspects of occurrence and spread of the disease that are pertinent to effective control (Chin, 1999). In 1953, when uniform national surveillance for TB was initiated, there were more than 84,000 TB cases in the United States. From 1953 through 1984, the number of TB cases decreased by an average of 6% each year, and in 1985 the number of TB cases reached an all-time low of 22,201 (CDC, 1995b). With the introduction of effective antibiotics in the 1940s to 1960s, we enjoyed a 73% decline in the number of TB cases, and as a nation we thought the problem of TB had been solved (Ginsberg, 1998; Grimes & Grimes, 1997). The decrease in the number of TB cases is seen as contributing to the medical and political complacency that has resulted in lax control efforts and now to the resurgence of TB.

In 1986 the number of TB cases began to rise and continued to accelerate through 1990. From 1991 to 1994 the United States experienced four consecutive years of declining TB cases. However, by 1996 rates were staying the same or increasing again in almost half the states. Cases were increasingly being reported among members of racial and ethnic minorities, children, and foreign-born persons living in the United States. Compounding the effects of these demographic changes was the appearance of multidrug-resistant TB strains. The rising incidence of TB and multidrug-resis-

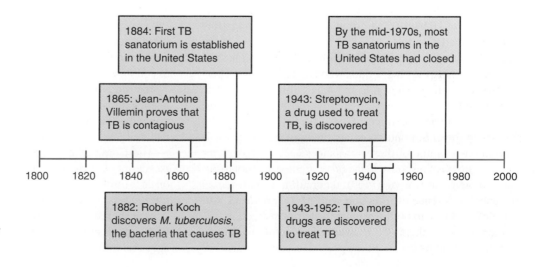

FIGURE 15–3. Timeline of major events in the history of tuberculosis.

tant TB has changed the TB situation considerably over the past decade and continues to be a major public health challenge (Snider & Castro, 1998).

POPULATIONS AT RISK

Minority populations tend to be at greater risk for TB. The proportion of TB cases among nonwhites compared with whites climbed to 73% of all cases in 1993, although, as a group, the nonwhite population makes up only 26% of the U.S. population. The overall case rate for whites in 1993 was 3.6 per 100,000, whereas among Asians/Pacific Islanders it was 44.5; among non-Hispanic blacks, 29.1; among Hispanics, 20.6; and among American Indians and Alaskan Natives, 14.6 (CDC, 1995b). In 1993, the percentages of TB disease cases were predominantly among the following groups of people: foreign-born persons (29%), the elderly (23%), homeless people (5%), and individuals infected with HIV (5%), in addition to low-income people, persons with alcohol or drug abuse problems, the underserved, the malnourished, people in correctional facilities, people with other medical conditions, those recently infected with TB, and individuals working where people at risk for TB are grouped together such as homeless shelters, drug treatment centers, and health care facilities. TB rates are highest among refugees and immigrants, and noncompliance with treatment among all groups is a major factor in continued transmission of the disease and development of multidrug-resistant organisms.

HIV infection is the strongest known risk factor for the development of TB. Immune-suppressed individuals such as those with AIDS can develop fulminant active TB within weeks of exposure to the mycobacterium, and the disease progresses much faster than in those with normal competent immune systems. Consequently, a suspected case of TB in a person with AIDS is usually treated immediately without waiting for sputum test or chest x-ray results. During the last 20 years, the incidence of HIV infection has shifted from a predominantly homosexual, white, middle-class male population to a more impoverished, heterosexual, inner-city minority population with a high prevalence of *M. tuberculosis* infection. Consequently, the incidence of HIV-related TB mortality has risen.

The risk of HIV-infected groups for TB infection is further complicated by false-negative reactions (anergy) of the tuberculin skin test due to the HIV-infected client's impaired immunity. Anergy testing is done when an HIV-infected person has a negative reaction to the tuberculin skin test. The recommended substances for anergy testing are mumps, *Candida,* or tetanus extracts (CDC, 1995c). Most healthy persons in the U.S. population can be assumed to be sensitized to one or more of these substances and will have a reaction. A positive response to the other antigen, but not to purified protein derivative (PPD) tuberculin, is considered evidence of absence of infection with *M. tuberculosis.* Absence of response to both warrants further investigation.

Increasing numbers of TB cases among children are especially worrisome because they point to escalated transmission in the United States. Cases in children most often result from recent infection, which is in contrast to cases among older adults that may develop as a result of infection occurring many years previously. TB among children suggests rising case rates among persons of reproductive age, who have contact with and transmit infection to susceptible children. This underscores the need to investigate the household and community contacts of the child for untreated disease. Likewise, when adult active TB cases are identified, it is essential to evaluate child contacts of the case.

Among children with active TB, minority groups account for a vast majority of the cases. Girls have a much higher incidence during elementary and high school years than do boys of the same age. Susceptibility in children and adolescence peaks during infancy and again in puberty. Infants show decreased ability to localize infection and have limited stores of acquired antibodies. It is unclear whether the increased susceptibility in adolescents is the result of increased contacts with infected persons, rapid hormonal changes and growth spurts, suboptimal diets, or a combination of all of these. The occurrence of TB infection and disease in children provides important information about its spread in homes and communities. For example, when children have TB infection or disease, we know it was transmitted relatively recently; the person who transmitted the TB may still be infectious; and other adults and children in the household or community have probably been exposed to it and, if infected, they may develop TB disease in the future (CDC, 1995b).

PREVENTION AND INTERVENTION

Tuberculin testing, the standard method for evaluating TB infection, is a simple skin test that measures by visible reaction whether the body has had immunologic experience with *M. tuberculosis* (Table 15–5). From there, evaluation procedures differentiate between classification status of the disease, ranging from 0 to 5. The two most used terms are infected, classification 2, and with the disease, classification 3 (Table 15–6). Thus, the skin test is not diagnostic of disease. There are two widely available skin test products. The tine test, a multiple-puncture type of test, delivers a premeasured dose of PPD under the skin by puncture. The Mantoux test delivers 0.1 mL of PPD by intradermal injection. The Mantoux (the dose is measured at time of injection) is generally considered the more reliable test, because the dose of the tine test and the technique of administration may be highly variable.

Interpretation of the tuberculin test is critical to subsequent evaluation of clients' status. The interpretation of this screening method must be as sensitive as possible while maintaining specificity for exposure.

The Committee on Infectious Disease of the American Academy of Pediatrics in 1988 developed guidelines based on cost-effectiveness for routine periodic skin testing only in high-risk populations. Such populations include children of American Indians and native Alaskans; children in neighborhoods where case rates are higher than the national average; children of immigrants from Asia, Africa, the Middle

TABLE 15–5. Classifying the Tuberculin Skin Test Reaction

5 or more millimeters	10 or more millimeters	15 or more millimeters
An induration of **5 or more millimeters** is considered **positive** for ■ People with HIV infection ■ Close contacts ■ People who have had TB disease before ■ People who inject illicit drugs and whose HIV status is unknown	An induration of **10 or more millimeters** is considered **positive** for ■ Foreign born persons ■ HIV-negative persons who inject illicit drugs ■ Low-income groups ■ People who live in residential facilities ■ People with certain medical conditions ■ Children younger than 4 years old ■ People in other groups as identified by local public health officials	An induration of **15 or more millimeters** is considered **positive** for ■ People with no risk factors for TB

(From: Centers for Disease Control [1995a]. *Self-study modules on tuberculosis: Transmission and pathogenesis of tuberculosis.* Atlanta, GA: Public Health Practice Program Office Division of Media and Training Services.)

East, Latin America, and the Caribbean; and children from households with one or more cases of active TB. Routine periodic screening was recommended for all children at 12 to 16 months of age, 4 to 6 years of age, and 14 to 16 years of age. Adults should be tested periodically once negative status has been determined. Frequency of testing depends on risk of exposure and symptoms, if any. Once a person is known to be a positive reactor to a skin test, the tuberculin test is not a valid means of assessing TB infection, and subsequent evaluation calls for a chest x-ray to identify tuberculous lesions.

Community health nurses working with ethnically diverse populations may meet clients who, after relating vaccination and/or TB histories, may have records of or recall receiving bacille Calmette-Guérin (BCG) vaccination. BCG is an antituberculosis vaccination first developed in 1906, which has been widely used on a global scale since 1921 in all countries except the Netherlands and the United States. Through collaborative efforts with the nations of the world, the World Health Organization in 1990 was able to meet its goal of immunizing 80% of the world's infants with the BCG vaccine. This rate hovered around 90% in 1997. BCG boosters for children at ages 5 to 7 and 11 to 14 are recommended in many countries (World Health Report, 1998).

BCG vaccine is an attenuated strain of *M. bovis* and may induce a positive TB skin test, although skin test reactivity tends to diminish with time. It is not used in the United States because it destroys this country's one control measure of a positive PPD to identify classification 3 individuals who should receive treatment for the TB infection. The BCG vaccine's efficacy is questionable. Also, protection begins to wane by 5 years, and by 10 years after vaccination, most recipients

do not have protection or measurable reactions. Another reason BCG has not been used in this country is that it has never been cloned, and vaccine products made in different locations may vary widely in effectiveness, providing from 0% to 80% effectiveness protection for inoculated individuals (American Thoracic Society, 1994). Because of these shortcomings, BCG is recommended in the United States *only* for infants and children with negative skin tests who (1) are at high risk of intimate and prolonged exposure to persistently untreated or ineffectively treated people with infectious pulmonary TB, who cannot be removed from the source of exposure and cannot be placed on long-term preventive therapy, or (2) are continuously exposed to persons with TB who have bacilli resistant to both isoniazid and rifampin (American Thoracic Society, 1994). Ideally, the development of a vaccine against TB with remarkably improved efficacy (ideally similar to the >90% efficacy currently achieved by other vaccines combating infectious diseases) is needed to eliminate this disease (Miller & Castro, 1996).

In 1987, the Secretary of the Department of Health and Human Services established the Advisory Committee for Elimination of Tuberculosis. This committee was charged with developing a strategy for eliminating TB from the United States by the year 2010. As a part of this effort, the CDC published guidelines for eliminating TB (CDC, 1989) and for preventing TB transmission in health care facilities (CDC, 1994b). To accomplish this goal, specific populations must be protected against the potential of exposure to people with latent infection. Public education and outreach are needed to develop positive working relationships with the target communities, involving them in successful program planning and implementation.

TABLE 15–6. Classification System for TB

Class	Type	Description
0	No exposure to TB Not infected	No history of exposure, negative reaction to the tuberculin skin test
1	Exposure to TB No evidence of infection	History of exposure, negative reaction to a tuberculin skin test given at least 10 weeks after exposure
2	TB infection No TB disease	Positive reaction to the tuberculin skin test, negative smears and cultures (if done), no clinical or x-ray evidence of TB disease
3	Current TB disease	Positive culture for *M tuberculosis* (if done), **or** A positive reaction to the tuberculin skin test and clinical or x-ray evidence of current TB disease
4	Previous TB disease (not current)	Medical history of TB disease, **or** Abnormal but stable x-ray findings for a person who has a positive reaction to the tuberculin skin test, negative smears and cultures (if done), and no clinical or x-ray evidence of current TB disease
5	TB suspected	Signs and symptoms of TB disease, but evaluation not complete

(From: Centers for Disease Control. [1995a]. *Self-study modules on tuberculosis: Transmission and pathogenesis of tuberculosis.* Atlanta, GA: Public Health Practice Program Office Division of Media and Training Services.)

Successful interventions will also require TB control programs to focus resources on high-risk people, including contacts of people recently diagnosed as having TB. Also targeted for prevention efforts are members of racial and ethnic minorities and people born in countries where TB prevalence is high. People with TB infection who have conditions placing them at increased risk of active TB, such as HIV infections, also require special attention. The American Nurses Association has developed two position statements on Tuberculosis and Public Health Nursing (1997b) (Display 15–3) and Tuberculosis and HIV (1997a) (Display 15–4), supporting the management of TB and TB/HIV.

A well-functioning TB control program is the best way to prevent TB and to prevent the emergence of drug resistance. Such programs:

- Follow standard public health practices
- Achieve prompt sputum conversion in people with active disease
- Investigate contacts of people with active cases to identify and treat other cases and people recently exposed
- Achieve a high completion-of-therapy rate within a year of diagnosis
- Have adequate funding and a dedicated TB control infrastructure (maintaining the amount of funding that was available for TB control programs annually from 1994 to 1998 of over $140 million a year)
- Avoid block grants or "privatization" of public health disease control functions (despite supporters of such change) (Horsburgh, 1998)

One of the most effective ways to achieve a high completion-of-therapy rate is through the WHO-supported directly observed treatment short-course (DOTS, frequently referred to as DOT) as the treatment strategy for detection and cure (World Health Report, 1998). It has become clear that the DOTS strategy can achieve high cure rates in any country

that is determined to succeed. The treatment success rate of cases in DOTS global areas was 78%, compared with 45% in non-DOTS areas. The use of DOTS expanded nearly tenfold from 1993 to 1997, cure rates nearly doubled, and drug resistance was lower in places where DOTS had been used (World Health Report, 1998). The American Thoracic Society (1994) proposes treating all patients with directly observed therapy because it reduces the sources of infection in the community.

This labor-intensive approach has proved effective for the most difficult of TB cases in the United States. The more difficult clients are those who do not realize their personal or social responsibility for health and those who do not have the resources to focus on health when there are other stressors or diversions in their life. Clients such as alcohol and drug abusers, transient homeless people, and low-income people thus may be the source cases for new cases of TB. DOTS therapy ensures that clients take a daily or intermittent dose of prescribed medication, locating them wherever they may be—neighborhood bars, sleeping on the sidewalk, a homeless shelter, or in a drug rehabilitation center. Most health departments and TB control programs have a percentage of their clients receiving DOTS therapy, using licensed staff or community health workers to administer the TB drug regimen (Brickner & McAdam, 1995). These ancillary staff members are often former program participants, trained and supervised by professional health workers (American Nurses Association, 1997b). A program like DOTS needs sustained political commitment with the governments of nations recognizing the long-term benefits of providing the resources and staff necessary to ensure its proper implementation.

Commitment and flexibility on the part of health providers and services can substantially enhance medication compliance. Significant improvement in compliance has been demonstrated with programs designed to provide DOTS therapy for all clients, using community-based health workers who meet

DISPLAY 15–3. ANA Position Statement on Tuberculosis and Public Health Nursing—Summary

The ANA advocates a nursing care management model as a proven strategy for TB control and supports:

- The use of a nursing case management model in TB control to coordinate patient services; facilitate the safe delivery of TB medications to patients in the community; ensure completion of therapy; and limit the transmission of the disease by identifying newly infected and diseased persons through contact investigation procedures.
- The utilization of unlicensed assistive personnel working under the supervision and direction of nurses.
- The enhancement of nursing's role in surveillance, assessment, treatment, and evaluation activities with priority given to nursing management of patients on treatment, education, and infection control practices that will promote prevention in the community and among health care workers.
- Collaboration with other agencies to encourage research on the development and implementation of different treatment models of care to provide a full range of available treatment options for clients with TB.
- Nursing research initiatives on the effectiveness of different treatment modalities in improving treatment outcomes, including the use of directly observed therapy and other adherence strategies.
- Innovative demonstration projects to document effective strategies for surveillance and screening methods with at-risk populations.
- Accelerated research to document the most effective control measures that will prevent the transmission of TB to nurses providing treatment.

(From American Nurses Association [1997b]. Position statement—Tuberculosis and public health nursing. Http://www.nursing-world.org/readroom/position/blood/bltbhl.htm. 9/17/98, 1–3.)

DISPLAY 15–4. ANA Position Statement on Tuberculosis and HIV—Summary

The ANA supports:

- Closely monitoring the HIV-infected person for TB symptoms and screening for TB. All individuals found to be HIV positive should be offered an appropriate TB test.
- Policy development to support linkages of TB with HIV, primary care and substance abuse screening, education, and treatment in accessible and convenient programs.
- The provision of joint testing services for TB and HIV which employ confidentiality and pre- and post-test counseling services.
- The ethical responsibility of nurses to engage in ongoing assessment related to communicable diseases, such as TB.
- Education for all nurses about the epidemiology, transmission, prevention strategies, and symptoms of TB.
- Employers' provision of protective equipment and appropriate safe work environment for nurses to prevent the transmission of communicable diseases such as TB.
- Federal and state resources being applied to alleviate conditions of social deprivation.
- Funding for increased research to expand knowledge of HIV/TB transmission and treatment.
- Increased participation of nurses in research for safe workplace protective equipment and technology to reduce the risk of communicable disease transmission.
- Continued nursing input into federal, state and local agencies and legislative processes about TB and HIV disease concerns.
- The HIV positive nurse to:
  —Know their TB status by following CDC-recommended guidelines for ongoing assessment,
  —Self-limit their nursing practice based on a case-by-case assessment of their TB status,
  —Self-restrict their contact with patients, coworkers, and visitors if symptoms associated with air-borne communicable disease are present,
  —Adhere to prescribed medication regimen for TB to decrease the opportunity for transmission of the disease.

(From American Nurses Association [1997a]. Position statement—Tuberculosis and HIV. http://www.nursingworld.org/readroom/position/blood/blhvtb.htm 9/17/98, 1–4.)

with clients in residences, at job sites, and at other local venues. In addition, new variations on the standard treatment regimens are being researched. Approaches include allowing individuals to take larger medication doses on a twice-weekly schedule, or providing an observed medication program for a limited period, followed by a course of self-administered medication with periodic reevaluation by health care providers.

MULTIDRUG-RESISTANT TUBERCULOSIS

Epidemiologists and communicable disease specialists cite a number of factors contributing to the development and spread of TB strains resistant to one or more of the standard arsenal

of TB drugs. Strains now exist that are resistant to as many as 9 of 11 standard antituberculosis drugs (see The Global Community). Chief among the factors contributing to drug resistance seems to be the political and social response to declining rates of TB over past decades, resulting in cuts in

TABLE 15–7. 6-Month Regimen Options[1] for Pulmonary and Extrapulmonary TB in Adults and Children

	Initial Phase		Continuation Phase		
	Drugs	**Interval and Duration**	**Drugs**	**Interval and Duration**	**Comments**
1	INH RIF PZA EMB[2] or SM	Daily for 8 weeks	INH RIF	Daily or 2 or 3 times weekly[3] for 16 weeks[4]	▪ EMB or SM should be continued until susceptibility to INH and RIF is shown. ▪ In areas where less than 4% of cases are resistant to INH (first drug susceptibility test only), EMB or SM may not be necessary for patients with no individual risk factors for drug resistance.
2	INH RIF PZA EMB[2] or SM	Daily for 2 weeks, then 2 times weekly[3] for 6 weeks	INH RIF	2 times weekly[3] for 16 weeks[4]	▪ Patients prescribed this regimen should be given directly observed therapy. ▪ After the initial phase, EMB or SM should be continued until susceptibility to INH and RIF is shown, unless drug resistance is unlikely.
3	INH RIF PZA EMB[2] or SM	3 times weekly[3] for 6 months[4]			▪ Patients prescribed this regimen should be given directly observed therapy. ▪ Continue all four drugs for 6 months.[5] ▪ This regimen has been shown to be effective for INH-resistant TB.

From Centers for Disease Control. [1995d]. *Self-study modules on tuberculosis: Treatment of tuberculosis infection and disease.* Atlanta, GA: Public Health Practice Program Office Division of Media and Training Services.)

Note: If a patient's drug susceptibility results show resistance to INH, RIF, PZA, EMB, or SM, or if the patient has symptoms, positive smears, or positive cultures after 3 months, consult a TB medical expert.

[1]For adults who have smear- and culture-negative pulmonary TB and for adults and children for whom PZA is contraindicated, different regimen options are necessary. Consult a medical expert for further information.

[2]Ethambutol is not recommended for children who are too young to be monitored for changes in their vision. However, ethambutol should be considered for all children who are too young to be monitored for changes in their vision. However, ethambutol should be considered for all children who have TB that is resistant to other drugs but susceptible to ethambutol.

[3]All patients prescribed an intermittent regimen should be given directly observed therapy.

[4]For infants and children with miliary TB, bone and joint TB, or TB meningitis, treatment should last at least 12 months. For adults with these forms of extrapulmonary TB, the patient's response to therapy should be monitored closely. If response is slow or inadequate, treatment may be prolonged on a case-by-case basis.

[5]There is some evidence that SM may be discontinued after 4 months if the isolate is susceptible to all drugs.

INH = isoniazid RIF = rifampin PZA = pyrazinamide SM = streptomycin EMB = ethambutol

funding for surveillance, treatment, and research and a premature sense that TB was beaten. Federal surveillance of drug-resistant TB strains was discontinued in 1986 because of budgetary constraints. On an individual case basis, noncompliance with therapy for the full recommended period is the most common means by which resistant organisms are acquired. Public health services with limited resources have been unable to provide the intensive follow-up necessary to ensure that people essentially feeling well remain on medication (which may produce unpleasant although usually mild and manageable side effects) for the 6 months considered necessary to achieve cure (CDC, 1995d) (Table 15–7). Public health officials face a challenge to network effectively to provide continuous case management for highly mobile and often disenfranchised infected minority populations.

The reality of drug-resistant strains of TB significantly complicates the crisis of AIDS. Thus, when candidates for drug therapy are identified, it is essential to provide program support to ensure that the maximum number of individuals comply with their medication regimen for the full duration of therapy. Isoniazid therapy for individuals infected with TB, but without evidence of active disease, has been shown to be highly effective in preventing progression to infectiousness and clinical symptoms. Isoniazid is also a key component of treatment for active disease. Adverse effects of isoniazid therapy are often overestimated, leading to inappropriate withdrawal of therapy.

HIV/AIDS

Human immunodeficiency virus (HIV) is a retrovirus that attacks the body's immune system. Two types have been identified: type 1 (HIV-1) and type 2 (HIV-2). These viruses are serologically and geographically relatively distinct, but have similar epidemiologic characteristics. The pathogenicity of HIV-2 appears to be less than that of HIV-1 (Chin, 1999).

It is transmitted through sexual contact, the sharing of HIV-contaminated needles and syringes, transfusion of infected blood or its components, and from infected mother to child during the perinatal period (Bryson, 1996). **Acquired immunodeficiency syndrome (AIDS)** is a severe, life-threatening condition representing the late clinical stage of infection with HIV in which there is progressive damage to the immune and other organ systems, particularly the central nervous system. Most people infected with HIV remain symptom-free for long periods, but viral replication is active during all stages of infection. AIDS eventually develops in almost all HIV-infected people from months to 17 years after infection, with a median of 10 years (CDC, 1998). The early diagnosis of HIV infection is important in order to begin treatments that are available to slow the declining function of the immune system. Preventive measures for *Pneumocystis carinii* pneumonia (PCP), toxoplasmis of the CNS, disseminated *M. avium* complex (MAC) disease, TB, and bacterial pneumonia are available, and HIV clients need to be aware of this. Because of its effect on the immune system, HIV affects the diagnosis, evaluation, treatment, and follow-up of such concurrent diseases.

INCIDENCE AND PREVALENCE

Only 20 years ago, HIV/AIDS was recognized as an emerging disease and has rapidly established itself throughout the world and into a global pandemic. It has infected tens of millions in less than 20 years and is now prevalent in virtually all parts of the world (World Health Report, 1998). It is estimated there are 30.6 million adults and children living with HIV/AIDS in 1998, with 2.3 million deaths in 1997 and a global number of AIDS deaths since the beginning of the epidemic of 11.7 million (UNAIDS, 1998). By the year 2000, it is estimated that over 40 million people will be living with HIV/AIDS (World Health Report, 1998).

Current estimates based on various studies are that over 1 million people in the United States are infected with HIV, and 670,000 have been diagnosed with AIDS since first reported in 1981 (CDC, 1998; UNAIDS, 1998). The number of AIDS cases in the United States climbed each year until 1996, when it dropped into second place among leading causes of death in the 25-to-44 age group of people for the first time in 4 years (U.S. Dept. of Health and Human Services, 2000).

Annual costs of HIV/AIDS care in the United States have been in the billions of dollars. More people are being drawn into the health care system at an earlier point for intervention of long duration. Consequently, it is expected that AIDS-related care costs will continue to grow. Combination therapy with at least three antiretroviral drugs was introduced in 1995 and became widespread in 1996 (UNAIDS, 1998). It is not yet known how long these therapies will prolong life, and they do not work for everyone, but their use is having a visible impact on AIDS incidence and AIDS mortality. The new antiviral drugs have delayed the onset of AIDS in HIV-infected people and have improved the quality of life for many HIV-infected people in North America (World Health Report, 1998). In Western Europe, AIDS cases fell from 23,954 in 1995 to 14,874 in 1997, a 38% drop. In the United States, we experienced a first-ever annual overall decrease in new cases in 1996, a 6% drop. An even larger decrease was expected in 1997. Unfortunately, among African Americans, new AIDS cases rose by 19% among heterosexual men and 12% among heterosexual women. The Hispanic community experienced 13% more cases among men and 5% more among women than a year earlier (UNAIDS, 1998). This may be, in part, because these communities find it hard to access the expensive new drugs that can stave off the onset of AIDS.

POPULATIONS AT RISK

AIDS was first recognized as a distinct syndrome in 1981 and, during the early years, was seen as a disease of male homosexuals, intravenous drug abusers, and/or people with a history of multiple blood transfusions. The at-risk population for AIDS now includes people with large numbers of sexual partners, adolescents, injecting drug users and their sexual partners, homosexual men and their male or female partners, people who exchange sex for drugs or money, and people already infected with HIV (U.S. Department of Health and Human Services, 2000). Sexual transmission of HIV is closely associated with other STDs, particularly those that have an ulcerative phase, including syphilis. With belated but growing awareness of the AIDS epidemic on a global scale, it is becoming recognized as a universal threat to the health and well-being of individuals and of populations. Worldwide, over two thirds of all the people now living with HIV—nearly 21 million men, women, and children—live in Africa south of the Sahara desert. Also, 83% of the world's AIDS deaths have been in this region (UNAIDS, 1998). Four out of five HIV-positive women in the world live in Africa, whereas 87% of the affected children live there. This is happening for several reasons: more women of childbearing age live in Africa than elsewhere; African women have more children on average that those in other continents; nearly all children in Africa are breastfed, which is a way to transmit HIV; and the new drugs are far less readily available in developing countries. AIDS is seen in the United States as a potential health threat to all sexually active people and their offspring. Heterosexually acquired AIDS increased significantly in the 1990s, especially among women and minority populations, with blacks and Hispanics accounting for 65% of AIDS cases reported in 1997 (Brooks, 1999; Chin, 1999).

Adolescents and young adults are considered to be at particular risk for HIV infection because many of them engage in high-risk behavior, believing themselves to be invulnerable to infection. In addition to the considerable risks posed by potential HIV infection, other adverse outcomes related to early initiation of sexual activity include higher levels of all STDs (World Health Report, 1998).

PREVENTION AND INTERVENTION

National HIV prevention and intervention efforts depend on two important factors: (1) self-perception of risk and (2) adoption of risk-reducing behaviors in response to awareness of the risk. Consequently, education about HIV/AIDS, including safe sex and injecting drug use, has become the key to prevention. Public health workers seek to identify and intervene with the at-risk population, providing counseling and prevention education as well as testing services. The primary purposes of counseling are to prevent further spread of HIV infection and, when possible, to slow progression of HIV infection to AIDs. HIV counseling can help uninfected people initiate and sustain behaviors to reduce their risk of infection; help infected people adopt behaviors to reduce the risk of transmission to others; encourage spouses and partners of infected people to adopt safe behaviors; and help infected people take better care of themselves. Properly using condoms, reducing the number of sexual partners, and abstaining from injecting drug use decrease, but do not eliminate, the risk of HIV infection (U.S. Department of Health and Human Services, 2000).

HIV infection and AIDS are important topics of concern to community health nurses for a number of reasons. They present an intriguing service delivery problem requiring complex and sophisticated multidisciplinary interventions. Sexual behaviors, illegitimate drug use, end-of-life issues, and other psychosocial aspects provide very human dimensions to a problem also demanding of nursing, medical, social, epidemiologic, political, and economic resources.

Care of people with HIV infection presents a special opportunity for community health nurses to meet an important and visible challenge in modern society. People with HIV/AIDS are living longer, requiring nursing care that is widely integrated with other community services. This population requires knowledgeable, skilled, often aggressive therapeutic and preventive nursing services for acute as well as chronic illness, supported by an interdisciplinary network of providers. Three major goals of care with this population are: (1) promoting general health and resilience, (2) preventing infections of all sorts, and (3) delaying the onset of clinical symptoms with antiviral therapy. To meet these goals, the community health nurse's role involves getting HIV-positive clients engaged in wellness programs such as promoting nutritional health, exercise, drug management, and preventing opportunistic infections. Stress reduction is essential for these clients; the nurse can facilitate relaxation activities, client and family counseling, and support groups to assist clients' coping abilities. An important part of nursing care with these clients is use of "universal precautions," which refers to the CDC recommendations to prevent infections

that are transmitted by direct or indirect contact with infected blood or body fluids (bloody body secretions, semen, vaginal secretions, tissue, cerebrospinal fluid [CSF], and synovial, pleural, peritoneal, pericardial, and amniotic fluids). Nurses can also make important contributions to the evolution of HIV/AIDS care and services by participating in the debates that occur and will likely continue over the ethical dimensions of the AIDS crisis, including HIV screening, contact investigation, and AIDS-related discrimination, which are discussed later in this chapter.

The therapeutic management of HIV infection and AIDS is evolving and is, in fact, largely experimental. Attempts at vaccine development are ongoing and include experimentation with vaccines for those already infected to increase resistance to multiplication of the viral agent and development of clinical symptoms. Nurses wishing timely updates on clinical and medical aspects of AIDS case management are urged to refer to recent issues of the CDC's *Morbidity and Mortality Weekly Report,* as well as professional journals devoted to disseminating information to practitioners working with AIDS patients.

CLIENTS WITH HIV AND TUBERCULOSIS

HIV infection is associated with an increased possibility to develop primary TB after exposure to source cases (Barnes et al., 1996). The connection between TB and HIV/AIDS is dramatic, with one third of the incidence in the last 5 years attributed to HIV. The weakened immune system makes a person infected with the tubercle bacillus 30 times more likely to become ill with TB. For example, 60% to 80% of people with AIDS in India, Myanmar, Nepal, and Thailand develop TB (World Health Report, 1998).

People with HIV infection should be given high priority for preventive therapy, regardless of their age. For HIV-infected people, preventive therapy consists of isoniazid daily for 12 months (the usual regimen for preventive therapy is 6 months) (CDC, 1995d). These clients must be monitored closely for effectiveness of the preventive therapy and tolerance to isoniazid. This drug has the capacity to develop adverse reactions, or negative side effects. Isoniazid may cause hepatitis or damage the liver. Close monitoring and regular follow-up can detect early symptoms, such as nausea, vomiting, abdominal pain, fatigue, and dark urine. Any combination of these symptoms would initiate liver function tests.

As mentioned earlier, HIV-positive clients may not have the ability to react to a skin test for TB because of a weakened immune system. Therefore, other methods to determine TB status are employed. If it is determined that TB disease is present, the HIV-infected client begins a regimen of drugs according to the schedule in Table 15–7. They should be closely monitored for response to treatment; if they do not seem to be responding, they should be reevaluated (CDC, 1995d).

Community health nurses have a responsibility to help HIV-infected clients experience a successful TB treatment regimen. Caregiving includes observing for adherence to treatment, administering medications (either directly through DOTS or through DOTS supervision of ancillary staff), observing for signs and symptoms of adverse reactions, monitoring for overall health and well-being, educating, and making referrals as needed.

Other Sexually Transmitted Diseases

As we have been discovering throughout this chapter, human history has been shaped by disease. All historical events have played a part in creating the preconditions for epidemics. Of all the communicable diseases, perhaps none are as closely interrelated with human activities and attitudes than sexually transmitted diseases (STDs). Many have occurred in epidemic proportions, and most have been among us for centuries. They are mentioned in the Bible and in ancient Chinese and Greek medical texts (Gelbart, 1998). Gonorrhea was the most common STD until the 15th century, when a new and deadly disease called syphilis invaded Europe. It spread to the New World and remained a major problem through the 1940s. Since then, other STDs such as chlamydia, genital herpes, human papilloma virus (HPV), and hepatitis have taken over the headlines. Most likely, new ones will emerge as we enter a new millennium.

Sexually transmitted diseases are those infections spread by transfer of organisms from person to person during sexual contact. STDs are of critical importance in any discussion of communicable disease control because, as a single class of disease, they include more than 25 infectious organisms and account for 87% of all cases among the top 10 most frequently reported diseases to the CDC and state health departments (CDC, 1996). Each year, 15 million Americans are infected with an STD, including 3 million teenagers (U.S. Department of Health and Human Services, 2000). The total direct and indirect costs to society of the principal STDs are an estimated $17 billion annually (Institute of Medicine, 1997).

The U.S. STD rate exceeds that of all other industrialized countries in the world, letting us know that we have not gone fast enough or far enough in our national attempt to control STDs. The STDs discussed in this section include gonorrhea, syphilis, chlamydia, genital herpes, and human papillomavirus (HPV; genital warts). AIDS, of course, is an STD, as is hepatitis B, although transmission of these diseases can also occur through intravenous drug use, transfusion of blood products before 1986, or accidental or intentional needlestick injury. These diseases are discussed separately in this chapter.

Of further concern to community health nurses is the fact that women and children suffer an inordinate amount of the STD burden. Leaving aside for the moment the risk of AIDS and subsequent death, the most serious complications of STDs are pelvic inflammatory disease (PID), sterility, ectopic pregnancy, blindness, cancer associated with HPV, fetal and infant death, birth defects, and mental retardation. The medically underserved, particularly the poor and mar-

ginalized and ethnic and racial minorities, shoulder a disproportionate share of this problem, experiencing higher rates of disability and death than the population as a whole. Some notable disproportionately affected groups include sex workers, adolescents and adults in detention, and migrant workers (U.S. Department of Health and Human Services, 2000). Sexual violence and sexual coercion are significant problems for America's young women. Studies show that not all sexually experienced young females enter a sexual relationship as a willing partner (Abma, Driscoll & Moore, 1998).

Healthy People 2010 identifies the availability and quality of public services for STD as key factors in reducing the spread of STDs and preventing complications (U. S. Department of Health and Human Services, 2000). Effective health promotion approaches in the community must include STD prevention in the curricula of middle and secondary schools. The initiation of sexual activity early in life results in an increased number of sexual partners over a person's lifetime and thus establishes the behavioral link to higher levels of STDs (Miller, Monson & Norton, 1995).

In addition to the need for more innovative and effective sexual health promotion approaches in school settings, a number of recommendations have been made for improvements in current delivery systems (U.S. Department of Health and Human Services, 2000). The number of clinics offering STD screening, diagnosis, treatment, counseling, and referral services should increase substantially to improve access to comprehensive services. Certainly, consideration, planning, and the allocation of resources should be directed to the quality-of-life issues that operate in young adults' lives and contribute to inappropriately early initiation of unprotected sexual activity. Case management by providers often does not conform to the CDC recommendations in the nature of medical treatment, follow-up strategies to confirm cure, or notification and treatment of sexual partners. This in turn may contribute to inadequate treatment, continued transmission, higher risk of complications, and the increase in drug-resistant strains of gonorrhea and other diseases. *Healthy People 2010* (U.S. Department of Health and Human Services, 2000) strongly recommends expansion of contact tracing efforts. Treating individuals who present with symptoms is only half the job. The partner or partners of infected people must be notified and also require treatment for effective and lasting "cure" of the case.

Adolescent and young adult females and males who have multiple sex partners over a specified period (eg, several months) are at increased risk for gonorrhea, syphilis, and chlamydia. Increased numbers of sex partners over a lifetime are associated with a greater cumulative risk for acquiring viral infections such as hepatitis B, genital herpes, HPV, and HIV. Nineteen of the national health objectives for the year 2010 (U.S. Department of Health and Human Services, 2000) focus on activities, services, and behaviors that will reduce sexually transmitted diseases.

Changes in behavior will require diverse and multidisciplinary interventions over an extended period of time. Such interventions must integrate the efforts of parents, families, schools, religious organizations, health departments, community agencies, and the media. The goals of educational programs should be to provide adolescents with the knowledge and skills they need to refrain from sexual intercourse, and to increase the use of condoms as well as other contraceptive measures among those unwilling to postpone onset of sexual activity (U.S. Department of Health and Human Services, 2000). Studies have suggested that parent–child conversations about sexual matters have been associated with delays in initiation of sexual activity and with the increased use of contraceptives by adolescents who engage in sexual intercourse. Additional recommendations to promote sexual health in adolescent populations included (1) innovations for early detection and treatment of STDs among teenagers, (2) specialized training for clinicians providing health services for adolescents, (3) school education combined with accessible clinical services, and (4) behavioral interventions to prevent exposure to and acquisition of STDs.

GONORRHEA

The U.S. gonorrhea rate has decreased by 56% between 1990 and 1997, going from 278 per 100,000 to 122.7, making the 1997 rate the lowest ever reported in the United States. Its causative agent is the gonococcus bacteria *Neisseria gonorrhoeae.* Among women, 15 to 19 year olds had the highest rate, whereas among men, 20 to 24 year olds had the highest rate. However, even in this group, gonorrhea has decreased by 49% since 1990. Incidence has decreased in all ethnic and racial groups from a high of 468 cases per 100,000 in 1975, and by 1997 we had reached the *Healthy People 2000* target of 100 cases per 100,000. Nevertheless, among African-Americans, even with a 58% decrease in cases, the reported rate was 812 in 1997. The target for 2010 is 19 cases per 100,000 (Chin, 1999; U.S. Department of Health and Human Services, 2000). Antimicrobial resistance continues to be a concern when treating the disease. Overall, 29% of isolates collected in the United States in 1996 were resistant to penicillin, tetracycline, or both. Globally, the prevalence patterns for gonorrhea in developing countries are 10 to 15 times those in developed countries, and drug-resistant strains of gonococcal infections provide added concern (World Health Report, 1998).

Frequently, the numbers of cases of gonorrhea are influenced by the disease reoccurring in the same individual, usually related to sexual lifestyle choices. Successful interventions with people with repeat infections could prove to be the most cost-effective way of managing the disease. Helping people avoid repeat infections will most likely begin with a thorough personal history, including partner characteristics and willingness to also be treated. It will also require a more comprehensive multiagency approach focusing on some of the other social, economic, and environmental issues that demand attention for successful, lasting behavior change.

Gonorrhea commonly presents in men as a purulent drainage from the penis, accompanied by painful urination,

within 2 to 7 days after an infecting exposure. In females, symptoms may be so mild as to go unnoticed. Progression of untreated gonorrhea may lead to serious reproductive system involvement and subsequent infertility. The recommended treatment regimen for gonorrhea has been ceftriaxone, ciprofloxacin, ofloxacin, or cefixime in a single dose, followed by a regimen effective against concurrent chlamydial infection, doxycycline twice daily by mouth for 7 days. This will also cure incubating syphilis and inhibit emergence of antimicrobial-resistant gonococci (Chin, 1999). Because treatment failure with the combined ceftriaxone/doxycycline regimen is rare, a follow-up test of cure is not considered essential except for pregnant women, who should have a culture as test of cure.

SYPHILIS

Syphilis is the first STD for which control measures were developed and tested. Incidence has decreased in recent years (from more than 50,000 cases in 1990 to 8,539 cases in 1997), exceeding the *Healthy People 2000* target of 4.0 cases per 100,000. In the United States, syphilis and congenital syphilis are highly focal both geographically and demographically. In 1997, 75% of U.S. counties reported no cases of syphilis. Rates have decreased by over 80% for all racial and ethnic groups. Only in the South do rates remain above the year 2000 target, with 6.6 cases per 100,000. The target for 2010 is 0.2 cases per 100,000 (U.S. Department of Health and Human Services, 2000).

Syphilis presents in several forms during the life cycle of the disease. Approximately 3 weeks after exposure, a primary lesion called a *chancre* characteristically appears as a painless ulcer at the site of initial invasion of the causative organism, *Treponema pallidum,* a spirochete. After 4 to 6 weeks, the chancre heals without treatment, to be replaced by the development of more generalized secondary skin eruption, classically appearing on the soles of the feet and palms of the hands, often accompanied by constitutional symptoms. Secondary manifestations resolve spontaneously, followed by a latent period, which may last from weeks to years. Unpredictably, severe, systemic involvement with disability or even death may occur (Chin, 1999).

Treatment of early primary, secondary, and early latent syphilis is generally accomplished through antibiotic therapy. The specific treatment is a long-acting penicillin G (benzathine penicillin), 2.4 million units given in a single intramuscular (IM) dose on the day of diagnosis. Clients should be reexamined serologically at 3 and 6 months post-treatment to ensure cure; however, the single dose treatment is effective therapy even if the client fails to return (Chin, 1999).

Community health nurses need to provide the same level of support to clients diagnosed with syphilis as they give other clients diagnosed with STDs. Occasionally, older clients may recall the horrors of untreated syphilis and the significant numbers of cases before the 1970s. They will need added assurance of the effectiveness of their treatment and education about the changes in the prevalence of this STD.

CHLAMYDIA

Chlamydia is the most common sexually transmitted bacterial infection in the United States, causing an estimated 4 million acute infections annually, 2.6 million of which are in women. Yet until recently, chlamydia was probably the least recognized of the STDs. Only as recently as 1996 was chlamydia required to be reported by 49 states, up from 5 states in 1984. People with uncomplicated infection are quite often symptom free until late and serious complications occur. Women and children typically are the most adversely affected, particularly in terms of sequelae, including PID, ectopic pregnancy, infertility, infant conjunctivitis, and infant pneumonia (Chin, 1999; U.S. Department of Health and Human Services, 2000).

Screening programs have been extremely effective in reducing chlamydia burden in groups that are screened regularly. In one area, it was reduced by 65% within 7 years of introducing screening, and chlamydia complications such as PID were reduced by as much as 56% within 1 year of introducing screening. One of the *Healthy People 2010* goals is to reduce the prevalence of *Chlamydia trachomatis* infections among young people (15 to 24 years of age) to no more than 3.0%. In 1997 for all races and ethnic groups, the percentage was 4.4% for females in family planning clinics and 12.2% (female) and 15.7% (male) in STD clinics (U.S. Department of Health and Human Services, 2000).

Control of chlamydial infections of the cervix is considered key to effective reduction in the rates of PID, particularly among teenage women. Although chlamydia can be successfully treated with relatively inexpensive therapy, efforts to identify infected asymptomatic people have been hindered by the lack of a widely available, inexpensive, easy to perform diagnostic test (a problem shared by a number of the communicable diseases, including TB). In addition, lack of compliance with the required 7-day treatment regimen of doxycycline twice a day, or tetracycline four times a day, is a major barrier to effective control (Chin, 1999). Prophylactic treatment of sexual partners is recommended. Because no antibiotic-resistant strains of chlamydia have been detected, the CDC does not presently recommend any follow-up to ensure cure (CDC, 1998).

GENITAL HERPES

Genital herpes is caused by the herpes simplex virus (HSV), usually type 2, and occurs mainly in adults. Primary and recurrent infections occur, with or without symptoms. In women, sites of primary disease are the cervix and the vulva. Recurrent disease generally involves the vulva, perineal skin, legs, and buttocks. In men, lesions appear on the penis, and in the anus and rectum of those engaging in anal sex.

Since the late 1970s, the prevalence has increased 30%. Approximately one in five adult Americans has serologic evidence of infection with genital herpes (HSV-2). Prevalence is increasing most dramatically among young white teens. The HSV-2 prevalence among 12- to 19-year-old whites is now five times higher than it was 20 years ago. Seventeen percent of young adults aged 20 to 29 have HSV-2 (U.S. Department

of Health and Human Services, 2000). The *Healthy People 2010* goal is to reduce this to 14%.

Control efforts for genital herpes are hampered because as many as three fourths of genital herpes infections are transmitted by people who are unaware of their own infection and because no cure for the condition exists. Symptomatic management is usually accomplished by treatment of the primary and recurrent episodes of genital herpes with acyclovir used orally (the most convenient to use), intravenously, or topically. Acyclovir has been shown to reduce shedding of the virus, diminish pain, and accelerate healing. However, mutant strains of herpes virus resistant to acyclovir have been reported.

VIRAL WARTS

Condyloma acuminata, verruca vulgaris, papilloma venereum, and the common wart are all forms of a viral disease manifested by a variety of mucous membrane and skin lesions (Chin, 2000). All are transmitted by direct contact, but condyloma acuminata, or genital warts, caused by HPV are usually sexually transmitted.

Researchers have identified more than 70 types of papilloma viruses, and at least 20 of these types of the virus commonly infect the anogenital area. Several of the subtypes of HPV (HPV-16, 18, 31, and 45) are associated with cervical dysplasia and genital cancers, which can occur 5 to 30 years after the initial infection, accounting for 80% of cervical cancers (World Health Report, 1998). The CDC estimates that 20 million Americans carry the virus and that as many as a million new cases are diagnosed each year, accounting for approximately 5% of all STD clinic visits. The reduction of HPV infection remains an objective in the *Healthy People 2010* document (U.S. Department of Health and Human Services, 2000).

In college populations HPV is epidemic, with outbreaks usually occurring after vacation and semester breaks. As many as half of all sexually active college women may be infected with HPV (Gerchufsky, 1996). Most cases occur in the 20- to 24-year-old population, appearing more frequently in women than in men. In people who are sexually active around age 15, the risk of HPV is double than in those who become sexually active after age 20. Genital HPV infection can be transmitted to newborns during passage through the birth canal, causing a sometimes fatal respiratory papillomatosis if lesions develop in the lungs. Many people believe that pregnant women with HPV should have cesarean deliveries to prevent this possibility.

Many people infected with HPV are asymptomatic and transmit the infection unknowingly. Genital HPV infections are difficult to treat and commonly reoccur. No culture method is available to diagnose HPV, so diagnosis is commonly made on clinical presentation. HPV's tell-tale cauliflower-like, fleshy growths occur in and around the genitalia, around the anus and within the anal canal, and are usually painless. The warts usually regress within months to years. If treatment is recommended (not in pregnant women), it involves treating visualized warts with a topical solution of podophyllin or by cryotherapy. If the genital lesions are widespread, 5-fluorouracil has been helpful. The goal of therapy is removal of the warts and relief of symptoms (Chin, 1999).

Hepatitis Viruses

Five viral hepatitis infections are discussed in this section, hepatitis A, B, C, D, and E. Each constitutes a serious liver disease caused by a different hepatitis virus. Progress is being made to develop immunizations against various types of hepatitis. Nevertheless, the number of people being infected with hepatitis is globally epidemic. Nationally, we are making substantial progress in eliminating some hepatitis viruses.

HEPATITIS A

Hepatitis A occurs worldwide and is sporadic and epidemic, with cyclic recurrences affecting children and young adults most frequently. Most recent major U.S. epidemics cycled in 1961, 1971, and 1989. Case-rates are high in Central and South America, the Caribbean, Mexico, Asia (except Japan), Africa, and southern and eastern Europe.

The hepatitis A virus (HAV) is the infectious agent and is identified by IgM antibodies against hepatitis A virus in the serum of acutely or recently ill clients. The disease is transmitted person to person by the fecal–oral route and distinguishes itself by abrupt onset that includes fever, malaise, anorexia, nausea and abdominal discomfort, which is followed by jaundice in more severe cases. Mild illnesses last 1 to 2 weeks, but more severe cases last a month or more. The case-fatality rate in the United States is low (<1/1,000), but higher rates have been reported in children under 5 years of age (1.5/1,000) and among people over 50 years of age (27/1,000) (Chin, 1999). The *Healthy People 2010* target for hepatitis A is to reduce new cases to no more than 4.5 cases per 100,000 (U.S. Department of Health and Human Services, 2000).

Where environmental conditions are poor, infection is common and occurs at an early age. In the United States, most cases are transmitted in day care centers among diapered children, in household and sexual contacts of acute cases, and among travelers to countries where the disease is endemic. At times, there are common-source outbreaks related to contaminated water, food contaminated by infected food handlers, raw or undercooked shellfish from contaminated water, and contaminated produce such as lettuce and strawberries. In 1996, a vaccine against hepatitis A was licensed. This provides the opportunity to eliminate this disease as a pubic health problem in the United States. The vaccine is recommended for high-risk groups and is recommended for children over age 2 living in communities with high rates of HAV. Only 15% of cases are found in high-risk groups, and, until the vaccine strategy becomes more wide-scale, as in routine vaccines for all children, this disease will not be eliminated.

Community health nurses have an important role in the prevention and control of this disease, which includes case-finding, education, and identifying at-risk populations for the hepatitis A vaccine (eg, international travelers).

HEPATITIS B

The hepatitis B virus (HBV) infection is a global problem, with 66% of the world's population living in areas where there are high levels of infection. More than 2 billion (one third of the world's population) people worldwide have evidence of past or current HBV infection, and 350 million are chronic carriers of the virus. This virus causes 60% to 80% of all primary liver cancer, which is one of the three top causes of cancer deaths in east and southeast Asia, the Pacific Basin, and sub-Saharan Africa.

In the United States, cases are related to exposure common in certain high-risk groups, including injected drug users, heterosexuals with multiple partners, homosexual men, and clients and staff in institutions for the developmentally disabled. Occupationally acquired HBV can be traced to exposure of contaminated blood or serous fluids among health care workers, such as surgeons, dentists, employees in hemodialysis centers, and operating room and emergency room staff.

The symptoms of HBV may be unnoticeable to fulminating and include anorexia, vague abdominal discomfort, nausea and vomiting, and rash, often progressing to jaundice. Diagnosis is confirmed by specific antigens and/or antibodies in serum.

Vaccination is the most effective way of preventing HBV transmission. Following WHO recommendations, 90 countries have integrated hepatitis B vaccine into their national immunization programs. By these means, the WHO's target is to reduce new HBV carriers in children by 80% by the year 2001. Even at $1.50 for the three-dose series, vaccination is more expensive than the combined cost of required vaccines for six other diseases. WHO and UNICEF strategized to help the poorest and neediest countries to procure the vaccine. Effective implementation of this strategy could effectively eliminate transmission of hepatitis B by the year 2025 (World Health Report, 1998).

Healthy People 2010 targets hepatitis B in five objectives: (1) reduce to no more than 400 chronic hepatitis B virus infections in infants (as a baseline there were 1,682 chronic infections in 1995); (2) reduce to 2.4 cases per 100,000 hepatitis B rates in people less than 25 years of age; (3) reduce hepatitis B cases per 100,000 among adults 25 to 39 and 40 and older to 5.1 and 3.8, respectively, per 100,000; (4) reduce by 75% hepatitis B cases in high-risk groups; and (5) decrease deaths from hepatitis B–related cirrhosis and liver cancer (U.S. Department of Health and Human Services, 2000).

Community health nurses have an important role in the prevention and control of hepatitis B. Most importantly, this role includes teaching that encourages immunization compliance and for people, especially those in high-risk lifestyles or occupations, to consistently follow universal precautions.

HEPATITIS C

Hepatitis C virus (HCV) was first identified in 1989 and has already become a major public health problem. Incidence of

HCV is not well known, but prevalence studies on the disease lead the WHO to estimate that 3% of the world's population is infected with HCV (World Health Report, 1998). About 170 million people are chronic carriers at risk of developing liver cirrhosis and liver cancer. In the United States, four times as many people have contracted HCV as have contracted HIV infection. Approximately 30,000 new acute infections and 8,000 to 10,000 deaths occur each year, becoming a leading reason for liver transplantation.

Symptoms are similar to hepatitis A and B and may be unrecognizably mild to fulminating. Diagnosis depends on the demonstration of antibody to the hepatitis C virus, which has been established as a screening test for blood donors in 1992 (Chin, 1999). Before this test, HCV was the most common cause of post-transfusion hepatitis worldwide, accounting for approximately 90% of this disease in the United States. Incidence of the disease in the United States is highest in injected drug users, hemophilia patients, and hemodialysis patients, but is found more frequently among heterosexuals with multiple sexual partners, homosexual men, and health care workers than the general public.

Healthy People 2010 objectives target two areas of improvement for hepatitis C: (1) increase the percentage of people with chronic hepatitis C virus infection who are identified by state and local health departments, and (2) decrease the number of new cases to 1 per 100,000 from 2.4 per 100,000 in 1996. Chronic liver disease is the tenth leading cause of death among adults in the United States, with 40% to 60% of the deaths related to HCV (8,000 to 12,000 deaths a year) (U.S. Department of Health and Human Services, 2000).

A community health nurse's role includes case-finding, encouraging testing for people who received blood transfusions before 1992, and reinforcing universal precautions. There is no vaccine, and the current interferon-alpha therapy has been shown to have an overall beneficial effect only in about 25% of chronic hepatitis C cases. A recent study that combined interferon injections with an antiviral pill, Ribavirin, showed that response rates doubled or tripled over interferon alone (Kahn, 1998).

HEPATITIS D

Hepatitis D virus (HDV), sometimes called hepatitis delta virus, is worldwide, with variable prevalence. It occurs epidemically or endemically in populations at high risk of HBV. Highest incidence occurs in parts of Russia, Romania, southern Italy, Africa, and South America. Severe epidemics have been observed in tropical South America, the Central African Republic, and in the United States in Massachusetts (Chin, 1999).

Diagnosis is made by detection of total antibody to HDV. Symptoms resemble those of hepatitis B, which may be severe and are always associated with a coexisting hepatitis B virus. Delta hepatitis may be self-limiting, or it may progress to chronic hepatitis. The role of the community health nurse would be similar to that with hepatitis B.

HEPATITIS E

Outbreaks of hepatitis E virus (HEV) have occurred widely, primarily in countries with inadequate environmental sanitation, occurring as water-borne epidemics. It is transmitted by way of contaminated water and person to person by the fecal–oral route. The attack rate is highest in young adults, with the disease being uncommon in children and the elderly. In the United States and most other developed countries, hepatitis E has only been documented in people traveling to HEV-endemic areas, such as India, Myanmar, Iran, Bangladesh, Ethiopia, Nepal, Pakistan, Central Asian republics of the former Soviet Union, Algeria, Libya, Somalia, Mexico, Indonesia, and China.

This disease runs a clinical course similar to hepatitis A, with a similar case-fatality rate, except in pregnant women, where the rate may reach 20% among those infected during the third trimester of pregnancy. Education for primary prevention is the greatest role of the community health nurse, but epidemiologic investigation of suspected cases is an important activity if needed.

Influenza

Influenza derives its importance from the rapidity with which epidemics evolve, the widespread morbidity, and the seriousness of complications, namely pneumonias (Chin, 1999). Influenza has been recognized since 412 BC and was first described by Hippocrates. It existed throughout the early centuries, and about 30 possible pandemics have been documented in the past 400 years. Three have occurred in the 20th century—in 1918, 1957, and 1968. The 1918 "Spanish flu" was the most devastating, killing more than 20 million people worldwide from 1918 to 1920 (World Health Report, 1998). This pandemic occurred because the new virus was easily transmitted from person to person.

The WHO Network for Global Influenza Surveillance, which involves 110 national influenza centers worldwide, maintains constant vigilance for new influenza viruses. Sources of influenza virus include swine, birds, and poultry. In 1997, a new influenza virus called A(H5N1) was identified in chickens in Hong Kong before emerging in humans. As a precautionary measure, the infected poultry were destroyed to eliminate the risk of further transmission. Globally, we were expecting a pandemic event, which did not materialize.

FluNet is a prototype World Wide website for the electronic submission of influenza data from participating national laboratories. Only designated users can submit data, but the results—graphics, maps, and tables of influenza activity on a global scale—are available to the general public. As new data arrive and are verified, the maps and tables are revised to give users an up-to-date overview of the influenza situation. FluNet has speeded up the sharing of information on influenza patterns and virus strains and is becoming an essential tool in preparing for and preventing influenza pandemics. We do not know when or where the next flu epidemic or pandemic will occur, but the emergency response plans have to be prepared in advance, and the recent Hong Kong scare became a practice. Collaborating Influenza Surveillance Centers have created a task force of experts on influenza to develop a plan for the global management and control of a pandemic. The world's public health leaders are trying to prevent another 1918 pandemic of influenza.

Influenza is identified as an acute communicable viral disease of the respiratory tract characterized by fever, headache, myalgia, prostration, coryza, sore throat, and cough. When a new subtype appears, all children and adults are equally susceptible, except those who have lived through earlier epidemics caused by the same subtype. Influenza immunization is available that has been closely matched to the circulating strains of the virus. Killed-virus vaccines provide 70% to 80% protection in healthy young adults. In the elderly, immunization may be less effective in preventing illness but reduces the severity of disease and the incidence of complications by 50% to 60% and death by approximately 80% (Chin, 1999).

The vaccine should be given every year *before* influenza is expected in the community (November to March in the United States). For those living or traveling outside of the United States, timing of the immunization should be based on the seasonal patterns of influenza where they are traveling.

Community health nurses have a major role in primary prevention. Influenza shot clinics are frequently planned and organized by or with the local public health agency, with the injections administered by community health nurses. People can get immunized at worksites, shopping malls, pharmacies, and senior centers. Private physicians and health maintenance organizations (HMOs) provide immunization for their patients/members. Often, the community health nurse participates in this primary prevention activity during the fall of each year.

It is extremely important for older adults and people with chronic illnesses, respiratory diseases, and suppressed immune systems to get immunized each year. People working in critical professions, like the health care industry, and people in congregate living situations, such as assisted living centers or skilled nursing facilities, also should be immunized.

In 1995, adult immunization rates for influenza continued to increase toward the *Healthy People 2000* goal of 60%. Influenza vaccine coverage rates were up from 33% in 1989 to 58% in 1995. The target rates for African Americans and the Hispanic population remain substantially below the general population and the year 2000 targets (U.S. Dept. of Health and Human Services, 1991). *Healthy People 2010* has set an objective to monitor the national impact of influenza vaccinations on influenza-related hospitalizations and mortality among high-risk populations by annually collecting, analyzing, and reporting data from at least one medical care organization in all nine influenza surveillance regions of the country. They will use, as a baseline, 1997/1998 data or 63% vaccinated (U.S. Department of Health and Human Services, 2000). As a target for 2010, 90% of adults will be immunized. If successful, we will see a dramatic decline in morbidity requiring hospitalization and influenza-related mortality rates.

Pneumonia

Community-acquired pneumonia is a significant cause of morbidity and mortality. It is the sixth leading cause of death and the first leading cause of infectious death in the United States. An increased incidence of pneumonia often accompanies epidemics of influenza. There are an estimated 3 million cases per year, with approximately 20% requiring hospital admission (Kollek, 1998). Pneumonia hospital admissions and mortality are far more common in people over age 65 and the mortality rate is approximately 50% (Mick, 1997). In the 1980s, acute respiratory infections in developing countries, mainly pneumonia, were the major killers of children under age 5. These children often suffered several conditions at once, such as being dehydrated from diarrhea, being malnourished, and acquiring pneumonia. The WHO and UNICEF worked out clinical guidelines to approach these conditions collectively, and this integrated case management approach seems to be improving the plight of children in developing countries. Incidence of pneumonia is highest in winter. It is spread by droplet, by direct oral contact, and through **fomites,** which are any inanimate objects freshly soiled with respiratory discharges. People most susceptible to pneumonia are the elderly and people with a history of chronic diseases, a compromised immune system, and any condition affecting the anatomic or physiologic integrity of the lower respiratory tract.

Symptoms of pneumonia include a sudden onset with a shaking chill, fever, pleural pain, dyspnea, a productive cough of "rusty" sputum, and tachypnea. The onset is less abrupt in the elderly and may need diagnosis confirmed by x-ray. In infants and young children, fever, vomiting, and convulsions may be the initial symptoms.

Primary prevention is the best course of action and includes a pneumonia vaccine, especially to high-risk people, which includes the groups of people mentioned above. Reimmunization is recommended every 6 years to this group. The vaccine is not effective in children younger than 2 years of age and not recommended for the healthy population from 2 to 65 years of age. For these people, education about preventing pneumonia is a major part of the community health nurse's role.

Secondary prevention includes the early diagnosis and prompt treatment of people affected. Antimicrobials, such as penicillin and erythromycin, are the first drugs of choice for treating pneumonia.

GLOBAL ISSUES IN COMMUNICABLE DISEASE CONTROL

Our small planet has many common concerns. Communicable disease control is one of them. A new issue is the increasing number of emerging communicable diseases occurring globally. New diseases bring new challenges in case-finding, surveillance, and control. To conquer these challenges, community health nurses are assisted by the steps of the nursing process.

Globally Emerging Communicable Diseases

Emerging diseases either have newly appeared or are rapidly increasing in incidence or geographic range (Gordon, 1996). Most emerging diseases are not caused by genuinely new pathogens; rather, ecologic, environmental, and demographic factors place nonimmune people in increased contact with a pathogen or its host or promote the pathogen's dissemination. As mentioned earlier in this chapter, the shrinking of our world with the current volume, speed, and reach of international travel makes the emergence of communicable diseases truly a global problem. The following is a brief profile of some old and new emerging infectious diseases.

Ebola hemorrhagic fever, a severe acute viral illness with sudden onset of fever, malaise, myalgia and headache, pharyngitis, vomiting, diarrhea, and a maculopapular rash, has been confined to countries in tropical Africa. It was identified in 1976, in the Democratic Republic of the Congo where the case-fatality rate has ranged from 50% to 90%. Person-to-person transmission occurs by direct contact with infected blood, secretions, organs or semen. People of all ages are susceptible.

Legionnaires' disease (Legionellosis) is a bacterial form of a potentially fatal pneumonia caused by bacteria that contaminate water and air-conditioning systems. It was first identified in Philadelphia, Pennsylvania, in 1976. It is characterized by anorexia, malaise, myalgia, and headache; within a day, there is a rapidly rising fever associated with chills, a nonproductive cough, abdominal pain, and diarrhea. The case-fatality rate has been as high as 39% in hospitalized clients and higher in those with compromised immune systems. The disease occurs most frequently with increasing age, with most patients over 50 years of age. Primary prevention is easily accomplished by draining cooling towers when not in use, mechanically cleaning them, and using appropriate biocides.

Hantavirus is an old virus with a newly recognized clinical illness. It first occurred in Manchuria before World War II. In 1951, it was recognized in Korea and is considered a major, expanding public health problem in China, with 40,000 to 100,000 cases reported annually. It was first seen in the United States in 1993 in the four-corner area of the country where Utah, Colorado, New Mexico, and Arizona meet, and 28 people died. Since 1993, 217 cases have been identified in 30 states (Gordon, 1996; Leslie et al., 1999). The severe form of the disease is endemic in Eurasia and Scandinavia. Deer mice appear to be the reservoir, and transmission is by way of aerosolization of infected droppings. It is an acute viral disease characterized by abrupt onset of fever, low back pain, varying degrees of hemorrhagic manifestations, renal involvement, hypotension, and shock. Prevention is focused on rodent control and surveillance for the infection in wild rodents.

E. coli O157:H7 was first identified as a pathogen in 1982 in the United States. An outbreak of severe bloody diarrhea was traced to contaminated hamburgers. In January 1993, a large outbreak affected 700 people who ate undercooked hamburgers in the Puget Sound area of Washington. Other outbreaks have been caused by unpasteurized milk and apple cider made from apples contaminated by cow manure. Children under the age of 5 are most susceptible and are at greatest risk of developing hemolytic-uremic syndrome. *E. coli* infections are recognized to be an important problem in Europe, South Africa, Japan, South America, and Australia. Humans may serve as a reservoir for person-to-person transmission. Primary prevention can be accomplished by following federal guidelines requiring commercially prepared meat to be cooked to an internal temperature of 140°F and by safe and hygienic cooking practices at home, keeping raw meats separated from fruits, vegetables, and cooked meats on cutting boards—separate ones should be used and cleansed with hot soap and water and rinsed using a bleach solution.

Lyme disease was first discovered in the United States in the 1970s when an unusually high incidence of children developed rheumatoid arthritis in Lyme, Connecticut. It is an infection caused by a spirochete called *Borrelia burgdorferi* and is characterized by a distinctive skin lesion, systemic symptoms, and neurologic, rheumatologic, and cardiac involvement occurring over a period of months to years. A bite from a tick that dogs and cats can have carries the bacteria and can pass the disease on to humans. All 48 mainland states have reported cases, but it is most prevalent in the Northeast. Until 1996, the number of cases soared each year and then decreased in the dryer year, 1997. Lyme disease is treatable and is not communicable person to person. Two different vaccines for Lyme disease are being tested. Primary prevention includes educating the public about the mode of transmission, being aware of high-risk areas—wooded, bushy, and tall-grass areas—and checking for ticks after an outing. If a tick is found, it should be removed with forceps (tweezers), trying not to crush the tick's body so that no fluid escapes.

Dengue fever, an acute febrile viral condition, is not transmitted person to person but through the bite of an infected mosquito. Symptoms include sudden onset beginning with fever, severe headache, myalgia, arthralgia, retro-orbital pain, anorexia, GI disturbances, and rash. Children have milder symptoms than adults. Prevalence has increased due to increasing worldwide urbanization during the last few decades. Dengue and dengue hemorrhagic fever (DHF) have been reported from over 100 countries in the world, except in Europe. These two diseases often occur in massive epidemics, most recently in 1996 when severe epidemics were reported in 27 countries in the Americas and in southeast Asia. Outbreaks of DHF have recently been reported in Brazil, Cuba, India, and Sri Lanka. The WHO strategy of control is based on prevention of transmission by controlling the vector mosquito, which starts with eliminating areas for breeding, such as small pools of stagnant water, even in empty flowerpots or abandoned tires.

Global Response to Communicable Diseases

As discussed throughout this chapter, communicable diseases are not limited to specific regions of the world; they are the problem of all people. In 1996, WHO focused on completing the unfinished business of eradication and elimination of specific diseases; tackling "old" diseases such as TB and malaria, and the problem of antimicrobial resistance; and combating newly emerging diseases. WHO continues to focus on safeguarding the gains already achieved, which depends largely on sharing health and medical knowledge, expertise, and experience on a global scale. During the 50 years of its existence, WHO has taken a three-pronged approach to communicable diseases: case-finding, surveillance and control, and elimination and eradication.

Case-finding is an important beginning to communicable disease control and eventual eradication. Because of the changing nature of the world's demography, use of space, and accelerating technology, old or once unknown diseases are reemerging or are being seen on our planet for the first time. Differentiation of one set of symptoms from the symptoms of another disease is an essential first step in case-finding. Once a disease has been identified, all cases need to be found through the traditional case-finding methods of contact investigation. Each contact leads to another piece of information and becomes communicable disease detective work.

Once a disease has been identified and is known to exist in a particular community, the steps of surveillance and control begin. Questions—How is the disease spread? What needs to be done to reduce the impact of the source? Do the infected need to be isolated? Does the disease respond to antimicrobial therapy?—need to be answered and acted upon. Weekly, monthly, and yearly documentation of the disease frequency and distribution is gathered and shared globally. Control measures then begin. Some developing countries may need more technical and financial support to achieve control. The cost of locating cases, eliminating vector pools, and providing immunizations and/or treatment can be a burden beyond the capabilities of poorer nations.

Effective surveillance and control can lead to the goal of elimination and eradication of a disease in many cases. We have been successful with smallpox and are closing in on polio. Within the next 25 years other diseases, such as measles and TB, have the potential for elimination. Global collaboration, using the strengths from all nations, is needed to achieve these goals.

USING THE NURSING PROCESS FOR COMMUNICABLE DISEASE CONTROL

As we mentioned in Chapters 11 and 14, the nursing process has steps similar to the research process and the epidemiologic process when approaching any health problem or condition. Therefore, using the nursing process to achieve communicable disease control should be an important and natural process for community health nurses.

Assessment

The first step of the nursing process, assessment, aligns itself with case-identification and case-finding in communicable disease control. The community health nurse must use all assessment skills and tools available during contact with clients in order to not overlook the possibility of a communicable disease. Assessment must be comprehensive, including physical, social, and environmental data. There is no place for assumption. At times, a nurse can become "lulled" into usual patterns of inquiry, and the oversight may prove fatal to the client.

> "Baby Josephine is irritable," says the mother. "Well, babies sometimes are," the nurse says. "How are you feeding her? Show me how you hold her. Does she sleep well? Rock her in the rocking chair before bedtime. Burp her more frequently. I'll check back with you in 2 weeks." Does the nurse record the baby's temperature, look at her for a rash, compare present weight with last weight, ask about bowel habits or vomiting, inquire about illnesses in the family, check on breastfeeding technique or watch while the mother demonstrates formula preparation, inspect the family's water source, ask about other foods the baby is eating, and so forth?

Broader inquiry into a simple statement from the mother may lead to the discovery of a life-threatening, undiagnosed communicable disease.

Assessment in the broader community health nursing role may involve assessing a community's need for communicable disease surveillance and new or improved control programs. Nurses are in the community and can get a feel for the increasing or decreasing numbers of communicable diseases. They are often the first ones to know of a new outbreak of communicable disease in the community.

Planning

The planning step in the nursing process involves different activities depending on whether the planning is for an individual, family, group, or entire community. At the individual level, the nurse may assist a client with a communicable disease to get immunizations or definitive treatment, or assist the client in ways to care for the communicable disease symptoms that provide relief and comfort, and reduce the chance of transmitting the disease to others in the family or community. When working with families, the nurse's actions are similar to those with individual clients and include assisting the family in getting available and needed immunizations, controlling the disease if infected, limiting it to the people already exposed, and getting appropriate treatment and meaningful rehabilitation, if needed. With groups and communities, planning includes the collaboration of many different groups. Whether an immunization clinic is proposed or a flu shot day for senior citizens planned, there are location, staff, and supplies to prepare, which may include writing grants, establishing contracts, and training and orienting staff, before implementation can begin.

Implementation

During this step, the nurse actually takes the action that was identified as being needed during assessment and planned for with clients and others in collaboration. In the implementation step, the nurse may actually deliver the service or may supervise other staff or volunteers. On a large scale, such as with the implementation of a new immunization clinic, recognizing this will be an ongoing service has to be considered in an agency's budget, staff turnover issues, relief when there is absence, and continuous formative (during the implementation process) evaluation of the services so that minor changes to improve day-to-day operation can be introduced. Implementing plans with small groups or families may involve arranging for transportation to get several people immunized or seen by a primary care provider. It may include gathering stool samples to bring to a laboratory from a family recovering from a *Salmonella* infection. Education on primary prevention of future infections is an essential part of the implementation phase. Agency record keeping, state-required contact investigation, and reporting cases of communicable diseases are essential in this phase. Figure 15–4 provides an example of a reporting form.

Evaluation

Evaluation is an essential step in the nursing process with all conditions, diseases, and services community health nurses provide. When dealing with communicable diseases, it is most important to determine whether actions have achieved the established goals. Have the outcomes been accomplished? Are people in the families immunized? Are all family members free of the disease? Do families know how to prevent this and other diseases from occurring or recurring? Does the community have the communicable disease services it needs? Is the community free of the disease? What needs to be done now to keep the community safe from communicable diseases? Are there funding issues, programs nearing completion that need support, or growth of services needed that can be addressed before a critical need? These are sample questions that need answers during evaluation. The community health nurse concerned with the health and safety of the community follows the steps of the nursing process to achieve healthy community goals.

ETHICAL ISSUES IN COMMUNICABLE DISEASE CONTROL

When working to effectively control communicable diseases in communities and population groups, it is important to ensure that the activities undertaken are ethically sound and justified. It is important in communicable disease control to consider the ethical aspects of access to disease prevention and treatment services; enforced compliance with preventive measures; screening programs; privacy, confidentiality, and discrimination; and issues involving the health worker employee who is infected with or is a carrier of an infectious agent.

Health Care Access in Communicable Disease Control

Access to health care means that people needing services find them available, acceptable, and appropriate, unrestricted by barriers to use. Such access has been advocated as an essential public health value, yet the global economy has been experiencing rising inequality, with income gaps between countries and within countries continuing to widen (World Health Report, 1998).

It would be misleading to say that rates of communicable diseases in population subgroups provide reliable indicators of health care access. The issue is significantly compounded when health care providers miss opportunities to vaccinate and when parents who have the means fail to seek out services to ensure immunizations are up to date. It is clear that in the absence of access to health care services, opportunities for people to receive the information and the services necessary to prevent transmission and progression of infectious diseases are sharply curtailed.

Enforced Compliance

Legally, the responsibilities of public health officials in communicable disease control include the police power to enforce compliance with treatment or restrict the activity of infectious people to protect the welfare of others (Chin, 1999). In disease prevention, completely voluntary measures to encourage healthier lifestyles tend to be ineffective.

Regulations that enforce compliance with disease prevention strategies are a justifiable restriction if the measures proposed are demonstrably effective and grounded in ethical principles (Robbins, Towne, Gotschlich & Schneerson, 1997). Coercion must be of the mildest sort compatible with achieving the goals of the regulation. Information must be provided to allow consumers to see the consequences of deleterious habits and the value choices that must be made. Inducements should be favored over disincentives. Remediable conditions that make choice less than free should be ameliorated (through

CONFIDENTIAL MORBIDITY REPORT

NOTE: For STD, Hepatitis, or TB, complete appropriate section below. Special reporting requirements and reportable diseases on back.

DISEASE BEING REPORTED: _____

Patient's Last Name

Social Security Number ___ — ___ — ___

Ethnicity (✔ one)
- ❏ Hispanic/Latino
- ❏ Non-Hispanic/Non-Latino

First Name/Middle Name (or initial)

Birth Date Month | Day | Year | **Age**

Race (✔ one)
- ❏ African-American/Black
- ❏ Asian/Pacific Islander (✔ one)
  - ❏ Asian-Indian ❏ Japanese
  - ❏ Cambodian ❏ Korean
  - ❏ Chinese ❏ Laotian
  - ❏ Filipino ❏ Samoan
  - ❏ Guamanian ❏ Vietnamese
  - ❏ Hawaiian ❏ Other _____

Address: Number, Street   **Apt./Unit Number**

City/Town   **State**   **Zip Code**

Area Code Home Telephone   **Gender** M / F   **Pregnant?** Y / N / Unk   **Estimated Delivery Date** Month | Day | Year

Area Code Work Telephone   **Patient's Occupation/Setting**
- ❏ Food service ❏ Day care ❏ Correctional facility
- ❏ Health care ❏ School ❏ Other _____

- ❏ Native American/Alaskan Native
- ❏ White _____
- ❏ Other _____

DATE OF ONSET Month | Day | Year

Reporting Health Care Provider

Reporting Health Care Facility

REPORT TO

DATE DIAGNOSED Month | Day | Year

Address

City   **State**   **Zip Code**

DATE OF DEATH Month | Day | Year

Telephone Number ( )   **Fax** ( )

Submitted By   **Date Submitted (Month/Day/Year)**

(Obtain additional forms from your local health department.)

SEXUALLY TRANSMITTED DISEASES (STD)

Syphilis
- ❏ Primary (lesion present)
- ❏ Secondary
- ❏ Early latent < 1 year
- ❏ Latent (unknown duration)
- ❏ Neurosyphilis
- ❏ Late latent > 1 year
- ❏ Late (tertiary)
- ❏ Congenital

Syphilis Test Results
- ❏ RPR Titer: _____
- ❏ VDRL Titer: _____
- ❏ FTA/MHA: ❏ Pos ❏ Neg
- ❏ CSF-VDRL ❏ Pos ❏ Neg
- ❏ Other _____

Gonorrhea
- ❏ Urethral/Cervical
- ❏ PID
- ❏ Other _____

Chlamydia
- ❏ Urethral/Cervical
- ❏ PID
- ❏ Other _____

- ❏ PID (Unknown Etiology)
- ❏ Chancroid
- ❏ Non-Gonococcal Urethritis

STD TREATMENT INFORMATION
- ❏ Treated (Drugs, Dosage, Route) Date Treatment Initiated Month | Day | Year
  _____
  _____
- ❏ Untreated
- ❏ Will treat
- ❏ Unable to contact patient
- ❏ Refused treatment
- ❏ Referred to _____

VIRAL HEPATITIS

		Pos	Neg	Pend	Not Done
❏ Hep A	anti-HAV IgM	❏	❏	❏	❏
❏ Hep B	HBsAg	❏	❏	❏	❏
❏ Acute	anti-HBc	❏	❏	❏	❏
❏ Chronic	anti-HBc IgM	❏	❏	❏	❏
	anti-HBs	❏	❏	❏	❏
❏ Hep C	anti-HCV	❏	❏	❏	❏
❏ Acute	PCR-HCV	❏	❏	❏	❏
❏ Chronic					
❏ Hep D (Delta)	anti-Delta	❏	❏	❏	❏
❏ Other		❏	❏	❏	❏

Suspected Exposure Type
- ❏ Blood transfusion
- ❏ Other needle exposure
- ❏ Sexual contact
- ❏ Household contact
- ❏ Child care
- ❏ Other _____

TUBERCULOSIS (TB)

Status
- ❏ Active Disease
  - ❏ Confirmed
  - ❏ Suspected
- ❏ Infected, No Disease
  - ❏ Convertor
  - ❏ Reactor

Site(s)
- ❏ Pulmonary
- ❏ Extra-Pulmonary
- ❏ Both

Mantoux TB Skin Test Month | Day | Year
Date Performed _____
Results _____ mm   ❏ Pending ❏ Not Done

Chest X-Ray Month | Day | Year
Date Performed _____
❏ Normal ❏ Pending ❏ Not Done
❏ Cavitary ❏ Abnormal/Noncavitary

Bacteriology Month | Day | Year
Date Specimen Collected _____
Source _____
Smear: ❏ Pos ❏ Neg ❏ Pending ❏ Not Done
Culture: ❏ Pos ❏ Neg ❏ Pending ❏ Not Done
Other test(s) _____

TB TREATMENT INFORMATION
- ❏ Current Treatment
  - ❏ INH ❏ RIF ❏ PZA
  - ❏ EMB ❏ Other _____
  - Date Treatment Initiated Month | Day | Year
- ❏ Untreated
  - ❏ Will treat
  - ❏ Unable to contact patient
  - ❏ Refused treatment
  - ❏ Referred to _____

REMARKS

FIGURE 15–4. Communicable disease reporting form—contact investigation.

education, by restraints on misleading advertisement, reducing peer or group pressure, and treating emotional problems). Regulation should be confined to actions with direct public impact and be limited severely in matters that are personal and private.

Screening for Communicable Diseases

As discussed earlier in this chapter, screening programs for communicable diseases are conducted to detect existing or potential public health problems. One can argue that they are morally and ethically justified if they protect and serve infected people as well as those who might be at risk for exposure. However, other issues arise that must be addressed. Are screening resources allocated to areas where they will have the most benefit in preventing disease and premature death? Should people receiving the screening service take on the burden of diagnosis if treatment is unavailable because of cost or access? Are screening costs justified in light of scarce health care dollars?

Until recently, there was no ethical justification for an HIV screening program for the infected. Since the advent of several drugs, taken in combination, that postpone the development of AIDS in the HIV-positive population and improve the quality of life, determining one's HIV status has immense value. Prevention of transmission of the virus continues to require voluntary changes in behavior of infected people, and there has always been an ethical justification for HIV screening for that reason. If screening was to become mandatory, identification of the estimated 1 million or more HIV-infected people in the United States would exceed the capacity of the health care system to provide services. However, people who engage in high-risk behaviors owe it to themselves to be screened for HIV so the life-prolonging drugs can be started and precautions can be taken to not infect others.

Confidentiality, Privacy, and Discrimination

To carry out communicable disease interventions, client needs for confidentiality and privacy must be ensured. Screening and other interventions must take place in a physical setting that does not allow overt differentiation between those clients with positive and negative results. As agency and national data systems and programs continue to evolve, it is essential to make confidentiality and data protection measures clear priorities. Studies have reported between 60 and 100 people having access to an average hospital record. Anonymity is frankly incompatible with early intervention. Two areas of current practice that may benefit from closer ethical scrutiny in regard to protection of privacy are contact investigation in sexually transmitted disease programs and school-based screening for pediculosis.

Human society has had a long-standing aversion to infectious diseases that is still true today. Ostracism in the past of

people with leprosy and other contagious conditions has shifted to discrimination against people with TB, AIDS, head lice, and other current forms of communicable disease. Such discrimination should be of as much concern to those in public health as in the legal sector.

Passage of the Americans with Disabilities Act in 1990 has resulted in legal protections for people diagnosed with communicable diseases who suffer discrimination regardless of status of infectiousness. The objectives of *Healthy People 2010* encourage community-based agencies to expand communicable disease services, among other strategies, by offering expanded contact follow-up services (U.S. Dept. of Health and Human Services, 2000). Such expansion should occur only with careful planning for the ethical standards that will spell out the protections due each individual client while still effectively advancing the cause of disease prevention.

The issue of confidentiality has always been a major concern in contact investigation. It continues to be a source of debate in balancing the values of protection of the individual with protection of the public's health. Not only must the identity of the individual be protected to the maximum extent possible, but also any breaches of confidentiality must be clearly justified on the basis of a threat to the safety of any individual. That is, failure to provide essential information must jeopardize the well-being of the exposed person or contact. It is important to ensure that accessible services exist for the exposed partner or contact in the event that, as a result of screening intervention, they are burdened with the emotional, physical, and financial consequences of diagnosis.

Infected Health Care Workers

Health workers have historically been at high risk when caring for clients with communicable diseases, be it plague, typhus, or TB. Advances in treatment strategies for these clients, however, have consistently resulted in a safer working environment for their caregivers and those exposed to body fluids and various contaminated fomites. Trends in increasing community-based rather than inpatient care for communicable diseases have further contributed to equalizing the risk faced by health workers and the general population.

Yet the pendulum swings. HIV infection, multidrug-resistant TB, and nosocomial infections, particularly with MRSA, now threaten caregivers in significant ways, and the ethical implications of these issues are considerable and evolving. Legislation is proliferating requiring health care workers who are known to be HIV-positive to report to their local and state health authorities. MRSA is a growing problem in many facilities where health care workers are undergoing screening for colonization by the organisms, patients with MRSA are being refused admittance, and the work activities of colonized workers are curtailed. Strategies for health care workers' protection and disease prevention must be mandated and enforced to a greater extent.

SUMMARY

Communicable diseases pose a major threat to the public's health and have done so since the beginning of humankind. Such diseases are transmitted globally as the result of mobile populations, increased urbanization, and international travel. These diseases are transmitted through direct contact from one person to another or indirectly through contaminated objects (air, water, food) or a vector (animal or insect). Communicable diseases affect large groups of people and have worldwide significance.

Ideally, prevention of communicable diseases is accomplished through the primary prevention methods of mass media, one-on-one education, and immunization. Knowledge of the vaccine-preventable diseases (VPD), schedule of VPDs, a community's immunization status, herd immunity, barriers to immunization coverage, planning and implementing immunization programs, adult immunizations, and the immunization needs of international travelers, immigrants, and refugees have been discussed. Secondary prevention activities of screening and the criteria for screening tests, and contact investigation and case-finding are the steps to be taken when primary prevention activities have failed. Tertiary prevention is needed to ensure additional people are not infected. This is accomplished through isolation and quarantine, universal precaution practices among health care workers, and the safe handling and control of infectious wastes.

Becoming familiar with major communicable diseases affecting our nation is essential baseline information for community health nurses. TB, resurging since the 1980s, may be the biggest public health problem in the new millennium. Nurses need to be aware of the populations at risk, how the disease is prevented, appropriate interventions during diagnosis, and treatment. Issues compounding the control of TB are twofold: there are increasing multidrug-resistant strains of TB, and the number of people with TB and HIV/AIDS is increasing, making diagnosis and treatment more complicated.

A second major disease, HIV/AIDS, was first identified in the 1980s. In a short 20 years, 30 million people worldwide have been infected. With the success of antiviral drugs, this disease is almost becoming a chronic disease for clients in industrialized nations, and they can experience 10 to 15 years of life after diagnosis. Africa is being deeply affected by the massive numbers of women and children who are HIV-positive, without access to the life-prolonging drugs available to people in developed nations.

Sexually transmitted diseases (STDs) threaten the health and lives of millions of citizens. At risk are the sexually active, particularly adolescents and young adults, as well as minorities, women of childbearing age, and children. Control of STDs can be accomplished through effective screening, treatment, contact investigation, and aggressive public education. Several common ones have been discussed, including gonorrhea, syphilis, chlamydia, genital herpes, and anogenital warts.

Five hepatitis viruses have been discussed in this chapter. Hepatitis is more common than HIV and can lead to life-threatening events, such as cirrhosis and liver cancer. Yet these diseases do not get the attention they need. Most of the public is unaware of the types of hepatitis, prevention, transmission, and treatment. Vaccines for two of the forms are now available, and hepatitis B vaccine is required in the routine childhood vaccine schedule.

Influenza and pneumonia are "old" diseases causing increased morbidity and mortality in the United States. Unfortunately, these diseases are occurring in our frailest citizens, the very young and the very old, when there are vaccines to prevent them. A national objective for 2010 is to increase the immunized population, achieving a herd immunity, to prevent such preventable diseases.

There are several emerging or new diseases occurring globally. Such diseases as Ebola, hantavirus, *E. coli*, Legionnaires' disease, Lyme disease, and dengue fever sound very new to older residents in the United States; however, they are occurring in increasingly alarming numbers. It may not be unusual for community health nurses to come across these diseases in their practice.

Internationally, WHO has been working for 50 years to make the world a healthier place to live. By providing all nations with the technical support, resources, and education they need, WHO is aggressively tackling communicable diseases. Case-finding, surveillance, control, elimination, and eradication are the steps toward meeting the WHO goals for communicable diseases.

Community health nurses use the nursing process in their important role with regard to all populations at risk for communicable diseases. Nurses concerned with communicable disease control must recognize who is at risk, where the potential reservoirs and sources of infectious disease agents are located, what environmental factors promote their spread, and what are the characteristics of vulnerability of community members and groups—particularly those subject to intervention. Community health nurses must work collaboratively with other public health professionals to establish immunization and education programs, to improve community infection control policies, and to develop a broad range of services to populations at risk.

Ethical issues in communicable disease and infection control include access to health care, enforced compliance, the justifiability of screening, preservation of confidentiality and privacy, avoidance of discrimination against infected people, and problems posed by infected health workers.

ACTIVITIES TO PROMOTE CRITICAL THINKING

1. Interview a professional in your local or state health department who works in communicable disease

CLINICAL CORNER | Salmonella: A Cultural Conflict

You are a nurse working for the Brownsville Department of Health. One of your responsibilities is epidemiologic follow-up on reports of communicable disease. Today, you will be performing your second visit on the following clients:

- Tai: a 17-year-old boy
- Nguyen: a 15-year-old girl

Tai and Nguyen are cousins. Both clients became infected with *Salmonella* from undercooked pork, after a church picnic. Both are from Vietnamese families who immigrated to the United States 7 years ago.

During your initial visit, you spoke with the parents of Tai and Nguyen and educated them about the following:

1. Medication administration
2. Strict handwashing
3. Proper bowel habits
4. Food preparation and handling
5. Treatment of gastrointestinal sequelae
6. Collection of stool specimens
7. Modes of transmission
8. Assessment indicating exacerbation of signs and symptoms

The information you presented related to *Salmonella* was taken from recommendations from the Board of Health. In your education of the parents, you were careful to impress on them the potential deleterious consequences of non-compliance with these standards. You warned them that other family members would be placed at risk if there was deviation from the recommended practices.

Upon your return visit today, you are presented with the following scenarios:

Tai

Tai's family has followed your directions meticulously. His father tells you that the family has declined an invitation to an upcoming church social "because they're the ones who made my boy sick . . . they don't cook things right and I'm not taking my family there any more," he states. The parents also advise you that they have stopped giving Tai herbal teas and are instead providing him with rehydration drinks as recommended by his physician.

Additionally, Tai's parents have prohibited their children from visiting their cousins "because they don't take good care of themselves." Tai's mother tell you, "Their kids don't even wash their hands after using the toilet and you said that would make us all sick."

Nguyen

Your visit with Nguyen and her parents reveals the following information. Nguyen has refused to provide a stool specimen. Her parents speak little English and rely on Nguyen for interpretation. "They think you were mad at them last time," Nguyen informs you. "They got upset and scared." Nguyen goes on to tell you that "We're not drinking that stuff you told us about . . . my mom says that the tea has worked for our people for generations, so it's good enough for me." Nguyen adds that her parents have used spooning techniques to provide her with relief from gastrointestinal problems.

Questions

1. Is there a "good" and a "bad" client in this scenario?
2. Did you achieve desired nursing outcomes based on your intervention with Tai's family? Why or why not?
3. What might you have done differently to ensure the provision of culturally appropriate education with these families?
4. How might mutual goals have been developed?
5. What issues does this scenario elicit regarding:
   Fears and anxiety in this role
   Lack of immediate resources (eg, supervisor)
   Social justice
   Building partnerships within your communities
   Globalization of public health
6. In your role as the community health nurse, what activities might you be involved with in the prevention as well as reduction of the spread of communicable diseases within the aggregate of Vietnamese immigrants in your community?

---

control. Determine (a) how he or she conducts communicable disease surveillance, (b) what diseases must be reported in your state, and (c) which communicable diseases are posing the greatest threat to the health of your states' citizens.

2. Compare a recent issue of *Mortality and Morbidity Weekly Report* with the same issue published a year earlier in terms of cases of specific notifiable diseases in the United States. Which diseases appear to be increasing? Decreasing? Select one disease

and read at least one recent publication on this subject to determine the reasons for its rise or decline.

3. Determine through your local health department what percentage of preschool children are immunized in your city or county. Is this a safe level of herd immunity? Propose some recommendations for preserving or raising this level.

4. Select one high-risk population discussed in this chapter and list the factors that make this group

vulnerable to communicable disease. Use at least one other published source to enhance your understanding. Propose one nursing intervention (such as a specific screening or educational program) and outline how it might be accomplished.

5. Interview a professional who works in STD services and/or with the HIV-infected population. Determine what methods he or she uses for contact investigation. How does he or she preserve privacy and confidentiality? What measures have proved most effective in reaching contacts? What is your evaluation of the success?

6. Access the CDC through the Internet (http://www.cdc.gov) and browse around its various services. Are there special travelers warnings in certain countries at this time? What are some of the CDC's current concerns regarding communicable diseases? Select a communicable disease and identify the number of cases presently reported. Return to the same website in a month. Has the incidence of the disease increased or decreased? (See Clinical Corner.)

REFERENCES

Abma, J., Driscoll, A., & Moore, K. (1998). Young women's degree of control over first intercourse: An exploratory analysis. *Family Planning Perspectives, 30*(1), 12–18.

American Academy of Pediatrics. (1997). *1997 Red Book: Report of the committee on infectious diseases.* Elk Grove Village, IL: American Academy of Pediatrics.

American Nurses Association. (1997a). *Position statements— Tuberculosis and HIV.* Available: http://www.nursingworld.org/readroom/position/blood/blhvtb. htm.

————. (1997b). *Position statement—Tuberculosis and public health nursing.* Available: http://www.nursingworld.org/readroom/position/blood/bltbhl. htm.

American Thoracic Society. (1994). Treatment of tuberculosis and tuberculosis infection in adults and children. *American Journal of Respiratory Critical Care Medicine, 149,* 1359–1374.

Annas, G. J., & Grodin, M. A. (1998). Human rights and maternal–fetal HIV transmission prevention trials in Africa. *American Journal of Public Health, 88*(4), 560–563.

Barnes, P. F., El-Hajj, H., Preston-Martin, S., et al. (1996). Transmission of tuberculosis among the urban homeless. *Journal of the American Medical Association, 275*(4), 305–307.

Brickner, P. W., & McAdam, J. M. (1995). Tuberculosis, HIV disease and directly observed therapy. *Journal of Public Health Management and Practice, 1*(4), 52–54.

Brooks, J. (1999). *The minority AIDS crisis. Closing the gap* (pp. 1–3). Washington, DC: U.S. Department of Health & Human Services, Office of Minority Health.

Bryson, Y. J. (1996). Advances in the prevention and treatment of perinatal infection. *Improving the Management of HIV Disease, 4*(3), 7.

Centers for Disease Control and Prevention. (2000). *Recommended childhood immunization schedule—United States, January–December.* Atlanta: CDC.

————. (1998). 1998 guidelines for treatment of sexually transmitted diseases. *Morbidity and Mortality Weekly Report, 47*(RR-1).

————. (1997). Status report on the Childhood Immunization Initiative: National, state, and urban area vaccination coverage levels among children aged 19–35 months—United States, 1996. *Morbidity and Mortality Weekly Report, 46,* 657–664.

————. (1996). Ten leading national notifiable infectious diseases—United States, 1995. *Morbidity and Mortality Weekly Report, 45*(1), 883– 884.

————. (1995a). *Self-study modules on tuberculosis: Transmission and pathogenesis of tuberculosis.* Atlanta, GA: Public Health Practice Program Office, Division of Media and Training Services.

————. (1995b). *Self-study modules on tuberculosis: Epidemiology of tuberculosis.* Atlanta, GA: Public Health Practice Program Office, Division of Media and Training Services.

————. (1995c). *Self-study modules on tuberculosis: Diagnosis of tuberculosis infection and disease.* Atlanta, GA: Public Health Practice Program Office, Division of Media and Training Services.

————. (1995d). *Self-study modules on tuberculosis: Treatment of tuberculosis infection and disease.* Atlanta, GA: Public Health Practice Program Office, Division of Media and Training Services.

————. (1994a). General recommendations on immunization: Recommendations of the Advisory Committee on Immunization Practices (ACIP). *Morbidity and Mortality Weekly Report, 43* (RR-1).

————. (1994b). Guidelines for preventing the transmission of *Mycobacterium tuberculosis* in health care facilities, 1994. *Morbidity and Mortality Weekly Report, 43*(RR-13).

————. (1989). A strategic plan for the elimination of tuberculosis in the United States. *Morbidity and Mortality Weekly Report, 38*(S-3), 1–25.

Chin, J. E. (Ed.). (1999). *Control of communicable diseases manual* (17th ed.). Washington, DC: American Public Health Association.

Dugger, B. (1997). Antimicrobial drug resistance: A danger to world health. *Journal of Intravenous Nursing, 20*(2), 101–108.

Eng, T. R., & Butler, W. T. (Eds.). (1997). *The hidden epidemic: Confronting sexually transmitted diseases.* Washington, DC: National Academy Press.

Falvo, D. R. (1994). *Effective patient education: A guide to increased compliance.* Gaithersburg, MD: Aspen.

Flora, J., & Cassady, D. (1990). Roles of media in community-based health promotion. In N. Bracht (Ed.), *Health promotion at the community level.* Newbury Park, CA: Sage.

Gannon, J.C. (2000). The global infectious disease threat and its implication for the United States. NIE–99–170. Available: http://www.odci.gov/cia/publications/pubs.html.

Gelbart, M. (1998, January 21). New illness, old attitude. *Nursing Times, 94*(3), 28–30.

Gerchufsky, M. (1996, May). Human papilloma virus. *Advance for Nurse Practitioners,* 21–25.

Ginsberg, A. M. (1998). The tuberculosis epidemic: Scientific challenges and opportunities. *Public Health Reports, 113,* 128–136.

Glanz, K., & Yang, H. (1996). Communicating about risk of infectious diseases. *Journal of the American Medical Association, 275*(3), 253–256.

Gordon, S. M. (1996). Recognizing and treating new and emerging infections encountered in everyday practice. *Cleveland Clinic Journal of Medicine, 63*(3), 172–178.

Grimes, D. E., & Grimes, R. M. (1997). Tuberculosis: What nurses need to know to help control the epidemic. In B. W. Spradley & J. A. Allender (Eds.), *Readings in community health nursing* (5th ed.). Philadelphia: J. B. Lippincott.

Hamlin, J. S., Wood, D., Pereyra, M., & Grabowsky, M. (1996). Inappropriately timed immunizations: Types, causes, and their relationship to recordkeeping. *American Journal of Public Health, 86*(12), 1812–1814.

Horsburgh, C. R. (1998). Editorial: What it takes to control tuberculosis. *American Journal of Public Health, 88*(7), 1015–1016.

Kahn, C. (1998, December 12). Our fight to stop those deadly bugs. *Parade Magazine,* pp. 12–13.

Kollek, D. (1998, September 28). *Community acquired pneumonia* (pp. 1–10). Available: http://www.hamcivhos.on.ca/esp/pneumo1.htm.

Leslie, M., et al. (1999). Update: Hanta virus pulmonary syndrome—United States, 1999. *Morbidity and Mortality Weekly Report, 48*(24), 521–525.

Mackenzie, E. R. (1998). *Healing the social body: A holistic approach to public health policy.* New York: Garland Publishing.

Maibach, E., & Parrott, R. L. (Eds.). (1995). *Designing health messages: Approaches from communication theory and public health practice.* Thousand Oaks, CA: Sage.

Manning, A. (1995, September 18). Painful, flu-like tropical illness can be deadly. *USA Today,* pp. D1–D2.

Mick, D.J. (1997). Pneumonia in elders. *Geriatric Nursing, 18*(3), 99–102.

Miller, B., & Castro, K. G. (1996). Sharpen available tools for tuberculosis control, but new tools needed for elimination. *Journal of the American Medical Association, 276*(23), 1916–1917.

Miller, B., Monson, B., & Norton, M. (1995). The effects of forced sexual intercourse on white female adolescents. *Child Abuse and Neglect, 19,* 1289–1301.

O'Donnell, L. N., et al. (1995). Video-based sexually transmitted disease patient education: Its impact on condom acquisition. *American Journal of Public Health, 85*(5), 817–822.

Ostroff, S. M., & Kozarsky, P. (1998). Emerging infectious diseases and travel medicine. *Infectious Disease Clinics of North America, 12*(1), 231–241.

Robbins, J. B., Towne, D. W., Gotschlich, E. C., & Schneerson, R. (1997) "Love's labours lost": Failure to implement mass vaccination against group A meningococcal meningitis in sub-Saharan Africa. *Lancet, 350,* 880–882.

Satcher, D. (1996). CDC's first 50 years: Lessons learned and relearned. *American Journal of Public Health, 86*(12), 1705–1708.

Scutchfield, F. D., & Keck, C. W. (1997). *Principles of public health practice.* Albany, NY: Delmar.

Selekman, J. (1998). Infectious diseases and the immunizations of today and tomorrow. *Pediatric Nursing, 24*(4), 309–315.

Snider, D. E., & Castro, K. G. (1998). The global threat of drug-resistant tuberculosis. *New England Journal of Medicine, 338*(23), 1689–1690.

Tenover, F. C., & Hughes, J. M. (1996). The challenges of emerging infectious diseases. *Journal of the American Medical Association, 275*(4), 300–304.

USAIDS (1998). *Report on the global HIV/AIDS epidemic.* Geneva: UNAIDS/World Health Organization.

U.S. Department of Health and Human Services. (2000). *Healthy people 2010* (conference edition in two volumes). Washington, DC: U.S. Government Printing Office.

———. (1991). *Healthy people 2000: National health promotion and disease prevention objectives* (S/N 017-001-00474-0). Washington, DC: U.S. Government Printing Office.

World Health Organization. (1997). *WHO report on the tuberculosis 3 epidemic 1997.* Geneva, Switzerland: Author.

World Health Report (1998). *Report of the director-general.* Geneva: World Health Organization.

INTERNET RESOURCES

Center for International Health Information

　http://www.cihi.com

Centers for Disease Control and Prevention

　http://www.cdc.gov

American Public Health Association

　http://www.apha.org/

WHO Network for Global Influenza Surveillance

　http://www.whoinfluenza@who.ch

SELECTED READINGS

Anderson, C. (1995). Childhood sexually transmitted diseases: One consequence of sexual abuse. *Public Health Nursing, 12*(1), 41–46.

Brooke, P. S. (1997). Legally speaking: HIV and the law. *RN, 60*(5), 59–64.

Centers for Disease Control and Prevention. (1998). AIDS among persons aged >50 years—United States, 1991–1996.

———. (1998). Recommendations for prevention and control of tuberculosis among foreign-born persons. *Morbidity and Mortality Weekly Report, 47*(RR-16).

———. (1997). Immunization of health-care workers. *Morbidity and Mortality Weekly Report, 46*(RR-18).

———. (1996). Prevention of varicella. *Morbidity and Mortality Weekly Report, 45*(RR-11).

———. (1994). Addressing emerging infectious disease threats: A prevention strategy for the United States. *Morbidity and Mortality Weekly Report, 43*(RR-5).

Cerrato, P. L. (1996). Always a death sentence? *RN, 59*(8), 22–27.

Cosivi, O., Grange, J. M., Daborn, C. J., et al. (1998). Zoonotic tuberculosis due to *Mycobacterium bovis* in developing countries. *Emerging Infectious Diseases, 4*(1), 1–17.

Coward, D. D. (1994). Meaning and purpose in the lives of persons with AIDS. *Public Health Nursing, 11*(5), 331–336.

Curtis, S., & Taket, A. (1996). *Health & societies: Changing perspectives.* London, England: Arnold.

Halverson, P. K., Mays, G. P., Miller, C. A., Kaluzny, A. D., & Richards, T. B. (1997). Managed care and the public health challenge of TB. *Public Health Reports, 112,* 22–28.

Hussar, D. A. (1998). New drugs 98: Part 1. *Nursing 98, 28*(1), 53–59.

Jackson, E. K. (1995). Climate change and global infectious disease threats. *The Medical Journal of Australia, 163*(4), 570–574.

Kegeles, S. M., Hays, R. B., & Coates, T. J. (1996). The Empowerment project: A community-level HIV prevention intervention for young gay men. *American Journal of Public Health, 86*(8), 1129–1136.

Lilienfeld, D. E., & Stolley, P. (1994). *Foundations of epidemiology* (3rd ed.). New York: Oxford University Press.

Lisanti, P., & Zwolski, K. (1997). Understanding the devastation of AIDS. *American Journal of Nursing, 97*(7), 27–34.

Malotte, C. K., Rhodes, F., & Mais, K. E. (1998). Tuberculosis screening and compliance with return for skin test reading among active drug users. *American Journal of Public Health, 88*(5), 792–796.

McKenna, M. T., McCray, E., Jones, J. L., et al. (1998). The fall after the rise: Tuberculosis in the United States, 1991 through 1994. *American Journal of Public Health, 88*(7), 1059–1063.

Nokes, K., Wheeler, K., & Kendrew, J. (1994). Development of an HIV assessment tool. *Image—The Journal of Nursing Scholarship, 26*(2), 133–138.

Raviglione, M., Dye, C., Schmidt, S., & Kochi, A. (1997). Assessment of worldwide tuberculous control. *Lancet, 350,* 624–629.

Salsberry, P. J., Nickel, J. T., & Mitch, R. (1994). Immunization status of 2-year-olds in middle/upper- and lower-income

populations: A community survey. *Public Health Nursing, 11*(1), 17–23.

Sellers, D. E., McGraw, S. A., & McKinlay, J. B. (1994). Does the promotion and distribution of condoms increase teen sexual activity? Evidence from an HIV prevention program for Latino youth. *American Journal of Public Health, 84*(12), 1952–1959.

Sikkema, K. J., Heckman, T. G., Kelly, J. A., et al. (1996). HIV risk behaviors among women living in low-income, inner-city housing developments. *American Journal of Public Health, 86*(8), 1123–1126.

Strausbaugh, L. J. (1998). Emerging infectious diseases: No end in sight. *American Journal of Infection Control, 26,* 3–4.

Tulsky, J. P., White, M. C., Dawson, C., et al. (1998). Screening for tuberculosis in jail and clinic follow-up after release. *American Journal of Public Health, 88*(2), 223–226.

Ungvarski, P. J. (1997). Update on HIV infection. *American Journal of Nursing, 97*(1), 44–51.

UNICEF. (1994). *The state of the world's children, 1994.* New York, NY: Oxford University Press.

USAID. (1998). *The USAID polio eradication initiative 1997 report to Congress.* Arlington, VA: Center for International Health Information.

———. (1997, December). *Accomplishments in HIV/AIDS programs.* Washington, DC: Author.

Wilkinson, D., Davies, G. R., & Connolly, C. (1996). Directly observed therapy for tuberculosis in rural South Africa, 1991 through 1994. *American Journal of Public Health, 86*(8), 1094–1097.

Yu, E. S. H., Xie, Q., Zhang, K., et al. (1996). HIV infection and AIDS in China, 1985 through 1994. *American Journal of Public Health, 86*(8), 1116–1122.

Zuber, P. L., McKenna, M. T., Binkin, N. J., et al. (1997). Long term risk of tuberculosis among foreign-born persons in the United States. *Journal of the American Medical Association, 278,* 304–307.

Environmental Health and Safety

KEY TERMS

- Contaminant
- Deforestation
- Demographic entrapment
- Desertification
- Ecologic perspective
- Ecosystem
- Environmental health
- Environmental impact
- Environmental justice
- Extinction
- Global warming
- Pollution
- Toxic agent
- Wetlands

LEARNING OBJECTIVES

Upon mastery of this chapter, you should be able to:

- Discuss the importance of applying an ecologic perspective to any investigation of human–environment relationships.
- Explain the concepts of prevention and long-range environmental impact and their importance for environmental health.
- Discuss at least five global environmental concerns, and describe hazards associated with each area.
- Relate the effect of the above hazards on people's health.
- Discuss appropriate interventions for addressing the above environmental health problems, including community health nursing's role.
- Describe how national health objectives for the year 2010 target environmental health.
- Describe strategies for nursing collaboration and participation in efforts to promote and protect environmental health.

In 1998, a study reported in the *American Journal of Public Health* (Morgan, Corbett & Wlodarczyk, 1998) revealed that the air pollution levels in Sydney, Australia, were associated with increased hospital admissions for respiratory distress and heart disease. In addition, there was an association with the daily mortality in that city (Morgan, Corbett, Wlodarczyk & Lewis, 1998). Another study found that children living in neighborhoods near a battery factory in Managua, Nicaragua, had higher lead levels than children living elsewhere in the city and were at an increased risk of lead poisoning (Bonilla & Mauss, 1998). In Colorado, lifeguards in an indoor swimming pool developed granulomatous lung disease from water spray, which ventilation system improvements did not prevent (Rose et al., 1998). Our environment—the conditions within which we live and work, including the quality of our air, water, food, and working conditions—strongly influences our health status. Consequently, the study of environmental health has tremendous meaning for community health nurses. Broadly defined, **environmental health** is concerned with assessing, controlling, and improving the impact people make on their environment and the impact of the environment on them. The field of environmental health is concerned with all those elements of the environment that influence people's health and well-being. The conditions of workplaces, homes, or communities, including the many forces—chemical, physical, and psychological—present in the environment that affect human health, are important considerations.

Different environments pose different health problems and benefits. Consider the effects of acid rain, soil erosion, and insect invasions on a rural community or the effects of industrial toxic wastes, auto emissions, and airport noise on urban residents. The health effects of a hot, dry climate are different from those of an arctic area, and the environmental conditions of an industrialized nation are dramatically different from those of a developing country.

This chapter describes conceptual and theoretical approaches to environmental health, examines historical perspectives, global environmental health issues, and the primary environmental areas of concern to community health nurses. The primary environmental areas include air pollution, water pollution, unhealthy and contaminated food, waste disposal, insect and rodent control, and safety in the home, worksite, and community.

CONCEPTS AND THEORIES CENTRAL TO ENVIRONMENTAL HEALTH

Assessing environmental health means more than looking for illness or disease-causing agents; it also means examining the quality of the environment. Do the conditions of both the manmade and the natural environment combine to provide a health-enhancing milieu? Are people's surroundings safe and life sustaining? Are they clean and aesthetically enriching? Is the environment not only physically but also psychologically health enhancing? To answer these questions and gain greater understanding, the nurse needs to consider conceptual and theoretical approaches essential to assessing and controlling environmental health.

Preventive Approach

The study of environmental health has become increasingly complex as people's influence on the environment has increased. With the unprecedented advances in science and technology that have taken place in the past few decades, society's ability to affect the environment has expanded and the implications are not fully comprehended. New forms of energy, new synthetic chemical substances, and genetic engineering research bombard us with such rapidity that it is nearly impossible to anticipate all the potential side effects on the environment and, in turn, on people's health. For each advance and "improvement," the toll to be paid is frequently unknown.

Thus, the concept of prevention is vital to environmental health. Scientists must use foresight as they design innovations; government, business, and citizens must play watchdog; and those concerned with human and environmental health must monitor new developments and intervene to prevent problems from occurring. Health practitioners need to

determine causal links between people and their environment with an eye to improving the health and well-being of both. Nurses, in particular, must be aware of environmental factors that have the potential to either promote or adversely affect the health of communities. All three (primary, secondary, and tertiary) levels of prevention must be employed, but most important is primary prevention. Preventing a disease or *hazard* (a source of danger and risk particularly affecting human health) from occurring at all has the greatest benefit to the community.

Although small-scale preventive and health-promoting measures, such as safety education in the home or workplace, are important, it is the larger environmental problems that ultimately place many, if not all, members of a given community at risk. Community health nurses can develop an understanding of these environmental threats as well as the collaborative skills needed to work with other members of the public health team to prevent or alleviate them.

Ecologic Perspective

It is important to consider issues of environmental health from an **ecologic perspective,** keeping in mind the total relationship or patterns of relationships between people and their environment. Even when environmental health efforts focus on a specific health hazard or single environmental factor that poses a health threat, a broad view of human/environment relationships must be maintained. One cannot isolate a single causal factor in most cases, because there may be many causal relationships. An outbreak of food poisoning, for example, may be attributed to the *Salmonella* organism. However, it is most likely also associated with improper food handling and restaurant standards, which, in turn, may be affected by inadequate inspections and monitoring. The multiple relationships present in any environmental situation have been referred to as a *web* and the multiple causes of a problem as a *web of causation* (see Chapter 14).

An **ecosystem** is a community of living organisms and their interrelated physical and chemical environment; no one factor, whether organism or substance, can be viewed in isolation from the rest of its environment. Within an ecosystem, any manipulation of one element or organism may have hazardous effects on the rest of the system. Thus, no one factor, whether organism or substance, can be viewed in isolation. For example, in produce processing, there are several points at which contamination can occur: at production and harvest—growing, picking, and bundling; during initial processing—washing, waxing, sorting, and boxing; during distribution—trucking; and during final processing—slicing, squeezing, shredding, and peeling. In a number of instances from 1990 to 1996, several different pathogens were associated with cases of food-borne diseases from produce grown in the United States and Central America (Tauxe, 1998) (Table 16–1). Pathogens may have been introduced in the ir-

TABLE 16–1. Emerging Food-Borne Diseases 1990–1996

Year	Pathogen	Vehicle	No. of Cases	No. of States	Source
1990	S. Chester	Cantaloupe	245	30	Central America
1990	S. Javiana	Tomatoes	174	4	United States
1990	Hepatitis A	Strawberries	18	2	United States
1991	S. Poona	Cantaloupe	>400	23	United States/Central America
1993	E. coli O157:H7	Apple cider	23	1	United States
1993	Salmonella montevideo	Tomatoes	84	3	United States
1994	Shigella flexneri	Scallions	72	2	Central America
1995	S. Hartford	Orange juice	63	21	United States
1995	E. coli O157:H7	Leaf lettuce	70	1	United States
1996	E. coli O157:H7	Leaf lettuce	49	2	United States
1996	Cyclospora	Raspberries	978	20	Central America
1996	E. coli 0157:H7	Apple juice	71	3	United States

(Tauxe, R.V. [1998] Emerging food-borne diseases: An evolving public health challenge. URL. http://www.cdc.gov/ncidod?EID/vol3no4/tauxe.htm.)

rigation water, manure, or from lack of field sanitation during production and harvest; from contaminated wash water and handling at initial processing; from contaminated ice and dirty trucks during distribution; or in the final processing from dirty wash water, improper handling, or cross-contamination. By taking an ecologic approach in studying environmental health, the community health nurse acknowledges that people can affect their environment and the environment can affect them. Preventive and health promotive measures may be applied to all aspects of the environment as well as to the people in it. Humans share this planet with millions of other living creatures and must consider the ecologic balance and anticipate the far-reaching consequences of their actions before introducing environmental change with contaminants or toxic agents. A **contaminant** is organic or inorganic matter that enters a medium, such as water or food, and renders it impure. A **toxic agent** is a poisonous substance in the environment that produces harmful effects on the health of humans, animals, or plants.

Using a model similar to the epidemiologic triad introduced in Chapter 14, Curtis and Taket (1996) present a triangle of human disease ecology. This model stresses the links between habitat, population, and behavior (Fig. 16–1). *Habitat* includes aspects of the environment in which people live, including housing, workplaces, communication systems, flora, fauna, climate, topography, services, and economic and political structures of societies and local communities. *Population* factors include the characteristics of the population (age, gender, and genetic predisposition), which help to determine health status and disease susceptibility. *Behavioral* factors include health-related beliefs and behaviors, which are shaped by a range of social and economic factors. The triangular relationship among these factors suggests that there are no real boundaries between them and that the health of populations is a result of the interaction of all factors. It

also indicates that action on one part of the system in isolation is unlikely to be effective without complementary action on other relevant factors.

Environmental justice is a movement that has sought to ensure that no particular part of the population is disproportionately burdened by the negative effects of pollution (American Public Health Association, 1999). Industrial plants, waste facilities, and other potential polluters are more likely to be situated in poorer communities, and pollutants from these facilities can make the neighboring people ill. In one slum neighborhood in Bhopal, India, at least 3,500 people died and 200,000 were injured in 1984 when isocyanate was released from a pesticide factory (Beaglehole & Bonita, 1997). The impact of this disaster continues to be felt, although accurate records of the numbers of people whose health has been permanently affected do not exist. It is very possible that, as poor countries industrialize and embrace Western development and consumerism, there will be more disasters.

In the United States, it is not unusual to identify commu-

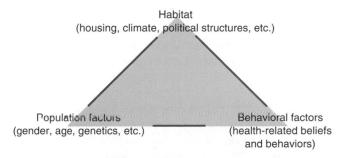

FIGURE 16–1. The triangle of human disease ecology. (Adapted from Curtis, S., & Taket, A. [1996]. *Health and societies: Changing perspectives.* London: Arnold.)

nities that are exposed to higher levels of pollutants than others. Members of these communities are not well equipped to deal with pollution problems because of their limited involvement in the political process. In addition, they may not be aware of their exposure to pollutants and may be more vulnerable to health problems because of poor nutrition and inadequate health care.

Aesthetics is the appreciation of beauty that is culturally pleasing to the person observing the person, place, or thing. Even accounting for cultural differences, there are some things, such as a woodland path, a rocky beach, or a colorful sunset, that most people would find aesthetically pleasing. How does the aesthetics or beauty of our environment affect us? People themselves are the best sources for ideas regarding those things that they cherish as being beautiful. However, an environment that is free of waste material, clutter, and foul smells and that includes well-landscaped surroundings can contribute to the inhabitants' well-being.

The benefits of aesthetically pleasing surroundings are difficult to measure. Nevertheless, we know how good it makes us feel when we experience it, that we would like to linger there longer, and that we would like to not let it disappear. If people were able to feel this way about their home, their neighborhood, and their community, the world would be a more harmonious and healthier place.

Long-Range Environmental Impact

When studying environmental health, it is important to consider the effect of positive or negative changes on the environment and on the people, animals, and plants living in it. This **environmental impact** must be viewed not only in terms of its consequences for people living now but also in terms of its long-range impact on the human species. One must consider the health of future generations as well as present ones. Considerations should include food and fuel limitations of the natural environment, attendance to conservation by balancing present and future needs, and preventing the consequences of environmental abuse. This last point broadens the focus even more. Certainly, one should determine how current practices and toxins are hurting humans, but it is also imperative to discover what threats they pose to the biosphere and thus to future generations—their long-range environmental impact. For example, carbon monoxide gas given off by factories and automobiles is toxic and can be lethal, causing dizziness, headaches, and lung diseases in humans who inhale it at certain concentrations. It has also been found to reduce the atmosphere's ozone layer, which protects us against ultraviolet irradiation. Thus, it poses a serious ecologic threat for the future. A study by the Institute of Medicine (1999) calls for more research to help policy makers weigh the possible environmental risks of any new industrial or business facility against its potential job and tax benefits for local citizens.

EVOLUTION OF ENVIRONMENTAL HEALTH

Environmental influences on people's health span all of human history. People's interactions with their environment and the conditions of that environment have shaped their mental, emotional, and physical health since the beginning of time. From ancient tribal practices of burial of excreta to modern-day sewage treatment, humans have been concerned with how the environment would provide for their needs and affect their well-being.

Global Perspective

In an effort to promote human health, people have taken steps to control, alter, and adapt to their environment. Demonstrations of this concern go back to Biblical times, when the Israelites observed strict rules governing food preparation, practiced sanitation, and quarantined people with infectious diseases, such as leprosy.

As populations became more settled and urbanized, many different environmental health concerns developed. Community actions to deal with these developments have been recorded as far back as 2500 BC. Archaeologists have discovered remnants of sophisticated water and waste systems in ancient cities of northern India and in the Middle Kingdom of Egypt. Early Roman engineers built aqueducts for supplying fresh water, and they developed management operations for overseeing water and sewage systems (McGrew, 1985).

A major environmental issue in the medieval world was the spread of infectious diseases brought about by the growth of cities, increased trade, and wars. Plague, spread by rodents, appears in the writings of Dionysius in the 3rd century (Blumenthal & Ruttenber, 1994). The most severe infectious diseases were outbreaks of leprosy and bubonic plague during the 13th and 14th centuries (McGrew, 1985). As leprosy spread and peaked in Europe in the early 13th century, people recognized a connection between the environment and the spread of the disease. They instituted epidemic control by isolating people with signs of the disease and checking newcomers to the community. Thus, long before science had discovered the true cause of these diseases, people were instinctively changing or avoiding harmful environmental circumstances in an effort to promote health. Simple city ordinances restricted locals from washing their clothes or tanners from cleaning their skins in rivers that supplied drinking water. A law passed in London in 1309 governed the disposal of wastes into the Thames River. Similarly, people passed rules governing the sale of old or spoiled meat to local residents, and "in Basel, leftover fish were displayed at a special inferior food stall and sold only to strangers" (McGrew, 1985, p. 139). This early concern for sanitary conditions became a major focus in public health, reaching its peak between 1840 and 1880.

The social hygiene movement called for societal transformation to create a truly healthful environment (McGrew, 1985, p. 139). During the mid- to late-1800s, Florence Nightingale in England and Dr. Ignace Semmelweiss in Vienna pioneered the promotion of clean hospital and surgical conditions to prevent illness. Oliver Wendell Holmes made the connection between exposure to sepsis and maternal infection in Boston in 1843. John Snow first documented environmental spread of disease in London in 1850 when he linked the spread of cholera with contaminated drinking water (Moeller, 1992). The work of Pasteur and Koch demonstrated the role of bacteria in disease. All of these, in addition to greater use of the microscope, shed further light on the relationship of the environment to health.

Awareness of environmental impact on health was first documented in a "Report on an Inquiry into the Sanitary Conditions of the Labouring Population of Great Britain" by Edwin Chadwick in 1842 (Turnock, 1997). This document addressed the necessity for a healthy environment. About the same time, a similar report in the United States called "Report of the Sanitary Commission of Massachusetts," by Lemuel Shattuck, provided original insights into environmental health issues, including smoke prevention, pest control, sanitation programs, and food regulations (Pickett & Hanlon, 1990). These documents marked the first organized concern for public health and environmental health controls. Since that time, the focus has gradually expanded from sanitation to the problems generated by advances in technology, chemical production, and pollution, which are discussed in this chapter.

An important international agency, the World Health Organization (WHO), was created in 1948 and has helped to identify and address world health problems, including issues of environmental concern. Because many modern technological discoveries cause far-reaching health hazards that affect the environment and the health of the entire global population, this organization and others like it will play increasingly important roles in the future (WHO, 1998).

National Perspective

In the United States, all levels of government have worked diligently to assess, prevent, and correct environmental health hazards. The major environmental health efforts of the federal government have come primarily since the early 1970s. Local governments assume responsibility for proper waste disposal, pure water supply, and efficient sanitary and safety conditions within the community. State governments, represented by different agencies, handle broader issues that deal with the creation of state regulations, policies, and supervision of local health efforts (Williams & Torrens, 1999). The federal government is charged with establishing and enforcing health standards and regulations. During the past 20 years, the public concern for people's health in relation to the environment, as well as concern for the environment itself, has stimulated increased government actions. The Environmental Protection Agency (EPA) was established in 1971 and was given extensive authority over all environmental concerns and protection of public health. Other related agencies included incorporation of the Food and Drug Administration (FDA) within the Public Health Service in 1968, the Occupational Safety and Health Administration (OSHA) for regulation and the National Institute for Occupational Safety and Health (NIOSH) for research, both established in 1970. The Public Health Service under the U.S. Department of Health and Human Services has helped to focus environmental control efforts through development of objectives published in 1979 and again in 1991. Its 1991 document, *Healthy People 2000,* lists objectives in major target areas. In the new follow-up document, *Healthy People 2010,* objectives for improvement in environmental health parameters continue (U.S. Department of Health and Human Services, 1991, 2000) (Display 16–1).

Private business has become more conscious of health and safety issues as those issues have been enhanced by legislation such as the Products Liability Law and monitored by the Products Safety Commission. Private business and industry have often been accused of having total disregard for the health of the environment and its effect on human health, but this image seems to be changing slowly. Many companies, confronted by concerned environmentalists or consumer protection groups that have formed in recent years, have been forced to change their practices. Boycotts of products, listings of environmentally conscientious firms, and general public outrage have put a stop to many harmful practices. A number of companies have been concerned for some time with the environmental impact of their business operations; they have sought not only reduction of health hazards but also ways to promote environmental and public health. Timber companies, for example, have actively engaged in reforestation projects. Private business has been a major contributor to many nonprofit, environmentally concerned projects and agencies, such as the Sierra Club (Display 16–2).

Maintaining a healthy environment and balanced ecology and promoting the health of those living in it remain challenging. Past efforts to accomplish these goals have been only partially successful. However, increased public awareness and concern for future generations have exerted tremendous pressure to create new and more effective measures.

MAJOR GLOBAL ENVIRONMENTAL CONCERNS

The global perspective, and specifically the national perspective, of environmental health provides us with a picture of humankind's attempts to protect populations. However, for much of our world's history, protecting people, other living beings, or the earth itself has not been a priority or even a con-

DISPLAY 16–1. *Healthy People 2010* Objectives Related to Environmental Health

In 1998, it was reported by the U.S. Department of Health and Human Services, in the *Healthy People 2010 Objectives for Public Comment*, using midpoint data, that the following progress (or lack of it) was made in the following areas:

1. Reduce asthma morbidity, measured by reduced asthma hospitalizations, to no greater than 43 per 10,000 population
   Special target populations: Blacks, nonwhites, and children
   1999: 94 per 10,000
2. Reduce prevalence of serious mental retardation among school-aged children to no more than 124 per 10,000 children.
   1995: 1991–1994 prevalence was 131 per 10,000.
3. Reduce outbreaks of water-borne disease from infectious agents and chemical poisoning to no more than 2 per year.
   Special target populations: People served by public or investor-owned water systems.
   1987–1996 average: 6 outbreaks per year.
4. Reduce the prevalence of blood lead levels among children to zero. Target: total elimination.
   Special target population: Inner-city, low-income, black children
   1991–1994: 4.4% of children aged 1 to 5 years had blood lead levels exceeding 10 μg/dL.
5. Reduce the proportion of people exposed to air that does not meet the Environmental Protection Agency (EPA) health-based standards for harmful air pollutants. Target air pollutants include ozone, carbon monoxide, nitrogen dioxide, sulfur dioxide, particulates, and lead.
   1997: ozone, 43%; particulate matter, 12%; carbon monoxide, 19%; nitrogen dioxide, 5%; sulfur dioxide, 2%; lead, <1%. 2010 target: 0%.
6. Increase to at least 20% the proportion of homes in which homeowners/occupants have tested for radon concentrations and concentrations have been found to pose minimal risk or have been modified to reduce risk to health, as a means to reduce the incidence of lung cancer.
   1998: An estimated 17% of the nation's homes had been tested for radon concentrations.
7. Reduce air toxic emissions to decrease the risk of adverse health effects caused by airborne toxics.
   Baseline 1993: 8.1 million tons of toxics were released into the air. Target: 2.0 tons—a 75% improvement.
8. Increase recycling of municipal solid waste.
   1996 baseline: 27% of total municipal solid waste generated was recycled. Target: 38% of municipal solid waste generated recycled.
9. Increase the proportion of people to at least 95% who receive safe drinking water supplies that meet the regulations of the Safe Drinking Water act.
   1995: 73% of community water systems met safe drinking water standards, which is the same as the baseline year of 1998; however, the EPA continues to issue additional safe standard levels.
10. Reduce potential risks to human health from surface water. This will be measured by a decrease in the proportion of surface waters (lakes, streams, and so forth) that do not support beneficial uses, such as fishing and swimming. This is a developmental objective with no percentages set; however, in 1994 40% of the nation's surface waters were too polluted for fishing or swimming.
11. Provide testing for lead-based paint in at least 50% of homes built before 1950.
    1998: 16% of people living in homes built before 1950 reported that the house paint had been analyzed for lead content.
12. Increase the number of new homes constructed to be radon resistant.
    1997: 1.4 million new homes. Target: 2.1 million additional new homes.
13. Eliminate significant health risks from hazardous waste sites on the Environmental Protection Agency's National Priority List. This will be measured by performing site cleanups sufficient to eliminate specified health threats. The year 2010 target is 98%.
    1995: 90% of the recommendations were followed among the 1,232 hazardous waste sites.
14. Increase or maintain the number of territories, tribes, states, and the District of Columbia that monitor environmental diseases. (These diseases include lead poisoning, other heavy metal poisoning, pesticide poisoning, carbon monoxide poisoning, heatstroke, hypothermia, acute chemical poisoning, methemoglobinemia, and respiratory diseases due to environmental factors.)
    1999 baseline: 4–41 jurisdictions. Target: 2010: 10–51 jurisdictions.
15. Reduce the proportion of children aged 6 and younger who are regularly exposed to tobacco smoke at home.
    1994: 27% of household with children under age 6 expose their children to tobacco smoke at least 4 days per week. Target: 10%.

(U.S. Department of Health and Human Services [2000]. *Healthy People 2010* [conference edition in two volumes]. Washington, DC: Government Printing Office.)

DISPLAY 16–2. Selected Environmental Health Acts/Agencies/Activities Influencing Health in the United States

Date	Act/Agency/Activity
1850	The Shattuck Report
1872	The American Public Health Association was founded
1872	The American Forestry Association was established
1890	Yosemite National Park in California became the first national park in the United States
1936	The National Wildlife Federation was founded
1970	The Environmental Protection Agency was formed
1970	The Clean Air Act
1970	Poison Prevention Packaging Act
1970	Occupational Health and Safety Act (OSHA)
1970	National Institute of Occupational Safety and Health (NIOSH) formed
1970	Hazardous Materials Transportation Control
1970	National Environmental Policy Act
1970	First annual Earth Day was held
1971	Lead-Based Paint Poisoning Prevention Act
1972	Federal Water Pollution Control Act Amendments
1972	Noise Control Act
1974	Safe Drinking Water Act (amended in 1996)
1976	Resource Conservation and Recovery Act
1976	Toxic Substances Control Act
1977	Clean Water Act
1979	U.S. Department of Health and Human Services helped to focus environmental control efforts
1980	Low Level Radiation Waste Policy Act
1980	Comprehensive Environmental Response, Compensation, and Liability Act (Superfund)
1991	*Healthy People 2000* set environmental health objectives as a priority
1992	The United States, the European community, and 153 other nations signed the United Nations Framework Convention on Climate Change (UNFCCC), an agreement pledging to reduce greenhouse gases to the 1990 level by the year 2000
1995	*Healthy People 2000: Midcourse Review and 1995 Revisions* gave update on environmental health progress
1996	The Food Quality Protection Act
1996	The World Health Organization, scientists, and United Nations officials called for stronger efforts to combat global warming
2000	*Healthy People 2010* used the 1995 review and revisions and input from professionals from around the country to establish 2010 environmental health goals

---

cern. Because of this history, there are major global environmental concerns now facing the world, including overpopulation, ozone depletion and global warming, deforestation, wetlands destruction, desertification, energy depletion, inadequate housing, aesthetics, and environmental justice issues.

Overpopulation

Human population took hundreds of thousands of years to grow to 2.5 billion in 1950; since then, in less than 50 years, it has more than doubled to 5.9 billion (Population Action International, 1998). This exponential population growth "will lead to either a levelling off because of actions taken now, or a dramatic reduction because of environmental disaster, if no action is taken" (Beaglehole & Bonita, 1997). Uncontrolled population growth is indisputably a public health issue (McMichael, 1995).

The world's population is still increasing by over 80 million people a year, This rate is expected to continue until 2010, at which point, it will gradually decline to about 40 million a year by 2050 (Population Action International, 1998; WHO, 1998). However, even with a worldwide trend toward smaller families, we will continue to add at least another 2 billion people to our small planet in the next 50 years.

The burden of the population growth is being carried by the poorest developing countries where 90% of the growth is occurring, such as in Africa and India. Over 95% of future population growth is also expected to occur in these regions. Between one third and one half of the population in most developing countries is under age 15, in part because advances in public health have lowered mortality among all age groups, but especially among infants and children.

In some nations, the population is projected to shrink. If low fertility rates continue in Germany, Italy, Russia, and Spain, their populations will decrease 5% to 15% by 2025. In contrast, countries such as Nigeria, Zaire, and Jordan have high fertility rates, and it is likely they will see their population more than double over the same period of time.

What do these statistics and trends mean for the health of populations and the ecosystem? When a population exceeds the ability of its ecosystem to either support it or acquire the support needed, or when it exceeds its ability to migrate to other ecosystems in a manner that preserves its standard of living, the population is said to be experiencing **demographic entrapment.** Such a population faces the four tragedies of entrapment. Depending on cultural, political, and ecologic factors, it can starve, die from disease, slaughter itself or others, or be supported indefinitely by aid from others (King & Elliott, 1995).

GOVERNMENT'S ROLE

The government has a responsibility to prevent a population from exceeding the limits of the nation's resources and boundaries. The possible methods of preventing, or solutions to, overpopulation are controversial, depending on one's culture, religious beliefs, or personal values and convictions. Ideally, the political system governing a country has a responsibility to provide a well-formed infrastructure of health and safety services for its population; economic development that provides employment, housing, and services; and political strength to provide stability to the nation. Many countries with unstable political systems are unable to deal effectively with overpopulation issues.

NURSE'S ROLE

Public health professionals, including community health nurses, have a responsibility in the area of overpopulation, both globally and locally. Productive interventions include teaching families that birth spacing improves child and maternal survival and that a planned family is the best environment for a child's development; preventing high-risk pregnancies such as those among teens and females with HIV/AIDS; preventing the growing epidemic of HIV/AIDS; providing family planning education to prevent worldwide deaths from unsafe abortions; and providing prenatal care—because healthy mothers equal healthy children. These are four key areas where public health efforts can reap major rewards for families (Population Action International, 1997).

Air Pollution

For many centuries, people have known that air quality affects human health. In Europe and America in the 1800s and early to mid-1900s, documented episodes of concentrated air pollution due to thermal atmospheric inversion caused many reported deaths (Moeller, 1992). **Pollution** refers to the act of contaminating or defiling the environment to the extent that it negatively affects people's health. Air pollution is now recognized as one of the most hazardous sources of chemical contamination. It is especially prevalent in highly industrialized and urbanized areas where concentrations of motor vehicles and industry produce large volumes of gaseous pollutants.

Air pollution is a global problem. Decades of environmentally insensitive industrial development in eastern Europe and the Soviet Union, as it was known then, have caused serious life- and health-threatening air pollution in recent years. In the Czech Republic, one of the most heavily polluted countries, air pollution may be responsible for up to 3% of all deaths (Beaglehole & Bonita, 1997). There is evidence that tens of thousands of people in these countries have developed respiratory

and cardiovascular problems from air-borne contaminants, and 75% of the children in many industrial areas of these countries have respiratory disease. A study of low-level air pollution in Helsinki, Finland, demonstrated that symptoms of ischemic cardiac and cerebrovascular diseases may be provoked by pollutants in concentrations lower than those given as guidelines in many countries and lower than previously shown (Ponka & Virtanen, 1996). A similar study on hospital admissions in Sydney, Australia, found that the levels of air pollution in Sydney were associated with increased hospitalization for respiratory and heart disease among those 65 years and older during 1990 to 1994 (Morgan, Corbett & Wlodarcyzk, 1998). In the United States from 1970 to 1997, overall emissions of the six major pollutants the federal government measures (carbon monoxide, nitrogen oxides, hydrocarbons, particulate matter, sulfur dioxide, and lead) decreased 31%. However, some 107 million Americans lived in counties with significant pollution problems in 1997.

Air-borne pollutants have adverse effects on many areas of human life; costs to property, productivity, quality of life, and especially human health are enormous. The list of diseases and symptoms of ill health associated with specific air pollutants is lengthy, ranging from minor nose and throat irritations, respiratory infections, and bronchial asthma to emphysema, cardiovascular disease, lung cancer, and genetic mutations (Fig. 16–2).

As with other toxic chemicals, it is often difficult to establish a cause–effect relationship between air pollution and illness. A relatively short, high level of exposure is normally easier to identify. There have been a number of poignant examples. One acute episode in Donora, Pennsylvania, in 1948 caused 20 deaths with 1,190 people sick (almost 43% of the area's population). Another occurred in London in 1952, when an atmospheric inversion trapped coal-burning smoke and fog over the city for nearly a week. Four to eight thousand people, mostly the elderly and those vulnerable from respiratory and cardiac diseases, died as a result (EPA, 1997a). Although these disasters and others like them are dramatic and frightening, the effects of long-term exposure to low levels of pollution, such as exposure from passive smoking at work, are perhaps even more threatening (Wells, 1998). They are definitely more difficult to record, measure, understand, define, correlate, and control. It may be impossible to ever document their total effects.

Certain geographic areas are more susceptible to the ill effects of air pollution because of weather conditions or physical terrain. The episode in London occurred when a lack of wind combined with low temperatures to create a temperature inversion—a phenomenon in which air that normally rises is trapped under a layer of warm air, allowing air contaminants to build up to intolerable levels. Los Angeles, another city troubled by air pollution, is surrounded by mountains that prevent winds from clearing away smoke and fumes. A further condition occurs in urban areas where city buildings create a "heat island effect" in which warm air traps pollution in the atmosphere around the city (Blumenthal & Ruttenber, 1994). Thus, in examining the effects of air pollution, it is necessary to take into account the climate conditions and topography of an area.

DUSTS, GASES, AND NATURALLY OCCURRING ELEMENTS

Dusts can contain numerous types of chemical irritants and poisons. Many hazardous dusts are associated with the workplace; for example, coal miners have developed black lung disease from inhaling coal dust, and a respiratory disease called silicosis is caused by exposure to silica dust (common in mining, sandblasting, and tunnel work). Dusts are also associated with farming and grain elevator work, as well as highway construction. Asbestos fibers, which are found in insulation and fireproofing materials, textiles, and many other products, have been associated with lung cancer. Although people who smoke are at 30 times greater risk of developing lung cancer than those who do not smoke, passive smoking is estimated to cause approximately 3,000 lung cancer deaths in nonsmokers each year (EPA, 1993b).

Although much air pollution results from some type of human activity, naturally occurring elements, such as pollen from plants and flowers, ash from volcanic eruptions, or airborne microorganisms, can also have ill effects on health. A long list of gaseous pollutants, including sulfur oxides and nitrogen oxides produced by industrial emissions, pose additional problems for community health. Such gases cause respiratory disease, asphyxiation, and other problems in humans and can harm plant and animal life as well. Other gases, including chlorine, ozone, sulfur dioxide, and carbon monoxide, are all harmful to individual health as well as to the broader environment and the ecosystem.

Another gas that has been a topic of concern in recent years is radon. This colorless, odorless, radioactive gas is formed by the breakdown of uranium in soil and rock. It has been associated with up to 30,000 deaths each year and is the second leading cause of lung cancer in the United States (EPA, 1993a). Radon enters buildings through cracks in basement walls or through sewer openings. Furnaces and exhaust fans can help pull radon into a house, although the highest levels tend to be found in basements where the gas enters. Home testing for radon was recommended by the EPA and the U.S. Public Health Service starting in 1988. Sealing the cracks in basement walls and covering dirt floors can substantially reduce radon levels. In addition, the EPA estimates that 20% of America's school children are exposed to radon in their schools (Miller, 1996).

ACID RAIN

The emission of hazardous chemicals into the earth's atmosphere has a serious effect on the environment. Air pollutants

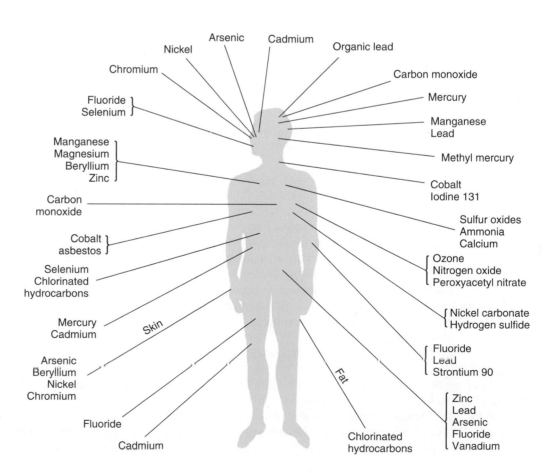

FIGURE 16–2. Body system targets of major air pollutants.

such as sulfur dioxide from power plant emissions or nitrogen oxides from motor vehicle exhaust combine with water vapor to produce sulfuric and nitric acid, known as "acid rain," in many parts of the northern United States (Kilburn, 1998). Although acid rain does not seem to pose any direct danger to humans, it kills small forms of life and endangers the forest and fresh water ecologies. An increased accumulation of carbon dioxide in the atmosphere from fuel combustion is altering the climate and causes a condition called the "greenhouse effect."

OZONE DEPLETION AND GLOBAL WARMING

Two new and very threatening environmental hazards of stratospheric ozone layer depletion and global warming are closely related. **Global warming** is the trapping of heat radiation from the earth's surface that increases the overall temperature of the world, causing a greenhouse effect (Beaglehole & Bonita, 1997). This warming is caused by carbon dioxide and other gases that enter the atmosphere through a depleting ozone layer and become trapped. The direct health effects of ozone depletion include an increase in the risk of skin cancer and cataracts. Greater indirect effects, from the global warming, could result through damage to the food chain, an increase in the global population exposed to vector-borne diseases, raised ocean levels, and a variety of effects on crop production (Patz et al., 1996; McMichael, Haines, Slooff & Kovat, 1996). For example, scientific studies based on mathematical models indicate that a global mean temperature increase of 1°C to 2°C would enable mosquitos to extend their range to new geographic areas, leading to 45% to 60% increases in cases of malaria by 2050 (WHO, 1998). In addition, there are already at least 25 million people, sometimes called environmental refugees, who can no longer support their families in their homelands because of drought, soil erosion, desertification, deforestation, and other environmental problems (Myers & Kent, 1995).

In the past, changes in the earth's climate resulted from natural causes and enabled the evolution of species over hundreds of thousands of years. The accumulation of stratospheric ozone shields the earth from damaging ultraviolet light, filtering and reducing the extent of radiation that reaches the earth. Today, human activities are affecting our climate in serious and immediate ways (EPA, 1997b). It is being destroyed as a result of chemical interactions between air pollutants, primarily chlorofluorocarbons (CFCs). Most of the ozone-destroying chemicals and greenhouse gases come from the wealthier countries.

GOVERNMENT'S ROLE

Government regulation of air pollution has been relatively slow. In 1963, the federal government passed the first series of Clean Air Acts. These set standards for air quality and industrial emissions and delegated funds to assist in pollution control programs. Although progress has been made, further public health efforts are needed to help identify pollution sources and related health hazards (see Display 16–2).

Even if our air is cleaner than it was 30 years ago, there is work yet to be done. The EPA has new rules to force reductions in nitrogen oxide emissions by 2003 at a cost of $1.7 billion for the power industry. The automobile is a continued target as a source of pollutants, and new steps will include reducing sulfur in gasoline, tightening emission standards, and removing a loophole that allows sports utility vehicles to defy emission standards (Borenstein, 1998).

The EPA (1997b) has identified 10 ways people can help stop global warming. These are suggestions the community health nurse can use and pass along to clients:

1. Reduce home energy usage (eg, keep heat lower in the winter and air conditioning higher in the summer, shut off lights in rooms not occupied, and unplug appliances when not in use).
2. If considering buying or building a new house, make sure it is energy-efficient.
3. Buy products that feature reusable, recyclable, or reduced packaging to save the energy required to manufacture new containers.
4. When buying a car, consider a fuel-smart car, one that gets more miles to the gallon than your current vehicle.
5. Consider transportation alternatives such as mass transit, car pooling, bicycling, and telecommuting. When you do drive, keep your car tuned up and its tires properly inflated to save on fuel costs.
6. Insulate your home to save money and energy, caulk windows and doors, and tune up your furnace and air conditioner.
7. Encourage your utility company to do its part by offering energy from clean sources (landfill gas recovery, high-efficiency natural gas-fired power plants, or renewable sources such as solar and wind).
8. Get involved at work by ensuring your company has joined EPA programs such as Green Lights, ENERGY STAR Buildings, and Waste Wi$e recycling programs, and by buying office equipment with an ENERGY STAR label (this label indicates high efficiency, saving energy and money, performing better, and helping prevent air pollution).
9. Plant trees—trees absorb carbon dioxide, a greenhouse gas, from the air. Join family members, neighbors, or community service groups in planting trees in your yard, along roadways, and in parks.
10. Educate others—let friends, family, and clients know about these practical, energy-saving steps they can take to save money while protecting the environment.

NURSE'S ROLE

Community health nurses can influence air quality through detection, community education, and lobbying for appropriate legislation. People are exposed to numerous impurities in the air in their homes and workplaces. Nurses can promote health by helping to detect indoor pollutants and inform people of existing or potential dangers. Many household products and building materials emit vapors that can cause problems. Cigarette and cigar smoke are common indoor pollutants that can have ill effects on nonsmokers as well as smokers (Wells, 1998). Infants and other vulnerable persons are at risk to such exposure (Association of Maternal and Child Health Programs, 1998). Carbon monoxide poisoning may result from stove and furnace emissions or car exhaust accumulating in a garage. Radon gas trapped in basements or tightly insulated homes is also a major concern (Kilburn, 1998; Miller, 1996). Nurses can assist with prevention or elimination of these health hazards by ensuring a well-ventilated (oxygenated) indoor environment and properly maintained heating equipment and by looking for possible sources of pollution.

Water Pollution

Water is such an essential element to human survival that the available quantity and quality of water within a community become a prime environmental health issue. Water has many uses other than consumption by humans. It serves as a means of transportation. It cleans and cools the body or other objects. It is the basis for many forms of recreation and sports such as swimming and boating, and it provides a vehicle for disposing of human and industrial wastes and controlling fires. Apart from serving human needs, water also serves as a medium for sustaining other living organisms, as a home to plant and animal life, and as a means of carrying and distributing necessary nutrients in the environment. Although nursing's environmental health role concerns the safe consumption of water by humans, it is important, taking an ecologic perspective, to keep in mind water's other uses and users.

Drinking water comes from two main sources: surface water, such as lakes and streams, and underground sources, called groundwater, collected in areas known as aquifers; it comes to the surface through wells and springs. In general, underground sources are thought to be less subject to contamination than are surface sources, which are open to runoff from agricultural pesticides or industrial wastes. However, groundwater too may be contaminated when seepage occurs. In the Middle Ages, disease epidemics spread as people drank water contaminated by human waste; this is still a problem in developing countries today and, at times, in other countries when there is flooding. Well water, for example, may contain fecal contaminants from improper septic tank drainage. Toxic agents may affect groundwater and include buried hazardous wastes or nitrate contamination of wells in rural areas (Conway, 1998).

In most industrialized nations, lack of sufficient water for drinking has not been a serious issue. Areas with limited water supplies have devised facilities to store water during high-flow periods so it would be available to satisfy the year-round needs of a given community. Adequate water supply to meet agricultural demands still has not been achieved, however.

The major concern with regard to water is its purity. Water can be contaminated and made unsafe for drinking in many different ways. Three are discussed here.

1. Water may be infected with bacteria or parasites that cause disease. *Giardia lamblia* is a parasite shown to enter the water supply by contamination from human or wild animal feces. It can cause giardiasis, a gastrointestinal disease that results in diarrhea and malabsorption of nutrients. For example, beavers in the northern Cascade Mountains often contaminate water (Blumenthal & Ruttenber, 1994). Humans using the area for recreation must treat the water with iodine before drinking it. Water may also be contaminated with bacteria such as *Vibrio cholerae,* resulting in cholera, or with viruses leading to hepatitis A (Moeller, 1992).

2. Toxic substances such as pesticides introduced by humans into water systems are another source of water pollution. These may contaminate streams, lakes, and wells (Conway, 1998). Industrial pollutants may also enter drinking water through oil spills, careless dumping, or buried hazardous wastes that seep into underground water sources. Such wastes not only harm the quality of the water, but also have been implicated in diseases such as leukemia. They can also contaminate local fish and shellfish, making them unfit for consumption. Mercury poisoning from contaminated seafood on the Atlantic coast is a case in point: by 1988, one third of the nation's shellfish beds had been closed because of pollution.

3. Pollutants may upset the ecosystem, affecting natural organisms that help purify water systems (Nadakavukaren, 1995). Power plants or other industries dissipate excess heat into lakes and streams and cause water temperatures to rise. This thermal pollution kills off beneficial organisms in the water.

In response to the various potential water pollutants, most cities and local communities with public or semipublic water systems in operation have set up water testing and treatment purification centers to ensure safe drinking water (Conway, 1998). Unfortunately, testing for bacteria and toxins often does not occur until after illness has been reported. Another major problem arises in rural areas where most water supplies are private and thus not assured of systematic testing and treatment. Testing water for coliforms as indicator organisms has proved useful. Water frequently is treated with chlorine to disinfect it, but this too has led to risk of chloroform exposure.

Recreational uses of water, such as public swimming, have health implications. Lakes, oceans, rivers, and even hot tubs often carry infectious agents and result in a number of health problems, including swimmers' itch, diarrheal diseases, and granulomatous pneumonitis (Moeller, 1992; Rose et al., 1998). Many disease outbreaks have been caused by polluted water systems serving campgrounds, parks, and other public areas.

The marine ecosystem can be altered by any changes that affect the oceans, such as water temperatures at the surface, nutrient levels, winds, currents, and precipitation patterns. This can lead to possible increases in diseases transmitted from fish and shellfish, toxic "red tides," and a dormant form of cholera that develops when pH, temperature, salinity, and nutrient levels are insufficient (EPA, 1997a). In addition, research has shown that coming in contact with marine waters contaminated with domestic sewage can cause nonenteric illnesses, including febrile respiratory illness from fecal streptococci, and ear ailments from fecal coliform exposure among swimmers in the United Kingdom (Fleisher et al., 1996).

GOVERNMENT'S ROLE

Most of the responsibility for maintaining water quality rests with state and local governments. The federal government took a needed step in 1974 by passing the Safe Drinking Water Act, which gave the EPA authority to establish water standards and to ensure that these standards were upheld. The federal government also provided funds to assist state and local governments in this effort. However, policies related to groundwater quality protection need continued monitoring. In 1998, the EPA developed a Right-to-Know report, which tells consumers about contaminants in their drinking water. These long-awaited rules set the minimum requirements for healthy drinking water and helped to ensure the safety of drinking water supplies (Fouse & Zimmerman, 1998). Saltwater intrusion caused by changes in sea level is threatening drinking water supplies in many communities along the East Coast. The state of Florida has resorted to building desalinization plants (EPA, 1997a).

Globally, because of enormous health problems in developing nations due to unclean water, WHO declared the 1980s as the International Clean Water Decade and established a goal to have safe drinking water for all by the year 1990 (Blumenthal & Ruttenber, 1994). This goal was not met; only 50% of the world's population had a safe water supply in 1980, 55% in 1985, and 66% by 1990 (WHO, 1998). Efforts to address water purity globally continue to assume high priority; however, the focus is shifting from drinking water quality alone toward overall improvement of the environment.

NURSE'S ROLE

What role can community health nurses play in the effort to keep water safe? As nurses work in a community, they can help by examining household or city drinking water. Is there a strange odor or discoloration? Are particles or sediment visible in the water? Being aware of drinking water quality and possible contaminants in a given locality alerts the nurse to consider possible causal relationships if a prob-

lem exists. Asking clients to observe and report changes in water quality further assists the nurse in the monitoring process. When such changes occur, the proper authorities, such as health department officials, should be notified and water samples tested. Community health nurses can also be alert to increased incidence of illnesses that might be water related. For example, if several children exhibit similar symptoms, the nurse might inquire as to whether all have been swimming in the same pool or drinking from the same water fountain. Although water quality monitoring is ultimately the responsibility of environmental health authorities, it behooves the nurse, as a collaborating member of the health team, to observe and report any information that would further the goal of safe and healthy water for communities.

Deforestation, Wetlands Destruction, and Desertification

Deforestation is the clearing of tropical and temperate forests for cropland, cattle grazing, or urbanization. Elimination of these natural habitats is dooming some species of insects and animals to **extinction,** the loss of a species from the earth forever. **Wetlands** are natural inland bodies of shallow water, such as marshes, ponds, river bottoms, and flood plains, that filter contaminated surface waters and support wildlife reproduction and growth (Nadakavukaren, 1995). They can be as small as a neighborhood seasonal stream bed or as large as the Everglades in Florida. At one time, the Everglades covered the lower 20% of the state, but the U.S. Army Corps of Engineers converted thousands of acres into housing developments 50 years ago. The destruction of this major U.S. wetland has caused numerous species of wildlife to disappear from the area or become extinct. There is discussion to reclaim some of the land and convert it back to much-needed wetlands. **Desertification** refers to the conversion of fertile land into desert, which is unable to support crop growth or wildlife (Miller, 1996).

Any natural or manmade process that changes these life-supporting regions into land for other use or barren wastelands upsets the ecosystem of the area. The destruction of forests and the upturning of earth for urban sprawl uncovers organisms hidden for eons that humans and animals can now be exposed to. In addition, the ozone once absorbed by these lost trees now contributes more gases, which increases global warming. Deforestation, in turn, contributes to desertification because forests provide protection for the surrounding topsoil by way of the roots, fallen leaves, and undergrowth. When this protection is lost, landslides and other geographic changes occur. Global temperature increases that cause the drying up of riverbeds create desert areas that are unable to support the people who once inhabited the area. Drought, famine, and starvation often follow in such areas. The loss of the forests and wetlands along with increasing desertification affect millions of people each year, with potential for catastrophic environmental damage in the future.

GOVERNMENT'S ROLE

Our government has the power to make decisions that save the wetlands and forests in the United States. The decision to save these lands is made when constituents express their concern loudly enough for the congressperson or senator to hear and then respond positively. Often, industrial and housing developers are more influential and their business interests win. If the importance of the wetlands and forests is not recognized where decisions are made, then they will be lost to industry.

NURSE'S ROLE

Community health nurses can make a difference in this area. Perhaps no other person knows a community more intimately than the community health nurse. This role gives a valid voice of concern at the local level. By using leadership and collaborative skills, the nurse can initiate grassroots efforts to save wetlands and forests in the community. Chapters 10 and 13 provide you with information for bringing about change, beginning at the local level.

Energy Depletion

Most of the energy sources we use today are not renewable. Wood has been used for thousands of years and was our first fuel. It is still a primary source of home heating for most of the world's population (and contributes to deforestation and to air pollution). Natural gas for heat and fuel can be a highly efficient energy source, but pipelines must be built for hundreds or thousands of miles in some cases, a luxury smaller and poorer countries cannot afford. Coal takes thousands of years to create, and worldwide sources will soon be depleted. Some countries do not have coal as a natural resource and have similar problems with natural gas.

Nuclear energy has been used for 30 years or more. This source of energy has been controversial since first used, yet it has proved to be an effective power product. Nevertheless, there have been some near disasters and real disasters caused by human error. In 1979, a nuclear power plant on Three Mile Island near Harrisburg, Pennsylvania, had a near disaster in one of its cooling towers; fortunately, the nuclear core was never exposed. This scare caused many people in the United States to lobby against nuclear power plants in their communities. The largest radiation disaster occurred in April 1986 at the Chernobyl nuclear power plant in Ukraine. Five million people in Ukraine, Belarus, and the Russian Federation were exposed to ionizing radiation. Twenty-eight of the 444 people at the plant who were directly exposed died within 3 months, and 300 were hospitalized. Psychological effects among peo-

ple living in the surrounding areas resulted from the lack of information immediately after the accident, the stress and trauma of compulsory relocation, a break in social ties, and fear that radiation exposure could cause health damage in the future. There has been an increase in the incidence of childhood thyroid cancer, particularly in Belarus. Ultimately, it is estimated that the aftereffects of this nuclear disaster will cause 6,600 more deaths from cancer and leukemia (Beaglehole & Bonita, 1997). The area remains unsafe to enter today, more than 15 years later.

GOVERNMENT'S ROLE

Other renewable sources of energy need to be discovered, rediscovered, or tapped. Newer and more "environmentally friendly" energy sources are used experimentally in limited areas. They include landfill gas recovery, solar power, and wind. There are a few examples in the United States of how these sources can make a difference (EPA, 1997b):

- A National Wind Coordinating Committee established by utility companies, consumers groups, state and federal regulators, and the U.S. Department of Energy has instituted experimental projects in six northeastern, midwestern, and southeastern sites. The resulting savings in energy costs were expected to reach $484 million.
- The U.S. Department of Energy is working closely with industry to develop photovoltaic systems for harnessing the rays of the sun to generate power. During the 1996 Olympics in Atlanta, the swimming competitions took place under lights powered by photovoltaics.
- The U.S. Department of Energy is working to address the need for growing and harvesting crops that can be turned into biomass fuels and to reclaim waste products from agricultural crops and forestlands for generating electricity. Two demonstration projects are presently in progress—the Vermont Gasifier Project and the Hawaii Biomass Gasifier Facility.
- The U.S. Department of Energy also is involved in geothermal projects. One includes the development of a pipeline that involves geysers in California. Another is from a consortium of more than 70 utility companies, promoting the use of geothermal heat pumps.

It will take a global effort to create an awareness and the accompanying technology needed to use these energy sources in enough areas to make an environmental difference.

NURSE'S ROLE

A community health nurse may not have a direct role in the creation of new energy sources or use of a particular source. However, he or she can educate people about energy conservation, discuss alternative energy sources presently available in the community, and encourage people to become interested in and knowledgeable about the importance of the potential for energy depletion in the future.

Inadequate Housing

Housing is of central importance to quality of life. Ideally, it minimizes disease and injury and contributes much to physical, mental, and social well-being. Perhaps we cannot appreciate the kind of housing people in most of the world call home. Because of lack of exposure to developing countries and poor countries, most Americans think of poor housing as being a smaller than desirable house, without a fresh coat of paint, needing some repairs, and with an unkempt yard; or as an apartment in a poor neighborhood with graffitied walls, unpredictable plumbing, and unsafe elevators. This is unfortunate enough in a country such as the United States but is far above the substandard living conditions in which most of the world lives.

At least 600 million people in Africa, Asia, and Latin America living in urban areas live in life- and health-threatening homes and neighborhoods. Most live in overcrowded dwellings, with four or more persons to a room in tenements, cheap boarding houses, or shelters built on illegally occupied or subdivided land. In Chile, just 30 minutes outside of Santiago, there are shantytowns in fields that resemble piles of trash at a dump. These "homes" have no water or electricity. Tens of millions are homeless and sleep in public or semi-public places—such as pavement dwellers and those sleeping in bus shelters, train stations, or parks (WHO, 1998).

GOVERNMENT'S ROLE
WHO identifies nine features of the housing environment that have important direct or indirect effects on the health of their occupants. WHO considers the home and its surrounding environment as being "the health burden of poor housing" (WHO, 1998):

1. The structure of the shelter (does it protect the occupants from extremes of heat or cold, and insulate against noise and invasion by dust, rain, insects, and rodents?)
2. The extent to which the provision for water supplies is adequate—both from a qualitative and a quantitative point of view
3. The effectiveness of provision for the disposal (and subsequent management) of excreta and liquid and solid wastes
4. The quality of the housing site, including the extent to which it is structurally safe for housing and provision is made to protect it from contamination (provision for drainage is among the most important aspects)
5. Overcrowding, which can lead to household accidents and increased transmission of air-borne infections such as acute respiratory infectious diseases, pneumonia, and tuberculosis
6. The presence of indoor air pollution associated with fuels used for cooking and/or heating
7. Food safety standards—including the extent to which the shelter has adequate provision for storing food to protect it against spoilage and contamination
8. Vectors and hosts of disease associated with the domestic and peridomestic environment
9. The home as a workplace—where the use and storage of toxic or hazardous chemicals and unsafe equipment may present health hazards

NURSE'S ROLE
In this area of environmental health and safety, the community health nurse has great influence. Much of the nurse's commitment to the community focuses on assessment, planning, intervention, and evaluation of a client's home and surrounding environment. The role may call for client education about home improvements, advocacy for routine maintenance of rental housing conditions, or assisting clients who live on the streets or in shelters to locate and secure more permanent and adequate safe housing.

Unhealthy or Contaminated Food

This section describes how the supply of food, particularly the quality of that food, is affected by the environment, and what health hazards are associated with food. The community health nurse needs to ask: "How does the environment influence the safety of food for human consumption?" Three types of hazardous foods must be considered when examining food as a possible health problem: inherently harmful foods, contaminated foods, and foods with toxic additives.

INHERENTLY HARMFUL FOODS
Poisonous foods, such as certain types of mushrooms or inedible berries, do not pose a serious threat to most people. The general public can identify and avoid harmful plants and substances, so poisonings are rare. There are, however, numerous household plants and outdoor flowers, shrubs, and trees that are poisonous if consumed. Children are at risk because some bear berries or colorful flowers that capture the child's interest, including:

Asparagus fern
Azalea
Begonia
Chrysanthemum
Holly
Honeysuckle
Jade plant
Jerusalem cherry
Medicine aloe
Mistletoe
Mountain-ash
Oak
Oleander
Philodendron
Poinsettia

Poison ivy
Rhododendron
Rubber plant
Schefflera
Spider plant

CONTAMINATED FOODS

Contaminated foods pose a more serious health problem. Food may contain harmful bacteria such as *Salmonella enteritidis, Staphylococcus aureus,* or *Clostridium botulinum,* causing outbreaks of disease. Of these, salmonellosis is the most common. An estimated 5 million *Salmonella* infections alone occur annually in the United States (Chin, 1999). Salmonellosis is characterized by sudden onset of headache, abdominal pain, diarrhea, nausea, vomiting, fever, and dehydration. The acute enterocolitis may develop into septicemia or a severe focal infection, such as endocarditis, meningitis, pneumonia, or pyelonephritis. Infants, elderly, and debilitated persons are at greatest risk for death. Blumenthal and Ruttenber (1994) reported that nationally in 1 year, 33% of poultry, 15% of pork, and close to 10% of beef products were contaminated with *Salmonella* because of inadequate processing and shipping methods. Cooking destroys the organism, but problems may be caused by eating undercooked foods, such as rare roast beef, or handling raw meats. *Shigella* infections transmitted by the fecal–oral route cause bloody diarrhea, fever, nausea, vomiting, and cramps. More than 32,000 cases were reported in the United States in 1995 (National Institutes of Health, 1998). *Shigella* can be transmitted by as few as 10 organisms, making personal hygiene and proper food preparation imperative. Parasitic transmission generally takes the form of trichinosis, caused by ingesting *Trichinella spiralis* in undercooked pork. Various types of worm infestations have created serious health problems, particularly in developing countries. Viral food transmission is rare. Different types of chemical food contamination result from improper food handling or processing. Examples include dirty machines used in food processing factories, pesticides and herbicides used by farmers to grow their crops, and mercury in fish that live in polluted water (WHO, 1998).

Food-borne diseases are costly. It is estimated that the yearly cost of all food-borne diseases in the United States is $5 to $6 billion in direct medical expenditures and lost productivity (National Institutes of Health, 1998) (see Research: Bridge to Practice).

International trade and travel and changes in demographics, consumer lifestyles, food production, and microbial adaptation create the emergence of new food-borne diseases. This globalization of the food supply means that people are exposed, through foods purchased locally, to pathogens native to remote parts of the world. As a result of international travel, people are exposed to food-borne hazards in a foreign country and bring the disease into their own country after their return, possibly exposing others in a location thousands of miles from the original source of the infection (National Institutes of Health, 1998).

FOODS WITH TOXIC ADDITIVES

A third health hazard from food comes from the intentional introduction of additives to food products. Because present-day consumers demand convenience foods and timesaving devices, and businesses want to produce food items with long shelf-lives, enhanced flavor, and lasting, vibrant colors, many foreign chemicals and synthetic products have been added to foods. Animals that are raised for food, such as chickens, pigs, and beef cattle, are often fed or injected with substances to speed their growth. As consumers shift toward healthier eating, they do not know and are only starting to question the effects these additives may have over time. For example, red dye #2 once was added to improve the color of certain food products but has since been proved carcinogenic. Preservatives and chemical flavorings such as saccharin have also proved hazardous in large doses. It is still questionable what small doses may do with prolonged use. Recently, questions have been raised about potential long-range effects of NutraSweet, a sugar substitute. Furthermore, such natural flavor enhancers as salt and processed sugars appear in excessive quantities in some canned and packaged foods and are linked to unhealthy dietary consequences such as hypertension or obesity. In small doses these additives may not be harmful, but when additives are consumed in combination over prolonged periods of time, they may create serious health consequences.

GOVERNMENT'S ROLE

It is the legal responsibility of food producers, processors, and manufacturers to guarantee the quality and safety of food products. However, conflicting motives, such as concern over loss of profit, often lead to careless or inadequate monitoring. Governmental regulatory agencies exist on the local, state, and federal levels to set standards and control the quality of food sold to the public. Such public health authorities as the U.S. Food and Drug Administration and the Departments of Agriculture and Health and Human Services are all necessary to help ensure the purity of commercial food products. Included in their jurisdiction is the supervision of the food service industry. Licensing requirements, sanitation standards, and inspections serve as control measures.

Governmental agencies cannot cover all the bases, however. Inadequate inspection of the quality of commercial fish sold for food, for example, has led to numerous outbreaks of hepatitis A and other illnesses. With the wide variety of possible contaminants and potential dangers, consumers' best protection is to supervise their own food quality (see Related Phone Numbers and Internet Resources at the end of the chapter).

NURSE'S ROLE

Community health nurses can have a significant impact through health education. Most bacterial and viral food-

RESEARCH Bridge to Practice

Mahon, B.E., Slutsker, L., Hutwagner, L., Drenzek, C., et al. (1999). Consequences in Georgia of a nationwide outbreak of Salmonella infections: What you don't know might hurt you. *American Journal of Public Health, 89*(1), 31–35.

Various food items, such as bottled juices, frozen hamburgers, and ice cream are produced in enormous volumes in central locations and then widely distributed. Contamination of any of these foods during the production phase can cause widespread outbreaks of food-borne diseases. Such outbreaks can present public health challenges, including locating and informing at-risk populations about how to avoid illness and retrieving the contaminated food for safe disposal. Two methods are generally used: mass media messages to the public and product recall at the distribution point. However, products that have already been purchased are very difficult to retrieve.

The case discussed here was the largest common-vehicle *Salmonella* outbreak ever recognized in the United States, with 41 states reporting a total of 224,000 cases. The source of contamination was probably tanker trucks that delivered ice cream premix to the factory for freezing. These trucks also were routinely used to haul liquid raw eggs, a common source of *Salmonella* serotype Enteritidis, the causative agent. Notifying possible consumers was not as difficult as it usually is because the product was sold only by direct home delivery and the company had the names and addresses of all customers that bought ice cream from them. They were notified by mail, and a delivery-truck-recall process was begun in addition to several weeks of national media coverage.

For this study, a telephone survey of 1% of the ice cream purchasers in Georgia began 13 to 17 days after news media warnings began. Contact was made to 211 of the 250 randomly selected customers, and interviews were conducted with respondents for 179 households that met the age and other study criteria. They were asked if they had heard about the outbreak and, if they did, how did they hear about it. Of the 179 respondents, 163 had heard about the warning before the interview. Many customers misunderstood or were skeptical of the media warnings. After first hearing the warning, 36% of the respondents did not understand that the implicated ice cream should not be eaten. Worse, in 31% of the households that had heard the warning, a family member had eaten the product anyway. The letters mailed by the ice cream company were reportedly reached by only 21% of those questioned, making this a suboptimal warning method.

What was learned during this study was that television as a media source gets the warning out the fastest, but the public health message is often lost. Word of mouth from friends and family members is an effective warning method. Individual contacts through visits, letters, or telephone calls are slow but may reach persons otherwise missed. Most importantly, public health officials should help ensure the thoroughness of communications and the retrieval of the contaminated product. The researchers in this study examined four other investigations of warnings during acute outbreaks of food-borne diseases, and all showed that communication to the target population was late, incomplete, or inaccurate. Not knowing what we need to know may indeed hurt us.

borne diseases can be prevented if people know and practice proper cooking and storage of food as well as proper personal hygiene (Display 16–3).

Nurses can teach the basics of keeping perishable products sufficiently refrigerated, discarding foods that may be old or spoiled, cooking foods thoroughly, and bringing water to a full boil when appropriate to be certain of eliminating microbes. Nurses can emphasize washing and cleaning produce and tools used in food processing, including the preparer's own hands. Finally, nurses can educate people to watch for signs of contamination. A dented can, for example, may signal the presence of living bacteria using the oxygen within the container and contaminating its contents. Nurses can raise public awareness regarding the conditions of supermarkets, restaurants, and other food handlers. They can also help promote community standards, enabling legislation, and policies for safer food supplies.

Waste Disposal

The United States generates more solid and hazardous waste per capita than any other industrialized nation. On average in 1990, each person in the United States produced 4.3 lb of combustible or landfilled maintained waste. In 1995, it was 4.4 lb. This equals 1,600 lb of municipal solid waste each year (Fig. 16–3). More frightening is the fact that U.S. industry produces the equivalent of over 1 ton of *hazardous* waste per person each year (Moeller, 1992). In addition, some 8.1 million tons of air toxics were released into the air

---

DISPLAY 16–3. **Ten Golden Rules for Safe Food Preparation**

To prevent and control food-borne disease, the World Health Organization has developed the following rules:
1. Choose food processed for safety.
2. Cook food thoroughly.
3. Eat cooked food immediately.
4. Store cooked food carefully.
5. Reheat cooked foods thoroughly.
6. Avoid contact between raw foods and cooked foods.
7. Wash hands repeatedly.
8. Keep all kitchen surfaces meticulously clean.
9. Protect foods from insects, rodents, and other animals.
10. Use pure water.

(Chin, J. [Ed.] [1999]. *Control of communicable diseases in man* [17th ed.]. Washington, D.C.: American Public Health Association)

in 1993. The year 2010 target is 2.0 tons (U.S. Department of Health and Human Services, 2000).

With the vast amounts of waste produced in the form of household garbage, human excreta, and agricultural and industrial byproducts, including hazardous chemical and radioactive substances, it is no wonder that waste management and disposal has become an important and pressing topic in recent decades. New technology has effectively addressed some of the problems, but there is still much need for improvement. Solid and hazardous wastes pose a wide range of public health concerns. Therefore, it is imperative that health officials, including nurses, become aware of the possible health hazards that these wastes present to individuals and to communities.

DISPOSAL OF HUMAN WASTE

One of the oldest environmental health hazards comes from improper disposal of human excreta. Although industrialized nations successfully address the problem, it continues to be widespread in developing nations and in rural, poverty-stricken communities. Human wastes, particularly feces, provide a perfect environment in which bacteria and disease-causing parasites can live and reproduce. Therefore, conta-

minated drinking water, food grown in contaminated soil, and, of course, direct contact with the water or soil can cause infections. For example, hookworm, a problem in the United States in the early part of the 20th century, usually enters the body through the skin of bare feet (Blumenthal & Ruttenber, 1994).

DISPOSAL OF GARBAGE

Dumping, burning, and burying are the most common solid-waste disposal methods. Dumping is problematic because garbage dumps provide perfect conditions for the breeding of rats, flies, and other disease-carrying organisms and may potentially be a source of water contamination from runoff. Dumps also are eyesores that take up valuable land resources. Burning, although it reduces the volume of garbage, produces noxious odors and pollutes the air. Sanitary landfills have generally replaced dumps as a more effective way to dispose of refuse by burying it. With proper handling, including covering and daily sealing (to prevent insect and rodent breeding), this method has proved satisfactory for handling of solid waste.

DISPOSAL OF HAZARDOUS WASTE

Disposal of toxic chemical and radioactive wastes produced by industry is another grave concern. The threat is serious because one cannot be certain of all the effects of these wastes or whether present methods of disposal are foolproof. Furthermore, many of these wastes escape containment or accidentally leak into water systems and into the soil to contaminate drinking water and food.

Primary methods of hazardous waste disposal include burial in double-lined cells in landfills, surface impoundments for special treatment and storage, waste-injected underground steel and concrete lined wells, solid waste piles, and land treatment facilities. Some hazardous wastes are incinerated before disposal. With the disposal of hazardous waste, it is always a concern that storage containers may not be leakproof, and interference with dump sites or storage facilities may expose the environment to these toxic substances. Examples of chemical contamination have been discovered in communities such as Elizabeth, New Jersey; Times Beach, Michigan; and Love Canal, New York, where residents developed cancer and other health problems because of exposures to toxic chemicals (Blumenthal & Ruttenber, 1994). There is also the continuing problem of securing disposal sites for the increasing volume of hazardous wastes. Communities seek the advantages of new technology but do not wish to bury the resulting wastes in their backyards. In many instances, legislators and public officials have faced serious conflict in their efforts to locate acceptable toxic waste dump sites.

With burgeoning industry and new technology in the world today, society has developed more sophisticated means of energy production, more labor-saving devices, and more practical and innovative products. This massive new product development has created a problem for the en-

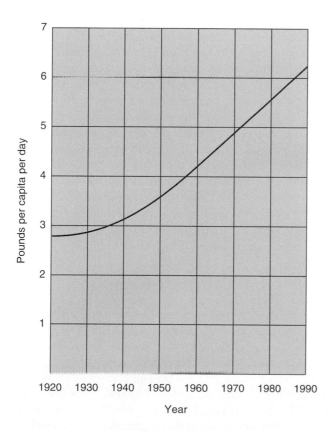

FIGURE 16–3. United States trend in per capita refuse production.

vironment—how to handle the vast amount of waste created from discardable goods, byproducts of production, and the "throwaway" mentality. For example, over 18 billion disposable diapers, which alone are estimated to be 2% of municipal wastes, are used each year in the United States. Until the late 1990s, the diapers were made of durable plastics and are estimated to resist deterioration up to 5 centuries after burial in a landfill. They are now made of treated paper with an absorbent gel within the diaper, and they biodegrade quickly in landfills. However, surveys show that 99% of disposable diaper users discard them directly into the trash instead of flushing fecal material down the toilet (Nadakavukaren, 1995). Consequently, a large amount of raw, untreated sewage is ending up in landfills with the potential for serious problems in the future. Not only does the development of such products take an enormous toll on natural resources, but the quantity and nature of the resulting wastes also pose serious health hazards and environmental problems. Improper disposal of domestic products, such as toxic insect sprays, some household cleaners, partially used paint cans, used auto oil, and termite fumigation chemicals, causes health dangers (Calvert et al., 1998).

GOVERNMENT'S ROLE

The government's role is to establish standards for safe waste disposal and to monitor and enforce compliance. In most modernized urban areas, the public sewage system handles waste by treating raw sewage and disposing it into a body of water. In most instances in the United States, state health departments oversee proper waste treatment and disposal. In rural areas where people usually have private septic systems, the supervision of proper waste handling is difficult and not as consistent. Health workers in rural settings should be alert to the potential dangers posed by inconsistent monitoring.

More research is needed to determine the effects of various disposal methods and to improve disposal practices. It is imperative that people learn not only to dispose of wastes safely—to protect humans, the environment, and future generations—but that they also look seriously at other options. More emphasis must be placed on transforming waste into usable products, increasing the amount and kinds of recycling done, and reducing the amount of refuse produced in the first place.

NURSE'S ROLE

Community health nurses can encourage the above actions by educating the public and lobbying for enabling legislation. Nurses can promote greater sensitivity among citizens to the problems of accumulating waste with its potential health hazards, encourage clients to buy products that can be recycled, and discourage use of aerosol spray containers, plastics, and other nonrecyclable items.

Insect and Rodent Control

All human communities are affected by the insects and rodents living in their environment. On the least dangerous level, they can cause irritation, such as from mosquito or flea bites, and discomfort, such as from infestations of bedbugs or lice. They can also pose a direct threat to health through such things as attacks by diseased rats or squirrels. They can consume and, in turn, contaminate food. However, by far the most serious health hazard they impose is through their role as *vectors*, nonhuman carriers of disease organisms that can transmit these organisms directly to humans (Blumenthal & Ruttenber, 1994).

The most common vectors are mosquitos, flies, ticks, roaches, fleas, rats, mice, and ground squirrels. All of these agents can serve as reservoirs for germs that they then transmit through physical contact with humans or by contaminating human foodstuffs or water. Table 16–2 summarizes some of the diseases spread by vectors. Cases of vector-spread diseases range from the 14th-century bubonic plague epidemic spread by rat fleas, which killed a quarter of the European population, to the outbreak in 1999 in New York of encephalitis caused by West Nile virus spread by mosquitos.

GOVERNMENT'S ROLE

Vector surveys, research, and control are usually left to local and state health departments. These agencies have also implemented community awareness and pest control programs. Once vectors have been found, health workers can attempt to control them through many methods. Approaches used in the past include trapping rodents, poisoning, spraying with pesticides, and eliminating areas where vectors breed, by draining or filling marshes to control mosquito populations, for example. It is essential in planning any approach to consider the possible health hazards to humans or other living organisms and the effect the method will have on the ecosystem—how it may upset the ecologic balance. Many years ago, WHO advocated that the most basic, yet effective, approach is to improve sanitary conditions and practices to the extent that the condition no longer exists that will encourage the multiplication of insects and rodents (WHO, 1986).

NURSE'S ROLE

The community health nurse can contribute through awareness of the presence and possible health threat of rodents and insects. By remaining alert to the presence of rodents and insects in homes, schools, and communities, nurses can take measures to educate affected persons and notify proper authorities when corrective action is needed. They can assist this effort by surveying homes and neighborhoods for exposed rubbish or conditions that might attract insects and rodents. They can also promote preventive efforts through education and influencing policy makers.

Vector	Disease	Pathogen
MOSQUITOES		
Anopheles sp	Malaria	*Plasmodium* sp (protozoa)
Culex sp	Filariasis	*Wuchereria bancrofti* and *malayi* (nematodes)
Culex sp	Encephalitis	Arbovirus
Aedes aegypti	Yellow fever	Arbovirus
Aedes aegypti	Dengue	Arbovirus
BITING FLIES		
Deerfly	Filariasis	*Loa loa* (nematode)
Black fly	River blindness	*Onchocerca volvulus* (nematode)
Tsetse fly	Sleeping sickness	*Trypanosoma gambiense* and *rhodesiense* (protozoa)
Sand fly	Kala-azar	*Leishmania donovani*
	Tropical ulcer	*Leishmania tropica*
	Cutaneous leishmaniasis	*Leishmania mexicana*
	Espundia	*Leishmania braziliensis* (protozoa)
	Phlebotomus fever	Arbovirus
OTHER INSECTS		
Gnats	Filariasis	*Mansonella ozzardi* (nematode)
Rat flea	Plague	*Yersinia pestis* (bacteria)
	Murine typhus	*Rickettsia mooseri*
Body louse	Epidemic typhus	*Rickettsia prowazekii*
	Trench fever	*Rickettsia quintana*
Tick	Rocky Mountain spotted fever	Rickettsia rickettsii
Tick	Colorado tick fever	Arbovirus
Mite	Riskettsialpox	Rickettsia akari

TABLE 16–2. Some Insect Vectors and Diseases Transmitted By Them

(Blumenthal, D & Ruttenber, J. [1994]. *Introduction to environmental health* [2nd ed]. New York: Springer.)

Safety in the Home, Worksite, and Community

As we have seen, the environment of the home, the workplace, and the community at large significantly affects people's health. This section addresses five additional problems that affect people's safety: exposure to toxic chemicals, radiation exposure, injury hazards, noise pollution, and psychological hazards.

EXPOSURE TO TOXIC CHEMICALS

The number of natural and synthetic chemicals in the environment and the threats they pose to human and environmental health are overwhelming. Approximately 55,000 different chemicals are in use in the United States. Of these, about 1,500 constitute the greatest threat of hazardous exposures, but only about 450 have established threshold limit values and adequate toxicity testing. Several hundred new chemicals come into use each year that are basically untested (Schecter, 1998). This section presents a general overview of the different categories of environmental chemicals, where they are found, the dangers they impose, and community health nurses' role in forestalling or detecting those dangers.

Toxic chemicals include those that do not contain carbon, are not derived from living matter, and are usually of mineral composition. Substances such as zinc, cadmium, lead, iron, calcium, sodium, potassium, magnesium, and copper often play an important and healthful role in human physiology, but they become toxic if a person is exposed to large quantities. A toddler's accidental ingestion of several chewable vitamins with iron can cause mild gastrointestinal distress or—if many are ingested—devastating physiologic damage (Deason, 1995).

Lead is a toxic agent frequently found in occupational or industrial settings. Workers must be careful to avoid inhaling lead fumes and exposing their families to lead dust on their clothing. Lead was once widely used in paint and can still be found in leaded gasoline and batteries. According to the Agency for Toxic Substances and Disease Registry (ATSDR), lead is ranked first among the top 10 hazardous substances. Lead poisoning usually produces symptoms of cerebral or central nervous system disorders. It is especially dangerous in children, whose high metabolic activity makes them more susceptible (Lanphear, 1998). In-utero lead exposure is another concern (Amaya & Ackall, 1996). Even low-level exposure to lead has a dangerous cumulative effect. This has been observed, for example, in children who play near roadways where dirt has absorbed lead from gasoline. Low levels of lead have been detected in household dust and even drinking water (American Nurses Association, 1997). Community health nurses need to check with clients for possible exposure and examine client homes for lead-based paint, now restricted in residential use. In particular, nurses can warn parents to keep their young children from eating paint chips from windowsills, walls, or furniture painted with lead-based paint and to keep them away from lead-infused dirt near roads and from dust and debris when older buildings are being torn down or renovated.

Mercury is also highly toxic. It is used in many scientific instruments, electronic equipment, crop fungicides, and the processing of dental fillings. Inorganic mercury can be changed through bacterial action in industrial processes to more toxic organic compounds, as in the bleach used for paper manufacturing. Toxic mercurials then escape into the environment and contaminate the food chain. In Minanata Bay, Japan, for example, many persons were crippled with nervous system disorders caused by eating mercury-contaminated seafood.

Other harmful metals include aluminum, which recently has been associated with certain mental disorders and has been found in high levels in the brain tissue of patients with Alzheimer's disease (Schecter, 1998). Chromium, nickel, and arsenic are included among other toxic compounds.

Many toxic chemicals are byproducts of the petroleum industry, including many alcohols, ethers, hydrocarbons such as benzene, medicines, and plastics that contain carbon. Ingestion or exposure may cause cancer, liver and kidney disease, birth defects, and many other health problems. Pesticides for household and crop use, particularly DDT (dichlorodiphenyltrichloroethane), have created major health hazards (Blumenthal & Ruttenber, 1994). DDT, a very dangerous chemical used for pest control, was banned in 1972 in the United States because of environmental and health concerns. However, it is still present in the environment and continues to be used illicitly, posing a danger to farmers and migrant farmworkers in particular. It has also been used legally in certain countries to control malaria.

Exposure to toxic chemicals can have far-reaching effects on humans. People may come in contact with them in their homes through building materials, cleaning products, or airborne dust. Another source is the workplace, where many different compounds are created and used each day. Toxic substances also may be transferred home from the workplace in motor vehicles and on clothing or shoes. In the greater community, pollutants in the air and food chain create further hazards. Toxic chemicals can cause illness when they are inhaled, come into contact with the skin (as in industrial accidents where chemicals are spilled), or are ingested (as when a child drinks from a liquid cleaning solvent bottle). Table 16–3 lists some common workplace carcinogens.

EXPOSURE TO RADIATION

Radiation is technically defined as a process by which energy is propagated through space or matter (Thomas, 1993). Natural radiation from the sun, soil, and minerals can be found in virtually all areas of the earth's environment. The largest natural source of radiation exposure is airborne radon. Radiation in its manmade form has numerous beneficial uses in science and industry for lasers, radiographs that help in the diagnosis of disease, and in the production of nuclear energy. It is found in many home electronic devices, such as television sets, smoke detectors, and microwave ovens (see Levels of Prevention).

Regardless of its source, radiation is a threat to human health in the workplace and in the general environment. The extent of danger depends on the dose and type of radiation. For example, casualties among miners can be attributed to their prolonged and intense exposure to radioactive minerals such as uranium. Prolonged exposure may cause skin ulcers, damage to cells, cancer, premature aging, kidney dysfunction, and genetic disorders in the children of those whose cells have been damaged. Naturally occurring radioactive materials are present in tobacco and further threaten the health of smokers. A two-pack-per-day cigarette smoker receives more than ten times the long-term dose-rate limit for radiation exposure (Moeller, 1992).

A certain amount of natural radiation exposure from the sun is important for the absorption of vitamin D. However, intentional exposure by sunbathing, still a popular activity, must be tempered with the use of lotions with sunscreen. The highest screening protection factor (SPF) lotions are allowed to offer is a factor of 30. This should be used by people of all ages when exposed to the sun for more than 10 to 15 minutes in the winter or summer. Sunscreen is more important at higher elevations and when participating in outdoor snow activities, such as skiing, because the snow reflects the sun's rays (Display 16–4).

A major area of concern centers on the problems associated with nuclear energy and nuclear weapons. The production of radioactive wastes, the threat of accidental exposure from unsafe reactors, and possible fallout from weapons testing generate real fears. These fears have been confirmed by the nuclear-reactor accidents at Three Mile Island and Chernobyl, which allowed radioactive ions to escape into the atmosphere. Accidents of this type are uncommon, however, and the safe operation of nuclear power plants exposes communities to much less radiation than other sources, such as medical or natural radiation.

INJURY HAZARDS

An environmental characteristic that must be considered in assessing health risks is a community's level of physical safety. How likely is it that injuries will occur? This is a very important question when one considers that in the United States the leading cause of death from age 1 through 34 is unintentional injury. In 1997, 95,644 Americans died from unintentional injuries (U.S. Dept. of Health and Human Services, 2000). Groups at highest risk are the young and the elderly, the poor, minorities, and rural residents.

TABLE 16–3. Occupational Carcinogens

Carcinogen	Cancer Site	Examples of Exposed Occupations
4-Aminodiphenyl Auramine B-napthylamine Magenta Benzidine	Bladder	Dye manufacturing, rubber manufacturing
Arsenic	Skin, lung, liver	Metal smelting, arsenic pesticide production, metal alloy workers
Asbestos	Lung, mesothelium, gastrointestinal tract	Asbestos miners, insulators, shipyard workers
Benzene	Leukemia (blood-forming organs)	Petrochemical workers, chemists
Bischloromethyl ether (BCME)	Lung	Organic chemical synthesizers
Cadmium	Prostate	Cadmium alloy workers, welders
Chromium/chromates	Lung, nasal sinuses	Chromate producers, metal workers
Coke oven emissions	Lung, kidney	Coke oven workers
Foundry emissions	Lung	Foundry workers
Leather dust	Nasal cavity, nasal sinuses, bladder	Shoe manufacturing
Nickel	Lung, nasal passages	Nickel smelting, metal workers
Radiation (x-rays)	Leukemia (blood-forming organs), skin, breast, thyroid, bone	Radiologists, industrial radiographers, atomic energy workers
Radon gas	Lung	Uranium and feldspar miners
Soots, tars, and oil Petroleum (aromatic hydrocarbons)	Skin, lung, bladder, scrotum	Roofers, chimney sweepers, shale oil workers
Ultraviolet light	Skin	Outdoor workers
Vinyl chloride	Liver, brain, lung	Polyvinyl chloride synthesizers, rubber workers
Welding fumes	Lung	Welders
Wood dust	Nasal passages	Hardwood workers, furniture makers

(Blumenthal, D. & Rutenber, J. [1994]. *Introduction to environmental health* [2nd ed]. New York: Springer.)

Not surprisingly, motor vehicle crashes cause approximately 42,000 deaths per year. The second-ranked cause of injury death is from falls. Deaths from poisoning, drowning, and residential fires follow in ranking, respectively. Alcohol plays a major role in many of these injuries and subsequent deaths, particularly with motor vehicle crashes and drownings (U.S. Department of Health and Human Services, 2000). Additionally, many unintentional injuries occur in the home (see Chapter 30 for home-safety assessment).

Another area of safety concern is injury and death from violence. Individuals, families, schools, and communities are frequently at risk for violent acts stemming from domestic quarrels and abuse, dysfunctional behavior, and crime. Violence and the injuries and deaths it causes are becoming one of the most urgent health problems in the United States. In 1995, 35% of injury-related deaths were intentional, primarily homicides and suicides. Use of handguns and domestic abuse make women, children, and the elderly particularly at risk for injury and death (Powell, Jacklin, Nelson & Bland, 1998). Community health nurses have a responsibility to assess situations for the threat of potential physical harm and work with other professionals to design preventive measures. The subject of violence is discussed further in Chapters 25 and 36.

EXPOSURE TO NOISE POLLUTION

People in the United States are bombarded by noise from many sources. Household appliances, traffic, radios, machinery, and voices are typical noise sources. Noise is measured three ways. First, noise is measured by the magnitude of the noise, or *decibels*. A whisper may measure 10 to 20 decibels, and a fire engine siren may measure 80 to 100 decibels. Another way to measure is by the high and low tones of the noise, referred to as *frequency*. A male voice is usually a lower frequency than a female voice; a drum is a lower frequency than a flute. A third factor is the *time history,* or length of time one has been exposed to the noise.

Noise has been cited as a major environmental health problem. Extremely loud noises, such as pneumatic drills or loud rock music, can cause temporary or permanent hearing loss (Moeller, 1992). Other noises, perhaps from machinery at the workplace or residential exposure to airport traffic, can lead to general annoyance; headaches; sleep, speech, and task interference; alterations in emotions; stress; lowered body resistance to disease; ulcers; and aggravation of exist-

LEVELS OF PREVENTION

RADON IN HOMES

GOAL
Increase to at least *20%* the proportion of homes in which homeowners/occupants have tested for radon concentrations and that have been found to pose minimal risk or have been modified to reduce risk to health, as a means to reduce the incidence of lung cancer. (Baseline: *11%* in 1994).

PRIMARY PREVENTION
Conduct community education regarding the nature and dangers of inhaling the solid, radioactive decay products of radon gas. Require home testing for radon concentrations. Require sealed basement construction to avoid release of radon into building from underlying soil.

SECONDARY PREVENTION
Circulate air with electric fans in homes where radon concentrations are low. Use fan in combination with a positive-ion generator to more effectively reduce inhaled concentrations of air-borne radon decay products. Periodic testing to ensure minimal levels of radon concentrations.

TERTIARY PREVENTION
Require building modifications where radon concentrations are high (ten or more times remedial action level). Seal cracks in basement floors and walls. Install subslab exhaust systems below basement floors.

(From U.S. Department of Health and Human Services, 2000.)

ing physical disorders (Moller, 1998). The effects vary in severity depending on the intensity and duration of the noises and the disposition of the people concerned.

There are three methods of control. First, the source of the noise can be relocated, such as by having the teen band practice in the garage instead of the family room, or replaced, such as by fixing or replacing a broken toy or appliance. Another method is to do something about the path of the noise. A barrier, enclosure, or muffler may be effective. This is often seen along highways where 8- to 10-foot walls have been built between the highway traffic noises and housing developments. An automobile muffler serves a similar purpose of "muffling" the engine's sound. A third method of control is to relocate the receiver. For instance, if parents are annoyed by the loudness and music choice of their teenager, they may want to go to another room in the house. Finally, the receiver can use hearing protectors such as ear plugs. For example, airline ground-crew members wear highly sophisticated hearing protectors.

Community responses to noise pollution take many forms. There are usually community standards for noise abatement after 10 PM and before 8 AM. Police will respond if a neighbor complains about a loud neighborhood party. As highways creep into suburban neighborhoods, barriers are erected in the form of walls or noise-absorbing trees and shrubbery.

Standards for the decibel levels of appliances and tools are set by manufacturers, following OSHA standards. Packaging instructions indicate whether hearing protectors should be used with the tool or piece of equipment.

EXPOSURE TO BIOLOGIC POLLUTANTS

Biologic pollutants are or were living organisms that promote poor indoor air quality (U.S. Consumer Product Safety Commission, 1996). Some common indoor biologic pollutants include animal dander (minute scales from hair, feathers, or skin), dust mite and cockroach parts, fungi, infectious agents (bacteria and viruses), and pollen. Breathing indoor air contaminated with biologic pollutants can cause health problems or make existing health problems worse, especially among infants, young children, the elderly, and those with chronic illnesses. The effects range from allergic symptoms (conjunctival inflammation, rhinitis, sneezing, nasal congestion, itching, dyspnea, coughing, wheezing, chest tightness, headache, and malaise) to infections and toxicity (Last, 1998).

Home conditions that promote this type of pollution are damp homes or parts of homes, which encourage the growth and buildup of the biologic pollutants. It is estimated that

DISPLAY 16–4. The TAN Commandments

1. Don't sunbathe.
2. Wear protective clothing and a wide-brimmed hat when in the sun for more than 15 minutes.
3. Don't spend time in the sun without a sun-screening lotion.
4. Use a sun-screening lotion with the highest SPF available (SPF 30).
5. Reapply sun-screening lotion periodically, especially after swimming or perspiring.
6. Stay out of the sun when the sun's rays are the most direct, usually between 10 AM and 2 PM.
7. Remember that even on cloudy days you can burn—use sun-screening lotion and/or protective clothing.
8. Be aware that sun exposure can be dangerous in any season. Wear sun-screening lotion and/or protective clothing when gardening in the spring, swimming in the summer, hiking in the fall, or skiing in the winter.
9. Although people of all ages and races can be affected by the sun's rays, infants and children are especially vulnerable because their skin is more sensitive and the sun's effects are cumulative. Be especially vigilant in protecting children with hats, clothing, and sun-screening lotion.
10. Take additional precautions if living or vacationing at higher altitudes, where the effects of sun exposure are greater.

30% to 50% of all structures, mostly in warm, moist climates, have damp conditions. In addition, there are particular items and areas in homes where biologic pollutants are commonly found and where proper cleaning or care is especially important. These include:

- Humidifiers and/or dehumidifiers
- Bathrooms without vents or windows
- Kitchens without vents or windows
- Refrigerator drip pans
- Laundry rooms with an unvented dryer
- Unventilated attics
- Damp basement floors with carpeting
- Bedding
- Closets on outside walls
- Heating/air conditioning systems
- Book shelves, curio cabinets, and other areas that accumulate dust
- Dog and cat bedding, litter boxes, bird cages, fish tanks, and so forth
- Areas with water damage (around windows, the roof, or the basement)

The most important role of the community health nurse is to assess clients' homes for possible biologic pollutants and then provide them with the information they need to correct or improve the situation. If clients are renting a house or apartment and the dampness is due to structural conditions or to owner negligence, the nurse may act as an advocate for clients to remedy the potentially hazardous situation. Display 16–5 includes a list of assessment questions the nurse should include during home visits when clients may have been exposed to biologic pollutants.

PSYCHOLOGICAL HAZARDS

A discussion of environmental health and safety would not be complete if it overlooked the psychological hazards that people must face in their environments. Environment plays a significant role in the mental health of a community. The psychological variables that affect people often lead to physiologic illnesses. Such elements as noise, overcrowding, traffic, lack of privacy, unavailability of work, lack of natural beauty, and boredom can be detrimental to peoples' well-being.

Another psychological hazard is urban crowding. Early studies on crowding done by J. B. Calhoun demonstrated serious effects on behavior. When healthy, naturally clean laboratory mice were forced to live in overcrowded conditions, they experienced dramatic behavior changes. Gross insanitary conditions led to aggressive behavior, strong mice attacking the weak, symptoms of regression and mental disturbance, mating decline, and neglect or cannibalization of weaker offspring. Although this is an extreme example, it perhaps provides some insight into the conditions of urban areas and the psychological stress that urban conditions may create (Nakamura, 1999).

The daily psychological stresses of the modern world are innumerable. Excessive stimulation comes from rapid soci-

etal changes created by new technology, an accelerated pace of living, increased work production demands, and other causes. All can create potential health hazards.

GOVERNMENT'S ROLE

The government plays an active role in promoting public safety. Standards and regulations have been set at the federal level regarding toxic chemicals, radiation exposure, occupational safety practices, noise abatement, and other safety issues. State and local governments seek to enforce business, industry, and community compliance with these standards. Health departments and other government agencies assist with monitoring of chemical use and production as well as promotion of public education programs to alert people to the presence and potential dangers of toxic chemicals and expo-

---

DISPLAY 16–5. Assessment Questions to Detect Biologic Pollutants in Homes

- Does anyone in the family have frequent headaches, fevers, itchy watery eyes, a stuffy nose, dry throat or a cough?
- Does anyone complain of feeling tired or dizzy all the time?
- In anyone wheezing or having difficulties breathing on a regular basis?
- Did these symptoms appear after you moved to this home/apartment?
- Do the symptoms disappear when you go to school or work or go away on a trip, and return when you come back home?
- Have you (or your landlord or apartment manager) recently remodeled your home or done any energy conservation work, such as installing insulation, storm windows, or weather stripping?
- Does your home feel humid?
- Can you see moisture on the windows or on other surfaces, such as walls and ceilings?
- What is the usual temperature in your home? Is it very hot or cold?
- Have you recently had water damage?
- Do you have a basement? Is it wet or damp?
- Is there any obvious mold or mildew in the basement, closets, in bathrooms?
- Does any part of your home have a musty or moldy odor?
- Is the air stale?
- Do you have pets? (Consider all—including fish, turtles, snakes.)
- Do you have house plants? Do they show signs of mold?
- Do you have air conditioners or humidifiers that have not been properly cared for or cleaned?
- Does your home have cockroaches or rodents?

(Adapted form U.S. Consumer Product Safety Commission, 1996.)

sure to radiation in the environment. Research is examining the biologic effects of chemicals and radiation. The medical and dental fields have developed simple safety procedures, such as having patients wear lead aprons during radiographs and having technicians stand behind metal walls. The U.S. Public Health Service holds responsibility for monitoring nuclear plants and other possible sources of radiation to protect the public.

Because the government holds companies liable for the safety of their products, industry now invests considerable resources into researching and designing safe goods. Many products have been modified to make them more safe, such as childproof caps on medication bottles, flame-retardant children's clothing, and seat belts and airbags in automobiles. Industry must also warn consumers if a product is inherently dangerous, as when toys have sharp edges or parts are small enough to be ingested by toddlers. Bright orange frowning faces on bottles that contain harmful substances have helped to warn consumers and reduce the number of poisonings. Children learn to avoid poisonous plants and other potential hazards through school and community education efforts.

Community safety organizations, government agencies, and public health officials all play their part in assessing community safety and taking measures to prevent accidents. Organizations such as the Consumer Protection Agency and consumer advocates such as Ralph Nader continue to watchdog environmental safety. Federal and state legislation to enforce speed limits has helped to reduce the number of automobile crashes, and supervision of recreational and occupational areas has led to discovery of health hazards and promoted the development of safety programs. State-established boating safety regulations and the assigning of adequate lifeguards to monitor busy swimming beaches are measures that help to reduce the number of recreational accidents. Community surveys of intersections where multiple traffic crashes have occurred have led to installation of traffic signals and a reduction of crashes.

The role of government in reduction or control of violence and psychological hazards has been less effective. Certain federal-level agencies, such as the National Institute for Mental Health, the National Institute for Occupational Safety and Health, and the Departments of Labor, Commerce, and Transportation, influence standards and regulations affecting psychological well-being. Legislation regarding firearm use and penalties associated with domestic abuse and physical violence have become more stringent. Nonetheless, both violence and psychological hazards continue to be serious public health problems that are preventable and deserve greater attention.

NURSE'S ROLE

It is difficult to monitor all the possible contacts a person or community may be experiencing with toxic chemicals or radiation, but such monitoring is necessary in order to estimate health risks and establish correlations. Multiple exposures in small doses from many different sources may add up. Are clients' homes well ventilated? Is the burning of fossil fuels polluting the air with sulfur oxides? Does home, school, or worksite insulation contain asbestos? Are all household chemical agents stored in a childproof place? Monitoring difficulties arise from the many opportunities for exposure to toxic chemicals or radiation, cumulative exposure over time, and the fact that disease symptoms may not appear until years after exposure, when the agent may no longer be in the immediate environment. The best protection is to promote and monitor the safe use and disposal of chemical hazards and limit radiation exposure to prevent health problems from occurring.

Community health nurses can promote environmental safety and prevent injuries in many ways. Six target area settings in which to concentrate preventive measures are highways, homes, worksites, schools, farms, and recreational sites. Working with the police, fire personnel, social services, schools, drug rehabilitation counselors, and many other community groups, the nurse can help to develop programs targeted at preventing drunk driving, firearm misuse, failed smoke detectors, unsafe playground equipment, and much more. In homes, nurses can encourage safe storage of toxic materials. Railings can be installed on stairways and in bathrooms used by the elderly. Gates at the tops of stairways and window guards can prevent small children from falling. Nonskid decals can be used in bathtubs to prevent slipping.

Safety education offers one of the most vital preventive measures. When people are made aware of possible dangers and unsafe areas, they can avoid injuring themselves. Local community programs to educate people on the dangers of driving while intoxicated, to instruct them on the proper handling of home machinery such as chainsaws, or to encourage safe use of fireworks during holiday celebrations can also help to reduce injuries. In the event that an injury does occur, educating the public about appropriate actions to take can help to reduce its potential impact. Promoting first-aid and CPR classes can be beneficial.

Community health nurses need to be aware of the effects noise can have on hearing health and overall well-being. This will help the nurse identify specific health problems caused by increased noise. Teaching employers, employees, teachers, and children about the potential harm of repeated loud noises in their environment, even the noise from a headset that is turned to a high decibel level, is essential.

Education as a preventive measure against injuries applies particularly in the case of natural disasters. Although a tornado or earthquake cannot be prevented, people can be prepared in the event that one does occur. By running fire drills in schools and workplaces, informing people of the location of safe and unsafe places to take shelter during an electrical storm or hurricane, and of what to do in an earthquake or flood, nurses can help to forestall or minimize tragic events (see Chapter 20).

It is necessary for community health nurses to be aware of psychological hazards in the environment, to recognize the potential they have for affecting both psychological and physiologic health, and to encourage stress reduction wherever possible. Some specific ways that community health nurses can promote a psychologically healthy environment include active lobbying for control and prevention of domestic abuse and violence, neighborhood crime prevention, reduction of workplace stressors, and development of educational and support programs to reduce lifestyle stressors.

STRATEGIES FOR NURSING ACTION IN ENVIRONMENTAL HEALTH

Each of the preceding sections has discussed actions and given examples of ways that the community health nurse can be involved in environmental health. To summarize, the nurse has a two-part challenge: (1) to help protect the public's health from potential threats in the environment and (2) to help protect and promote the health of the environment itself so it can be life and health enhancing for its human inhabitants. The following strategies for collaboration and participation provide a summary of the nurse's role and can assist the nurse in addressing this two-part goal:

1. Learn about possible environmental health threats. The nurse has a responsibility to keep abreast of current environmental issues and know the proper authorities to whom problems should be reported.
2. Assess clients' environment and detect health hazards. Careful observation and an environmental checklist can assist in this assessment.
3. Plan collaboratively with citizens and other professionals to devise protective and preventive strategies. Remember that environmental health work is generally a team effort.
4. Assist with the implementation of programs to prevent health threats to clients and the environment.
5. Take action to correct situations in which health hazards exist. Nurses can use direct intervention, as with an unsafe home situation, notify proper authorities, or publicly protest when corrective measures are beyond their sphere.
6. Educate consumers and assist them to practice preventive measures. Examples of preventive measures include radon testing in homes or well-water testing in rural communities.
7. Take action to promote development of policies and legislation that enhance consumer protection and promote a healthier environment.
8. Assist with and promote program evaluation to determine effectiveness of environmental health efforts.
9. Apply environmentally related research findings and participate in nursing research.

SUMMARY

Environmental health is a discipline encompassing all the elements of the environment that influence the health and well-being of its inhabitants. Public health workers, including community health nurses, need to monitor and determine causal links between people and their environment with a concern as to how they may promote the health and well-being of both.

An ecologic perspective of environmental health is important to understand the human–environment relationship and how the health of one impacts the health of the other. Prevention and strategic or long-range concerns are also important in considering environmental health because what is done today may impact the health of many generations in the future.

There are major global environmental concerns such as overpopulation, ozone depletion and global warming, deforestation, desertification and wetlands destruction, energy depletion, air pollution, water pollution, unhealthy or contaminated food, waste disposal, insect and rodent control, biologic pollutants, and safety in the home, worksite, and community. Each has its own set of problems, concerns, and solutions.

Both public and private sectors are involved in regulating, monitoring, and preventing environmental health problems and have accomplished much during the past 30 years. Much, however, is still left to be done, and new problems continue to develop. The community health nurse is an important member of the team of health professionals promoting and protecting the reciprocal relationship between the environment and the public's health. The nurse can follow several important strategies to accomplish the two-part goal of (1) protecting the public's health from environmental threats and (2) promoting a healthy and health-enhancing environment.

ACTIVITIES TO PROMOTE CRITICAL THINKING

1. You are planning a visit to a young family who live in an older home. You know that older homes may have radon, lead pipes and lead-based paint, asbestos

insulation, and other safety, fire, and health threats, such as those from biologic pollutants. Using the nursing process, design a plan for (a) determining whether any of these threats are present, (b) what actions should be taken if the dangers exist, (c) how to assist the family in taking corrective action, and (d) evaluating successful removal of existing threats.

2. Data from the local health department show that, in the past year, five people from the same rural portion of the county died of cancer. What collaborative actions would be appropriate for you to take to determine whether there is an environmental relationship? What other members of the health team should be involved in the investigation? Write a letter to the mayor and the county commissioners to justify why nurses should be involved in this study.

3. Select an article from the mass media (newspaper, weekly news magazine, and so forth) that deals with an "environmental health" problem. Analyze and critique the article by answering the following questions: What are the characteristics of the community involved? What appear to be the sources of the problem? What evidence is provided in the

article to substantiate the cause? Does the news coverage describe health effects? What population is at risk? Does the coverage provide adequate information for consumers to understand the problem and seek any needed assistance? What suggestions do you have for improving the article?

4. Design a list of items to include in a checklist for assessing clients' home, school, or worksite environments. Consider each of the environmental areas of concern described in this chapter and what potential health threats might be present in each area. Review this list with an environmental health expert for accuracy and completeness. Use the list as a teaching tool with two different sets of clients and evaluate its effectiveness for assessment and diagnosis of environmentally related health hazards.

5. Identify an environmental health problem in your community or state. Become informed about this problem by talking with experts in the area, reading recent literature and research reports, and searching the Internet for information about the problem. Meet with a senator or congressperson who has been involved in legislation related to the problem and learn what he or

---

CLINICAL CORNER — Occupational Environmental Health and the Nurse's Role

Scenario

Metropolis Tool Company is a manufacturing plant that employs 1,200 workers. Most of the employees work in assembly or data entry jobs. Recently, there have been increasing complaints of work-related stress, with employees citing pressure to perform and produce at higher levels as the root of the stress. You are an occupational health nurse working for the company.

It has come to your attention that there has been a significant increase in insurance claims for the following conditions:

- Stress-related migraine headaches
- Early pregnancy leave for women experiencing low maternal weight gain

Metropolis Tool Company has been in business for over 29 years. Recently, competition in the manufacturing industry has increased, and the company's executives are looking for ways to cut expenses. Insurance premiums cost the company a considerable amount, and rates will increase if the number of claims continues to rise. Your employer recently became aware of the problems leading to increased utilization of disability. He approached you and asked you to "fix" these problems in an expenditious manner.

Available assessment data that may be related to the problems include:

- The plant recently moved to rotating shifts and is now operating around the clock

- Staff layoffs are predicted within 6 months
- Increasing corporate competition has led to higher productivity standards

Questions

1. Discuss additional assessment data needed and how you will go about gathering these data.
2. Describe your role related to the issue of environmental health and safety.
3. Discuss interventions that your program may perform at the following levels of prevention:
- Primary
- Secondary
- Tertiary
4. Your supervisor in your role of occupational health nurse is a company vice president. He is very knowledgeable about business but knows little about health issues. Where will you turn to obtain information to assist you in addressing the problems identified in this scenario?
5. How will you evaluate the effects of your interventions?
6. What issues does this scenario elicit regarding:
Fears and anxiety in this role
Lack of immediate resources (supervisor)
Social justice
Building partnerships within your communities
Globalization of public health

she plans to do about it. Summarize what you have learned and present it in writing as a letter to the editor of your city newspaper. (See Clinical Corner.)

REFERENCES

Amaya, M., & Ackall, G. (1996, 3rd quarter). Perinatal lead exposure. *Reflections*, 18–19.

American Nurses Association. (1997). *Position statements: Lead poisoning & screening*. Available: http://www.nursingworld.org/readroom/position/social/sclead.htm.

American Public Health Association. (1999). More research needed to guide policy on environmental justice. *Nation's Health, 29*(3), 4.

Association of Maternal and Child Health Programs. (1998). *AMCHP fact sheet: Tobacco*. Washington, DC: Author.

Beaglehole, R., & Bonita, R. (1997). *Public health at the crossroads: Achievements and prospects*. Cambridge, England: Cambridge University Press.

Benenson, A. S. (Ed.). (1995). *Control of communicable diseases in man* (16th ed.). Washington, DC: American Public Health Association.

Blumenthal, D., & Ruttenber, J. (1994). *Introduction to environmental health* (2nd ed.). New York: Springer.

Bonilla, C. M., & Mauss, E. A. (1998). A community-initiated study of blood lead levels of Nicaraguan children living near a battery factory. *American Journal of Public Health, 88*(12), 1843–1845.

Borenstein, S. (1998, December 29). Air-pollution report card improves, but still falls short of an "A" grade. *The Fresno Bee*, p. B3.

Calvert, G. M., et al. (1998). Health effects associated with sulfuryl fluoride and methyl bromide exposure among structural fumigation workers. *American Journal of Public Health, 88*(12), 1774–1780.

Chin, J. (Ed.). (1999). *Control of communicable diseases manual* (17th ed.). Washington, DC: American Public Health Association.

Conway, J. B. (1998). Water quality management. In R. B. Wallace (Ed.), *Maxcy-Rosenau-Last public health and preventive medicine* (14th ed.). Stamford, CT: Appleton & Lange.

Curtis, S., & Taket, A. (1996). *Health and societies: Changing perspectives*. London, England: Arnold.

Deason, J. G. (1995). Acute iron ingestion in a 2-year-old child. *Journal of Emergency Nursing, 21*, 9–11.

Environmental Protection Agency. (1997a). *Climate change and public health*. Washington, DC: Office of Policy, Planning and Evaluation.

———. (1997b). *Cool facts about global warming*. Washington, DC: Office of Policy, Planning and Evaluation.

———. (1993a). *Radon: The health threat with a simple solution. A physician's guide*. Washington, DC: Office of Policy, Planning and Evaluation.

———. (1993b). *Second-hand smoke*. Washington, DC: Office of Policy, Planning and Evaluation.

Fleisher, J. M., et al. (1996). Marine waters contaminated with domestic sewage: Nonenteric illnesses associated with bather

exposure in the United Kingdom. *American Journal of Public Health, 86*(9), 1228–1234.

Fouse, D., & Zimmerman, C. (1998, August 4). EPA's new right-to-know rules for drinking water will help protect the nation's health. *APHA News*.

Institute of Medicine. (1999). *Toward environmental justice: Research, education and health policy needs*. Washington, DC: National Academy Press.

Kilburn, K. H. (1998). Pulmonary responses to gases and particles. In R. B. Wallace (Ed.), *Maxcy-Rosenau-Last public health and preventive medicine* (14th ed.). Stamford, CT: Appleton & Lange.

King, M., & Elliott, C. (1995). Double think—a reply. *World Health Forum, 16*, 293–298.

Lanphear, B. P. (1998, September 11). The paradox of lead poisoning prevention. *Science, 281*, 1617–1618.

Last, J. M. (1998). Housing and health. In R. B. Wallace (Ed.), *Maxcy-Rosenau-Last public health and preventive medicine* (14th ed.). Stamford, CT: Appleton & Lange.

Mahon, B. E., Slutsker, L., Hutwagner, L., Drenzek, C., et al. (1999). Consequences in Georgia of a nationwide outbreak of *Salmonella* infections: What you don't know might hurt you. *American Journal of Public Health, 89*(1), 31–35.

McGrew, R. (1985). *Encyclopedia of medical history* (pp. 137–141). New York: McGraw-Hill.

McMichael, A. J. (1995). Contemplating a one child world. *British Medical Journal, 311*, 1651–1652.

McMichael, A. J., Haines, A., Slooff, R., & Kovat, S. (Eds.). (1996). *Climate change and human health*. Geneva, Switzerland: World Health Organization.

Miller, G. T. (1996). *Living in the environment* (8th ed.). Belmont, CA: Wadsworth.

Moeller, D. W. (1992). *Environmental health*. Cambridge, MA: Harvard University Press.

Moller, A. R. (1998). Effects of the physical environment: Noise as a health hazard. In R. B. Wallace (Ed.), *Maxcy-Rosenau-Last public health and preventive medicine* (14th ed.). Stamford, CT: Appleton & Lange.

Morgan, G., Corbett, S., & Wlodarczyk, J. (1998). Air pollution and hospital admissions in Sydney, Australia, 1990–1994. *American Journal of Public Health, 88*(12), 1761–1766.

Morgan, G., Corbett, S., Wlodarczyk, J., & Lewis, P. (1998). Air pollution and daily mortality in Sydney, Australia, 1989 through 1993. *American Journal of Public Health, 88*(5), 759–764.

Myers, N., & Kent, J. (1995, June). *Environmental exodus: An emergent crisis in the global arena*. Washington, DC: Project of the Climate Institute.

Nadakavukaren, A. (1995). *Our global environment: A health perspective* (4th ed.). Prospect Heights, IL: Waveland Press.

Nakamura, R. M. (1999). *Health in America: A multicultural perspective*. Boston: Allyn and Bacon.

National Institutes of Health. (1998). *Foodborne diseases*. Bethesda, MD: National Institute of Allergy and Infectious Diseases (NIAID) Office of Communications.

Patz, J. A., Epstein, P. R., Burke, T. A., et al. (1996). Global climate change and emerging infectious diseases. *Journal of the American Medical Association, 275*, 217–223.

Pickett, G., & Hanlon, J. (1990). *Public health: Administration and practice* (9th ed.). St. Louis: Times Mirror/Mosby.

Ponka, A., & Virtanen, M. (1996). Low-level air pollution and hospital admissions for cardiac and cerebrovascular diseases in Helsinki. *American Journal of Public Health, 86*(9), 1273–1280.

Population Action International. (1998). *Fact sheet. What birth dearth? Why world population is still growing.* Washington, DC: Author.

———. (1997). *Fact sheet. How family planning protects the health of women and children.* Washington, DC: Author.

Powell, K. E., Jacklin, B. C., Nelson, D. E., & Bland, S. (1998). State estimates of household exposure to firearms, loaded firearms, and handguns, 1991 through 1995. *American Journal of Public Health, 88*(6), 969–972.

Rose, C. S., et al. (1998). "Lifeguard lung": Endemic granulomatous pneumonitis in an indoor swimming pool. *American Journal of Public Health, 88*(12), 1795–1800.

Schecter, A. J. (Ed.). (1998). Environmental health. In R. B. Wallace (Ed.), *Maxcy-Rosenau-Last public health and preventive medicine* (14th ed.). Stamford, CT: Appleton & Lange.

Tauxe, R. V. (1998). *Emerging foodborne diseases: An evolving public health challenge.* Available: http://www.cdc.gov/ncidod/EID/vol3no4/tauxe.htm.

Thomas, C. (Ed.). (1993). *Taber's cyclopedic medical dictionary* (17th ed.). Philadelphia: F. A. Davis.

Turnock, B. K. (1997). *Public health: What it is and how it works.* Gaithersburg, MD: Aspen.

U.S. Consumer Product Safety Commission. (1996). *Biological pollutants in your home.* Washington, DC: U.S. Government Printing Office.

U.S. Department of Health and Human Services. (2000). *Healthy people 2010* (conference edition in two volumes). Washington, DC: U.S. Government Printing Office.

———. (1991). *Healthy people 2000: National health promotion and disease prevention objectives* (S/N 017-001-00474-0). Washington, DC: U.S. Government Printing Office.

Wells, A. J. (1998). Lung cancer from passive smoking at work. *American Journal of Public Health, 88*(7), 1025–1029.

Williams, S. J., & Torrens, P. R. (1999). *Introduction to health services* (5th ed.). Albany, NY: Delmar.

World Health Organization. (1998). *The World Health Report 1998.* Geneva, Switzerland: WHO.

———. (1986). *Health and the environment.* WHO Regional Publications, European series, No. 19 (pp. 12–16). Vienna, Austria: Author.

RELATED PHONE NUMBERS

Environmental Protection Agency Indoor Air Quality Information Clearinghouse
1-800-438-4318
Environmental Protection Agency's Ozone Hotline
1-800-296-1996
FDA's Food Information and Seafood Hotline
1-800-FDA-4010
Local American Lung Association
1-800-LUNG-USA
National Institute of Occupational Safety and Health
1-800-35-NIOSH
National Lead Information Center
1-800-LEAD-FYI

National Pesticides Telecommunications Network
1-800-858-PEST
U.S. Consumer Product Safety Commission
1-800-638-CPSC
USDA's Meat and Poultry Hotline
1-800-535-4555

INTERNET RESOURCES

Environmental Protection Agency (EPA)

http://www.epa.gov/globalwarming

Food and Drug Administration (FDA)

http://www.fda.gov/

FDA, Office of Health Affairs

www.fda.gov/oc/oha

National Food Safety Initiative

http://v./cfsam/fda/gov/~7Edms/fs-toc html

Partnership for Food Safety Education

www.fightbac.org

Population Action International

http://www.populationaction.org

SELECTED READINGS

Aschengrau, A., Ozonoff, D., Coogan, P., et al. (1996). Cancer risk and residential proximity to cranberry cultivation in Massachusetts. *American Journal of Public Health, 86*(9), 1289–1296.

Beauchat, L. R., & Ryu, J. (1998). Produce handling and processing practices. *Emerging Infectious Diseases, 3*(4), 459–465.

Bonneaux, L. (1994). Rwanda: A case of demographic entrapment. *Lancet, 344,* 1689–1690.

Durch, J. S., Bailey, L. A., & Stoto, M. A. (1997). *Improving health in the community: A role for performance monitoring.* Washington, DC: National Academy Press.

Evans, R. G., Barer, M. L., & Marmor, T. R. (1994). *Why are some people healthy and others not?* New York: de Gruyter.

Goldman, R. R. (1996). *Public health nursing in a multi-cultural society: Lead poisoning from non-traditional sources.* Los Angeles: Los Angeles County Department of Health Services.

Hall, J. M., & Stevens, P. E. (1992). A nursing view of the U.S.-Iraq war: Psychosocial health consequences. *Nursing Outlook, 40,* 113–120.

Harris, M. J., & Kotch, J. B. (1994). Unintentional infant injuries: Sociodemographic and psychosocial factors. *Public Health Nursing, 11*(2), 90–97.

Kleffel, D. (1996). Environmental paradigms: Moving toward an ecocentric perspective. *Advances in Nursing Science, 18*(4), 1–10.

Loescher, L. J., Emerson, J., Taylor, A., et al. (1995). Educating preschoolers about sun safety. *American Journal of Public Health, 85*(7), 939–943.

Lum, M. R. (1995). Environmental public health: Future direction, future skills. *Family and Community Health, 18*(1), 24–35.

Mascola, M. A., Van Vunakis, H., Tager, I. B., et al. (1998). Exposure of young infants to environmental tobacco smoke: Breast-feeding among smoking mothers. *American Journal of Public Health, 88*(6), 893–896.

Neufer, L. (1994). The role of the community health nurse in environmental health. *Public Health Nursing 11*(3), 155–162.

Phillips, L. (1995). Chattanooga Creek: Case study of the public health nursing role in environmental health. *Public Health Nursing, 12*(5), 335–340.

Schuster, E. A., & Brown, C. L. (1995). *Exploring our environmental connections.* NLN Press Publication. Sudbury, MA: Jones and Bartlett.

Stevens, P. E., & Hall, J. M. (1992). Applying critical theories to nursing in communities. *Public Health Nursing, 9,* 2–9.

Tiedje, L., & Wood, J. (1995). Sensitizing nurses for a changing environmental health role. *Public Health Nursing, 12*(6), 359–365.

U.S. Food and Drug Administration. (1998). FDA approves meat irradiation for pathogen control. *Public Health Reports, 113,* 105.

Wagner, K. D. (1998). *Environmental management in healthcare facilities.* Philadelphia: W. B. Saunders.

Walker, B. (1994). Impediments to the implementation of environmental policy. *Journal of Public Health Policy, 15*(2), 186–202.

Wartenberg, D. (1998). Residential magnetic fields and childhood leukemia: A meta-analysis. *American Journal of Public Health, 88*(12), 1787–1794

Theoretical Basis of Community Health Nursing

KEY TERMS

- Bioterrorism
- Community-oriented, population-focused care
- Genetic engineering
- Global economy
- Migration
- Model
- Relationship-based care
- Technology
- Tenet
- Theory

LEARNING OBJECTIVES

Upon mastery of this chapter, you should be able to:

- Discuss two essential characteristics of nursing service when a community is the client: community-oriented, population-focused care, and relationship-based care.
- Describe the contributions of at least six models of nursing practice to community health.
- Explain the benefits of applying eight tenets of public health nursing to community health nursing.
- Identify at least five social issues that influence contemporary community health nursing care.

When you open the door of a senior center where you will be promoting cardiovascular fitness through teaching, advocating for exercise equipment, and changes in the on-site meal program, how might theories of community health nursing contribute to your success? When you approach your city council about the need to increase staffing of public health services, what models of community health nursing practice might support your argument? What, really, do we mean by *theories, models,* and *tenets,* and what is their relevance to day-to-day community health nursing practice? These are the key issues we will explore in this chapter. First, though, let's take a fresh look at some of the fundamental characteristics of community health nursing that we began to explore back in Chapter 1.

WHEN THE CLIENT IS A COMMUNITY: CHARACTERISTICS OF COMMUNITY HEALTH NURSING PRACTICE

Nursing exists to address people's health care needs, and nurses fulfill this purpose through their work in various specialty areas. Specialties are characterized by the unit of care for which the specialty is responsible and by the goal of the specialty. Each specialty requires a particular area of knowledge and set of skills for excellence in practice.

Community health nursing, as we have emphasized throughout this text, is a specialty for which the unit of care is a specific community or aggregate for which the nurse has accepted responsibility to help improve health. The goal of this specialty is health improvement of that community. The skills required for excellence in community health nursing practice include, among others, skills in epidemiology, research, teaching, community organizing, and interpersonal, relational care (see The Global Community).

In summary, then, we could say that community health nursing is characterized by community-oriented, population-focused care and is based on interpersonal relationships. Let's examine each of these characteristics in more depth.

Community-Oriented, Population-Focused Care

As we saw in Chapter 1, a *community* is a group of people who have some characteristic(s) in common, are bound by time, interact with one another, and feel a connection to one another. Members of an Internet-based support group for people with colitis, for example, are a community. They share similar experiences and concerns, and they often influence one another's behavior. For instance, they may recommend food choices or complementary therapies to one another. Members of a class of community health nursing students are also a community. Because they begin and end their studies in a particular month and year, they are bound by time, and they certainly share certain values, such as helping people, and feel a sense of connection to one another.

Community orientation implies a process that is actively shaped by the unique experiences, knowledge, concerns, values, beliefs, and culture of a given community. For example, when an outbreak of hepatitis occurs, the community health nurse does more than simply treat infection in individuals. The nurse also:

- Uses disease-investigation skills to locate possible sources of infection
- Determines how the community's knowledge, values, beliefs, and prior experiences with infectious disease

may influence their interpretation of the outbreak, response, and treatment preferences
- Uses the knowledge and suggestions gathered from the community to develop, in collaboration with other health professionals, a community-specific program to prevent future outbreaks

A community-oriented nurse who provides education to a group of students at a Catholic college about sexually transmitted diseases will consider community values regarding sexual behavior. Similarly, a community-oriented nurse who provides nutritional counseling to a community of Hispanic seniors will consider the meaning of food in this culture, the types of foods most commonly consumed, and the cooking methods most commonly used.

A *population,* as we saw in Chapter 1, is any group of people who share at least one characteristic, such as age, gender, race, a particular risk factor, or disease. Thus, smokers and breast cancer survivors are two populations. The concept of population may also include delineation by time, as in all children born in the year 2000. The nurse's place of employment commonly limits the population that the nurse serves. For example, a nurse who works for a county health department is limited professionally to caring for the population of that county.

A *population focus* implies that nurses use the population-based skills such as epidemiology and research in community assessment and community organizing as interventions. For example, a population-focused nurse employed by an autoworkers' union may study all cases of repetitive-use injury occurring in the auto industry in the United States in the past 5 years, develop a program for reducing repetitive-use injury, and lobby industry executives for adoption of the program.

Community-oriented, population-focused care employs population-based skills and is shaped by the characteristics and needs of a given community. Community health nurses provide community-oriented, population-focused care when they count and interview homeless people sleeping in a park and, based on these data, help develop a program providing food, clothing, shelter, health care, and job training for this population.

Relationship-Based Care

Relationship-based care incorporates the value of establishing and maintaining a reciprocal, caring relationship with the community. It is a necessary and feasible aspect of community health nursing practice. According to a Pew Commission report on relationship-centered care, "Developing and maintaining relationships with the community forms the foundation for effectively caring for the community's health" (Tresolini & Pew, 1994, p. 32). A reciprocal, caring relationship with the community involves listening, participatory dialogue, and critical reflection, and it may also involve sociopolitical elements of practice such as advocacy, community empowerment, and movement to action (Shields & Lindsey, 1998).

Community health nurses provide relationship-based care

THE GLOBAL COMMUNITY

Z. Ladhani, personal communication, July 20, 1999.

Nurses from Aga Khan University provided pre- and postnatal checkups for women in urban slums in Karachi, Pakistan. After an analysis of the clinic's records, the nurses validated consistently high rates of anemia among these women. The nurses used this information to help develop and promote a program to reduce anemia that included screening all pregnant women and new mothers both at the clinic and in the community, providing iron prescriptions and pills at low cost, and teaching the women about the importance of iron intake, sources of iron-rich foods, how and when to take the pills, and normal side effects of iron supplementation. This program was successfully implemented and reduced anemia among pregnant women and new mothers so significantly that it became part of primary health care programs in other urban slum areas in Pakistan.

when they meet regularly with a group of female inmates to learn about their physical and psychosocial health care needs and the needs of their families, and then advocate for this population with prison officials and other professionals in the community. They also provide relationship-based care when they work with parents of children with cancer, a psychologist, and a hospital chaplain to learn about the needs of these families and to facilitate the development of a self-help group. In both these examples, community health nurses are working to establish and maintain ongoing relationships with other professionals in the community and with their community of clients.

THEORIES AND MODELS FOR COMMUNITY HEALTH NURSING PRACTICE

A **theory** is a set of systematically interrelated concepts or hypotheses that seek to explain or predict phenomena. For example, the "big bang theory" seeks to explain the series of events that occurred in the earliest moments in the history of our universe. In contrast, a **model** is a description or analogy used as a pattern to enhance our understanding of some reality. For example, the fluid mosaic model of the eucaryotic cell wall is a verbal and visual description that enhances our understanding of cell-wall structure and function. Both theories and models have been developed to describe, clarify, and guide nursing practice. Here, we will briefly discuss nine theories or models that have particular relevance to the practice of community health nursing.

Nightingale's Theory of Environment

Florence Nightingale's environmental theory has great significance to nursing in general and to community health nursing specifically, because it focuses on preventive care to populations. During her work organizing and supervising a nursing service for soldiers in the Crimean War, Nightingale kept meticulous records that suggested that disease was more prevalent in poor environments and that health could be promoted by providing adequate ventilation, pure water, quiet, warmth, light, and cleanliness. The crux of her theory, then, was that poor environmental conditions are bad for health and that good environmental conditions reduce disease (Nightingale, 1992).

There is no consensus as to the specific conditions that should be ensured so people can be healthy. Some people believe that in addition to a clean environment, social services such as public transportation, education, and health care are necessary. In thinking about services that promote the health of communities, it is useful to consider:

- Why these services were created
- Who benefits from the services
- Who pays for the services

- The cost to the people using the services
- The public's perception of the services

For example, if ventilation in a city's homeless shelter is inadequate, the community health nurse who plans to advocate for capital improvements to the shelter will need to consider who pays for the shelter as well as the public's perception of the shelter.

Orem's Self-Care Model

Dorothy Orem, a nurse administrator and educator, focused on the concept of *self-care,* learned, goal-oriented actions to preserve and promote life, health, and well-being. She described people needing nursing care as those who lack ability in self-care (Orem, 1991). When a demand for self-care exceeds the client's ability, then the client experiences a self-care deficit and nursing intervention becomes appropriate. The goal of nursing actions is to help people recognize their self-care demands and limitations and increase their self-care ability. Nursing care also functions to meet clients' self-care needs until they are able to do so for themselves.

Orem further describes three types of requirements that influence people's self-care abilities:

- Universal requirements, common to all human beings, are self-care activities essential to meet physiologic and psychosocial needs.
- Developmental requirements are activities necessary to help people progress developmentally.
- Health-deviation requirements are activities needed to help people deal with a diminished level of wellness.

Although Orem's theory focused primarily on individuals, it can be applied to community health nursing. Populations and communities can be considered to have a collective set of self-care actions and requirements that affect the well-being of the total group. When an aggregate's demands for self-care exceed its ability, then the aggregate experiences a self-care deficit and community health nursing intervention is indicated. According to this theory, the goal of community health nursing is to promote a community's collective independence and self-care ability.

For example, a riverside community that ingests large quantities of fish contaminated with heavy metals might have self-care deficits related to awareness of dangers of eating local fish and the risk to various subpopulations such as pregnant women and young children. The community health nurse should help the community become aware of the risk and identify other food sources. The nurse should also help the community lobby government and industry to reduce pollution and clean up the river.

Neuman's Health Care Systems Model

Betty Neuman, a leader in mental health nursing and nursing education, proposed a systems model (Neuman, 1982, 1995) that we have adapted here to view clients as aggregates. In this model, people are seen as open systems that constantly and reciprocally interact with their environment. Each system is greater than the sum of its parts, and wellness exists when the parts of the system interact in harmony with each other and with the system's environment (Beckman et al., 1994). Four sets of variables, or influences, make up each system's "whole." These are physiologic, psychological, sociocultural, and developmental variables. Given these variables, each system will have a unique response to stressors, those tension-producing stimuli that may cause disequilibrium or illness.

A system's response to stressors may be envisioned as a series of concentric circles (Fig. 17–1). In the center is a core of basic survival abilities, such as a community's ability to make the best use of its natural resources. Surrounding this core are three boundaries. The innermost boundary is a flexible line of resistance and it encompasses internal defenses, such as a community's collective sense of responsibility for raising healthy children. The second boundary is the system's normal line of defense, such as a community's police force or voluntary fire brigade. The third boundary is a dynamic, flexible line of defense, a buffer that prevents stressors from invading the system's normal line of defense. An example is regular maintenance of a community's roads and bridges.

In Neuman's model, stressors can originate from the internal environment or the external environment. Examples of internal stressors include a high proportion of low-income residents or an inadequate system of water purification. External stressors might include natural disasters, war, or a downturn in the global economy. The role of community health nursing, then, is to assist communities in remaining stable within their environment (Beckman et al., 1994).

Rogers' Model of the Science of Unitary Man

In 1970, Martha Rogers developed a nursing model based on systems theory. Her model emphasized that the whole is greater than the sum of its parts (ie, to focus on the parts of a community, such as its health care or housing, does not provide an adequate picture of its totality).

Rogers also incorporated developmental theory into her model by describing the development of "unitary" persons or systems according to three principles: (1) life proceeds in one direction along a rhythmic spiral, (2) energy fields follow a certain wave pattern and organization, and (3) human and environmental energy fields interact simultaneously and mutually, leading to completeness and unity. Using this model, the community health nurse can focus on community–environment interaction: The community functions interdependently with others and with the environment. Thus, community health nursing's goal is to promote holistic and healthful community–environment interaction.

Pender's Health Promotion Model

As we have noted throughout this text, health promotion is a priority in the practice of community health nursing. Pender defines health promotion as action "directed toward increasing the level of well-being and self-actualization of a given individual or group" (Pender, 1987, p. 57). It is a proactive

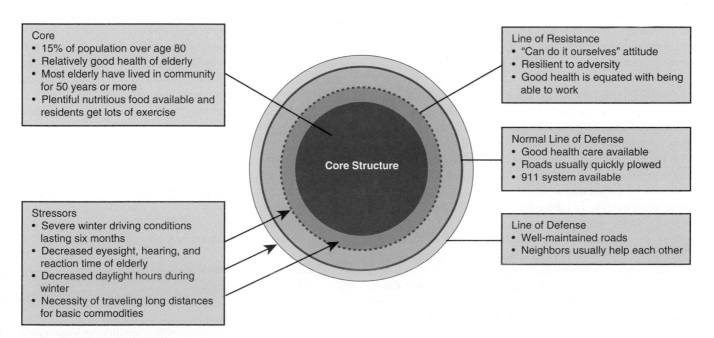

FIGURE 17–1. Neuman's health care systems model applied to a rural county regarding traffic safety issues concerning the elderly. (Source: Derryl Block.)

set of behaviors in which people act on their environment rather than react to stressors arising from the environment.

Pender's *health promotion model* seeks to explain this proactive behavior. The model is based on social learning theory that stresses cognitive processes that help regulate behavior, such as the perceptions people have that directly influence their motivation to begin or continue health-promoting behaviors. These include, for example, people's perceived control of their health, their perceived health status, the perceived benefits of health-promoting behaviors, and the perceived barriers to engaging in health-promoting behaviors.

Five types of modifying factors influence people's perceptions about pursuing health-promoting behaviors. These include:

- Demographic factors, such as age, race
- Biologic characteristics, such as height and weight
- Interpersonal influences, such as the expectations of others
- Situational factors, such as availability of healthful foods
- Behavioral factors, such as stress-coping patterns

Using Pender's model, a community health nurse might interview the residents of a low-income housing project for their perceptions about improving their health and safety, and conduct research into demographic, situational, and other factors that might influence the residents' motivation and ability to change their circumstances.

Roy's Adaptation Model

Sister Callista Roy's model describes people as open and adaptive systems that experience stimuli, develop coping mechanisms, and produce responses. These responses, which may be adaptive or maladaptive, provide feedback that influences the amount and type of stimuli they can handle next time (Andrews & Roy, 1991; Roy & Andrews, 1999).

Roy describes two response processes. The *regulator* process receives stimuli from the internal and external environments, and then processes this combination of information to produce a response. The *cognator* process considers perceptions, learning, judgment, and emotion when formulating a response to stimuli. For example, a regulator process might begin with a community's desire to keep adolescents from smoking (internal stimuli) and new state regulations prohibiting the sale of tobacco products to minors (external stimuli). These combined stimuli lead to a city ordinance against minors purchasing cigarettes (coping mechanism) that results in lowered levels of smoking (response) among this population. A cognator process might begin with the stimulus of heavy rainfall in a riverside community. Residents' perceptions of the amount of rainfall, their memories of past floods, their insights about preventing or managing flooding, and their emotions of anxiety will all contribute to their plans for evacuation, sandbagging, and soliciting county or state assistance.

When applying Roy's model to community health nursing, it is important to remember that communities are made up of many parts and are influenced by many variables. Thus, their adaptation levels are constantly changing. The community health nurse must assess a community's coping mechanisms and help members to use their collective abilities to promote adaptation. If a community is doing nothing to respond to increased numbers of teen pregnancies, for example, nursing actions can be designed to encourage more healthful coping patterns and adaptive responses.

Milio's Framework for Prevention

Nancy Milio, a nurse and leader in public health policy and public health education, developed a *Framework for Prevention* that includes concepts of community-oriented, population-focused care (Milio, 1976, 1981). Milio's basic treatise is that behavioral patterns of populations—and individuals who make up populations—are a result of habitual selection from limited choices. She challenged the common notion that a main determinant for unhealthful behavioral choice is lack of knowledge. Governmental and institutional policies, she said, set the range of options for personal choice making. Milio's framework describes a sometimes-neglected role of community health nursing, examining the determinants of a community's health, and attempting to influence those determinants through public policy.

Salmon White's Construct for Public Health Nursing

Marla Salmon White, a leader in public health nursing administration, nursing education, and public health policy in the United States, proposed a model to guide community health nursing practice. In *Construct for Public Health Nursing,* White (1982) described public health as an organized societal effort to protect, promote, and restore the health of people, and public health nursing as focused on achieving and maintaining public health.

The model describes three practice priorities. Not surprisingly, these are prevention of disease and poor health, protection against disease and external agents, and promotion of health. Three general categories of nursing intervention include:

- Education directed toward voluntary change in the attitudes and behavior of the subjects
- Engineering directed at managing risk-related variables
- Enforcement directed at mandatory regulation to achieve better health

The scope of practice spans individual, family, community, and global care. Interventions target determinants in four categories: Human/biologic, environmental, medical/technological/ organizational, and social. Thus, for White, a community health nurse working to reduce the transmission of tuberculosis collaborates on education, engineering, and enforcement in a population of individuals and families living in a given community. The nurse collaborates on a variety of interventions, from medications to teaching to social support, to prevent further disease in the community and promote global health.

Block and Josten's Ethical Theory of Population-Focused Nursing

Derryl Block and LaVohn Josten, public health nurse educators, developed an ethical theory of population-focused nursing that is based on the intersecting fields of public health and nursing. Block and Josten suggest three essential elements of population-focused nursing that stem from these two fields: an obligation to population, the primacy of prevention, and the centrality of relationship-based care. The first two elements stem from public health, and the third is integral to all of nursing (Block & Josten, 1999).

This theory has important applications for community health nursing. According to Block and Josten, obligation to population and emphasis on prevention are not sufficient for community-oriented, population-focused nursing. As we noted earlier in the chapter, community health nursing practice must include relationship-based care as well.

TENETS OF PUBLIC HEALTH NURSING APPLIED TO COMMUNITY HEALTH NURSING

The word **tenet** stems from a Latin verb meaning "to hold," and thus can be defined as any principle or doctrine held as true. Community health nursing's goal of promoting and protecting the health of communities is facilitated by adhering to the eight tenets of public health nursing described below and summarized in Display 17–1 (Quad Council, 1999).

Tenet 1: Use a Comprehensive and Systematic Process

The first tenet requires the use of a comprehensive and systematic process to assess population health, plan or develop policies, and ensure their implementation. A process is comprehensive when it considers all determinants of health. Additionally, when a sample of the population is being assessed or treated, a systematic process includes people who truly represent the entire population.

Tenet 2: Work in Partnership With the People

The second tenet requires the community health nurse to work in partnership with the community. The nurse and the community each bring their own values, beliefs, and expertise to the partnership. Policy development and assurance are

---

DISPLAY 17–1 Tenets of Public Health Applied to Community Health Nursing

1. The process of population-based assessment, policy development, and assurance is systematic and comprehensive.
2. In all processes, partnerships with representatives of the people are essential.
3. Primary prevention is given priority.
4. Creating healthful environmental, social, and economic conditions in which people can thrive guides selection of intervention strategies.
5. The practice incorporates an obligation to actively reach out to all who might benefit from an intervention or service.
6. The dominant concern and obligation are for the greater good of all of the people or the population as a whole.
7. The stewardship and allocation of available resources are supported to gain the maximum population health benefit from the use of those resources.
8. The health of the people is most effectively promoted and protected through collaboration with members of other professions and organizations.

(Quad Council of Public Health Nursing Organizations [1999]. *Scope and standards of public health nursing practice.* Washington, DC: American Nurses Publishing.)

---

more likely to be accepted and applied if there is mutual consideration of and respect for these elements. Developed policies need to be communicated in language that reflects an understanding of the community. Thus, an essential part of establishing a partnership with a community is getting to know the members and groups within that community.

Tenet 3: Focus on Primary Prevention

The third tenet of public health nursing underscores the importance of primary prevention in promoting the health of people. Most fields of medicine, as well as acute care nursing, are primarily concerned with illness, including efforts to prevent complications and reoccurrence of the illness. In contrast, community health nursing has an obligation to prevent health problems from occurring and to promote a higher level of wellness. Community health nurses take initiative to seek out high-risk groups, potential health problems, and situations that contribute to health problems. They then institute preventive programs. For example, if community assessment revealed a large number of new mothers in the community suffering from postpartum depression, community health nurses would address secondary prevention through establishing mental health programs. However, they would also attend to primary prevention by working to change the conditions in the community that increase the risk for postpartum depression.

Tenet 4: Promote a Healthful Environment

The fourth tenet recognizes the importance of ensuring that people live in conditions conducive to health. Therefore, it is aligned with Nightingale's environmental theory of health. People are less likely to be healthy if they live in a community with high unemployment, crowded housing, and dirty air, or where it is difficult to obtain inexpensive, healthful food. They are also less likely to be healthy if their community's norms include acceptance or even encouragement of activities such as smoking, binge drinking, drug use, or unsafe sex. Changing any of these conditions requires commitment, perseverance, patience, resourcefulness, and a long-range view (see Voices From the Community).

Tenet 5: Target All Who Might Benefit

The fifth tenet involves outreach strategies to meet the obligation to serve all people who might benefit from an inter-

vention. This tenet requires the nurse to examine policies or programs to determine whether they are accessible and acceptable to the entire population in need, and to advocate for needed changes if necessary.

In one community, families with young children had a high (80%) rate of compliance with regulations requiring the use of infant and toddler car seats, but continuing assessments revealed that over 90% of the seats were being used incorrectly. For example, the harness straps were too loose, the seats were not properly installed, or the model of seats in use had been recalled for safety problems. A coalition of community health nurses and law enforcement officials implemented a summer-long, monthly car seat checkup service in the parking lot of a local mall, and advertised the service in a media campaign. In evaluating the program, the coalition acknowledged that the campaign had not affected the transport of children born after the intervention time period had expired, nor residents who were out of town for the summer, nor had it increased the knowledge of car seat safety among expectant parents or the community in general.

The questions in Display 17–2 help the nurse evaluate a planned program's success in reaching people who might benefit. These questions should guide the design, implementation, and evaluation of outreach strategies.

Tenet 6: Give Priority to Community Needs

The sixth tenet deals with the ethical obligation of the community health nurse to give priority to the needs and preferences of the whole community over one individual. This means that the nurse must consider interventions that will lead to the greatest good for the most people. For example, programs that make mammograms for early detection of breast cancer available to all women regardless of income level are given priority over bone marrow transplantation for women with advanced metastatic breast cancer.

Voices From the Community

In a mostly rural upper Midwest region, community health nurses and other health care workers conducted a survey of over 2000 randomly selected adult residents about their perceptions of the most important health concerns of their community and of the state and nation (Block, Hutton & Braum, 1999). The issue of insurance costs and access to insurance was most commonly mentioned, with 43% of the residents citing it as a most important state/national health concern and 21% of residents naming it as a most important local health concern. The high cost of health care was the next most commonly mentioned issue. This included the high cost of medications and dental care and of caring for certain populations such as the elderly, poor, and single mothers. The high cost of care was mentioned by 30% of the residents as the most important state/national health concern and by 19% of the residents as a most important local concern.

These results were surprising because many community health nurses in the region expected more residents to mention issues of tobacco, cancer, heart disease, and protecting the environment.

1. How do the Tenets of Public Health Nursing Applied to Community Health Nursing pertain to this survey?
2. How might the community health nurses use the results of this survey to help plan population-focused care for this region?

DISPLAY 17–2 Determining Whether Programs Serve Intended Populations

- Is the service offered in a manner that encourages utilization, which might include:
   Are the services located conveniently?
   Do the hours of the service fit with the work or school life of the people?
   Are the services offered in a manner that is respectful of the values, beliefs, mores, and traditions of the people?
   What kind of marketing strategies have been used to inform the people of the service?
- What is the satisfaction level of users of the service?
- Why are some people not using services?

Tenet 7: Promote Optimum Allocation of Resources

The seventh tenet addresses resource-allocation decisions. In most communities, the available resources are not sufficient to meet all the needs of all the people. The nurse must ensure that the community is using limited resources in a way that leads to the greatest improvement in health. To promote optimum allocation of resources, the nurse must:

- Know the latest research on the effectiveness of various programs in addressing needs
- Collect information about the short- and long-term costs of programs
- Evaluate existing programs and policies for ways to improve or discontinue them
- Communicate this information to community decision-makers so they can make resource-allocation decisions that are most likely to improve the community's health

Tenet 8: Collaborate With Others in the Community

The eighth tenet underlines the importance of collaboration with other nurses, health care providers, social workers, educators, spiritual leaders, business leaders, and government officials within the community. This interdisciplinary collaboration is essential to establish and maintain effective programs. Programs planned and implemented in isolation can lead to fragmentation, gaps, and overlaps in health services. For example, without collaboration, a well-child clinic may be started in a community that already has a strong developmental screening program but does not have community prenatal services. Without collaboration, programs may also fail to be effective. For instance, a Saturday-morning cardiovascular fitness program designed without consultation with spiritual leaders may be totally ineffective in a devout Jewish community, where members devote Saturdays to religious observances.

SOCIETAL INFLUENCES ON COMMUNITY-ORIENTED, POPULATION-FOCUSED NURSING

Society is constantly changing. The community health nurse needs to stay abreast of these changes for the following reasons:

- Social changes influence a community's health. Thus, community health nurses need to continually adapt their strategies to respond to changing conditions. For example, increased international air travel means increased levels of communicable disease in a small city with a new international airport. Community health nurses in this city must be proactive in

developing strategies to control the spread of communicable disease.
- Social changes affect the availability of resources necessary to ensure that effective intervention strategies are available. For example, a downturn in the stock market may prompt closure of a community business that once generously supported local community services.

Contemporary community health nurses must be especially aware of the mutual interaction between nursing and technology. By **technology,** we refer to the application of science for changing processes of production or industry. Ideally, technological innovations lead to an improvement of processes for creating products or services. The last century was filled with technological innovations that simultaneously disrupted old patterns of production and created new opportunities for increasing production. Two technological changes highly relevant to contemporary community health nursing are communication technology and genetic engineering.

Communication Technology

Changes in communication technology present new opportunities and challenges for community-oriented, population-focused care. Because of advances in satellite and telecommunications chip technology, communication is possible anywhere in the world where resources are available to purchase equipment and services. This means that a community health nurse, whether working in the Australian Outback or at a public health clinic in Anchorage, Alaska, can contact clients, consultants, and agencies worldwide—again, if resources are available to take advantage of the technologies.

In addition, Internet technology has made it possible to access local, state, national, and international data for community assessment, planning, and evaluation. Nurses requiring data for a new intervention strategy, for example, can search the Internet for information from consumer groups, researchers, and other experts worldwide. To keep apprised of emerging issues and trends in public health, the nurse can join numerous Internet-based electronic discussion groups or listservs (electronic discussions distributed by way of e-mail). The challenge to the nurse is to manage the volume of information and to weigh its worth.

Health care consumers face similar opportunities and challenges. For most diseases and disabilities, information is available on the Internet, and consumers are increasingly searching the Net for health-related data. Little is known about the effects of this increased access on people's health (Coiera, 1998). Certainly, the validity and reliability of information on the Internet vary widely. Research is necessary to understand how people decide what information to use from the Internet, how they use it, and how its use affects their health. As health educators, community health nurses can provide guidelines for people to consider when deciding how to use health information found on the Internet (Pemberton & Goldblatt, 1998) (Display 17–3). Additionally,

---

DISPLAY 17–3 Determining Worth of Health Information on the Internet

- What are the credentials and affiliation of the author?
- Is it easy to determine who is the publisher or sponsor of the web site? Evaluate how the publisher or sponsor might gain economically through your use of the information.
- Is the date of publication of the web site included? Is the information current?
- Are both sides of an issue described? Does the author discuss pros and cons of information presented?
- What references are included to substantiate the information in the article?

---

community health nurses need to participate in studies to determine whether regulation of health information on the Internet is feasible and desirable.

At the same time, community health nurses need to be actively involved in creating their own Internet sites to provide health information specific to their targeted communities. Technologies can include interactive chat sessions, listserv discussions, and asynchronous communications in which community health nurses interact with community members to improve their health.

The Internet is also a superb vehicle for rapidly tracing the international spread of infectious diseases. For example, the World Health Organization, in collaboration with the *Institute National de la Sante et de la Recherche Medicale,* has developed an Internet site for countries to report epidemiologic and laboratory data on influenza (Flahault et al., 1998).

Genetic Engineering

Genetic engineering can be defined as gene manipulation in a laboratory setting (Tortora, Funke & Case, 1998). The development of the field was made possible by the discovery of certain enzymes that can "cut" DNA from two or more different sources into pieces that can be recombined in a test tube. Gene manipulation also required the development of methods for inserting these recombinant DNA molecules into cells by using so-called *vectors,* such as viruses (Tortora, Funke & Case, 1998).

Genetic engineering allows scientists to alter the herbicide-, pest-, and stress-resistance of crops and to increase the nutrition and attractiveness of the foods we eat. Genetic engineering also allows scientists to develop new kinds of medicines and to cure diseases by replacing absent or faulty genes. Mapping the DNA sequence that makes up the "genetic blueprint" of human beings provides new opportunities for protecting human health (Ellsworth & Manolio, 1999). In addition to increasing our understanding of the contribution

of genetic material to health and disease, it creates new opportunities for early identification, prevention, and treatment of people at risk for disease. For example, it is anticipated that techniques for DNA screening of newborns will allow for early detection of risk for certain diseases and disabilities, and thus for early interventions (Reilly & Page, 1998). However, despite the enthusiasm of many commercial industries, genetic engineering has generated much controversy.

The controversy emerges from a number of different concerns. One concern is the inability to know for sure the long-term consequences of genetically altering foods or organisms such as bacteria, insects, or human beings. For example, the release of a genetically altered weed or insect could be catastrophic if that weed or insect reproduces prolifically and damages the ecosystem. Fears of negative effects of the engineered gene transfers between species in genetically engineered food include allergic reactions, spread of diseases across crop species, and new diseases because of unpredictable mutations in the genetic code. The potential scientific capacity to alter methods of reproduction of humans raises concerns about creating unintended consequences for the human race. Another source of concern is that science is "playing God." For some people, the possibility of being able to select the gender or intelligence or eye color of a child raises concerns about interfering with nature and creates conflict with people's religious or ethical views. Additionally, genetic screening could be used to deny rights and opportunities to people. For example, someone who is found to carry a gene that increases the risk for heart disease might be denied health insurance coverage. Another source of concern is the distrust many people have of governments, large commercial enterprises, and/or the scientific community. Some people believe that they are not being told the truth about scientific or other issues, and because genetically altering food or humans can affect the survival of individuals, groups, or society as a whole, this distrust results in people being very opposed to any type of genetic engineering.

In dealing with these concerns, it will be the community health nurses' responsibility to be aware of the latest scientific information for educating communities so they can make decisions that best fit their value systems. Advocating for the highest scientific rigor in genetic engineering research will also be an important role of community health nurses. Community health nurses will need to advocate for research that not only maps the DNA sequence but also identifies interventions that can change the outcomes for people identified by genetic screening as being at risk. Nurses also need to balance what is good for the community as a whole against potential costs to people at risk, advocating for policies and regulations that ensure such a balance.

Global Economy

Hundreds of years ago, communities' economies were largely local. If a drought led to a reduction in crop yield in one region, for example, only that region and perhaps its closest neighbors would be affected. Since World War II, however, there has been a consistent trend toward international trade, investment, travel, and ownership of information and ideas (Moller, 1999). This increasingly **global economy** is evidenced by the recent creation of the European Economic Community and passage of the North American Free Trade Agreement. It has contributed to a strong economy for many developed nations, including the United States, but has also led to increased instability of all economies as problems in markets in distant countries affect markets worldwide.

This interrelationship of economies was made clear in the southeast Asian monetary crisis in the late 1990s. When key markets in southeast Asia experienced downturns, the economies of the United States and other investor nations suffered as well. In the United States damage was limited to industries conducting business directly with southeast Asian countries, such as agriculture and the computer industry, but the toll worldwide in increased poverty and decreased opportunities can only be guessed at.

A global economy also means that rich countries in need of skilled workers can recruit them from developing countries, causing a shortage of skilled labor in those countries that need it most. In recruiting countries, if new immigrant groups are seen as a threat to the local culture or economy, ethnic, racial, and religious tensions may increase (Moller, 1999). Even people with well-paying jobs may react negatively because they see their world changing and their own future more uncertain. At the same time, when citizens in developing nations perceive their country or its citizens as suffering unjustly because of unfair economic changes, there may be an increase in nationalism and even international terrorism.

Finally, the economic trends of the late 20th century have contributed worldwide to greater disparities in wealth, health, and *relative poverty,* a measurement of an individual's income against the average for the society in which that individual lives. The disparity in wealth is indicated by the fact that the world's 358 wealthiest people have a net worth equal to that of the world's 2.3 billion poorest people (United Nations, 1996). In the United States, economic disparity has been fueled by an increasing demand for skilled workers and a decreasing demand for unskilled laborers. When the demand for skilled workers, such as software engineers, exceeds the supply, these workers can demand increased wages. This pushes up the cost of housing, health care, products, and services even to those unskilled laborers whose wages have decreased. Another factor in the United States was the tremendous growth of the stock market, which contributed to the wealth of those people already wealthy enough to invest in it. Those who were "just getting by," however, were largely left behind by the "bull market" of the 1990s.

Reducing income disparities and their effects is a challenge for all people who work in service of humanity. Community health nurses have an obligation to read the latest research so they can better understand the relationship of poverty to health. At the same time, they need to advocate for policies that will reduce adverse effects of poverty and income disparities. Chapter 32 addresses health issues related to poverty.

Migration

Migration is the act of moving from one region or country to another, temporarily, seasonally, or permanently. Throughout history, people have migrated from place to place to seek improved opportunities or to escape intolerable conditions in their home country. The late 20th century saw a dramatic increase in the number of *refugees* who migrated from their homes to escape invasion, oppression, or persecution. The 20th century also saw an increased reliance on migrant farmworkers, people who move from one region to another seasonally, following the crops.

The health care needs of migrants and migrant refugees are enormous. Environmental factors are a primary source of decreased health and include inadequate waste disposal, crowded and often unsanitary living conditions, lack of access to healthful foods, and even air pollution from an increased concentration of vehicles used for moving refugees. Potential health effects associated with migration suggest that community health nurses need to ensure that surveillance systems are in place to detect emerging health problems, and that programs are developed to prevent health problems or to treat existing conditions. The specific health care needs of migrant farmworkers are discussed in Chapter 33.

Bioterrorism

Terrorism is one way a small group who perceives that they have been unfairly treated can exert influence on a larger group or nation (Moller, 1999). Groups wishing to harm other countries need sophisticated skills for most conventional weapons, but some methods of *bioterrorism* may be cheaper and easier to use (Noah, Sobel, Ostroff & Kildew, 1998). **Bioterrorism** is the use of living organisms, such as bacteria, viruses, or other organic materials, to harm and/or intimidate others in order to achieve political ends. Some of the possible biologic agents used include the *Bacillus anthracis* bacteria, smallpox virus, *Brucella,* and botulism toxins (Wise, 1998).

Because of escalating concerns about bioterrorism, public health workers increasingly recognize the need for skills in dealing with a bioterrorist attack. They need to:
- Ensure that adequate surveillance systems are in place for early detection
- Educate emergency and other health personnel about symptoms, treatment, and prevention of further spread
- Establish coordinated response plans with health and law-enforcement officials (Centers for Disease Control and Prevention, 1999)

Perhaps more importantly, community health nurses need to be involved in primary prevention of bioterrorism through advocating for the elimination of biologic weapons and addressing issues' "root causes" such as poverty, hunger, housing, clean water, and health care (Cohen, Gould & Sidel, 1999).

Climate Changes

Climate changes can be considered societal changes because they may be influenced by economics. Since the Industrial Revolution, the earth's atmosphere has received increased amounts of carbon dioxide, methane, and nitrous oxide created by manufacturing industries, automobile emissions, and consumer products. Many scientists believe that these increases have contributed to climate changes that are expected to affect sea levels, the production of food, fiber, and medicines, and the spread of infectious diseases (Martens, Slooff & Jackson, 1997). Conversely, it has been estimated that significant increases in fuel efficiency and other efforts to reduce pollution could avoid 8 million deaths around the world (Working Group on Public Health and Fossil-Fuel Combustion, 1997). Population-focused nurses need to educate the public about the potential dangers of continuing to contaminate the environment, and to advocate for changes in public policy that promote reducing air and water contaminants. Chapter 16 explores health-related environmental issues in detail.

SUMMARY

Community health nursing is a community-oriented, population-focused nursing specialty that is based on interpersonal relationships. The unit of care is the community or population rather than the individual, and the goal is to promote healthy communities.

Theories and models of community health nursing aid the nurse in understanding the rationale behind community-oriented care. Florence Nightingale's environmental theory emphasized the importance of improving environmental conditions to promote health. Orem's self-care model provides a framework within which the community health nurse can promote a community's collective independence and self-care ability. Neuman's health care systems model describes the nurse's role as one of assisting clients to remain stable within their environment, whereas Rogers' model of the science of unitary man focuses on client–environment interaction and holistic health. Pender's model focuses on the promotion of health behaviors in people. Nursing's goal is to enhance the likelihood of people engaging in health-promoting behaviors by assessing and influencing perceptual and modifying factors. Roy's adaptation model describes the nurse's goal as promoting healthful coping mechanisms and adaptive responses to stressors. Milio's framework for prevention indicates that

health-related behaviors are a result of habitual selection from limited choice. Salmon White's construct for public health nursing prescribes education, engineering, and enforcement with individuals, families, communities, and nations. Finally, Block and Josten's ethical theory of population-focused nursing focuses on the nurse's obligation to population, emphasis on prevention, and requirement for relationship-based care.

The eight tenets of public health nursing applied to community health nursing provide a framework within which the nurse works to promote and protect the health of populations. They emphasize the primacy of prevention, the need for outreach, and the importance of working in collaboration for the greatest good of the greatest number of people.

Nurses need to anticipate and adapt to societal changes in order to fulfill their mission of promoting the health of all people. Contemporary societal influences on community health nursing include communication technology, genetic engineering, the global economy, migration, bioterrorism, and climate changes.

ACTIVITIES TO PROMOTE CRITICAL THINKING

1. Interview a community health nursing director to determine what population-focused programs are offered in your locality. Explore nursing's role in the assessment, development, implementation, and evaluation of these programs. Discuss with the director how community health nurses might expand their population-focused interventions.

2. Describe a situation in community health nursing practice where use of an educational intervention would be most appropriate. Do the same with engineering and enforcement interventions. Discuss what made you match each situation with that intervention.

3. Assume you have been asked to make a home visit to a 75-year-old man living alone whose wife recently died. Besides assessing his individual needs, what additional factors should you consider for assessment and intervention that would indicate an aggregate or community focused approach?

4. Select one of the societal influences on community or population. How would the theories or models for community health nursing practice that were discussed in this chapter guide your practice concerning that societal issue? Choose three models or theories to discuss.

5. Explore one of the societal influences on community or population using the Internet. Using the information in Display 17–3, try to determine the worth of the information on at least one Internet site.

REFERENCES

Andrews, H. A., & Roy, C. (1991). *The Roy adaptation model: The definitive statement*. Norwalk, CT: Appleton-Lange.

Beckman, S. J., Boxley-Harges, S., Bruick-Sorge, C., Harris, S. M., Hermiz, M. E., Meininger, M., & Steinkeler, S. E. (1994). Betty Neuman: Systems model. In A. Marriner-Tomey (Ed.), *Nursing theorists and their work* (3rd ed., pp. 269–304). St. Louis: Mosby.

Block, D. E., Hutton, S. J., & Braun, B. (1999). Health concerns of adults: Qualitative data of the Bridge to Health Survey. *American Journal of Health Behavior, 23*(3), 163–171.

Block, D. E., & Josten, L. (1999, June). *The ethical basis of population focused nursing: Graduate student and faculty reflections*. Paper presented at the Association of Community Health Nursing Educators Spring Institute, Nashville, TN.

Blum, H. L. (1974). *Planning for health*. New York: Human Sciences Press.

Catalano, R. A., Lind, S. L., Rosenblatt, A. B., & Attkisson, C. C. (1999). Unemployment and foster home placements: Estimating the net effect of provocation and inhibition. *American Journal of Public Health, 89*(6), 851–855.

Centers for Disease Control and Prevention. (1999). Bioterrorism alleging use of anthrax and interim guidelines for management—United States, 1998. *Morbidity and Mortality Weekly Report, 48*(4), 69–74.

Cohen, H. W., Gould, R. M., & Sidel, V. W. (1999). Bioterrorism initiatives: Public health in reverse? *American Journal of Public Health, 89*(11), 1629–1631.

Coiera, E. (1998). Information epidemics, economics, and immunity on the Internet. *British Medical Journal, 317,* 1469–1470.

Davis, D. R. (1998). Technology, unemployment, and relative wages in a global economy. *European Economic Review, 42,* 1613–1633.

Diatta, M. A., & Mbow, N. (1999). Releasing the development potential of return migration: The case of Senegal. *International Migration, 37*(1), 243–266.

Ellsworth, D. L., & Manolio, T. A. (1999). The emerging importance of genetics in epidemiologic research. I. Basic concepts in human genetics and laboratory technology. *Annals of Epidemiology, 9*(1), 1–16.

Flahault, A., Dias-Ferro, V., Chaberty, P., Esteves, K., Valleron, A. J., & Lavanchy, D. (1998). FluNet as a tool for global monitoring of influenza on the Web. *Journal of the American Medical Association, 280*(15), 1330–1332.

Frank, J. W., & Mustard, J. F. (1995). The determinants of health from a historical perspective. *Daedalus, Journal of the American Academy of Arts and Sciences, 123*(4). Available: http://children.metrotor.on.ca/taskforce/must.html.

Institute of Medicine, Committee for the Study of the Future of Public Health. (1988). *The future of public health*. Washington, DC: National Academy Press.

Josten, L. E., Block, D., Vincent, P., Savik, K., & Wedeking, L. (1997). Linking high risk, low income women to public health services. *Journal of Public Health Management and Practice, 3*(2), 27–36.

Kamel, W. W. (1997). Health dilemmas at the borders—a global challenge. *World Health Forum, 18*(1), 9–16.

Lantz, P. M., House, J. S., Lepkowski, J. M., Williams, D. R.,

Mero, R. P., & Chen, J. (1998). Socioeconomic factors, health behaviors, and mortality: Results from a nationally representative prospective study of U.S. adults. *Journal of the American Medical Association, 279*(21), 1703–1708.

Leavell, H. R., & Clark, E. G. (1965). *Preventive medicine for the doctor in his community: A epidemiologic approach* (3rd ed.). Norwalk, CT: Appleton and Lange.

Lynch, D. (1992). *Titanic: An illustrated history*. New York: Hyperion.

Marriner-Tomey, A. (1994). *Nursing theorists and their work* (3rd ed.). St. Louis: Mosby.

Martens, W. J. M., Slooff, R., & Jackson, E. K. (1997). Climate change, human health, and sustainable development. *Bulletin of the World Health Organization, 75*(6), 583–588.

Milio, N. (1981). *Promoting health through public policy*. Philadelphia: F. A. Davis.

———. (1976). A framework for prevention: Changing health damaging to health-generating life patterns. *American Journal of Public Health, 66*(5), 435–439.

Miller, B. A. (1998). Trends: Immigration and technology. *Journal of the American College of Dentists, 65*(4), 36–38.

Minnesota Public Health Nursing Directors Association. (1994). *Public health nursing core functions*. (Available from Minnesota Department of Health, 717 SE Delaware Street, Minneapolis, MN 55455).

Moller, J. O. (1999). The growing challenge to internationalism. *The Futurist, 33*(3), 22–27.

Murray, C. J. L., & Lopez, A. D. (1997). Alternative projections of mortality and disability by cause 1990–2020: Global Burden of Disease Study. *The Lancet, 349,* 1498–1504.

Nesvadbova, L., Rutsch, J., & Sojka, S. (1997). Migration and its health and social problems in the Czech Republic. Part I. *Central European Journal of Public Health, 5*(4), 188–192.

Neuman, B. (1995). *The Neuman systems model* (3rd ed.). Norwalk, CT: Appleton-Lange.

———. (1982). *The Neuman systems model: Application to nursing education and practice*. Norwalk, CT: Appleton-Lange.

Nightingale, F. (1992). *Florence Nightingale's notes on nursing* (edited with an introduction, notes, and guide to identification by V. Skretkowicz). London: Scutari Press (originally published 1859).

Noah, D. L., Sobel, A. L., Ostroff, S. M., & Kildew, J. A. (1998). Biological warfare training—infectious disease outbreak differentiation criteria. *Military Medicine, 163*(4), 198–201.

Noddings, N. (1994). *Caring: A feminine approach to ethics and moral education*. Berkeley, CA: University of California Press.

Orem, D. E. (1991). *Nursing: Concepts of practice* (4th ed.). St Louis: Mosby.

———. (1985). *Nursing: Concepts of practice* (3rd ed.). New York: McGraw-Hill.

———. (1980). *Nursing: Concepts of practice* (2nd ed.). New York: McGraw-Hill.

Pemberton, P. J., & Goldblatt, J. (1998). The Internet and the changing roles of doctors, patients and families. *Medical Journal of Australia, 169*(11–12), 594–595.

Pender, N. J. (1987). *Health promotion in nursing practice* (2nd ed.). Norwalk, CT: Appleton-Lange.

Quad Council of Public Health Nursing Organization (1999).

Scope and standards of public health nursing practice. Washington, DC: American Nurses Publishing.

Reilly, P. R., & Page, D. C. (1998). We're off to see the genome. *Nature Genetics, 20,* 15–17.

Roy, C., & Andrews, H. A. (1999). *The Roy adaptation model.* Stamford, CT: Appleton-Lange.

Saunders, P. (1998). Poverty and health: Exploring the links between financial stress and emotional stress in Australia. *Australian and New Zealand Journal of Public Health, 22*(1), 11–16.

Shields, L. E., & Lindsey, A. E. (1998). Community health promotion nursing practice. *Advances in Nursing Science, 20,* 23–36.

Syme, S. L. (1998). Social and economic disparities in health: Thoughts about intervention. *The Milbank Quarterly, 76*(3), 493–505.

Szwarcwald, C. L., Bastos, F. I., Viacava, F., & Tavares de Andrade, C. L. (1999). Income inequality and homicide rates in Rio de Janeiro, Brazil. *American Journal of Public Health, 89*(6), 845–850.

Tortora, G. J., Funke, B. R., & Case, C. L. (1998). *Microbiology.* San Francisco: Benjamin/Cummings Publishing.

Tresolini C. P., & Pew-Fetzer Task Force on Psychosocial Health Education. (1994). *Health professions education and relationship-centered care.* San Francisco: Pew Health Professions Commission.

United Nations Development Programme (1996). *Human development report.* New York: Oxford University Press.

White, M. S. (1982). Construct for public health nursing. *Nursing Outlook, 30*(9), 527–530.

Wise, R. (1998). Bioterrorism: Thinking the unthinkable. *The Lancet, 351*(9113), 1378.

Working Group on Public Health and Fossil-Fuel Combustion. (1997). Short-term improvements in public health from global-climate policies on fossil-fuel combustion: An interim report. *The Lancet, 350*(9088), 1341–1349.

SUGGESTED READINGS

Adams, L. A. (1997). Vulnerable populations: A community oriented perspective. *Family and Community Health, 19*(4), 1–18.

Anderson, E. T., & McFarlane, J. (1996). *Community as partner: Theory and practice in nursing.* Philadelphia: Lippincott-Raven.

Block, D. E., Peterson, J., Finch, M., Kinney, A., Miller, P., & Cherveny, J. (1998). The Bridge to Health Project: A collaborative model for assessing the health of the community. *Journal of Public Health Management and Practice, 4*(3), 43–49.

Clark, P. N. (1998). Research issues. Nursing theory as a guide for inquiry in family and community health nursing. *Nursing Science Quarterly, 11*(2), 47–48.

Frank, J. W., & Mustard, J. F. (1995). The determinants of health from a historical perspective. *Daedalus, Journal of the American Academy of Arts & Sciences, 123*(4). Available: http://children.metrotor.on.ca/taskforce/must.html.

Jezewski, M. A. (1995). Staying connected: The core of facilitating health care for homeless persons. *Public Health Nursing, 12*(3), 203–210.

Josten, L., Wedeking, L., Block, D. E., Savik, K., & Vincent, P. (1997). Linking high risk, low income pregnant women to public health services. *Journal of Health Care Management and Practice, 3*(2), 27–36.

Keller, L. O., Strohschein, S., Lia-Hoagberg, B., & Schaffer, M. (1998). Population-based public health nursing interventions: A model from practice. *Public Health Nursing, 15*(3), 207–215.

Shields, L. E., & Lindsey, A. E. (1998). Community health promotion nursing practice. *Advances in Nursing Science, 20,* 23–36.

CHAPTER

18

The Community as Client: Assessment and Diagnosis

KEY TERMS

- Assets assessment
- Client myth
- Community as client
- Community collaboration
- Community diagnoses
- Community needs assessment
- Community subsystem assessment
- Comprehensive assessment
- Descriptive epidemiologic study
- Familiarization assessment
- Individualism
- Location myth
- Location variables
- Outcome criteria
- Population variables
- Problem-oriented assessment
- Skills myth
- Social class
- Social system variables
- Survey

LEARNING OBJECTIVES

Upon mastery of this chapter, you should be able to:

- Describe the meaning of community as client.
- Discuss how a key American value and three myths can undermine a nurses's intention to move beyond an individualistic focus to practice population-based community health nursing.
- Articulate specific considerations of each of the three dimensions of the community as client.
- Express the meaning and significance of community dynamics.
- Compare and contrast five types of community needs assessment.
- Discuss community needs assessment methods.
- Describe four sources of community data.
- Discuss the significance of community diagnoses formation.
- Explain the characteristics of a healthy community.

As we have seen in earlier chapters, community health nurses work with clients at several levels: as individuals, families, groups, subpopulations, populations, and communities. Table 18–1 presents the characteristics of these levels and describes typical nursing involvement at each.

Although community health nurses work at all six levels of practice, working with communities is a primary mission for two important reasons. First, the community directly influences the health of individuals, families, groups, subpopulations, and populations who might be a part of it. For example, if a city fails to take aggressive action to stop air pollution, the health of all its citizens will be adversely affected. Second, provision of most health services occurs at the community level. Community agencies help develop specific health programs and disseminate health information to many types of groups and populations.

The community health nurse, then, must work with the community as the client (McKnight & Van Dover, 1994). The **community as client** refers to the concept of a community-wide group of people as the focus of nursing service. Understanding the concept of the community as client is a prerequisite for effective service at every level of community nursing practice, as described in Chapter 17.

TABLE 18–1. Variations in Scope of Community Health Nursing Practice

	Client	Example	Health Characteristics	Nursing Assessment	Involvement
Individual	Individual	Kim Murphy	One person with various needs	Individual health assessment	A dyad; interaction with the individual
	Family	Murphy family (seven members)	A small group based on kin ties; specific roles	Family health assessment	Family visits; interaction with members as a group
	Group	Parenting group; Al-Anon club	Two or more people; face-to-face communication; inter-dependency	Assessment of group effectiveness in fulfilling its functions	Group participation; having a role in meetings
Aggregate	Subpopulation	Unmarried pregnant adolescents in a school district	Large group sharing one or more characteristics (subset of a larger group)	Assessment of collective health problems and needs	Study of and planning for meeting specific health needs
	Population	Homeless people in Chicago	An aggregate of people who share one or more personal or environmental characteristics	Study of health needs and vital statistics	Membership in organizations such as a health planning council
	Community	East Harlem, New York City; gay community in the United States	A large aggregate sharing geographic location or special interests	Study of community health characteristics and competence	Researching the community; planning and setting up services

FACTORS OPPOSED TO THE CONCEPT OF COMMUNITY

A variety of factors can undermine a community health nurse's efforts to practice at the level of community. These include the American value of individualism and the myths that the value perpetuates about nursing practice.

The Value of Individualism

Every society has a small number of core values that give meaning to life and provide motivation for its people. The very existence of a society and its way of life depend on a deep commitment to these shared values. People learn them early in life and come to take them for granted as the way things ought to be. Throughout the United States, individualism is one of these core values. **Individualism** refers to a belief that the interests of the individual are or ought to be paramount.

Nearly every social observer who has written about American society has identified this value. "Protect the rights of the individual"; "Equal justice for all under the law"; "Life, liberty, and the pursuit of happiness for all individuals" are familiar cries. More than 50 years ago, the sociologist Robert Lynd described this value: "Individualism, 'the survival of the fittest,' is the law of nature and the secret of America's greatness; and restrictions on individual freedom are un-American and kill initiative" (Lynd, 1939, p. 60).

This basic premise underlies most American institutions. Individual effort and success are rewarded from kindergarten through graduate school by educational policies that evaluate and reward individual achievement. In the workplace, despite the recent focus on team building, individual awards, promotions, and bonuses are still the primary motivators. The criminal justice system punishes individual crimes far more harshly than corporate crimes: A woman who stole $5 in a Southern state was punished by several years in prison, whereas a large oil company that stole millions by overcharging customers paid a relatively small fine. Health care is also dominated by a commitment to the treatment of individuals. The vast majority of researchers, personnel, and health care institutions focus on the care of individual illness rather than promotion of community health.

This value profoundly influences the entire practice of nursing. All nurses are first educated to focus on the *individual* client in clinical nursing. However, in community health practice the focus must shift to the community.

Myths Perpetuated by an Individualistic Focus

Three pervasive myths seem to hinder the nurse from focusing on aggregates or communities: the location myth, the skills myth, and the client myth.

LOCATION MYTH
The **location myth** defines community health nursing by describing it in terms of where it is practiced—in a specific setting or location such as outside of the hospital. This myth silently influences nurses to define their practice based not on the nature of the service given but on the location of its delivery. This myth promotes the belief that community health nursing emphasizes care of individuals. Instead, community health nursing focuses on assessing and treating the health needs of

population groups and aggregates wherever that might occur—in the hospital, at home, in the workplace, or in the community (McKnight & Van Dover, 1994; Williams, 1997).

SKILLS MYTH

The **skills myth** states that community health nurses employ only the skills of basic clinical nursing when working with community clients. This myth leads many nurses to assume that their clinical skills are completely adequate for population-focused practice. It can lead them to overlook a large and sophisticated body of knowledge and competencies required for defining problems and developing solutions for populations (Williams, 1997). Community health nurses need skills drawn from the public health sciences in measurement and analysis (epidemiology and biostatistics), skills in social policy based on the history and philosophy of public health, and skills in management and organization for public health (McKnight & Van Dover, 1994; Milbank, 1976). At the baccalaureate level, nurses can begin to build these skills; they can strengthen and refine them at the masters and doctoral levels.

CLIENT MYTH

Community health nursing involves working with populations, but the **client myth** says that the primary clients are individuals and families. This myth can hinder the nurse from a broader focus on the health of aggregates and groups at risk, which is central to community health nursing practice. It is population-focused practice that distinguishes community health nursing from other nursing specialties (American Public Health Association [APHA], 1996; Williams, 1997).

DIMENSIONS OF THE COMMUNITY AS CLIENT

Chapter 1 defined a *community* as having three features: (1) a location, (2) a population, and (3) a social system (Lynd, 1939). This three-dimensional view especially suits the idea of a local community that can vary by expanding or constricting the geographic boundary (Figure 18–1). For example, one might define the community of Seattle, Washington, as all the people living within the city limits, or the community of greater Seattle as the city, its suburbs, and the other small towns located on its perimeter. A community health nurse might want to restrict the size of the community to a specific district within Seattle for study or services. Regardless of size or geographic boundaries, all these communities still share the three common denominators of an identified location, population, and social system. It is useful to think of these three dimensions of every community as a rough map one can follow for assessing needs or planning for service provision. Further guidance in assessing the health of a community is provided in the Community Profile Inventory (Tables 18–2, 18–3, and 18–4). In considering each di-

mension, one should pay particular attention to the questions that must be asked to assess the health of a community.

Location

Every physical community carries out its daily existence in a specific geographic location. The health of a community is affected by this location, including the placement of health services, the geographic features, climate, plants, animals, and the human-made environment. The location of a community places it in an environment that offers resources and also poses threats (Barker et al., 1994; Neuman, 1995). The healthy community is one that makes wise use of its resources and is prepared to meet threats and dangers. In assessing the health of any community, it is necessary to collect information not only about these location variables but also about how the community relates to them. Do groups cooperate to identify threats? Do health agencies cooperate to prepare for an emergency such as flood or earthquake? Does the community make certain that its members are given available information about resources and dangers? Table 18–2 describes the location perspective of the Community Profile Inventory, including the six **location variables**—community boundaries, location of health services, geographic features, climate, flora and fauna, and the human-made environment.

COMMUNITY BOUNDARIES

To talk about the community in any sense, one must first describe its boundaries (Shamansky & Pesznecker, 1981). All measurements of wellness and illness within a community

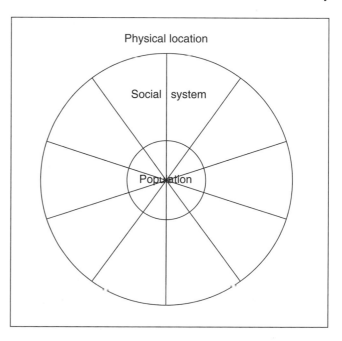

FIGURE 18–1. The community has (1) a physical location, represented here by the square boundary; (2) a population, shown here by the central circle; and (3) a social system, divided here into subsystems.

TABLE 18–2. Community Profile Inventory: Location Perspective

Location Variables	Community Health Implications	Community Assessment Questions	Information Sources
			(For all—various Internet sites)
Boundary of community	Community boundaries serve as basis for measuring incidence of wellness and illness, and for determining spread of disease.	Where is the community located? What is its boundary? Is it a part of a larger community? What smaller communities does it include?	Atlas State maps County maps City maps Telephone book City directory Public library
Location of health services	Use of health services depends on availability and accessibility.	Where are the major health institutions located? What necessary health institutions are outside the community? Where are they?	Telephone book Chamber of commerce State health department County or local health departments Maps Public library
Geographic features	Injury, death, and destruction may be caused by floods, earthquakes, volcanoes, tornadoes, or hurricanes Recreational opportunities at lakes, seashore, mountains promote health and fitness.	What major landforms are in or near the community? What geographic features pose possible threats? What geographic features offer opportunities for healthful activities?	Atlas Chamber of commerce Maps State health department Public library
Climate	Extremes of heat and cold affect health and illness. Extremes of temperature and precipitation may tax community's coping ability.	What are the average temperature and precipitation? What are the extremes? What climatic features affect health and fitness? Is the community prepared to cope with emergencies?	Weather atlas Chamber of commerce State health department Maps Local government Weather bureau Public library
Flora and fauna	Poisonous plants and disease-carrying animals can affect community health. Plants and animals offer resources as well as dangers.	What plants and animals pose possible threats to health?	State health department Poison control center Police department Emergency rooms Encyclopedia Public library
Human-made environment	All human influences on environment (housing, dams, farming, type of industry, chemical waste, air pollution, and so forth) can influence levels of community wellness.	What are the major industries? How have air, land, and water been affected by humans? What is the quality of housing? Do highways allow access to health institutions?	Chamber of commerce Local government City directory State health department University research reports Public library

depend on defining the outer limits of the unit under consideration. Nurses need to be clear, for example, that a target community of the elderly includes a description of age and location (eg, all persons 65 and older in a city or county). Some communities are distinctly separate, such as an isolated rural town, whereas others are closely situated to one another, such as suburbs of a large metropolis. Thus, it is important for the nurse to know the nature of each one's location and explicitly define its parameters.

LOCATION OF HEALTH SERVICES

If the members of a town must travel 300 miles to the nearest clinic or dental office, the health of the community will be affected. When assessing a community, the community health nurse will want to identify the major health centers

and know where they are located. In one city, for example, the alcoholism treatment center for indigent alcoholics was located 30 miles outside the city. This location presented transportation problems and profoundly affected who volunteered for treatment and how long they remained at the center. If a well-baby clinic is located on the edge of a high-crime district, this location may deter parents from using it. It is often enlightening to plot the major health institutions, both inside and outside the community, on a map that shows their proximity and relation to the community as a whole.

GEOGRAPHIC FEATURES

Communities have been constructed in every conceivable physical environment, and that environment certainly can affect the health of a community (see further discussion in Chapter 16 on environmental health). A healthy community takes into consideration the geography of its location, identifies the possible problems and likely resources, and responds in an adaptive fashion (Neuman, 1995). For example, both Anchorage, Alaska, and San Francisco, California, are located on a geologic fault line and subject to major earthquakes. In such places, the health of the community is partly determined by its preparedness for an earthquake and its ability to cope when such a crisis occurs. In Ontario, Canada, a series of lakes called the Lac la Croix is a valuable food resource for the Ojibway Indian communities because they depend on fish from the lakes for their livelihood. In recent years, acid rain generated from coal-burning power plants in the United States and Canada has begun to affect the lakes and the fish. A major food supply has thus become contaminated for the Ojibway Indian communities.

CLIMATE

The climate also has a direct influence on the health of a community (Kilbourne, 1998). When Buffalo, New York, is blanketed with deep winter snows, members of this community are sometimes immobilized for days. Deaths from coronary occlusions increase as people attempt to shovel their walks and uncover their cars. The intense summer heat of another location, such as Phoenix, Arizona, can create other health problems. Skin cancer, for example, is highest in the Sun Belt states. A healthy community will encourage physical activity among its members, but the climate, in turn, affects this activity. Although long, cold winters can restrict activity, one community, St. Paul, Minnesota, holds an annual Winter Carnival. Sporting events, parades, ice sailing, dogsledding, a treasure hunt, and hot air balloon races bring thousands of Minnesotans outdoors at a time when they might otherwise be confined by the weather.

FLORA AND FAUNA

Plant and animal populations in a community are often determined by location. The way a community responds to these populations, whether wild or domesticated, can affect the health of the community. In the Sierra foothill communities of central California, black widow and tarantula spiders, scorpions, and rattlesnakes form insect and reptile populations that pose potential health threats. The poison from a single bite may cause injury and death. In western Washington State, a bushy, attractive plant known as deadly nightshade thrives in backyards and vacant lots, but its appealing black berries are extremely poisonous. The community health nurse will want to know about the major sources of danger from plants and animals affecting the community under study. Are there community agencies that provide educational information about these dangers? Does the populace understand their significance? Are emergency services, such as a poison control center, available to community members?

HUMAN-MADE ENVIRONMENT

Every community is located in the midst of an environment created and transformed by human ingenuity. People build houses and factories, dump wastes into streams or vacant lots, fill the air with gases, and build dams to control streams. All these human alterations of the environment have important implications for community health (Blumenthal & Ruttenber, 1994). A community health nurse might improve the health of a community by working for legislation to prevent disposing of waste chemicals into water or landfills. Such legislation could have avoided the disaster at New York State's Love Canal, where toxic wastes continued to seep into residential areas for many years, severely affecting the community's health.

Agricultural activity can alter the environment through chemical fertilizers and pesticide applications creating potential health hazards to the community. Many farm communities attract migrant workers whose economic and health needs often pose a challenge to community resources (see Chapter 33). Thus, a community's physical location has many health implications.

Population

When one considers the community as the client, the second dimension to examine is the population of the total community. Population consists not of a specialized aggregate, but of all the diverse people who live within the boundaries of the community.

The health of any community is greatly influenced by the population that lives in it. Different features of the population suggest health needs and provide a basis for health planning (Dever, 1997). A healthy community has leaders who are aware of the population's characteristics, know its different needs, and respond to those needs. Community health nurses can better understand any community by knowing about its **population variables,** which are its size, density, composition, rate of growth or decline, cultural characteristics, social class, and mobility. Table 18–3 presents the population perspective section of the Community Profile Inventory.

SIZE

The town of Dover, Delaware, with approximately 10,000 people, and the city of Los Angeles, California, have radically different health problems. If a single case of *Salmonella* poisoning occurred in Dover, health officials would likely learn of it. It would be relatively easy to trace the course, check the few restaurants in town, and interview people about sanitation practices. However, many cases might occur in Los Angeles without the health department's knowledge. Moreover, if these cases were discovered, tracing the source of contamination might involve a long and complicated search. This is only one small way in which population size might affect the health of a community, but it also would influence the presence of slums, heterogeneity of the population, and almost every conceivable area of health need and service. Knowing a community's size provides community health nurses with important information for planning.

TABLE 18–3. Community Profile Inventory: Population Perspective

Population Variables	Community Health Implications	Community Assessment Questions	Information Sources
			(For all—various Internet sites)
Size	The number of people influences number and size of health care institutions. Size affects homogeneity of the population and its needs.	What is the population of the community? Is it an urban, suburban, or rural community?	State health department Census data Maps City or town officials Chamber of commerce
Density	Increased density may increase stress. High and low density often affect the availability of health services.	What is the density of the population per square mile?	Census data State health department
Composition	Composition of the population often determines types of health needs.	What is the age composition of the community? What is the sex composition of the community? What is the marital status of community members? What occupations are represented and in what percentages?	Census data State health department Chamber of Commerce U.S. Department of Labor Statistics
Rate of growth or decline	Rapidly growing communities may place excessive demands on health services. Marked decline in population may signal a poorly functioning community.	How has population size changed over the past two decades? What are the health implications of this change?	Census data State health department
Cultural differences	Health needs vary among sub-cultural and ethnic populations. Utilization of health services varies with culture. Health practices and extent of knowledge are affected by culture.	What is the ethnic breakdown of population? What racial groups are represented? What subcultural populations exist in the community? Do any of the subcultural groups have unique health needs and practices? Are different ethnic and cultural groups included in health planning?	Census data State health department Social and cultural research reports Human rights commission City government Health planning boards
Social class	Class differences influence the utilization of health services. Class composition influences cost of public health services.	What percentage of the population falls into each social class? What do class differences suggest for health needs and services?	State health department Census data Sociological reports
Mobility	Mobility of the population affects continuity of care. Mobility affects availability of service to highly mobile populations.	How frequently do members move into and out of the community? How frequently do members move within the community? Are there any specific populations, such as migrant workers, that are highly mobile? How does the pattern of mobility affect the health of the community? Is the community organized to meet the health needs of mobile groups?	State health department Census data Health agencies serving migrant workers Farm labor offices Program serving transients and the homeless

DENSITY

In some communities, thousands of people are crowded into high-rise apartments. In others, such as farm communities, people live at great distances from one another. We do not yet know the full impact of living in high-density communities, but some research has already shown that crowding affects individual and community health. A classic study of Ohio farmers living in low-density communities suggested that the absence of stress from crowding may have contributed to their reduced rate of coronary artery disease (Nagi, 1959).

A low-density community, however, may have problems. When people are spread out, health care provision may become difficult. There may not be enough resources in the form of taxes to support public health services. Rural communities often suffer from inadequate distribution of health care personnel, ranging from private physicians to community health nurses (see Chapter 31). A healthy community will take into consideration the density of its population. It will organize in ways to meet the differing needs created by its density levels (eg, it will recognize differences in density between the inner city and the suburbs and allocate services accordingly).

COMPOSITION

Communities differ in the types of people who live within their boundaries. A retirement community in Florida whose members are mostly over 65 years of age has one set of interests and concerns. A city with a large number of women in the childbearing years will have another set of concerns. A healthy community is one that takes full account of, and provides for, differences in age, sex, educational level, and occupation of its members, all of which may affect health concerns. For example, in a town where 75% of the workers are employed by a textile mill, the community lives under the threat of brown lung disease, caused by cotton dust. Understanding a community's composition is an important early step in determining its level of health.

RATE OF GROWTH OR DECLINE

Community populations change over time. Some grow rapidly, such as the unparalleled recent growth of Las Vegas as a popular place to live, placing extreme demands on the provision of health and other services. Others, because of economic change, may decline. Any significant fluctuation in population size can affect the health of the community. As people leave to find new employment or better living conditions, overall consumption of goods and services drops. Community morale may suffer, and community leadership may decline. Even a stable community may have problems (eg, members may resist needed change because they see little fluctuation in their population).

CULTURAL CHARACTERISTICS

A community may be composed of a single cultural group, such as an Ojibway Indian reservation in Wisconsin. A community may also be made up of many cultures or subcultures. If a city has a large Hispanic population, a grouping of Native Americans living in the inner city, and a cluster of Vietnamese refugees, the cultural differences among these members will influence the health of the community. These differences, for example, can create conflicting or competing demands for resources and services or create intergroup hostility. A healthy community is aware of such cultural differences and acts to promote understanding between subcultural groups.

SOCIAL CLASS AND EDUCATIONAL LEVEL

Social class refers to the ranking of groups within society by income, education, occupation, prestige, or a combination of these factors (Bond & Bond, 1993). There is no absolute agreement on the income amounts or other criteria used to designate social class categories (upper, middle, lower) other than the government formula used to compute poverty level. Although class distinctions are not clearly defined, class rankings based on occupation, education, and wealth (income plus assets) seem to correlate with many different social patterns and are used frequently in research. Occupational level, in particular, has proved to be a reliable measure, with extraordinarily similar rankings among all societies for which there are data. It appears that people with higher occupational levels experience higher incomes, have more education, exert more political influence, and are more highly esteemed by others.

Educational level, which is closely associated with social class, is a powerful determinant of health-related behavior. Years of formal education are strongly related to age-adjusted mortality in countries as disparate as Hungary, Norway, and England (Institute of Medicine, 1997). In the United States, "adults with less than a high school education can be at increased risk of health problems because of illiteracy, low-paying jobs that do not provide health insurance, lack of health information, and poor living conditions" (Institute of Medicine, 1997, p. 157). People with higher educational attainment tend to be healthier, respond more readily to health professionals' interventions, and are more likely to modify their behavior in positive, health-enhancing ways. These modifications may include smoking cessation, weight control, exercise, dental care, and use of immunizations. People in the lower economic strata of society frequently have the worst health and are more difficult to reach with health information; they also tend to have a higher incidence of communicable diseases. Generally, health promotion and preventive health services are most needed by low-income groups and people with fewer years of education, although most members of a community will benefit from community health efforts.

It is generally known that social classes have different health problems, resources for coping with illness, and ways of using health services (Bond & Bond, 1993). A healthy community recognizes these differences and creates health care services to meet these varied needs.

MOBILITY

Americans are a mobile population. People move to go to college, take new jobs, or seek new climates after retirement. This mobility has a direct effect on the health of communities. If the population turnover is extensive, continuity of services may suffer. Leadership for improving the health of the community may change so frequently that concerted action becomes difficult. High turnover may require special attention to health education about local conditions.

Population groups may arrive and depart in seasonal swings; migrant farm workers, tourists, and college students can affect a community. The community health nurse will want to identify those populations that are seasonally mobile. They not only present special health needs but may also place

TABLE 18–4. Community Profile Inventory: Social System Perspective

Social System Variables	Community Health Implications	Community Assessment Questions	Information Sources
Health system Family system Economic system Educational system Religious system Welfare system Political system Recreational system Legal system Communication system	Each system must fulfill its functions for a healthy community. Collaboration among the systems to identify goals and problems affects health of community. Undue influence of one system on another may lower the health of the community. Agreement on the means to achieve community goals affects community health. Communication among organizations in each system affects community health.	What are the functions of each major system? What are the major subsystems of each system? What are the major organizations in each subsystem? How well do the various organizations function? Are the subsystems in each major system in conflict? Is there adequate communication among the major systems? Is there agreement on community goals? Are there mechanisms for resolving conflict? Do any parts of the total system dominate the others? What community needs are not being met?	(For all—various Internet sites) Chamber of Commerce Telephone book City directory Organizational literature Officials in organizations Community self-study Community survey Local library Key informants

an added burden on a community. If a town of 3,000 people has an annual influx of 10,000 students who disappear in the summer, residents must prepare to meet this population change. In contrast, the small island towns in the San Juan Islands in Puget Sound, Washington, can get such high summer rents that some low-income, year-round residents camp in tents during those months because they are unable to pay the high rents. Thus, the lives of many families are disrupted each year. A healthy community neither ignores nor overreacts to this kind of mobility; rather, it identifies the nature of population change, determines the needs created by such change, and organizes to meet those needs.

Social System

In addition to location and population, every community has a third dimension—a social system. The various parts of a community's social system that interact and influence the system are called **social system variables.** These variables include the health system, family systems, economic system, educational system, religious system, welfare system, political system, recreational system, legal system, and communication system (Dever, 1997). Whether assessing a community's health, developing new services for the mentally ill within the community, or promoting the health of the elderly, the community health nurse needs to understand the community as a social system. A community health nurse working in a tiny village in Alaska needs to grasp the social system of that village no less than a nurse working in New York City. Table 18–4 guides the nurse in assessing a community's social system variables.

THE CONCEPT OF A SOCIAL SYSTEM

A social system is an abstract concept and can be more readily understood by first considering the people who make up the community's population. Each person enacts multiple roles, such as parent, spouse, employee, citizen, church member, or political volunteer. Certain roles tend to be more closely connected, such as supervisor and staff nurse or customer and sales clerk, and the patterns and interactions that emerge among roles form the basis of organizations. Some organizations are informal (eg, an extended family group). Other organizations, such as a city police department or a software business, are more formal. However, all organizations are constructed from roles that are enacted by individual citizens. Organizations, in turn, interact with one another, forming linkages. For example, a medical equipment company and a laboratory establish contracts (linkages) with a home care agency. When a group of organizations are linked and have similar functions, such as all those providing social services, they form a community system or subsystem (Fig. 18–2). It is important to remember that the various community systems have a profound influence on one another. Because this interaction among parts determines the health of the whole, it is the total social system that concerns community health nurses.

THE HEALTH CARE DELIVERY SYSTEM AS PART OF THE SOCIAL SYSTEM

Although community health nurses must examine all the systems in a community and how they interact, the health system is of particular importance. Studying the health system in a community can be compared to assessment of an individual client. The latter involves a head-to-toe examination

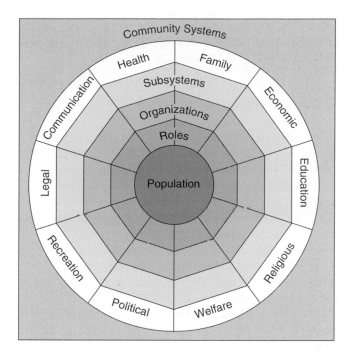

FIGURE 18–2. The community as a social system. Each of the ten major systems of a community includes a number of subsystems that are made up of organizations. Members of the community occupy roles in these organizations.

looking for indications of wellness and illness in the respiratory, musculoskeletal, glandular, skin, and circulatory systems, among others. Initial assessment of a community also begins with a survey of its ten major systems. Before asking about how well the specific parts are functioning, such as whether the police are doing their job or whether the mayor is an effective leader, the nurse would inquire first about the political system as a whole: What are its constituent parts? Are there gross signs of health or illness? To answer questions about a system's level of functioning, one must first know its function (ie, the job it has to do as part of the larger system). The nurse might ask, for example, "How well does the communication system keep citizens informed about important matters?" This question implies that this system has a basic function, information dissemination. The nurse might also ask, "Does the educational system offer equal education to all children of the community?" This question implies that this system's function is to offer learning opportunities to everyone in a particular age group.

The major function of the health system is to promote the health of the community. Community assessment does not merely ask whether, but also how well, the system is functioning. What is the level of health promotion as carried out by the health system of a community? To answer this question, which can be applied to any system, one needs a clear notion about the subsystems, organizations, and roles that make up the system. Any evidence of inadequate functioning becomes a warning signal for more careful assessment. For

---

CLINICAL CORNER | Centerville: Interaction of Social System Variables

The health department of the city of Centerville reported more than 75 pregnancies in 1 year among teenage girls, a large number for the size of this community. The situation placed a marked strain on the families of the girls and caused increased demands for services from the health system. Because the vast majority of these pregnancies were unplanned, they presented a problem for the unmarried teenage parents, their families, and, eventually, the community. What would happen to the babies of these girls? Evidence from research suggested that, in the future, the girls were likely to have larger families, depend more frequently on the welfare system, and have a higher number of health problems than women who were not teenage mothers (Nakamura, 1999).

How should the community respond to this situation? The way it did respond gave clues to the overall health of the community. For one thing, the problem had been ignored, a sign of defense rather than adaptation. When it came to public attention, it divided various groups. Families blamed the schools; school officials, in turn, blamed the changing sexual mores represented in motion pictures and television shows. Some members of the health system asked Planned Parenthood to set up a clinic in the town to provide

family planning education and services as a preventive measure. Almost immediately, however, the religious system entered the picture with groups forming to picket Planned Parenthood facilities because of the association's stand on abortion. Planned Parenthood set up its clinic in an old restaurant on the edge of the business district. Individuals from the religious and economic system (local businesspeople) joined to file suit to prevent Planned Parenthood from occupying the old building. Within months, every major system of this community was involved in the problem, yet it was as far from solution as ever. Indeed, the original problem had almost fallen by the wayside as community members fought over the issues of abortion and the Planned Parenthood headquarters. Vandals set several fires that destroyed part of the building. Pickets daily called attention to what they considered to be an unwanted health agency. Moreover, in the midst of the trouble, more teenagers, some with parents who were deeply involved in the conflict, became pregnant.

What were the signs that this was an unhealthy community? How should the situation be handled? What role could community health nursing play in helping to resolve the problem of teen pregnancies?

example, a high rate of teenage pregnancies in a city may signal inadequate functioning of several systems—perhaps the family, educational, religious, and health systems. Thus, a closer look is in order. What community values influence sexual behavior among adolescents? What sex education programs are available to this population? Does the health system provide information and counseling?

The components of the health system, described in Figure 18–3, include eight major subsystems, each with one or more organizations. Although the community health nurse must be aware of all the systems in a community, the health system is of central importance.

COMMUNITY DYNAMICS

The discussion to this point may have suggested that the community is a rigid structure composed of a geographic location, a population, and a social system. Yet every community has a dynamic or changing quality. Think of the diagram in Figure 18–2 as a wheel that turns as the community changes. Three factors in particular affect community dynamics: (1) citizen participation in community health programs, (2) the power and decision-making structure, and (3) community collaboration efforts of the community (Corrigan & Udas, 1996; Lynd, 1939).

Citizen Participation

In some communities, citizens show little concern about public health issues and rely on health officials to take the entire responsibility. When such apathy abounds, community health nurses will need to promote community education and awareness. In other communities participation may be widespread but either uninformed or obstructive, as when citizens hamper or block the development of some programs. It is much more difficult to work in a community where groups have become polarized by issues such as abortion and fluoridation. Assessing the type and extent of citizen participation will be a necessary first step in community work.

The goal of encouraging responsible participation touches on the concept of self-care discussed in earlier chapters. One goal of community nurses when working with families or groups is to encourage people to participate and take responsibility for their own health care. They have the right to make decisions, to have adequate information, and to consult

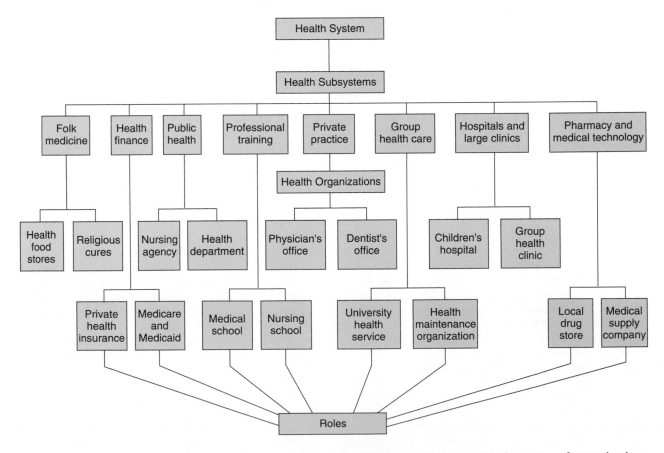

FIGURE 18–3. Components of the health system. This figure shows some representative types of organizations for each of the major subsystems. In turn, each of these organizations also has members with many different roles, and the health of the entire system depends, in part, on how well these roles are carried out.

widely about their own health. The nurse's role is to encourage the full development of a self-care attitude. On a community level, self-care occurs when citizens become committed to the goal of a healthy community. Such a commitment includes responsible involvement in assessing, planning, conducting, and evaluating programs to meet community needs. Community self-care is community health nursing's goal.

Power and Decision-Making Structure

The second dynamic factor, the power and decision-making structure of a community, is a central concern to anyone wishing to bring about change. The description of the community as a social system may suggest that power and decision-making reside primarily in the political system, but this is not the case. In their classic work, Sanders and Brownlee (1979, p. 421) have argued against oversimplifying the decision-making process: "In its naivest, simplest terms this [oversimplification] blandly states that (1) every community has an identifiable power clique and (2) that if you get the members on your side, all of your problems will be solved."

Decision-making in any community is much more complex than this description. Sanders and Brownlee suggest that power is distributed unevenly among members of organizations in various community systems. A key leader may have influence in more than one system, but that power will be diffuse. Seldom does a public health official have power in the religious system or a member of the clergy in the legal system. A dominant leader is one who has specific power, but only within a single community system. An organizational leader will have power, but generally within a single organization, not often in the entire system. Sanders and Brownlee also say that key and dominant leaders will often work through other, less powerful leaders, called functionaries, issue leaders, and spokespersons. (This text explores the topic of leadership and types of leaders in Chapter 10.)

Although power and decision-making in any community are complex, Sanders and Brownlee do suggest several propositions to use as general guidelines for understanding this aspect of a community's dynamics.

1. Because communities differ widely in their power structures, do not assume that what is known about one community will be true of another.
2. The leaders within the health system have different degrees of power and varying spheres of influence; a knowledge of these differences is prerequisite to effective community work.
3. Those leaders whose power is limited to the health system or organizations often have a network of contacts with similar leaders in other systems. Many of the decisions are made informally through this network.
4. Power does not automatically flow through the established bureaucratic channels. Locate the informal patterns of power and decision-making.

5. Beware of leaders who speak authoritatively on issues outside their sphere of power. Their power may be more apparent than real.
6. Leaders from the health system may become key leaders with power that extends far beyond the health system.
7. Learn to distinguish between political, economic, and social power; then use the appropriate combination needed to promote community health issues.
8. Do not overestimate the support of key leaders or power cliques; their support may be helpful but still may leave much organizational work to be done.
9. Try to encourage participation in the decision-making process at every level, from average citizen to key leader.
10. One can assume that leaders in one part of a community are ignorant of needs and problems in other parts of the system. When one contacts such leaders, recognize that they will have to be educated in community health issues.

Community Collaboration Efforts

The third component of a functioning community social system is the degree to which the community collaborates. We mentioned earlier that people in a community have different roles. The owner of a bakery is a high school baseball coach and a member of a church choir. Another person works as a legal secretary, is a Girl Scout leader, and volunteers at the local hospital. These two people interact with most of the major systems in the community. Each person has a different level of power and influence within each role. Knowing that people have many roles within a community, the community health nurse can use this information to enhance collaboration when working toward a health goal in the community.

Community collaboration refers to the ability of the community to work together as a team of citizens, professional and lay people alike, in order to meet an identified need in the community. Centerville had a low level of community collaboration. Healthy communities have a tradition of collaborating that is a part of their infrastructure. They use the skills of the community members to enhance the health of the community for all people. There are broad principles that underpin collaboration efforts (Connell, Kubisch, Schorr & Weiss, 1995; Hooper-Briar & Lawson, 1994):

1. Central to client and community well-being is a recognition that public policy issues are beyond the scope of any single person's or profession's jurisdiction and responsibility. Community members need to be involved to change the status quo, regardless of professional identity or lack thereof.
2. The community needs results-based accountability that emphasizes programs' or projects' effectiveness as the goal.

3. Cultural competence is the norm. All programs (design, delivery, and evaluation) require respect for ethnic and linguistic identity and the reduction of marginalization, invisibility, and devaluation of people.
4. Ethical behavior is fundamental in collaborative relationships.
5. People work in teams, across traditional lines of programs, agencies, disciplines, and professions.
6. Funding strategies need to be decategorized to give more flexibility at the community level as a better way of allocating resources for where they are needed.

Collaboration, a skill community health nurses must be prepared with when working with communities, is discussed in detail in Chapter 8.

TYPES OF COMMUNITY NEEDS ASSESSMENT

After considering the importance of community dynamics, the community health nurse is ready to determine the community's needs. Assessment is the first step of the nursing process, which for nurses means to collect and evaluate information about a community's health status to discover existing or potential needs as a basis for planning future action (Barton, Smith, Brown & Supples, 1993).

Assessment involves two major activities: (1) collection of pertinent data and (2) analysis and interpretation of data. These actions overlap and are repeated constantly throughout the assessment. Thus, while assessing a community's ability to enhance its health, the nurse may simultaneously collect data on community lifestyle behaviors and interpret previously collected data on morbidity and mortality.

Community needs assessment is the process of determining the real or perceived needs of a defined community of people. In some situations, an extensive community study becomes the first priority. In others, all that is needed is a study of one system or even one organization. At other times, community health nurses may need to familiarize themselves with an entire community without going into any depth—in other words, to perform a cursory examination, or conduct a "windshield survey." An asset assessment focuses on the strengths of a community and not its deficits. The type of assessment will depend on variables such as the needs that exist, the goals to be achieved, and the resources available for carrying out the study. Although it is difficult to determine the type of assessment needed in advance, the decision will be facilitated by understanding several different types of community assessment.

Familiarization or "Windshield Survey"

A familiarization assessment is the most necessary. **Familiarization assessment** involves studying data already available on a community, and gathering a certain amount of first-hand data, to gain a working knowledge of the community. Such an approach, sometimes called a "windshield survey," is used in nursing students' community assessment courses and among new staff members in community health agencies (Kulig & Wilde, 1996; Ammerman & Parks, 1998). Nurses drive (or walk) around the community; find health, social, and governmental services; obtain literature; introduce themselves as working in the area; and generally become familiar with the community. This type of assessment is needed whenever the community health nurse works with families, groups, organizations, or populations. Familiarization provides a knowledge of the context in which these aggregates exist and may enable the nurse to connect clients with the community and its resources.

Problem-Oriented Assessment

A second type of community assessment, **problem-oriented assessment,** begins with a single problem and then assesses the community in terms of that problem. Suppose that Jean, the nurse who explored services available for the Angelos' deaf child, had discovered that there were none. Confronted with this problem, one family with one deaf child, she could make a problem-oriented community assessment. Her first step would be to seek to discover the incidence of childhood deafness, both in the community and in the state. Second, the nurse might begin interviewing officials in the schools and health institutions to find out what had been done in the past to assist deaf children. She could check the local library to locate available resources on the subject of deafness, such as the journal *The Deaf American.* Are there interpreters available for adults who use sign language? How do hospitals and courts approach deafness? Are there any clubs or other organizations for deaf adults? Are there school programs for the deaf, and where are they located?

The problem-oriented assessment is commonly used when familiarization is not sufficient and a comprehensive assessment is too expensive. This type of assessment responds to a particular need. The data collected will be useful in any kind of planning for a community response to the problem.

Community Subsystem Assessment

In the **community subsystem assessment,** the community health nurse focuses on a single dimension of community life. For example, the nurse might decide to survey churches and religious organizations to discover their roles in the community. What kinds of needs do the leaders in these organizations believe exist? What services do these organizations offer? To what extent are services coordinated within the religious system and between it and other systems in the community?

The community subsystem assessment can be a useful way for a team to conduct a more thorough community assessment. If five members of a nursing agency divided up the

CLINICAL CORNER   **The Angelo Family and a Familiarization Assessment**

A community health nurse named Jean visited the Angelo family on the outskirts of Philadelphia. During the initial visit, she gathered information, learning that the family was Italian American and that there were four children, ranging in age from 13 to 3. The father had been out of work for 6 months; the mother worked on weekends as a maid in a motel; the oldest boy had been in trouble with the juvenile authorities; a younger child was deaf; and their house appeared rundown. Jean assessed this family, trying to determine its coping ability and its level of health. Furthermore, because community health nursing is population focused, her concern was not only for the Angelo family but also for the population of families with similar problems that this family represented.

However, the nurse's assessment was almost impossible without further knowledge of the community. Was theirs an Italian-American neighborhood with specific cultural influences? What was the extent of unemployment in this city? What were the services for the deaf? Were all the houses in this part of town old and in need of repair? Once the nurse began working with the family, familiarity with the community became even more imperative. She discovered that, as a result of the Angelos' low income, family conflicts were intense. The family members seldom got out; they made almost no

use of the community's recreational system. Before she could help them make use of it, however, the nurse had to find out what resources were available. As she familiarized herself with the community, she discovered Friends of the Deaf, which sponsored a group for parents of deaf children. The nurse could now help Mr. and Mrs. Angelo become part of that group. A quick survey of the religious system in the community revealed two job-transition support groups, one of which would welcome Mr. Angelo. In the meantime, the nurse chose to find out about the welfare system and how this family and other similar families could benefit from its services. Even her own attitude changed as she studied the community. For instance, she discovered that a strike had closed down the plant where Mr. Angelo worked for 20 years, and so could view his and others' unemployment from a broader perspective. Using a familiarization assessment helped this nurse to enhance her practice.

Whatever role nurses play in community health promotion, they will want to be making a continuous study, an ongoing assessment. Whether nurses become client advocates, work with the local government, or operate from a nursing agency serving the elderly, a familiarization assessment is prerequisite for their work.

---

ten systems in the community, and each person did an assessment of two systems, they could then share their findings and create a more comprehensive picture of the community and its needs.

Comprehensive Assessment

The **comprehensive assessment** seeks to discover all relevant community health information. It begins with a review of existing studies and all the data presently available on the community. A survey would compile all the demographic information on the population, such as its size, density, and composition. Key informants would be interviewed in every major system—education, health, religious, economic, and others (Torres, 1998). Then, more detailed surveys and intensive interviews would yield information on organizations and the various roles in each organization. A comprehensive assessment would not only describe the systems of a community but also how power was distributed throughout the system, how decisions were made, and how change occurred (Soriano, 1995; Witkin & Altschuld, 1995).

Because comprehensive assessment is an expensive, time-consuming process, it is seldom performed. Indeed, in many cases, such a thorough research plan might be a waste of resources and might repeat, in part, other studies. Performing

a more focused study based on prior knowledge of needs is often a better strategy. Yet knowing how to conduct a comprehensive assessment has an important influence over the approach to a more focused study.

Community Assets Assessment

The final form of assessment presented here is the **assets assessment.** It "focuses on the strengths and capacities of the community rather than the problems alone," (Ammerman & Parks, 1998). Based on a model developed by McKnight and Kretzmann in the 1980s (McKnight, 1987), it provides tools to conduct a complete functional community assessment and serves as a guide to the community for the nurse. The previous methods mentioned are more needs oriented and deficit based, or are "pathology" models, where the assessment is done in response to needs, barriers, weaknesses, problems, or scarcity in the community. This may result in a fragmented approach to solutions for the community's problems rather than a focused approach to the community's possibilities, strengths, and assets.

The assets assessment begins with what is present in the community. The capacities and skills of community members are identified, focusing on creating or rebuilding relationships among local residents, associations, and institutions to multiply power and effectiveness. This approach requires that the assessor look for the positive, or see the glass as "half full." The nurse can then become a partner in community intervention efforts, rather than merely provide services.

Asset assessment has three levels: (1) an inventory of specific skills, talents, interests, and experiences of individual community members; (2) an inventory of local citizen associations and organizations; and (3) an inventory of local institutions (Ammerman & Parks, 1998). The key, however, is linking these assets together to enhance the community from within.

COMMUNITY ASSESSMENT METHODS

Community health needs may be assessed through a variety of methods. However, regardless of the assessment method employed, data must be collected. Data collection in community health requires the exercise of sound professional judgment, effective communication techniques, and special investigative skills. Four important methods mentioned here are surveys, descriptive epidemiologic studies, community forums/town meetings, and focus groups.

Surveys

A **survey** is an assessment method in which a series of questions is used to collect data for analysis of a specific group or area. Surveys are commonly used and provide a broad range of data that are helpful when used in conjunction with other sources or when other sources are not available (Urrutia-Rojas & Aday, 1991). To plan and conduct community health surveys, one's goals should be to determine the presence of selected environmental, socioeconomic, and behavioral conditions or needs that affect disease control and wellness promotion (Dever, 1997). Thus, the nurse may choose to conduct a survey to determine such things as health care use patterns and needs, immunization levels, demographic characteristics, or health beliefs and practices. The survey method involves three phases needed to ensure an adequate design and appropriate collection of data.

1. Planning Phase
   a. Determine what and why information is needed.
   b. Determine precise data to be collected.
   c. Select population to be surveyed (individuals, a household, a city block).
   d. Select survey method/instrument approach to be used (ie, interviews, telephone calls, questionnaires).
   e. Determine sampling size (a percentage of the total population in question).
2. Data Collection Phase
   a. Identify and train data collectors (eg, interviewers).
   b. Pretest and adjust instrument.
   c. Supervise actual collection, planning for nonresponses or refusals.

3. Data Analysis and Presentation Phase
   a. Organize data for tabulation and analysis.
   b. Apply appropriate statistical methods.
   c. Determine relationships and significance of analysis.
   d. Report the results. Include implications, recommendations, and next steps needed, providing feedback to the population surveyed through a community forum (discussed below) (Polit & Hungler, 1999; Torres, 1998).

Descriptive Epidemiologic Studies

A second assessment method is a **descriptive epidemiologic study,** which examines the amount and distribution of a disease or health condition in a population by person (who is affected?), place (where does the condition occur?), and time (when do the cases occur?). In addition to their value in assessing the health status of a population, descriptive epidemiologic studies are useful for suggesting what persons may be at greatest risk and where and when the condition might occur. They are also useful for health planning purposes and for suggesting hypotheses of disease etiology. Their design and use are detailed in Chapter 14.

The choice of assessment method varies depending on the reasons for data collection, goals and objectives of the study, and available resources. It also varies with the theoretical framework or philosophical approach the nurse uses to view the community (Torres, 1998). That is, the community health nurse's theoretical basis for approaching community assessment will influence her or his purposes and the selection of methodology for conducting the assessment. For example, Neuman's health care systems model forms the basis for the "community-as-partner" assessment model developed by Anderson and McFarlane (1996), and an asset assessment approach guides community interventions using the Assets Model developed by McKnight and Kretzmann (Ammerman & Parks, 1998; McKnight & Van Dover, 1994). Additional methodology resources for assessing community health are available in the list of References and Selected Readings at the close of this chapter.

Community Forum/Town Hall Meetings

The community forum or town hall meeting is a qualitative assessment method designed to obtain community opinions. It is an approach that is completed in the neighborhood of the people involved, perhaps in a school's gymnasium or an auditorium. The participants are selected to participate by being invited by the group organizing the forum. Members come from within the community, representing all segments of the community that are involved with the issue. For instance, if a community is contemplating building a swimming pool, the people invited to the community forum would include potential users of the pool (residents of the community without pools and special groups such as Scouts, elders, and disabled citizens), community planners, health and safety personnel, and any other key people with vested interests. They are asked to give their views on the pool: Where should it be located? Who will use it? How will the cost of building be assumed? What are the drawbacks to having the pool? Any other pertinent issues the participants may raise are included. This method is relatively inexpensive, and results are quickly obtained (Krueger, 1994). A drawback of this method is that the most vocal community members or those with the greatest vested interest in the issue are heard, not giving a representative voice to others in the community also affected by the proposed decision.

This method is frequently used to elicit public opinion on a variety of issues, including health care concerns, political views, or feelings on an issue in the public eye, such as the verdict in a high-profile murder case. Frequently, local cable television channels air important city commissioner or school board meetings, or local news programs may hold town meetings, soliciting public opinion on regional issues. Various other methods of opinion gathering include e-mailing a television news program with a particular view, or using a toll-free number set up especially for a "yes" or "no" vote on an issue. We are seeing more of these electronic methods of data gathering and will continue to see more in the future as people enter chat rooms from home on personal computers (Snider, 1994). These "electronic town meetings" are designed to elicit grassroots opinions from local community members.

Focus Groups

This fourth assessment method is similar to the community forum or town hall meeting in that it is designed to obtain grassroots opinion. However, it has some differences. First, it is a small group process—usually 5 to 15 people (Polit & Hungler, 1999). The members chosen for the group are homogeneous in regards to demographic variables. For example, the focus group may be made up of female community health nurses, young women in their first pregnancy, or retired businessmen. Leadership skills are used along with the small group process to promote a supportive atmosphere and to accomplish set goals (Krueger, 1994). The interviewer guides the discussion according to a predetermined set of questions or topics.

The group usually meets for 1 to 3 hours and may be one of a series. For example, community health nurses from each of six different agencies in a three-county area may meet with the same interviewer in the course of a month, or groups of pregnant women being served by three different agencies may meet over a series of weeks. Each group usually meets only once, but assessment data can be collected from several groups over a period of time. A major advantage of a focus group is its efficiency and low cost, as with the community forum or town hall meeting format. A focus group can be organized "to represent a microcosm of an aggregate, to capture contingents or interest groups within a community, or to

sample for diversity in the population by organizing several groups" (Stevens, 1996, p. 175). However, in each method, there may be some people who are uncomfortable expressing their views in a group situation (Polit & Hungler, 1999).

SOURCES OF COMMUNITY DATA

There are many places the community health nurse can look to obtain data that will enhance and complete a community assessment. Data sources can be primary or secondary and are from international, national, state, and local sources.

Primary and Secondary Sources

Community health nurses make use of many sources in data collection. They begin by talking with community members, including the formal leaders, informal leaders, and community inhabitants because they can frequently offer the most accurate insights and comprehensive information. This is primary data because it is obtained directly from the community. A secondary source of data are people who know the community well and the records they create. This includes health team members, client records, community health statistics, Census Bureau data, reference books, research reports, and community health nurses. Secondary data may not totally describe the community or reflect community self-perceptions; thus, they may need augmentation or further validation.

International Sources

International data are collected by several agencies, including the World Health Organization (WHO) and the six regional offices and health organizations of WHO, such as the Pan-American Health Organization. In addition, the United Nations and global specialty organizations that focus on certain populations or health problems, such as the United Nations Children's Fund, are major sources of international health-related data. WHO publishes an annual report of their activity (World Health Organization, 1998), and, by using the Internet, international statistics of diseases and illness trends can be elicited. Such information from these official sources can give the nurse in the local community information about the immigrant and refugee populations she or he serves.

National Sources

There are official and nonofficial sources of national data community health nurses should access when needed. Official sources develop documents based on data compiled by the government. The following are the major agencies:

U.S. Public Health Service (USPHS). This is the main agency from which data can be retrieved, and its agency, the National Center for Health Statistics, was specifically established for the collection and dissemination of health-related data. USPHS also published *Healthy People 2000* and the newer document *Healthy People 2010* (U.S. Department of Health and Human Services, 1991, 2000). These two major documents were designed to focus America's attention on the major health-related markers in the country and include realistic goals for national, state, and local agencies to work toward over the next decade.

U.S. Bureau of the Census. This agency undertakes a major survey of American families every 10 years, gathering data on health, socioeconomic, and environmental conditions. Since 1990, this information has been available on CD-ROM, allowing several variables to be viewed in combination and to develop a community profile more easily.

National Institutes of Health (NIH). This system of 17 biomedical research agencies focuses on improving the health of our nation. These agencies prevent, diagnose, and treat diseases and conduct and disseminate research findings.

Nonofficial agencies have data sources generated from research they conduct that focuses on the populations or disease/condition they were developed to serve. Each agency collects data at the national level; however, the more accessible arm for services functions at state and local levels. Examples of these agencies include the American Cancer Society (ACS), the American Association of Retired Persons (AARP), and Mothers and Students Against Drunk Drivers (MADD and SADD). Information from such national sources as these allows community health assessment teams to compare their local data with national and state statistics and trends.

State Sources

The most significant state source of assessment data comes from the state health department. This official agency is responsible for collecting state vital statistics and morbidity data. As a resource to local health departments, their support services are invaluable and they are the main source of state health-related data. Nonofficial agencies have state chapters or headquarters and compile their information at the state level. Local nonofficial agency chapters have documents of compiled state and national data on the population, disease, or condition they focus on.

Local Sources

There are many sources of information at the local level. Some key sources are the visitor's bureau, city Chamber of Commerce, city planner's office, health department, hospitals, social service agencies, county extension office, school districts, universities or colleges, libraries, clergy, business and service organizations, and community leaders and key informants. Some of these sources compile their own statistics, but all have views of the community particular to their discipline, interest, or knowledge base.

Frequently, some agencies at the local level develop city or county resource directories. These are updated periodically and are valuable resources for community health assessment teams and for community health nurses.

Not to be overlooked is the usefulness of area maps. These are valuable tools for the community health nurse. Maps can be modest (a free fold-up map from the Chamber of Commerce) or large and detailed, purchased from a discount or stationery store. Often, within the community health agency, a large map is located on one of the walls. This might be just for obtaining directions to clients and services, or it might be a "working" map. Working maps are used to plot such things as the numbers and types of diseases known to be in the community, the location of clients presently being visited and the nurses serving them (by using pins with different colored heads), or locating places in the community that provide services especially needed by clients. The most useful working map for community assessment data is a map used to plot where people with known diseases or conditions live. For instance, red pins are placed in the map at every location where a person with tuberculosis lives, yellow pins are used to locate clients with hepatitis, and so on. This gives a picture of the health of the community. It can monitor trends in illnesses that might be associated with population mobility trends (Fig.18–4).

DATA ANALYSIS AND DIAGNOSIS

This stage of assessment requires analyzing the information gathered, drawing inferences or possible conclusions about the data's meaning, validating those inferences to determine their accuracy, and forming a nursing diagnosis.

The Process of Analysis

First, the data must be validated. Are they accurate? Several validation procedures may be used: (1) data can be rechecked by the community assessment team, (2) data can be rechecked by others, (3) subjective and objective data can be compared, and (4) community members can consider the findings and verify them.

Validated data are then separated into categories such as physical, social, and environmental.

In many instances database sheets are used, providing a structure for organizing data. Next, each category is examined

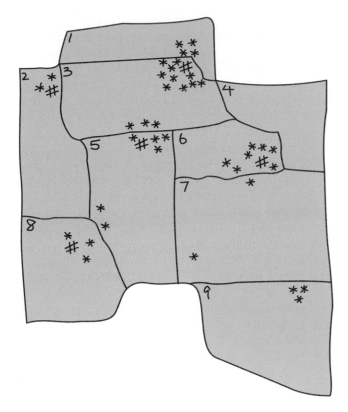

FIGURE 18-4. A sample working map. Reported cases of tuberculosis in Harvard County, June through December 2000. * = cases of tuberculosis; # = cities over 5000 population; 1–9 = census tracts.

There are computer programs designed to analyze community assessment data. For large, complex, or ongoing community assessment plans, this may be the best method. For one-time smaller assessments, the paper-and-pencil method may be sufficient and less unwieldy. Some communities may hire an outside professional assessment service. These teams often use the latest technology when analyzing data. Not all communities can afford such a service, and if key leaders become familiar with the assessment, analysis, and diagnostic process, an investment in a computer program would be worthwhile. Regardless of the analysis method used, data interpretation remains a critical phase of the process.

There is an ever-present danger in data interpretation of making inaccurate assumptions and diagnoses. The importance of validation cannot be overemphasized. Before making a diagnosis, all assumptions must be validated. Are they sound? Community members should participate actively in validation efforts by clarifying perceptions, explaining the circumstances surrounding the situation, and acting as sounding boards for testing assumptions. Other resources are also used, such as the health team members and community leaders, to explore and confirm inferences. Data collection, data interpretation, and nursing diagnosis are sequential activities, with validation serving as the bridges between them (Table 18 5). When performed thoroughly, these steps lead to accurate diagnoses.

Community Diagnosis Formation

to determine its significance. At this point, there may be a need to search for additional information to clarify the meaning of the present data. Only now can inferences be made, and a tentative conclusion about the meaning of the data can be reached.

The next step in the nursing process is a nursing diagnosis. Neufeld & Harrison (1994) used the classic work of Mundinger and Jauron (1975) in developing nursing diagnoses, and proposed using nursing diagnoses in the community

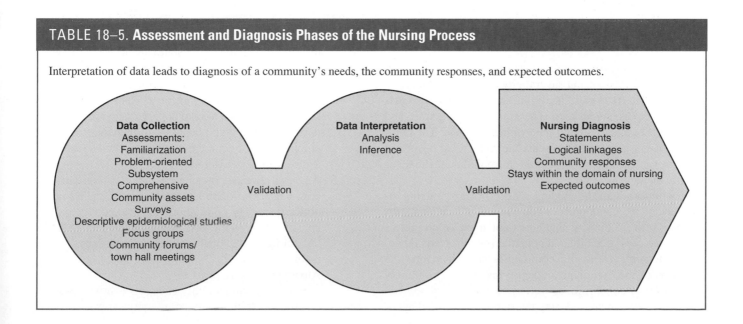

TABLE 18-5. Assessment and Diagnosis Phases of the Nursing Process

Interpretation of data leads to diagnosis of a community's needs, the community responses, and expected outcomes.

Data Collection
Assessments:
Familiarization
Problem-oriented
Subsystem
Comprehensive
Community assets
Surveys
Descriptive epidemiological studies
Focus groups
Community forums/
town hall meetings

Validation

Data Interpretation
Analysis
Inference

Validation

Nursing Diagnosis
Statements
Logical linkages
Community responses
Stays within the domain of nursing
Expected outcomes

by substituting the term *patient* with client, family, group, or aggregate. Their definition is:

> **The statement of a [client's] response which is actually or potentially unhealthful and which nursing intervention can help to change in the direction of health. It should also identify essential factors related to the unhealthful response (Neufeld & Harrison, 1996, p. 221).**

Neufeld and Harrison built on this work by including a wellness diagnosis by using the phrase "healthful response" in lieu of the phrase "unhealthful response." Their wellness diagnosis is:

> **The statement of a client's [community's] healthful response which nursing intervention can support or strengthen. It should also identify the essential factors related to the healthful response (Neufeld & Harrison, 1996, p. 221).**

By substituting the term *community* for client, family, group, or aggregate, the nursing or wellness diagnosis can be applied to the community as a whole. These diagnoses identify the conclusion the nurse draws from interpretation of collected data and describes a community's healthy or unhealthy responses that can be influenced or changed by nursing interventions. Change comes about in collaboration with other community and health team members.

In community health, nurses do not limit their focus to problems; they consider the community as a total system and look for evidence of all kinds of responses that may influence the community's level of wellness. Responses encompass the whole length of the health–illness continuum from specific deficits, such as a lack of senior centers or day care programs, all the way to opportunities for maximizing a community's health by promoting improvement of police protection or the safety of the roadways. Thus, the statement of community response, the diagnosis, can focus on a wide range of topics.

Community Diagnoses

Data have been gathered using a variety of sources. The data have been validated using several procedures. The data have been recorded, tabulated, analyzed, and synthesized so patterns and trends can be seen. The use of charts, graphs, and tables assists in visualizing the synthesized data. The community assessment team presents the findings to peers and uses their expertise to assist in the formulation of the community diagnoses.

Continuing with the nursing process format, nursing diagnoses for the community are developed. **Community diagnoses** refer to nursing diagnoses about the community's ineffective coping ability and potential for enhanced coping. The statements about the community should include the strengths of the community, identifying where community solutions may come from as well as the community's weaknesses or problem areas. Using the standard nursing diagnosis format, community level diagnoses can be developed (Carpenito, 1999). These diagnoses are used as tools as the community begins to plan, intervene, and evaluate outcomes they work toward. Diagnostic categories for individuals, such as a knowledge deficit of senior services or high-risk injury, can frequently be applied at the community level. Acceptable community level nursing diagnoses, adapted from Neufeld and Harrison (1996):

1. Portray a community focus
2. Include the community response (clause #1) and the related factors (clause #2) that have potential for change by community health nursing
3. Include response and related factors that are logically consistent

A wellness diagnosis may:

4. Include maintenance or potential change responses (due to growth and development) when no deficit is present

Community nursing diagnoses must also:

5. Include statements that are narrow enough to guide interventions
6. Have logical linkages between community responses (clause #1) and related factors (clause #2)
7. Use a community response instead of a risk, goal, or a need statement
8. Include factors within the domain of community health nursing intervention.

Examples of wellness and deficit community nursing diagnoses and several diagnoses for a specific community follow:

1. Wellness Nursing Diagnosis for an Assisted Living Community of Elders. The senior residents of an assisted living center have the potential for achieving optimal functioning related to (host factors) their expressed interest in exercise, diet, and meaningful activities, and to (environment factors) their access to exercise opportunities, nutritional information, and social outlets.
2. Deficit Community Nursing Diagnosis for a Rural Farmworker Community. The inhabitants of (name of the town) in (name of the state) are at risk for illness and injury related to (host factors) exposure to pesticides and a lack of motivation to add or use safety devices on farm machinery, lack of safety knowledge, choice to take unnecessary risks, and to (environment factors) lack of family income to purchase newer equipment, plus long hours leading to stress and exhaustion.
3. Anytown, Kansas, is experiencing an increase in crime, many new community members, and a small police force. The community has worked together constructively in the past, communicates well, and has strong recreational outlets for community members:

   Anytown, Kansas, has:

   > Expressed vulnerability and feels overwhelmed related to threats to community safety

Has failed to meet its own expectations related to inadequate law enforcement services

Expressed difficulty in meeting the demands of change related to an influx of new community members

A successful history coping with a previous crisis of teenage pregnancy

Positive communication among community members

A well-developed program for recreation and relaxation

These diagnoses will guide the communities toward maximizing or improving their health as they plan, implement, and evaluate changes that will be measured by outcome criteria they established for themselves. **Outcome criteria** are measurable standards community members will use to measure their success as they work toward improving the health of their community.

The nursing diagnosis changes over time because it reflects changes in the community health status; therefore, diagnoses need to be periodically reevaluated and redefined. The changing diagnosis can be a useful means of encouraging a community toward improved health because it gives community members a clear standard against which to measure their progress (see Research: Bridge to Practice).

WHAT IS A HEALTHY COMMUNITY?

What is a healthy community? If health practitioners are going to assess a community, develop nursing diagnoses for the community, set goals based on outcome criteria for community health, plan to improve the health of a community, and work toward goals, they require some criteria of a healthy community. Just as health for individuals is relative and changes, all aggregates exist in a relative state of health. New needs emerge every day; the system is threatened or weakened and must respond to maintain equilibrium.

Because of their complexity, criteria for healthy communities must be discussed cautiously. At present, there is not wide agreement on such criteria, but four important characteristics of a competent or healthy community were outlined by Cottrell (1976) and are still relevant today:

1. They can collaborate effectively in identifying community needs and problems.
2. They can achieve a working consensus on goals and priorities.
3. They can agree on ways and means to implement the agreed-upon goals.
4. They can collaborate effectively in the required actions.

These general requirements take one closer to an understanding of a healthy community. However, one must still determine the factors that enable a community's systems to work together in these ways. Cottrell suggests several essential conditions for community competence: (1) commitment of members, (2) self-awareness and awareness of others among groups, (3) clarity of situational (positional) definitions, (4) articulateness of various subgroups, (5) effective communication, (6) conflict containment and accommodation, (7) participation (community involvement), (8) management of relations with the larger society, and (9) machinery for effective decision-making. Drawing from this list and other sources (Carlson, 1997; Kang, 1997), the following descriptors can serve as a guide for assessing a healthy community:

1. A healthy community is one in which members have a high degree of awareness that "we are a community."
2. A healthy community uses its natural resources while taking steps to conserve them for future generations.
3. A healthy community openly recognizes the existence of subgroups and welcomes their participation in community affairs.
4. A healthy community is prepared to meet crises.
5. A healthy community is a problem-solving community; it identifies, analyzes, and organizes to meet its own needs.
6. A healthy community has open channels of communication that allow information to flow among all subgroups of citizens in all directions.
7. A healthy community seeks to make each of its systems' resources available to all members of the community.
8. A healthy community has legitimate and effective ways to settle disputes that arise within the community.

RESEARCH Bridge to Practice

Problem-Oriented Community Needs Assessment

Barker, J., Bayne, T., Higgs, Z., Jenkin, S., Murphy, D., & Synoground, G. (1994). Community analysis: A collaborative community practice project. *Public Health Nursing, 11*(2), 113–118.

A concern in many communities is lack of access to health care. To determine the factors that adversely affect access to care, a group of nurses and community members in Washington State conducted a community analysis. Focusing on the problem of access, they developed a questionnaire to obtain information from providers regarding barriers to access. As a result, four community diagnoses were formulated. One was an "insufficient database for community-wide planning" due to lack of certain specified data. Two was "inadequate low-income housing" in the county caused by certain specified conditions. Three was "insufficient community resources for low-income clients." Four was "lack of use of existing community services" by low-income clients due to certain specified barriers. Analysis of these data will be combined with data derived from a subsequent survey of consumers to be used in community-wide planning.

9. A healthy community encourages maximum citizen participation in decision-making.
10. A healthy community promotes a high level of wellness among all its members.

SUMMARY

A major mission of community health nursing practice is to promote the health of aggregates of people. This focus conflicts with the strong value of individualism in the United States, which often distracts nurses from a broad focus. An individualistic focus has led to three pervading myths: (1) that community health nursing involves only clinical nursing in the community setting, (2) that community health nursing employs only the skills of basic nursing, and (3) that the primary client in community health nursing is the individual. In reality, community health nursing is practiced in many settings, employs not only basic nursing expertise but adds many important concepts and skills from public health, and focuses primarily on promoting the health of populations and aggregates, not only individuals.

Any geographic community has three important dimensions to consider when assessing its health needs: location, population, and social system. Location may be further analyzed by considering such variables as its boundary, location of health services, geographic features, climate, flora and fauna, and human-made environment. Population, the second dimension, should be analyzed by determining population size, density, composition, rate of growth or decline, cultural differences, social class, and mobility, to help better understand the community. The third important dimension of a community is its social system, which includes ten major systems (health, family, economic, education, religious, welfare, political, recreation, legal, and communication) and many subsystems. Each subsystem is composed of organizations whose members assume various roles. A Community Profile Inventory guides the community health nurse in making thorough assessments of all these important facets of a community.

Initial assessment of a community begins with a survey of the major systems to determine how well they are functioning. Evidence of malfunctioning in any part becomes a stimulus for further and more detailed analysis.

Community dynamics, the driving forces that govern a community's functioning, also must be considered when assessing community health. Three factors, in particular, affect community dynamics: citizen participation in community health programs, community collaboration efforts, and the power and decision-making structure. Community health nurses need to encourage community self-care by promoting the community's involvement in, commitment to, and responsibility for, its own health. Nurses also need to recognize the sources of community influence in order to use the system effectively to promote community health.

There are primarily five different types of community assessment: (1) familiarization assessment, which studies available data, perhaps adding some firsthand data, to gain a general understanding of the community; (2) problem-oriented assessment, which focuses on a single problem and studies the community in terms of that problem; (3) community subsystem assessment, which examines a single facet of community life; (4) comprehensive assessment, which surveys the entire community in depth; and (5) a community asset assessment that expects a change of thinking where the positive aspects of a community are the focus.

There are many methods for assessing a community's health. Four important ones are surveys, descriptive epidemiologic studies, community forum/town hall meetings, and focus groups. Once data have been collected from all available sources, they must be analyzed. This process can be done by hand or through the use of computer programs. When completed, the community health nurse can begin to form community-level nursing diagnoses. They need to be based on accurately analyzed data and can be deficit focused or wellness focused, either maximizing or improving the health of the community.

A healthy community has a number of characteristics that community health nurses look for when assessing its overall wellness. Among them are a sense of unity, ability to collaborate and communicate effectively, a problem-solving orientation, ability to use yet conserve resources, and ability to handle crises and conflict.

ACTIVITIES TO PROMOTE CRITICAL THINKING

1. Explain to a colleague why it is important to understand and work with the community as a total entity.
2. How does defining community as client change the community health nurse's practice? List some specific examples of how this concept can be applied.
3. If you were part of a health planning team concerned about the health needs of the elderly in your community, what are some location, population, and social system variables you would want to assess? Name some of the sources from which you might collect the data.
4. Discuss under what circumstances you might choose to conduct a problem-oriented community health assessment. What method would you consider using to conduct this assessment, and how would you carry it out?
5. Interview someone from your state or local health department who has recently conducted a community needs assessment survey. Analyze the process they used, comparing that with the steps for conducting a survey described in this chapter.

6. Use the Internet to contribute your ideas in response to a health-related survey taken by a television show, newspaper, or magazine, or share your opinions in a health-related chat room.

REFERENCES

American Public Health Association. (1996, March). *The definition and role of public health nursing. A statement of APHA Public Health Nursing Section,* 1–5. Washington, DC: Author. Available: www.apha.org.

Ammerman, A., & Parks, C. (1998). Preparing students for more effective community interventions: Assets assessment. *Family and Community Health, 21*(1), 32–45.

Anderson, E., & McFarlane, J. (1996). *Community as partner: Theory and practice in nursing* (2nd ed.). Philadelphia: Lippincott-Raven.

Barker, J., Bayne, T., Higgs, Z., Jenkin, S., Murphy, D., & Synoground, G. (1994). Community analysis: A collaborative community practice project. *Public Health Nursing, 11*(2), 113–118.

Barton, J., Smith, M., Brown, N., & Supples, J. (1993). Methodological issues in a team approach to community health needs assessment. *Nursing Outlook, 41*(6), 253–261.

Blumenthal, D., & Ruttenber, J. (1994). *Introduction to environmental health* (2nd ed.). New York: Springer Publishing.

Bond, J., & Bond, S. (1993). *Sociology and health care: An introduction for nurses and other health care professionals* (2nd ed.). Philadelphia: W.B. Saunders.

Carlson, L. K. (1997). The nest step: Creating healthier communities. In B. W. Spradley & J. A. Allender (Eds.), *Readings in community health nursing* (5th ed., pp. 177–185). Philadelphia: Lippincott-Raven.

Carpenito, L. J. (1999). *Handbook of nursing diagnosis* (8th ed.) Philadelphia: Lippincott Williams & Wilkins.

Connell, J., Kubisch, A., Schorr, L., & Weiss, C. (1995). *Roundtable of comprehensive community initiatives for children and families.* Washington: Aspen Institute.

Corrigan, D., & Udas, K. (1996). Creating collaborative, child- and family-centered, education, health, and human services systems. In J. Sikula, T. Buttrey, & E. Guyton (Eds.), *The handbook of research on teacher education: A project of the Association of Teacher-Educators* (2nd ed., pp. 893–921). New York: Macmillan.

Cottrell, L. S., Jr. (1976). The competent community. In B. H. Kaplan, R. N. Wilson, & A. H. Leighton (Eds.), Further explorations in social psychiatry (pp. 195–209). New York: Basic Books.

Dever, G. E. A. (1997). *Improving outcomes in public health practice: Strategy and methods.* Gaithersburg, MD: Aspen.

Ervin, N. E., & Kuehnert, P. L. (1993). Application of a model for public health nursing program planning. *Public Health Nursing, 10*(1), 25–30.

Hooper-Briar, K., & Lawson, H. (1994). *Serving children, youth, and families through interprofessional collaboration and service integration: A framework for action.* Oxford, OH: The Danforth Foundation and the Institute for Educational Renewal, Miami University.

Institute of Medicine. (1997). *Improving health in the community: A role for performance monitoring.* Washington, DC: National Academy Press.

Kang, R. (1997). Building community capacity for health promotion: A challenge for public health nurses. In B. W. Spradley & J. A. Allender (Eds.), *Readings in community health nursing* (5th ed., pp. 221–232). Philadelphia: Lippincott-Raven.

Kilbourne, E. M. (1998). Illness due to thermal extremes. In R. B. Wallace (Ed.), *Maxcy-Rosenau-Last public health and preventive medicine* (14th ed.). Stamford, CT: Appleton & Lange.

Krueger, R. A. (1994). *Focus groups: A practical guide for applied research* (2nd ed.). Thousand Oaks, CA: Sage.

Kulig, J. C., & Wilde, I. (1996). Collaboration between communities and universities: Completion of a community needs assessment. *Public Health Nursing, 13*(2), 112–119.

Lynd, R. (1939). *Knowledge for what? The place of social science in American culture.* Princeton, NJ: Princeton University Press.

McKnight, J. (1987). *The future of low-income neighborhoods and the people who reside there: A capacity-oriented strategy for neighborhood development.* Chicago: Center of Urban Affairs and Policy Research, Northwestern University.

McKnight, J., & Van Dover, L. (1994). Community as client: A challenge for nursing education. *Public Health Nursing, 11*(1), 12–16.

Milbank Memorial Fund Commission. (1976). *Higher education for public health: A report.* New York: Prodist.

Mundinger, M. O., & Jauron, G. D. (1975). Developing a nursing diagnosis. *Nursing Outlook, 23*(2), 94–98.

Nagi, S. Z. (1959, October). Factors related to heart disease among Ohio farmers. *Ohio Agricultural Experiment Station Research Bulletin,* 842.

Nakamura, R. M. (1999). *Health in America: A multicultural perspective.* Boston: Allyn and Bacon.

Neufeld, A., & Harrison, M. J. (1996). Educational issues in preparing community health nurses to use nursing diagnosis with population groups. *Nurse Education Today, 16,* 221–226.

———. (1994). Use of nursing diagnosis with population groups. *Nursing Diagnosis, 5*(4), 165–171.

Neuman, B. (1995). *The Neuman systems model* (3rd ed.). Stamford, CT: Appleton & Lange.

Polit, D. F., & Hungler, B. P. (1999). *Nursing research: Principles and methods* (6th ed.). Philadelphia: Lippincott Williams & Wilkins.

Sanders, I. T., & Brownlee, A. (1979). Health in the community. In H. E. Freeman, S. Levine & L. G. Reeder (Eds.), *Handbook of medical sociology* (3rd ed., pp. 412–433). Englewood Cliffs, NJ: Prentice-Hall.

Shamansky, S., & Pesznecker, B. (1981). A community is . . . *Nursing Outlook, 29,* 182–185.

Snider, J. H. (1994). Democracy on-line: Tomorrow's electronic electorate. *The Futurist, 28*(5), 15–19.

Soriano, F. I. (1995). *Conducting needs assessments: A multidisciplinary approach.* Thousand Oaks, CA: Sage.

Stevens, P. E. (1996). Focus groups: Collecting aggregate-level data to understand community health phenomena. *Public Health Nursing, 13*(3), 170–176.

Torres, M. I. (1998). Assessing health in an urban neighborhood: Community process, data results and implications for practice. *Journal of Community Health, 23*(3), 211–226.

Urrutia-Rojas, X., & Aday, L. A. (1991). A framework for community assessment: Designing and conducting a survey in a

Hispanic immigrant and refugee community. *Public Health Nursing, 8*(1), 20–26.

U.S. Department of Health and Human Services. (1998). *Healthy people 2010 objectives: Draft for public comment.* Washington, DC: U.S. Government Printing Office.

————. (1991). *Healthy people 2000: National health promotion and disease prevention objectives* (S/N 017-001-00474-0). Washington, DC: U.S. Government Printing Office.

Williams, C. A. (1997). Community health nursing—What is it? In B. W. Spradley & J. A. Allender (Eds.), *Readings in community health nursing* (5th ed.). Philadelphia: Lippincott-Raven.

Witkin, B. R., & Altschuld, J. W. (1995). *Planning and conducting needs assessments: A practical guide.* Thousand Oaks, CA: Sage.

World Health Organization (1998). *The world health report.* Geneva: WHO.

INTERNET RESOURCES

Agency for Toxic Substances and Disease Registry
http://www.atsdr1.atsdr.cdc.gov:8080

CDC's National Center for Health Statistics
http://www.cdc.gov/nchswww/

Health Finder
http://www.healthfinder.gov

Hispanic Health Link
http://www.cossmho.org

National Health Information Center
http://nhic-nt.health.org

National Institute of Environmental Health Sciences
http://www.niehs.nih.gov

National Institutes of Health
http://search.info.nih.gov

National Library of Medicine
http://www.nlm.nih.gov

National Safety Council
http://www.ncs.org

Office of Disease Prevention
http://www.odphp.osophs.dhhs.gov

SELECTED READINGS

Aubel, J., & Samba-Ndure, K. (1996). Community participation: Lessons on sustainability for community health projects. *World Health Forum, 17,* 52–57.

Baker, E. L., Melton, R. J., Stange, P. U., et al. (1994). Health reform and the health of the public: Forging community health partnerships. *Journal of the American Medical Association, 272*(16), 1276–1282.

Blane, D. (1995). Editorial: Social determinants of health—Socioeconomic status, social class, and ethnicity. *American Journal of Public Health, 85,* 903–905.

Carey, M. (1994). The group effect in focus groups: Planning, implementing and interpreting focus group research. In J. Morse (Ed.), *Critical issues in qualitative research methods* (pp. 225–241). London, England: Sage.

Conley, E. (1995). Public health nursing within core public health functions: "Back to the future." *Journal of Public Health Management Practice, 1,* 1–8.

Cowley, S., Bergen, A., Young, K., & Kavanagh, A. (1996). Establishing a framework for research: The example of a needs assessment. *Journal of Clinical Nursing, 5,* 53–61.

Fowler, J. (1994). How to build a healthy community. Healthcare Forum's Health Communities Action Kits, Module 3. *The Healthcare Forum.* Available: http://www.well.com/user/bbear/hc_how_to.html.

Higginbotham, N., Heading, G., Pont, J., et al. (1993). Community worry about heart disease: A needs survey of the Coalfields and Newcastle areas of the Hunter region. *Australian Journal of Public Health, 17*(4), 314–321.

Hugman, J., & McCready, S. (1993). Profiles make perfect practice. *Nursing Times, 89*(27), 46–49.

Kuehnert, P. L. (1995). The interactive and organizational model of community as client: A model for public health nursing practice. *Public Health Nursing, 12*(1), 9–17.

McEwen, J., Russell, E. M., & Stewart, S. (1995). Needs assessment in Scotland: Collaboration in public health. *Public Health, 109,* 179–185.

Parks, C., & Straker, H. O. (1996). Community assets mapping: Community health assessment with a different twist. *Journal of Health Education, 27,* 321–323.

Sen, R. (1994). Building community involvement in health care. *Social Policy, 24,* 32–43.

Timmereck, T. C. (1995). *Planning, program development, and evaluation: A handbook for health promotion, aging, and health services.* Boston: Jones & Bartlett.

White, J. E., & Valentine, V. L. (1993). Computer assisted video instruction and community assessment. *Nursing and Health Care, 14*(7), 349–353.

Wickizer, T., Von Korff, M., Cheadle, A., Maeser, J., Wagner, E., Pearson, D., Beery, W., & Psaty, B. (1993). Activating communities for health promotion: A process evaluation method. *American Journal of Public Health, 83*(4), 561–567.

Wolf, E. M., Young, B. R., & Cotton, K. L. (1994). Collaborative needs assessment for mental child health program development. *Journal of Mental Health Administration, 21,* 161–169.

Planning, Intervention, and Evaluation of Health Care in Communities

KEY TERMS

- Coalition
- Community development
- Evaluation
- Goals
- Implementation
- Interaction
- Objectives
- Partnerships
- Planning
- Setting priorities

LEARNING OBJECTIVES

Upon mastery of this chapter, you should be able to:

- Describe the nursing process components of planning, implementing and evaluating as they apply to community health nursing.
- Discuss methods the community health nurse uses to interact with the community.
- Identify the four phases of developing a plan for meeting the health needs in the community.
- Identify actions taken when implementing health promotion activities with aggregates.
- Describe the process of evaluating aggregate health interventions.
- Discuss characteristics of the nursing process affecting nursing practice with the community as client.
- Describe the role of the community health nurse as a catalyst for community development.

Since the beginning of your nursing program, you have been familiar with one of the classic organizing systems underlying nursing practice—the nursing process. Does it continue to provide the community health nurses with the structure they need to work effectively with families and aggregates that have complex health care needs? Are there additional models and tools that can guide you when you work in the community? These are some of the questions addressed in this chapter as we continue to explore the usefulness of the nursing process in the community.

Consisting of a systematic, purposeful set of interpersonal actions, the nursing process provides a structure for change that remains a viable tool employed by the community health nurse. In Chapter 18, we examined the first two steps of this process: assessment and nursing diagnosis. This chapter examines the last three steps of the nursing process: planning, implementation, and evaluation as applied to the aggregate level. These five components give direction to the dynamics for solving problems, managing nursing actions, and improving the health of communities and community health nursing practice.

Three characteristics support the use of the nursing process in community health nursing. First, the nursing process is a problem-solving process that addresses community health problems at all aggregate levels and aims to prevent illness and to promote the public's health. Second, it is a management process that requires analysis of a situation, making decisions, planning, organizing, directing and controlling service efforts, and evaluating outcomes. As a management tool, the nursing process addresses all aggregate levels. Third, it is a change process that works to improve various levels of health-related systems and the way people behave within those systems.

In this chapter, we also explore two other models for planning, intervening, and evaluating health care delivered to aggregates. The models highlighted are the Health Planning Process and the Omaha Classification System, which was developed specifically for use in community health settings. In addition, we will briefly explore the usefulness of the North American Nursing Diagnosis Association (NANDA) nursing diagnoses with families and aggregates as services are planned, implemented, and evaluated.

NURSING PROCESS COMPONENTS APPLIED TO COMMUNITY AS CLIENT

In community health, the nursing process involves a series of components, or steps, that enable the nurse to work with aggregates to achieve their optimal health. Process, the moving element of this tool, means forward progression in an orderly fashion toward some desired result. Nursing theorists attach different labels to the components, but all agree on the basic sequence of actions: assessment, diagnosis, planning, implementation, and evaluation.

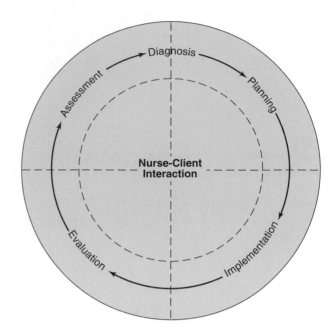

FIGURE 19–1. Nursing process components. Nurse–client interaction, a preamble structure, forms the core of the process. As a nurse and client maintain a reciprocal exchange of information and trust through interaction, they can effectively assess client needs; diagnose needs; and plan, implement, and evaluate care.

Interacting With the Community

All steps of the nursing process depend on **interaction,** reciprocal exchange, and influence among people. Although nurse–client interaction is often an implied or assumed element in the process, for community health nursing, it is an essential first consideration. Whether listening to a group of elderly people, teaching a class of expectant mothers, lobbying in the legislature for the poor, or working with parents to set up a dental screening program for children—all involve relationships, and relationships require interaction. This mutual give and take between nurse and clients, whether a family, a group of mothers on a Native American reservation, or a population of school children, is an expected and much needed skill, integrated throughout the nursing process (Fig. 19–1).

NEED FOR COMMUNICATION
Interaction Requires Communication. When a community health nurse initially contacts a group of community leaders, for example, any information the nurse may have in advance can give only partial clues to that group's needs and wants. Unless they begin by talking and listening, the steps in the nursing process will go awry. By open, honest sharing, the nurse (and possibly others on the health team) will begin to develop trust and establish lines of effective communication. For instance, the nurse explains who he or she is and why he or she is there. The nurse encourages the group members to talk about themselves. Nurse and group members together discuss their relationship and clarify the desired nature of that alliance. Does the group want help to identify and work on its health needs? Would its members like this nurse to continue regular contacts? What will their respective roles be? Effective communication, as a part of interaction, is essential to develop understanding and facilitate a free exchange of information between nurse and clients.

Interaction Is Reciprocal. It is a two-way sharing of information, ideas, feelings, concerns, and self. Nurses must avoid the temptation either to do all the talking or merely to listen while group members monopolize the conversation. There is a dynamic exchange between two systems, with the community health nurse (and other collaborating health professionals) representing one system and the client group representing the other. Whether the client is a parent group, a homeless population, or an entire community, this exchange involves a two-way sharing between the nurse and client group. The key elements of interaction are mutuality and cooperation.

Consider the following example: A dozen junior high school boys, most of whom were on the football team, met for several weeks with the school nurse to discuss physical fitness, nutrition, and other health topics. After their agreed-upon goals had been accomplished, the nurse wondered whether further meetings were needed. The nurse raised the question and offered several topics, such as taking drugs and preventing injuries, for possible future sessions. The boys were not interested in these suggestions but, after more discussion, said they did want help with talking to girls. Renewed interaction was necessary as a first step in reapplying the nursing process and redefining the goals for the group.

Interaction Paves the Way for a Helping Relationship. As nurse and client interact, each is learning about the other. There is a period of testing before trust can be fully established. For the school nurse, establishing interaction had been more difficult at the time of the initial contact with the boys. They had been reluctant to talk, felt embarrassed to discuss personal subjects with an adult they did not know, and yet had strong interests in bodybuilding and personal appearance, strong enough to attract them to these optional sessions. Interaction began with a friendly exchange on nonthreatening topics and gradually deepened as the boys seemed ready to discuss personal subjects. Now it was relatively simple to talk about a new "problem" (and start the nursing process over again) because a helping relationship had already been developed. The nurse had a track record. The boys trusted, respected, and liked the nurse, so they were happy to interact around a newly stated need.

AGGREGATE APPLICATION

Because community health practice focuses largely on the health of population groups, interaction goes beyond the one-to-one approach of clinical nursing (Williams, 1977). The challenge that the community health nurse faces is a one-to-aggregate approach. A group of parents concerned about teenage alcoholism, handicapped people needing access ramps, and a neighborhood's elderly population frightened by muggings and theft are all aggregates of people with different concerns and opinions. As defined in previous chapters, an *aggregate* refers to a mass or grouping of distinct individuals who are considered as a whole. Each person in an aggregate is influenced by the thinking and behavior of the other group members. Nursing interaction with an aggregate as the client demands an understanding of group behavior and group-level decision-making, and it requires interpersonal communication at the group level. Thus, the task of interacting is more complex with an aggregate than with an individual, but it also can be challenging and rewarding. Once community health nurses address themselves to understanding aggregate behavior, they can capitalize on the potential of group influence to make a far-reaching impact on the health of the total community. Chapter 8 examines communicating and working with groups more closely.

Forming Partnerships and Building Coalitions

A further health-planning consideration is that aggregate-level nursing practice requires teamwork. The job of planning for the health of an entire community or a community subsystem requires that the nurse collaborate with other professionals. Usually, the nurse is part of an organized team, separate from the agency that employs the nurse, which comes together to improve the health of the community. Each group member brings expertise and a particular view of the problem. These interprofessional work groups are formed as either partnerships or coalitions.

Partnerships are agreements between people (and agencies) to benefit a joint purpose. A partnership can be large, involving a multinational corporation and several high schools or a city government and the county jail system, or the partnership could be more modest, involving a group of senior citizens and a preschool program or a Girl Scout troop and a community recycling program. Community-wide partnerships require more planning and coordination than do small partnerships. For example, a college's nursing program may need two additional temporary and part-time faculty members during a time with increased student enrollment in their community health nursing course. The county public health department is interested in more new graduate nurses coming to work in their agency. The nursing program and the health department form a partnership and design a plan to solve both of their problems. The health department selects two masters-prepared staff nurses to become clinical instructors for two community health nursing undergraduate clinical laboratories one day a week for two semesters. The benefits to both partners and the people involved include: The nursing program solves a temporary staffing problem; the staff nurses use their expertise with the students, which enhances their practice and the students' experience; and the health department has oriented and introduced a pool of students to their agency and its services who may choose to work there after graduation, boosting their staffing.

A **coalition** is an alliance of individuals or groups working together to influence outcomes of a specific problem (Chausmer, 1997). Coalitions are an effective means to achieve a collaborative and coordinated approach to solving community problems. Steps to coalition building include defining goals and objectives, conducting a community assessment, identifying key players or leaders, and identifying potential coalition members.

Once these steps have been achieved, the leader needs to keep the coalition active. This is best done by knowing the coalition members, running effective meetings, staying in touch with the members, and keeping the members involved (Display 19–1).

All sound public health practice depends on pooling resources, including people, in ways that will best serve the public. Whether health service is aimed at families, a group, subpopulation, population, or community, the consumers of that service are equally important members of the team. In planning for a community's health, the community (represented by appropriate individuals and agencies) must be involved. Community health nurses cannot lose sight of the need for client involvement at all levels and in all stages of community health practice.

DISPLAY 19–1. Coalition Contributions

A suburban community with a large teenage population is interested in preventing motor vehicle injuries. Assessment reveals a high incidence of injury to adolescents with alcohol consumption as a factor. The local paramedics and police have been interested in the problem for a number of months. Local police, alcohol store owners, area parents, school counselors and nurses, Alcohol Abuse Council professionals, and high school Students Against Driving Drunk (SADD) members are all interested in educating teens about alcohol and motor vehicles. In this situation, there is a need and an interest. Forming a coalition may help to reduce the amount of adolescent drinking and motor vehicle use, thus reducing the high incidence of injury to the teens in this community (Chausmer, 1997).

PLANNING TO MEET THE HEALTH NEEDS IN THE COMMUNITY

Planning is a logical, decision-making process of designing an orderly, detailed program of action to accomplish specific goals and objectives. Planning for community health is based on assessment of the community and the nursing diagnoses formulated, but assessment and diagnosis alone do not prescribe the specific actions necessary to meet clients' needs. Knowing that the group of mothers at the well-child clinic needed emotional support did not tell the nurse what further action was indicated. A diagnosis of culture shock (adjustment deficit to a contrasting culture) for a family newly arrived from Cuba does not reveal what action to take. The nurse must plan (see Levels of Prevention).

Using a Model

Planning for community health caregiving and programs can be enhanced by the use of conceptual frameworks and models. A model helps to identify target population characteristics for intervention, clarify program goals, and specify nursing interventions and client outcomes (Ervin & Kuehnert, 1993). A planning model also enables the nurse to test ideas and adjust solutions before actual implementation. Finally, use of a model enhances the planning process and promotes effectiveness of services as well as professional standards of practice (Ervin & Kuehnert, 1993).

In addition to a model, a systematic approach to planning guides the community health nurse to (1) list needs in order of priority, (2) establish goals and objectives, and (3) record the plan. As they do in the rest of the nursing process, community health nurses collaborate with clients and other appropriate professionals in each of these planning activities.

THE HEALTH PLANNING PROCESS

The health planning process is a four-stage system used when designing new health-related programs or services in the community. It is used by health educators when designing educational programs, by administrators in community health agencies to initiate new services, or when other nonnurses develop services. The nursing process is very similar to the health planning process (Table 19–1). Each model helps to promote service effectiveness in addition to maintaining standards of practice. Community health nurses familiar with both the health planning process and the nursing process should be able to work in collaboration with community health professionals using either model.

THE OMAHA SYSTEM

The Omaha System was developed in the 1970s by the Visiting Nursing Service of Omaha as a framework for caregiving. The Omaha system includes three schemes: problem classification, intervention, and the problem rating scale for outcomes. The Omaha system involves 40 client problems grouped into four domains: environmental, psychosocial, physiologic, and health behaviors with modifiers and signs and symptoms (Martin, 1994; Martin & Scheet, 1992) (Display 19–2). Although the Omaha System is a useful tool in the community with individuals, families, and small groups, it has limits because, in its present structure, use does not adapt well to the care of populations, the primary focus of community health nursing.

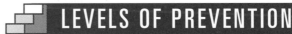

LEVELS OF PREVENTION

HEALTH PLANNING FOR COMMUNITY AS CLIENT

GOAL
To reduce the incidence of child abuse in a given community by 50% within 2 years.

PRIMARY PREVENTION
Assess factors contributing to child abuse; identify families in the community at greatest risk (parents with history of child abuse, families under great stress, and so forth); institute family life education programs through schools and community groups; develop community resources to support health promotion and protection programs.

SECONDARY PREVENTION
Develop early detection programs through schools, clinics, and physicians' offices; promote enforcement of child protection laws; establish programs to provide prompt treatment for abused children and abusing parents.

TERTIARY PREVENTION
Establish rehabilitation programs for abused children including safer home placement, physical and emotional treatment, self-esteem building. Rebuild the family unit if appropriate or possible.

TABLE 19–1. Comparison Between the Health Planning Process and the Nursing Process

Health Planning Process	Nursing Process
1. ASSESSMENT STAGE	**1. ASSESSMENT**
	Determine data needed and collect data.
	Interpret data and identify needs.
	Set goals based on needs.
2. ANALYSIS AND DESIGN	**2. DIAGNOSIS**
	Analyze findings and set specific objectives.
	Design alternative interventions.
	Analyze and compare pros and cons of various solutions.
	Formulate nursing diagnoses.
	3. PLANNING
Create a plan.	List needs in order of priority.
	Establish goals and objectives.
	Write an action plan.
3. IMPLEMENTATION STAGE	**4. IMPLEMENTATION**
	Describe how to operationalize the plan.
	Design a method for monitoring progress.
4. EVALUATION STAGE	**5. EVALUATION**
	Examine costs and benefits of proposed solution.
	Judge the potential outputs, outcomes, and impact of plan.
	Modify to achieve the best plan.
	Present plan to sponsoring group or agency.
	Obtain acceptance (and funding).

DISPLAY 19–2. Components of the Omaha System

Domains
Environmental
Psychosocial
Physiologic
Health-related behaviors

Sample Problems
Communication with community resources
Health care supervision
Hearing
Income
Neighborhood/workplace safety
Personal hygiene
Respiration

Typical Modifiers
Health promotion
Potential deficit
Potential impairment
Deficit
Impairment
Individual
Family

Samples of Signs and Symptoms
Inadequate money management
Difficulty buying necessities
Dissatisfaction with services
Absent/abnormal response to sound
Inability to coordinate multiple appointments/regimens
Other (specify)

(Adapted from Martin, K.S. & Scheet, N.J. [1992]. *The Omaha system: A pocket guide for community health nursing,* Philadelphia: W.B. Saunders.)

The Omaha system addresses situations encountered by clients in the community more accurately than the present taxonomy of the NANDA nursing diagnoses. NANDA focuses on diagnoses for ill individuals with limited opportunity to design wellness nursing diagnoses with a health-promoting focus or diagnoses for more complex situations that aggregates in the community present. However, there has been recent development of NANDA family diagnosis categories, such as altered family processes, parental role conflict, and compromised family coping (North American Nursing Diagnosis Association, 1999). As health care continues to move into the community in the 21st century, there may be further development in both the Omaha system and NANDA diagnoses to assist community health nurses in assessing, planning, implementing, and evaluating care with aggregates.

Setting Priorities

Setting priorities involves assigning rank or importance to clients' needs to determine the order in which goals should be addressed (Rohrer, 1996). One way to order needs is to group them into three categories—immediate, intermediate, and long-range—and then assign a priority to those in each group. Immediate needs are more urgent but not necessarily more important. For example, a community health nurse and a group of senior citizens wanted a class on exercise techniques, yet did not have a place to meet. Obviously, their goal, to learn about appropriate exercises, was more important than finding a place to meet; however, they had to first find a place to meet (immediate need) in order to accomplish their long-range goal. Some needs are ranked as immediate because they are potentially hazardous or life-threatening, such as lack of eye protection in a school welding class. Other needs are ranked first because they are of the greatest concern to clients. For example, a group of elderly people who were fearful of crime selected neighborhood safety as their highest priority although they had identified many other needs.

Establishing Goals and Objectives

Goals and objectives are crucial to planning. The diagnosis that identifies needs must be translated into goals to give focus and meaning to the nursing plan. **Goals** are broad statements of desired end results, and **objectives** are specific statements of desired outcomes stated in behavioral terms that can be measured and include target dates. Objectives, as used here, are like stepping stones to help one reach the end results of the larger goal. For the elderly group concerned about crime in their neighborhood, their need, goal, and objectives were defined in the following manner:

Need: The group of elderly people has altered coping ability related to their fear of crime.

Goal: Within 6 months, this group of elderly people will be free to walk the streets of their neighborhood without any incidents of criminal assault.

Objectives:

1. By the end of the 1st month, a safety committee (composed of seniors, nurses, police, and other appropriate community members) will be established to study the crime patterns in the neighborhood.
2. The safety committee will develop strategies for crime reduction and elder protection to be presented to the city council for approval by the end of the 3rd month.
3. Safety strategies, such as increased police surveillance and escort services, will be implemented by the end of the 5th month.
4. By the end of the 6th month, nursing assessment of the seniors will demonstrate that they report feeling free to walk the streets.
5. Within the 6th month, there will be no reported incidents of criminal assault.

Development of objectives depends on a careful analysis of all the ways one could accomplish the larger goal. One should first select the courses of action best suited to meeting the goals, and then build objectives. For the group of elderly people, other alternatives, such as staying indoors or always walking in pairs, were considered and rejected. Their choice was to find a way to make their environment safe and enjoyable.

Some rules of thumb are helpful when writing objectives. (1) Each objective should state a single idea. When more than one idea is expressed, as in an objective to obtain equipment and learn procedures, completion of the objective is much more difficult to measure. (2) State each objective so it describes one specific behavior that can be measured. For instance, the fourth objective describes that the seniors will report feeling free to walk outdoors within 6 months. It describes a behavior that can be measured at some point in time. One can more readily evaluate objectives that include specifics such as what will be done, who will do it, and when it will be accomplished. Then everyone knows exactly what has to be done and

within what time frame. Writing measurable objectives makes a tremendous difference in the success of planning.

Planning means thinking ahead. The nurse looks ahead toward the desired end product and then decides on all the intermediate actions necessary to meet that goal. Sometimes, an objective itself describes the intermediate actions. At other times, the nurse may wish to break down an objective further into several activities. For example, with the second objective, the safety committee was charged with developing strategies, presenting them to the city council, and gaining approval. Good planning requires this kind of detail.

Making decisions is an important part of planning. Decisions must be made while establishing priorities. Selecting goals and, from a variety of possible solutions, choosing the best courses of action to meet the goals require decisions. Further decision-making is involved in selecting objectives and, when indicated, the specific actions to accomplish the objectives.

To facilitate planning and decision-making, the community health nurse involves other people. Clients, of course, must be included at every step. They, after all, are the ones for whom the planning is being done and without whose insights and cooperation the plan may not succeed. At times, the involvement of other nurses is important. Team meetings, nurse-supervisor conferences, or nurse-expert consultant sessions are all useful resources for planning. In addition, the community health nurse will frequently wish to confer with members of other health and professional disciplines. Interdisciplinary team conferences are valuable for gaining a broader perspective and enlisting wider support for the evolving plan.

Recording the Plan

Recording the plan is the next step. Up to this point, the planning phase has been a series of intellectual exercises done jointly with clients and perhaps with other health team members. The nurse has probably written notes on the decisions made about priorities, goals, objectives, and actions, but now the nurse needs to clearly record the plan. One way to record the plan is to list items in columns with space for the nurse to record specifics. It is also helpful to share copies of the plan with clients. In many instances, having copies of the plan promotes clients' sense of being equal partners in the responsibility of meeting goals. It may also encourage clients to contribute more ideas once they see the plan in writing.

Regardless of the type of plan format used, certain items must be included in the written plan:

1. *A database* comprises all the subjective and objective information collected about clients—physical, psychological, social, and environmental. It includes background health information (past and present); aggregate health assessment; and group history or group systems review. The database is best kept with a format that allows space for ongoing entries and analysis. Various computer programs and applications can assist this process (Dever, 1997).
2. *Aggregate needs* are the specific areas related to

clients' health that have been identified for intervention. Preferably, they are areas that both clients and nurse agree require action. They are drawn from the nursing diagnosis. Goals are statements that describe the resolution of needs. For clarity in planning, both a written need statement and a written goal statement are helpful.

3. *Objectives* are the specific statements that describe in behavioral and measurable terms what the nurse and clients hope to accomplish. It is often necessary to construct several objectives, sometimes around different categories of needs, to achieve comprehensive results. These objectives provide the nurse planner with specific targets at which to aim and around which to design actions.

4. *Planned actions* are the specific activities or methods of accomplishing the objectives or expected outcomes. Plans should include appropriate actions by nurse, clients, and other people.

5. *Outcome measurement* is the judging of the effectiveness of goal attainment. How and when was each objective met, and if not met, why not? It is essential to include this type of outcome evaluation in the written plan. Progress notes are not the same as outcome measurement. Progress notes are useful, periodic summaries that give a running account of what is occurring, but the outcome measurement requires analysis of these occurrences and conclusions to be drawn. Progress notes and outcome measurement may be combined if space is allowed on the plan format. Generally, it is best to enter progress notes on a separate space.

IMPLEMENTING PLANS FOR PROMOTING THE HEALTH OF AGGREGATES IN THE COMMUNITY

Implementation is putting the plan into action and actually carrying out the activities delineated in the plan, either by the nurse and other professionals or by clients. Implementation is often referred to as the action phase of the nursing process. In community health nursing, implementation includes not just nursing action or nursing intervention but collaborative implementation by the clients and perhaps other professionals. Certainly, the nurse's professional expertise and judgment provide a necessary resource to the client group. The nurse is also a catalyst and facilitator in planning and activating the action plan. However, a primary goal in community health is to help people learn to help themselves toward their optimal level of health (see The Global Community). To realize this goal, the nurse must constantly involve clients in the deliberative process and encourage their sense of responsibility and autonomy. Other health team members, too, may participate in carrying out the plan. Therefore, all are partners in implementation.

THE GLOBAL COMMUNITY

Implementing a Program for Youth in Mexico

Low-income youth in Mexico's overcrowded cities face significant health and social problems. Many have poor relationships with their families, are unable to find work, and spend all day in the streets. Some have turned to selling drugs or have jointed gangs, often because they have no positive ways to channel their energy. Poor nutrition, dental caries, sexually transmitted diseases, drug addiction, violence, and crime are among this population group's problems. Starting in 1982, an organization called Centro Juvenil Promocion Integral (CEJUV) offered programs and activities for young people between 14 and 28 years of age in Mexico City, Cuernavaca, and Juarez (Kellogg Foundation, 1994). Using an integrated approach, CEJUV continues to provide young people assistance with such things as studies and homework, career counseling, vocational training, sports activities, health education programs, and community celebrations to promote intergenerational dialogue. CEJUV's purpose is to provide alternative educational experiences for low-income youth by involving them in volunteer activities in their neighborhoods. Many young Mexicans are discovering new capabilities and building bridges to a more promising future.

Preparation

The actual course of implementation, outlined in the plan, should be fairly easy to follow if goals, expected outcomes, and planned actions have been designed carefully. Professionals and clients should have a clear idea of the who, what, why, when, where, and how. Who will be involved in carrying out the plan? What are each person's responsibilities? Do all understand why and how to do their parts? Do they know when and where activities will occur? As implementation begins, nurses should review these questions for themselves as well as clients. This is the time to clarify any doubtful areas and thus facilitate a smooth implementation phase.

Even the best planning, though, may require adjustments. For example, some nurses offering a health fair for seniors discovered that the target group did not have transportation to the site because the volunteering bus company had withdrawn its offer. Instead, the nurses arranged for volunteers from local churches to pick up the seniors and deliver them afterward to their homes. Thus, implementation requires flexibility and adaptation to unanticipated events.

Activities or Actions

The process of implementation requires a series of nursing actions or activities to be taken:

1. The nurse applies appropriate theories, such as systems theory or change theory, to the actions being performed.
2. The nurse helps to facilitate an environment that is con-

ducive for carrying out the plan, such as a quiet room in which to hold a group teaching session or engaging local officials' support for an environmental cleanup project.

3. The nurse, along with other health team members, prepares clients for the service to be received by assessing the clients' knowledge, understanding, and attitudes and carefully interpreting the plan to clients. This interaction nurtures open communication and trust between nurse and clients. Professionals and clients (or if a larger aggregate, its representatives) form a contractual agreement about the content of the plan and how it is to be carried out.

4. The plan is carried out or modified and then carried out by professionals and clients. Modification requires constant observation and interchange during implementation because these actions determine the success of the plan and the nature of needed changes.

5. The nurse and the team monitor and document the progress of the implementation phase by process evaluation, which measures the ongoing achievement of planned actions.

The Research: Bridge to Practice display describes a study undertaken to determine effective interventions for promoting wellness in the elderly.

EVALUATING IMPLEMENTED AGGREGATE HEALTH PLANS

Evaluation, the final component of the nursing process, is the last in a sequence of actions leading to the resolution of client health needs. As described before, evaluation refers to measuring and judging the effectiveness of that goal attainment. The nursing process is not complete until evaluation takes place. Too often, emphasis is placed primarily on assessing client needs and planning and implementing service. How effective was the service? Were client needs truly met? Professional practitioners owe it to their clients, themselves, and to other health service providers to evaluate.

Evaluation is an act of appraisal in which one judges value in relation to a standard and a set of criteria (Timmreck, 1995). For example, when eating dinner in a restaurant, diners evaluate the dinner in terms of the standard of a satisfying meal. Their criteria for "a satisfying meal" may include qualities such as a wide variety of choices on the menu, reasonable price, tasty food, nice atmosphere, and good service. They also evaluate the meal for a purpose. Does this restaurant serve their purpose of providing a satisfying meal at reasonable prices for future dining experiences? Evaluation requires a stated purpose, specific standards and criteria by which to judge, and judgment skills.

Purpose

The ultimate purpose of evaluating interventions in community health nursing is to determine whether planned actions

RESEARCH Bridge to Practice

Laferriere, R. H., & Hamel-Bissell, B. (1994). Successful aging of oldest old women in the Northeast Kingdom of Vermont. *IMAGE, 26*(4), 310–23.

In addition to studying problems, community health nurses also examine wellness responses to learn more effective health promotion interventions. One population with a clear wellness response is that segment of the elderly who have aged successfully. A nursing study conducted in rural northeast Vermont focused on "oldest old" women (over 85 years of age) to determine why, despite certain health problems, they maintained a high level of morale and adjusted successfully to the challenges of aging.

Using ethnographic methodology, the researchers obtained life histories from six of these women (ages ranged from 87 to 93 years) by means of participant observation and extensive interviewing. All lived alone and remained in their own homes with limited assistance. From the data, four dominant themes were identified with successful aging: (1) "being a woman with family and friends," which emphasized close and supportive relationships, (2) "living off the land," which emphasized their enjoyment of raising their own food and the outdoors, (3) "dealing with the difficult times," which showed their ability to face hardships of all sorts with practicality and self-reliance, and (4) "working hard and staying active," which emphasized the purpose and meaning that work gave to their lives as well as a sense of accomplishment and control over their lives.

The researchers concluded that the ingredients for successful aging with these women were challenge, commitment, control, and resiliency, combined with an adequate social support system. They recommended implementing nursing health promotion with this age group emphasizing maximum independence and self-reliance while encouraging strong social support systems.

met client needs; if so, how well they were met; and, if not, why not. For example, an evaluation was conducted to determine the effectiveness of a group health promotion program with elderly, low-income women (Ruffing-Rahal, 1994). Criteria for evaluation focused on health practices, psychological and spiritual well-being, and social integration. No significant increases in outcomes were demonstrated for the intervention group over the 6-month period of weekly interventions. However, the evaluation suggested that the program had a preventive-maintenance effect for the participants by shielding them against factors that might otherwise cause beneficial health outcomes to be slowly eroded away.

Criteria

Sometimes, plans may include individual goals and criteria and group goals and criteria. Goals are the outcomes desired, and criteria are the smaller increments or steps necessary to take to achieve the larger achievement, the goal. For example, several diabetic women attending a clinic had a problem with obesity. A community health nurse working in the clinic helped them form a weight loss group. Each member developed individual weight loss goals to accomplish within a year. The women planned ways to meet their individual goals, by identifying specific criteria such as daily calorie limits (eg, 1500 calories per day) and regular exercise programs (eg, 20-minute exercise sessions, three times a week). They evaluated their individual goals by determining whether they met these criteria.

To maximize group support and encourage healthy behavior patterns during weight loss, the nurse suggested having a group goal and objectives to measure group success.

Group Goal: The group will stay healthy while accomplishing 90% of member weight loss goals.

Group Objectives:

1. By the end of the year, the group will lose at least 90% of the sum of the expected individual weight losses.
2. The group will have no diabetes-related infections during the year.
3. All of the group members will be exercising at least once a week by the end of the year.
4. No more than 10% of the group will have had an illness that kept them in bed more than 1 day during the year.

The prepared set of criteria helped the group evaluate its success.

The above examples emphasize the relationship of good planning to evaluation. When nurse and clients prepare clear, specific goals and objectives, there is no question about how or what to evaluate. It will be obvious that the goal is either met or not met.

Judgment Skills

Evaluation requires judgment skills by which the nurse compares real outcomes with expected outcomes and looks for discrepancies (Schalock, 1995). When actual client behavior matches the desired behavior, then the goal is met. If goals are not met, the nurse will need to examine several possible explanations for the failure. They may include inadequate data collection, incorrect diagnosis, unrealistic plan, or ineffective implementation. Circumstances, community motivation, or both may have changed. There may not have been enough community participation in one or more parts of the process. After determining the cause of the failure, the nurse can reassess, plan, and initiate corrective action.

Types of Evaluations

To determine the success of their planning and intervention, community heath nurses use two main types of evaluation: structure-process evaluation and outcomes evaluation. Each type of evaluation has importance to the success of any plan.

STRUCTURE-PROCESS EVALUATION

Structure-process evaluation concentrates mainly on the formation and operation of a plan or program as determined by established performance standards (Des Harnais & McLaughlin, 1994). It is part of the structure-process-outcome model of quality improvement developed by Donabedian and discussed in Chapter 12. However, in practice, agencies and professionals may develop two different evaluation systems, one for structure-process and the other for outcomes measurement.

Structure refers to the tools and resources in the health care environment that are beyond one's control. They include the physical and organizational structure of the agency and/or community resources as a foundation to providing health care services (Doheny, Cook & Stopper, 1996; Schmele, 1996). Such resources as staff qualifications, caseload, licensing, certification, compliance with state regulations, and available funding are part of the structural component. When conducting a structure-process evaluation, questions to be answered include: Are all professional staff licensed? Do they hold the appropriate certification? Does the facility meet state and local health department standards? Are there adequate and accessible resources in the community to meet client referral needs?

Process criteria refer to how caregiving is performed. These criteria focus on the delivery of services designed to achieve community health care outcomes. Process evaluation questions include: Are agency policies and procedures being followed? Are caregivers skilled in the latest technologies or caregiving practices required by the client mix? Do the staff nurses have adequate time for documentation? Is documentation done appropriately?

OUTCOMES EVALUATION

The third part of the Donabedian model is outcomes evaluation (Donabedian, 1966). Although the term *outcomes evaluation* became recognized with Donabedian's conceptual framework in the 1960s, it has more recently been used independently to identify quality measurement of the end results of service—the effect and the impact of services.

First, the *effect* or the degree to which an outcome has been met informs the agency or program leader of its impact on clients' health. As an example, one manufacturing company had an 80% adherence rate of employees who wore proper protective devices (goggles, safety shoes, and hard hats) within the plant. This was a concern to union representatives and the health and safety team, as well as the company management. They were concerned that 20% of their employees were at risk of injury, which would cause pain, suffering, loss of worktime, disruption to the manufacturing process, and reduction in profitability. The occupational health nurse along with the safety officer began a month-long safety campaign, which included safety mini-classes, posters, and incentives for departments having 100% safety equipment adherence. Three months after the program, 95% of the employees were adhering to the safety regulations. This 15% increase was attributed to the effect of the safety program.

The *impact* of a program determines how closely it is able to attain its goals. In the above example, the objective of the safety campaign was to increase safety equipment adherence. This was significantly increased as a result of the program. However, if the goal of the program was to decrease accidents and save the company money, this could only be determined by additional information. Were there fewer accidents causing injury? Were there fewer days lost to injury? Did the company save money related to employee safety adherence? Depending on these outcomes, the objective of the program was met, but the overall goal of the program may or may not have been met. The impact of the program is unknown without additional data.

Quality Measurement and Improvement

In community health nursing, evaluation is also performed to measure the quality of services, programs, and nurse performance (Newman et al., 1990; Schmele, 1996). Programs to measure quality are called by a variety of names—quality management programs (or systems), total quality management (TQM) programs, or quality assurance programs. Regardless of their title, they reflect nursing's increasing concern with measuring and improving quality. A sound quality management system includes the following:

1. An organizational entity created for assessing quality
2. Establishment of standards or criteria against which quality is assessed
3. A routine system of gathering information
4. Assurance that such information is based on the total population or representative sample of clients or potential clients

5. A process that provides the results of review to clients, the public, providers, and sponsoring organizations, as well as methods to institute corrective actions

With the burgeoning emphasis on accountability in health services, community health nursing is being challenged to devise better ways of documenting service effectiveness and cost-efficiency. A variety of methodologies and tools exists and is constantly being broadened to facilitate these evaluative processes (Irwin & Fordham, 1995; Pearson et al., 1991).

NURSING PROCESS CHARACTERISTICS APPLIED TO COMMUNITY AS CLIENT

The nursing process provides a framework or structure on which community health nursing actions are based. Application of the process varies with each situation, but the nature of the process remains the same. Certain elements of that nature are important for community health nurses to emphasize in their practice (Fig. 19–2).

Deliberative

The nursing process is deliberative—purposefully, rationally, and carefully thought out. It requires the use of sound judgment based on adequate information. Community health nurses often practice in situations that demand independent thinking and making difficult decisions. Furthermore,

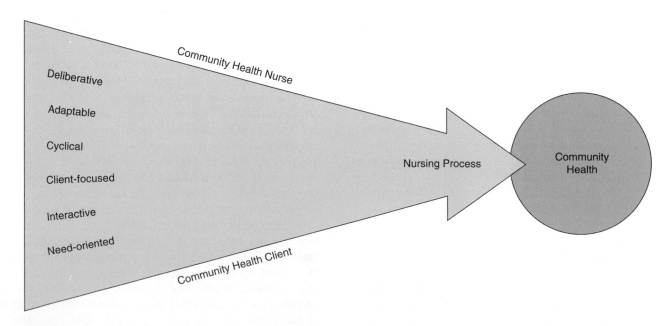

FIGURE 19–2. Nursing process characteristics emphasized in community health nursing practice.

thoughtful, deliberative problem solving is a skill needed for working with the community health team to address the needs and problems of aggregates in the community. The nursing process is a decision-making tool to facilitate these determinations (see Chapter 12 for more details).

Adaptable

The nursing process is adaptable. Its dynamic nature enables the community health nurse to adjust appropriately to each situation and to be flexible in applying the process to aggregate health needs. Furthermore, its flexibility is a reminder to the nurse that each client group, each community situation is unique. The nursing process must be applied specifically to that situation and that group of people. Based on assessment and sound planning, the nurse adapts and tailors services to meet the identified needs of each community client group.

Cyclic

The nursing process is cyclic or in constant progression. Steps are repeated over and over in the nurse–aggregate client relationship. The nurse in any given situation engages in continual interaction, data collection, analysis, intervention, and evaluation. As interactions between nurse and client group continue, various steps in the process overlap with one another and are used simultaneously. The cyclic nature of the nursing process enables the nurse to engage in a constant information feedback loop. That is, information gathered and lessons learned at each step of the process promote greater understanding of the group being served, the most effective way to provide quality services, and the best methods of raising this group's level of health.

Client Focused

The nursing process is client focused; it is used for and with clients. Community health nurses use the nursing process for the express purpose of addressing the health of populations (Koch et al., 1994). They are helping aggregate clients, directly or indirectly, to achieve and maintain health. Clients as total systems, whether groups, populations, or communities, are the target of community health nursing's use of the nursing process.

Interactive

The nursing process is interactive wherein nurse and clients are engaged in a process of ongoing interpersonal communication. Giving and receiving accurate information are necessary to promote understanding between nurse and clients and foster effective use of the nursing process. Furthermore, as the consumer movement, client's rights, and the self-care concept have gained emphasis, client groups and community health nurses have increasingly joined forces to assume responsibility for promoting community health. The nurse–aggregate client relationship can and should be a partnership, a shared experience by professionals (nurses and others) and client groups.

Need Oriented

The nursing process is need oriented. Long association with problem solving has tended to limit the nursing process' focus to the correction of existing problems. Although problem solving is certainly an appropriate use of the nursing process, the community health nurse can also use the nursing process to help anticipate clients' needs and prevent problems. The nurse should think of nursing diagnoses as ranging from health problem identification to primary prevention and health promotion opportunities. This focus is needed if the goals of community health—to protect, promote, and restore the people's health—are to be realized.

THE COMMUNITY HEALTH NURSE AS CATALYST FOR COMMUNITY DEVELOPMENT

Regardless of the agency focus, inherent in the community health nurse role is improvement or development of the community. With individual clients, if they become healthier, they will bring their healthier state into the community. If a family's health is improved, their greater wellness will improve the quality of their involvement in the community. If groups within the community, such as pregnant teens or third graders, improve their health status by following up with prenatal care or brushing their teeth on a regular basis, this will have a positive effect on the community's health. Using community developmental theory, the community health nurse acts as a catalyst to promote safe and healthy communities.

Community Development Theory

Community development is the process of collaborating with community members to assess their collective needs and desires for a positive change and to address these needs through problem solving, use of community experts, and resource development (Glick, Hale, Kulbok & Shettig, 1996). A community development perspective assumes that community members participate in all aspects of change—assessment, planning, development, the delivery of the services, and evaluation. Using this approach, the focus is on healthful community changes generated from within the community in partnership with the inhabitants rather than being disseminated by health care providers (Goeppinger, 1993).

The outcomes are more positive when community members have a greater sense of "ownership" of health programs and services that address their needs (Bragg, 1997; Glick, Hale, Kulbok & Shettig, 1996). This enhances empowerment within the community and enables members to "effectively control and participate in transforming their lives and environment" (Bragg, 1997, p. 44). This implies that health care agency infrastructures are appropriate in addition to services that are planned and delivered in an acceptable manner to the community.

When applying community development theory, the change agent, often the community health nurse, is considered a partner rather than an authority figure who is responsible for the community's health. To achieve acceptance as a partner, the nurse must listen and learn from the community members because they are the "experts" regarding their health care needs, culture, and values. They have mastered adaptation to the community and have firsthand knowledge of prevention methods and interventions that are appropriate to their norms (Glick, Hale, Kulbok & Shettig, 1996). An example of this can be seen in a study conducted by an interprofessional research team among 690 women in 18 impoverished inner-city neighborhoods in five cities. Significant changes in health behaviors to prevent human immunodeficiency virus (HIV) infection occurred among the women after they attended HIV risk reduction workshops and community HIV prevention events implemented by women who were popular opinion leaders among their peers (Sikkema et al., 2000).

On a global perspective, the Conference on Primary Health Care held at Alma-Ata in 1978 concluded that, globally, people have little control over their own health care services and that the emphasis should be on health problems identified by the members of the community in attaining wellness (World Health Organization, 1998). The World Health Organization has been providing leadership in the use of community development methods in the 20-plus years since Alma-Ata to improve global health.

Building Healthy and Safe Communities

What makes a community healthy? It is more than the health care services available in a community. It is the feeling of safety. It is being well informed, which gives the power to make choices. It is establishing lasting bonds with one another. It is having strong families. It is having a sense of meaning in one's life (Fowler, 1994).

Experts agree that the health of a community depends on its interconnectedness:

Linda Bergthold (a principal in a human resource and benefits consulting firm)—"A healthy community would be dense with empowering organizations at the local level and is a community that has identified its own priorities and has set out to build them."

Hazel Henderson (anti-economist)—"A healthy community means shifting our value system away from compulsive individualism toward re-balancing the needs of communities."

Sean Sullivan (National Business Coalition)—"Housing, education, crime, or the community's vision of itself are not things that usually show up in conversations of healthcare reformers about ways of reducing healthcare costs . . . or that managed competition will have much impact on."

Drew Altman (Kaiser Family Foundation)—"A good job and a strong family is the best health and human services program" (Fowler, 1994).

Community health nurses have a rich history in promoting health in communities. They are uniquely positioned to act as catalysts in the community to approach major health problems that affect populations and eventually the health of the community. Health problems such as infant mortality and acquired immunodeficiency syndrome (AIDS) are difficult to resolve at the individual level and require community collaboration and action (Rinehard et al., 1996).

The philosophical basis of community health nursing is grounded in the public health mission of promoting healthy communities by collaborating with clients where they live, work, and go to school. The goal of community health nursing is to position the nurse as a central person in the community to improve accessibility of care for consumers (Rinehard et al., 1996).

A component of a healthy community is that the community is a safe community. Community member involvement is essential to the success and stability of any safety programs, as it is in any community health program (National Highway Traffic Safety Administration, 1998). For communities to be safe, involvement by community participants who are recent immigrants, ethnic minorities, parents of infants, elders, bicyclists, joggers, skaters, and schoolchildren is essential. People in these groups perceive the world and the way their peers move through it in ways that can provide valuable insights for problem identification, program design and development. These participants can act as "key informants," providing qualitative data that can help prioritize the identified problems.

The community health nurse is in a position to initiate, promote, coordinate, and, at times, provide the beginning leadership as health and safety programs are developed in communities (El-Askari et al., 1998). Ideally, citizen participation will be developed and citizen control will emerge (Fig. 19–3).

SUMMARY

The effectiveness of community health nursing practice depends on how well the nursing process is used as a tool for enhancing aggregate health. The nursing process means appropriately applying a systematic series of actions with the goal of helping clients achieve their optimal level of health. These actions or components of the process include assessment, diagnosis, planning, implementation, and evaluation; this chapter focuses on the last three.

Interaction is integrated throughout the nursing process. Because nurse and clients must first establish a relationship of reciprocal influence and exchange before any change can take place, interaction could be considered the most essential step in the process. Effective communication is inherent in assessing needs and establishing trust between nurse and clients as partners in the nursing process.

The first two steps of the nursing process, assessment and formulation of nursing diagnoses, are covered in detail in Chapter 18. The third step, planning, includes designing a specific course of action to address the target group's diagnosis. It involves ranking a group's or aggregate's needs, establishing goals and measurable objectives, designing activities to meet the objectives, and developing a plan. The plan also includes a means to evaluate each objective.

Models are useful to community health nurses to organize service delivery. Two models are discussed, the health planning model and the Omaha system. They are discussed in light of the basic tool of the nursing process and with the help and limitations of the NANDA nursing diagnoses. Community health nurses can judge the value of these models and tools when planning services with community members.

The fourth step, implementation, activates the plan and sees it through to completion. During implementation, the nurse applies appropriate theory, provides a facilitative environment, prepares clients for service, carries out or modifies and carries out a plan (with clients), and documents the implementation.

The last and very important step is evaluation, which measures and judges the effectiveness of the evaluations. Well-prepared goals and objectives are essential for adequate evaluation. If goals are not met, the failure may result from inadequate assessment or planning. Determining the cause of the failure can lead to corrective action. Evaluation does not end the nursing process; rather, it documents what has been accomplished and what yet needs to be done so the process, a continuing cycle, can start again.

Certain characteristics are important to the nursing process and should be emphasized by community health nurses in their practice. The process is deliberative, requiring and aiding the exercise of judgment in making decisions. It is adaptable, encouraging flexibility in practice. It is cyclic, fostering a constant, ongoing use of the process. It is client focused, helping the nurse to keep the proper target of clients' health in view. It is interactive, promoting nurse–client communication and client participation. Finally, it is need oriented, focusing on the clients' current and future needs including prevention and health promotion to help clients achieve optimal health.

Using the nursing process in the community would not be complete without looking at the role of the community health nurse as a catalyst for community development. Community development theory is the foundation that supports citizen empowerment and use of the key players in the community to plan for the health and safety of the community.

ACTIVITIES TO PROMOTE CRITICAL THINKING

1. You have been using the nursing process with individuals to effect change in their health status. Now, consider how you can expand that application to aggregates. Select a population group in your community, such as preschoolers, unwed mothers, a group of refugees, or elderly homebound people.

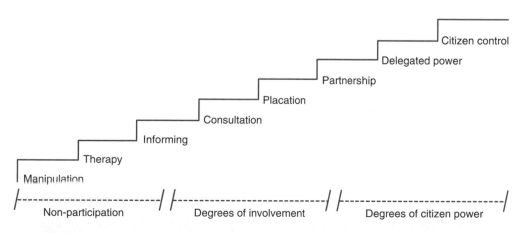

FIGURE 19–3. Eight steps of citizen participation. (Adapted from Arnstein, S.R. [1969]. A ladder of citizen participation. *Journal of the American Institute of Planners,* July, 217–224.)

CLINICAL CORNER   Evaluating Outcomes of a Home Care Postpartum Program

Scenario

As a nurse working as the liaison between Capitol City Hospital and its home health agency, you are given the job of reviewing your early postpartum discharge program. Your program has been in effect for 18 months. Client satisfaction is high. The program has increased revenue for the hospital because many clients choose to deliver at Capitol City Hospital because of the early discharge program.

The protocol for your early discharge program includes a postpartum home visit by an RN from the home health agency. These visits are provided as a service to the client. In some cases, visits are billable to insurance companies. Medicaid authorizes payment for one postpartum visit.

You have gathered the following information about the early discharge program:

I. Protocol: Standard is one visit within 48 hours after discharge which includes:
   A. Education
      1. Newborn care
      2. Breastfeeding
      3. Warning signs warranting follow-up (mother and baby)
         —Infection
         —Hemorrhage
      4. Comfort
      5. Parenting
      6. Sexuality
         —Resumption of sexual activity
         —Contraception
      7. Community resources
      8. Nutrition
      9. Well and sick baby care
   B. Assessment
      1. Infant: Jaundice (heel stick performed if necessary)
         Mother: Hemorrhage, perineal lacerations, hematomas
         Both: Nutrition
         —Weight
         —Hydration
         —Breastfeeding
      2. Elimination
II. Cost:
   A. Fully reimbursed by some insurance companies
   B. All mother/baby dyads receive postpartum visits, regardless of insurance coverage

   C. Optional or additional methods of reimbursement have not been explored by the agency
   D. Agency makes money on reimbursed visits, loses money on non-reimbursed, but additional revenue generated by clients choosing the hospital because of the positive public perception program is thought to balance out cost of nonreimbursed visits.

Outcomes. Outcomes of postpartum early discharge with accompanying home visit (as compared to traditional length of postpartum stay)
   I. Positive
      A. Higher percentage of successful (at least 2 months) breastfeeding
      B. Higher rate of immunization compliance
      C. Fewer inappropriate emergency room visits
      D. High client satisfaction
      E. Lower levels of maternal stress reported to pediatricians
   II. Negative
      A. Higher incidence in jaundice in babies whose mothers participated in the early discharge program

Questions

1. What, if any, additional information do you need to make a recommendation regarding the program?
   ■ How will you obtain this information?
2. As the nurse making a recommendation for the continuation or termination of the postpartum early discharge program, what are your recommendations?
   ■ Should the program be abandoned?
   ■ Should the program be maintained?
3. What, if any, alterations would you make in the following areas:
   ■ Funding
   ■ Protocol
      —Client education
      —Assessment
      —Timing of Visit
4. Outcome measurements are critical to demonstrate the efficacy of this program.
   ■ What will you evaluate?
   ■ How often?
   ■ Why?

a. How might you start the interaction phase with these potential clients?
b. What specific areas would you want to assess? Make a list of hypothetical indicators that suggest a need.
c. Invent a diagnosis for this group that would be

supported by the data you collected in your assessment.
d. What alternative courses of action should you consider for addressing this need? Select the most appropriate one.

e. Start a plan for implementation, including an overall goal and at least one objective.

f. List the activities needed to meet your objective(s), and describe how you might carry them out.

g. How would you evaluate your nursing interventions with this population group?

2. Search your own community for examples of healthy community practices in the form of programs, partnerships, coalitions, and so forth. Explore one, and assess the degree of community involvement in the form of citizen leadership and control.

3. Use the Internet to locate community health nursing articles highlighting examples of community development where the community health nurse assumes the role of catalyst. (See Clinical Corner.)

REFERENCES

Arnstein, S. R. (1969, July). A ladder of citizen participation. *Journal of the American Institute of Planners,* 217–224.

Bragg, M. (1997). AN empowerment approach to community health education. In B. S. Spradley & J. A. Allender (Eds.), *Readings in community health nursing* (5th ed., pp. 504–510). Philadelphia: Lippincott-Raven.

Chausmer, K. (1997). *Tips for coalition building. Safe communities.* Washington, DC: The National Highway Traffic Safety Administration: U.S. Department of Transportation.

Des Harnais, S., & McLaughlin, C. P. (1994). The outcome model of quality. In C. P. McLaughlin & A. D. Kaluzny (Eds.), *Continuous quality improvement in health care: Theory, implementation and applications* (pp. 47–69). Gaithersburg, MD: Aspen.

Dever, G. E. A. (1997). *Improving outcomes in public health practice: Strategy and methods.* Gaithersburg, MD: Aspen.

Doheny, M., Cook, C., & Stopper, C. (1996). *The discipline of nursing: An introduction* (4th ed.). Stamford, CT: Appleton & Lange.

Donabedian, A. (1966). Evaluating the quality of medical care. *Milbank Quarterly, 44,* 166–206.

El-Askari, G., Freestone, J., Irizarry, C., et al. (1998). The healthy neighborhoods project: A local health department's role in catalyzing community development. *Health Education and Behavior, 25*(2), 146–159.

Ervin, N. E., & Kuehnert, P. L. (1993). Application of a model for public health nursing program planning. *Public Health Nursing, 10*(1), 25–30.

Fowler, J. (1994). How to build a healthy community. *Healthy communities action kit, Module 3.* The Healthcare Forum. Available: http://www.well.com/user/bbear/hc_how_to.html.

Glick, D. F., Hale, P. J., Kulbok, P. A., & Shettig, T. (1996). Community development theory: Planning a community nursing center. *Journal of Nursing Administration, 26*(7/8), 44–50.

Goeppinger, J. (1993). Health promotion for rural populations. *Family Community Health, 16*(1), 1–10.

Irwin, P., & Fordham, J. (1995). *Evaluating the quality of care.* Philadelphia: Churchill Livingstone.

Koch, C. K., et al. (1994). Population-oriented nursing: Preparing tomorrow's nurses today. *Journal of Nursing Education, 33*(5), 236–237.

Martin, K. (1994). The Omaha system: A data base for ambulatory and home care. In M. E. C. Mills, C. A. Romano & B. R. Heller (Eds.), *Information management in nursing and health care* (pp. 39–44). Springhouse, PA: Springhouse Publishers.

Martin, K. S., & Scheet, N. J. (1992). *The Omaha system: A pocket guide for community health nursing.* Philadelphia: W. B. Saunders.

National Highway Traffic Safety Administration. (1998). Citizen involvement and safe communities. *Building Safe Communities, 1*(5), 1–2.

Newman, D. L., et al. (1990). What is evaluation: Nurse decision-makers' perceptions of program evaluation. *Journal of New York State Nurses Association, 21*(3), 10–14.

North American Nursing Diagnosis Association. (1999). *Nursing diagnoses: Definitions and classification 1999–2000.* Philadelphia: Author.

Pearson, M. A., et al. (1991). Program evaluation application of a comprehensive model for a community-based respite program. *Journal of Community Health Nursing, 8*(1), 25–1.

Rinehard, S. C., Christopher, M. A., Mason, D. J., et al. (1996). Promoting healthy communities through neighborhood nursing. *Nursing Outlook, 44*(5), 223–228.

Rohrer, J. E. (1996). *Planning for community-oriented health systems.* Washington, DC: American Public Health Association.

Ruffing-Rahal, M. A. (1994). Evaluation of group health promotion with community-dwelling older women. *Public Health Nursing, 11*(1), 38–48.

Schalock, R. L. (1995). *Outcome-based evaluation.* New York: Plenum Press.

Schmele, J. A. (1996). *Quality management in nursing and health care.* Albany, NY: Delmar.

Sikkema, K. J., Kelly, J. A., Winett, R. A., et al. (2000). Outcomes of a randomized community-level HIV prevention intervention for women living in 18 low-income housing developments. *American Journal of Public Health, 90*(1), 57–63.

Timmreck, T. (1995). *Planning, program development, and evaluation: A handbook for health promotion, aging, and health services.* Boston: Jones & Bartlett.

Williams, C. A. (1977). Community health nursing—What is it? *Nursing Outlook, 25,* 250–253.

World Health Organization (1998). *Primary health care in the 21st century is everybody's business.* Geneva: WHO.

SELECTED READINGS

American Nurses' Association (1986). *Standards for community health nursing practice.* Kansas City, MO: Author.

Barker, J. B., et al. (1994). Community analysis: A collaborative community practice project. *Public Health Nursing, 11*(2), 113–118.

Barriball, K., et al. (1992). The demand for measuring the impact of nursing interventions: A community perspective. *Journal of Clinical Nursing, 1*(4), 207–212.

Billingham, K. (1997). A public health approach to nursing in the community. *Nursing Standard, 11*(35), 43–46.

Bracht, N. (1999). *Health promotion at the community level* (2nd ed.). Thousand Oaks, CA: Sage.

Burns, J. (1993). Caring for the community. *Modern Health Care, 23*(45), 30–33.

Chaskin, R. J., Joseph, M. L., & Chipenda-Dansokho, S. (1997). Implementing comprehensive community development: Possibilities and limitations. *Social Work, 42*(5), 435–444.

Denham, A., Quinn, S. C., & Gamble, D. (1998). Community organizing for health promotion in the rural south: An exploration of community competence. *Family Community Health, 21*(1), 1–21.

Elizur, Y. (1996). Involvement, collaboration, and empowerment: A model for consultation with human-service agencies and the development of family-oriented care. *Family Process, 35,* 191–210.

Feikema, R. J., Segalavich, J. H., & Jeffries, S. H. (1997, March/April). From child development to community development: One agency's journey. *Families in Society: The Journal of Contemporary Human Services,* 185–195.

Glick, D. F., et al. (1994). Grant writing: An innovative project for teaching community health program planning. *Journal of Nursing Education, 33*(5), 238–240.

Halbert, T. L., et al. (1993). Population-based health promotion: A new agenda for public health nurses. *Canadian Journal of Public Health, 84*(4), 243–245.

Kemp, C. (1994). Community health clinical experiences: The primary care setting. *Public Health Nursing, 11*(1), 2–6.

Marrelli, T. M., & Hilliard, L. S. (1996). *Home care and clinical paths: Effective care planning across the continuum.* St. Louis: Mosby.

McKnight, J., & Van Dover, L. (1994). Community as client: A challenge for nursing education. *Public Health Nursing, 11*(1), 12–16.

Peckham, S., et al. (1994). Community development approaches to health needs assessment. *Health Visitor, 67*(4), 124–125.

Penner, S. (1994). HIV/AIDS and mental illness: The case for community health planning. *Psychosocial Rehabilitation Journal, 17*(4), 127–136.

Speers, M. A., & Lancaster, B. (1998). Disease prevention and health promotion in urban areas: CDC's perspective. *Health Education & Behavior, 25*(2), 226–233.

Wickizer, T., VonKorff, M., Cheadle, A., et al. (1993). Activating communities for health promotion: A process evaluation method. *American Journal of Public Health, 83*(4), 561–567.

Yura, H., & Walsh, M. B. (1988). *The nursing process: Assessing, planning, implementing, evaluating* (5th ed.). Norwalk, CT: Appleton and Lange.

Communities in Crisis: Disasters, Group Violence, and Terrorism

LEARNING OBJECTIVES

Upon mastery of this chapter, you should be able to:

- Describe disasters in terms of a variety of characteristics, including causation, number of casualties, scope, and intensity.
- Discuss a variety of factors contributing to a community's potential for experiencing a disaster.
- Identify the four phases of disaster management.
- Describe the role of the community health nurse in preventing, preparing for, responding to, and supporting recovery from disasters.
- Compare and contrast the most common types of group violence.
- Discuss a variety of factors contributing to a community's potential for experiencing group violence.
- Describe the role of the community health nurse in preventing and responding to group violence.
- Distinguish terrorism from other types of group violence.
- Describe the role of the community health nurse in preventing and responding to acts of terrorism.

W hat would you do if your local news station broadcast an announcement that your community was directly in the path of a hurricane that earlier in the day had caused extensive damage and loss of life in a neighboring state? What would you do if you were shopping at a local mall and you suddenly heard an explosive noise followed by shouts and cries for help, then noticed that a pungent odor was filling the air? As distant as these scenarios might seem from your own life, disasters, group violence, and terrorism are ever-present possibilities, and nurses and other health care professionals have an obligation to respond appropriately. This chapter will further your understanding of the role of the community health nurse in responding to disasters, group violence, and terrorism.

DISASTERS

A **disaster** is any event that causes a level of destruction that exceeds the abilities of the affected community to respond without assistance. According to this definition, a crash of a private plane over the Pacific Ocean, in which no bodies are recovered and no environmental impact is felt, is not considered a disaster because no specific community-based response is required or even possible. However, if a plane with 150 passengers crashes over land and destroys several homes in its path, the community affected may be unable to cope with the injuries, deaths, and property destruction without assistance. Thus, we would say that this community has experienced a disaster.

The geographic distribution of certain disasters varies because, in some parts of the world, certain types of disasters are simply more common. For example, we tend to associate California with earthquakes and Florida with hurricanes. Similarly, we are not surprised to hear of drought in Ethiopia or flood in India during the monsoon season. When certain types of disasters are anticipated, communities are usually better prepared for them. For instance, California has strict building codes to prevent destruction of structures in the event of earthquakes, but most California homes lack the basements and insulation that characterize homes in regions often visited by winter storms. Similarly, residents of North Dakota are better prepared for blizzards than for heavy rains, which probably explains in part the devastation caused in some North Dakota communities by the floods of 1997.

Because the local media in the United States do not typically report on disasters unless they result in mass casualties, you may be unaware of the frequency and variety of both natural and technological disasters worldwide. Here is a brief sampling of major disasters that occurred in just the first few months of 2000:

- In the Philippines, eruption of the Mayon volcano forced 70,000 people from their homes.
- In Madagascar, two cyclones forced 600,000 people to flee their homes.
- In Mozambique, floods claimed more than 1,000 lives and left 950,000 homeless.
- In Zambia, heavy flooding destroyed crops, leaving over 15,000 people at risk for starvation.

Characteristics of Disasters

We often characterize disasters as being caused by natural events, such as the earthquakes in Turkey in 1999 or the floods in Mozambique in February of 2000. However, disasters may also be caused by human technology and activity, such as the bombing of the Federal Building in Oklahoma City in 1995, the displacement of thousands of Kosovars during their war with Serbia in 1999, or the rioting in Seattle during the World Trade Organization meeting in 1999. Other technological disasters include nuclear reactor meltdowns, industrial accidents, oil spills, construction accidents, and air, train, bus, and subway crashes.

A **casualty** is a human being who is injured or killed during or as a direct result of an accident. Although major disasters sometimes occur without any injury or loss of life, it is common to characterize disasters by the number of casualties involved. When casualties number more than 2 people

but fewer than 100, then the disaster is characterized as a *multiple-casualty incident*. Whereas multiple-casualty incidents may strain the health care systems of small or midsized communities, *mass-casualty incidents,* those involving 100 or more casualties, often completely overwhelm the resources of even large cities. Preparedness for mass-casualty incidents is essential for all communities.

The possibility of preparedness is another characteristic that varies with different types of disasters. For instance, the path of hurricanes can sometimes be tracked, allowing for early evacuation of residents in the storm's path. Communities can also minimize devastation from flooding through building reservoirs or refusing building permits in flood-prone areas. During rainy weather, communities can begin sandbagging. In fire-prone areas, communities can post notices to heighten awareness of fire danger in dry seasons and enforce regulations to cut back vegetation near the sides and roofs of structures in forested areas. On the other hand, some disasters strike without warning. For example, the Oakland Hills fires in 1991 were largely unanticipated, leaving residents stalled in traffic jams on narrow mountain roads as the fires approached.

The **scope** of a disaster is its range of effect, either geographically or in terms of the number of victims. The collapse of a 500-unit high-rise apartment building has a greater scope than the collapse of a bridge which only two cars were crossing at the time of collapse.

The **intensity** of a disaster is the level of destruction and devastation it causes. For instance, an earthquake centered in a large metropolitan area and one centered in a desert may have the same numeric intensity rating on the Richter scale, yet have very different intensities in terms of the destruction they cause.

Victims of Disasters

Because disasters are so variable, there is no one typical victim of disasters, nor can anyone predict whether he or she will ever become a victim of a disaster. However, once disaster strikes, it is common to characterize victims by their level of involvement. **Direct victims** are the people who experience the event, whether a fire, volcanic eruption, war, or bomb. They are the dead and the survivors, and even if they are without physical injuries, they are likely to experience health effects from their experience. Some may be without shelter or food, and many will experience serious psychological stress long after the event is over.

Depending on the cause and characteristics of the disaster, some direct victims may become displaced persons or refugees. **Displaced persons** have to leave their homes to escape the effects of the disaster. Usually, displacement is a temporary condition and involves movement within the person's own country. A common example is relocation of residents of flooded areas to schools, churches, and other shelters on higher ground. Typically, the term **refugee** is reserved for people who are forced to leave their homeland because of war or persecution. For example, in early 2000, thousands of refugees fled Chechnya to escape advancing Russian troops opposed to the republic's separatist attempts. Often, the displacement of refugees is permanent. For example, many young people who fled Argentina during the "disappearances" of 1976 to 1982 did not return when a democratic government regained power in 1983.

Indirect victims are the relatives and friends of direct victims. Although these people do not experience the stress of the event itself, they often undergo extreme anguish when trying to locate their loved ones or accommodate their emergency needs. When bodies are not found or are unable to be identified, indirect victims experience even greater anguish and may not be able to move beyond their loss. For example, many of the mothers of the young Argentinians who disappeared in the 1970s still march in downtown Buenos Aires daily, demanding public acknowledgment of the murders of their daughters and sons.

Factors Contributing to Disasters

It is useful to apply the host, agent, and environment model to our understanding of factors contributing to disasters, because manipulation of these factors can be instrumental in planning strategies to prevent or prepare for disasters.

HOST FACTORS
In terms of disasters, the *host* is the human being who experiences the disaster. Host factors that contribute to the likelihood of experiencing a disaster include age, general health, mobility, psychological factors, and even socioeconomic factors. For instance, elderly residents of a mobile-home community may be unable to evacuate independently in response to a tornado warning if they no longer have a license to drive. Impoverished residents of a low-income apartment complex in a large city may notice that their building is not compliant with city fire codes but may avoid alerting authorities for fear of being forced to move to more expensive housing.

AGENT FACTORS
The *agent* is the natural or technological element that causes the disaster. For example, the high winds of a hurricane and the lava of an erupting volcano are agents, as are radiation, industrial chemicals, and bombs.

ENVIRONMENTAL FACTORS
Environmental factors are those that could potentially contribute to or mitigate a disaster. There are many possibilities, but some of the most common include a community's level of preparedness; the presence of industries that produce harmful chemicals or radiation; the presence of flood-prone rivers, lakes, or streams; average amount of rainfall or snowfall; average high and low temperatures; proximity to fault lines, coastal waters, or volcanoes; level of compliance with

local building codes; and presence or absence of political unrest.

Agencies and Organizations for Disaster Management

Among disaster-relief organizations, perhaps none is as famous as the Red Cross, the name commonly used when referring to the American Red Cross, the Federation of Red Cross and Red Crescent Societies, and the International Committee of the Red Cross. The American Red Cross was founded in 1881 by Clara Barton and was chartered by the U.S. Congress in 1905. It is authorized to provide disaster assistance free of charge across the country through its more than 1 million volunteers.

The Federal Emergency Management Agency (FEMA), established in 1979, is the federal agency responsible for assessment of and response to disaster events in the United States. It also provides training and guidance in all phases of disaster management.

The World Health Organization's Emergency Relief Operations provide disaster assistance internationally, and the Pan American Health Organization works to coordinate relief efforts in Latin America and the Caribbean. In addition, various international nongovernmental organizations, such as Doctors Without Borders, the International Medical Corps, Operation Blessing, religious groups, and other volunteer agencies provide needed and emergency care.

Governments often send their military personnel and equipment in response to international disasters. For example, in March of 2000 the governments of South Africa, England, Germany, France, and the United States, among other nations, responded to the floods in Mozambique with helicopters, planes, boats, and supplies.

When natural or technological disasters within the United States are accompanied by civil disturbances, looting, or violent crime, the resources of local police departments may be overwhelmed. In such cases, the National Guard is often called in to restore order.

Phases of Disaster Management

In developing strategies to address the problem of disasters, it is helpful for the community health nurse to consider each of the four phases of disaster management: prevention, preparedness, response, and recovery.

PREVENTION PHASE
During the *prevention phase,* no disaster is expected or anticipated. The task during this phase is to identify community risk factors and develop and implement programs to prevent disasters from occurring. Task forces typically include representatives from the community's local government, health care providers, social services providers, police and fire departments, major industries, local media, and citizens' groups.

Programs developed during the prevention phase may also focus on strategies to mitigate the effects of disasters—such as earthquakes, hurricanes, and tornadoes—that cannot be prevented.

PREPAREDNESS PHASE

Disaster *preparedness* involves planning to save lives and minimize injury and property damage. It includes plans for communication, evacuation, rescue, and victim care. Any plan must also address acquisition of equipment, supplies, medicine, and even food, clean water, blankets, and shelter. Semiannual disaster drills and tests of the Emergency Broadcast System are examples of appropriate activities during the preparedness phase.

RESPONSE PHASE

The *response phase* begins in the moments immediately after the onset of the disastrous event. Preparedness plans take effect immediately, with the goal of saving lives and preventing further injury or damage. Activities during the response phase include rescue, triage, on-site stabilization, transportation of victims, and treatment at local hospitals. Response also requires care of the dead and provisions to notify and care for the families and friends of the dead. Supportive care, including food, water, and shelter for victims and relief workers, is also an essential element of the total disaster response.

RECOVERY PHASE

During the *recovery phase,* the community takes actions to repair, rebuild, or relocate damaged homes and businesses and restore health and economic vitality to the community. Psychological recovery must also be addressed. The emotional scars from witnessing a traumatic event may last a lifetime, and both victims and relief workers should be offered mental health services to support their recovery.

Role of the Community Health Nurse

The community health nurse has a pivotal role in each phase of preventing, preparing for, responding to, and supporting recovery from a disaster. After a thorough community assessment for risk factors, the community health nurse may initiate the formation of a multidisciplinary task force to address disaster prevention and preparedness in the community.

PREVENTING DISASTERS

Disaster prevention may be considered on three levels: primary, secondary, and tertiary. These are applied to a natural disaster in the Levels of Prevention display.

Primary Prevention. Primary prevention of disasters means keeping the disaster from ever happening, taking actions to completely eliminate its occurrence. Although it is obviously the most effective level of intervention both in terms of promoting clients' health and containing costs, as we have seen,

LEVELS OF PREVENTION

TORNADO

PRIMARY PREVENTION

Increase community awareness and preparation through education. Each person is as prepared as possible physically and emotionally and knows what to do and where to go whether at home, work, school, or elsewhere in the community.

SECONDARY PREVENTION

Get to safety before the impact—either the southwest corner of the basement or an interior room away from windows and under heavy furniture. Leave a damaged building cautiously if able and not seriously injured. Do not return to the house if it is damaged. Beware of hazards such as live wires, broken gas lines, and fallen debris.

TERTIARY PREVENTION

Remain safe during immediate recovery period. Accept help from others. Go to friends, family members, and community services for support. Accept counseling and other services to restabilize life physically, emotionally, spiritually, and financially.

it is not always possible. Tornadoes, earthquakes, and other disasters often strike without warning, despite all our technological devices for prediction and tracking.

When possible, primary prevention of disasters can be practiced in all settings—in the workplace and home with programs to reduce safety hazards, and in the community with programs to monitor risk factors, reduce pollution, and encourage nonviolent conflict resolution. Primary disaster prevention efforts should take into account a community's physical, psychosocial, cultural, economic, and spiritual needs.

The second aspect of primary disaster prevention is anticipatory guidance. Disaster drills and other anticipatory exercises help relief workers experience some of the feelings of chaos and stress before a disaster occurs. It is much easier to do this at a time when energy and intellectual processes are at a high level of functioning. Anticipatory work can thus dissipate the impact of a disastrous event.

Secondary Prevention. Secondary disaster prevention focuses on earliest possible detection and treatment. For example, a mobile-home community is devastated by a tornado, and the local health department's community health nurses work with the American Red Cross to provide emergency assistance. Secondary prevention corresponds to immediate and effective response.

Tertiary Prevention. Tertiary disaster prevention involves reducing the amount and degree of disability or damage resulting from the disaster. Although it involves rehabilitative work, it can help a community recover and reduce the risk of further disasters. In this sense, it is a preventive measure.

PREPARING FOR DISASTERS

The disaster plan of a community, business, or hospital need not be lengthy. Two weeks after the Oklahoma City bombing, one hospital distilled its 44-page manual into a 5-page disaster response guide. However, the plan should contain information on the elements discussed in this and the following section (Display 20–1).

Personal Preparation. Before we discuss the preparation of a disaster plan for a community, we should consider the need for all nurses to address their own personal preparedness to respond in a disaster. Display 20–2 describes the tragic outcome of one nurse's lack of preparation when she attempted to provide nursing care at the scene of the Oklahoma City bombing in 1995. Personal preparedness means that the nurse has read and understood workplace and community disaster plans and has developed a disaster plan for her or his own family. The prepared nurse also has participated in disaster drills and knows CPR and first aid. Finally, nurses preparing to work in disaster areas should have with them a copy of their nursing license, driver's license, durable clothing, basic equipment such as their stethoscope, a flashlight, and a cellular phone.

Assessment for Risk Factors and Disaster History. As noted earlier in the chapter, the community health nurse is uniquely qualified to perform a community assessment for risk factors that may contribute to disasters. In addition, the nurse should review the *disaster history* of the community. Have earthquakes, tornadoes, hurricanes, floods, blizzards, riots, or other disasters occurred frequently in the past? If so, what (if any) were the warning signs? Were they heeded? Were people warned in time? Did evacuation efforts remove all people in danger? What were the community's on-site responses, and how effective were they? And what programs were put in place to rehabilitate the community?

Establishing Authority, Communication, and Transportation. In addition to assessing for preparedness, the effective disaster plan establishes a clear chain of authority, develops lines of communication, and delineates routes of transport.

DISPLAY 20–1. Elements of a Disaster Plan

A disaster plan should address all of the following elements:

Chain of authority
Lines of communication
Routes and modes of transport
Mobilization
Warning
Evacuation
Rescue and recovery
Triage
Treatment
Support of victims and families
Care of dead bodies
Disaster worker rehabilitation

DISPLAY 20–2. Nurses at Disaster Sites: Help or Hindrance?

On April 19, 1995, 37-year-old Rebecca Anderson, a registered nurse working in Oklahoma City, after hearing a televised report of the bombing of the Federal Building, responded to the site wearing jeans and a sweatshirt. Amidst firefighters and other rescue workers in hardhats and other protective gear, she was allowed to enter the scene. Within a short time, Rebecca was struck on the back of the head by a concrete slab that fell from the building's wreckage. She died 5 days later of massive cerebral edema. Nurses can learn the following lessons from this tragedy:

- Never enter a disaster scene unless you are directed to do so by an emergency medical technician, fire, or law enforcement official.
- Contact local hospitals and clinics to offer your help; your medical expertise is more useful in the clinical environment.
- Take courses in first aid and emergency care. Contact your local Red Cross for a list of courses.
- Contact your local health department to learn more about your community's disaster plan and how you can contribute in the event of a disaster in your area.

Establishing a clear and flexible chain of authority is critical for successful implementation of a disaster plan. Usually, the chain is hierarchical, with, for example, the community's governmental head, such as the mayor, initiating the plan, alerting the media to broadcast warnings, authorizing the police to begin evacuations, and so on. Within each branch, the hierarchy continues (eg, at the local hospital, the hospital administrator may be responsible for alerting nurse managers to call in additional personnel, and so on). Flexibility is essential because key authority figures may themselves be victims of the disaster. If the home of the chief of police is destroyed in an earthquake, his or her second-in-command must have equal knowledge of the community's disaster plan and be able to step in without delay.

Effective communication is often a point of breakdown for communities attempting to cope with major disasters. After the bombing in Oklahoma City in 1995, phone lines were damaged and cellular sites were overwhelmed, making communication possible only through hand-held radios or by way of couriers on foot. At times of heightened chaos and stress, as well as physical damage to communication facilities and equipment, misinformation and misinterpretation can flourish, leading to delayed treatment and even increased loss of life. Again, clarity and flexibility are the watchwords for establishing lines of communication. How will warnings be communicated? What backups are available if the normal communication systems are destroyed in the disaster? How will communication between the relief workers at the disaster site, the hospital personnel, the police, and the governmental authorities be maintained? What role will local media play, both in keeping information flowing to the outside world and in broadcasting needs for assistance and supplies? Finally, how will the friends and family members of victims be informed of the whereabouts or health status of their loved ones? The characteristics of effective communication during disasters are summarized in Display 20–3.

Closed or inefficient routes of transportation can also increase injury and loss of life. For example, if a single, narrow, mountainous road is the only means of transporting firefighters to or evacuating residents from the scene of a forest fire, then disaster planners should propose widening the road or clearing a second road. Disaster planners must also consider what routes emergency vehicles will take when transporting disaster victims to local and outlying hospitals and health care workers to the disaster site. What if the chosen routes are inaccessible because of flood waters, advancing fires, mountainslides, or building rubble? Are alternative routes designated?

Mobilizing, Warning, and Evacuating. For many natural disasters, local weather service personnel, public-works officials, police officers, or firefighters will have the earliest information indicating an increasing potential for a disaster. These officials typically have a plan in place for providing community authorities with specific data indicating increased risk. They may also advise the mayor's office or other community leaders of their recommendations for warning or

evacuating the public. Additionally, they may recommend actions the community can take to mitigate damage, such as spraying rooftops in the path of fires, sandbagging the banks of rising rivers, or imposing a curfew in times of civil unrest.

Disaster plans must specify the means of communicating warnings to the public, as well as the precise information that should be included in warnings. Planners should never assume that all citizens can be reached by radio or television or that broadcast systems will be unaffected by the disaster. Broadcast media may indeed be a primary means of communicating warnings, but alternative strategies, such as police or volunteers canvassing neighborhoods with loudspeakers, should also be in place. Obviously, in multilingual communities, messages should be broadcast in multiple languages. Not only homes but also businesses must be informed. Information that should be communicated includes the nature of the agent; the exact geographic region affected, including street names if appropriate; and the actions citizens should take to protect themselves and their property.

An evacuation plan is an essential component of the total disaster plan. The plan should cover notification of the police, local military personnel, or voluntary citizens' group of the need to evacuate, as well as methods of notifying and transporting the evacuees. A plan should also be made for responding to citizens who refuse to evacuate. For example, will police authorities forcibly remove an elderly citizen from his home to a shelter? Also, will evacuation plans include household pets? If farms or ranches are in the path of fires or floods, will animals be evacuated?

RESPONDING TO DISASTERS

At the disaster site, police, firefighters, nurses, and other relief workers effect a coordinated response to rescue, triage, and treat disaster victims.

Rescue. One of the first obligations of relief workers is to remove victims from danger. This job typically falls to firefighters and personnel with special training in search and rescue. Depending on the disaster agent, protective gear, heavy equipment, and special vehicles may be needed, and dogs trained to sniff for dead bodies may be brought in (Fig. 20–1). Usually, the immediate disaster site is not the best place for the disaster nurse, who can be far more effective in triage and treatment of victims. One of the lessons of the Oklahoma City bombing was that the greatest need for medical professionals was at the local hospitals, not at the disaster site.

Rescue workers face the logistically and psychologically difficult task of determining when to cease rescue efforts. Some factors include increasing danger to rescue workers, diminishing numbers of survivors, and diminishing possibilities for survival. For example, after a plane crash on a snowy mountain, rescue efforts may cease after a certain number of days if it is deemed that anyone who might have survived the crash would subsequently have died from exposure.

Triage. Whereas emergency nurses daily determine which clients require priority care, the community health nurse may be at a loss as to where to start if faced with multiple victims

---

DISPLAY 20–3. Effective Communication During Disasters

To be effective, communication during disasters must elicit action. Communication that elicits action provides information that is:
- Believable
- Current
- Unambiguous
- Authoritative
- Predictive of the probability of future events (what is going to happen next?)

Effective communication is:
- Interactive—it allows for and addresses questions
- Conclusive—it eliminates room for speculation and catastrophizing
- Urgent—but without resorting to fear tactics
- Clear, simple, and repetitive
- Characterized by solutions and suggestions for success
- Personal—it uses people's names if possible and addresses their real and perceived needs

Finally, because rumors can hinder effective action or provoke premature action, effective communication includes rumor control. It provides suggestions for constructive activity, reducing time and energy spent on rumor generation and perpetuation.

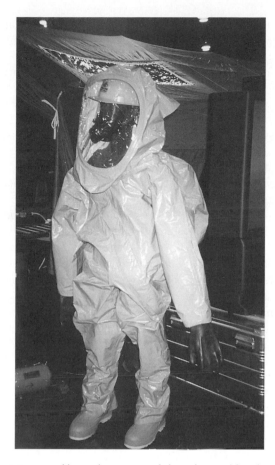

FIGURE 20–1. Hazardous materials suit used by the military and most fire departments. (Photo by Cynthia Tait.)

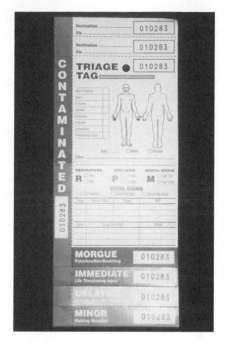

1. **Red:** Urgent/Critical
   Victims in this category have injuries or medical problems that will likely lead to death if not treated immediately (e.g., an unconscious victim with signs of internal bleeding).
2. **Yellow:** Delayed
   Victims in this category have injuries that will require medical attention; however, time to medical treatment is not yet critical (e.g., a conscious victim with a fractured femur).
3. **Green:** Minor/Walking Wounded
   Victims in this category have sustained minor injury or are presenting with minimal signs of illness. Prolonged delay in care most likely will not adversely effect their long-term outcome (e.g., a conscious victim with superficial cuts, scrapes, and bruises).
4. **Black:** Dead/Non-salvageable
   Victims in this category are obviously dead or have suffered mortal wounds because of which death is imminent (e.g., an unconscious victim with an open skull fracture with brain matter showing). Life-saving heroics on this group of victims will only delay medical care on more viable victims.

FIGURE 20–2. Victim triage tag recommended by the California Fire Chiefs Association. There are four basic categories that are all applied when a medical system is overwhelmed with victims. (Photo by Cynthia Tait.)

of a disaster. Knowing the principles and practice of triage allows the nurse to offer her or his nursing skills in the most effective manner.

The French word **triage** describes the process of sorting multiple casualties in the event of a war or major disaster. It is required when the number of casualties exceeds immediate treatment resources. The goal of triage is to effect the greatest amount of good for the greatest number of people. Figure 20–2 shows the four basic categories of the international triage system, as well as a triage tag.

Prioritization of treatment may be very different in a mass-casualty event as opposed to an average day in a hospital emergency department. For example, normally a person presenting to a hospital emergency room with a myocardial infarction would receive immediate treatment and have a significant chance of recovery. On a disaster site, a victim without a pulse or respirations would most likely be placed in the nonsalvageable category.

Immediate Treatment and Support. Disaster nurses provide treatment on-site at emergency treatment stations, in shelters, or at local hospitals and clinics. In addition to direct nursing care, interventions on-site might include arranging for transport once victims are stabilized and managing the procuring, distributing, and replenishing of all supplies. Disposable

items might be in short supply, requiring resterilization procedures that may be unfamiliar to a nurse not accustomed to field work, and a challenge for even an experienced nurse because of the field environment. Either on-site or in a shelter, provision and/or distribution of food and beverages, including infant formulas and rehydration fluids, may also be managed by the nurse, as may arranging for adequate, accessible, and safe sanitation facilities. Finally, the nurse often must arrange for psychological and spiritual care of victims of disasters.

Some victims who seem physically uninjured may, in fact, be suffering from major injuries but be unable to relate their symptoms to a relief worker because of shock or anxiety over injured, dead, or missing loved ones. For instance, a father pulling debris away from his collapsed house after a tornado may be so worried about a missing child that he does not realize he has a broken arm.

Other victims may be so emotionally traumatized by the disaster that they act out, disrupting efforts to assist them and other victims and even engaging in dangerous activities. This may cause relief workers to focus on their emotional care; however, such victims must be assessed for head trauma and internal injuries, because their behavior may have a physical cause. If they are physically able, giving such victims a simple, repetitive task to perform may distract them and restore, to a small extent, their sense of being able to control their environment.

Care of Bodies and Notification of Families. Identification and transport of the dead to a morgue or holding facility are crucial, especially if contagion is feared. Toe tags make documentation visible and accessible. Records of deaths must be made and maintained, and family members should be notified of their loved ones' deaths in as timely and compassionate a manner as possible. When feasible, a representative from each of the area's faith communities should be available to assist families awaiting news of loved ones who are missing. As was stated earlier, when notification of indirect victims is not possible because the victims' bodies are badly damaged or not found, the family's recovery from their loss is often delayed.

SUPPORTING RECOVERY FROM DISASTERS

Disasters do not suddenly end when the rubble is cleared and the victims' wounds are healed. Rather, recovery is a long, complex process that often includes long-term medical treatment, physical rehabilitation, financial restitution, and psychological and spiritual support.

Long-Term Treatment. Long-term treatment may be required for many victims of disasters, straining the local rehabilitative-care facilities and resources. Children who were victims may have to deal with lifelong disabilities or scars from their ordeal, and their families may be without adequate financial support for their child's medical care. Elderly citizens who may formerly have been in excellent health but who sustained serious injuries in the disaster might suddenly find that they can no longer live independently and must move to a long-term care facility. After floods, landslides, fires, or earthquakes, extensive property damage may cause some residents or businesses to relocate rather than rebuild on land they now deem disaster-prone. For these reasons, if a disaster creates numerous victims in a small community, it may alter the entire social fabric of that community permanently.

Long-Term Support. Victims of disasters may be in need of funding to reopen businesses, such as stores, restaurants, and other services needed by the community, or to repair or rebuild their homes. Insurance settlements, FEMA funding, and private donations may assist in financing community rehabilitation. Health care workers may be required to assist victims in filling out necessary paperwork because, immediately after a disaster, some victims may be unable to concentrate on anything beyond fulfilling their immediate needs and those of their family.

Psychological support is often required after a disaster, both for victims and for relief workers. Post-traumatic stress disorder (PTSD), a syndrome that may be marked by flashbacks, nightmares, disinterest in daily affairs, hypervigilance, survivor's guilt, or decreased concentration, may occur in some individuals. Less dramatically, many victims, especially elderly persons displaced from their homes, may quietly lose their will to live and drift into apathy and malaise. Individuals whose belief in God was unshakeable before the incident may now wonder how God could have let this happen, especially if they have lost a loved one. These victims often require not only empathic listening but also long-term skilled spiritual counseling before they can begin to regain their former faith. In assessing a community's citizens for counseling needs after a disaster, the nurse should not forget to include children. Often, children do not have words to express their feelings or fears and may act out in ways adults find difficult to understand, unless age-appropriate psychological intervention is provided.

Need for Self-Care. Self-care, including stress education for all relief workers after a disaster, helps to lower anxiety and put the situation into proper perspective. **Critical incident stress debriefing (CISD)** provides victims with a mechanism for emotional reconciliation. The ideal time for professional debriefing is between 24 and 72 hours after the disaster event. Positive effects of CISD include:

- Accelerating the healing process
- Equipping participants with positive coping mechanisms
- Clearing up misconceptions and misunderstandings
- Restoring or reinforcing group cohesiveness
- Promoting a healthy, supportive work atmosphere
- Identifying individuals requiring more extensive psychological assistance

CISD addresses all components of the human response to trauma, including physiologic effects, emotions, and cognition. Studies have shown that CISD has allowed individuals to regain a sense of normalcy to their lives much sooner than those not receiving CISD.

GROUP VIOLENCE

The rates of group violence and violent crime decreased in many U.S. cities at the end of the 1990s; the actual number of violent crimes peaked in 1993, at almost 4.2 million. By 1998, that number had dropped to less than 2.8 million (U.S. Bureau of Justice, 1999). However, violent crime is still an emotional and powerful public issue, often influencing our votes, our choices of where to live, work, shop, and vacation, and our decisions about where and how to educate our children. Indeed, the American Public Health Association (APHA) has worked for many years to "turn the spotlight on violence as a public health issue," calling gun violence in particular "both a public health emergency and a grave threat to the goal of equality and social justice" (APHA, 2000).

Types of Group Violence

We will discuss the problem of family violence in Chapter 25 and workplace violence in Chapter 29. Here, we look at how group violence and violent crimes affect schools and communities.

SCHOOL VIOLENCE

Violence among school-aged children is reaching alarming proportions in the United States. The 1990s saw multiple school shootings in small towns and large cities from the Southeast to the Northwest. Unfortunately, the trend seems to be continuing. In March 2000, people across the United States were shocked to learn of the shooting of a 6-year-old Michigan girl by a first-grade classmate at their elementary school. Currently, 10% of public schools report one or more serious violent crimes annually (homicide, rape, assault with a weapon, and so forth), and the leading crime reported by elementary schools is physical assault without a weapon (Riner, 1999). In 1997, the U.S. High School Risk Behavior Survey revealed that 18.3% of students had carried a weapon onto school property at least once and 5.9% had carried a gun in the past year. Approximately 33% of high school students have been victims of stolen or damaged property and 36.6% had been in at least one physical fight in the past 12 months. The reality of these statistics is validated when one considers that *daily:*

- 100,000 children take guns to school
- 6,250 teachers are verbally or physically threatened
- 260 teachers are assaulted
- 14,000 students are assaulted on school property
- 160,000 children miss school because of their fear of violence

GANG VIOLENCE

The California Attorney General defines a **gang** as a loose-knit organization of individuals between the ages of 14 and 24 that has a name, is usually territorial or claims a certain territory as under its exclusive influence, and is involved in criminal acts. Its members associate together and commit crimes against other gangs or against the general population. Specifically, gangs are most commonly involved in drug distribution, aggravated assault, robbery, burglary, and motor vehicle theft (U.S. Department of Justice, 1999). Large cities are the most likely to have gang problems, whereas rural counties are the least likely.

Gangs often require members to display symbols of their allegiance to one another. These symbols also serve to identify them to other gangs. They may include certain colors, special caps or coats, tattoos, handshakes or other signs, and terminology unique to the gang. Gangs may also require members to participate in "rites of passage" or "hazing" events to test their loyalty. Many of these activities involve committing a crime. Gang members usually share the same ethnicity or at least the same belief system. Finally, many gangs today have sophisticated websites and are capable of equally sophisticated crimes.

Gang members consider themselves family and turn to each other or the group for support. Often, members are searching for emotional intimacy in the gang as a substitute for a dysfunctional family that is unwilling or unable to provide that intimacy. Gangs also provide discipline and a structured environment to young people who, because of absent or unresponsive parents, may have a strong desire for an external locus of authority and a set of predictable rules and regulations.

RIOTS

A **riot** is a violent disturbance created by a large number of people assembled for a common purpose. It may or may not involve criminal activities, such as willful destruction of cars, stores, and other property, **looting** (stealing goods), **arson** (the deliberate burning of buildings), **lynching** (executing without due process of law), or physical attacks on the perceived "enemy" or on law enforcement officers.

Riots often erupt during times of war, political instability, racial inequity, and economic injustice. For example, in the United States, the decades of the 1960s and 1970s were marked by frequent demonstrations against the Vietnam War, which occasionally escalated from peaceful marching and protests to full-scale riots. Riots have also been sparked during protests of racial inequities and are especially common after announcements of legal decisions that are perceived as racist. For example, when the officers accused of assaulting Rodney King in Los Angeles were acquitted in April of 1992, violent riots caused 53 deaths, 2,000 arrests, and more than a billion dollars in property damage. Internationally, riots often erupt over inflated food prices or unequal distribution of food or supplies. In 1999, for example, there were widespread riots in India over the inflated price and limited availability of onions, a staple in the Indian diet.

VIOLENT CRIMES

Violent crimes include those involving physical or psychological injury or death or the threat of injury or death. These crimes are often accompanied by destruction to or loss of property. For example, armed robbery is considered a violent crime, whether or not anyone is injured during the crime.

Assault and Battery. Legally, **assault and battery** refers to the threat to use force against another person, and the accomplishment of that threat. More loosely, *assault* can be used to refer to any violent attack, such as an "assault with a deadly weapon" or "sexual assault." We will discuss domestic assault in Chapter 25.

One type of group assault that is becoming more prevalent is assault on the homeless. These assaults are usually perpetrated on individual homeless men, often by groups of three or more young men who beat the victim severely and sometimes fatally, sometimes for no other reason than that he asked them for money. Alcohol and drugs are often, though not always, factors.

Rape. Legal definitions of **rape** vary, but the key elements include some form of sexual contact and a lack of consent. Consent is considered lacking under conditions of force, deception, or coercion or when the victim is of minor age, drugged, unconscious, mentally retarded, or physically restrained.

A variety of different types of rape are also commonly described. One of the most common is *date rape,* in which the assailant and victim meet by mutual consent, but the assailant forces the victim to engage in a sexual act against the victim's will. *Stranger rape* is sudden and usually violent, involving the use of a knife, gun, or violent physical force. *Statutory rape* refers to sexual intercourse with a female who has not reached the statutory age of consent; in many states, this age is 14. Rape may also be perpetrated by a group, as when a group of college males drugs and then rapes a female student or when a youth gang assaults and rapes a woman jogging on their "turf" after dark.

Homicide. **Homicide** is the killing of one person by another. Like the rates for group violence overall, the homicide rate is declining. In 1980, there were 10.2 homicides per every 100,000 population; by 1998, this rate had fallen to 6.3 per 100,000 (U.S. Bureau of Justice, 1999). However, homicide is still the leading cause of death for African-American youth ages 15 to 24. Their rate is an alarming 114.6 per 100,000 (Singh, Kochanek, & MacDorman, 1996). In addition, the 21st century has already witnessed numerous instances of multiple homicides in schools, universities, restaurants, and workplaces. For example, on March 1, 2000, a gunman in Pennsylvania went on a shooting spree at his apartment complex and at two fast-food restaurants, killing two people and critically wounding three.

Genocide. The most notorious historical example of **genocide,** the killing of a group of people because of their racial, political, or cultural differences, was the murder of millions of Jews, Catholics, gypsies, homosexuals, intellectuals, and other "undesirables" by the Nazis before and during World War II. Tragically, genocide continues today. Recent examples include the mass "ethnic cleansings" in Bosnia, Rwanda, and Kosovo in the last decade of the 20th century.

Factors Contributing to Group Violence

The U.S. Department of Justice has identified a number of host causes or correlates of delinquency, including feelings of alienation or rebelliousness and lack of societal bonding (Wilson & Howell, 1993). Environmental factors include:

- Parental conflict, lack of supervision, child abuse, or inconsistent parenting
- Negative school experiences, including early academic failure and lack of commitment to school
- Negative peer influence, including peers who engage in criminal activity
- Socioeconomic factors, such as high rates of substance abuse in the community, living in a high-crime neighborhood, and economic deprivation

The roots of youth gang problems are multifactorial. They may be related to lack of social opportunities, social disorganization, institutional racism, cultural misadaptation, deficiencies in social policy, and the availability of criminal opportunities.

Additionally, frequent exposure to violence in the news, at sporting events, on television programs, in movies, on the Internet, in video games, and in violent pornography has been linked to an increase in aggression. Children seem to be especially vulnerable, and the link seems to be especially strong when the subject matter glorifies violence as the ideal and appropriate solution to personal problems. For example, Dr. James Garbarino of Cornell University, author of *Lost Boys: Why Our Sons Turn Violent and How We Can Save Them* (1999), observes that children " . . . have ample opportunities to see on television and in the movies how you threaten people, what it means to shoot someone, and ample opportunities to learn about revenge and how desirable it is in this society. For the nation to be shocked and appalled . . . is either a kind of denial or hypocrisy" (Goode, 2000).

Simple access to weapons cannot be discounted as a factor in criminal activity. The United States imposes fewer restrictions on the manufacture, sale, and licensure of guns than any other first-world nation and, as a correlate, is faced with higher rates of gun-related injuries and murders. Indeed, many of the youths involved in school shootings in the United States in the 1990s had easy access to guns belonging to parents, other relatives, or neighbors, whereas weapons such as simple bombs can be made from instructions found on the Internet. Increasingly, rifles and assault weapons rather than handguns are being used in acts of group violence. These weapons allow for more rapid firing of more bullets than handguns and tend to cause significantly higher numbers of casualties. The murders of 12 students and 1 teacher in the assault in 1999 at Columbine High School in Colorado, for example, were only made possible by the easy acquisition and use of these more sophisticated weapons (see Research: Bridge to Practice).

Both agent and environmental factors can contribute to rape. Some of the more common include an increased history of childhood sexual abuse among rapists, a patriarchal value system in which males are expected to prove their masculinity by dominating or "conquering" women, and an environment in which violence is explicitly or implicitly accepted or encouraged. In two different surveys of college-age men, conducted 10 years apart, an average of more than 40% of the men surveyed said that they would rape a woman if they were

RESEARCH Bridge to Practice

Safety and Home Firearm Storage Patterns

Schuster, M.A., Franke, T.M., Bastian, A.M., Sor, S., & Halfon, N. (2000). Firearm storage patterns in US homes with children. *American Journal of Public Health, 90*(4), 588–594.

The researchers involved with this study used data from the 1994 National Health Interview Survey (NHIS) and the Year 2000 Objectives supplement to look at the presence of firearms in the home and firearm storage patterns among families with children. The NHIS is an annual survey covering demographics, health, health care utilization, and insurance. One section of the Year 2000 supplement covers firearms.

Respondents from the 6,990 sample homes with children younger than 18 years old (representing more than 22 million children in more than 11 million homes) reported that they had at least one firearm (69% reported having more than one firearm), with 43% keeping at least one unlocked firearm. Overall, 9% kept firearms unlocked, unloaded, and stored with ammunition; thus, 1.4 million homes with 2.6 million children stored firearms in a manner accessible to children.

The percentage of children living in homes with firearms increases with the child's age, from 28% for children younger than 1 year old to 38% for children aged 13 to 17 years old. The types of firearms these families had included 53% with a handgun, 61% with a shotgun, 65% with a rifle, and 2% with another type of firearm.

Although only a small percentage of families (9%) report storing firearms unlocked and loaded, this percentage represents 946,000 homes with 1,708,000 children who have access to a firearm ready to use. An additional 911,000 children live in homes where firearms are stored unlocked, unloaded, and with ammunition. With the accessibility of firearms increasing in households as children age, loading firearms by older children is a possibility.

Community health nurses, of course, do not control what goes on in the homes of families with children. Ultimately, families will decide what they believe is best. We can, however, make sure that when families make these decisions, they are informed about the risks associated with firearms and how to reduce those risks. Special efforts may be warranted to address firearm safety issues directly with adolescents.

---

certain they could not be caught and punished. Most also reported believing that the woman would enjoy it (Sampselle, 1991).

Healthy People 2010 Goals for Reducing Group Violence

The *Healthy People 2010* (U.S. Dept. of Health and Human Services, 2000) document lists a number of goals focused on reducing youth violence, including:

- Reduce physical assaults among people aged 12 and older to less than 25.5 per 1,000 persons, from a baseline in 1998 of 31.1 per 1,000 persons

- Reduce to 33.3% the prevalence of physical fighting among adolescents in grades 9 through 12 from a baseline in 1997 of 36.6%
- Reduce to less than 6% the prevalence of weapon carrying by adolescents in grades 9 through 12 from a baseline in 1997 of 8.5%

In addition, *Healthy People 2010* calls for a reduction in work-related homicides to no more than 0.4 per 100,000 workers from a baseline in 1998 of 0.5 per 100,000. It also calls for a reduction in workplace assault to no more than 0.6 per 100 workers from a baseline in 1987 to 1992 of 0.85 per 100.

Role of the Community Health Nurse

Community health nurses can play a key role in reducing group violence by interacting with students, parents, churches, law enforcement officials, local politicians, and community organizers.

PREVENTING GROUP VIOLENCE

The typical model for preventing or reducing group violence includes activities such as assessing the problem, developing policy based on established objectives, conducting research, procuring funding, and promoting offender accountability. For example, an increase in rapes on one university campus might prompt the nursing department to facilitate a university-wide open forum to discuss the issue, identify possible factors, initiate research, and develop solutions. Programs might include outreach to all students currently enrolled at the university through dormitory teaching sessions, church-group activities, involvement of team coaches for university sports, and even participation by teachers and student advisors.

Research has shown that violence can be reduced in elementary and secondary schools by increasing supervision and surveillance. Examples of successful actions some schools have taken are listed in Display 20–4.

Community health nurses can influence the reduction of school violence by establishing strong cooperative relationships between adults and students (Riner, 1999). Examples of such involvement include:

- Speaking about school violence at middle and high school assemblies, PTA meetings, parenting meetings, neighborhood-watch meetings, church meetings, and so forth
- Participating in local and national crime-prevention councils
- Joining professional nursing organizations that engage in campaigns to reduce violence
- Writing, producing, or promoting public service announcements that aim to reduce violence
- Promoting the inclusion of articles about group violence in local newspapers, community newsletters, church bulletins, and so forth
- Offering ongoing anger management and conflict resolution courses

DISPLAY 20-4. Actions Schools Can Take to Reduce Violence

Schools can take the following actions to reduce their risk for violence:

- Improve environmental design
- Install surveillance cameras, metal detectors, and pay phones or dial-free access connections to emergency services
- Increase security personnel
- Decrease access by outsiders to campus
- Institute school-wide safety plans, drills, and codes
- Train administrators and teachers to identify potentially violent or psychologically impaired students
- Identify students who are associated with gangs
- Expel students who are caught with weapons on campus
- Suspend or expel students for threatened or real acts of violence
- Institute a policy that allows for searching students and lockers
- Hold parents accountable for students' actions and make them financially responsible for any damages incurred

To reduce gang membership and associated violence, positive social development starting from infancy and focusing intensively on interactions within the school system is crucial. The school nurse or community health nurse working within education can sponsor programs to nurture social values and ethics and to help students dissociate from delinquent peers and role models. After-school programs in which youths have an opportunity to play sports; volunteer with the poor, the sick, or the elderly; or challenge their learning in math clubs, on debate teams, and so forth can improve self-esteem and reduce the seduction of gang membership.

The community health nurse can also provide proactive leadership in preventing gang activity. Community mobilization and local organization are key components. Additionally, understanding both the roots of specific gang issues as well as the community conditions that contribute to the problem is necessary for finding solutions and alternatives to youth gang involvement.

An effective school gang-suppression strategy should include:

- Development of guidelines for appropriate teacher and staff response to a variety of gang behaviors and delinquency
- Application and enforcement of rules and regulations that support positive relationships and communication between school personnel, parents, students, and community agencies
- Development of parenting and gang-awareness classes
- Establishment of training programs for increasing

knowledge of gangs and the community resources available for assistance

Finally, while community health nurses cannot prevent riots as such, they can be familiar persons in their neighborhoods, encouraging the sharing of feelings of anger or hostility or the exchange of information about criminal activities. Also, the nurse is usually familiar with the normal environment in the neighborhood—the flow of people, the usual level of friendliness of neighbors and business owners, and the usual activities. The nurse can use this familiarity to detect when there is something unusual in the "feeling" of the neighborhood. Part of a continuous community assessment includes gathering such subconscious impressions or intuitions. If cues from the community indicate increased tensions or exaggerated negative feelings toward particular persons or groups, the nurse can share this information with the proper authorities. Many neighborhoods are served by community centers where there are social workers, educators, neighborhood-watch groups, probation officers, and other community service workers who are excellent resources with whom the nurse can share perceptions.

ASSESSING A COMMUNITY'S LEVEL OR POTENTIAL FOR VIOLENCE

School nurses are in an ideal position to identify behaviors that indicate an increased potential for youth violence and to initiate age-appropriate therapies. The following indicators can be used to identify potentially violent youths. It is crucial to identify these behaviors early and to teach others to watch for them (National Crime Prevention Council, 1999):

- Depression or mood swings
- Obsession with violent or pornographic games, Internet sites, television shows, or movies
- Absence of age-appropriate anger-management skills
- Artwork, writing, or language that displays violence, profanity, anger, association with gangs, or social isolation
- Evidence of cruelty to animals
- History of bullying or fighting
- Self-perception as a victim
- Obsession with violence or weapons

All riots begin with an altercation between two or more people that then accelerates out of control. Thus, in assessing a community's potential for a riot, the nurse needs to be keenly and continually aware of interactions between individuals and smaller groups within the community. In some sharply divided communities, even disagreements at a school-board meeting or town-council meeting can escalate into localized riots. In communities where drug dealing is common, riots between gangs can occur when drug deals "go bad" or when police conduct large "sting" operations. Communities fraught with poverty, high levels of unemployment, or ethnic or racial divisions also experience a high level of tension that can erupt into violence over seemingly minor events, such as a routine arrest of individuals in a barroom brawl. Even the number and quality of constructive after-school activities for older children and teens can be a predictor of group violence, because restless teens roaming neighborhood streets, drinking alcohol, and "looking for fun" often end up engaging in violent fights and group crimes. In all these areas, the community health nurse has an obligation to assess for the potential for group violence.

RESPONDING TO GROUP VIOLENCE

Community models for addressing the problem of group violence should involve as many community members as possible. Not only key legislators and law enforcement officials but also former criminals and even current gang members and youth and adult offenders should be included. Community religious leaders, educators, members of social and cultural organizations, and even criminologists can contribute significantly to developing effective plans for action that the entire community can endorse. The community health nurse also should be integrally involved in these community actions to reduce group violence.

SUPPORTING RECOVERY FROM GROUP VIOLENCE

Although the community health nurse should leave investigation and suppression of violent crime to law enforcement officials, an effective interface for community rehabilitation may involve education, community mobilization, and outreach. Comprehensive case management is paramount. Multiagency cooperation is required to provide needed services for mental health, drug treatment, family counseling, job training and placement, reentry to school or workforce, forming more positive social alliances, and providing expanded economic opportunities.

Counseling is the primary rehabilitative intervention for victims of rape and may be necessary not only immediately after the attack but months or even years later, as new responses and reactions arise. In addition, options for pregnancy prevention and the prevention of sexually transmitted disease need to be discussed. Possible exposure to human immunodeficiency virus (HIV) is another harrowing aspect of rape with which women need medical and psychological support to cope.

TERRORISM

The turn of the 21st century has proved that society has become a global community. This is particularly evident in the increased incidence and sophistication of terrorist threats and acts around the world. Incidents such as the bombing of the New York World Trade Center in 1993 have emphasized the need for increased preparedness within our communities. Terrorist bombings increased 400% between 1984 and 1994, resulting in 256 deaths, 3,215 injuries, and $575 million in property damage (Buck, 1998).

Terrorism is the unlawful use of force or violence against persons or property to intimidate or coerce a government or civilian population in the furtherance of political or social objectives. Terrorists typically use nuclear, biologic, or chemical (NBC) agents and explosives/incendiary devices against their targets. Common biologic agents include anthrax, botulinum, bubonic plague, Ebola, and smallpox. For example, the U.S. Office of Technology Assessment (U.S. Army Chemical and Biological Defense Command, 1998) speculates that the release of 220 lb of anthrax spores from a cropduster over the Washington, DC, area on a calm, clear night could kill 1 to 3 million people.

Factors Contributing to Terrorism

Political factors are the most common contributors to terrorism. Anti-American sentiment runs high in many foreign countries, especially those that perceive the United States as a threat to their military, economic, social, or religious self-determination. Terrorism against American military installations abroad, in airports, in planes, at American embassies, and even on American soil has occurred frequently in the last decade as an expression of political unrest.

Within the United States, violence-prone members of militia movements, violent anti-abortion activists, racial desegregation advocates, and other radical groups have performed terrorist acts, such as the bombing of health clinics offering abortions. As another example, in the fall of 1984, members of a religious cult in Oregon that had been denied permission to build on their land decided to try to reduce voter turnout in an upcoming election by sprinkling *Salmonella* bacteria on salad bars in local restaurants. They hoped that with a reduced voter turnout, representatives friendlier to their group would win the election. Their attack failed to affect the election and killed no one; however, 751 people became sick.

Role of the Community Health Nurse

Community health nurses should be alert to the signs of possible terrorist activity. They must look and listen within their communities for antigroup sentiments and report any untoward activities accordingly. Specific indicators of possible chemical or biologic terrorism include unusual dead or dying animals; unexplained serious illnesses or deaths; unusual liquid, spray, vapor, or odor; and low-lying clouds or fog unrelated to weather. Unusual swarms of insects might also indicate usage of biologic agents for terrorism. Less subtle forms of terrorism include bombings, mass shootings, and hijackings.

Although prevention of terrorist incidences is primarily the responsibility of the Department of Defense and law enforcement agencies, community health nurses must be ready to handle the secondary and tertiary effects of such attacks. Realizing that terrorist attacks may result in large numbers of casualties, the community health nurse must be prepared to act safely, access information rapidly, and use resources effectively. Specifically, the community health nurse may be

---

CLINICAL CORNER | **Communities in Crisis—Disaster, Group Violence, Terrorism**

A 1999 shooting at a high school in Colorado left 15 people dead. National attention was focused on the issue of violence among teens. The public and the media looked to public health experts for answers to the problem of increasing violence in this population. Community health nurses are among those whose aim is to assess and address the problems surrounding individual and group violence in their communities.

Imagine that, as a community health nurse, you have just been named the head of a multidisciplinary task force whose objective is to prevent teen violence within your community. Your project has been funded for 3 years. Having worked in other nursing roles in your community over the past 10 years, you have developed excellent partnerships with resources within your community. After reading the information about your community, respond to the questions that follow.

Community Information

A desert suburban community of 40,000 individuals, primarily commuting to high-tech jobs in a nearby city. The average household income is $56,000 per year. The divorce rate in the community is 63%. The number of teens whose primary caregiver returns home after

5:30 PM is 78%. Ethnicity is as follows: 52% Anglo, 30% Asian, 12% Hispanic, 4% Black, and 2% other.

Identified problems among teens include racial division, gang violence, high school dropout rate of 17%, high incidence of methamphetamine use. The incidence of violent crimes in this community is 28% higher than in neighboring communities.

Besides organized sports, there are very few extracurricular activities available through the school or within the community.

Questions
1. Faced with this daunting task, where will you begin your efforts?
2. With what agencies and individuals will you need to develop partnerships to maximize the efficacy of the task force?
3. Brainstorm about possible ways you will capitalize on the use of technology in your efforts to reduce the risk of violence in the community.
4. How will you disseminate the information you obtain to advance the cause of globalization of public health?
5. What ethical issues will you anticipate as you begin your efforts?

---

called on to provide direct care to victims, to volunteer as a hospital-community liaison, to set up and administer mass immunizations, to make home visits to affected families, or to serve on committees responding to terrorist acts. Formulating, updating, and following a disaster plan is one of the most effective community-based strategies to minimize injury and mortality from terrorism.

SUMMARY

A disaster is any event that causes a level of destruction that exceeds the abilities of the affected community to respond without assistance. Disasters may be caused by natural or technological events and may be classified as multiple-casualty incidents or mass-casualty incidents.

The scope of a disaster is its range of effect, and the intensity is the level of destruction it causes.

Victims of disasters include direct victims, those injured or killed, and indirect victims, the loved ones of direct victims. Displaced persons are those forced to flee their homes because of the disaster, and refugees are specifically those who are forced to leave their homelands, usually in response to war or political persecution.

Host factors that contribute to the likelihood of experiencing a disaster include age, general health, mobility,

psychological factors, and even socioeconomic factors. The disaster agent is the fire, flood, bomb, or other cause. Environmental factors are those that could potentially contribute to or mitigate a disaster.

In developing strategies to address the problem of disasters, it is helpful for the community health nurse to consider each of the four phases of disaster management: prevention, preparedness, response, and recovery.

Primary prevention of disasters means keeping the disaster from ever happening, taking actions to completely eliminate its occurrence. Secondary prevention focuses on earliest possible detection and treatment. Tertiary prevention involves reducing the amount and degree of disability or damage resulting from the disaster.

In addition to assessing for preparedness, an effective disaster plan establishes a clear chain of authority, develops lines of communication, and delineates routes and modes of transport. Plans for mobilizing, warning, and evacuating are also critical elements of the disaster plan.

At the disaster site, police, firefighters, nurses, and other relief workers effect a coordinated response to rescue victims from further injury, triage victims by seriousness of injury, and treat victims on-site and in local hospitals. Care and transport of dead bodies must also be managed, as well as support for the loved ones of the injured, dead, or missing.

Long-term support includes both financial assistance and physical and emotional rehabilitation.

Self-care, including stress education for all relief workers after a disaster, helps to lower anxiety and put the situation into proper perspective. Critical incident stress debriefing (CISD) provides victims with a mechanism for emotional reconciliation and healing.

Problems of group violence include school violence, gangs, riots, and violent crimes. A gang is an organization of youths that has a name, is usually territorial or claims a certain territory as under its exclusive influence, and is involved in criminal acts.

The roots of group violence are multifactorial, including inadequate parenting, socioeconomic and racial injustices, exposure to violence in media, cartoons, pornography, and easy access to weapons.

Healthy People 2010 goals for reducing violence include reductions in physical assaults and weapon carrying among school children, and reduction of work-related assaults and homicides.

The role of the community health nurse in preventing and reducing group violence includes effective community organization and program development, as well as policy making to address the family and environmental factors that contribute to increased risk of group violence.

Terrorism is the unlawful use of force or violence against persons or property to intimidate or coerce a government or civilian population in the furtherance of political or social objectives. The community health nurse should be alert to the signs of possible terrorist activity, and be prepared to address the secondary or tertiary effects of such attacks. (See Clinical Corner.)

ACTIVITIES TO PROMOTE CRITICAL THINKING

1. Think about your own community and its residents. What are some host factors that might increase its risk of experiencing a disaster? What environmental factors might be significant? In each case, identify the likely agent. What interventions could be included in a disaster plan to reduce these risk factors?
2. The nightly news shows that at least 200 people have been injured in an explosion in a neighboring community. At the disaster site, victims are still being recovered from the wreckage, and local hospitals are overwhelmed with patients with fractures, lacerations, and burns. You want to offer your assistance as a registered nurse, but how should you go about volunteering your services?
3. Your local high school is complaining of an increasing gang presence. Members have been recruiting and intimidating students, and fights with

knives have broken out repeatedly in the past month. A random search of lockers revealed two guns and eight knives, and as many as 25% of students are remaining out of school because of parents' fears of violence. Describe one possible response of a community health nurse to address the problem of gang violence in this situation.
4. Access one or more of the Internet sites listed in this chapter. Report on the change in statistics for either disasters, group violence, or terrorism since the year 2000. Have rates increased or decreased? What factors might be involved in this change?

REFERENCES

American Association of Colleges of Nursing. (1999). *Violence as a public health problem: Position statement*. Washington, DC: Author.

American Public Health Association. (2000, February). *The nation's health* (p. 13). Washington, DC: Author.

Anteau, C. M., & Williams, L. A. (1998, March). What we learned from the Oklahoma City bombing. *Nursing 98*.

Bromet, E., & Dew, M. A. (1995). Review of psychiatric epidemiologic research on disasters. *Epidemiological Review, 17*, 113–119.

Buck, G. (1998). *Preparing for terrorism: An emergency services guide*. Albany, NY: Delmar Publishers.

Burgess, A. W., & Fawcett, J. (1996). The comprehensive sexual assault assessment tool. *Nurse Practitioner, 21*(4), 66–86.

Everly, G., Jr. (1995). *Innovations in disaster and trauma psychology. Volume One: Applications in emergency services and disaster response*. Ellicott City, MD: Chevron Publishing.

Farrell, A. D., Meyer, A. L., & Dahlberg, L. L. (1996). Richmond youth against violence: A school-based program for urban adolescents. *American Journal of Preventive Medicine, 12*(5, Suppl), 13–21.

Feiner, B. (1996, March). Basic instinct: The delicate balance of safety versus heroism. *EMS Magazine,* 19.

Garbarino, J. (1999). *Lost boys: Why our sons turn violent and how we can save them*. New York: Free Press.

Gellert, G. A. (1998). *Confronting violence*. Washington, DC: American Public Health Association.

Goode, E. (2000, March 2). Struggling to make sense out of boy-turned-killer. *New York Times*.

Hadley, S. M., Short, L. M., & Zook, E. (1996). WomanKind: An innovative model of health care response to domestic abuse. *Women's Health Issues, 5*(4), 189–198.

Hopmeier, M. J. (1998, August). Terrorism scenarios: If they come true, this can happen to you! *Responder*.

Logue, J. N. (1996). Disasters, the environment, and public health: Improving our response. *American Journal of Public Health, 86*(9), 1207–1210.

Maniscalco, P. M., & Christen, H. T. (1999, January). EMS incident management: Emergency medical logistics. *EMS Magazine,* 693–701.

Moralejo, D. G., Russell, M. L., & Porat, B. L. (1997,

July/August). Outbreaks can be disasters: A guide to developing your plan. *Journal of Emergency Nursing, 27*(7/8), 56–60.

National Crime Prevention Council. (1999, October 25). Watch for signs—Take action. Available: http://www.ncpc.org/2schvio/htm#signs.

Nawar, M. (1998). Workplace violence: One nurse's night of fear. *American Nurse, 30*(5), 15.

Noji, E. K. (1997). *The public health consequences of disasters.* New York: Oxford University Press.

Osattin, A., & Short, L. M. (1998). *Intimate partner violence and sexual assault: A guide to training materials and programs for health care providers.* Atlanta, GA: National Center for Injury Prevention and Control, CDC.

Pan American Health Organization. (1995). *Guidelines for assessing disaster preparedness in the health sector.* Washington, DC: Author.

Riner, M. E. (1999, November 1). Stopping school violence in its tracks. *Nurseweek, 12*(22), 18–19.

Sampselle, C. (1991). The role of nursing in preventing violence against women. *Journal of Obstetric, Gynecologic, and Neonatal Nursing, 20*(6), 481.

Schuster, M. A., Franke, T. M., Bastian, A. M., Sor, S., & Halfron, N. (2000). Firearm storage patterns in US homes with children. *American Journal of Public Health, 90*(4), 588–594.

Singh, G. K., Kochanek, K. D., & MacDorman, M. F. (1996). Advance report of final mortality statistics, 1994. *Monthly Vital Statistics Report, 45*(3S), 96–120.

U.S. Army Chemical and Biological Defense Command. (1998). *Domestic preparedness program: Hospital provider course.* McLean, VA: Booz-Allen & Hamilton, Inc. and SAIC, Inc.

U.S. Department of Health and Human Services (2000). *Healthy people 2010* (conference edition in two volumes). Washington, DC: U.S. Government Printing Office.

U.S. Department of Justice, Office of Juvenile Justice and Delinquency Prevention. (1999, March). *Highlights of the 1997 National Youth Gang Survey.* Washington, DC: Author.
———. (1994, October). *Gang suppression and intervention: Community models: Research summary.* Washington, DC: Author.

Visher, C. A. (1994). Understanding the roots of crime. *National Institute of Justice Journal, 228,* 9–15.

Wilson, J. J., & Howell, J. C. (1993). *A comprehensive strategy for serious, violent, and chronic juvenile offenders.* Washington, DC: U.S. Department of Justice, Office of Juvenile Justice.

INTERNET RESOURCES

Action Committee Against Violence
http://www.gov.calgary.ab.ca

Almanac of Disasters
http://www.disasterium.com

Disasters
http://www.expage.com

MADV—Domestic Violence Resources
http://www.silicom.com

National Coalition Against Domestic Violence NCADVE.htm
http://www.healthtouch.com

National Crime Prevention Council
http://www.ncpc.org

National School Board Association
http://www.keepschoolssafe.org

National School Safety Center
http://www.nssc1.org

National Youth Gang Center
http://www.iir.com/nygc/

NBC Domestic Preparedness
http://www.nbc.prepare.org

Pan American Health Organization
http://www.paho.org/english/disaster.htm

Partnerships Against Violence Network (PAVNET)
http://www.healthfinder.gov

United Nations Declaration of Human Rights "A Life Free from Violence"
http://www.undp.org

Violence protection: Family services
http://www.clerkofcourts.com

Youth Crime Watch of America
http://www.ycwa.org

SELECTED READINGS

Bonnie, R. J., Fulco, C. E., & Liverman, C. T. (Eds.). (1999). *Reducing the burden of injury: Advancing prevention and treatment.* New York: Population Council.

Brenner, S. A., & Noji, E. K. (1995). Tornado injuries related to housing in the Plainfield tornado. *International Journal of Epidemiology, 24,* 144–149.

Chandler, K. A., Chapman, C. D., Rand, M. R., & Taylor, B. M. (1998). *Students' reports of school crime: 1989 and 1995.* NCES publication 98-241/NCJ-169607. Washington, DC: U.S. Department of Education.

Corder, C., & Brobl, K. (Eds.). (1999). *It couldn't happen here: Recognizing and helping desperate kids.* Washington, DC: Child Welfare League of America.

Elders, J. (1994). Violence as a public health issue for children. *Childhood Education, 70,* 260–262.

Ellickson, P. L., & McGuigan, K. A. (2000). Early predictors of adolescent violence. *American Journal of Public Health, 90*(4), 566–572.

Friedman, E. (1994). Coping with calamity: How well does health care disaster planning work? *Journal of the American Medical Association, 272,* 1875–1879.

Gerrity, E. T., & Flynn, B. W. (1997). Mental health consequences of disasters. In E. K. Noji (Ed.), *The public health consequences of disasters* (pp. 101–121). New York: Oxford University Press.

Kleck, G. (1997). *Targeting guns: Firearms and their control.* New York: Adeline De Gruyter.

Leor, J., Poole, W. K., & Kloner, R. A. (1996). Sudden cardiac death triggered by an earthquake. *New England Journal of Medicine, 334,* 414–419.

McFarlane, A. C. (1995). Stress and disaster. In S. E. Hobfol & M. W. de Vries (Eds.), *Extreme stress and communities: Impact and intervention* (pp. 247–265). Boston: Kluwer Academics.

Meyer, M., & Graeter, C. (1995). Health professional's role in disaster planning. *American Association of Occupational Health Nurses Journal, 43*(5), 251–262.

O'Carroll, P. W., Friede, A., Noji, E. K., et al. (1995). The rapid implementation of a statewide emergency health information system during the 1993 Iowa flood. *American Journal of Public Health, 85,* 564–567.

Rosner, D. (2000). When does a worker's death become murder? *American Journal of Public Health, 90*(4), 535–540.

Saner, H., & Ellickson, P. L. (1996). Concurrent risk factors for adolescent violence. *Journal of Adolescent Health, 19,* 94–103.

Schultz, C. H., Koenig, K. L., & Noji, E. K. (1996). A medical disaster response to reduce immediate mortality after an earthquake. *New England Journal of Medicine, 334,* 438–444.

Wallace, D., & Wallace, R. (1998). Scales of geography, time, and population: The study of violence as a public health problem. *American Journal of Public Health, 88,* 1853–1858.

The Global Community: International Health Concerns

KEY TERMS

- Bilateral agencies
- Chronic disease
- Disability-Adjusted Life Year (DALY)
- Eradication, elimination, and control of communicable disease
- Global Burden of Disease (GBD)
- Global nursing
- Health for All
- Integrated management of childhood illness (IMCI)
- Multilateral agencies
- New and emerging diseases
- Non-governmental organizations (NGOs)
- Pluralistic medical systems
- Primary health care
- Private voluntary organizations (PVOs)
- United States Agency for International Development (USAID)
- World Bank (WB)
- World Health Organization (WHO)

LEARNING OBJECTIVES

Upon mastery of this chapter, you should be able to:
- Discuss the interrelationship of global health issues.
- Describe the pluralistic medical systems of the world.
- Differentiate between multilateral and bilateral agencies.
- Explain the role of non-governmental agencies.
- Describe the purpose of the World Health Organization.
- Discuss the United States Agency for International Development (USAID).
- Analyze the implications of the Health for All movement.
- Be familiar with specific global health concerns.
- Describe what is meant by the Global Burden of Disease and Disability-Adjusted Life Year.
- Differentiate between eradication, elimination, and control of communicable disease.
- Identify new and emerging diseases.
- Increase awareness of the role of the global nurse.
- Summarize global nursing opportunities.

The pictures taken of the earth from space a number of years ago were a graphic illustration that we belong to one small planet of interdependent nations. This interdependence relates to virtually all areas of life, including health. As systems theory suggests, what happens in one country affects many others in important ways. For example, the 1999 war in Kosovo forced refugees not only into neighboring countries but also into host countries overseas as well. The polio-immunization level of 2-year-olds in Kosovo was only at 53%; therefore, when a case of suspected polio was registered in that country in August 1999, the risk of a major outbreak in the area was high (WHO, 1999a). As another example, air travel can transport health problems from a country halfway around the world to new communities in less than a day. In New York in the fall of 1999, sixty-one severe cases and seven deaths were reported from a mysterious viral illness later identified as the West Nile virus, which had not previously been reported in the U.S. Researchers now speculate that the virus may have traveled to the U.S. in smuggled exotic birds. The virus was closely related genetically to strains found in the Middle East (CDC, 2000). Global health issues become ours when they spread within our borders, when we commit resources to a country in need, or when we make a personal commitment to improving the health of a population beyond our shores.

Much of this text focuses on community health nursing at the local, state, or national level. We hope that this chapter will help you recognize the contributions of community health nurses internationally, and perhaps prompt you to investigate international nursing as a career option. Health care on a global level carries with it the allure of travel to foreign countries and offers the nurse exclusive views of the world and humanity. In addition, it provides a unique opportunity to improve the health of the world that we inhabit, to help create a healthy planetary community. A sense of justice commonly compels nurses to enter international health: many are concerned about the intolerable conditions that one-third of the world suffers, especially when they realize that they are benefiting from the misfortunes of the poor (Lanza, 1996). Whatever their reasons for choosing global health, it is clear that nurses make a profound contribution to the health of disenfranchised populations around the world.

In this chapter, we will see how health issues are addressed throughout the world in terms of international responses, ideology, community development, and the establishment of health priorities. Some health care systems and agencies will be described, illustrating both their differing goals and structures and their similar struggles and challenges. The main health concerns facing our world will then be discussed. Lastly, career and service opportunities for nurses will be suggested.

INTERNATIONAL HEALTH CARE SYSTEMS

Pluralistic medical systems are found in practically all developing countries. They often consist of traditional healing systems, lay practices, household remedies, transitional health workers, and Western medicine (Kloos, 1994). Traditional healing may be all that is available to populations in most rural areas and also in cities. Other than traditional birth attendants, it is not customary for national health systems to integrate traditional healing into the national health system, with the exception of the U.S., China, India, and some African countries. Western medicine was introduced to developing countries during colonial times, and systems were operated either by colonial administrations or by missions. After independence, health systems varied in their development. Some continued the colonial practices; others followed tax-financed government insurance or socialist health care systems. Curative health care expanded rapidly in urban areas, and the level of health care was raised in those locales. In the late 1970s, the Primary Health Care (PHC) approach was adopted in nearly all of the developing countries as they sought to serve all populations, both urban and rural. It is common for such countries to expend only 3% to 4% of government budgets on health, whereas middle-income countries tend to expend 5% to 6% (Kloos, 1994).

Entrepreneurial, Welfare-Oriented, Comprehensive, and Socialist Systems

A country's health care system is based on its political economy. The world's economic recession in the 1980s was a barrier to the development of effective health services. Roemer (1991) developed the first typology of health systems based on political ideology. He categorized them as (1) entrepreneurial, (2) welfare-oriented, (3) comprehensive, or (4) socialist. He further describes each category in the type of country in which it is found: industrialized, transitional, or very poor. Variations in these systems can be explained by differential growth of the economies and by differences in the redistribution of wealth and political will. It is commonly understood that economic growth is needed for increasing the standard of living, and countries that also emphasize redistribution are characterized by better education, lower infant mortality, and higher life expectancy than countries focusing on growth alone. Therefore, the four types of health care systems have further variation depending on whether they are in industrialized, transitional, or very poor countries.

The entrepreneurial health system is typically found in industrialized countries. These countries have a free-market economy and abundant resources, place large amounts of money into health care, and there is a decentralized government. Such countries have a highly individualistic perspective. The U.S. system of health care delivery is typical of the entrepreneurial system.

The welfare-oriented system is driven by statutory programs to support the cost of medical care for all, or nearly all, of the population. Such a program is commonly referred to as "national health insurance." Over one-half of the health-related expenditures are from government sources, but most physicians and dentists also remain in private practice. Western Europe, Japan, and Australia subscribe to the welfare-oriented health system.

A comprehensive system is a step further from the welfare-oriented type. There are substantial modifications in delivery and financing resulting in universal entitlements. This system abandons the separate and complex sources of financing found in the previous two systems. The Scandinavian countries, as well as Great Britain and New Zealand, utilize a comprehensive health care delivery system.

The socialist system came about through social revolution that totally abolished free-market economies and replaced them with socialism. Under socialism, the health care system is also socialized. The first overthrow of capitalism was in Russia in 1917, then Eastern Europe, Albania, Bulgaria, Czechoslovakia, East Germany, Hungary, Poland, Romania, Yugoslavia, and later China. A socialist health care system views health services as a social entitlement and a government responsibility, emphasizes prevention, engages in central planning for health resources and services with one central health authority, gives priority to industrial workers and children, and bases health care work on scientific principles. Non-scientific or cultist practices are not permitted.

The four health systems that have been described apply to industrialized countries. Roemer applies the same typology to transitional and very poor countries. Countries that are in the process of development are referred to as transitional. Such countries and their health care systems are moving effectively toward economic and social development. The global median gross national product (GNP) of these countries is $1500 per capita.

Very poor countries are even less economically developed and have lower GNPs per capita than the industrialized or transitional countries. Examples of very poor countries are Ethiopia, Kenya, Ghana, Burma, Sri Lanka, Mozambique, and China.

Other countries that do not easily fit into the above health care system matrix are the oil-rich developing countries. In just a few years, the wealth in such countries exploded upward from low levels typical of Africa and some Asian countries to those of high industrialized countries or higher. Examples are Gabon, Libya, Saudi Arabia, and Kuwait. The governments of these countries use their income to extend and improve health services for the general population. Entrepreneurial or socialist systems are not found in these countries. Gabon and Libya are classified as welfare-oriented as they have different schemes of social insurance for health services for large amounts of the population. Saudi Arabia and Kuwait are universal and comprehensive as they use government funding to provide complete health services to everyone.

Health systems are affected by broader social trends. The major social influences are urbanization, industrialization, education, government structure, international trade, and demographic changes. Since 1940 to 1990, all national health systems have undergone significant changes (Roemer, 1991). These changes are due to increasing organization of health systems, expansion of resources (personnel, facilities, equipment), population demands for and increased use of health services, growth in health-related expenditures, collectivized financing, cost control, efficiency improvement, technology, preventive and primary health care, quality assurance, increased public responsibility, and community participation (Roemer, 1991).

GLOBAL HEALTH AGENCIES

Many different international agencies cooperate on world health matters. Historically, this cooperation has been erratic; fortunately, in the last few years, it has improved greatly through the efforts of both intergovernmental and non-governmental organizations.

Multilateral and **bilateral organizations** are mainly intergovernmental. The United Nations, the World Health Organization, and the World Bank are examples of **multilateral agencies.** These agencies are multi-national organizations that support development efforts of governments and organizations in less-developed nations of the world. The U.S. Agency for International Development, the Peace Corps, and the U.S. Centers for Disease Control and Prevention are examples of agencies that usually deal directly with other individual governments and are therefore called bilateral agencies.

In contrast, **non-governmental organizations** (NGOs) are those not under government sponsorship or control. The U.S. government designates these as **private voluntary organizations** (PVOs). They include humanitarian and professional organizations concerned with global health. Examples of PVOs are the Global Health Council, the Center for International Health and Cooperation, CARE, the Carter Center, and the International Council of Nurses. NGOs are found in most countries.

The World Health Organization

The **World Health Organization** (WHO) promotes health on a global basis. Its mandate includes acting as the directing and coordinating authority on international health work and maintaining effective collaboration with United Nations specialized agencies and other national and international bodies responsible for health development (Wenzel, 1998). Fostering equitable human development, lifting populations out of poverty, and assisting men and women to realize their potential are all goals that the WHO shares with its 191 member countries (Display 21–1).

The WHO's primary function is to provide technical support for sustainable health care systems and advice to members on strategies to meet their health care needs. It thus serves as a catalyst to mobilize the resources of national governments, financial institutions and endowments, and bilateral partners for health development (WHO, 1999b). The WHO is assisted in carrying out its mission by United Nations agencies, the private sector, NGOs, and leading service, training, and research centers worldwide.

In her address to the 1999 International Health Conference of the Global Health Council, Dr. Gro Harlem Bruntdland, the WHO's Director General, noted that, "We are leaving a century of remarkable human progress. The health gains of the 20th century count as one of the biggest social transformations of our times. Living conditions have dramatically improved for the large majority of human beings. But the century also left a legacy. More than a billion fellow human beings have been left behind in the health revolution." She noted that, "Health is key to reversing the downward

---

DISPLAY 21–1. Definition of Health

Health is a state of complete physical, mental, and social well-being and not merely the absence of disease or infirmity.

Source: World Health Organization Constitution

spiral linking poverty, malnutrition and environmental degradation. Good health enhances the capabilities of the poor, builds social and human capabilities which, in turn, advance the productivity of people, communities and societies. This is what development is all about" (GHC, 1999a). Dr. Brundtland identified the burdens of excess mortality and morbidity that disproportionately affect poor people. Her organization primarily gives attention to known interventions that can achieve the greatest health gain possible with available resources.

HISTORY

The WHO began in 1945 when three physicians serving as delegates from Brazil, China, and Norway to the founding General Assembly of the United Nations met at a San Francisco restaurant. Over lunch, they discussed the notion of global health as a peacekeeping strategy, and envisioned a world body that would take the leading role in promoting global health. Just 1 year later, the WHO constitution was adopted in New York by the representatives of 61 countries (Wenzel, 1998). Although it has been closely associated with the United Nations since its inception, the WHO has had its own charter. It has taken the primary technical responsibility not only for its own programs funded by regular and extra budgetary funds, but also for health-related initiatives sponsored and funded by United Nations agencies and other international bodies.

CENTRAL AND REGIONAL ORGANIZATION

The WHO's headquarters is in Geneva, Switzerland. It has a decentralized form of governance featuring six regional offices, each governed by a committee of delegates from that region's member countries. For example, the regional office in New Delhi, India serves Southeast Asian members. Special offices have recently been established in Addis Ababa, Ethiopia to work with the Organization of African Unity, and in Moscow to work with Eastern European countries and the newly independent states of Central Asia.

WORLD HEALTH ASSEMBLY

The World Health Assembly is the highest governing body within the WHO. Made up of delegates from the 191 member countries, it meets annually to review progress and performance of the WHO and to give direction to its efforts. In 1999, the 52nd World Health Assembly resolved to promote equitable, accessible, and sustainable health care systems in developing countries based on primary health care (see the discussion in the next section). The Assembly urged its members to take steps to meet the needs of the most vulnerable of their populations, including freeing the poor from the burden of infectious diseases and preventing non-communicable diseases (WHO, 1999c).

MAJOR PROGRAMS

Among the WHO's highest achievements has been the eradication of smallpox. When smallpox was endemic in 31 countries in 1967, 13 million cases were estimated world-

wide. It is projected that 20 million people would have died in the next two decades if smallpox had not been eradicated. Other important accomplishments include reduction of malaria, standardization of data-collection systems, adoption of international standards for the control and reporting of morbidity and mortality, and publication of classic works for the prevention and management of disease (Whaley & Hashim, 1995). In addition, the work of the WHO has been credited with preventing hundreds of millions of cases of tropical diseases.

As the 21st century begins, new eradication/elimination programs are under way for polio, leprosy, river blindness, guinea worm, and measles. In addition, initiatives have begun that include:

- reducing transmission and incidence of HIV/AIDS
- launching a "Roll Back Malaria" program
- stopping the transmission of tuberculosis
- increasing access to essential pharmaceuticals
- reducing the poor quality of some pharmaceuticals
- preventing and treating iron deficiency
- reducing maternal morbidity and mortality
- promoting healthful lifestyles for all age groups, including elders
- establishing "Health Promoting Schools"

To achieve some of these initiatives, the WHO is involved in a number of significant partnerships. For example, the initiative for establishing Health Promoting Schools is a collaborative effort of the WHO, the United Nations Educational, Scientific and Cultural Organization (UNESCO), and the United Nations Children's Fund (UNICEF). School Health Education is comprehensive when it:

- views health as more than the absence of disease;
- utilizes all available opportunities for health education (formal and informal, traditional and alternative, inside and outside school);
- harmonizes the health messages that are delivered;
- enables students to promote conditions supportive of health services;
- encourages the development of a healthy environment (WHO, 1992).

Another example of such partnerships is the Human Reproduction Program, a global research program on reproductive health. It collaborates with two programs of the United Nations as well as the World Bank. Similarly, the WHO has joined with several other organizations to fight hunger and improve food standards, and has collaborated in a "Solar Alert" campaign to alert people about the harmful effects of solar radiation (WHO, 1999d) (Display 21–2).

World Bank

The World Bank is a major health-related agency that collaborates with the WHO and other global health organizations in health development. Founded in 1944, its goal is "a world free of poverty." Thus, its mission is threefold:

DISPLAY 21–2. Health Promotion

Health is created and lived by people within the settings of their everyday life; where they learn, work, play and love. Health is created by caring for oneself and others, by being able to take decisions and have control over one's life circumstances; and by ensuring that the society one lives in creates conditions that allow the attainment of health by all its members.

(World Health Organization. [1997]. Promoting health through schools: Report of a WHO expert committee on comprehensive school health education and promotion. *WHO Technical Report Series, 180,* 5. Geneva: WHO.)

- to fight poverty with passion and professionalism for lasting results
- to help people help themselves and their environment by providing resources, sharing knowledge, building capacity, and forging partnerships in the public and private sectors
- to be an excellent institution that is able to attract, excite, and nurture committed staff with exceptional skills to know how to listen and learn.

The Bank's Population, Health, and Nutrition Department works to alleviate poverty and promote development through investments and partnerships with other organizations concerned with global health (World Bank, 1998) (Display 21–3).

The United States Agency for International Development

The **United States Agency for International Development** (USAID) is an independent, executive-branch, bilateral agency that provides economic and humanitarian assistance overseas. Under guidance from the Secretary of State, it focuses its efforts on participatory development activities, working in partnership with PVOs. Its activities are purported to lead to direct economic benefits to the U.S. as well as to the countries it serves (Fredericks, 1999).

The American International Health Alliance (AIHA) operates under a cooperative agreement with the USAID. It es-

DISPLAY 21–3. World Bank

The fight against poverty is not a fight for glory. It is about equity and social justice, about the environment and resources we all share, and about peace and security. It is a fight for a better life for all of us and for our children who will live in this very interconnected world.

James D. Wolfensohn, 1999

tablishes and manages hospital partnerships between health care institutions in the U.S. and their counterparts in Europe and Central Asia. AIHA is reportedly the U.S. hospital sector's most coordinated response to health care issues in those areas and, in 1997, oversaw 44 health partnerships (AIHA, 1997).

Non-governmental Organizations

Non-governmental organizations operate in most countries of the world. Some of the organizations most significant to the work of community health nursing are discussed here.

GLOBAL HEALTH COUNCIL
The Global Health Council (formerly the National Council for International Health) is a leading private, voluntary American NGO. It focuses on advocacy, alliance building, and communicating best practices for global health development. It also works to increase awareness of international health problems to U.S. citizens, legislators, public agencies, and the academic community. Its membership includes hundreds of private and public organizations around the world as well as several thousand professionals involved in global health. It is staffed by a multi-disciplinary, cross-cultural board of directors, health professionals, student interns, volunteers, and members (GHC, 1999b).

CENTER FOR INTERNATIONAL HEALTH AND COOPERATION
The Center for International Health and Cooperation (CIHC) was founded in 1992 to promote healing and peace in countries shattered by war, regional conflicts, and ethnic violence. Former U.S. Secretary of State Cyrus Vance, former U.N. Secretary General Boutros Boutros-Ghali, and many other distinguished men and women volunteer their services to the Center and bring exceptional experience, knowledge, statesmanship, and insights to bear on the complex problems and opportunities associated with humanitarian efforts in international conflicts. The belief is that health and other basic humanitarian endeavors often provide the only common ground for initiating dialogue and cooperation among warring parties.

CARE
The Cooperative for American Remittances to Europe (CARE) was founded in 1945 when 22 American organizations joined together to rush life-saving "care packages" from individual American citizens, churches, clubs, and businesses to survivors of World War II. Millions of CARE packages followed in the next two decades. In the 1950s, CARE expanded its program to developing nations, using surplus American food to feed the hungry. In the 1960s, it pioneered primary health care. Now called the Cooperative for Assistance and Relief Everywhere, CARE has responded to famines and disasters worldwide with emergency food, supplies, and

rehabilitative efforts. In addition, it delivers programs in education, health, population, water and sanitation, agriculture, environmental preservation, economic development, and community building (CARE, 1999) (Display 21–4).

THE CARTER CENTER
Former President Jimmy Carter and his wife Roselyn founded the Carter Center in 1986 in order to help countries through a nongovernmental mechanism. The Center works in disease-prevention programs, as well as in agriculture, throughout the world. Two of their programs seek to eradicate Guinea worm in Africa and parts of Asia and river blindness in Africa and Latin America (Carter Center, 2000).

INTERNATIONAL COUNCIL OF NURSES
The International Council of Nurses (ICN) represents the global interests and concerns of the nursing profession. Founded in 1899, its current membership includes nursing organizations from 120 countries and 1.5 million nurses. ICN's mission is to maintain the role of nursing in health care through its global voice (Vance, 1999).

Since nurses and midwives constitute up to 80% of the qualified health care work force in most national health care systems, they represent a powerful force for bringing health care to all people. Nurses' contributions to health services cover the whole spectrum of primary care, promotion, and prevention, as well as health research, program planning, implementation, and innovation (ICN, 1999).

HEALTH FOR ALL: A PRIMARY HEALTH CARE INITIATIVE

In 1977, the World Health Assembly determined that the major social goal of governments and the WHO should be the attainment by all people by the year 2000 of a level of health that would allow them to lead a socially and economically productive life. This desire for **"Health for All"** was formally expressed in the *Declaration of Alma-Ata* in 1978. This document was produced by a WHO/UNICEF conference in Alma-Ata, Kazakhstan, in the former Soviet Union, attended by representatives of 134 nations. The *Declaration* promoted an ecological/social concept of health and offered political and economic guidelines for achieving primary health care

for all (Carlaw & Ward, 1988). The United States' *Healthy People 2000* initiative is based on the WHO Health for All model, as were the previous *Healthy People* agendas.

The Health for All initiative is a comprehensive approach to serving the most needy and remote populations through partnerships between the country's health-services system and local communities. The communities take the leading responsibility for identifying their own priority health concerns and planning and implementing their own primary health care service. They receive supportive guidance from their country's central health authority, generally their Ministry of Health (Carlaw & Ward, 1988). These **primary health care** services include prevention, health promotion, and curative and rehabilitative care provided by the people themselves (WHO, 1989a) (Display 21–5).

Functions

Article VII of the *Declaration of Alma-Ata* lists the eight basic functions of primary health care:
- Education concerning prevailing health problems and the methods of preventing and controlling them
- Promotion of food supply and proper nutrition
- An adequate supply of safe water and basic sanitation
- Maternal and child health, including family planning
- Immunization against major infectious diseases
- Prevention and control of locally endemic diseases
- Appropriate treatment of common diseases and injuries
- Provision of essential drugs

Primary health care goes beyond the health sector and, to be effective, must involve all related sectors concerned with national and community development, including agriculture, animal husbandry, food, industry, education, housing, public works, communication, and others (Article VI, section 4).

DELIVERY SYSTEMS
Community-based primary health care calls for a partnership between health professionals and communities, and thus represents a striking change in responsibility and authority. The community becomes the initiator of action; the basic unit of primary health care in most developing countries is a voluntary health service created at the village level. At least two components are commonly included: a local committee and

---

DISPLAY 21–4. Care

Every CARE package is a personal contribution to the world peace our nation seeks. It expresses America's concern and friendship in a language all peoples understand.

President John F. Kennedy, 1962

DISPLAY 21–5. Primary Health Care

Primary health care is not more medicine for the poor. Primary health care is essentially a call for a partnership in health, based on the concepts of equity and social justice, to enable communities, both rural and urban, to take intelligent responsibility for upgrading their health environment and health status.

Raymond W. Carlaw, 1988

a group of community health workers (CHWs). The committee accepts responsibility for health matters. The CHW is selected from the village and is approved by the committee to serve the village people in health matters. CHWs usually give 1 to 2 hours of health service per day, for which they may or may not be compensated by the community.

The CHW is trained in the fundamentals of promoting health and preventing and treating the most common diseases. This includes basic first aid, advice and assistance on simple treatments, and health teaching on personal hygiene, safe water supplies, safe disposal of human waste and refuse, and nutrition. The village midwife receives training in obstetrics and child care. This person provides basic antenatal, intrapartum, and postnatal care and makes referrals as required. In some countries, traditional medical practitioners receive formal training and return to their villages to continue their services with new knowledge and skills to enhance their effectiveness. (See Figure 21–1 for an illustration of the organizational pattern of community-based primary health care.)

ACHIEVEMENTS AND DETERRENTS
Primary health care programs have resulted in the following significant and quantifiable improvements in the health status of people worldwide:
- The worldwide infant mortality rate has decreased from 90 in 1000 live births in 1975 to 59 in 1995—a 34% decrease.
- Immunization coverage for children under 1 year of age has rise from 20% to 80% between 1980 and 1990.
- Access to safe drinking water in developing countries increased from 38% to 66%, and adequate sanitation from 32% to 38%, from the mid-1970s to 1990.

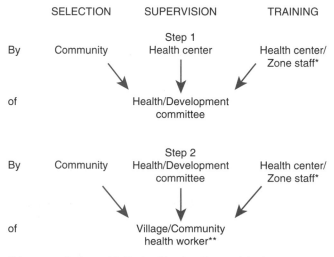

*Nurse, sanitarian, midwife, health education assistant
**Assistant midwife, traditional birth attendant, traditional practitioner

FIGURE 21–1. Community-based primary care. (Carlaw, R. [1988]. Community-based primary health care: Some factors in its development. In R.W. Carlaw & W. B. Ward (Eds.), *Primary health care: The African experience* [p. xx–xi]. Oakland, CA: Third Party Publishing Company.)

Some of the major deterrents to sustaining effective primary health care services include inadequate supervision and follow-up, failure to restock medical supplies on a regular basis, shortage of personnel, limited training, poor record keeping, and lack of cooperation on the part of health centers and nearby hospitals in receiving referrals from community health workers. Natural environmental phenomena such as rain and floods and poor or absent communication facilities periodically isolate areas. Other problems arise when expensive drugs are dispensed in place of less expensive generic brands or are given first to family friends of the health care workers in some cases, and when health centers fail to refer patients back to the referring community health worker.

However, in acknowledgment of significant global accomplishments, there was a renewal of the strategy of Health for All by the WHO's members in 1994. Future action regarding primary health care calls for strengthened collaboration across governmental agencies and NGOs in both the public and private sectors. Only then will the world have a realistic chance of achieving all of the goals set out in the *Declaration of Alma-Ata* (Display 21–6).

GLOBAL HEALTH CONCERNS

Most of the agencies discussed in this chapter strive not only to fulfill a country's health-program priorities but also to protect the rest of the world from the spread of communicable

---

DISPLAY 21–6. WHO's Ten Goals Toward Health for All

- To increase the span of healthy life for all people in such a way that health disparities between social groups are reduced.
- To ensure universal access to an agreed upon set of essential health-care services of acceptable quality, comprising at least the eight essential elements of primary health care.
- To ensure survival and healthy development of children.
- To improve the health and well being of women.
- To ensure healthy population development.
- To eradicate, eliminate, or control major diseases constituting global health problems.
- To reduce avoidable disabilities through appropriate preventive and rehabilitative measures.
- To ensure continued improvements in nutritional status for all population groups.
- To enable universal access to safe and healthy environments and living conditions.
- To enable all people to adopt and maintain healthy life-styles and health behavior.

(Lanza, R. [1996]. *One world: The health and survival of the human species in the 21st century.* Santa Fe, NM: Health Press.)

disease. To do so, reliable data on the global incidence and spread of communicable disease are crucial. Such information is also critical for sound policy decisions related to the prevention of disease and injury. In any given year, only about 30% of deaths worldwide are medically certified, and until recently there were only limited standardized assessments of comparable information on morbidity, mortality, and disability in populations throughout the world. Therefore, at the request of the World Bank, in 1992 the WHO initiated a study on the global burden of disease (Murray & Lopez, 1996).

The Global Burden of Disease

The WHO's study of the **global burden of disease** (GBD) verified with quantifiable data numerous long-held assumptions about the disparities in the burden of disease worldwide, especially disparities in the burden of disease in children. Among other findings, it revealed that:

- Ninety-eight percent of all deaths in children younger than 15 years are in the developing world.
- Eighty-three percent of deaths for those aged 15 to 59 years are in the developing world.
- The probability of death before age 15 ranges from 22% in sub-Saharan Africa to only 1.1% in countries with established market economies
- Five of the ten leading causes of death are communicable, perinatal, and nutritional maladies that largely affect children.

Display 21–7 lists the top 30 causes of death worldwide (Murray & Lopez, 1997).

In addition to causes of mortality, the GBD study quantified the burden of disease with a measure that could be used for cost-effectiveness analysis. In order to compare across conditions and risk factors, a measure called the **Disability-Adjusted Life Year** (DALY) was developed. DALYs are the combination of years of life lost due to premature mortality and years of life lived with disability adjusted for the severity of disability. The three leading causes of DALYs in 1990 were acute respiratory infections, diarrheal diseases, and conditions related to the perinatal period (Table 21–1) (Murray & Lopez, 1997). The GBD study grouped diseases and injuries into three clusters: Group 1 represents communicable diseases, maternal causes, conditions arising in the perinatal period, and nutritional deficiencies; Group 2 consists of noncommunicable diseases; and Group 3 lists all types of injuries (Table 21–2).

The information obtained from the GBD and its analysis guide current decisions related to investments in health, research, human resource development, and physical infrastructures. Reassessment of global and regional information on diseases and injury is expected to occur every 3 to 5 years.

Eradication, Elimination, and Control of Communicable Diseases

A primary global health concern is communicable disease, and a primary goal is the **eradication, elimination, and con-**

DISPLAY 21–7. Thirty Leading Causes of Death Worldwide in 1990

RANK/CAUSE OF DEATH

- Ischemic heart disease
- Cerebral-vascular disease
- Lower respiratory infection
- Diarrheal diseases
- Perinatal disorders
- Chronic obstructive pulmonary disease
- Tuberculosis (HIV seropositive excluded)
- Measles
- Road traffic accidents
- Trachea, bronchus, and lung cancers
- Malaria
- Self-inflicted injuries
- Cirrhosis of the liver
- Stomach cancer
- Congenital anomalies
- Diabetes mellitus
- Violence
- Tetanus
- Nephritis and nephrosis
- Drowning
- War injuries
- Liver cancer
- Inflammatory heart diseases
- Colon and rectal cancers
- Protein-energy malnutrition
- Esophagus cancer
- Pertussis
- Rheumatic heart disease
- Breast cancer
- HIV

(Murray, C.J. & Lopez, A.D. [1997]. Mortality by cause for eight regions of the world: Global Burden of Health Disease Study. *Lancet, 349,* 1269–1347.)

---

trol of the leading communicable diseases worldwide. Eradication means the interruption of person-to-person transmission and a limitation of the reservoir of infection such that no further preventive efforts are required; it indicates a status whereby no further cases of a disease occur anywhere. At times the term elimination is used when a disease has been interrupted in a limited, defined geographic area. In 1991, the WHO defined elimination as a reduction of prevalence to a level below one case per million population in a given area. In contrast, the term control indicates that a specific disease has ceased to be a public health threat. Control programs are aimed at reducing the incidence and/or prevalence of communicable and some non-communicable conditions.

Although eradication is always the desired effect, it usually requires extensive funding and much international cooperation to achieve such a goal. The successful eradication of smallpox from the world in 1977, as mentioned earlier, came about because of the leadership of the WHO and was a tremendous accomplishment in public health. In 1967, small-

TABLE 21–1. Seventeen Leading Causes of DALYs in the World in 1990 and Projected to 2020

Disease or Injury	Rank: 1990	Rank: 2020 Baseline Scenario
Lower respiratory infections	1	6
Diarrheal diseases	2	9
Conditions arising during the perinatal period	3	11
Unipolar major depression	4	2
Ischemic heart disease	5	1
Cerebral-vascular disease	6	4
Tuberculosis	7	7
Measles	8	25
Road traffic accidents	9	3
Congenital anomalies	10	13
Malaria	11	24
Chronic obstructive pulmonary disease	12	5
Falls	13	19
Iron-deficiency anemia	14	39
Protein-energy malnutrition	14	37
War	16	8
Self-inflicted injuries	17	14
Violence	19	12
HIV	28	10
Trachea, bronchus, and lung cancers	33	15

(Murray, C.J. & Lopez, A.D. [1996]. Evidence-based health policy—lessons from the Global Burden of Disease Study. *Science, 274,* 740–743.)

pox was endemic in 31 countries, with 10 to 15 million individuals infected. Remarkably, within 10 years there were no cases in the world (Whaley & Hashim, 1995). A vital lesson that this multi-region effort taught us was that, if global eradication programs are to be successful, interdependence is

necessary (Foege, 1998). These programs are dependent on commitment from involved governments, international bodies, non-governmental organizations, and the affected communities themselves.

Eradication programs currently in progress as the 21st century begins are aimed at poliomyelitis, guinea worm, river blindness, leprosy, and measles. Additionally, efforts have increased to reduce, control, and prevent malaria, tuberculosis, HID/AIDS, diarrheal diseases, and respiratory infections.

POLIOMYELITIS

In 1988, the World Health Assembly adopted the goal of global eradication of poliomyelitis by the end of the year 2000. At the time of the inception of the campaign, there were an estimated 35,000 annual cases of polio in the world (WHO, 1999e). By 1991, the disease was eliminated from the western hemisphere. Polio is now close to elimination worldwide, but wars and funding limitations have interrupted eradication efforts. Eight out of ten of the world's infants are immunized against polio; however, 50 countries are still considered to be polio-endemic. National immunization days and house-to-house vaccinations are strategies that will help eliminate the disease. The estimated cost of eradication is $1.25 billion (Hull, 1999).

GUINEA WORM

Guinea worm is expected to be the next disease after smallpox to be eradicated. This parasitic disease infects a person through drinking water and migrates through the body, with the worm usually emerging from the feet. Farmers are the most commonly affected. Although there is no cure once the parasite is ingested, the eradication strategy includes interruption of transmission, surveillance, and certification (WHO, 1998b). Interruption of transmission includes measures such as protecting drinking water by keeping infected feet out of it, filtering drinking water, and chemically treating water to eliminate the vector.

TABLE 21–2. Distribution of Death by Specific Causes in 1990

Group 1	Group 2	Group 3
Infectious and parasitic diseases	Malignant neoplasms	Unintentional injuries
Respiratory infections	Other neoplasms	Intentional injuries
Maternal disorders	Diabetes mellitus	
Perinatal disorders	Endocrine disorders	
Nutritional deficiencies	Neuropsychiatric disorders	
	Sense organ disorders	
	Cardiovascular disorders	
	Respiratory disorders	
	Digestive disorders	
	Genitourinary disorders	
	Skin disorders	
	Musculoskeletal disorders	
	Congenital anomalies	
	Oral disorders	

(Murray, C.J. & Lopez, A.D. [1996]. Evidence-based health policy—lessons from the Global Burden of Disease Study. *Science, 274,* 740–743.)

RIVER BLINDNESS

Twenty years ago, river blindness afflicted hundreds of thousands of people annually in West Africa alone, leading to a loss of livelihood and autonomy. In 1991, the River Blindness Program, a collaborative effort involving both public and private organizations, set a primary objective of supporting the delivery of ivermectin, the medication used to treat river blindness, to at least 80% of those living in endemic areas, and to maintain coverage for 10 to 15 years (Miri, 1998). Vector-control activities were also to be supported. The program has been successful, and the impending elimination of river blindness is a landmark in public- and private-sector collaboration.

LEPROSY

Since 1985, multi-drug therapy has reduced the global prevalence of leprosy by 85%, and there remain only a few endemic countries (WHO, 1999f). However, the WHO estimates that nearly 2 million patients worldwide have yet to be detected. Most often, these patients live in remote areas that lack health services as well as the necessary drugs. These factors have thus far prevented effective eradication of this age-old disease. Nonetheless, with continued effort, it is hoped that this disease will disappear.

MEASLES

Over 40 million people contract measles every year, and about 1 million children subsequently die from the disease. Most of those deaths occur in sub-Saharan Africa and India. The **Integrated Management of Childhood Illness** (IMCI) is an intervention that is likely to have the greatest impact in reducing measles. This implementation promotes wider immunization coverage; rapid referral of serious cases; prompt recognition of secondary conditions; improved nutrition, including breastfeeding; and vitamin A supplementation (WHO, 1998c).

MALARIA

With 50% of the world's population living in malaria-endemic areas, 200 million new cases are diagnosed yearly and 2 million deaths are reported (Kaneko, 1998). Malaria was originally targeted for eradication as far back as 1954. Although there was success in a number of places, malaria has not been eradicated in most of the developing world, and a number of areas have reverted to control programs rather than eradication. High endemicity, dependence on pesticides such as DDT, resistance of multi-drug therapy, lack of human and economic resources, and a tenacious vector have all contributed to this lack of worldwide success. Perhaps the major contributors to lack of success have been failure to integrate the malaria eradication effort into basic health services, inadequate efforts to exploit the effective involvement of communities, and an absence of necessary sustainable political commitment and funding. These difficulties led the World Health Assembly to switch to a control strategy in 1993 (Trigg & Kondrachine, 1998). Today, methods of control include early case finding and treatment, reduction of contact with mosquitoes, destruction of adult mosquitoes and larvae, source detection, destruction of malaria parasites, and community education programs (Jamison et al., 1993).

In May 1999, the World Health Assembly launched a "Roll Back Malaria" program committed to halving malaria-related deaths throughout the world by 2010. As this text goes to press, the search for an effective anti-malaria vaccine has taken a significant step forward through development of a recombinant gene candidate vaccine at the CDC in Atlanta. Human trials may begin in 2001. India and Kenya also have vaccine studies under way (WHO, 1999g).

Illustrating the spillover effect of disease from an endemic country to a non-endemic country are statistics on malaria in the United Kingdom. Of the estimated 2000 annual reported cases in a 10-year period, researchers found that 46% of the infected people had traveled to West or Central Africa on oil-related business (Nathwani & Spiteri, 1997).

HIV/AIDS

Today, 34.3 million people are estimated to be living with HIV/AIDS. According to the United Nations, 33.0 million are adults, 15.7 million are women, and 1.3 million are children under 15 (UNAIDS/WHO, 2000). More than 95% of all HIV-infected people now live in developing countries, as did 95% of those who have died from AIDS. It is predicted that life expectancy in those countries is likely decline by as much as 27%. The disease attacks young adults in productive age groups, leaving young children as orphans and elderly adults without caregivers. The epidemic threatens to upset and destabilize entire societies in Africa. Control efforts in developing countries have focused on strengthening the safety of blood used for replacement therapy, supporting advocacy efforts, and education. Currently under debate is the possibility of exporting antiviral drug regimens for HIV-positive individuals that have worked in developed countries to the developing world. Although this possibility is cost-prohibitive at the moment, there is discussion about drug manufacturers making these life-lengthening regimens more financially feasible for poor countries (CDC, 1998).

TUBERCULOSIS

We are currently experiencing a worldwide tuberculosis (TB) epidemic (Display 21–8).

- Someone in the world is newly infected with TB every second.
- 7 to 8 million people around the world become sick with TB each year.
- Nearly 2 million TB cases per year occur in sub-Saharan Africa.
- Nearly 3 million TB cases per year occur in Southeast Asia.
- Over a quarter of a million TB cases per year occur in Eastern Europe.
- TB kills 2 to 3 million people each year.
- TB accounts for more than one-quarter of all preventable adult deaths in developing countries.
- Nearly 1% of the world's population is infected with TB each year.

DISPLAY 21–8. Tuberculosis

Tuberculosis kills more youth and adults than any other infectious disease in the world today. It is a bigger killer than malaria and AIDS combined and kills more women than all the combined causes of maternal mortality. It kills 100,000 children each year.

(World Health Organization. [1999]. Tuberculosis. *WHO Fact Sheet No. 104.* Geneva: WHO.)

- Overall, one-third of the world's population is infected with the TB bacillus.
- Five to 10% of people who are infected with TB become sick or infectious at some time during life.

In the year 2000, more people died of TB than in any other year in history. HIV and TB form a lethal combination, each speeding the other's progress. TB is the leading cause of death among people who are HIV positive. Poorly managed TB programs are threatening to make TB incurable, and the movement of people is helping spread the disease. In industrialized countries, at least one-half of TB cases are among foreign-born people. For a more detailed discussion of TB, see Chapter 15.

DIARRHEAL DISEASES

The incidence of diarrheal diseases is somewhat elusive as it depends on which definition of diarrhea is used, the frequency of surveillance, and the population (Martines et al., 1993). Recent studies have used the definition of more than three stools passed during a 24-hour period for those older than 3 months. Sometimes public health professionals use the term to mean dysentery, although this is usually characterized by the presence of blood in the stool with or without looseness or specified frequency. Diarrhea can be caused by a host of enteric pathogens, among other things. Generally, these pathogens are most significant in developing countries. Poverty, poor personal and domestic hygiene, infected water, low maternal education, and lower occupational status have been associated with diarrheal morbidity and mortality (Martines et al., 1993). The risk is highest among infants who are not breastfed. In 1993, an estimated 3.2 million children below 5 years of age died from diarrhea (WHO, 1995). The reduction of mortality is largely due to the promotion of oral rehydration therapy, a simple treatment administered by mother to child that replaces fluid and electrolytes. WHO recommendations for prevention of diarrheal disease include the promotion of personal and domestic hygiene, improvement of water supply and sanitation facilities, promotion of breastfeeding, improvement in weaning practices, rotavirus immunization (as available), cholera immunization, and measles immunization.

ACUTE RESPIRATORY INFECTIONS

The most common illness in the world, and a leading cause of mortality in the developing world, is acute respiratory infection (ARI). Four million annual deaths are attributed to ARI among children under 5 years of age, usually from pneumonia (Stansfield & Shepard, 1993). Global commitment to a reduction of ARI was realized by a resolution at the World Summit for Children in 1990 that called for a one-third reduction in deaths from ARI. This has been difficult because of the varying clinical symptoms and causative organisms of pneumonia. Risk factors include low birth weight, poverty, crowding, lower educational levels, poor nutrition, inadequate child care practices, and a lack of health education about ARI. Additional risk factors include smoking and indoor and outdoor air pollution. Indoor air pollution is twenty times higher in villages in developing countries than in homes where two packs of cigarettes are smoked per day (Stansfield & Shepard, 1993). The source is largely indoor cook stoves that use organic fuel. Immunizations, birth spacing, and improvement in nutrition and living conditions (including use of smokeless cooking stoves) will all assist in better control of ARI. A threat to the reduction of pneumonia, however, is the increase in drug-resistant organisms. (See Levels of Prevention.)

Other Global Health Concerns

IMMUNIZATION

In 1974 the WHO launched the Expanded Program of Immunization (EPI). At that time, fewer than 5% of infants in the developing countries were fully immunized (Phillips, 1990). Millions of children have been saved yearly from mortality and morbidity partly because of global immunization programs. The intent of the program was to protect all children in the world against six major childhood diseases: diphtheria, pertussis, tetanus, measles, polio, and tuberculosis. Eight out of ten of the world's children are protected today. This was accomplished through good management and training for health staff and the development of an effective "cold chain" to maintain vaccine stability and potency. This program continues today and has linked up with other programs to promote widespread use of vaccines.

MATERNAL AND PERINATAL MORBIDITY AND MORTALITY

WHO estimates that 500,000 women die yearly from complications of pregnancy and birth. Ninety-nine percent of these deaths are in the developing world. Women living in parts of Africa face a 1-in-16 risk of death because they do not receive needed prenatal care. In Europe and North America the risk is 1 in 4,000 (WHO, 1999h). The demise of a mother profoundly affects the well-being of the entire family.

Early pregnancy, high fertility, and close child spacing are frequent in developing countries and are known to be major determinants of poor health for mothers and children. Poverty, illiteracy, poor nutrition, low weight gain, maternal age (under 20 or over 34 years of age), infections, smoke in the home, smoking, and poor health care are some of the major determinants associated with high health risks to mothers and children in the poorest nations of the world.

Prevention strategies include better general health for women through poverty alleviation, education, guidance in

LEVELS OF PREVENTION

GOAL
Prevention of acute respiratory infection in children in developing countries

PRIMARY PREVENTION
Good prenatal care; advocacy of breastfeeding, child spacing, and adequate nutrition; teaching good hygiene and child care practices, including immunizations and when to seek medical attention; the elimination of indoor contaminants such as smoke from cook stoves without chimneys and cigarette or pipe smoking. Elimination of poverty and household crowding and an increased level of education.

SECONDARY PREVENTION
If acute respiratory infection develops, ventilate room to eliminate indoor smoke and allow fresh air in, diagnose, and treat early with antibiotics (if indicated and available) and give symptomatic care. Teach caregiver signs and symptoms of complications.

TERTIARY PREVENTION
Restore child to optimal level of functioning through the recovery period. Educate on the prevention of recurrence and spread of disease.

---

family planning, prenatal care including food supplementation, local and regional care with referrals for complications, training of traditional birth attendants, and effective postpartum care (Walsh et al., 1993) (see Research: Bridge to Practice).

TOBACCO-RELATED MORBIDITY AND MORTALITY

Tobacco is expected to develop into the single largest killer and burden of disease in the next century, with deaths increasing from 3.5 million per year today to 10 million per year after the year 2010. WHO predicts that by the year 2030 tobacco will be the leading cause of disease burden in the world, causing about one in eight deaths, with 70 percent of them in developing countries (WHO, 1999i).

The Tobacco Free Initiative, launched by WHO in July 1998, will implement the General Assembly's resolution to prevent and control the global spread of tobacco use in the 21st century. Work has also begun on a convention on tobacco control that will address the global problem of tobacco advertising and promotion, agricultural diversification, smuggling, taxes, and subsidies. WHO plans to have the convention process completed by 2003.

Cigarette smoking is increasing rapidly in the developing world as their economies improve and tobacco companies target them. In an anecdotal note, the authors of this chapter witnessed this very event. While working with the WHO in Ethiopia in 1994, at the end of its protracted civil war, we saw very little tobacco use. Over the last few years, we have returned to the area and were struck by the markedly increased availability and use of tobacco as the economy and living standards have improved.

RESEARCH Bridge to Practice

Tarkka, M.T., Paunonen, M. & Laippala, P. (1999). Social support provided by public health nurses and the coping of first-time mothers with child care. *Public Health Nursing, 16*(2), 114–119.

First-time mothers find the initial months post-partum can be a stressful time for them. The new mother has many tasks to accomplish, including adapting and responding to the newborn. Previous studies have shown that a mother's coping is related to the characteristics of both mother and child. The purpose of this study conducted in Finland was to examine factors related to the first-time mother's coping with care of the child (referred to as child care) when the infant was 3 months old. In that country, child welfare services are available for all families after delivery. For the first 6 months post-partum, the family attends the child welfare clinic approximately once a month. In Finland, all mothers can stay at home approximately a year as they can obtain government-granted maternity insurance.

Using a questionnaire developed from the literature and instruments from previous studies, the researchers collected data on a sample of 271 first-time mothers during a 6-month period. The dependent variable was coping with child care. Child care was assessed by rating 13 tasks or situations according to how well the mothers perceived themselves to be coping with that task or situation. All the infants were 3 months of age at the time. A Spearman correlation coefficient and stepwise regression analysis was used to assess coping with child care. A positive correlation was found between the mother's competence, attachment to the child, health, depression, spousal relationship, sense of isolation and role restriction, and the mother's coping with child care. The mother's competence and her coping showed the strongest correlation. A positive correlation was also found between the infant's mood, demandingness and acceptability, and the mother's coping with child care. The child's demandingness and coping had the strongest correlation. Social support (such as that from the mother's social network, plus the affect and affirmation from the public health nurses) and coping with the child care also showed a positive correlation. Using the multivariate method, predictors were the mother's competence, health, depression, and attachment to her child; child's mood and ease or difficulty of care; and the affect and affirmation from the public health nurse. In summary, the results showed that a mother's coping with child care is affected by characteristics of both mother and child as well as social support, including the public health nurse at the child welfare clinic.

1. What affect do you think home visits by a public health nurse, as opposed to counseling in a clinic, might have on a new mother's coping with the care of an infant?
2. What factors do you think might affect a new mother's coping with a child care in rural Africa? In the United States?
3. What affect do you think a socialist medical health care system might have on a new mother's coping with child care?

ACCIDENTS AND INJURIES

Accidents and injuries are another global health concern. Worldwide, injury ranks fifth among the leading causes of death, and the annual medical and social costs of injury are estimated to exceed $500 billion (WHO, 1998e). One of every four to nine persons incurs a disabling injury each year in developing countries. Because of their socioeconomic and political disadvantages, they live with daily risks that are unacceptable in industrial countries. Injuries result from exposure to damaging mechanical, electrical, thermal, or chemical energy or by a sudden change in an essential life-sustaining element such as a lack of oxygen. Fatal injuries in developing countries are usually the result of motor vehicle collision, burns, poisonings, drownings, and falls. Nonfatal injuries include laceration by cutting and piercing instruments, animal injuries, minor motor vehicle collisions, and falls (Stansfield et al., 1993).

In 1998, policy makers from fifty countries convened in Stockholm to "respond to the urgent need for promoting accident and injury prevention and to mitigate their consequences on the health of people" (WHO, 1998e). They developed a "Manifesto for Safe Communities" that made recommendations to formulate public policy for safety, create supportive environments, strengthen community action, and broaden public services. Improvements in the area of accident and injury are expected.

CHRONIC DISEASE

Despite the programs of control, many infectious diseases continue in the world. Compounding that challenge is the more recent emergence of chronic diseases in the developing world. For countries in development, an interesting transition occurs. As infectious diseases decrease with development work, it is found that life expectancy lengthens, and the population experiences the degenerative diseases that are seen in developed countries. The concept of epidemiologic transition explains the replacement of infectious disease morbidity and mortality with that of **chronic disease.** This phenomenon is occurring in many countries today.

Diseases of the circulatory system, cancer, and diabetes are important causes of mortality in the developed world, and over 50% of all deaths due to these causes actually occur in developing countries (Hakulinen et al., 1986). This requires a change in the response of the health care system in terms of provision of care and planning and allocation of resources. Addressing these concerns is considered a cost-effective investment in a nation's human capital.

ENVIRONMENTAL ILLNESS

In addition to disease and injury, the environment that people live in is also one of today's major health concerns. Our air, climate, soil, and water all affect health, and environmental hazards are found throughout the world. The Blumenthal classification lists classes of environmental hazards. They include:

- infectious agents (such as bacteria and viruses)
- respiratory fibrotic agents (such as coal dust)
- asphyxiates (such as carbon monoxide)
- poison (such as pesticides)
- physical agents (noise)
- psychological agents (stressful synergisms such as crowding combined with noise)
- mutagens (such as dioxin)

- teratogens (such as cadmium)
- carcinogens (such as cigarette smoke) (Whaley & Hashim, 1995)

Humans come in contact with pollutants in two basic ways: by direct exposure to the source or by direct release of the pollutant into air or water. In places such as Peru, Egypt, and Thailand, raw sewage is directly released into rivers that are used for drinking and bathing. Such practices often result in diarrheal diseases, including cholera. For example, in 1991 a cholera outbreak was identified at the port of Chancoy in Peru; it rapidly spread along the coast, over the Andes, and into the Amazon basin, resulting in 400,000 reported cases and 4000 reported deaths in 13 countries (Whaley & Hashim, 1995).

Annually, over 5 million people die from illnesses linked to unsafe drinking water, poor household hygiene, and improper human and animal waste disposal. Every 8 seconds a child dies of a water-related disease. One-half of the population in the developing world suffers from one or more of the six main diseases associated with water and sanitation—diarrhea, ascariasis, dracunculiasis, hookworm, schistosomiasis, and trachoma—and one-fourth of the world's population is without proper access to water and sanitation.

Water-related diseases arise from the ingestion of pathogens in contaminated water or food and from insects or other water-associated vectors. Improvement of water and sanitation is estimated to reduce morbidity and mortality rates by 20% to 80% (WHO, 1996a). No single type of intervention has greater overall impact on national development and public health than does the provision of safe drinking water and proper disposal of human excreta. However, overall progress in reaching people unserved by adequate water and sanitation services has been poor since 1990 (Display 21–9).

Another worldwide concern is the depletion of the ozone layer (discussed in Chapter 16). Reduction of the ozone layer could result in increasing cataract and cancer rates (especially melanoma and basal cell carcinoma). It is believed that human activities are contributing to depletion of the ozone layer; these activities include the use of chlorofluorocarbons (CFCs) (found in the manufacture of air conditioners, refrigerators, and aerosol propellants, among others) and methylbromides (found in pesticides and herbicides). Efforts are under way to phase out CFCs in 13 countries, including the United States.

MALNUTRITION

No discussion of global health issues would be complete without discussing the problem of protein-energy malnutrition of the poor, mainly in developing countries. The consequences affect child growth, cognitive development and school performance as well as labor productivity for adults. More than 500 million people cannot meet their daily energy and protein requirements, partly as a consequence of infectious diseases, inadequate intake, or both. Interventions include education, child spacing, sanitation and clean water, access to food, increased income to acquire food, food supplementation for children and women, food fortification, and other policies (Pinstrup-Anderson et al., 1993).

DISPLAY 21-9. Sanitation

Every eight seconds a child dies of a water-related disease. Every year more than five million human beings die from illnesses linked to unsafe drinking water, unclean domestic environments and improper excreta disposal.

(World Health Organization [1996]. Water and sanitation. *WHO Fact Sheet No. 1122*. Geneva: WHO).

NEW AND EMERGING DISEASES

Most of the diseases discussed thus far have been with us for many years, some for thousands of years. Nonetheless, 20 years ago public health specialists thought most infectious diseases would soon play a minor role in heath. Unfortunately, they are still the world's leading cause of death, killing at least 17 million people a year (WHO, 1996b).

A contributing factor in infectious disease mortality is a host of **new and emerging diseases** and a resurgence of some that were previously thought to be under control. Since 1973, the world has seen the emergence of a number of previously unknown diseases; among them are HIV/AIDS, Ebola hemorrhagic fever in Central Africa, Lassa fever, hantavirus, Lyme disease, Legionnaires' disease, and toxic shock syndrome. See Table 21-3 for a list of diseases that have emerged since 1973.

The development of antimicrobial-resistant organisms, mainly due to overuse and misuse of antibiotics, has fueled a resurgence of some diseases that were under control, such as tuberculosis. TB medications are no longer effective in up to 20% of patients in some parts of the world. Two leading antimalaria medicines have become ineffective in many Asian countries, and a third is effective in only half of the world. With international travel increasing by 50% every decade, prospects for containing future outbreaks are decreasing (WHO, 1996b). Another cause is urbanization, which serves to concentrate large numbers of people in small geographic areas. Still another is the fact that vectors or pathogens that transmit the disease have become resistant to control measures.

ARMED CONFLICTS AND POLITICAL UPHEAVALS

Armed conflicts and political upheavals strongly influence both health status and health care needs of a country. They are extremely complex social phenomena, of which the most rooted causes are inequity, cultural and religious intolerance, and ethnic discrimination (Mulli, 1996). According to the Carter Center, there are over 100 conflicts in the world today, mostly civil wars (D. Congelio, personal communication, September 9, 1999). At any given time there are 30 major armed conflicts. An armed conflict is defined as major when the number of deaths has reached 1000. Political violence appears to be increasing in much of the developing world (Zwi & Ugalde, 1989). Typically, armed conflicts and upheavals initially cause governments and agencies to place a high pri-

ority on health care, but their ability to sustain health care is reduced as time goes on. The health infrastructure becomes vulnerable due to the instability. Often opposing factions raid hospitals and clinics. Health services are disorganized and experience decreased resources. Epidemics are almost inevitable. As conflict goes on, the medical needs of the combatants often take priority over the civilians, usually leaving thousands of children injured, orphaned, and at risk for disease. Additionally, conflict disrupts food cultivation, harvest, and distribution, leaving populations at risk for malnutrition and setting the stage for disease. Refugees from such events have special health and social needs. Often refugee camps will be developed by international organizations on the fringe of such conflicts to temporarily assist refugees with shelter, food, and the rudiments of health care. Such camps strain the neighboring countries. Recovery after conflict is a long-term project. Any post-conflict recovery effort has to deal with the disabled, mental illness, prisoners, widows, orphans, abandoned children, homeless and displaced persons, refugees, and the unemployed (Mulli, 1996). Additionally, land mines continue to injure or kill long after hostilities have ceased.

Human Development and Health

The relationship between development and health has been mentioned in previous sections. Development, in the broad sense, usually means investment by a country with the intent to improve its per capita income or gross national product. An improved economy is expected to bring better diets, housing, social change, and a reduction in infectious diseases. Development can mean increased labor productivity, satisfaction of basic human needs, and modernization, including education and social and infrastructure changes. It can mean improving the status of women or other particular social groups. The United Nations Development Program (UNDP) is under the mandate of the United Nations Charter and is committed to the ideal that development is inseparable from the quest for peace and human security. UNDP's mission is to assist countries in their own efforts to obtain sustainable human development by helping build their own capacity to design and carry out development programs. It has long been thought to be a truism that there is a reciprocal relationship between development and health. A healthy population favors economic development, whereas an unhealthy population favors poverty and underdevelopment (Phillips, 1990). Indeed, this is the foundation on which the World Bank is based and which it implements as it loans money to developing nations for development work. Recall, too, that the WHO was founded on the concept that health was a necessary ingredient for socioeconomic development and peace.

THE ROLE OF NURSES IN GLOBAL HEALTH

The role of nurses in global health is multifaceted. Nurses can be involved in many of the organizations that have been men-

TABLE 21–3. Examples of Emerging Pathogens Identified Since 1973

Year	Microbe	Disease
1973	Rotavirus	Major cause of infantile diarrhea globally
1976	*Cryptosporidium parvum*	Acute and chronic diarrhea
1977	Ebola virus	Ebola hemorrhagic fever
1977	*Legionella pneumophilia*	Legionnaires' disease
1977	Hantaan virus	Hemorrhagic fever with renal syndrome
1977	*Campylobacter jejuni*	Enteric diseases distributed globally
1980	Human T-lymphotropic virus 1 (HTLV-1)	T-cell lymphoma-leukemia
1981	Toxin producing strains of *Staphylococcus aureus*	Toxic shock syndrome
1982	*Escherichia coli* 0157:H7	Hemorrhagic colitis; hemolytic uremic syndrome
1982	HTLV-II	Hairy cell leukemia
1982	*Borrelia burgdorfei*	Lyme disease
1983	HIV	AIDS
1983	*Helicobacter pylori*	Peptic ulcer disease
1988	Hepatitis E	Enterically transmitted non-A, non-B hepatitis
1990	Guanarito virus	Venezuelan hemorrhagic fever
1991	*Encephalitozzon hellem*	Conjunctivitis, disseminated disease
1992	*Vibrio cholerae* 0139	New strain associated with epidemic cholera
1992	*Bartonella henselae*	Cat-scratch disease; bacillary angiomatosis
1994	Sabia virus	Brazilian hemorrhagic fever
1995	Hepatitis G virus	Parenterally transmitted non-A, non-B hepatitis
1995	Human herpesvirus-8	Associated with Kaposi sarcoma in AIDS patients
1996	TSE-causing agent	New variant Creutzfeldt-Jakob disease
1997	Avian Influenza (Type A [H5N1])	Influenza

(World Health Organization. [1998d]. Examples of pathogens recognized since 1973. *WHO Fact Sheet No. 97*, 4. Geneva: WHO.)

tioned in this chapter, either through paid employment or volunteering. **Global nursing** falls along the full spectrum from nurse policy maker in international organizations to the point of service as an instructor of a village health worker or even working at one of the levels of primary health care. To find out more about specific opportunities, the nurse should contact the organization of interest (see the listing of selected organizations at the end of the chapter). Some of the larger organizations such as WHO require graduate education and at least 5 years of experience, but many organizations do not. Nurses can participate in a large number of smaller organizations that are involved in health programs. Among such groups seeking nurses are the U.S. Peace Corps, religious and lay organizations, private and governmental agencies, as well as societies and foundations. The Global Health Council provides information on career opportunities in global health for community health nurses and others. It also offers career seminars and has noted some suggestions made by global health experts for nurses interested in entering the field. These include:

- Accept unpaid work in return for valuable experience (internships/volunteer assignments)
- Work on project administration/project management or analytical work
- Talk with others who have worked overseas
- Volunteer at local non-governmental offices or private volunteering organizations as a means of demonstrating your commitment to social action programs

- Become involved with many cross-cultural opportunities in the U.S.
- Get on mailing lists of projects and organizations of interest to you
- Organize informational interviews with people in your area of interest to establish a connection
- Take a few risks (GHC, 1999b)

University student nurses can also contact their campus office of global affairs for opportunities available overseas. (See Voices From the Community.)

On a global basis, there are more community health nurses than any other professional group providing health services to people everywhere. They also are involved with and provide a wider range of services in multiple settings than any other health care professionals. They are responsible for health and medical services, teaching, and research in medical centers, health clinics, schools, work places, and other community settings in the most remote areas of the least developed countries to the most sophisticated of the world's renowned centers of excellence. In the most needy places in the world, nurses are the primary providers of preventive and curative services. This includes providing training, guidance, and professional supervision to traditional midwives and practitioners. No other group is as involved in working with mothers, who are the most influential persons in all societies for development of health knowledge, beliefs, attitudes, and practices that people take with them throughout their lives.

Their roles may be long-term in primary, secondary, or tertiary prevention, or they may serve in short-term capacities as consultants for special projects or programs. Health care workers and community leaders in developing countries view nurses, especially community health nurses, as experts who can guide them with everything from technical procedures to development of health policy. In developing countries, nurses will often find a cadre of other foreign workers or volunteers with whom they can collaborate. Cultural understanding and respect will help the nurse build partnerships not only with the local community but also with professional colleagues.

Recently former President Jimmy Carter and his wife, Roselyn, were awarded the highest civilian honor by President Clinton in recognition of their worldwide peace and health work through the Carter Center. Carter's comments encapsulate what global nursing is like when he described such work as "satisfying, a joy, a pleasure, a challenge, an adventure." Global nursing can be all of those things (see The Global Community).

Voices From the Community

Global health nurses always receive far more than they give.

Cydne, former Peace Corps nurse

The developing world may be poor in materiality, but it is rich in hope and spirit.

Edith, missionary nurse

Nurses working in foreign lands make a big difference through their training and support of local nurses and others. Their professional dedication to quality health care and promotion of healthful living among their patients, families and communities serves as an effective role model and has a profound impact on the well-being of the people they work with.

Tom, physician

Living overseas for many years was a challenging and rewarding experience. Raising a family was not always easy, but our six children, now adults, value the exposure they had to other cultures and the many interesting friendships they made.

Inez, spouse of a global health administrator

Nurses play an important role ministering to the health care needs of not only the indigenous population, but also the sometimes sizable population of expatriates and their families.

Jennifer, teacher

THE GLOBAL COMMUNITY

Susan Purdin, RN, MPH, was the 1999 recipient of the Best Practices in Global Health Award from the Global Health Council. She has worked in the field of global health for 10 years and has worked in over a dozen countries. Susan is currently with the Reproductive Health for Refugees Consortium as the global technical advisor and is based in Nigeria. Her insight in global health work is valuable for nurses who are interested in the field and is summarized below.

A lifelong interest in health led her to nursing and to study for a MPH. She found that a career in global health could combine her interests in nursing and travel. She found there is wonder in the similarities and differences among the people in the world, and a great joy in learning from the accomplishments of health workers in each location as they tackle human problems with innovations born of good intentions coupled with hard work.

Susan finds that international health workers transfer effective measures to prevent and control illness from one location to another in a very practical way. They expose the local population to other caring people from other cultures, which brings insight to the universality of humanity in a world where we often recognize only differences. Any detrimental effects of international workers tend to be a matter of process more than content. Practices that disregard local cultural sensitivity either in professional or private arenas cause problems, and rarely solve the ones they had targeted.

"International volunteering is great. There is plenty of work to be done, too little money, and a lot of learning available. The volunteer has to have a sensitive, almost self-effacing, approach. We always learn more than we teach."

Her advice to BSN graduates interested in the field:

- Learn a second language.
- Work with people from a culture other than your own, for example, in a local clinic serving an immigrant population.
- Work in a setting with low-income people.
- Live in an unfamiliar (foreign) situation for at least a year.
- Get overseas experience—Peace Corps or other.
- Be willing to work for low pay.
- Understand that the way something is done in the U.S. is not the only right way to do things.
- Be willing to volunteer for a few months to demonstrate your ability to be effective in the field—an "audition" before being hired.
- Clarify your expectations with the employer, and be sure you understand theirs.
- Consider an MPH with an international emphasis after a couple of years of work experience.

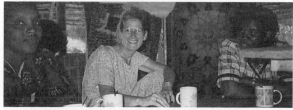

Susan Purdin in Nyagatare, Rwanda.

SUMMARY

Our world is a complex one of interdependent nations. Health is an important part of that interdependency. What occurs in one country can have a profound health effect on other parts of the world, sometimes within less than 24 hours. Community health nurses often gravitate toward global practice due to their interest in the world's larger community and the relationship of health to others, and also because of a sense of justice for disenfranchised populations. Community health nurses make important contributions to international health.

The world's communities deliver health care in different ways depending on their political economy. The entrepreneurial, welfare-oriented, comprehensive, and socialist systems vary in the manner countries provide for the health of their citizens. There are variations of these systems depending on whether the county is considered industrialized, transitional, or very poor. Many global health agencies assist less developed nations with areas of health. Some of these are intergovernmental and multilateral, such as the United Nations and the World Health Organization; others are bilateral, such as the U.S. Agency for International Development and the Peace Corps. Many non-government organizations (or private voluntary organizations) also assist with global health. Each of these agencies plays a role in keeping the world healthy. WHO's "Health of All" movement utilizing primary health care has made a difference in many poor and remote populations.

The Global Burden of Disease Study gave us important quantifiable information about morbidity and mortality in the world, as well as disability measurements. A primary global health concern is the eradication, elimination, or control of communicable disease. In addition, there are other global health concerns such as immunization, maternal and perinatal morbidity and mortality, tobacco-related diseases, chronic disease, environmental illness, and malnutrition. In addition to these age-old health problems, there are new, emerging, or re-emerging diseases. Armed conflicts and political upheavals also adversely affect health—an important consideration in world health because there are a number of major armed conflicts at any given time. There is important synergy between development and health as healthy populations promote economic development. Community health nurses are well represented in the global health arena. We provide important primary, secondary, and tertiary levels of prevention throughout the world. Nurses will continue to be an important factor in the health of our interdependent nations.

ACTIVITIES TO PROMOTE CRITICAL THINKING

1. Go to the Internet and compare the three leading causes of mortality between several countries in sub-Saharan Africa, Asia, the former Soviet Union, and the United States. What do you think contributes to the differences?

2. Repeat the exercise above, but examine the three leading causes of morbidity in each country. What do you think contributes to the differences?

3. Determine what type of health care service each of these countries has. What relation do you think the health care delivery service of each country has to its mortality and morbidity?

4. Develop a plan to eradicate measles in the world.

5. What do you think the future holds for the "Health for All" movement? Why?

6. Collect newspaper articles on issues of global health during the semester. What role is politics playing in these health issues?

REFERENCES

AIHA (1997). Brief overview of AIHA, American International Health Alliance. Available at http://www.aiha.com/english/aiha/overview.htm. Accessed 1999.

CARE (1999). About CARE. Available at http://www.CARE.ORG/about/history.html. Accessed November 1, 1999.

Carlaw, R. (1988). Community-based primary health care: Some factors in its development. In R. W. Carlaw & W. B. Ward (Eds.), Primary health care: The African experience (pp. xx–xi). Oakland, CA: Third Party Publishing.

Carter Center (2000, February 23). Fighting disease and advancing health. Available at http://www.cartercenter.org/healthprograms.html. Accessed September 3, 1999.

Centers for Disease Control and Prevention (CDC) (1998, December 1). International projections & statistics. Available at http://www.hivpositive.com/f-HIVyou/f-Statistics/internat.htm. Accessed August 12, 1999.

Centers for Disease Control and Prevention (CDC) (2000, Feb. 1). CDC answers your questions about West Nile encephalitis. Available at http://www.cdc.gov/ncidod/dvbid/arbpr/West_Nile_QA.htm. Accessed February 24, 2000.

Foege, W. H. (1998). Smallpox eradication in west and central Africa revisited. *Bulletin of the World Health Organization, 76*(3), 233–235.

Fredericks, J. A. (1999, September 8). Joseph A. Fredericks, Acting Director, USAID Information Center. Washington, DC: United States Agency for International Development. Available at jfredericks@usaid.gov. Accessed September 9, 1999.

Global Health Council (GHC) (1999a). Speech delivered by Dr. Gro Harlem Brundtland, Director General World Health Organization. Washington, D.C.: Global Health Council. Available at http://www.ghc.org. Accessed November 4, 1999.

Global Health Council (GHC) (1999b, May 1). The Global Health Council, May 1, 1999. Available at http://www.golobalhealthcouncil.org/content.html. Accessed June 28, 1999.

Hull, H. F. (1999, October 5). Fighting stops for polio immunization. Geneva: World Health Organization. Available at http://www.who.int/inf/polio.html. Accessed October 26, 1999.

International Council of Nurses (ICN) (2000, March 9). The International Council of Nurses. *Nursing N Line.* Available at vatre@uni2a.unige.ch. Accessed March 9, 2000.

Jamison, D. T., Mosley, W. H., Measham, A. R. & Bobadilla, J. L. (Eds.). (1993). *Disease control priorities in developing countries.* New York: Oxford University Press.

Kaneko, A. (1998). Malaria on the global agenda: Control and chemotherapy of malaria in Vanuatu. *Rinsho Yori, 46*(7), 637–644.

Kloos, H. (1994). The poorer third world: Health and health care in areas that have yet to experience substantial development. In D. R. Phillips & Y. Verhasselt (Eds.), *Health and development* (pp. 199–215). New York: Routledge.

Lanza, R. (1996). *One world: The health and survival of the human species in the 21st century.* Santa Fe, NM: Health Press.

Martines, J., Phillips, M. & Feachem, R. G. (1993). Diarrheal diseases. In D. T. Jamison, W. H. Mosley, A. R. Measham, & J. L. Bobdilla (Eds.). *Disease control priorities in developing countries* (pp. 91–116). New York: Oxford University Press.

Mulli, J. C. (1996). War and health. In R. Lanza (Ed.), *One world: The health and survival of the human species in the 21st century* (pp. 149–160). Santa Fe, NM: Health Press.

Miri, E. S. (1998). Problems and perspectives of managing an onchocerciasis control programme: A case study from Plateau state, Nigeria. *Annals of Tropical Medicine and Parasitology, 68E*(92), 121–128.

Murray, C. J. & Lopez, A. D. (1996). Evidence-based health policy—Lessons from the Global Burden of Disease Study. *Science, 274,* 740–743.

Murray, C. J. & Lopez, A. D. (1997). Mortality by cause for eight regions of the world: Global Burden of Disease Study. *Lancet, 349,* 1269–1347.

Nathwani, D. & Spiteri, J. (1997). Information about anti-malarial chemoprophylaxis in hospitalized patients—Is it adequate? *Scottish Medical Journal, 42*(1), 13–15.

Phillips, D. R. (1990). *Health and health care in the third world.* New York: Longman Scientific & Technical with Wiley and Sons.

Pinstrup-Anderson, P., Burger, S., Habicht, J. P., Peterson, K. (1993). Protein-energy malnutrition. In D. T. Jamison, W. H. Mosley, A. R. Measham, & J. L. Bobdilla (Eds.), *Disease control priorities in developing countries* (pp. 391–420). Oxford: Oxford University Press.

Roemer, M. I. (1991). *National health systems of the world.* New York: Oxford University Press.

Stansfield, S. K. & Shepard, D. S. (1993). Acute respiratory infection. In D. T. Jamison, W. H. Mosley, A. R. Measham, & J. L. Bohadilla (Eds.), *Disease control priorities in developing countries* (pp. 67–90). Oxford: Oxford University Press.

Tarkka, M. T., Paunonen, M. & Laippala, P. (1999). Social support provided by public health nursing and the coping of first-time mothers child care. *Public Health Nursing, 16*(2), 114–119.

Trigg, P. I. & Kondrachine, A. V. (1998). Commentary: Malaria control in the 1990s. *Bulletin of the World Health Organization, 76*(1), 11–16.

UNAIDS Program and World Health Organization (2000). Report on global HIV/AIDS epidemic as of end 1999. Available at http://www.unaids.org/epidemic_update/report/Epi_report.htm glob.

Vance, C. (1999). Nursing in the global arena. In E. J. Sullivan (Ed.), *Creating nursing's future* (p. 335). St. Louis: Mosby.

Walsh, J. A., Feifer, C. N., Measham, A. R. & Gertler, P. J. (1993). Maternal and perinatal health. In D. T. Jamison, W. H. Mosley, A. R. Measham, & J. L. Bobdilla (Eds.). *Disease control priorities in developing countries* (pp. 363–390). Oxford: Oxford University Press.

Wenzel, E. (1998, September 27). WHO Constitution, Article 2. Available at http://.www.ldb.org/vl/top/whoconst.htm. Accessed August 12, 1999.

Whaley, R. F. & Hashim, T. J. (1995) *A textbook of world health: A practical guide to global health care.* New York: Parthenon Publishing Group.

World Bank (1998, September 27). Why do we need a World Bank? Available at http://www.worldbank.org/. Accessed November 1, 1999.

World Health Organization (1995, October). The treatment of diarrhea: A manual for physicians and other senior health workers. Available at http://www-micro.msb.le.ac.uk/335/Diarrhoea.html. Accessed November 1, 1999.

World Health Organization (1996a, November). Water and sanitation. *WHO Fact Sheet No. 112,* 2. Geneva: WHO. Available at http://www.who.int/inf-fs/fact112.html. Accessed October 26, 1999.

World Health Organization (1996b, June). Cities and emerging or re-emerging diseases in the XXIst century. *WHO Fact Sheet No. 122,* 1. Geneva: WHO. Available at http://www.who.int/inf-fs/fact122.html. Accessed October 26, 1999.

World Health Organization (1997). Promoting health through schools: Report of a WHO expert committee on comprehensive school health education and promotion. *WHO Technical Report Series, 180,* 5. Geneva: WHO.

World Health Organization (1998a, 27 November). Primary health care in the 21st century is everybody's business. *Press Release WHO/89,* 1–2. Geneva: WHO.

World Health Organization (1998b, March). Dracunculiasis eradication. *WHO Fact Sheet No. 98,* 1–2. Geneva: WHO.

World Health Organization (1998c, September). Reducing mortality from major killers of children. *WHO Fact Sheet No. 178,* 3. Geneva: WHO. Available at http://www.who.int/inf-fs/en/fact178.html. Accessed March 9, 2000.

World Health Organization (1998d). Examples of pathogens recognized since 1973. *WHO Fact Sheet No. 97,* 4. Geneva: WHO.

World Health Organization (1998e). Manifesto for safe communities: Safety—a universal concern and responsibility for all. Resolution adopted at the First World conference on Accident and Injury Prevention, September 20, 1998, Stockholm.

World Health Organization (1999a, 18 August). Vigilance needed as first cases of epidemic-prone diseases registered in Kosovo. *Press Release WHO/41,* 1–2. Geneva: WHO.

World Health Organization (1999b). Highlights of the 52nd World Health Assembly. *Bulletin of the World Health Organization, 77*(7), 612–613. Geneva: WHO.

World Health Organization (1999c, 25 May). World Health Assembly gives resounding support to WHO technical programs. *Press Release WHA/18,* 1–3. Geneva: WHO.

World Health Organization (1999d, 3 August). Solar alert '99. *Press Release WHO/40,* 1–2. Geneva: WHO.

World Health Organization (1999e, 5 April). Polio outbreak in Central Africa. *Press Release WHO/21,* 1–2. Geneva: WHO.

World Health Organization (1999f, 19 April). Leprosy elimination moves a step nearer: WHO focuses attention on a few remaining endemic countries. *Press Release WHO/25,* 1–2. Geneva: WHO.

World Health organization (1999g). Malaria vaccine progress. *Bulletin of the World Health Organization, 77*(4), 361–362. Geneva: WHO.

World Health Organization (1999h, 28 October). UN agencies issue joint statement for reducing maternal mortality. *Press Release WHO.* Geneva: WHO.

World Health Organization (1999i, 1 February). WHO Executive Board gives green light to framework convention on tobacco control. *Press Release WHO/6.* Geneva: WHO.

Zwi, A. & Ugalde, A. (1989). Towards an epidemiology of political violence in the Third World. *Social Science and Medicine, 28*(7), 633–642.

RELATED RESOURCES

Career Network. Global Health Council (GHC), 1701 K St., NW, Suite 600, Washington, D.C. 20006. Phone: (202) 833–5900. Fax: (202) 833–0075. Yearly price: $60—members, $120—non-members. Monthly.

International Employment Hotline. Will Cantrell, ed., PO Box 3030, Oakton, VA 22124. Phone: (703) 620–1972. Monthly.

Medical Ambassadors International, PO Box 6645, Modesto, CA 95357. Phone: (209) 524–0600. Protestant church sponsored.

American Red Cross and International Red Cross and Red Crescent Societies. E-mail: *www.red-cross.org.*

International Career Employment Opportunities. Rt. 2, Box 305, Standardsville, VA 22973. Phone: (804) 985-6444. Bimonthly.

International Jobs Bulletin. University Placement Center, Woody Hall B208, Southern Illinois University, Carbondale, IL 62901. Biweekly.

International Opportunities: A Career Guide for Students. Publisher: Kennedy Center for International Studies, Brigham Young University, 280 Herald, Clark Building, PO Box 24538, Provo, UT 84602-4538. $10.95. Phone: (800) 528-6279. Information on internships and employment opportunities with non-profit and voluntary organizations, private agencies, the United Nations, the U.S. Government, and educational organizations.

Monday Developments. Interaction, 1717 Massachusetts Ave., NW, 8th floor, Washington, DC 20006. Phone: (202) 667-8227. Employment opportunities listed. $65/year. Biweekly.

Options. Project Concern, 3550 Afton Rd., San Diego, CA 92123. Phone: (619) 279-9690. Information on professional volunteer opportunities in programs, hospitals, and clinics worldwide.

PDRC Placement Hotline. School for International Training, Brattleboro, VT 05302. Phone: (802) 257-7751

SELECTED READINGS

Abell, H. (1998, summer). Globalization causes a world of health problems. *Hesperian Foundation News,* 1–3.

Berman, P. (1997). National health accounts in developing countries: Appropriate methods and recent applications. *Health Economics, 6,* 11–30.

Chin, J. (Ed.) (2000). *Control of communicable diseases manual.* Washington, D.C.: American Public Health Association.

Deen, J. L., Vos, T., Huttly, S. R., & Tulloch, J. (1999). Injuries and noncommunicable diseases: Emerging health problems of children in developing countries. *Bulletin of the World Health Organization, 77*(6), 518–523.

Hammer, J.S., & Berman, P. (1995). Ends and means in public health policy in developing countries. *Health Policy, 32,* 29–45.

Hart, G. (1997). From "Rotten wives" to "Good mothers": Household models and the limits of economism. *IDS Bulletin, 28*(3), 14–25.

Hsiao, W. C. (1995). The Chinese health care system: Lessons for other nations. *Social Science and Medicine, 41*(2), 171–220.

Kalache, A. & Keller, I. (1999). The WHO perspective on active aging. *Promotion and Education Quarterly, VI*(4), 20–23.

Ministry of Health. (1998). *AIDS in Ethiopia—Background, projections, impacts and interventions.* P.O. Box 1234, Addis Ababa, Ethiopia.

Murray, C. & Chen, L. (1993). In search of a contemporary theory for understanding mortality and change. *Social Science and Medicine, 36*(2), 143–155.

Nyamu, J. (1998). Target: A stronger health sector—special initiative gives priority to preventive and primary care. *Africa Recovery, 11*(4), 18–20.

Schuler, S. R., Hashemi, S. M. & Riley, A. P. (1997). The influence of women's changing roles and status in Bangladesh's fertility transition: Evidence from a study of credit programs and contraceptive use. *World Development, 25*(4), 563–575.

Schuermann, L. (1999, September). American Society for Microbiology supports PAHO efforts to strengthen region-wide network of public health laboratories. *PAHO Today,* 3.

Van Grinneken, J. K., Lob-Levyt, J. & Gove, S. (1996). Potential Interventions for preventing pneumonia among children in development countries: Promoting maternal education. *Tropical Medicine and International Health, 1*(3), 283–294.

Varmus, H. & Satcher, D. (1997). Ethics are local: Engaging cross-cultural variation in the ethics for clinical research. *Social Science and Medicine, 35*(9), 1070–1091.

World Health Organization. (1978). *Alma-Ata 1978: Primary health care.* Geneva: WHO.

World Health Organization (1986). *The Ottawa charter for health promotion.* Geneva: WHO.

World Health Organization. (1998). *Fifty facts from the World Health Report 1998: Global health situations and trends 1955 to 2025.* Geneva: WHO.

Theoretical Bases for Promoting Family Health

KEY TERMS

- Adoptive family
- Blended family
- Cohabitating couples
- Commune family
- Commuter family
- Contemporary family
- Energy exchange
- Family
- Family culture
- Family functioning
- Family map
- Family structure
- Family system boundary
- Foster families
- Gangs
- Group-marriage family
- Group-network family
- Homeless family
- Intrarole functioning
- Kin-network
- Multigenerational family
- Nontraditional family
- Nuclear-dyad family
- Nuclear family
- Primary relationship
- Roles
- Single-adult family
- Single-parent family
- Stepfamily
- Traditional family
- Wider family

LEARNING OBJECTIVES

Upon mastery of this chapter, you should be able to:

- Analyze changing definitions of family.
- Discuss characteristics all families have in common.
- Identify five attributes that help explain how families function as social systems.
- Discuss how a family's culture influences its values, behaviors, prescribed roles, and distributions of power.
- Compare and contrast the variety of structures that make up families.
- Describe the functions of a family.
- Identify the stages of the family life cycle and the developmental tasks of a family as it grows.
- Analyze the role of the community health nurse in promoting the health of the family unit.

When you hear the word *family,* what do you think of? How would you define you own family? Is your grandfather a member of your family? Your niece? Your neighbor? A friend? A family pet? Although many different definitions exist, most family theorists agree that a **family** consists of two or more individuals who share a residence or live near one another; possess some common emotional bond; engage in interrelated social positions, roles, and tasks; and share a sense of affection and belonging (Murray & Zentner, 1997; Friedman, 1998).

The family is a separate entity with its own structure, functions, and needs. In every society throughout history, the family is the most basic unit; so too in community health (Kristjanson & Chalmers, 1997). It is the family, more than any other societal institution, that nurtures and shapes a society's members.

Today's community health nurse needs to understand and work with many types of families, each of which will have different health problems and needs. For example, a young single mother who is homeless seeks help in caring for her sick infant. A 55-year-old grandfather is caring for his elderly mother who was recently discharged from the hospital after a stroke. A group of parents, siblings, cousins, and children, all refugees from Laos, need instruction on the purchase and preparation of food. Why is it important for the community health nurse to understand and respect the unique characteristics, cultures, structures, and functions of each of these families? Do families, as basic units of a community, have characteristics that affect community health nursing service? The answer is an unqualified yes. As a community health nurse, effectiveness depends on knowing how to work with a family as a unit of care. This chapter examines the nature of families, family functioning, and family health. It draws from various theories to strengthen your understanding and appreciation of families as clients. This information will increase the effectiveness of your interventions with families at the primary, secondary, and tertiary levels of prevention (see Levels of Prevention).

Family functioning is defined as those behaviors or activities by family members that maintain the family and meet family needs, individual member needs, and society's views of family. The interdependence of family members involves a set of internal relationships that influence the effectiveness of family functioning (Friedman, 1998). There is a complex communication pattern of functioning among family members, and the quality of the pattern contributes to the health of a family.

Family health is concerned with how well the family functions together as a unit. It involves not only the health of each member and how they relate to other members, but also how well they relate to and cope with the community outside the family. In fact, family health, like individual health, ranges along a continuum from wellness to illness. A family may be at one point on that continuum now and at a much different point 6 months from now. Family health refers to the health status of a given family at a given point in time.

LEVELS OF PREVENTION

A HEALTHY FAMILY

GOAL
The family will provide the emotional and material resources necessary for its members' growth and well-being.

PRIMARY PREVENTION
Adults are well prepared for the responsibilities of their union and enter the relationship with the personal resources necessary to promote the growth and development of their family unit.

SECONDARY PREVENTION
At the earliest possible moment of recognition that problems exist in the relationships among or between family members, or if one family member has personal problems that affect the family as a whole, the family seeks out the appropriate resources that brings the family to the highest level of wellness possible.

TERTIARY PREVENTION
After the family suffers a crisis, the members recognize the need for help and accept that help, drawing on personal resources to rebuild relationships and heal the family unit, again bringing it to the highest level of wellness possible.

UNIVERSAL CHARACTERISTICS OF FAMILIES

Several observations can be made about families in general. First, each family is unique. The families mentioned earlier each have their own distinct problems and strengths. When you approach the door of a house or push the buzzer of an apartment, you cannot assume what the family inside will be like. Consequently, you will have to gather information about each particular family in order to achieve nursing objectives.

Second, every family shares some universal characteristics with every other family. These universal characteristics provide an important key to understanding each family's uniqueness. Five of the most important family universals for community health nursing are:
1. Every family is a small social system.
2. Every family has its own cultural values and rules.
3. Every family has structure.
4. Every family has certain basic functions.
5. Every family moves through stages in its life cycle.

No matter how many families a nurse might visit or serve in the course of a year, each one will have these universal features, and it is important for community health nurses to know each family's unique manifestation of these features as they affect that family's health. These five universals of family life, which provide the framework of this chapter, are based on systems theory, sociological theories, and theories of family development. While considering the universals of family life, this chapter will also cover the unique family features and structures that characterize our changing world (see The Global Community).

ATTRIBUTES OF FAMILIES AS SOCIAL SYSTEMS

Many Americans fall into the habit of viewing families merely as collections of individuals. Caused partly by our strong cultural emphasis on individualism, this error also occurs because we often encounter families through the individual members. When a community health nurse sits in a living room talking with a young mother about her new infant, it is difficult to keep in mind that all the other family members are present by way of their influence. Systems theory offers some insights about how families operate as social systems. Knowing the attributes of living systems or open systems can help strengthen an understanding of family structure and function. There are five attributes of open systems that help explain how families function: (1) families are interdependent, (2) families maintain boundaries, (3) families exchange energy with their environment, (4) families are adaptive, and (5) families are goal-oriented.

THE GLOBAL COMMUNITY

Southeast Asian Refugee Women: Disruption to Family Structure and Function

Fox, P. G., Cowell, J. M. & Johnson, M. M. (1995). Effects of family disruption on Southeast Asian refugee women. *International Nursing Review, 42*(1), 26–30.

Southeast Asia is an agricultural economy with a society that promotes strong family ties. Families are large and extended; its members have clearly defined roles and responsibilities. Religious roots in Buddhism and Confucianism also serve to maintain devotion and allegiance to the family as well as ancestors.

The Southeast Asian woman's dominant role is to meet the needs of her extended family, husband, and children. She is directed by cultural norms to accept the authority of her husband and the other men in her extended family. Since a woman's identity is attached to her family role, loss or separation from other family members, particularly her husband, is an emotionally stressful experience.

Over the past two decades over 1 million refugees have immigrated to the United States from Southeast Asia to escape war and economic and political oppression. Many of these refugees are women who suffer profound grief and chronic stress from the loss of their husbands and from lack of news of family members left behind. These women feel isolated in a foreign culture without their past supports and role identities. Additionally, the loss of family members forces these women into new gender roles without the benefit of traditional family assistance that is so important to them. Adjustment for them is difficult, and the stress may lead to illness.

Nurses need to assess the importance of the loss of family members on the lives of refugee women and design intervention programs that encourage social support networks, family viability, and ethnic community development.

Interdependence Among Members

All the members of a family are interdependent; each member's actions affect the other members. For example, consider the changes a father might make to reduce his risk of coronary heart disease. If he cuts back on working overtime, the family's income will be reduced. If he begins to eat different foods, food preparation and eating patterns in the family will be altered. If he starts a new exercise program three evenings a week, this may upset other family routines. Even his ability to carry out his usual roles as husband and father may be affected if, for instance, he has less time to help his children with their homework or share household chores with his wife.

It is possible to illustrate the pattern of interactions between members using a family map (Fig. 22–1). This tool can reveal a great deal about the interdependence of family members. The way parents relate to each other, for instance, influences the quality of their parenting. When the interactions

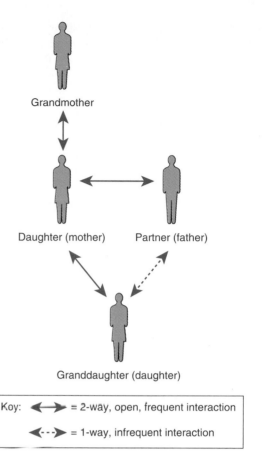

FIGURE 22–1. This map indicates that the mother is a key figure for family interaction. The maternal grandmother, father, and daughter communicate primarily to her rather than directly to one another.

between them are frequent, honest, and nurturing, they have more to offer their children. Marital, parent–child, and sibling relationships all significantly influence family functioning. They determine how well the family as a system handles conflict, provides a support system for its members, copes with crises, solves daily problems, and capitalizes on its own resources.

Family Boundaries

Families, as systems, set and maintain boundaries: ego-boundaries, generation boundaries, and family-community boundaries (Barker, 1992). These boundaries, which result from shared experiences and expectations, link family members together in a bond that excludes the rest of the world. Also, a greater concentration of energy exists within the family than between the family and its external environment, thereby creating a **family system boundary.**

For example, the Salazar extended family gathers for a Sunday afternoon backyard picnic. The distinctiveness of this family from all the others in the neighborhood is noticeable, as would that of any other family be. The elders in the family were born in Mexico, and they sit together reminiscing in Spanish. The food is traditional and plentiful. It is prepared and served by the women: Aunt Rosa's tamales, Cousin Teresa's tortillas, and flan for dessert from Grandma Lupe's own recipe. While the women prepare the foods, some of the men play ball while others listen to Uncle Gilberto play the guitar and discuss the future of the family grape-growing business. The children gather in small groups and play loudly. Several of them, prompted by their parents, will display their musical talent later in the day, by singing some old favorite songs and doing some traditional Mexican dances. Because of the things they have in common, the Salazars set and maintain boundaries that unite them and also differentiate them from others.

Energy Exchange

Family boundaries are semipermeable; although they provide protection and preservation of the family unit, they also allow selective linkage with the outside world. As open systems, in order to function adequately, families exchange materials or information with their environment (Friedman, 1998). This process is called **energy exchange.** All normally functioning living systems engage in such an input–output relationship. This energy exchange serves to promote a healthy ecological balance between the family system and the environment that is its immediate community.

A family's successful progress through its developmental stages depends on how well the family manages this energy exchange. For example, a childbearing family needs adequate food, shelter, and emotional support as well as information on how to accomplish its developmental tasks. The family also needs community resources such as health care, education, and employment, all of which are forms of environmental input. In return, the family contributes to the community by working and by consuming goods and services. When a family does not have adequate income or emotional support or does not use community resources, that family is not experiencing a proper energy exchange with its environment. An inadequate exchange can lead to dysfunctioning and poor health (Neuman, 1995).

Adaptive Behavior

Families are adaptive, equilibrium-seeking systems. In accordance with their very nature, families never stay the same. They shift and change in response to internal and external forces. Internally, the family composition changes as new members are added or members leave through death or divorce. Roles and relationships change as members advance in age and experience; normative expectations change as members resolve their tensions and differing points of view. Externally, families are bombarded by influences from sources such as school, work, peers, neighbors, religion, and

government; consequently, they are forced to accommodate to new demands. Adapting to these influences may require a family to change its behavior, goals, and even its values. Like any system, the family needs a state of quasi-equilibrium in order to function (Neuman, 1995). Thus, with each new set of pressures, the family shifts and accommodates to regain balance and a normal lifestyle.

There are times when a family's capacity for adaptation is stressed beyond its limits. At this point the system may be in danger of disintegrating; that is, family members will leave or become dysfunctional because of unresolved stress. This is an indication that families may need some form of intervention to help restore family equilibrium. These interventions may take the form of extended family mediation or external professional help.

Community health nurses play an influential role in family equilibrium-seeking. Neuman describes the major goal of nursing as keeping the individual and family client systems stabilized within their environment (Neuman, 1995). Chapter 23 explores the community health nurse's stabilizing interventions with families in detail.

Goal-Directed Behavior

Families as social systems are goal directed. Families exist for a purpose—to establish and maintain a milieu that promotes the development of their members. In order to fulfill this purpose, a family must perform basic functions such as providing love, security, identity, a sense of belonging, assistance with preparation for adult roles in society, and maintenance of order and control. In addition to these functions, each family member engages in tasks to maintain the family as a viable unit. Duvall and Miller (1985) describe specific functions and tasks for each stage of the family's development. These functions and tasks will be examined in more detail later in this chapter.

FAMILY CULTURE

Families are social systems with cultural dimensions; families are also tied biologically through kinship and socially through choice. This structure exists for a purpose. Duvall's definition nicely summarizes these aspects of the family: "The family is a unity of interacting persons related by ties of marriage, birth, or adoption, whose central purpose is to create and maintain a common culture which promotes the physical, mental, emotional, and social development of each of its members" (Duvall & Miller, 1985, p. 6).

Family culture is the acquired knowledge that family members use to interpret their experiences and to generate behaviors that influence family structure and function. The concept of family culture arises from a significant body of literature in the social and behavioral sciences of cross-cultural comparisons and in-depth analyses that demonstrate that each family has a "culture" that strongly influences its structure and function. Culture explains why families behave as they do (Leininger, 1991; Pender, 1996; Spector, 1996). Family culture also gives the community health nurse a basis for assessing family health and designing appropriate interventions.

Three aspects of family culture deserve special consideration: (1) family members share certain values that affect family behavior, (2) certain roles are prescribed and defined for family members, and (3) a family's culture determines its distribution and use of power.

Shared Values and Their Effect on Behavior

Although families share many broad cultural values drawn from the larger society in which they live, they also develop unique variants. Every family has its own set of values and rules for operation that we can speak of as family culture (Barker, 1992). Some values will be explicitly stated: "Family matters must always stay within the family." Such values may give rise to specific operating rules: "Don't tell anyone about our problems."

Like all cultural values, however, many family values remain outside the conscious awareness of family members. These values, often not verbalized, become powerful determinants of what the family believes, feels, thinks, and does. Family values include those beliefs transmitted by previous generations, religious influences, immediate social pressures, and the larger society. Values become an integral part of a family's life and are very difficult to change. A family that values free expression for every member engages comfortably in loud, noisy debates. Another family that values quietness, order, and control will not tolerate its members raising their voices. One family uses birth control based on beliefs about human life and parental responsibility; another family chooses not to use birth control because it holds a different set of values. How a family views education, health care, life style, courtship, marriage, childrearing, sex roles, or any of the myriad other issues requiring choices depends upon the cultural values of that family.

Prescribed Roles

Roles, the assigned or assumed parts that members play during day-to-day family living, are bestowed and defined by the family (Hanson & Boyd, 1996). For instance, in one family the father role assigned to the male adult may be defined as an authoritative one that includes establishing rules, judging behavior, and administering punishment for violation of rules. In another family, the father role may be defined primarily as that of a loving benefactor. If there is an absence of an immediate male parent, a grandfather, uncle, friend, or mother may take over the father role. Selection of specific roles to be played in any given family will vary depending on the family's structure, needs, and patterns of functioning. In a single-parent family, for example, the parent may need to assume the roles of mother, father, and breadwinner, as well as other roles.

Families distribute among their members' roles all the responsibilities and tasks necessary to conduct family living. The responsibilities of breadwinner and homemaker, for example, with their accompanying tasks, may belong to husband and wife, respectively, or may be shared if both husband and wife hold jobs outside the home. Older children may help younger ones with homework or entertain them. This releases parents for other tasks and increases the responsibility of older children.

Family members play several roles at the same time. This **intrarole functioning** can be exceptionally taxing. A woman, for instance, may play the role of wife to her husband, daughter to her mother who lives with her, and mother to each of her children. The mother role may involve taking on several additional roles and responsibilities and will vary with each child's needs. In a family in which the mother is seriously ill, many of the roles she held will have to be assumed by others. This places new demands on other family members during the treatment and healing process or throughout a terminal illness (Fitch, Bunston, & Elliot, 1999). A single parent often takes on the roles of both father and mother, but may distribute responsibilities and tasks more widely. A grandmother or child(ren) may assume responsibility for some chores and thus relieve the demands placed on the single parent. Among families, there is great variation in expectations for each role and the degree of flexibility in role prescriptions. Consequently, a family may place great demands on some members, although those same members may interpret the expectations placed on them and their roles differently. Confusion and conflict can develop unless roles are clarified.

Other roles of family members extend beyond the immediate family. There may be extended family members nearby who interact with the family on a regular basis or only on special occasions such as birthdays. If both parents are employed, they may have an expansive social network from work or from within the neighborhood. Friendships are often made with the parents of the childrens' friends, particularly if their children participate in the same extracurricular activities. Many families enjoy the fellowship of organized religious or cultural groups. This fellowship can be a source of support and comfort in addition to being an additional role function for the family members. Another intrarole function is that of community participant in activities separate from the family. These roles may revolve around local or regional politics, community improvement, volunteerism for non-profit agencies, or any other service outside the home the community may offer. These diverse role relationships should enrich and energize the participants. However, many people may become over-committed, thus creating an imbalance of role responsibilities that is draining and causes friction and stress. The community health nurse must work with families to achieve a balance of activities and roles to promote family health.

Power Distribution

Power, the possession of control, authority, or influence over others, assumes different patterns in each family. In some families, power is concentrated primarily in one member, whereas in others it is distributed on a more egalitarian basis. The traditional patriarchal family, in which the father holds absolute authority over the other members, is rare in American society. However, the pattern of husband as head of the household and dominant member of the family is still frequently seen. Whether male or female, the dominant partner holds the majority of the decision-making power, particularly over the more important family matters such as employment and finances. Other areas of decision-making, including choices about vacations, housing, leisure activities, household purchases, and childrearing, may be shared or delegated. With changing societal influences, however, the present trend among American families is toward egalitarian power distribution.

Rudolf Dreikurs (1964) long ago advocated that families form a "family council" for shared decision-making and distribution of tasks. Today many families practice joint decision-making and equal participation by all members. However, the community health nurse can suggest this activity for families not using such a method. Role-playing this technique can be incorporated on a home visit or as a teaching technique with an aggregate group. Specific educational interventions are discussed in Chapter 9.

Roles often influence power distribution within the family. Along with the responsibilities attached to a role, a family may assign decision-making authority. The mother role frequently includes decision-making regarding household management. A responsibility related to a son's role, such as lawn-mowing, may be enhanced as a learning activity, if he is allowed to decide when and how often he does the job.

Family power structure is also influenced by the amount of personal power residing in each member (Friedman, 1998). A mother or eldest son, for example, can exercise considerable influence over the family by virtue of personality and position rather than delegated authority. Even a child who throws temper tantrums can wield considerable power in a family.

FAMILY STRUCTURES

Globally, families—in all their varied forms—are the basic social unit. The meaning of family among the Hmong of northern Laos may include hundreds of people and make up a clan. In Mexico the families remain close, are large, and extend into multiple generations. In Germany and Japan families are small and tend to the needs of their elders at home, whereas in the United States, where families come from many cultural groups, all the variations coexist within communities.

For many people in the United States, the term *family* evokes a picture of a husband, wife, and child(ren) living under one roof with the male as breadwinner and the female as homemaker. This nuclear family was often seen as the norm for everyone. However, the pressures of changing social values and cultural lifestyles, such as women working outside the home, combined with the acceptance of alternative lifestyles, has changed the definition of family. Today definitions of family include a variety of households such as unmarried adults living together with or without children, single-parent households, divorced couples who combine households with children from previous marriages (the blended family), and even homosexual couples with or without children.

It must be considered a privilege to gain entrance into a family's home. This is a uniquely private space belonging to the family. The people who make up the members of this household interact, care for one another, and bond in ways that may never be fully understood by anyone outside of the family. Therefore, being granted entrance into this system gives the community health nurse an opportunity to work with the family that few other professionals experience. Each type of household requires recognition and acceptance by community health nurses who must help families achieve optimal health.

Families come in many shapes and sizes. The varying **family structures** or compositions comprise the characteristics of individuals who make up a family unit (age, gender, and number). A growing body of research on family structure and function shows that families have changed dramatically since the nuclear family was the dominant form. Family structures fall into two general categories: traditional and nontraditional.

Traditional Families

Traditional family structures are those that are most familiar to us and that are most readily accepted by society. They include the **nuclear family:** husband, wife, and child(ren) all living together in the same household. In nuclear families, the workload distribution between the two adults can vary. Both adults can work outside the home; one adult can work outside the home and the other may stay at home and assume primary responsibilities for the household; or partners can alternate, constantly renegotiating work and domestic responsibilities. A **nuclear-dyad family** consists of a husband and wife living together who have no children or who have grown children living outside the home. Traditional families also include **single-adult families** in which one adult is living alone either by choice to remain single or because of separation from spouse and/or children owing to divorce, death, or distance from children. Some traditional families are **multigenerational families** in which several generations or age-groups live together in the same household, for example, a household in which a widowed woman lives with her divorced daughter and two young grandchildren (Jendrick, 1994). Sometimes, particularly in close-knit ethnic communities, we see families forming a **kin-network** in which several nuclear families live in the same household, or near one another, and share goods and services. They may own and operate a family business, sharing the work and child-care responsibilities, incomes and expenses, and maybe even meals. Variations of this trend are increasing among all groups as children postpone leaving home because of economic conditions or educational plans, or an elderly parent may move into the adult child's home to recover from a recent illness.

Another deviation from the traditional nuclear family is the **blended family.** In this structure, single parents marry and raise the children from each of their previous relationships together. They may be the custodial parents who have the children with them except for planned visits with the noncustodial parent, or they may share custody so the children live in the blended arrangement only part-time. This family may include children from the couple's union in addition to the children brought into this relationship.

Single-parent families include one adult (either father or mother) caring for a child or children as a result of a temporary relationship or a legal separation, divorce, or the death of a spouse. In single-parent families, the parent may or may not be employed. Other nontraditional single-parent family situations are described in the next section.

One contemporary variant of the traditional family is the **commuter family.** Both partners in this family work, but their jobs are in different cities. The pattern is usually for one partner to live, work, and perhaps raise children in the "home" city while the second partner lives in the other city and commutes home for weekends or less frequently, depending on the distance. Sometimes this arrangement is short-term, as when one partner is transferred through work and the couple chooses not to move the rest of the family until the end of the school year. At other times, the commuting may continue for years. For example, the family home may be in a town where the cost of living is reasonable, and one parent works in a financially and personally rewarding career several hundreds of miles away and commutes home on weekends. In other instances, one parent may be in the military and be on assignment in another country for 6 months or longer, leaving the other parent alone for months at a time. Clearly these arrangements influence family roles and functions, challenging a family's ability to maintain healthy relationships. A traditional family in which one partner is required to travel a great deal of the time for business or in which one partner is caring for an ill family member at a distant location may experience similar problems and stressors. Table 22–1 lists a number of traditional family structures.

Nontraditional or Contemporary Families

The traditional nuclear family has been a fundamental part of the European cultural heritage shared by many Americans,

reinforced by religion, education, and other influential social institutions. Variations from this pattern often were treated as deviant and abnormal, even in studies of the family as recent as 1983 (Olson et al., 1983). However, unmarried people living together increased from 500,000 in 1970 to 2.8 million in 1989 (Saluter, 1992). There is every indication that this trend will continue in the 21st century (Harway & Wexler, 1996).

Society is accepting nontraditional definitions of family. The concept of **wider family** was initially presented by Marciano (1991) and is defined as a family that "emerges from lifestyle, is voluntary, and independent of necessary biological or kin connections" (p. 160). "With today's wide variety of family types and structures, the most advanced definition of family may be 'the family is who the client says it is'" (Bell & Wright, 1993, p. 391).

Families that do not fit the traditional nuclear model make up an increasing proportion of the American population. For instance:

- in 1960, legally married couples made up 75% of American households, but by 1990 that number had dropped to only 50% (U. S. Bureau of the Census, 1990)
- in 1995, 32% of the women in the United States were single (U.S. Department of Commerce, 1998)
- fewer than 20% of American families now have a working father, a full-time homemaker mother, and one or more children
- the number of couples who share a household without marrying increased more than five times between 1970 and 1989 (Saluter, 1992)
- as of 1990, approximately 25% (more than 20 million) of all families in the United States were headed by one adult, usually a woman
- the number of single households headed by men has increased to 3% of all families, an increase from 2.1% in 1980
- the proportion of children under 18 years of age who live with one parent increased from 12% in 1970 to 25% in 1990, and 40% of all children will live part of their lives before adulthood with a single parent (Coleman et al., 1998)

Divorce is also changing family structures; half of all marriages now end in divorce (higher for teenage marriages) and the median duration of marriages is approximately 7 years. Twenty women per 1000 divorce each year in the United States, a number staying fairly steady since 1990 but double the rate in other industrialized nations such as Germany (9 per 1000), Canada (11 per 1000), and Japan (10 per 1000) (U.S. Department of Commerce, 1998). Display 22–1 describes one nontraditional American family.

Some **nontraditional** and **contemporary family** structures are becoming more common and thus are generally accepted by society. Others are still generally regarded as illegitimate or even dangerous to society. Table 22–1 lists some of the more common nontraditional and contemporary family structures.

TABLE 22–1. The Traditional and Nontraditional American Family

Structure	Participants	Living Arrangements
TRADITIONAL		
Nuclear dyad	Husband Wife	Common household
Nuclear family	Husband Wife Children	Common household
Commuter family	Husband Wife Children (sometimes)	Household divided between two cities
Single-parent family	One adult (separated, divorced, widowed) Children	Common household
Divorced family (shared custody of children)	One adult parent, children part-time	Two separate households
Blended family	Husband Wife (His and/or hers, and possibly their children)	Common household
Single adult	One adult	Living alone
Multigenerational family	Any combination of the traditional family structures	Common household
Kin network	Two or more reciprocal households (related by birth or marriage)	Close geographic proximity
NONTRADITIONAL		
Unmarried single-parent family	One parent (never married) Children	Common household
Cohabitating partners	Two adults (heterosexual, homosexual, or "just friends") Children (possibly)	Common household
Commune family	Two or more monogamous couples Sharing children	Common household
Group marriage commune family	Several adults "married" to each other Sharing childrearing	Common household
Group network	Reciprocal nuclear households or single members	Close geographic proximity
Homeless families	Any combination of family members previously mentioned	The streets and shelters
Foster families	Husband and wife or single adult Natural children (possibly) Foster children	Common household
Gangs	Males and females usually of same cultural or ethnic background	Close geographic proximity (same neighborhood)
"Loose shirt" families	Parents work from home via the personal computer (word processing, e-mail, faxing, cellular telephone—"telecommuting")	Common household

The approach used by Scanzoni and colleagues (1989) is to consider the **primary relationship** of two or more persons interacting in a continuing manner within the greater environment. This primary relationship encompasses all the possible family structures. As long as 20 years ago, Stein (1981) suggested the notion of a "life-spiral" rather than a life-cycle pattern to more realistically describe the fluctuations of contemporary nontraditional families. The spiral more realistically depicts the fluid-like movement within family structures than a cycle that provides a picture of a continuous linear movement along a path. Traditional functions and structures of the family continue to evolve as new combinations of people live together and consider their relationship that of a "family."

One of the most common forms of nontraditional family seen today is the single-parent family headed by a woman. Sometimes this form is chosen by single women who decide to adopt or have children without being married. In most cases, though, this nontraditional form results from an unplanned pregnancy when there is no marriage. Statistics indicate that the single-parent family is being headed more and more frequently by teenagers, with pregnancies in junior high school common. Among teens 15 to 19 years old, 1 in 10 becomes pregnant each year, resulting in 1,100,000 pregnancies annually (Alpers, 1998). The implications for the role of the community health nurse are greatest with this population. For example, nurses work with young teens through

DISPLAY 22–1. **A Look at One Nontraditional American Family**

Baby boomer families experience divorce and other contemporary family phenomena in unique ways, as demonstrated in the following example (Riley & Riley, 1996):

> Our granddaughter, Susan (a Harvard alumna), cohabits with Ted (an astrophysicist at Harvard). They are not married, but they have a baby (our first great-grandson). Ted has been twice divorced and has a daughter nearly as old as Susan. Susan has close bonds to this daughter and to both of Ted's ex-wives and often travels from Massachusetts to Texas to visit them. The question is: How is Susan related to all these "ex's"? Even more intriguing: Suppose one of us were suddenly stranded alone in Texas and needed a supportive relationship. It is not unimaginable that Susan's grandparent might seek out one of Ted's ex-wives for help—indeed, might eventually develop a close relationship with her. And what would that relationship be called? (pp. 288–289)

schools or clinics to ensure healthy pregnancy progression; teach parenting skills to the youthful parents as well as grandparenting skills to the teen's parents; and ensure that the infant receives immunizations and primary health care services as needed, as well as family planning information for the new parents. On a broader scale, community health nurses collaborate with other professionals to assure that the community has resources for all levels of prevention that focus on primary prevention.

Many adult couples form a family alliance outside of marriage or through a private ceremony not legally recognized as marriage. **Cohabitating couples** may range from young adults living together to an elderly couple sharing their lives outside of marriage to avoid tax penalties or inheritance issues. Cohabitating couples may be heterosexual or homosexual; they may or may not share a sexual relationship. In some instances, these couples have their own biological or adopted children.

Another nontraditional family form is the **commune family,** a group of unrelated, monogamous (married or committed to one person) couples living together and collectively rearing their children. A **group-marriage family** involves several adults who share a common household and consider that all are married to one another; they share everything, including sex and child rearing. Group-marriage families usually center on one main male patriarch who designates responsibilities and dictates to the other members some religious or social ideology. The Branch Davidians who lived in a compound outside of Waco, Texas, until destroyed by the FBI in 1993 are a tragic example of this family type.

A **group-network family** is made up of nuclear families not related by birth or marriage but bound by a common set of values such as a religious system. These families live close to one another and share goods, services, and childrearing responsibilities. Some commune and group-network families select one of their members, usually a male, to be their leader, or head.

Many children are removed from their homes of origin due to family stresses of abuse, violence, or neglect. In most communities, these children are housed with families known as **foster families.** These families may take a variety of forms, but all foster families have had formal training to accept unrelated children into their home on a temporary basis while the parent(s) of the foster child(ren) receive the help necessary to reunify the original family. Although this arrangement is not ideal, most foster families provide a safe and loving home for these children in transition. Often the foster children have emotional and physical health problems, and they may never have experienced the positive structure that foster families provide. These problems, which can cause stress for everyone involved, are typically ones that the community health nurse can help to solve. In fact, the state of California recently appropriated $2.48 million to provide public health nursing expertise explicitly to meet the health care needs of children in foster care. This was matched (25%/75%) with federal funds at the local level, making $9.9 million available for health promotion of foster children. The nurses are located at local county welfare offices but are hired, funded, and supervised by local health departments (Department of Social Services, 1999).

Some families, because of their lack of marketable skills, negative economic changes, or chronic mental health problems, including substance abuse, find themselves without permanent shelter. These **homeless families** are increasing in numbers and their characteristics are changing. "Each year of this decade, homeless service providers have reported that single women with dependent children are the fastest growing segment of the homeless population, at approximately 20%" (Gillis & Singer, 1997, p. 30). The homeless population is also increasingly made up of nuclear families. Frequently the community health nurse provides services to shelters or drop-in clinics frequented by the homeless. Since this population is increasing, it has many implications for the nurse.

A destructive form of "family" occurring in many cities is gangs. **Gangs** are formed by young people searching for the emotional ties of family as a substitute for an absent or dysfunctional family. Gang members consider themselves family and rely on one another or the group for support that they are not receiving from members of their family of origin. Obviously, gangs are a dysfunctional and destructive form of family: typically, they draw their members into drugs and violence and cause frequent injury, abuse, and even death to gang members, their associates, and innocent bystanders. Gangs are discussed in more detail in Chapter 20. Many nurses serving urban areas may be working with families and groups who are involved with gangs and should be prepared to deal with the issues gangs create.

Implications for the Community Health Nurse

The variety of family structures raises three important issues for consideration. First, community health nurses can no longer hold to a myth that idealizes the traditional nuclear family. They must be prepared to work with all types of families and accept them as valid. Unless the community health nurse is able to accept traditional, nontraditional, and emerging family lifestyles and address the special problems and needs these lifestyles may present, she or he may not be able to help the family and may even create additional problems for them.

Second, the nurse must realize that the structure of an individual's family may change several times over a member's lifetime. A girl may be born into a kin-network, shift to a nuclear family when her parents move, and become part of a single-parent family when her parents are divorced. As she matures, she may become a single adult living alone, then become a part of a cohabitating couple, and still later marry and have children in a nuclear family. For the individual, each variant family form involves changes in roles, interaction patterns, socialization processes, and linkages with external resources. The community health nurse must learn to address the client's needs throughout these life changes, equipping people with the skills needed to deal with the inevitability of changing structures.

Finally, the nurse must realize that each type of family structure creates different issues and problems that, in turn, influence a family's ability to perform its basic functions. Each particular structure determines the kind of support needed from nursing or other human service systems (Eliopoulos, 1997). A single adult living alone, for instance, may lack companionship or a sense of being needed by other family members. A kin-network family provides broad, extended family support and security, but may have problems with power distribution and decision making. An unmarried couple raising a child may be parenting well, but may feel isolated from married couples in the community and need more peer support and socialization. Variations in structure create variations in family strengths and needs, an important consideration for community health nurses. Display 22–2 lists additional factors affecting families in America.

FAMILY FUNCTIONS

Families in every culture throughout history have engaged in similar functions: families always have produced children, physically maintained their members, protected their health, encouraged their education or training, given emotional support and acceptance, and provided supportive and nurturing

---

> ### DISPLAY 22–2. Facts Affecting Families in America
>
> - On any given night in the United States there are 500,000 to 600,000 homeless men, women, and children (Gillis & Singer, 1997).
> - 500,000 children are missing each year.
> - 3.3 million children live with their grandparents as the primary care providers (Jendrek, 1994).
> - 460,000 children were in foster homes in 1991 (Chira, 1994).
> - 10% of girls between 15 and 19 years old get pregnant each year, producing 1,100,000 pregnancies annually (Alpers, 1998).
> - 10.7% of white, 28.1% of Hispanic, and 31.9% of black families live below the poverty level (Northam, 1996).
> - There are 5 million migrant farmworkers in the United States, with an infant mortality 2.5 times higher than the national average; a life expectancy of 49 years, compared with the national average of 75 years; and a parasitic infection rate 11 to 59 times higher than in the general population (Sandhaus, 1998).
> - 10% of the population has significant problems related to substance abuse (Reilly, 1998).

---

care during illness. Some societies have experimented with separation of these functions, allocating activities such as child care, socialization, or social control to a larger group. The Israeli kibbutz and Chinese commune are examples. In American society, certain social institutions help perform some aspects of traditional family functions. Schools, for example, help socialize children; professionals supervise health care; and religious organizations influence values.

Six functions are typical of American families today and are essential for maintenance and promotion of family health: (1) providing affection, (2) providing security, (3) instilling identity, (4) promoting affiliation, (5) providing socialization, and (6) establishing controls (Duvall & Miller, 1985). These tasks help promote the growth and development of members. Understanding these functions, and how well individual families accomplish the functions, enables the community health nurse to work more effectively with the various families encountered at their level of functioning.

Providing Affection

The family functions to give members affection and emotional support. In Western societies, love brings couples together. In some other cultures, affection comes after marriage. Continued affection creates an atmosphere of nurturance and care for all family members that is necessary for health, development, and survival (Grace, 1995). It is common knowledge that infants require love to thrive. Indeed, human beings of any age require love as sustenance for growth and find it most often in the family. Families, unlike many other social groups, are bound by affectionate ties whose strength determines family happiness and closeness. Consider how the sharing of gifts on a holiday or the loving concern of a family for a sick member draws the family together.

Positive sexual identity and sexual fulfillment are also influenced by a loving atmosphere. Early students of the family emphasized sexual access and procreation as basic family functions. Now we recognize that families exist not only to regulate the sex drive and perpetuate the species but also to sustain life and foster human potential through a strong affectional climate.

Providing Security and Acceptance

Families meet their members' physical needs by providing food, shelter, clothing, health care, and other necessities; in so doing, they create a secure environment. Members need to know that these basics will be available and that the family is committed to providing them.

The stability of the family unit also gives members a sense of security. The family offers a safe retreat from the competition of the outside world, a place where its members are accepted for themselves. They can learn, make mistakes, and grow in a secure environment. Where else does the toddler, after repeated falls, receive the encouragement to keep trying to walk; or the child, teased by a bully, regain his courage; or a parent, feeling burned out by a job, find comfort and renewal? The dependability of the family unit promotes confidence and self-assurance among its members. This contributes to their mental and emotional health and equips them with the skills necessary to cope with the outside world.

Instilling Identity and Satisfaction

The family functions to give members a sense of social and personal identity. Like a mirror, the family reflects back to its members a picture of who they are and how valuable they are to others. Positive reflections provide the individual with a sense of satisfaction and worth, such as that experienced by a girl when her family applauds her efforts in a swimming meet or by a boy whose family praises the bird house he builds in Cub Scouts. Needs fulfillment in the home determines satisfaction in the outside world; it particularly affects other interpersonal relationships and career choices. Roles learned within the family also give members a sense of identity. A boy growing up and learning his family's expectations for the male role quickly develops a sense of the kind of person he must strive to be; often, he is expected to be strong, competitive, successful, and unemotional. As a girl grows up, she often learns what is expected of her from her mother: to defer her needs to the family, be flexible and nurturing, and have homemaking skills. In other families, all children may

have equal expectations of achievement and success. Families influence their members' positions in society by instilling values and goals. For some families the emphasis may be on higher education; for others it may be to work at a skill or trade. Still other families may be influenced by religious or political affiliations. Whatever the family influence, it is certain to shape each member's identity.

Promoting Affiliation and Companionship

The family functions to give members a sense of belonging throughout life. Because families provide associational bonds and group membership, they help satisfy their members' needs for belonging. Each person knows that he or she is integral—that he or she belongs—to the family. However, the quality of a family's communication influences its closeness. If communication patterns are effective, then affiliation ties are strong and needs for belonging are met. One family handles conflict over financial expenditures, for instance, by discussing differences and making compromises; this promotes affiliation. In another family, financial conflicts go unacknowledged: members keep spending selfishly and never discuss compromises.

The family, unlike other social institutions, involves permanent relationships. Long after friends from school, the old neighborhood, work, or the religious center have come and gone, there is still the family. The family provides its members with affiliation and fellowship that remains unbroken by distance or time. Even when scattered across the country, family members will gather to support one another and to share in a holiday, wedding, graduation, or funeral. It is to the family that its members turn in times of happiness, tragedy, or need. This family affiliation remains a resource for life.

Providing Socialization

The family functions to socialize the young. Families transmit their culture—their values, attitudes, goals, and behavior patterns—to their members. Members, socialized into a way of life that reflects and preserves that family's cultural heritage, pass that heritage on, in turn, to the next generation. From infancy on, children learn to control their bowels, eat with utensils, dress themselves, manage emotions, and behave according to sociocultural prescriptions for their age and sex. Through this process, members also learn their roles in the family. Lifestyles, the foods preferred, relationships with other people, ideas about child rearing, and attitudes about religion, abortion, equal rights, or euthanasia are all strongly influenced by the family. Although experiences outside of the family also have a strong influence, they are filtered through the perceptions acquired during early socialization.

The socialization process also influences the degree of independence experienced by growing children. Some families release their maturing members by degrees, preparing them gradually but steadily for adult roles. Other families promote dependent roles and find release painful and difficult.

Establishing Controls

The family functions to maintain social control. Families maintain order through establishment of social controls both within the family and between family members and outsiders. Members' conduct is controlled by the family's definition of acceptable and unacceptable behaviors. From minor etiquette rules, such as keeping elbows off the table, to larger issues, such as standards of home cleanliness, appropriate attire, children's behavior towards adults, or a teenager's curfew, the family imposes limits. It then maintains those limits by a system of rewards for conformity and punishments for violations. Children growing up in a family quickly learn what is "right" and what is "wrong" by family standards. Gradually family control shifts to self-control as members learn to discipline their own behaviors; later on, they will adopt or modify many of the same standards to use with their own children.

Division of labor is another aspect of the family's control function. Families allocate various roles, responsibilities, and tasks to their members in order to assure provision of income, household management, child care, and other essentials. Families also regulate the use of internal and external resources. The family identifies and directs the use of internal resources, such as member abilities, financial income, or material assets. For instance, if a man has artistic skills he may be chosen to landscape the yard; if a woman has more mechanical aptitude she may be designated to repair appliances. One family may choose to drive an old car rather than buy a new one in order to spend more on entertainment.

Families also determine the external resources used by their members. Some families take advantage of the religious, health, and social services available to them in the community. They seek regular medical care, encourage their children to use the public library, become involved in religious activities, or join a bowling league. Other families, either because they do not know about potential external resources available to them or because they do not recognize those resources as having any value, limit their members' use of them.

FAMILY LIFE CYCLE

Many of the characteristics and defined developmental stages of individual growth also apply to families. For example, it is known that families, while maintaining themselves as entities, change continuously. Families inevitably grow and develop as the individuals within them mature and adapt to the demands of successive life changes. A family's composition, set of roles, and network of interpersonal relationships change with the passage of time (Friedman, 1998). Family structures, too, vary with each stage of the family life cycle.

Consider the following example. The Jordans, a young married couple, concentrated on learning their respective roles of husband and wife and building a mutually satisfying marriage. With the birth of their first child, Scott, the family composition and relationships changed and role transitions occurred. The Jordans were not only husband and wife but also father, mother, and son; the family had added three new roles. Within the next 4 years, two daughters, Lisa and Tammy, were born. The introduction of each new member not only increased family size but also significantly reorganized family living. As Duvall and Miller (1985) point out, no two children are ever born into precisely the same family. The children entered school; Mrs. Jordan returned to work as a florist; and soon Scott was leaving for college. The Jordans, like every family, were moving through a predictable and sequential pattern of stages known as the *family life cycle*. Community health nurses can provide anticipatory guidance to families when they are knowledgeable about this cycle in families. For instance, while teaching prenatal care to a pregnant teen, the nurse helps the soon-to-be mother anticipate the responsibility and costs of raising her child by helping her calculate child care needs while she finishes school; the nurse suggests she figure out the monthly costs of breastfeeding versus buying formula, disposable diapers versus cloth or a diaper service, and the clothing, equipment, and medical costs of infant care. When working with the middle-aged parents of a brain-injured adult son living at home, the nurse discusses what arrangements the parents have made for their son's care when they are older and unable to give the care themselves, or when one or both of them die.

Stages of the Family Life Cycle

There are two broad stages in the family life cycle: one of *expansion* as new members are added and roles and relationships are increased, and one of *contraction* as family members leave to start lives of their own, or age and die. Within this framework of the expanding-contracting family are more specific phases, such as launching of children, retirement of parents, and so on. In some families the expanding and contracting is repeated as various members are added, return home with their children and perhaps a partner, or leave home permanently.

Family Developmental Tasks

To progress through the stages of the life cycle, a family must carry out its basic functions and the developmental tasks associated with those functions. Unlike individual developmental tasks, which are specific to each age level, family developmental tasks are ongoing throughout the life cycle. All families, for instance, must provide for the physical needs of their members at every stage. The manner and degree to which each function is carried out will vary, however, depending on how well members are meeting their individual developmental tasks and on the demands of each particular stage. Physical maintenance, for example, will be affected by parents' ability to accept responsibility and seek out the necessary resources to provide food, clothing, and shelter for their children. At early stages, children will usually be dependent on their parents for meeting these needs; at the school, teenage, and launching stages, however, children may increasingly contribute to home management and family income. The responsibility for these tasks shifts from parents to other family members as well.

Some functions require greater emphasis at certain stages. Socialization, for example, consumes much of a family's time during the early years of child development. These same functions and their associated developmental tasks can be further broken down into actions specific to certain stages. A family, for example, while carrying out its function of maintaining controls, sets clearly defined limits for children at the preschool stage: "Do not cross the street." "You may have dessert only after you finish your vegetables." "Bedtime is at eight." During the school stage, control activities may center on allocating responsibilities and division of labor within the family: "Feed the dog." "Clean your room." "Take out the trash." When a family reaches the teenage stage, its control function increasingly focuses on the relationships between family members and outsiders. The family may regulate some activities by setting limits such as, "Be home by midnight." In areas such as moral conduct, controls may involve family values and thus be more subtle. A family at this stage must recognize the need for young people to assume increasing responsibility for their own behavior with the complementary recognition of its own diminishing control over members. Duvall and Miller (1985) describe these activities as "stage-critical" family developmental tasks. Sample community health nursing actions with the family at different stages are included in Table 22–2.

EMERGING FAMILY PATTERNS

Up to this point, the discussion of the family life cycle has focused primarily on the nuclear family. Since the nurse encounters many nuclear families in community health, the family life cycle provides a useful means of analyzing their growth and development.

Because of recent societal changes, today's community health nurses are facing increasing numbers of adolescent unmarried mothers, gay and lesbian families, blended families, elderly couples, and individuals living alone. They need to know the impact these emerging family patterns have on society and available resources and equip themselves with an appropriate knowledge base to provide needed services.

Adolescent Unmarried Parents

Teen parenthood is an important social issue with distinct medical and nursing ramifications. Teens are still undergoing emotional development themselves. They have limited parenting skills and need a tremendous amount of education and support. Even with much media attention, availability of family planning methods, and a social environment open to discussing sexuality and pregnancy, teen pregnancy rates have remained high among all teens but especially among teens of color and in those living in lower socio-economic situations.

Infants born to teen mothers are at risk for low birth weight, developmental delay, and death by 1 year of age. The infant mortality rate among mothers under 15 years of age is twice as high as for women ages 20 to 24 and 20% higher among teens ages 15 to 19 than for women in their 20s (USDHHS, 2000). In addition, during childhood they face high rates of poverty, educational underachievement, and inadequate health care (Brown & Eisenberg, 1995).

Teen fathers are often left out of the bevy of services communities provide for the teen mother and infant. However, paternal involvement contributes positively to the physical, social, and cognitive development of children. Children with absent fathers are at increased risk for behavioral difficulties and poor academic performance. Being emotionally supportive of the mother and providing child care and financial support for the child affects the child directly and indirectly (Rhein, et al., 1997).

With these many high-risk factors for pregnant teens and their children, it is imperative that community health nurses be knowledgeable about needed services, available resources, and the accessibility of each. In addition, because of the high-risk nature of teen pregnancy, preventing pregnancy among teens should be a priority. Nurses must collaborate in caregiving with other professionals and key players in teens' lives to provide the supportive services such young families need.

Gay and Lesbian Families

An emerging family pattern is the gay or lesbian family. Whether the unions between two women or two men are legitimized in the eyes of the law (gay and lesbian marriages are legal in many states) or are based on strong emotional attachments, gay and lesbian adults are forming expanding families by including natural children from previous heterosexual relationships, creating new life through artificial insemination, or expanding through adoption.

This emerging family pattern is not as significant in numbers as the adolescent or blended family, but it is increasing,

TABLE 22–2. Selected Stage-Critical Family Developmental Tasks

Stage of Family Life Cycle	Family Position	Stage-Critical Family Developmental Tasks	Role of the Community Health Nurse
Forming a partnership	Female partner Male partner	Establishing a mutually satisfying relationship	Interact with family where they are at
Childbearing	Partner-mother Partner-father Infant child(ren)	Adjusting to pregnancy and the promise of parenthood	
		Fitting into the kin network	
		Having and adjusting to infants, and encouraging their development	Assist them in developing strong relationships
		Establishing a satisfying home for both parents and infant(s)	
Preschool-age	Partner-mother Partner-father Child, siblings	Adapting to the critical needs and interests of preschool children in stimulating, growth-promoting ways	Assist in preparing for family expansion through education and anticipatory guidance
		Coping with energy depletion and lack of privacy as parents	
School-age	Partner-mother Partner-father Child, siblings	Fitting into the community of school-age families in constructive ways	Encourage time for each other as adults in a relationship separate from parenting role
		Encouraging children's educational achievement	
Teenage	Partner-mother Partner-father Child, siblings	Balancing freedom with responsibility as teenagers mature and emancipate themselves	Provide anticipatory guidance for the school-age children as they grow into adulthood
		Establishing outside interests and careers as growing parents	
Launching center	Partner-mother-grandmother Partner-father-grandfather Child, sibling, aunt or uncle	Releasing young adults into work, military service, college, marriage, etc., with appropriate rituals and assistance	Provide anticipatory guidance for the contracting family as children leave home
		Maintaining a supportive home base	
Middle-aged parents	Partner-mother-grandmother Partner-father-grandfather	Rebuilding the relationship	Prepare adults for grandparenting role
		Maintaining kin ties with older and younger generations	
Aging family members	Widow or widower Partner-mother-grandmother Partner-father-grandfather	Adjusting to retirement	Assist aging adults with emotional and financial security as they approach retirement
		Coping with bereavement and living alone	
		Closing the family home or adapting it to aging	Prepare the aging adults with ways to cope with the losses of old age, including changes in space, work, health, status, and loss of friends and family members

and community health nurses may provide services to these clients in many communities. It is important to recognize that much progress has been made in accepting people with values and beliefs different from those of the mainstream. However, pervasive homophobia and heterosexism continues to exist in our society (Hartman & Laird, 1998). Nurses must confront their own biases and be able to set them aside in order to provide nonjudgmental and comprehensive care to these emerging families.

Gay and lesbian families have all the fears and concerns regarding parenting that any family a community health nurse may visit will have. In addition, they experience the stress that accompanies being stigmatized by much of society. The nurse can become a valued resource for the family and, through education and anticipatory guidance, assist the parents to come successfully through the growth and developmental stages of their children and any of the varied issues faced by families.

Divorced and Blended Families

Divorce and remarriage are more frequent occurrences today than in previous generations. Divorces have gone from fewer than 20% of all marriages in the 1960s to nearly 50% in the 1990s (Delaney, 1995). It is estimated that 40% of all children will experience living with divorced or single parents before they reach adulthood (Coleman et al., 1998).

TABLE 22–3. When Families Divorce

Phase	Emotional Responses	Transitional Issues
1. Stressor leading to marital differenced	Reveal the fact that the marriage has major problems	Accepting fact that marriage has major problems
2. Decision to divorce	Accepting the inability to resolve marital differences	Accepting one's own contribution to the failed marriage
3. Planning the dissolution of the family system	Negotiating viable arrangements for all members within the system	Cooperating on custody visitation, and financial issues
		Informing and dealing with extended family members and friends
4. Separation	Mourning loss of intact family Working on resolving attachment to spouse	Develop coparental arrangements/ relationships
		Restructure living arrangements
		Adapt to living apart
		Realign relationship with extended family and friends
		Begin to rebuild own social network
5. Divorce	Continue working on emotional recovery by overcoming hurt, anger or guilt	Giving up fantasies of reunion
		Staying connected with extended families
		Rebuild and strengthen own social network
6. Post-divorce	Separate feeling about ex-spouse from parenting role Prepare self for possibility of changes in custody as child(ren) get older, be open to their needs Risk developing a new intimate relationship	Make flexible and generous visitation arrangements for child(ren) and non-custodial parent and extended family members
		Deal with possibilities of changing custody arrangements as child(ren) get older
		Deal with child(ren)s reaction to parents establishing relationships with new partners

Adjusting to divorce involves a series of transitions and reorganizations for all family members. For children, it means coping with changing geographical locations, changing schools, and changing mental and physical health of family members, and adjusting to a single-parent household and possibly remarriage and the addition of new family members (Thompson, 1998). The children of divorce face the normal growth and developmental changes, in addition to (1) an absent father or mother, (2) interparental conflict, (3) economic distress, (4) parent adjustment, (5) multiple life stressors, and (6) short-term crisis.

Not all divorced adults stay single. Most remarry or cohabitate with another adult who may or may not have children. This new couple may have children from their union, creating an even more complex family. Merged or blended families require considerable adjustment and relearning of roles, tasks, communication patterns, and relationships (Friedman, 1998).

There are identifiable phases that occur in divorce, remarriage, and the blending of families; each phase has its own emotional transitions and developmental issues. Tables 22–3 and 22–4 show these phases.

Since this emerging family pattern has become so prominent in such a short period of time in history, it is very possible that the community health nurse is familiar with this pattern and may live in such a family himself or herself. Nursing skills needed when working with divorced or blended families includes listening and empathy, a nonjudgmental attitude, and being a rich resource for the family. Support groups for the adults and the children are excellent resources and provide invaluable services at a time of emotional instability in the family. Peer support groups for children and adolescents and support from within the schools should be utilized, if available, or started if they do not exist. The community health nurse can have a significant role in community-wide planning if there are services that are needed but unavailable.

Older Adults

Elderly couples or elderly individuals are the fastest growing segment of the population. It is estimated that this group will represent 20% of the population by 2030 (Miller, 1999). There are 76 million baby boomers heading toward maturity, and our society is already experiencing the beginning of this "age wave" (Dychtwald, 1997).

Most elders live independently well into their 80s and maintain healthy contacts with family and friends. Others feel isolated because of chronic health problems that limit mobility and an inability to interact or contribute meaningfully in society. Aging is a relatively new phenomenon, and many of these aging families do not understand or practice the appropriate stage-specific functions and developmental tasks that would help them adjust and experience positive aging (Miller, 1999).

The community health nurse needs to understand the complex dynamics of such situations and offer support and encour-

TABLE 22–4. **Remarriage and Blending Families**

Phases	Emotional Responses	Developmental Issues
1. Meeting new people	Allowing for the possibility of developing a new intimate relationship	Dealing with child(ren) and exfamily members reactions to a parent "dating"
2. Entering a new relationship	Completing an "emotional recovery" from past divorce Accepting one's fears about developing a new relationship Working on feeling good about what the future may bring	Recovery from loss of marriage is adequate Discovering what your want from a new relationship Working on openness in a new relationship
3. Planing a new marriage	Accepting one's fears about the ambiguity and complexity of entering a new relationship such as: New roles and responsibilities Boundaries; space, time, and authority Affective issues: guilt, loyalty, conflicts, unresolvable past hurts	Recommitment to marriage and forming a new family unit. Dealing with stepchild(ren) as custodial or non-custodial parent Planning for maintenance of coparental relationships with ex-spouses Planning to help child(ren) deal with fears, loyalty conflicts and memberships in two systems Realignment of relationships with exfamily to include new spouse and child(ren)
4. Remarriage and blending of families	Final resolution of attachment to previous spouse Acceptance of new family unit with different boundaries	Restructuring family boundaries to allow for new spouse or stepparent Realignment of relationships to allow inter-mingling of systems Expanding relationships to include all new family members Sharing family memories and histories to enrich members lives

agement as family members work through these problems. Often a nurse will serve an entire community of elders such as in a senior apartment complex, an assisted living center, or a community of older adults living in mobile homes where focusing on maintaining wellness is the focus. Keeping physically active, eating healthy meals regularly, receiving appropriate medical care and immunizations, and establishing and maintaining social contacts are some of the tasks elders should focus on to stay healthy well into old age. These are some of the areas in which the community health nurse can intervene through the roles of teacher, counselor, and clinician. Reaching age 100 is not an unusual occurrence today, and more people will live to see these advanced ages in the 21st century.

SUMMARY

The family as the unit of service has received increasing emphasis in nursing over the years. Today family nursing has an important place in nursing practice, particularly in community health nursing. Its significance results from recognition that the family itself must be a focus of service, that family health and individual health strongly influence each other, and that family health affects community health.

Community health nurses' effectiveness in working with families depends on their understanding of family theory and characteristics, in addition to the changing family structures of today.

Every family on the globe is unique; its needs and strengths are different from those of every other family. At the same time, each family is alike because of certain shared universal characteristics. Five of these universals have particular significance for community health nursing: every family is a small social system, has its own cultural values and rules, has structure, has certain basic functions, and moves through stages in its life cycle.

Every family is a small social system. All the members within a family are interdependent; what one does affects the others and, ultimately, influences total family health. Families, as social systems, set and maintain boundaries that unite them and preserve their autonomy while also differentiating them from others. Because these boundaries are semipermeable, families engage in an input–output energy exchange with external resources. Families are equilibrium-seeking and adaptive systems that strive to adjust to internal and external life changes. Also, like other systems, families are goal directed. They exist for the purpose of promoting their members' development.

Every family has its own culture, its own set of values and rules for operation. Family values influence member beliefs and behaviors. These same values prescribe the types of roles that each member assumes. A family's culture also determines its power distribution and decision- making patterns.

Every family has a structure that can be categorized as either traditional or nontraditional (contemporary). The most common traditional family structure is the nuclear family, consisting of husband, wife, and child(ren) living together. Other traditional structures include husband and wife living as a couple alone, single- parent families, single-adult families, multigenerational families, kin networks, and blended families. Nontraditional family structures incorporate many family forms, some accepted by society and others not easily accepted. These variations include commune families, group marriages, and group networks. Unmarried single-parent families, unmarried gay or straight couples living together with or without children, and umarried older adults living together are emerging nontraditional family structures that are becoming more common and thus becoming more recognized and accepted in some communities more than others. These variant family structures remind us that the nuclear family is now in the minority, that people experience many family structures during their lifetimes, and that a family's ability to perform its basic functions is influenced by its structure.

Every family has certain basic functions: (1) to provide its members affection and emotional support; (2) to promote security by providing an accepting, stable environment in which physical needs are maintained; (3) to provide its members a sense of social and personal identity and influence their placement in the social order; (4) to provide members with affiliation, a sense of belonging; (5) to socialize its members by teaching basic values and attitudes that determine their behavior; and (6) to establish social controls to maintain order. Community health nurses use this information to assess a family's functioning. This information enables the nurse to work with the family and assist them in improving the quality of their functioning.

Every family moves through stages in its life cycle. Families develop in two broad stages: a period of expansion when they add new members and roles, and a period of contraction when members leave. Some families demonstrate a spiraling pattern, with repeated expanding and contracting patterns.

There are emerging family patterns that influence the role of the community health nurse. The single adolescent parent needs the community health nurse's knowledge of family developmental theory, as do gay and lesbian families with natural or adopted children.

More complex interaction patterns and living arrangements are created by divorce, remarriage, and the blending of families and the unique relationships these arrangements create. Older adults are living longer and will soon make up 20% of the population. The multiple needs of elders from ages 65 years to over 100 are more varied than any population group. Community health nurses see many more families today in one of these four emerging family patterns. Therefore, understanding their different needs will help the nurse provide appropriate services.

ACTIVITIES TO PROMOTE CRITICAL THINKING

1. Within a small group of your peers, individually define *family* and then compare each of your definitions. How alike and how different is each definition? What in each person's background contributes to the differences in the definitions? Were each of the peers in nursing? If they weren't, how did that contribute to any differences in the definitions?

2. Analyze two families (other than your own) that you know well, one traditional and the other nontraditional (contemporary), and answer the following questions:
   a. If the major breadwinner in this family became permanently disabled and unable to work or lost his or her income, how would the family most likely respond—- immediately and in the long term?
   b. What are some of these family's rules for operating and the values underlying the rules?
   c. Structurally, what kind of family is each one?
   d. What are the strongest and weakest functions performed by these families, and why do you think this is so?
   e. In what developmental stage is each family, and how does it affect their functioning?

3. Talk with the members of a blended family and discuss with each member his or her relationships with step-children or siblings, half- siblings, and step-parents. What problems can they identify? What problems have they overcome? What do they see as the positive elements of the union?

4. Gay and lesbian couples often seek parenting opportunities. How do you feel about this? What makes you feel this way? What are the positive and negative aspects of a child being raised by a homosexual couple?

5. Use the Internet and find information at different websites on family structural patterns in other countries. Many families in developing and some industrialized countries live in clans, tribes, groups, and kin-networks. In what countries do you find such family structures? What are the benefits and drawbacks of such systems?

REFERENCES

Alpers, R.R. (1998). The importance of the health education program environment for pregnant and parenting teens. *Public Health Nursing, 15*(2), 91–103.

Barker, P. (1992). *Basic family therapy* (3rd ed.). New York: Oxford University Press.

Bell, J.M. & Wright, L.M. (1993). Flaws in family nursing education. In G. Wegner & R. Alexander (Eds.), *Readings in family nursing* (pp. 390– 394). Philadelphia: Lippincott.

Brown, S.S., & Eisenberg, L. (1995). *The best intentions: Unintended pregnancy and the well-being of children and families.* Washington, DC: National Academy Press.

Chira, S. (1994). Starting point: Meet needs of our young children. *Capitol Bulletin, 635.*

Coleman, M., Ganong, L.H., Killian, T.S., & McDaniel, A.K. (1998). Mom's house? Dad's house? Attitudes toward physical custody changes. *Families in Society: The Journal of Contemporary Human Services, 79*(2), 112–122.

Delaney, S.E. (1995). Divorce mediation and children's adjustment to parental divorce. *Pediatric Nursing, 21,* 434–437.

Department of Social Services (1999). *New foster care public health nurse program in county welfare department.* Sacramento, CA: Health and Human Services Agency.

Dreikurs, R. (1964). *Children: The challenge.* New York: Meredith.

Duvall, E.M., & Miller, B. (1985). *Marriage and family development* (6th ed.). New York: Harper & Row.

Dychtwald, K. (1997). The 10 physical, social, spiritual, economic and political crises the boomers will face as they age in the 21st century. *Critical Issues in Aging, 1,* 11–13.

Eliopoulos, C. (1997). *Gerontological nursing* (4th ed.). Philadelphia: Lippincott-Raven.

Fitch, M.I., Bunston, T., & Elliot, T. (1999). When mom's sick: Changes in a mother's role and in the family after her diagnosis of cancer. *Cancer Nursing, 22*(1), 58–63.

Fox, P.G., Cowell, J.M. & Johnson, M.M. (1995). Effects of family disruption on Southeast Asian refugee women. *International Nursing Review, 42*(1), 26–30.

Friedman, M.M. (1998). *Family nursing: Research, theory, and practice* (4th ed.). Stamford, CT: Appleton & Lange.

Gillis, L.M. & Singer, J. (1997). Breaking through the barriers: Healthcare for the homeless. *Journal of Nursing Administration, 27*(6), 30–34.

Grace, J.J. (1995). Families and nurses: Building partnerships for growth and health. *Journal of Obstetric, Gynecologic, and Neonatal Nursing, 24*(4), 298–300.

Hanson, S.M., & Boyd, S.T. (1996). *Family health care nursing: Theory, practice, and research.* Philadelphia: F.A. Davis.

Hartman, A. & Laird, J. (1998). Moral and ethical issues in working with lesbians and gay men. *Families in Society: The Journal of Contemporary Human Services, 79*(3), 263–276.

Harway, M., & Wexler, K. (1996). Setting the stage for understanding and treating the changing family. In M. Harway (Ed.), *Treating the changing family: Handling normative and unusual events.* New York: John Wiley & Sons.

Jendrick, M.P. (1994). Grandparents who parent their children: Circumstances and decisions. *The Gerontologist, 34*(2), 206–216.

Leininger, M. (Ed.) (1991). *Culture, care, diversity, and universality: A theory of nursing.* New York: NLN Press.

Marciano, T. (1991). A postscript on wider families: Traditional family assumptions and cautionary notes. *Marriage and Family Review, 17,* 159–163.

Miller, C.A. (1999). *Nursing care of older adults: Theory and practice* (3rd ed.). Philadelphia: Lippincott Williams & Wilkins.

Murray, R.B., & Zentner, J.P. (1997). *Health assessment and promotion strategies through the life span* (6th ed.). Stamford, CT: Appleton & Lange.

Neuman, B. (1995). *The Neuman systems model: Application to nursing education and practice* (3rd ed.). Stamford, CT: Appleton & Lange.

Northam, S. (1996). Access to health promotion, protection, and disease prevention among impoverished individuals. *Public Health Nursing, 13*(5), 353–364.

Olson, D., McCubbin, H.I., & Associates. (1983). *Families: What makes them work.* Beverly Hills, CA: Sage.

Pender, N.J.(1996). *Health promotion in nursing practice* (2nd ed.) Stamford, CT: Appleton & Lange.

Reilly, C.E. (1998). A satisfaction survey on distance education: A model for educating nurses in the cognitive treatment of patients with addictive disorders. *Journal of Psychosocial Nursing, 36*(7), 38–41.

Rhein, L.M., Ginsburg, K.R., Schwarz, D.F., et al. (1997). Teen father participation in child rearing: Family perspectives. *Journal of Adolescent Health, 21,* 244–252.

Riley, M.W., & Riley, J.W. (1996). Generational relations: A future perspective, In T.K. Hareven (Ed.), *Aging and intergenerational relations: Life course and cross-cultural perspectives.* Hawthorne, NY: Aldine de Gruyter.

Saluter, A.F. (1992). Marital status and living arrangements: March 1991. In *Current Population Reports, Population Characteristics.* Washington, DC: U.S. Bureau of the Census, series P-20, No.461.

Sandhaus, S. (1998). Migrant health: A harvest of poverty. *American Journal of Nursing, 98*(9), 52, 54.

Scanzoni, J., Polonko, K., Teachman, J., & Thompson, L. (1989). *The sexual bond: Rethinking family and close relationships.* Newbury Park, CA: Sage Publications.

Spector, R.W. (1996). *Cultural diversity in health and illness* (4th ed.). Stamford, CT: Appleton & Lange.

Stein, P.J. (Ed.). (1981). *Single life: Unmarried adults in social context.* New York: St. Martin's.

Thompson, P. (1998). Adolescents from families of divorce: Vulnerability to physiological and psychological disturbances. *Journal of Psychosocial Nursing, 36*(3), 34–39.

U.S. Department of Commerce. (1998). *Statistical abstract of the United States* (118th ed.). Washington, DC: U.S. Government Printing Office.

United States Department of Health and Human Services. (2000). *Healthy people 2010* (conference edition in two volumes) Washington, DC: U.S. Government Printing Office.

SELECTED READINGS

Acock, A.C., & Demo, D.H. (1994). *Family diversity and well-being.* Thousand Oaks, CA: Sage.

Ballard, N. (1996). Family structure, function, and process. In S.M.H. Hanson & Boyd, S.T. (Eds.), *Family health care nursing: Theory, practice, and research* (pp. 57–78). Philadelphia: F.A. Davis.

Berg, M.A. (1994). Health problems of sheltered homeless

women and their dependent children. *Health and Social Work,* *19*(2), 125–131.

Carnegie Council on Adolescent Development. (1996). *Great transitions: Preparing adolescents for a new century.* New York: Carnegie Corporation of New York.

Crosbie-Burnett, M., & Helmbrecht, L. (1993). A descriptive empirical study of gay male stepfamilies. *Family Relations, 42,* 256–262.

Elkind, D. (1995). The family in the postmodern world. *National Forum, 75*(3), 24–28.

Erikson, E. (1963). *Childhood and society* (2nd ed.). New York: Norton.

Forchuk, C. & Dorsay, J.P. (1995). Hildegard Peplau meets family system nursing: Innovation in theory-based practice. *Journal of Advanced Nursing, 21,* 110–115.

Ferguson, V.D. (1999). *Cuse studies in cultural diversity.* Sudbury, MA: NLN Press.

Gelles, R.J. (1995). *Contemporary families: A sociological view.* Thousand Oaks, CA: Sage.

Havighurst, R.J. (1972). *Developmental tasks and education* (3rd ed.). New York: McKay.

Jendrek, M.P. (1993). Grandparents who parent their grandchildren: Effects on lifestyle. *Journal of Marriage and the Family, 55,* 609–621.

Johnson, S.K., Craft, M., Titler, M., et al. (1995). Perceived changes in adult family members' roles and responsibilities

during critical illness. *Image: Journal of Nursing Scholarship, 27*(3), 238–243.

Klein, D.M., & White, J.M. (1996). *Family theories: An introduction.* Thousand Oaks, CA: Sage.

Loveland-Cherry, C. (1996). Family health promotion and health protection. In Bomar, P.J. (Ed.), *Nurses and family health promotion: Concepts, assessments, and interventions (2nd ed., pp. 22–35). Philadelphia: W.B. Saunders.*

Mathabane, G. (1992). Our biracial family. *American Baby, 54*(7), 58, 86, 88.

Niska, K., Snyder, M., & Lia-Hoagberg, B., (1998). Family ritual facilitates adaption to parenthood. *Public Health Nursing, 15*(5), 329–337.

Phillips, J.R. (1993). Changing family patterns and health. *Nursing Science Quarterly, 6*(3), 113–114.

Piaget, J. (1973). *The psychology of intelligence.* Totowa, NJ: Littlefield, Adams.

Pillemer, K., & Suitor, J.J. (1998). Baby boom families: Relations with aging parents. *Generations, 22*(1), 65–69.

Spradley, J.P. & McCurdy, D.W. (1989). *Anthropology: The cultural perspective* (2nd ed.). Chicago: Waveland Press.

Vaughan-Cole, B., Johnson, M.A., Malone, J.A., & Walker, B.L. (1998). *Family nursing practice.* Philadelphia: W.B. Saunders.

Yates, P. (1999). Family coping: issues and challenges for cancer nursing. *Cancer Nursing, 22*(1), 63–71.

Assessment of Families

LEARNING OBJECTIVES

Upon mastery of this chapter, you should be able to:

- Describe the effect of family health on individual health and community health.
- Describe individual and group characteristics of a healthy family.
- Identify five family health practice guidelines.
- Describe three conceptual frameworks that can be used to assess a family.
- Describe the 12 major assessment categories for families.
- List the five basic principles the community health nurse should follow when assessing family health.

In Chapter 22 we explored the theoretical basis of family formation and the variety of family structures. The next important step for you in the process of working with families as a unit of service is to develop your family assessment skills. This is foundational to the development of a data base on which to formulate nursing diagnoses, which leads to the planning, implementation, and evaluation of services.

Assessment is a challenging experience because families are complex and you are now in the family's environment, where they are "at home" and you may feel like the stranger. This is the reverse of how the family feels in the acute-care setting, where you may feel more at home.

Although community health nursing emphasizes the family as a unit of service, a gap exists between family nursing theory, development, and practice (Kristjanson & Chalmers, 1997). The problem derives in part from a health care system that fosters an individualistic orientation, often to the exclusion of the family. There is a proliferation of programs geared to individuals in specific age groups or with specific health problems. Many third-party payers and reimbursement policies impose limits on the kinds of services funded, most of which are for individuals. Even public health agencies tend to organize their services around individuals. Often in response to governmental requirements, they must keep statistical records on specific disease or service categories, thus reflecting an individual, rather than family or aggregate, orientation. Family-level problem-solving techniques are needed to deal with many important health issues, including health promotion, pregnancy and childbirth, acute life-threatening illness, chronic illness, substance abuse, and terminal illness (Cox & Davis, 1993; Harway & Wexler, 1996). Community health nurses need to focus their practice on families and aggregates, an approach that benefits both individual clients and the community at large.

EFFECTS OF FAMILY HEALTH ON INDIVIDUALS AND COMMUNITIES

The health of each family member affects the other members and contributes to the total family's level of health. Following her husband's stroke, for example, a woman may cope successfully with the resulting physical and emotional demands of his care but have inadequate reserves to effectively meet the needs of her children. The level at which a family functions—how well it is able to solve problems and help its members reach their potential—significantly affects the individual's level of health (Nelson & Edgil, 1998). A healthy family will foster individual growth and resistance to ill health and sustain its members during times of crisis such as serious illness, emotional dilemmas, divorce, or death of a family member. On the other hand, a family with limited capacity for problem-solving, self-management, or self-care is often unable to promote the potential of its members or assist them in times of need (Zerwekh, 1992; Reutter, 1997).

Family health standards and practices also influence each member's health. For instance, many individuals, even as adults, adhere to family patterns of eating, exercise, and communication. Family values influence decisions about health services, such as whether a child receives immunizations or uses preventive measures such as regular visits to the doctor or birth control. Family health patterns also dictate whether members participate in their own health care and follow through and comply with professional advice. It is clear that individuals influence family health and that the family can either obstruct or facilitate individual health. The family, then, becomes an important focus for community health nursing assessment and intervention.

Just as families influence individual health, they also influence the health of communities. Rarely do families live in isolation from one another. Even in the most uncommunicative of neighborhoods, one family's noisy children, another family's trash-littered yard, and another's barking dog all have an impact on the surrounding families. The level at which each family functions determines whether it can promote a healthier community and support other families and groups rather than merely remain a liability (Tapia, 1997).

Healthy families influence community health positively. Some families, for example, have become foster parents (Seaberg & Harrigan, 1997). Some have temporarily housed Southeast Asian or Cuban refugees and assisted them in finding employment. Others have formed community groups to encourage neighborhood safety and beautification. Many families are regularly involved in church, scouting programs, or various civic activities, such as parent-teacher-student associations, all of which work toward the common good.

Conversely, families with a low level of health have a negative influence on community health. Because they lack the resources to manage their own affairs, frequently they create problems and even health hazards for others. Garbage left to accumulate in a back yard, for example, attracts rats; loaded guns left unsecured may find their way into playmates' hands; abandoned appliances may become death traps for playing children; and children subjected to physical or emotional abuse may lash out at others. Regardless of socioeconomic level, a poorly functioning family becomes a drain on community resources and a threat to community health. Consider the large proportion of tax dollars and private funds that go into remedial programs for children with learning and behavioral difficulties caused by problems at home, for adults with mental health problems, for the chemically dependent, and for victims of family violence. Since family health affects the health of other families, groups, and communities, nurses who help families develop and maintain positive health patterns and practices are also promoting community health.

CHARACTERISTICS OF HEALTHY FAMILIES

How does the community health nurse determine family health status? Analysis of a family in terms of how it meets its basic functions does not give a satisfactory picture of its health status. More definitive criteria are needed. Although it is difficult to define a "normal" family, studies have given some standards to determine whether a family is healthy (Barker, 1992; Thompson, 1998). Over the years, research on families, and particularly on family health behavior, has produced a growing body of data with which to assess family health.

In looking at families over the years, researchers have found many similar characteristics. Otto (1973) found characteristics of family unity, loyalty and interfamily cooperation, support and security, role flexibility, and constructive relationships with community. Olson, McCubbin, and associates (1983) identified seven major family strengths important for family functioning and coping with crises: family pride, family support, cohesion, adaptability, communication, religious orientation, and social support. Becvar and Becvar (1996) found characteristics of (1) a legitimate source of authority that is supported and consistent over time, (2) a stable and consistent system of rules, (3) consistent and regular nurturing behaviors, (4) effective childrearing practices, (5) stable and well-maintained marriages, (6) a set of agreed-upon goals toward which the family and individual work, and (7) sufficient flexibility to change in the face of both expected and unexpected stressors. More recently, Parachin (1997) identified six signs of a healthy family: maintaining a spiritual foundation, making the family a top priority, asking—and giving—respect, communicating and listening, valuing service to others, and expecting—and offering—acceptance.

In this chapter we will explore the following six important characteristics of healthy families that consistently emerge in the literature (Olson, 1991; Friedman, 1998):

1. There is a facilitative process of interaction among family members.

2. They enhance individual member development.
3. Their role relationships are structured effectively.
4. They actively attempt to cope with problems.
5. They have a healthy home environment and lifestyle.
6. They establish regular links with the broader community.

Healthy Interaction Among Members

Healthy families communicate. Their patterns of interaction are regular, varied, and supportive. Adults communicate with adults, children with children, and adults with children. These interactions are frequent and assume many forms. Healthy families use frequent verbal communication. They discuss problems, confront each other when angry, share ideas and concerns, and write or call each other when separated. They also communicate frequently through nonverbal means, particularly those families from cultural or subcultural groups that are less verbal. There are innumerable ways—smiling encouragingly, embracing warmly, frowning disapprovingly, being available, withdrawing for privacy, doing an unsolicited favor, serving refreshments, giving a gift—to convey feelings and thoughts without words. The family that has learned to communicate effectively has members who are sensitive to one another. They watch for cues and verify messages in order to assure understanding. This kind of family recognizes and deals with conflicts as they arise. Its members have learned to share and to work collaboratively with each other.

Effective communication is necessary for a family to carry out its basic functions. To demonstrate affection and acceptance, to promote identity and affiliation, and to guide behavior through socialization and social controls, family members must communicate. Like the correlation between a high degree of communication and a high degree of effectiveness in organizational functioning, families' facilitative communication patterns promote the health and development of their members (Schwebel & Fine, 1994). Huntley and Konetsky (1992) found that healthy families were more likely than unhealthy families to negotiate topics for discussion, use humor, show respect for differences of opinion, and clarify the meaning of one another's communications.

Enhancement of Individual Development

Healthy families are responsive to their individual members' needs and provide the freedom and support necessary to promote each member's growth. If a father in a healthy family loses his job, his family will work to support his ego and help him use his energy constructively to adjust and find new work. The healthy family recognizes the growing child's need for independence and fosters it through increasing opportunities for the child to try new things alone. This kind of family can tolerate differences of opinion or lifestyle. It is able to accept each

member unconditionally and respect each one's right to be his or her own self. Within an appropriate framework of stability and structure, the healthy family encourages freedom and autonomy for its members (Friedman, 1998).

Patterns for promoting individual member development will vary from one family to another, depending on its cultural orientation. The way autonomy is expressed in an Italian-American family will differ from its expression in a Native American family, yet each family can promote freedom and autonomy. The result is an increase in competence, self-reliance, social skills, intellectual growth, and overall capacity for self-management among family members (Wright & Leahey, 1994).

Effective Structuring of Relationships

Healthy families structure their role relationships to meet changing family needs over time (Olson, 1991). In a stable social context, some families may establish member roles and tasks, such as breadwinner, primary decision maker, and homemaker, that are maintained as workable patterns throughout the life of the family. Families in rural areas, isolated communities, or religious and subcultural groups are more likely than others to retain role consistency because they face few, if any, external pressures or needs to change. The Amish communities in Pennsylvania and other Midwestern states have maintained marked differentiation in family roles for more than 100 years.

In a technologically advanced society such as the United States, however, most families must adapt their roles to be consistent with changing family needs created by external forces. As women enter the work force, for instance, family roles, relationships, and tasks must change to meet the demands of the new situation. Many husbands assume more homemaking responsibilities; fathers engage in childrearing; children, along with the adults in their families, share decision-making and a more equal distribution of power. The latter may be essential for the survival of a single-parent family in which the children must assume adult responsibilities while the parent is working to support the family (Kissman & Allen, 1993; Fuller, 1997).

Changing life cycle stages require alterations in the structuring of relationships. The healthy family recognizes its members' changing developmental needs and adapts parenting roles, family tasks, and controls to fit each stage (Huntley & Konetsky, 1992). For example, household chores of increasing complexity and responsibility are assigned as children become capable of handling them. Rules of conduct relax as members learn to govern their own behavior.

Active Coping Effort

Healthy families actively attempt to overcome life's problems and issues. When faced with change, they assume responsibility for coping and seek energetically and creatively to meet the demands of the situation (Olson et al., 1983; Glick, 1994).

Sometimes coping skills are needed for families to deal with emotional tragedies such as substance abuse problems, serious illness, or death. When it is known that a family member has a substance abuse problem, the family may seek counseling and treatment opportunities involving all family members. If a family member is seriously ill, the family may ask for and accept assistance from extended family members or community health care workers. In the event of a death in the family, receiving consolation and support from one another and from relatives and friends is an important step in the healing process. The healthy family recognizes the need for assistance, accepts help, and pursues opportunities to eliminate or decrease the stressors that affect them.

More frequently, healthy families cope with less dramatic, day-to-day changes. For instance, one family may cope with the increased cost of food by cutting down on meat consumption, substituting other protein foods, and eating less frequently at restaurants. Healthy families are open to their innovative members and support new ideas and ways to solve problems. One family may try to solve the problem of spending too much on transportation by cutting down on daily travel; this may cause additional problems if three members have jobs in different areas of town or need to go to school functions and meetings. Another family, responding to environmental concerns and a personal need for a healthier lifestyle, may explore and arrive at new ways to reach their destinations by walking, bicycling, skating, or car pooling to school or work. Healthy coping may go beyond finding a simple, obvious solution. Members may try to rearrange schedules to avoid frequency of trips to regular destinations and plan ahead to avoid last-minute trips to stores. Healthy families actively seek and use a variety of resources to solve problems. They may discover these resources within the family, or they may find them externally; they engage in self-care. For example, a professional couple faced with the unaffordable expense of daytime baby-sitting arranged their work schedules so that they could share child-care during the first 2 years and later joined a cooperative preschool that allowed their child to attend daily but required parental participation only 1 day a week. In another example, a single parent of five children who was also a full-time nursing student was able to finance two or three family outings each year by recycling aluminum cans that everyone in the family collected.

Healthy Environment and Lifestyle

Another sign of a healthy family is a healthy home environment and lifestyle. Healthy families create safe and hygienic living conditions for their members. For instance, a healthy family with young children will childproof their home by removing the potential hazards of exposed electric outlets and cleaning solvents from a child's reach. In families where there are older adults prone to falls, the family will install good lighting and sturdy handrails (Farren, 1999). A healthy home environment is one that is clean and reduces the spread of disease-causing organisms.

A healthy family lifestyle encourages appropriate balance in the lives of its members. In an ideal family, there is activity and rest sufficient for the energy needs of daily living; the diet offered is varied and nutritionally sound; physical activity maintains ideal weight while promoting cardiac health; preventive hygiene habits are taught and followed by family members; emotional and mental health is encouraged through a supportive network of caring others; and family members seek out and use health care services and demonstrate adherence with recommended regimens.

The emotional climate of a healthy family is positive and supportive of member growth. Contributing to this healthful emotional climate is a strong sense of shared values, often combined with a strong religious orientation (Olson et al., 1983; Parachin, 1997). A healthy family demonstrates caring, encourages and accepts expression of feelings, and respects divergent ideas. Members can express their individuality in the way they dress or decorate their rooms. The home environment makes family members feel welcome and accepted.

Regular Links With the Broader Community

Healthy families maintain dynamic ties with the broader community. They participate regularly in external groups and activities, often in a leadership capacity. We may see them join in local politics, participate in a church bazaar, or promote the school's paper drive to raise money for science equipment. They use external resources suited to their family's needs. For example, a farm family with teenagers, recognizing the importance of peer group influence on adolescents, becomes very active in the local 4-H club. Another family, in which the father is out of work, joins a job transition support group. Healthy families also know what is going on in the world around them. They show an interest in current events and attempt to understand significant social, economic, and political issues. This ever-broadening outreach gives families knowledge of external forces that might influence their lives. It exposes them to a wider range of alternatives and a variety of contacts, which increases their options for finding resources and strengthens their coping skills.

An unhealthy family has not recognized the value of establishing links with the broader community. This may be because of (1) a knowledge deficit regarding community resources, (2) previous negative experiences with the broader community services, or (3) a lack of connection with the community related to family expectations or cultural practices.

It is important for the community health nurse to assess the family for information regarding their relationship with the broader community in addition to structural and developmental family variations, family interaction, coping strategies, and lifestyle. With a comprehensive family assessment, the nurse has a base from which to begin a plan of care.

FAMILY HEALTH PRACTICE GUIDELINES

Family nursing is a kind of nursing practice in which the family is the unit of service (Friedman, 1998). It is not merely a family-oriented approach in which the family concerns affecting the health of an individual are taken into account. Family nursing asks how one provides health care to a collection of people. It does not mean that nursing must relinquish its service to individuals. On the contrary, one of the distinctive contributions of nursing as a profession is its holistic approach to individual needs. However, community health nurses rise to the challenge of adding a service to population groups that include families.

Five principles guide and enhance family nursing practice: (1) work with the family collectively, (2) start where the family is, (3) adapt nursing intervention to the family's stage of development, (4) recognize the validity of family structural variations, and (5) emphasize family strengths.

Work With the Family Collectively

To practice family nursing, nurses must set aside their usual focus on individuals and remind themselves that several people together have a collective personality, collective interests, and a collective set of needs. Viewing a group of people as one unit may seem less strange if you examine the way you often think about business organizations. For example, you may think of a particular corporation as conservative or liberal. You may hear that a women's group has taken a stand on abortion or that a government agency needs to become better organized. In each case, the group is viewed collectively, as a single entity with attributes and activities in common. So it is with families. A family has its own personality, interests, and needs.

As much as possible, community health nurses want to involve all the members during nurse–client interaction (Wright & Leahey, 1994; Wallace et al., 1999). This approach reinforces the importance of each individual member's contribution to total family functioning. Nurses want to encourage everyone's participation in the work that the nurse and the family jointly agree to do. Like a coach, the nurse wants to help them work together as a team for their collective benefit.

Consider how a nurse might work collectively with the Beck family (Display 23–1).

Start Where the Family Is

When working with families, community health nurses begin at their present, not their ideal, level of functioning. To discover where a family is, the community health nurse first conducts a family assessment to ascertain the members' needs and level of health and then determines collective interests, concerns, and priorities. The accompanying description of the Kegler family illustrates this principle (Display 23–2).

DISPLAY 23–1. The Beck Family

A community health nurse had an initial contact with Mr. and Mrs. Beck and their youngest child at the well-baby clinic. The 9-month-old child was over the 95th percentile for weight and at the 40th percentile for height. The nurse also noted that both parents were obese. The nurse asked about the eating patterns in the family and of the baby in particular and suggested a home visit to determine whether the Becks were interested in family nursing. The nurse explained the purpose of home visits (to assess all family members, coping patterns, eating patterns, and food purchasing choices) and the importance of including all family members and asked for a time that would be good for the family as a whole. The nurse explained that each person should be involved and committed to the agreed-upon goals; that, like a team of oarsmen, the family would have to pull together to accomplish the purpose of the visits. To help the Beck family improve its nutritional status, the nurse might suggest a session of brainstorming to uncover many causes of poor nutrition. More brainstorming might result in solutions and plans for action. On each visit the nurse would view the Becks as a group. Group responses and actions would be expected. Evaluation of outcomes would be based on what the family did collectively. The Becks were interested and a home visit date was made.

Adapt Nursing Intervention to the Family's Stage of Development

Although every family engages in the same basic functions, the tasks to accomplish these functions vary with each stage of the family's development. A young family, for instance, will appropriately meet its members' affiliation needs by establishing mutually satisfying relationships and meaningful communication patterns. As the family enters later stages, these bonds change with the release of some members into new families and the loss of others through death. Awareness of the family's developmental stage enables the nurse to assess the appropriateness of the family's level of functioning and to tailor intervention accordingly. Nurses are becoming adept at the assessment of families; however, it is the intervention that needs to be focused on (Robinson, 1994). A nurse's work with the Roberts family illustrates this need (Display 23–3).

Recognize the Validity of Family Structural Variations

Many families seen by community health nurses are nontraditional in structure, such as single-parent families and unmarried couples (Miller, 1992; Kissman & Allen, 1993).

DISPLAY 23–2. The Kegler Family

Marcia Kegler brought her baby, Tiffany, to the well-child clinic once but failed to keep further appointments. Concerned that the family might be having other difficulties, Sara Villa, a community health nurse, made a home visit. The mobile home was cluttered and dirty; the baby was crying in his playpen. Marcia seemed uninterested in the nurse's visit. She listened politely but had little to say. She repeated that everything was okay and that the baby was doing fine, explaining that he was just fussy because he was teething. As they talked, Marcia's husband Bob, a delivery van driver, stopped by to pick up a sports magazine to read on his lunch hour. The three of them discussed the problems of inflation and how expensive it was to raise a child. Sara reminded them that the clinic was free and that they could at least get good health care without extra cost. They agreed without enthusiasm. After Bob left, the nurse spent the remainder of the visit discussing infant care with Marcia, particularly emphasizing regular checkups and immunizations.

The next visit also focused on the baby, but Sara had an uncomfortable feeling that this family was not really interested in her help. After consulting her supervisor, the nurse did what she wished she had done in the first place. She asked to talk with Marcia and Bob together and explained frankly why she had come to their home and what she could offer in the way of counseling, teaching, support, and referral to other community resources. She then asked them what problems or concerns they had. The Keglers were more than responsive and described their financial difficulties and feelings of isolation from family and friends. They were new in the city, and both their families lived some distance away on farms. The neighbors were friendly but not close enough to confide in. They believed they would eventually overcome their problems if they just had "someone to lean on," as they put it.

Now Sara could address the Keglers' primary needs and concerns for friends and emotional support. The nurse began to address the Keglers' social needs first and introduced them to a young couples' group that met at the community center. Sara continued to make periodic home visits and shared additional information about community services that the Keglers might find helpful. She praised Marcia and Bob for following up on immunizations for Tiffany. Over time Sara saw differences in the family's interest in their relationship with the community and their connection to its services. Sara realized that before she could address the issue of Tiffany's health, she needed to address the emotional health of the parents.

DISPLAY 23–3. The Roberts Family

The Roberts, a couple in their early seventies, had recently moved to a retirement complex. They had received nursing visits following Mrs. Roberts' stroke 3 years previously but requested service now because Mr. Roberts was feeling "poorly" all the time. He thought that perhaps his diet and lack of activity might be the cause and hoped the nurse would have some helpful suggestions. The couple had eagerly awaited Mr. Roberts' retirement from teaching, planning to be lazy, travel, visit all their children, and do all those things they had never had time to do when they were young. Now neither of them seemed to have enough energy or the capacity to enjoy their new life. The move from their home of 28 years had been difficult; they were still trying to find space in the tiny apartment for their cherished books and mementos, although they had given many of them away.

Ronald Bell, a community health nurse, recognized that the Roberts were experiencing a situational crisis (leaving their home of 28 years), a developmental crisis (aging and entering retirement), and perhaps some underlying health problems. Many of the Roberts' expectations for this new life stage were unrealistic; they had not adequately prepared themselves for the adjustments that the loss of their home and retirement would demand. Through dscussion, Ronald was able to help the Roberts understand their situation and express their feelings. He completed physical assessments on the Roberts and encouraged regular follow-up with their health care provider. He also helped them join a support group of retired persons who were experiencing some of the same difficulties. Because this nurse was able to help the Roberts through their crisis in a supportive and nonjudgmental manner, he found them receptive later to discussing preparation for the inevitable loss and bereavement that would occur when one of them died. He was adapting his nursing intervention to this family's stage of development.

Other families are organized around nontraditional patterns; for example, both parents may have careers, a husband may care for children at home while his wife financially supports the family, or both parents may telecommute and work at home. These variant structures and organizational patterns have resulted from social and technological changes such as changes in employment practices, welfare programs, economic conditions, sex roles, status of women and minorities, birth control, incidence of divorce, even war. Such variations in family structure and organization lead to revised patterns of family functioning. Member roles and tasks often differ dramatically from our expectations, as in a family with a single parent who works full-time while raising children or a dual-career marriage in which both partners have undifferentiated roles. Community health nurses, many of whom are accustomed to traditional family patterns, must learn to understand and accept these variations in family structure and organization in order to address the needs of the families. (See Chapter 22 for more information on changing family structure.)

There are two important principles to remember. First, what is normal for one family is not necessarily normal for another. Each family is unique in its combination of structure, composition, roles, and behaviors. As long as a family carries out its functions effectively and demonstrates the characteristics of a healthy family, one must agree that its form, no matter how variant, is valid.

Second, families are constantly changing. Marriage transforms two people into a married couple without children. Adding children changes this family's structure. Divorce again alters structure and roles. Remarriage with the addition of children from another family changes the family again. Children grow up and leave the home while the parents, together or singly, are left to adjust to yet another family structure. Throughout the life cycle, a family seldom stays the same for very long. Each of these changes forces a family to adapt to its circumstances. Consider the young woman with a baby whose husband deserts her. She has no choice but to assume a single-parent role. Each change also creates varying degrees of stress and demands considerable adaptive energy on the family's part. Many family changes are predictable; they are part of normal life-cycle growth. Some are not. The nurse's responsibility is to help families cope with the changes while remaining nonjudgmental and accepting of the various forms encountered.

Homosexual unions may be difficult for some nurses to deal with, particularly if they conflict with the nurse's own set of religious or cultural ideas. Yet the nurse's responsibility remains the same—to help promote the collective health. Consider the nurse's work with James Cutler and Brian Hoag (Display 23–4).

Nurses should view all families as unique groups, each with its own set of needs, whose interests can best be served through unbiased care. The Global Community display discusses the effect of chronic pain in one family member on the family unit.

Emphasize Family Strengths

Too often, community health nurses tend to focus their attention on family weaknesses, looking for and referring to them as needs or problems. This negative emphasis can be devastating to a family and undermine any hopes of a truly therapeutic relationship between nurse and client. Instead, families need their strengths reinforced. Emphasizing a family's strengths makes people feel better about themselves. It fosters a positive self-image, promotes self-confidence, and often helps the family to address other problems.

DISPLAY 23–4. James Cutler and Brian Hoag

James Cutler and Brian Hoag have a 6-year monogamous relationship. A homosexual couple, they had been working with an attorney to privately adopt a child. The arrangements were completed and their 2-week-old son, Adrian, arrived in their home last week. Helen Jeffers, a community health nurse, receives a referral from a county hospital where Adrian was born. The request is for an assessment of the home situation and parenting skills. The baby tested positive for cocaine with Apgars of 6 and 8, with some initial difficulty sucking. Birth weight was 2900 gms. Discharge weight, at 3 days, was 2850 gm. At her first home visit, Helen finds a neat and orderly two-bedroom condominium, well-equipped with baby supplies. The infant had gained 200 gm and was being well cared for by two fatigued parents who have had limited contact with infants. James and Brian have many questions and are anxious learners. Helen plans with the couple to make weekly home visits to assess infant growth and development, provide support, and answer questions. She also suggests a neighborhood parenting class and finding a reliable babysitter, and she helps James and Brian develop an infant care work schedule. After 6 weeks of intervention, Adrian is thriving; Helen closes the case to home visits, feeling confident that the parents' goal of becoming knowledgeable and confident has been achieved.

One helpful communication technique is **strengthening.** Verbally or in writing, the nurse lists positive points about an otherwise negative situation. Examples include: the baby is kept warmly dressed (the clothing might be filthy, but the baby is warm); the 2-year-old is taking a nap (albeit on the dirty floor); the 5-year-old got to school three times last week (up from an average of two times a week in the previous month); or the mother is awake with a robe on at 1 PM (not asleep as on other home visits made in the early afternoon). Each represents a positive change. If there is nothing positive the nurse can honestly say, he or she may be able to say that the family seems to be managing as best they can. This strengthening technique helps the nurse approach clients positively rather than with a condescending or punitive approach. This is not to say that nurses should ignore problems. On the contrary, their assessment should explore all aspects of family functioning to determine both strengths and weaknesses. The nurse needs a total picture to achieve an adequate perspective in nursing care planning and to know when the family is ready and chooses to begin work on problems. Yet even as the nurse becomes more aware of a family's unhealthy behaviors, the emphasis should remain on the positive ones. Emphasizing strengths proves to the clients, in effect, that they are important to the nurse.

Family strengths are traits that facilitate the ability of the family to meet the members' needs and the demands made

THE GLOBAL COMMUNITY

Snelling, J. (1994). The effect of chronic pain on the family unit. *Journal of Advanced Nursing, 19,* 543–551.

A study conducted in England sought to explore the effect of chronic pain on the family unit. The researcher found that chronic pain caused social isolation, role tension, and marital conflict and reduced sexual activity among marital partners. Feelings of anger, anxiety, resentment, and despondency occurred in other family members. Additionally, it was found that the extent to which chronic pain negatively affected the partner and family members depended somewhat on how effective the family was in coping with a relative with chronic pain.

There are implications for community health nursing practice. Nurses seeing families in their homes or in outpatient settings are in a key position to enhance change. They are able to use and develop their knowledge of family dynamics to support and assist the family as it addresses unhealthy responses to the family member's pain. Helping the family members to share their knowledge and feelings may lead to more emotional stability and also to more realistic expectations of one another's behavior. Families need to be assessed for maladaptive coping techniques and taught effective coping techniques, such as seeking information, seeking support from others, humor, laughter, and finding meaning in the experience.

upon it by systems outside the family unit. Not all traits that appear positive are necessarily strengths, however. Before the nurse selects a trait to emphasize, it should be examined closely to determine whether that behavior is actually facilitating family functioning. A strong work orientation may be a strength when balanced with play and relaxation, but a family obsessed by work is experiencing this trait as a weakness. The differentiating factor between whether a trait is a strength or a weakness is the amount of free choice, as opposed to compulsive drive, being exercised.

Some traits a nurse may consider possible strengths are basic family functions, family developmental tasks, and characteristics of family health. For instance, a nurse might wish to commend a family that meets its members' physical, emotional, and spiritual needs; shows respect for various members' points of view; or fosters self-discipline in its children. A vivid illustration of this principle is found in the family nursing care of the Stevensons (Display 23–5).

FAMILY HEALTH ASSESSMENT

To assess a family's level of health in a systematic fashion requires three tools: (1) a conceptual framework upon which to base the assessment, (2) a clearly defined set of assessment

categories for data collection, and (3) a method for measuring a family's level of functioning.

Conceptual Frameworks

A **conceptual framework** is a set of concepts integrated into a meaningful explanation that helps one interpret human behavior or situations. Several conceptual frameworks have been used historically to study families (Hill & Hansen, 1960; Kantor & Lehr, 1975; Reiss, 1981). More recently,

DISPLAY 23–5. The Stevenson Family

The community health nurse, Keith Dow, made an initial home visit after referral by an outpatient physician who was concerned about possible child abuse. Alice Stevenson had brought her baby to the emergency room for treatment of a laceration on the baby's forehead. He had fallen off the table while she was changing him, she claimed. A bruise on his arm made the physician suspicious, but Alice explained it was caused by his older brother's rough play. The nurse opened the visit by stating that he was simply following up on the emergency room treatment and wanted to see how the baby was progressing. Keith made no mention of child abuse. He observed the mother and children closely, looking for small things to compliment Alice on (strengthening) while learning all he could about the family's background. Because the nurse appeared approving rather than suspicious or judgmental, Alice agreed to further visits. During a later visit, Alice admitted to the nurse that she had slapped the baby and her ring cut his forehead. She could not get him to stop crying, no matter what she did; she just could not endure it any longer, she said. There had been other times when she grabbed him roughly to pull him away from things he wasn't allowed to touch, causing bruises on his arms. Alice told the nurse that she had not planned this baby; when her husband found out she was pregnant, he had left her shortly before the baby was born. Like many abusive parents, Alice had unrealistic expectations of her children's behavior as well as very inadequate self-esteem (Ryan, 1997; Taylor & Kemper, 1998). Realizing that Alice would be particularly vulnerable to any criticism, the nurse concentrated on her strengths. Keith complimented her on how well she managed her home and dressed the children, on maintaining her job, and on reading to her 3-year-old son. It took many visits before Alice trusted the nurse, but in time they were able to discuss her feelings frankly and work toward improving this family's health. Keith got her to attend a support group for single parents and she began counseling. Emphasizing strengths had provided a bridge for Alice and assisted in bringing her into a helping relationship.

Beavers and Hampton (1990) and Olson (1991) have designed models to describe family functioning. Three, in particular, are mentioned here, as they are particularly useful in community health nursing: interactional, structural-functional, and developmental.

The **interactional framework** describes the family as a unit of interacting personalities and emphasizes communication, roles, conflict, coping patterns, and decision-making processes. This framework focuses on internal relationships but neglects the family's interaction with the external environment.

The **structural-functional framework** describes the family as a social system relating to other social systems in the external environment, such as church, school, work, and health care system. This framework examines the interacting functions of society and the family, looks at family structures, and analyzes how a family's structure affects its functioning.

The **developmental framework** studies families from a life-cycle perspective by examining members' changing roles and tasks in each progressive life-cycle stage. This framework incorporates elements from interactional and structural-functional approaches so that family structure, function, and interaction are viewed in the context of the environment through each stage of family development.

Others have combined these concepts in various ways to design family assessment and intervention models focusing on human-environmental interactions, interactional and structural-functional frameworks, self-care, responses to stressors, and a developmental framework.

The six characteristics of healthy families already discussed serve as an initial framework for assessing family health using a combination of interactional, structural-functional, and developmental concepts.

Data Collection Categories

Within a conceptual framework for assessing family health, the community health nurse selects specific categories for data collection. The amount of data that one can collect about any given family may be voluminous, perhaps more than necessary for the purposes of the assessment. Certain basic information is needed, however, to determine a family's health status and design appropriate nursing interventions. From many sources in the family health literature, particularly from Turk and Kerns (1985), Edelman and Mandle (1986), and Friedman (1998), a list of twelve data collection categories has been generated. Table 23–1 lists the 12 categories grouped into three data sets: (1) family strengths and self-care capabilities, (2) family stresses and problems, and (3) family resources. The 12 assessment categories are explained below.

1. Family demographics refers to such things as a family's composition, its socioeconomic status, and the ages, education, occupation, ethnicity, and religious affiliations of its members.
2. Physical environment data describe geography, climate, housing, space, social and political structures, food availability and dietary patterns, and any other elements in the internal or external physical environment that influence a family's health status.
3. Psychological and spiritual environment refers to information such as affectional relationships, mutual respect, support, promotion of members' self-esteem and spiritual development, and family members' life satisfaction and goals.
4. Family structure and roles include family organization, socialization processes, division of labor, and allocation and use of authority and power.
5. Family functions refer to a family's ability to carry out appropriate developmental tasks and provide for its members' needs.
6. Family values and beliefs influence all aspects of family life. Values and beliefs might deal with raising children, making and spending money, education, religion, work, health, and community involvement.
7. Family communication patterns include the frequency and quality of communication within a family and between the family and its environment.
8. Family decision-making patterns refer to how decisions are made in a family, by whom they are made, and how they are implemented.
9. Family problem-solving patterns describe how a family handles its problems, who deals with them, the flexibility of a family's approach to problem solving, and the nature of its solutions.
10. Family coping patterns encompass how a family handles conflict and life changes, the nature and quality of family support systems, and family perceptions and responses to stressors.
11. Family health behavior refers to familial health history, current physical health status of family members, family use of health resources, and family health beliefs.
12. Family social and cultural patterns comprise family discipline and limit-setting practices; promotion of members' initiative, creativity, and leadership; family goal setting; family culture; cultural adaptations to present circumstances; and development of meaningful relationships within and without the family.

Assessment Methods

Many different methods are used to assess families. These methods serve to generate information about selected aspects of family structure and function; thus the methods must match the purpose for assessment.

Three well-known graphic assessment tools are the eco-

TABLE 23–1. Categories of Data Collection for Family Health Assessment

Assessment Categories	Family Strengths and Self-Care Abilities	Family Stresses and Problems	Family Resources
1. Family demographics			
2. Physical environment			
3. Psychological and spiritual environment			
4. Family structure/roles			
5. Family functions			
6. Family values and beliefs			
7. Family communication patterns			
8. Family decision-making patterns			
9. Family problem-solving patterns			
10. Family coping patterns			
11. Family health behavior			
12. Family social and cultural patterns			

map, the genogram, and the social support network map or grid (Tracy & Whittaker, 1990; Meyer, 1993). The **eco-map** is a diagram of the connections between a family and the other systems in its ecological environment, originally devised to depict the complexity of the client's story. Developed by Ann Hartman in 1975 to help child welfare workers study family needs, the tool visually depicts the dynamic family–environment interactions. The nurse involves family members in the map's development. A central circle is drawn, representing the family; smaller circles on the periphery represent people and systems, such as school or work, whose relationships with the family are significant (Fig. 23–1). The map is used to discuss and analyze these relationships (Hartman, 1978; Meyer, 1993).

The **genogram** displays family information graphically in a way that provides a quick view of complex family patterns

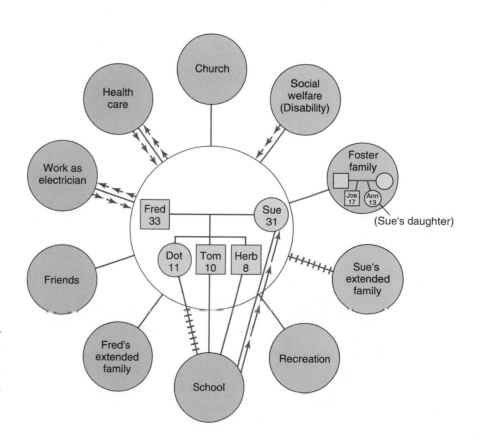

FIGURE 23–1. Ecomap of family's relationship to its environment. Lines indicate types of connections: *solid line,* strong; *dotted line,* tenuous; *lines with crossbars,* stressful. *Arrows* signify energy or resource flow, and absence of lines indicates no connection.

and a rich source of hypotheses about a family over a significant period of time, usually three or more generations (McGoldrick & Gerson, 1985). It diagrams family relationships by listing the family genealogy accompanied by significant life events (birth, death, marriage, divorce, illness), identifying characteristics (race, religion, social class), occupations, and places of family residence (Meyer, 1993). Again, this tool is used jointly with the family. It encourages family expression and sheds light on family behavior and problems (Fig. 23–2).

A **social network support map** or grid gives a detailed response regarding the quality and quantity of social connections. Strengths within the system can be elaborated with words, checks, and/or numbers (Tracy & Whittaker, 1990). The nurse uses this tool to help the family understand its sources of support and relationships and to form a basis for nursing care planning and intervention. Figures 23–3 and 23–4 show samples of a social network support map and grid.

Tapia (1997) depicted her concept of levels of family functioning through her model for family nursing. This model is based upon a continuum of five levels of family functioning:

- infancy (Level I—a very chaotic family)
- childhood (Level II—an intermediate family)
- adolescence (Level III—the normal family with many conflicts and problems)
- adult (Level IV—the family with solutions to its problems)
- maturity (Level V—the ideal independent family)

Tapia gives specific behaviors of families at each level, the family's expectation from the nurse, and, most importantly, the nurse's specific skill needed at each level of family functioning to best meet the family needs and help them reach a higher level of functioning. This visualization of family strengths, weaknesses, and expectations of the nurse and associated skills (Fig. 23–5) is a helpful tool for the novice nurse to assess levels of family functioning when working with a variety of families in the community.

Community health nurses also use several different family assessment instruments to gather data on family structure, functions, development, or combinations of all three. Public health nursing agencies generally develop their own tools, often in the form of questionnaires, checklists, flow sheets,

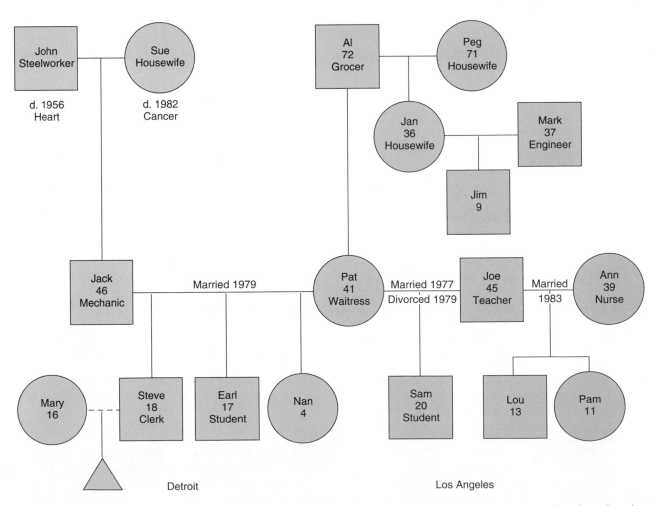

FIGURE 23–2. A genogram depicting three generations of family history. *Square,* male; *circle,* female; *triangle,* infant; *solid line,* married; *broken line,* not married.

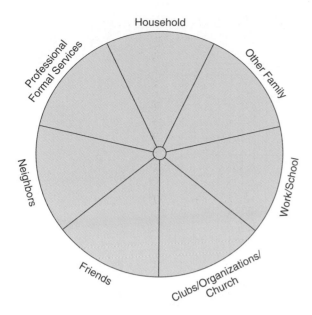

FIGURE 23–3. Social network support map.

or interview guides. The format varies to fit organizational needs. For example, most agencies have changed to computerized information management systems and adjusted data collection to be technologically compatible. Two sample assessment tools are shown in Figures 23–6 and 23–7.

Other methods, such as videotaping family interaction, structured observation, or analysis of life-changing events, use a variety of methods or tools. Examples include the Holmes-Rahe scale (Holmes & Rahe, 1967), which is a classic tool to measure a person's degree of stress, and the Self-Care Assessment Guide (Cleveland & Allender, 1999), which measures a family member's ability to provide self-care (Fig. 23–8). In a public health nursing agency or other community-based agencies, documentation is completed on individuals after family assessment information data are gathered. These tools provide useful information about stressors and self-care practices, including prescription medicines, over-the-counter (OTC) medicines, herbal remedies, nutritional supplements, and other complementary therapies. Such tools are useful adjuncts and are often used in combination to enhance breadth of data collection and understanding of the family.

GUIDELINES FOR FAMILY HEALTH ASSESSMENT

An assessment of family health will be most accurate if it incorporates the following five guidelines:

1. Focus on the family as a total unit.
2. Ask goal-directed questions.
3. Collect data over time.
4. Combine quantitative and qualitative data.
5. Exercise professional judgment.

Focus on the Family, Not the Member

Family health is more than the sum of its individual members' health. If the health of each person in a family was rated and those scores combined, it would not show how healthy that family is. To assess a family's health, the nurse must consider the family as a single entity and appraise its aggregate behavior (Wright & Leahey, 1994; CDC, 1998). As each criterion in the assessment process is considered, the community health nurse asks, "Is this typical of the family as a whole?" Assume that the nurse is assessing the communication patterns of a family. The nurse observes supportive interaction between two members in the family. What about the others? Further observation shows good communication among all but one member. It may be decided that, in spite of that one person, the family as a whole has good communication. When individual member behavior deviates from the aggregate picture, the nurse will want to note these differences. They can influence total family functioning and will need to be considered in nursing care planning.

Ask Goal-Directed Questions

The activities of any investigator, if fruitful, are guided by goal-directed questions. When solving a crime, a detective has many specific questions in mind. So, too, does the physician attempting a diagnosis, the teacher trying to discern a student's knowledge level, or the mechanic repairing a car. Similarly, the nurse determining a family's level of health has specific questions in mind. It is not enough to make family visits and merely ask members how they are. If relevant data are to be gathered, relevant questions must be asked. Figure 23–6 provides a sample set of questions that community health nurses may use to assess a family's health. Built upon the framework of the characteristics of a healthy family, these questions guide thinking and observations. They direct attention to specific aspects of family behavior to facilitate the goal of discovering a family's level of health. Consider the characteristic "Active Coping Effort." When visiting a family, the community health nurse watches for signs of their response to change and their problem-solving ability. The nurse asks, "Does this family recognize when it needs to make a change?" or "How does it respond when a change is imposed?" Perhaps a health problem has arisen, for instance, the baby has diarrhea. Does the family assume responsibility for dealing with the problem? Do family members consider a variety of ways to solve it? How do they respond to the nurse's suggestions? Do they seek out resources on their own, such as reading about causes of infant diarrhea, using home remedies, or consulting with the community health nurse, their doctor, or a nurse practitioner? How well do they use resources, once identified? Do they take a problem, try creative methods for solving it, and

	Area of Life 1. Household 2. Other family 3. Work/school 4. Organizations 5. Friends 6. Neighbors 7. Professionals 8. Other	Concrete support 1. Hardly ever 2. Sometimes 3. Almost always	Emotional support 1. Hardly ever 2. Sometimes 3. Almost always	Information/ advice 1. Hardly ever 2. Sometimes 3. Almost always	Critical 1. Hardly ever 2. Sometimes 3. Almost always	Direction of help 1. Goes both ways 2. You to them 3. They to you	Closeness 1. Not very close 2. Sort of close 3. Very close	How often seen 0. Does not see 1. Few times/yr. 2. Monthly 3. Weekly 4. Daily	How long known 1. Less than 1yr. 2. 1–5 yrs. 3. More than 5 yrs.
ID _____ Respondent _____									
Name #									
01									
02									
03									
04									
05									
06									
07									
08									
09									
10									
11									
12									
13									
14									
15									
1-6	7	8	9	10	11	12	13	14	15

Social Support Network Grid. SOURCE: Tracy and Whittaker 1990.

FIGURE 23–4. Social support network grid.

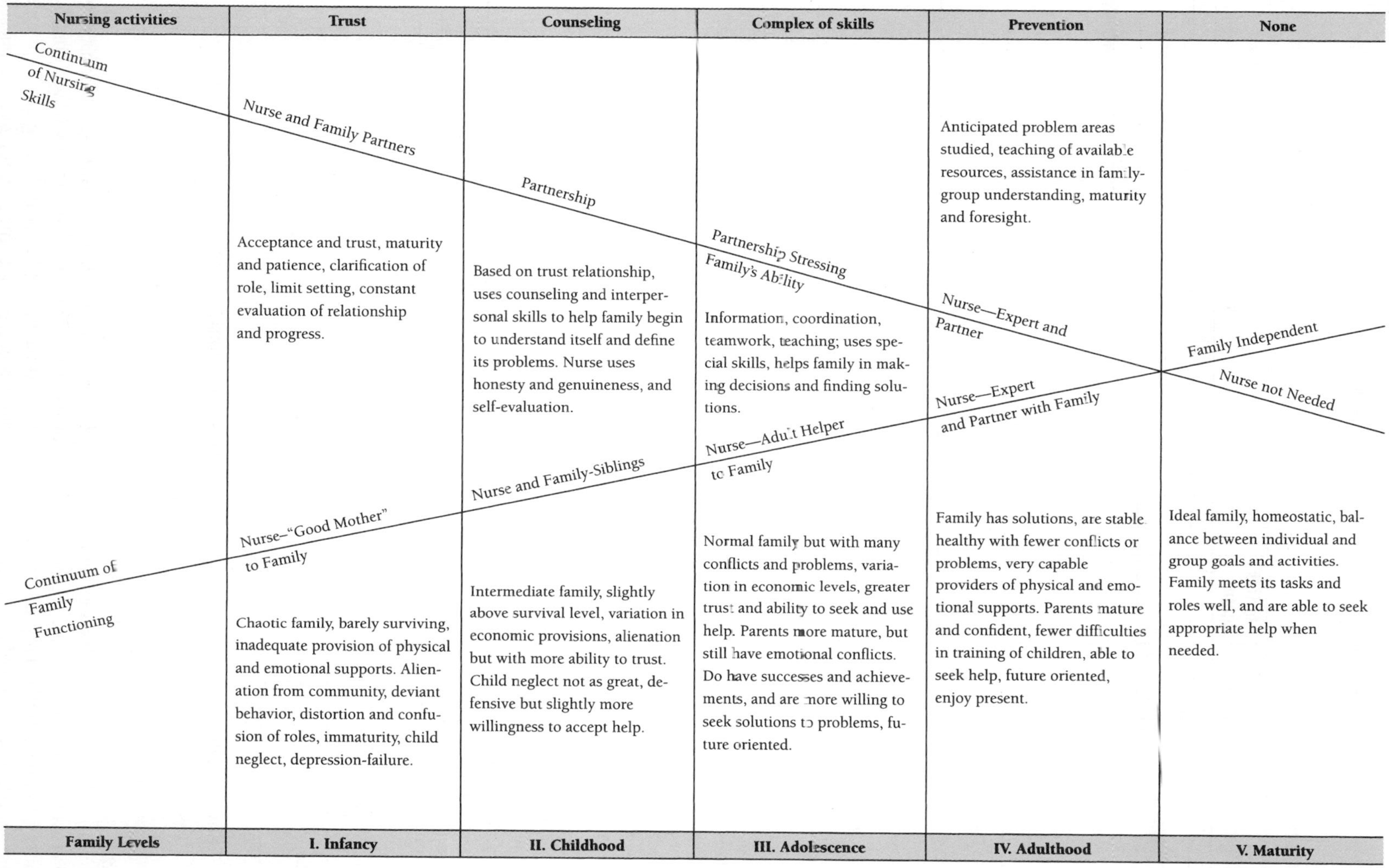

FIGURE 23-5. Model of family nursing.

Nursing activities	Trust	Counseling	Complex of skills	Prevention	None
Continuum of Nursing Skills	Nurse and Family Partners — Partnership — Partnership Stressing Family's Ability — Nurse—Expert and Partner			Nurse—Expert and Partner / Nurse—Expert and Partner with Family	Family Independent / Nurse not Needed
	Nurse—"Good Mother" to Family	Nurse and Family-Siblings	Nurse—Adult Helper to Family		
	Acceptance and trust, maturity and patience, clarification of role, limit setting, constant evaluation of relationship and progress.	Based on trust relationship, uses counseling and interpersonal skills to help family begin to understand itself and define its problems. Nurse uses honesty and genuineness, and self-evaluation.	Information, coordination, teamwork, teaching; uses special skills, helps family in making decisions and finding solutions.	Anticipated problem areas studied, teaching of available resources, assistance in family-group understanding, maturity and foresight.	Ideal family, homeostatic, balance between individual and group goals and activities. Family meets its tasks and roles well, and are able to seek appropriate help when needed.
Continuum of Family Functioning	Chaotic family, barely surviving, inadequate provision of physical and emotional supports. Alienation from community, deviant behavior, distortion and confusion of roles, immaturity, child neglect, depression-failure.	Intermediate family, slightly above survival level, variation in economic provisions, alienation but with more ability to trust. Child neglect not as great, defensive but slightly more willingness to accept help.	Normal family but with many conflicts and problems, variation in economic levels, greater trust and ability to seek and use help. Parents more mature, but still have emotional conflicts. Do have successes and achievements, and are more willing to seek solutions to problems, future oriented.	Family has solutions, are stable healthy with fewer conflicts or problems, very capable providers of physical and emotional supports. Parents mature and confident, fewer difficulties in training of children, able to seek help, future oriented, enjoy present.	
Family Levels	**I. Infancy**	**II. Childhood**	**III. Adolescence**	**IV. Adulthood**	**V. Maturity**

Family Assessment

Family Name _____

Family Constellation

Member	Birth Date	Sex	Marital Status	Education	Occupation	Community Involvement

Financial Status _____

Using the following scale, score the family based on your professional observations and judgement:

0 = Never   3 = Frequently
1 = Seldom   4 = Most of the time
2 = Occasionally N = Not observed

	score	date	score	date	score	date	score	date

Facilitative Interaction among Members

a. Is there frequent communication among all members?
b. Do conflicts get resolved?
c. Are relationships supportive?
d. Are love and caring shown among members?
e. Do members work collaboratively?

Comments _____

_____

Totals

Enhancement of Individual Development

a. Does family respond appropriately to members' developmental needs?
b. Does it tolerate disagreement?
c. Does it accept members as they are?
d. Does it promote member autonomy?

Comments _____

_____

Totals

FIGURE 23–6. Family assessment using questions based on characteristics of healthy families.

see it through to resolution? As the nurse focuses on these behaviors, he or she is asking goal-directed questions aimed at finding out the family's coping skills. This investigation will be one part of the nurse's assessment of the family's total health picture.

The set of questions presented in Figure 23–6 is one use-

ful way to appraise family health. Another more open-ended format is used by some community health nursing agencies. This approach, displayed in Figure 23–7, proposes assessment categories as a stimulus for nursing questions. When exploring family support systems, for example, the nurse asks, "What internal resources or strengths does this family

	score	date	score	date	score	date	score	date
Effective Structuring of Relationships a. Is decision making allocated to appropriate members? b. Do member roles meet family needs? c. Is there flexible distribution of tasks? d. Are controls appropriate for family stage of development?								
Comments _____ _____ Totals								
Active Coping Effort a. Is family aware when there is a need for change? b. Is it receptive to new ideas? c. Does it actively seek resources? d. Does it make good use of resources? e. Does it creatively solve problems?								
Comments _____ _____ Totals								
Healthy Environment and Life-style a. Is family life-style health promoting? b. Are living conditions safe and hygienic? c. Is emotional climate conductive to good health? d. Do members practice good health measures?								
Comments _____ _____ Totals								
Regular Links with Broader Community a. Is family involved regularly in the community? b. Does it select and use external resources? c. Is it aware of external affairs? d. Does it attempt to understand external issues?								
Comments _____ _____ Totals								

FIGURE 23–6. *(continued)*

have?" "Who, outside of the family, can they and do they turn to for help?" "What agencies, such as churches, clubs, or community services, do they use?" The open-ended style of this assessment tool allows a variety of questions to be raised aimed at determining family health.

Allow Adequate Time for Data Collection

Accurate family assessment takes time. An appraisal done on the first or second visit will most likely give only a partial picture of how a family is functioning. Time is needed to accumulate observations, make notes, and see all the family members interacting together in order to make a thorough assessment. To appraise family communication patterns, for instance, the nurse will want to observe the family as a group, perhaps at mealtime or during some family activity. They will need to feel comfortable in the nurse's presence in order to respond freely; it takes time and patience for such rapport to develop.

Consider one nurse's experience. Joe Burns had talked with the Olson family twice, first in the clinic and then at

---

FAMILY ASSESSMENT

Family Name

Family Constellation

Member names   Occupation   Educational background

Significant change in family life

Coping ability of family

Energy level

Decision-making process within the family

Parenting skills

Support systems of the family

Use of health care (include plans for emergencies)

Financial status

Other impressions

Signature of Nurse   Date

FIGURE 23–7. Open-ended family assessment.

home. Since Mr. Olson had not been present either time, Joe asked to see the family together and arranged an early evening visit. The Olsons were receiving nursing service for health promotion. They were particularly interested in discussing discipline of their young children and contracted with Joe for six weekly visits to be held in the late afternoon when Mr. Olson was home from work. Joe's assessment began on his first contact with the Olsons. He made notes on their chart and, guided by questions similar to those in Figure 23–6, kept a brief log. After the fourth visit, he filled out an assessment form to keep as a part of the family record. It was not until then that Joe felt he had collected enough data to make valid judgments about this family's level of health.

Combine Quantitative With Qualitative Data

Any appraisal of family health must be qualitative. That is, the nurse must determine the presence or absence of essential characteristics in order to have a data base for planning nursing action. To guide planning more specifically, the nurse can also determine degrees of the presence or absence of these signs of health. This is a quantitative measure. The nurse is not just asking whether a family does or does not engage in some behaviors, but how often. Is this behavior fairly

typical of the family, or does it occur infrequently? Figures 23–6 and 23–8 demonstrate ways to measure family health quantitatively. If the nurse were to use the tool in Figure 23–6 to assess the Beck family's ability to enhance individuality, for example, he or she could score their behavior on a scale from 0 to 4, 0 meaning never and 4 meaning most of the time. After several observations, the nurse would probably conclude that they responded appropriately to the members' developmental needs (*a* under "Enhancement of Individual Development") most of the time. Opposite *a* on the assessment form, the nurse would write the numeral 4 and the date of assessment.

The value of developing a quantitative measure is to have some basis for comparison. The nurse can assess a family's progression or regression by comparing its present score with its previous scores. Had the nurse conducted a family health assessment 6 months ago on the Keglers, for instance, and compared it with their present level of health, he or she would probably have discovered a drop in their scores in several areas. Many of their communication patterns, role relationships, and coping skills, in particular, would show signs of deterioration. A scored assessment gives a vivid picture of exactly which areas need intervention. For this reason, it is useful to conduct periodic assessments as a case is reopened or every 3 to 6 months if it is kept open longer. The nurse can

SELF-CARE ASSESSMENT GUIDE

Name _____ Birth date _____

_____

Address _____ Phone number _____

Names of health care providers visited in past year:

Name	Discipline	Address	Phone number	Times visited past year
1.				
2.				

Surgeries (Include date)

1. _____
2. _____

Major acute illnesses (Include date; indicate whether hospitalization was necessary)

1. _____
2. _____

Chronic illnesses (Include date)

1. _____
2. _____

Age of parents (If deceased, indicate date of death, age at death, and cause of death)

Mother _____ Father _____

Age of grandparents (If deceased, indicate age at death and cause of death)

MGM _____ MGF _____ PGM _____ PGF _____

Natural teeth Y N

Dentures or partials Y N

Dental care: ____ Brush teeth/Frequency _____
____ Floss teeth/Frequency _____

Women

Breast self-exam Y N Frequency _____
Mammograms Y N Frequency _____
Pap smears Y N Frequency _____

Men

Testicular self-exam Y N Frequency _____

TB skin test (Date) _____ Results _____

Immunizations

Adult DT (or tetanus) _____
Flu vaccine _____
Hepatitis vaccine _____
Other _____

Weight (At age 25) ____ Current weight ____ Normal weight ____

Height (At age 25) ____ Current height ____

Dietary practices (24-hour dietary recall)

First meal (Time) ____ Contents (Include amount) _____

_____

Second meal (Time) ____ Contents (Include amount) _____

_____

Third meal (Time) ____ Contents (Include amount) _____

_____

Snacks (Include time, contents, and amount) _____

_____

Usual food eaten (not mentioned above) _____
Foods not eaten at all (by preference) _____
Food allergies _____
Medicine allergies _____
Food taboos _____

Religious practices that affect health (prayer, special practices or services) _____

Exercise patterns (Include sample activities, duration, frequency, problems or side effects):

1. _____
2. _____

Medications and therapies

OTC drugs (Include name, length of treatment, frequency of use, side effects):

1. _____
2. _____
3. _____
4. _____

Prescription drugs (Include name, length of treatment, frequency of use, side effects):

1. _____
2. _____
3. _____
4. _____

Folk medicine/home remedies (eg, postpartum isolation, mustard poultice for chest congestion):

1. _____
2. _____
3. _____
4. _____

Complementary therapies (eg, biofeedback, imagery, herbalism)

1. _____
2. _____
3. _____
4. _____

Plan for self-care improvement

Overall goal _____

Areas needing modification (e.g., enhancement, moderation, deletion; include short- and long-term goal for each area):

1. _____
STG: _____
LTG: _____
2. _____
STG: _____
LTG: _____

Client role to reach long-term goals

Nurse's role(s) to reach long-term goals (eg, collaboration, teaching, evaluation)

_____

_____

Others' roles in reaching goals (Include discipline, name, address and phone number)

1. _____
2. _____

Comments

_____

_____

FIGURE 23–8. Self-care assessment guide. (Cleveland, L., & Allender, J. A. [1999]. Environment: Self-care issues. In L. Cleveland, D. S. Aschenbrenner, S. J. Veneable, & J. A. P. Yensen, *Nursing management in drug therapy.* Philadelphia: Lippincott Williams & Wilkins. Used with permission.)

RESEARCH Bridge to Practice

Nelson, D.B. & Edgil A.E. (1998). Family dynamics in families with very low birth weight and full-term infants: A pilot study. *Journal of Pediatric Nursing, 13*(2), 95–103.

The purpose of this pilot study was to determine differences in family health across six dimensions of functioning between families with a very-low-birth-weight infant (VLBW) and families with a full-term infant. The six dimensions include:

Individuation–Enmeshment

Clear communication–Unclear communication

Stability–Disorganization

Flexibility–Rigidity

Mutuality–Isolation

Role reciprocity–Role conflict

The conceptual framework includes an epidemiologic model and Barnhill's system theory of healthy family dynamics. The epidemiologic model included family data and five infant factors of rhythmicity, approachability, adaptability, intensity, and mood. Sixteen families with a VLBW infant and 25 families with a full-term infant were assessed for differences in family health across the above six dimensions.

There were no significant differences found in t-tests, multivariate analysis of variance (MANOVA), and Pearson product-moment correlation coefficients in the two dyads. However, using the Tukey HSD post hoc tests for main effect, significant differences related to the mother's position within the family were found. The position the mother maintained in the family significantly contributed to certain dimensions of family health.

Findings indicate that infants within both families had the ability to self-regulate and interact with the environment—a situation in which the promotion of optimal growth and development of the infant is possible. Approachability in the VLBW infants was related to promotion of family stability and role reciprocity, thus contributing to family health, indicating that the VLBW may not have such a limited repertoire of behaviors as suggested in some earlier studies. Among the full-term infants, rhythmicity, approach, and mood were found to be statistically significant on two dimensions of family health—clear communication and role reciprocity. More rhythmicity in the full-term infant correlated with clearer communication in the family, and greater approachability in the infant correlated with higher role reciprocity in the family. Also, the more positive the full-term infant's mood, the more role reciprocity existed within the family.

An interesting finding was the status and role of the mother in this study. When a mother lived with a friend or was a child within the family (living with her parents), two findings were statistically significant—individuation versus enmeshment and flexibility versus rigidity. More pathology or rigidity is present when the mother's position in the family is that of a child and therefore, perhaps, not one of a decision-making adult. Findings were more positive when the mother was married, which is supported of other studies' findings that marriage promotes family health.

Suggested interventions that a community health nurse could initiate and/or encourage based on these findings include supporting and empowering the mother, especially if living with parents or in-laws, to contribute to or make decisions concerning her infant (and family). Focus teaching on the mother and father–infant relationship; strengthening of

their relationship will promote family health. With both infants, stimulation encourages health; even for the VLBW infants, it was found that they interact using subtle signs that should not be overlooked, and their presence in the family helps to promote family health.

This pilot study produced interesting findings that need to be studied further, such as research that leads to the establishment of healthy functioning family practice models, identifying relationships between dimensions of family health, and identifying additional factors that promote family health.

---

monitor the progress of high-risk families through the early introduction of particular preventive measures, if a trend or regressive behavior in some area is seen. Periodic quantitative assessments also provide a means of evaluating the effectiveness of nursing action and can point to documented signs of growth.

Quantitative data serve another useful purpose. The nurse can compare one family's health status with that of another family as a basis for priority setting and nursing care planning. The difference in the levels of health between the Becks and the Keglers shows that the Keglers need considerably more attention right now. (See Research: Bridge to Practice.)

Exercise Professional Judgment

Although nurses seek to validate data, their assessment of families is still based primarily on their own professional judgment. Assessment tools can guide observations and even quantify those judgments, but ultimately any assessment is subjective. Even though it may be observed that a family makes good use of a community agency, the decision that the use of this external resource is contributing to their health is still a subjective one. This decision is not bad. Indeed, effective health care practice depends on sound professional judgment. However, nurses must, at the same time, be cautious about overemphasizing the value of an assessment tool. It is not infallible. It is only a tool and should be used as a guide for planning, not as an absolute and irrevocable statement about a family's health status. This caution is particularly important when dealing with quantitative scores, which may seem to be objective.

Ordinarily, it is best to conduct assessment of a family unobtrusively. The tool is not a questionnaire to be filled out in the family's presence; its purpose is to guide observations and judgments. Before going into a family's home, the community health nurse may wish to review the questions. He or she may find it helpful to keep the assessment tool in a folder for easy reference during the visit. Depending upon the nurse's relationship with a family, notes may be made during or immediately after the encounter. Like Joe, the nurse may choose to keep a short log—an accumulation of notes—until enough data have been collected to complete the assessment form.

Occasionally, a family with high self-care capability may be involved in the assessment. The nurse should introduce the idea

CLINICAL CORNER   A Family Assessment: Meeting Hector's Needs

You are a home health nurse working in Smithville. You have been given a referral for a new client, Hector. Hector is being released from the rehabilitation unit of Metropolis Hospital. Although he lives in Smithville, Metropolis Hospital was the only facility willing to accept a Medicaid client with a severe spinal cord injury.

Hector is a 19-year-old Hispanic man who sustained major injury to his spinal cord (T-4 injury) in a motorcycle accident. The injury occurred approximately 6 weeks ago. Hector has been diagnosed as paraplegic with some residual limitation of upper body strength and mobility.

Your job is to facilitate Hector's transition from the hospital to the home environment. You will be teaching Hector and his caregivers about the following:

1. Nutrition and fluid intake
2. Signs and symptoms warranting follow-up
3. Medication administration
4. Bowel and bladder care
5. Skin care
6. Activities of daily living (ADLs), self-care with sensory-motor deficits
7. Safety/injury prevention
8. Community resources
9. Rehabilitative services
10. Anticipatory guidance about grief, anger, and suicidal ideations; sexual function; fear of abandonment, role change, and social isolation; and altered family processes.

Following is a synopsis of information obtained during your initial visit with Hector and his family in their home.

Visit One. Hector lives in a migrant labor camp located on the outskirts of Smithville. His family has resided in the camp for 18 years. Living in the two-bedroom cabin-like home are:

- Hector
- Hector's uncle Manuel (32 years old). Manuel's job is seasonal; he has been offered a temporary job for a much higher salary, working out of state.
- Hector's brother Efran (16 years old). Efran is considering dropping out of high school in order to assist with the care of his family. His goal is to become an auto mechanic. He is fluent in both Spanish and English.
- Manuel's wife Micaela (29 years old). Micaela was a teacher in Mexico. She is extremely supportive of her family. She is concerned about the possibility of another pregnancy but does not believe in the use of birth control.
- Manuel and Micaela's children, Arturo (5 years old) and Jasmin (6 months old). Arturo begins a Head Start Program soon and will be gone for 5 hours each day. Jasmin is a healthy baby; she continues to be breast fed and is thriving at home.
- Hector's 74-year-old paternal grandmother (Abuela), who has recently arrived from Mexico and plans on assisting in Hector's care. Abuela has congestive heart failure and arthritis. She is not a legal resident of the U.S. and is not eligible for medical assistance. The whereabouts of Hector's mother are unknown; she moved from their village in Mexico shortly after Efran was born. She has remarried and started another family. She has had no contact with Hector or Efran. Hector's father lives in their home village in Mexico. Although he lived in the migrant camp in Smithville for many years, he recently remarried and has two young daughters in Mexico. Hector's father is aware of Hector's injury and has no plans to return to the U.S.

Your ability to speak fluent Spanish has enabled you to solicit the above information. Manuel has provided you with most of the information. He has been very involved in Hector's recovery through daily visits to the rehabilitation unit and frequent discussions with Hector's health care providers. Manuel tells you that "Hector is like a son to me...I have a responsibility to my older brother to watch over his son. My brother watched out for me when I was young...he even left school to work to help support our family." Manuel adds, "We don't have much but we will take care of Hector...we'll all work together."

You begin your discussion by explaining your role as home health nurse. You inform the family about the type of education and interventions you are able to provide. You ask Hector and the family to tell you what they have learned from the health care team at the rehabilitation unit and what plans have been developed by the family to address Hector's medical and psychosocial needs. As you begin the visit you notice that Hector's grandmother is sitting quietly in the corner of the room rocking Jasmin. You learn that Efran is working in the fields. Arturo is in school. Manuel, Micaela, and Abuela are participating in the home visit this morning. The conversation is as follows.

Nurse: Hector, can you tell me how you feel about being home?

Hector (looks at Micaela): Okay, I guess.

Micaela: He's a little scared, I think. He feels like it's going to be too much for us to deal with.

Nurse (looking at Hector): There's so much happening right now, so much to think about...

Hector: Uh-huh.

(Hector is maintaining eye contact with Manuel and Micaela only; since this is your initial visit to the home you feel that Hector may be more comfortable in the role of observer.)

CLINICAL CORNER | **A Family Assessment: Meeting Hector's Needs (Continued)**

Nurse (looking at Manuel and Micaela): Do you have any questions before we begin?

Micaela: They gave us a lot of information at the hospital... I'm most afraid about if the phone doesn't work and Hector needs help. What if something happens to Hector and I can't call anyone? That's the only thing I worry about.

Abuela: If anything happens to him I'll be right here with you, "mija." We can do this, we can take care of Hector if we work together.

Manuel: There is a store with a phone only two blocks away, if you needed to you could call from there. What I want to know is how we can get Hector into school or something that will help him to be around kids his own age. His English is good enough, he even finished high school. He needs to be ready to make a future for himself.

Hector (grins and looks at Manuel): Right, uncle, that is what I want, too.

You continue the conversation by revisiting Micaela's concerns about access to a telephone in case of an emergency. You ask specific questions about her concerns and use this as an opportunity to educate the family about circumstances warranting immediate follow-up. Together you decide that Micaela will develop a list of specific concerns that you will review together at a subsequent visit planned for 2 days from today.

Today's visit consists of:

I. Assessment
  A. Home environment
    1. Safety
    2. ADLs
  B. Knowledge of disease processes
  C. Fluid volume balance
  D. Nutritional resources of family
    1. Food availability
    2. Food preparation
  E. Insurance and financial status
II. Education
  A. Medications

B. Warning signs and symptoms and appropriate follow-up procedures
  C. Bowel and bladder care
  D. Hygiene prior to and following patient care

The plan for your visit in 2 days includes:

I. Referrals
  A. Community resources
  B. Educational opportunities
  C. Support groups (Spanish speaking)
  D. Peer group opportunities for Hector
II. Assessment
  A. Continuation of above
III. Education
  A. Continuation of above

Questions

1. What is the social structure of this family (traditional versus nontraditional)? Be specific about the type of traditional or nontraditional family system that exists in this scenario.
2. Discuss an example of triangulation in this scenario.
3. What essential functions are present within this family system?
4. What developmental stages appear to have been achieved?
5. What steps will you take in order to empower the family to make their own decisions?
6. List the strengths of the family.
7. Prioritize Hector's issues—medical and psychosocial.
8. Prioritize issues facing the other family members.
9. Identify mutual goals for this family:
   Immediate
   Mid-range
   Long-term
10. What community health nursing interventions will you utilize to achieve these mutual goals?

---

carefully and use professional judgment to determine when the family is ready to engage in this kind of self-examination.

SUMMARY

The family unit remains the focus of service in community health nursing. Family health and individual health strongly influence each other, and family health also affects community health. Thus, it is important for the nurse to be able to understand healthy family characteristics and to be able to use a variety of tools to conduct thorough family assessments.

Healthy families demonstrate six important characteristics:

1. There is a facilitative process of interaction among family members.
2. They enhance individual member development.
3. Their role relationships are structured effectively.
4. They actively attempt to cope with problems.
5. They have a healthy home environment and lifestyle.
6. They establish regular links with the broader community.

To assess a family's health systematically, the nurse needs a conceptual framework upon which to base the assessment, a clearly defined set of categories for data collection, and a method for measuring the family's level of functioning. The six characteristics of a healthy family provide one assessment framework that community health nurses can use. Assessment tools to aid the nurse in appraising the health of families include the eco-map, genogram, and social support network map or grid. There are also 12 main categories of family dynamics for which the nurse must collect data: family demographics, physical environment, psychological/spiritual environment, family structure and roles, family functions, family values and beliefs, family communication patterns, family decision-making patterns, family problem-solving patterns, family coping patterns, family health behaviors, and family social and cultural patterns.

Community health nurses enhance their practice with families by observing five principles: (1) work with the family collectively, (2) start where the family is now, (3) fit nursing intervention to the family's stage of development, (4) recognize the validity of family structural variation, and (5) emphasize family strengths.

During assessment, the nurse should focus on the family as a total unit, use goal-directed assessment questions, allow adequate time for data collection, combine quantitative with qualitative data, and exercise professional judgment.

ACTIVITIES TO PROMOTE CRITICAL THINKING

1. Construct an eco-map of your family. Ask a peer to do the same thing. Assess the balance between your family and the resources in its environment. How does it compare with your peer's? What changes are needed in each family system? Are you able to influence the changes that are needed?

2. Draw a genogram of your family and ask a peer to discuss it with you. Make your drawing of the genogram as complete as possible. Then analyze your thoughts and feelings. How did you feel while tracing your family history? Did you learn anything new about your family? Did any family trends or traits appear? Did any uncomfortable or suppressed information come to the surface? Do you have any new insights about your family?

3. Complete a social support network map or grid on yourself. Discuss it with a peer. Did any of the data surprise you? What areas need to be worked on?

4. Assess a family (other than your own) that you know well by completing a family assessment guide. You may use one of the forms in this chapter or a form available to you from some other source. Based on your assessment, determine as many nursing interventions that could be used to promote this family's health as practically as possible.

REFERENCES

Barker, P. (1992). *Basic family therapy* (3rd ed.). New York: Oxford.

Beavers, W.R. & Hampton, R.B. (1990). *Successful families: Assessment and intervention.* New York: Basic Books.

Becvar, D.S. & Becvar, R.J. (1996). *Family therapy: A systematic integration* (3rd ed.). Needham Heights, MA: Allyn and Bacon.

Centers for Disease Control and Prevention (CDC) (1998). *Assessing health risks in America: The behavioral risk factor surveillance system (BRFSS).* Washington, DC: U.S. Department of Health and Human Services.

Cox, R.P. & Davis, L.L. (1993) Social constructivist approaches for brief, episodic, problem-focused family encounters. *Nurse Practitioner, 18*(8), 45–49.

Edelman, C. & Mandle, C.L. (Eds.) (1986). *Health promotion throughout the life span.* St. Louis: Mosby.

Farren, M. (1999). Ensuring safety for the elderly client at home. In S. Zang & J.A. Allender (Eds.), *Home care of the elderly* (pp. 59–77). Philadelphia: Lippincott Williams & Wilkins.

Ford, L.C. (1973). The development of family nursing. In D. Hymovich & M. Barnard (Eds.), *Family health care.* New York: McGraw-Hill.

Friedman, M.M. (1998). *Family nursing: Research, theory and practice* (4th ed.). Stamford, CT: Appleton & Lange.

Glick, P.C. (1994). American families: As they are and were. In A. Skolnick & J. Skolnick (Eds.), *Family in transition* (8th ed., pp. 91–104). New York: Harper Collins.

Hartman, A. (1978). Diagrammatic assessment of family relationships. *Social Casework, 59*(10), 59–64.

Harway, M., & Wexler, K. (1996). Setting the stage for understanding and treating the changing family. In M. Harway (Ed.), *Treating the changing family: Handling normative and unusual events.* American Counseling Association. New York: John Wiley & Sons.

Hill, R., & Hansen, D. (1960). The identification of conceptual frameworks utilized in family study. *Marriage and Family Living, 22,* 299–311.

Holkup, P.A. (1998). Our parents, our children, ourselves: A therapy group to facilitate understanding of intergenerational behavior patterns and to promote family healing. *Journal of Psychosocial Nursing, 36*(2), 20–26.

Holmes, T. & Rahe, R. (1967). The social readjustment rating scale. *Journal of Psychosomatic Research, 11,* 213–217.

Huntley, D.K. & Konetsky, C.D. (1992). Healthy families with adolescents. *Topics in Family Psychology and Counseling, 1,* 62–71.

Kantor, D. & Lehr, W. (1975). *Inside the family: Toward a theory of family process.* San Francisco: Jossey-Bass.

Kissman, K., & Allen, J. (1993). *Single parent families.* Newbury Park, CA: Sage.

Kristjanson, L.J. & Chalmers, K.I. (1997). Preventative work with families: Issues facing public health nurses. In B.W. Spradley & J.A. Allender (Eds.), *Readings in community health nursing* (5th ed., pp. 377–388). Philadelphia: Lippincott-Raven.

McGoldrick, M. & Gersen, R. (1985). *Genograms in family assessment.* New York: Norton.

Meyer, C.H. (1993). *Assessment in social work practice.* New York: Columbia.

Miller, N. (1992). *Single parents by choice: A growing trend in family life.* New York: Plenum Press.

Nelson, D.B., & Edgil, A.E. (1998). Family dynamics in families with very low birth weight and full term infants: A pilot study. *Journal of Pediatric Nursing, 13*(2), 95–103.

Olson, D.H. (1991, November). *Three-dimensional (3-D) circumplex model: Theoretical and methodological advances.* Paper presented at the Theory Construction and Research Methodology Workshop at the annual convention of the National Council on Family Relations, Denver.

Olson, D., McCubbin, H.I., and Associates (1983). *Families: What makes them work.* Beverly Hills: Sage.

Otto, H.A. (1973). A framework for assessing family strengths. In A. Reinhardt & M. Quinn (Eds.), *Family-centered community nursing: A socio-cultural framework.* St. Louis: Mosby.

Parachin, V.M. (1997). Six signs of a healthy family. *Vibrant Life,* March/April, 5–6.

Reiss, D. (1981). *The family's construction of reality.* Cambridge, MA: Harvard University Press.

Reutter, L. (1997). Family health assessment: An integrated approach. In B.W. Spradley & J.A. Allender (Eds.), *Readings in community health nursing* (5th ed., pp. 329–342). Philadelphia: Lippincott-Raven.

Robinson, C.A. (1994). Nursing interventions with families: A demand or an invitation to change? *Journal of Advanced Nursing, 19*(5), 897–904.

Ryan, J.M. (1997). Child abuse and the community health nurse. In B.W. Spradley & J.A. Allender (Eds.), *Readings in community health nursing* (5th ed., pp. 371–376). Philadelphia: Lippincott-Raven.

Schwebel, A.I. & Fine, M.A. (1994). *Understanding and helping families: A cognitive-behavioral approach.* Hillsdale, NJ: Lawrence Erlbaum Associates.

Seaberg, J.R. & Harrigan, M.P. (1997). Family functioning in foster care. *Families in Society, 78*(5), 463–470.

Snelling, J. (1994). The effect of chronic pain on the family unit. *Journal of Advanced Nursing, 19,* 543–551.

Tapia, J.A. (1997). The nursing process in family health. In B.W. Spradley & J.A. Allender (Eds.), *Readings in community health nursing* (5th ed., pp. 343–350). Philadelphia: Lippincott-Raven.

Taylor, J.A., & Kemper, K.J. (1998). Group well-child care for high-risk families. *Archives of Pediatric and Adolescent Medicine, 152,* 579–584.

Thompson, P. (1998). Adolescents from families of divorce: Vulnerability to physiological and psychological disturbances. *Journal of Psychosocial Nursing and Mental Health Services, 36*(3), 34–39.

Tracy, E.M. & Whittaker, J.J.(1990). The social network map: Assessing social support in clinical practice. *Families in Society, 71,* 461–470.

Turk, D. C. & Kerns, R.D. (Eds.). (1985). *Health, illness and families: A life span perspective.* New York: John Wiley.

Wallace, H.M., Green, G., Jaros, K., Paine, L., & Story, M. (1999). *Health and welfare for families in the 21st century.* Boston: Jones and Bartlett.

Wright, L.M. & Leahey, M. (1994). *Nurses and families: A guide to family assessment and intervention* (2nd ed.). Philadelphia: F.A. Davis.

Zerwekh, J.V. (1992). Laying the groundwork for family self-help: Locating families, building trust, and building strength. *Public Health Nursing, 9*(1), 15–20.

SELECTED READINGS

Ahmann, E. (1994). Family-centered care: Shifting orientation. *Pediatric Nursing, 20,* 113–117.

Biller, H.B. (1993). *Fathers and families: Paternal factors in child development.* Westport, CT: Auburn House.

Bomar, P.J. (Ed.) (1996). *Nurses and family health promotion: Concepts, assessment, and interventions* (2nd ed.). Philadelphia: W.B. Saunders.

Broome, M.E., Knafl, K., Pridham, K., & Feetham, S. (Eds.) (1998). *Children and families in health and illness.* Thousand Oaks, CA: Sage.

Bulechek, G.M. & McCloskey, J.C. (Eds.) (1999). *Nursing interventions: Essential nursing treatments* (3rd ed.). Philadelphia: W.B. Saunders.

Cherry, B., & Giger, J.N. (1995). African-Americans. In J.N. Giger & R.E. Davidhizar (Eds.), *Transcultural nursing: Assessment and intervention* (2nd ed., pp. 165–203). St. Louis: Mosby.

Copeland, A.P., & White, K.M. (1991). *Studying families.* Newbury Park: Sage.

Cuellar, I., & Glazer, M. (1996). The impact of culture on the family. In M. Harway (Ed.), *Treating the changing family: Handling normative and unusual events.* American Counseling Association. New York: John Wiley.

Curtis, B. (1996). Managing a multitude. *Vibrant Life,* September/October, 20–21.

David, L.L. (1996). Dementia caregiving studies: A typology for family interventions. *Journal of Family Nursing, 2*(3), 30–55.

Elkind, D. (1995). The family in the postmodern world. *National Forum, 75*(3), 24–28.

Gillis, C.L. (1991). Family nursing research, theory and practice. *Image: The Journal of Nursing Scholarship, 23*(1), 19–22.

Glasser, P.H. & Glasser, L.N. (1970). *Families in crisis.* New York: Harper and Row.

Hall, R. (1992). *Families and groups.* Philadelphia: Saunders—Churchill Livingstone.

Hanson, S.M.H. & Boyd, S.T. (1996). *Family health care nursing: Theory, practice, and research.* Philadelphia: F.A. Davis.

Holman, A. M. (1983). *Family assessment: Tools for understanding and intervention.* Newbury Park, CA: Sage.

Jacobs, J. (1993). Families under siege. *Family Therapy Networker, 17*(1), 24–25.

Lotas, M., Penticuff, J., Medoff-Cooper, B., Brooten, D., & Brown, L. (1992). The HOME SCALE: The influence of socioeconomic status on the evaluation of the home environment. *Nursing Research, 41,* 338–341.

McCroskey, J., Sladen, A., & Meezan, W. (1997). *The family assessment form: A practice-based approach to assessing family functioning developed by the Children's Bureau of Southern California.* Washington, DC: Child Welfare League of America.

Minuchin, S. (1974). *Families and family therapy.* Cambridge: Harvard University Press.

Molina, C.W. & Aguirre-Molina, M. (Eds.) (1994). *Laotian health in the US: A growing challenge.* Washington, DC: American Public Health Association.

Murray, R.B., & Zentner, J.P. (1997). *Health assessment and promotion strategies through the life span* (6th ed.). Stamford, CT: Appleton & Lange.

Neuman, B. (1995). *The Neuman systems model* (3rd ed.). Stamford, CT: Appleton & Lange.

Pender, N. J. (1996). *Health promotion in nursing practice* (3rd ed.). Stamford, CT: Appleton & Lange.

Sameroff, A.J., Seifer, R., Baldwin, A., & Baldwin, C. (1993). Stability of intelligence from preschool to adolescence: The influence of social and family risk factors. *Child Development, 64,* 80–97.

Spector, R.E. (1996). *Cultural diversity in health and illness* (4th ed.). Stamford, CT: Appleton & Lange.

Stanhope, M. & Knollmueller, R.N. (1997). *Public and community health nurse's consultant: A health promotion guide.* St. Louis; Mosby.

Thomas, D.D. (1993). Minorities in North America: African-American families. In J.L. Paul & R.J. Simeonsson (Eds.), *Children with special needs: Family, culture, and society* (2nd ed., pp. 122–138). Philadelphia: Harcourt Brace Jovanovich.

United States Department of Health and Human Services. (1998). *Healthy people 2010 objectives: Draft for public comment.* Washington, DC: U.S. Government Printing Office.

Vaughan-Cole, B., Johnson, M.A., Malone, J.A., & Walker, B.L. (1998). *Family nursing practice.* Philadelphia: W.B. Saunders.

Vosler, N.R. & Robertson, J.G. (1998). Nonmarital co-parenting: Knowledge building for practice. *Families in Society, 79*(2), 149–157.

Planning, Intervening, and Evaluating Health Care to Families

KEY TERMS

- Home visit
- Mutual goals
- Nursing bag
- Outcome evaluation
- Referral
- Resource directory

LEARNING OBJECTIVES

Upon mastery of this chapter, you should be able to:

- Describe the components of the nursing process as applied to enhancing family health.
- Identify the steps in a successful family health intervention.
- Discuss the two foci of family health visits: education and health promotion.
- List at least six specific safety measures the community health nurse should take when traveling to and/or making a home visit.
- Describe useful activities and actions when intervening on family health visits.
- Describe three types of evaluations that are necessary following family health intervention.

Have you ever thought about how your family has influenced you? Did they influence you in your career choice, where you are attending school, your value system, your level of health, or the friends you have? How different do you think your life would be if you grew up in a family in which both of your parents were vegetarians as compared with growing up in a family in which your father took you out every fall to hunt for deer meat? Families are different—no two are alike. Community health nurses primarily work with families—in their own homes, classrooms, support groups, clinics, outpatient departments, neighborhood centers, homeless shelters, or relatives' homes.

Families are the main unit of service in the community and have been for over a century (Schoor & Kennedy, 1999). It is with the family in mind that the bulk of health care and related services are provided in the community. Immunization programs exist for infants and children; parks, recreation services, organized team sports, and social centers are there for the physical and emotional well-being of families. Pregnant women can attend childbirth education classes as well as receive medical care from their health care providers. Growing families can access parenting classes and support groups for developmental crises and management of chronic illness. For the older adults in the family, there are senior centers and a myriad of social and recreational activities that offer senior discounts. What is common among these people is the fact that they are members of families.

You have learned in other chapters that when families are assessed they come in all sizes, consist of members of many ages and biological relationships, and experience life filtered through unique cultures (Chapter 23), and that there are many theoretical approaches and roles to consider when caring for families (Chapter 22). In this chapter we will explore how community health nursing services are planned for and delivered to families in clinics, homes, work settings, or schools.

Just as each family is unique, so is each family's home and neighborhood. Some families live in homes that will look very much like yours, and you will feel comfortable almost immediately in those homes. However, you will find families living in places that do not feel so comfortable, including small, cluttered apartments, farm labor camps, sparsely furnished single rooms, houses in disrepair, mobile homes, high-rise inner-city apartments, rural cabins, and inner-city neighborhoods. Each setting brings a different challenge. Assessing, planning, implementing, and evaluating care to families in their own environment can be a daunting task to the novice community health nurse. This chapter focuses on the planning, implementing, and evaluating phases of the nursing process as used to enhance family health.

NURSING PROCESS COMPONENTS APPLIED TO FAMILIES AS CLIENTS

Assessing, planning, implementing, and evaluating nursing care are steps you have used as you delivered care to clients in acute care settings and in the extensive clinic system utilized by clients. Now these same steps are used with families and aggregates in community health nursing. The steps do not change, but because the context and client focus is different, external variables that you have not encountered previously must now be considered.

Working With Families in Community Health Settings

Family visits need not be limited to homes. At times family members may be visited in schools or at work during a lunch break, in a day care or senior center, in group homes, or at a myriad of after-work or after-school and recreational settings. The nurse must be very creative to accommodate various family schedules and routines. A general rule is: If a visit is all right with the family, school, or employer, it should be all right with the nurse (see Voices From the Community). Families appreciate the individualized effort and respond more postively when nurses are not put off by family member schedules but work with them.

When making visits in public places such as at work or school, be mindful of confidentiality and respect the family's wishes. They may agree to your visit during their lunch break in the department store on Tuesdays, which is the boss's day off, or at 2:00 PM after the lunch crowd in a fast-food restaurant when the client can take a break. Seek out a place for the visit where other employees or customers cannot overhear your conversation with the client.

Sometimes visiting where clients are during the day helps to enhance the family assessment. In families with a child in day care or an older adult in an adult day care program, your assessment of their ability to manage, participate, and inter-

Voices From the Community

I couldn't believe it when she (the community health nurse) said she could visit me during my lunch break. I have been so worried about Sammy's hearing and with my new work hours I kept missing her—I got her notes she left in the screen. She actually drove all the way out to my work to tell me about his hearing test at school and the teacher's classroom changes. I can't afford to lose this job—and she came here!

Beth 31, Sammy's mother

act can give insight into problems the family is referring to when you make a home visit.

Visiting children during the school day often gives insight into health problems the parents may be concerned about. This offers the community health nurse an excellent opportunity to consult with the principal, teachers, school nurse (see Chapter 28), counselor, and/or school psychologist. The community health nurse may suggest a team meeting of school professionals with the parents, coordinate the meeting, and act as the liaison during the meeting—always acting as a client advocate.

Working With Families Where They Live

Depending on the setting for your community health nursing practice, you will encounter most clients in their homes and in their neighborhoods. Some of you will see families in transition: living on the street, in a homeless shelter, or with other relatives. Regardless of the family's location, the client is the family; the family is the unit of service in family nursing (Friedman, 1998).

THE HOME VISIT
Working in the community and being able to visit families in their homes is a privilege. In this unique setting you are permitted into the most intimate of spaces we, as human beings, have. Our homes are our creations, our private spaces; they hold our personal treasures, our memories. To let a stranger into our home takes a certain amount of trust. To enter a client family's home also takes trust on the part of the nurse. Once the door is shut behind you, you are in the client's world. The rules have changed; they are the experts, you are the guest. You must respond to the family with this "switch" in mind. A **home visit** is conducted to visit clients where they live in order to assist them to achieve as high a level of wellness as possible. Later in this chapter we will discuss the components of a family health intervention included in a home visit and how the community health nurse can best use the phases of the nursing process to enhance family health.

NURSING SKILLS USED DURING HOME VISITS

There are many skills, in addition to expert nursing skills, that are needed when assessing, planning, implementing, and evaluting service in the home to families at a variety of levels of functioning (Tapia, 1997). Expert interviewing skills and effective communication techniques are essential to effective family intervention (see Chapter 8). When making home visits these special skills include the following.

Acute Observation Skills. The environment is new to you, and environmental observation and client observation are equally important. In addition to focusing on the family members' concerns and the purpose of your visit, you need to be observant about neighborhood and travel safety, home environmental conditions, number of household members, client demeanor and body language, and other nonverbal cues.

Traveling in new neighborhoods and attempting to locate some families can cause distress to even the most experienced nurse. Often clients are difficult to locate because the house or apartment number is missing, it is situated behind another house, it is a basement apartment without a number, or because of any other variety of architectual barriers unfamiliar to the nurse. Addresses on referrals may have numbers transposed, such as 123 Hickory instead of 132 Hickory. Perhaps there is a North Hickory–miles away from South Hickory—or there are different streets called Hickory such as Boulevard, Drive, Street, Road, Court, Lane, and Way. Then there is always the chance that the address is fictitious–given by clients who, for whatever reason, prefer to remain as anoymous as possible.

Assessment of Home Environmental Conditions. Observing the neighborhood and home environmental conditions reveals important assessment information that will guide the planning and intervention with families. While traveling to and arriving at the family home, you have been gathering information about resources and barriers encountered by the family. You use this information as planning with the family follows. It is important to remember that neighborhood conditions and even the physical appearance of the apartment or house may belie the family's values, resources, and goals. They have little individual control over the neighborhood and frequently the building they live in, especially if they are renting. For instance, the family may be a young couple with a baby who can afford $450 in rent; the only apartment available to them for that amount is in a low-income, deterioriating neighborhood occupied mostly by renters in dilapilated buildings owned by absentee landlords. These landlords do not live in the neighborhood and may own several buildings, mainly for profit. They are handled by managers who may not know the landlord and are employed through the owner's management company. Yet when you enter the apartment you see a well-furnished, neat, clean home that is opened to you, with pride, by the family.

In another situation, you may be planning to visit an older couple who live in their own home in an upscale suburban neighborhood. However, as you approach the house you see an overgrown yard and a house in need of painting and repairs.

When you enter the home, you can barely manage to squeeze through a pathway made in a living room piled ceiling-high with boxes, newspapers, and furniture. This continues throughout the house and even into a back bedroom where half the bed is covered with papers, books, and a few cats. An older woman is in the bed, and you notice that the husband who let you in moves very slowly and leaves you in the bedroom as he heads toward the back yard.

There are many environmental clues given in each of these situations that help the nurse begin an assessment that will lead to a plan to assist each family. Most neighborhoods and homes will not present you with such extremes. However, if you are unprepared for the extremes, when you are confronted by them they may overwhelm you and you may become so distracted that you cannot refocus wholly on the family and incorporate the importance of these data to the family into the plans.

Assessment of Household Members' Demeanor, Body Language, and Other Nonverbal Cues. You have knocked on the door or rung the doorbell and are in the home (Display 24–1). Once in the home or even when greeting the people in the doorway, you are gathering data and, being human, you may be forming opinions or making judgements about the family from the initial meeting. Know that they are doing the same thing. Be aware of all household members: acknowledge them, greet them. If some are absent on a visit, inquire about them. Make this a habit on all visits. Each member of the family is important and has opinions and health care needs, even if you only see parts of the family on each visit.

DISPLAY 24–1. How You Knock Helps Families Open the Door

At first this may seem trite, but how do you knock on the door when you visit a family? Do you use the "I don't want to be here and if they don't hear the knock I can quietly leave" type of knock that even Superman can't hear? Or do you knock like, "I'm a bill collector and YOU BETTER open this door!" During this knock the entire family is leaving through the back door! We suggest a knock that is loud enough to be heard, yet friendly and non-threatening. If necessary, practice "your knock" until you can create this beneficial combination.

With some families it is helpful to call towards the door as you knock or ring the bell with, "Mrs. Smith, this is Jenny from the Health Department—remember I was coming by today" or, "Ms. Jiminez, it's the student community health nurse, Terry Guara, and I brought those pamphlets for you" or, "Hello, it's James from the neighborhood clinic, we planned to meet today." Using such a greeting allows the family to know who is at the door and choose to open the door if they want. It will get you into more homes than the "quiet-as-a-mouse" or "bill-collector" knocks.

Be observant of family body language and demeanor. These nonverbal cues are giving you information that must not be overlooked. Observations such as, "You seem anxious today," or "Did I come at a bad time? You seem distracted" are openings that allow family members to express what is on their minds. If you are not open to family body language while making the visit, you may overlook these important cues and continue with your agenda, not realizing that the family is distracted by another, more pressing issue for them.

On a related note, it is important for the nurse to be aware of her or his own body language or demeanor. If you fidget with your car keys during the entire visit, noisily chew gum, give minimal eye contact while continuously looking at your paperwork, appear rushed, or refuse to sit on any of the family's furniture, your behavior will tell the family a great deal about you, including how you feel about being in their home.

PLANNING TO MEET THE HEALTH NEEDS OF FAMILIES DURING HOME VISITS

The greatest barrier to a successful family health visit is a lack of planning and preparing. A visit is not successful just because the nurse enters a home or other setting where clients are present. Making a successful family health visit takes much planning and preparation, involves many aspects while with the family, and requires accurate documentation and follow-up. In addition, safety measures must be followed, not only while traveling in the neighborhood but also in the home.

Components of the Family Health Visit

The structure of family health visits can be divided into four components that follow the nursing process (Display 24–2). Pre-visit preparation (assessment and planning) steps are necessary to ensure that the actual family health visit (implementation) is complete. The documentation and planning for the next visit (evaluation) concludes the responsibilities for one visit and prepares the nurse for the next action needed.

PRE-VISIT PREPARATION
Community health nurses design a plan for the initial family health visit based on a referral coming into the agency. A **referral** is a request for service from another agency or person. This request is formalized through the use of a form or information that the originating agency has transferred to the receiving agency. Referrals may be formal, from complementary agencies, or informal, through verbal or telephone referrals from friends or relatives when they feel someone is in need. Referrals are the source of new cases for agencies and need timely responses. Referrals could be from labor and delivery units referring low-birth-weight babies and teen mothers age 17 and under. They could be from social service agencies requesting a home assessment for a child being returned to parents after previously being removed from the home. A referral could come through a telephone call from a woman in a city 500 miles away, wanting a nurse to check on her mother who lives alone in your community and has recently exhibited slurred speech. Follow-up visits are made to these families based on need and agency protocol.

Nurses must have a physical place to work with access to a telephone and any other supportive resources deemed necessary, such as a source of educational material (pamplets, brochures, computer and related website addresses to access educational information), charting tools, and any other supplies ncessary for home visits. Nurses also need a **resource directory,** which is a published list of resources for the broader community, and/or a nurse-made directory of resources created over years of working with people in the community.

Some agencies issue a **nursing bag** to their nurses. This bag, traditionally black leather with two handles, serves to carry the materials a nurse may need on a home visit and can identify that the person carrying it comes from a certain agency. Not all agencies provide a nursing bag; thus, nurses become creative and devise their own carry-all for supplies—canvas totes, briefcases, or small molded plastic carriers. The supplies community health nurses need are minimal and may depend on the type of visit; some nurses have several totes for different kinds of visits. If the focus is educational, to do a Denver Developmental Screening Test (DDST), or to do a newborn assessment, each tote will have the appropriate materials in it. Basic supplies that all nurses should have available on any visit include disposable gloves, paper towels, and soap packets or a waterless hand cleanser. Nurses engaged in home health nursing are prepared with more supplies for each visit since the focus is on treatment in a majority of the visits (see Chapter 37).

Once the nurse is prepared, contact with the family is needed. For a home visit, ideally the referral contains a correct telephone for the family, a relative, or a neighbor. If the referral or chart does not contain this information, the nurse needs to make an unannounced visit. During this visit it is important to get a phone number of a relative or neighbor or of the client family if they did not have a phone previously and now have one. If there is a telephone number, the first and most important thing the nurse must do is introduce herself or himself; explain the reason for calling, why this family was selected for a visit, what the visit consists of; and find out when the visit would work best for the family and the nurse. Some people may become defensive or suspicious of your intentions. For example, a new young mother may think, "What did they see me doing wrong with my baby in the hospital?" In this kind of situation, it is very important that the nurse explain:

- that the visit is a service provided by the agency to all young mothers

DISPLAY 24–2. Guidelines for Making Home Visits: 30 Steps to Success

The following guidelines can be followed to evaluate yourself after making a home visit; or it can be a tool used when you are evaluated by another nurse (peer or instructor). Rate yourself using the following scale: 0 = does not apply, 1 = unsatisfactory, 2 = satisfactory.

Rating Assessment

_____ 1. Studies referral, record, or other available data about the family.

_____ 2. Gathers community resource information potentially appropriate to the family.

_____ 3. Obtains appropriate supplies or educational material in anticipation of family needs.

Planning

_____ 4. Contacts family to set up an appropriate time for the home visit.

_____ 5. Ascertains correct address and directions to the family for the home visit.

_____ 6. Formulates a written plan for nursing intervention with each family member.

_____ 7. Organizes a chart with forms and charting tools based on the focus of the visit.

_____ 8. Plans a route to the family's home that is the most direct, being resource efficient.

Implementation

_____ 9. Travels the community with safety, locating the family home with ease.

_____ 10. Knock on the door loudly enough to be heard and in a friendly manner.

_____ 11. Introduces self to family members in an appropriate manner.

_____ 12. Clearly states the reason for the visit.

_____ 13. Allows a few moments of socialization before beginning the visit.

_____ 14. Smiles, speaks in a pleasant, friendly tone of voice, and maintains eye contact.

_____ 15. Uses aseptic technique when providing nursing care.

_____ 16. Respects the dignity, privacy, safety, and comfort of family members.

_____ 17. Listens attentively to ascertain what family members are saying or implying.

_____ 18. Converses with family members during the home visit.

_____ 19. Communicates accurate and meaningful information to family members.

_____ 20. Responds to family members in a way that encourages them to continue talking.

_____ 21. Uses appropriate words of explanation for family member understanding.

_____ 22. Utilizes opportunities for incidental teaching.

_____ 23. Commends progress made by individual family members.

_____ 24. Explains nursing measures before, during, and after each procedure.

_____ 25. Shares the results of nursing measures with family members when indicated.

_____ 26. Closes the home visit by summarizing the main points of the visit.

_____ 27. Makes plans for the next visit, considering family member wishes.

Evaluation

_____ 28. Utilizes information gathered on the home visit to plan care for next visit.

_____ 29. Documents home visit in an appropriate and timely manner.

_____ 30. Completes a self-evaluation of the home visit.

- that the visit is paid for by taxes (or donations) or the client's HMO (if applicable), so there is no direct charge to the family
- we know that young mothers have lots of questions about their new babies
- having a nurse come to their home provides them with an opportunity to ask questions
- it is an opportunity for the nurse to show the mother things about her baby that she may not know

The nurse needs to ask explicit directions to where the family is staying. The referral may have a different address and the family may forget to tell you they are staying with an aunt until you ask for the directions.

MAKING THE VISIT

Upon locating and meeting the family, the following guidelines for initial contact should be utilized (Allender, 1998):

- Introduce yourself and explain the value to the family of the nursing services provided by the agency.
- Spend the first few minutes of the visit establishing cordiality and getting acquainted (a mutual discovery or "feeling out" time).
- Utilize acute observational skills.
- Be sensitive to verbal and nonverbal cues.
- Be adaptable and flexible (you may be planning a prenatal visit, but the woman delivered her baby the

day after you made this home visit appointment and there is a newborn now).

- Use a "sixth sense" to guide you regarding family responses, questions they ask, or your personal safety (trust your feelings).
- Be aware of you own personality, balance talking and listening, and watch your nonverbal behaviors.
- Be aware that most clients are not acutely ill and have higher levels of wellness than usually seen in acute care settings.
- Become acquainted with all family members and household members if you are making a home visit.
- Encourage each person to speak for himself or herself.
- Be accepting and listen carefully.
- Help the family focus on issues and move toward desired goals.
- After the body of the visit is over, review the important points, emphasizing family strengths.
- Plan with the family for the next visit.

Depending on the purpose of the visit, the length and primary focus will change. As a general guide, if the visit is shorter than 20 minutes, it probably should be folded into another visit (unless you are offering a piece of very important information, providing supplies, or have come by family request). On the other hand, if the visit exceeds 1 hour it should be conducted over two visits. Families have routines that are important to them and taking that large a portion of time out of their day may lead to resentment, putting future visits in jeopardy. Similarly, if nothing of value (according to the family) occurs on a visit, they will not continue to make themselves available for future visits. This be-

comes a balancing act for the family and the nurse and is an area where using your sixth sense and picking up on nonverbal cues is helpful (Zerwekh, 1997). In addition, home visits are an expensive way to provide community health nursing services, which are population based. The outcome of better health for family members must be demonstrated in order to support the value of such costly services (see Bridging Financial Gaps).

CONCLUDING AND DOCUMENTING THE VISIT

Making plans for the next visit and saying goodbye to the family members terminates the home visit. This is a good time to put away the paperwork, materials, and supplies from this visit and retrieve items needed for the next visit. It is always safer to open the car trunk in front of this home and get out what is needed for the next family's visit than to open your trunk in front of the next family's home. You do not want to give community members information about what is stored in your car's trunk while it is unattended and you are in the family's home.

Most typically, as soon as you return to your agency, you should complete the documentation of each home visit. However, some agencies provide their nurses with laptop computers with electronic charting forms, and charting is encouraged at the end of the visit before leaving for the next one. Sometimes time is allowed for the nurse to chart at home after the last visit of the day. For the most part, you will be expected to complete the charting by hand, using agency forms, as soon as is practically possible. Most agencies expect all charting to be completed by the end of each work day or no later than the end of the work week.

Agencies use a variety of forms that assist the nurse to

Bridging Financial Gaps

Karoly, L.A., Everingham, S.S., Hoube, J., et al. (1998). *Investing in our children: What we know and don't know about the costs and benefits of early childhood interventions.* MR—898. Santa Monica, CA: RAND.

A 1998 RAND study of nine early intervention models found the Prenatal and Early Childhood Nurse Home Visitation model (the Olds' model) yielded cost savings much greater than program costs; documented the program's high success rate in meeting its goals; and demonstrated significant benefits compared with other models. Benefits achieved are based on 15 years of research and evaluation of families served in Elmira, N.Y. The following benefits to families were found:

30 fewer months' use of welfare after the birth of the first child
2 years' interval or greater between the birth of the first and second child
69% fewer arrests among the mothers
44% fewer behavioral problems among the mothers due to substance abuse

79% fewer verified reports of child abuse and neglect through the first child's 15th birthday
56% fewer arrests among the 15-year-old children
69% fewer convictions and probation violations among the 15-year-old children
58% fewer sexual partners among these 15-year-old children
56% fewer days of consuming alcohol by the 15-year-old children
28% fewer cigarettes smoked by the 15-year-old children
　The following benefits to the community were found:
Cumulative costs (per child) of the program by age 15 = $5,000
Cumulative savings (per child) of the program by age 15 = $15,000*

Sources of the $10,000 net savings:
Welfare	= $5,600
Taxes	= $2,300
Criminal justice	= $2,000
Emergency room visits	= $100

*As these savings are projected over the child's life, the savings are much greater.

document fully and succinctly (Stanhope & Kronmueller, 1997). On some forms the nurse uses code numbers, letters, or checkmarks on developmental or disease-specific care plans devised in a checklist format. For example, a packet of four pages may be used to document a home visit when conducting a postpartum visit and newborn assessment: two narrative forms to chart the exceptions for mother and baby and a postpartum and a newborn assessment form where head-to-toe assessment information is documented. These forms have a place to document parent or client teaching according to expected parameters and a place for listing other professionals involved with the family. Similar developmentally focused forms may be used in the agency for high-risk infants, high-risk children, adolescents, and older adults. Other packets of forms may focus on chronic illnesses such as chronic obstructive pulmonary disease, hypertension, diabetes, alcoholism, AIDS, cancer, or whatever types of chronic illnesses are common in the agency client base.

Focus of Family Health Visits

The focus of family health visits differs, based on the mission and resources of the agency providing the service and the needs of the families being served. Some agencies provide education, recreational activities such as summer camps, and support groups for families of people with specific health problems such as Alzheimer's disease, asthma, diabetes, neurological disorders, etc. Other agencies may serve families by providing services directed toward those with special social or economic needs, such as immigrant families, people living in poverty, or the homeless. Home visits may be a part of the services when family members are unable to come to an agency and the service being provided is best conducted and received in the comfort and privacy of a family's home. Generally, family health visits are designed to be educational, to provide anticipatory guidance, and to focus on health promotion or prevention.

FAMILY EDUCATION AND ANTICIPATORY GUIDANCE

Family visits made through official agencies, such as county or city health departments, distribute their services based on the broader community's needs. For example, if there is a large population of teen pregnancies and high-risk infants, the health department may contract with hospitals and private doctors' offices to provide home or clinic visits to all teens or women with high-risk pregnancies and their newborns after delivery. On these visits the community health nurse teaches prenatal, postpartum, and newborn care and provides anticipatory guidance, information needed in the future regarding themselves or their children so they are prepared for what is to come, such as regular infant health care provider visits, immunizations, and safety. Another community may have a significant number of older adults who need to learn how to manage a chronic illness, enhance their nu-

trition, and practice safety measures to prevent injuries and falls.

FAMILY HEALTH PROMOTION AND ILLNESS PREVENTION

All populations, regardless of age, income, culture, or nation of origin, need the fundamental protection immunization gives, for themselves and the health of the larger community. In addition, providing the means for families to receive required immunizations is a responsibility of health departments. Usually immunization services are not brought into the home, but providing information about them, teaching the importance of following an immunization schedule, and following up on them is of paramount importance during home visits.

Teaching people how to prevent illness and how to remain healthy is basic to community health nursing (see Chapter 9). Even within the limitations of chronic illnesses, family members can be taught health promotion activities to live as healthfully as possible (Gorin & Arnold, 1998; Pender, 1996). Health promotion activities may include screening for hypertension and elevated cholesterol, performing physical assessment, and teaching about nutrition and safety.

Such activities can occur during a family health visit, with family members at their places of work, school, or recreation, or at self-help group meetings. Community health nurses often provide health promotion services to couples during prenatal classes by teaching about the expected changes during pregnancy and anticipatory guidance for safe infant care; by screening older adults at senior centers for hypertension or elevated cholesterol; and by teaching family members who attend groups, such as Alcoholics Anonymous or Gamblers Anonymous (see Chapter 35).

Personal Safety on the Home Visit

As mentioned earlier in this chapter, personal safety while traveling throughout the community is essential. In addition, continuation of personal safety while on the home visit must be considered.

Neighborhood, Travel, and Personal Safety. Upon leaving your "base of operation," such as the health department office, neighborhood clinic, homeless shelter, or campus classroom, have with you all the necessary tools to travel the community with safety. Most important, however, is to leave an itinerary of your planned travels, the phone numbers of the families you will attempt to visit, and your cellular phone number. Actually traveling in the community takes a variety of forms and means different things to different people.

If you are traveling in an agency or private car you need:
- a full gas tank
- a city/county map
- a cellular phone
- the family address(es)
- money for lunch or telephone calls (in case you are in an area where your phone does not work)

If you are using public transportation, plan to:
- have exact change for each bus trip
- carry a bus schedule
- exit the bus as near as possible to your client's home
- know where to get the bus for the return trip or to the next home visit
- carry a cellular phone

If you are walking or riding a bicycle to a home visit, you still need to travel safely. All the rules of the road pertain to you as a pedestrian and when on a bike. Do not jaywalk or ride the bicycle on the sidewalk; cross streets at crosswalks and at traffic lights. In some neighborhoods it is best to call ahead to the family you plan to visit, give them an approximate time of your arrival, and, if necessary, have them look out a window or door for your arrival. When walking in neighborhoods, walk with direction and purpose; do not look lost even if you are. Use neighborhood shopkeepers as resources for direction and information and as havens of refuge if you feel uncomfortable or threatened. If you need to ask for directions and you are not near any stores, look for another professional, such as a social worker, a public service employee (a postal worker or utility worker), or an apartment manager. If you need to approach a stranger for information, select a female. If you see a group of teens or adults that make you feel uncomfortable, cross the street, limit eye contact, and continue to the home you are intending to visit. Always avoid walking through alleys or along buildings that open onto alleys; stay on the middle of the sidewalk or closer to the street. It might be useful to carry a whistle on your key ring.

It is always safest to avoid compromising situations by staying alert and using safe traveling methods whenever you are in public, no matter how "safe" an area appears. However, if you are ever accosted by an individual or a group, immediately try to break free and run to a public place while making loud noises. Yell "Fire!" This response gets more attention than "Help." If a criminal wants your nursing bag, purse, or wallet, freely give it up—the contents are not worth your safety. Some nurses feel safer if they have attended self-defense classes, which are offered by police departments, as employee in-service programs in some agencies, and on some university campuses.

In some rough, inner-city neighborhoods, professionals visiting families travel only in pairs (usually with at least one male in the pair) or with a security guard or police escort. Know whether these resources are necessary or available to you before venturing into a crime-ridden community. In some inner-city neighborhoods, community health nurses refuse to visit people living on one block or in one apartment building. Know, and do not challenge, these important safety measures that are discovered by expert nurses and are followed for personal safety. They are unique to each community.

Arriving at the Home. Make sure you are at the right house, and do not go into the home until you are assured that the family you are intending to visit does live there and is home. For example, you may be planning to visit 16-year-old Jennifer and her 5-day-old infant, Marcus. However, when you knock on the door, it is answered by a 50-year-old man. Do not enter the home without asking whether Jennifer can come to the door or unless you see her in the house through the door, even though the man answering the door invites you in. Remain outside the home and only go inside after you talk to Jennifer at the door. This assures you the family members you want to visit are really home and that this is the right address.

Friction Between Family Members. During a home visit, two or more family members may begin to argue or physically fight with one another. Immediately remove yourself from the home visit and tell the family members that you will visit at another time when the family differences are resolved. You must let the family know that it is not a good time to visit when there are such distractions and you must leave. Depending on the type of altercation occurring, it may be appropriate to discuss the friction in the family on a later visit or call 911 from your cellular phone when you are out of the house. Never step in and offer to assist an adult family member when two people are physically fighting; you may be the next victim.

Family Members Under the Influence. If the focus of the visit is on two family members and a third member is demonstrating behaviors that indicate drug or alchohol use, you must use your judgment as to your best action. The agency you work for or the school you attend has guidelines you should follow. However, if the person goes to another room and falls asleep, it might be appropriate to continue the visit and perhaps discuss your observations with the remaining family members. On the other hand, if a person becomes abusive, remains in the room, or interrupts the home visit, it is best to terminate the visit and reschedule when this member is not under the influence or is not present. Again, you do not want to put yourself in the middle of a situation that may deteriorate rapidly, compromising your safety.

The Presence of Strangers. In some families, the coming and going of many extended family members, neighbors, and friends is commonplace and not distracting. However, too many people can create an uncomfortable environment for you. For example, what would you do if you arrived at a home and five teenage boys were sitting on the front porch steps so that you had to sidle your way through to knock on the door? What if you found three men sleeping on the living room floor in a small apartment of a teenage mother and her infant, or four neighbor children riding tricycles inside a house during a teaching visit to two young parents who did not seem fazed by the commotion? Such situations may not be indicative of danger, but they may make you feel vulnerable, uncomfortable, or distracted. It is best to ask the family when there would be a better time to visit, move the visit to another room, or go for a walk with the clients, continuing the visit while outside. In some way, take control of the environment so you feel safe and comfortable and your attention can focus on the family members who are a part of the visit. Certainly, inquire about the other people you see on the periphery of the home visit: ask about their relationship to the family, their general health, and if they should be included in the visit. Be prepared for the family to suggest that you ignore the other people and to say that they are transient family members whom you may never see again. On the other hand, it may be important to learn who they are as they may have unmet health care needs.

IMPLEMENTING PLANS FOR PROMOTING THE HEALTH OF FAMILIES

Once you have received a referral, contacted the family for a visit appointment, prepared for the visit, and met the family, you are ready to implement the plan. As the visit progresses, there are specific activities and actions that you can take to enhance the effectiveness of the visit and improve family health outcomes. These include contracting with the family and promoting the strengths of the family.

Assessing, Teaching, and Referring

The focus of each family visit is different. On a first visit initial assessment data must be obtained, in addition to working with the family to set goals they want to accomplish. On subsequent visits, actions and activities are taken to reach the goals. Specific actions fall mainly in the categories of assessing, teaching, and referring.

Assessing family health may be done informally through observation and occassional questioning, or it can take a more formal approach, with specific questions asked of each family member and including such information as health data, family history, etc. Physical data such as height, weight, pulses, temperature, and blood pressure are recorded on an assessment tool. (Chapter 23 describes family assessment in greater detail.)

With young children, growth and developmental assessment questionnaires or tests may be conducted to measure how well they are meeting growth and developmental tasks. One familiar test used for decades is the Denver Developmental Screening Test II (DDST). The results of this gross assessment screening test provide the nurse with information about the child's growth and developmental progress and are used to teach families anticipatory guidance and how to provide growth-enhancing experiences. This easily administered test can be purchased and comes with a training manual, test kit, and score sheets. There are also videos demonstrating the correct way to administer the DDST to children of different ages. The DDST items can be ordered from DDM, Inc., PO Box 6919, Denver, CO 80203.

If an adult family member has an identified disease process (diabetes, congestive heart failure, substance abuse, hypertension, chronic obstructive pulmonary disease, etc.) or a child has the potential for or has an identified health problem (a high-risk newborn, a drug-exposed infant, failure to thrive, a birth defect, etc.), a flow sheet developed by the agency can be used to guide you in obtaining standard assessment information during the home visit (Fig. 24–1). From this, an individualized approach to additional information can be developed. In addition, older adults may be assessed through observation of activities of daily living and instrumental activities of daily living (Farren, 1999) (see Chapter 30).

While on a home visit, the community health nurse should also conduct a home and family assessment that includes all aspects of the home environment, such as adequacy and permanancy. Education, employment and/or income, furnishings, support systems, and other agencies involved in the family care are different types of family resources that should be assessed (Murry & Zentner, 1997).

The assessment process is lengthy, time consuming, and ongoing. The nurse must gather the most essential assessment information on a first visit by selecting one or two concerns of priority to the family and nurse and focus assessment on these areas. Once gathered, this information will guide the nurse to additional assessments needed on subsequent visits. Once the selected assessment tools have been completed and reveal family information, these data are used to best assist the family during future visits by teaching them or by referring them to appropriate sevices available in the community.

Teaching health promotion activities to the family must be conducted only after they express an interest and recognize a need. If the family is not at a level of functioning to use anticipatory guidance and teaching, the nurse has other, more basic roles with the family, such as gathering resources and acting as a counselor (Tapia, 1997). If they are ready to learn ways to improve their health status, the nurse needs to assess the best teaching approach to use (see Chapter 9). Considerations of language barriers, previous knowledge and experience, family and community resources, and time available will influence the approaches used.

Often the community health nurse discovers that the family has needs beyond teaching and that there are others in the community with the skills and services to meet those needs. When this occurs, the nurse helps to initiate the referral process. Referring families is discussed in detail later in this chapter.

Contracting

Contracting is a method of formalizing the relationship between the family and the community health nurse and includes a verbal or written commitment on the part of the family and the nurse for the development and accomplishment of goals (see Chapter 8). Such a contract contains **mutual goals**—goals that the family and the nurse plan and take action on together. It is easy to go into a family's home, see exactly what is wrong, and set about "making it right" according to your values. You might think, "If only the family would wash their dishes each evening, keep the

Page 1

FLOW SHEET
HIGH RISK INFANT

Pt's Name _____ Address _____ Phone _____

At Birth: Weight _____ Length _____ Head Circ. _____ APGARS _____

	Date							
Irritability								
Lethargic								
Vomiting								
Diarrhea								
Feedings								
• Amount								
• Frequency								
• Suck								
Seizures/Convulsions								
Stools								
• Color								
• Consistency								
• Frequency								
Urine Output								
Edema								
Eyes Roll								
Temperature								
Pulse								
Respiration								
Weight								
Length								
Femoral Pulses								
Reflexes								
Muscle Tone								
Skin								
• Color								
• Condition								
Auscultate Chest								
Edema								
Output-Concentration								
Respiratory Function								
• Nasal Flaring								
• Grunting								
• Sternal Retracting								
• Tachycardia								
Head Circumference								
Chest Circumference								
Initials								

O - Normal   X - Problem (See Narrative)   C - Counseled for prevention

FIGURE 24–1. High-risk infant flow sheet.

Immunization (Circle & Date)

DPT 1 2 3 4 5 _____ PPD _____ MMR _____ Hib _____

Polio 1 2 3 4 5 _____ Hep B _____ Varicella _____

Instruction	Instruction Date	Pt. Understanding Date	Pamphlets Given Date	Comments	Initials
Review Disease Process					
Temperature Technique					
Feeding & Technique					
Bonding					
General Care					
• Bath					
• Hygiene					
• Formula Preparation					
• Cord Care					
Prevention of Infection					
Environment - Temperature Control					
Position					
Growth & Development					
Safety					
Stimulation					
Immunizations					
Referred to:					
Medical App./Date/M.D.					
S/S of Sick Child					

Initials	Signature

FIGURE 24–1. (*continued*)

floors uncluttered, put sheets on the bed, set an alarm and get up in the morning to get the children off to school, stop spending money on beer and cigarettes and buy milk and orange juice instead, etc., then most of their problems would be solved." It is easy to criticize from the outside and make blanket judgments and decisions about what others should do. As an observer, you may value clean dishes, swept floors, sleeping on sheets, getting your children to school, and drinking milk and orange juice. However, not all of these values are essential to the family's functioning. Instead, your role as a nurse is to influence the choices a family makes that influence their health, safety, and comfort. If the cluttered floors cause falls or the dirty dishes attract roaches and rats, you might find that intervening and teaching the family about the connection between these factors is important. If the family decides that a change in be-

havior is one of their goals and you agree to assist them with the change, this mutual goal could be formalized through a contract (Display 24–3).

Empowering Families

Throughout the family visit process, the nurse must remember that the ultimate goal is to assist the family to be independent of her or his services. This is accomplished through the approaches you use as you conduct the visit. How you structure the nurse–client relationship will also influence the direction of the outcomes. Four thoughts will help you clarify your working relationship with families.

- The family was functioning in a manner that worked for them before you ever met them.

DISPLAY 24-3. Sample Family Contract

Jane Doe, community health nurse, is agreeing to visit Sally Jones two times a month from 1/2/01–4/4/01 to work together towards helping Brian, aged 3, become toilet trained by April, 2001.

Jane Doe will:
1. Make 8 home visits during the next 4 months, focusing on toilet training
2. Bring Sally a pamphlet about successful toilet training and use it as a teaching guide
3. On each visit, reinforce progress and make suggestions for improvement
4. Praise the successful accomplishment of toilet training or renegotiate the contract

Sally Jones will:
1. Purchase a potty-seat and underpants for Brian during the first two weeks of working together
2. Read a story to Brian about toilet training and a little boy his age
3. Be consistent in following the successful toilet-training steps
4. Discuss her feelings about progress and setbacks with Jane Doe on each visit
5. Celebrate toilet training success; work with Jane to renegotiate the contract

Jane Doe, signature _____

Sally Jones, signature _____

Date _____

- If you ever feel obliged to do something for a family, consider who did this before you were available.
- Find family strengths even in the most deprived family situation.
- If you were in a similar situation would you manage as well, cope as well, or function as well as the members of this family?

Families have strengths that middle-class nurses may overlook or interpret as weaknesses. It is our job to recognize the strengths in families and help them recognize them as well. For example, some families borrow needed items (diapers, food, clothes) from each other, while some of us do not even recognize our next-door neighbors. Children from large families often learn to physically care for one another and entertain themselves, while our own family with only one or two children must constantly be entertained. A family's members may take public transportation or walk to accomplish errands, while we may take our car on the closest of errands and may never have been on a bus or subway. These are strengths that some middle-class families have forgotten or never developed.

At times, community health nurses want to help families by taking them to a doctor or to the store or bringing them a supply of formula or diapers. It might be a simple task since you will be driving by the clinic anyway or there are extra cans of formula in the agency office . . . but are you promoting their independence and self-sufficiency? It is a much better gift to promote family skills to plan ahead to meet their own transportation needs (neighbors, family members, loose change saved for the bus, or even walking) or to find ways to use their formula supplies wisely. For example, they could fill bottles to the amount the baby consumes so ounces are not wasted at each feeding; keep unused formula refrigerated so it is not wasted; be sure infants are not being overfed formula by assessing amounts consumed in 24 hours; progress to other foods and fluids at age-appropriate times; keep a can of powdered formula on hand for emergencies; or switch to powdered formula if using the more expensive premixed or concentrated formula types. Once they learn these skills, crises will occur less frequently or be managed more effectively.

Finally, always look for ways to genuinely praise families for managing under difficult situations. For example, on a home visit you can empower families by pointing out the positive aspects of their self-care and caregiving, rather than pointing out what they do not do or have. Verbally list these positive aspects in a natural and conversational manner. For example, a young woman greets you at the door holding her baby. You note that she has a dresser drawer for her baby to sleep in next to her mattress on the floor in a sparsely furnished one-room apartment. She has two baby bottles and a limited assortment of baby clothes. Later in this first visit you say, "Carlo looks so happy when you cuddle him in your arms, and you are considering his safety by letting him sleep in the dresser drawer next to your mattress. I notice you wash each bottle before making the formula, and you are keeping him warm in the sleeper and blanket. I think you are managing Carlo very well." In this brief scenario you are mentioning, in a positive way, bonding, infant health and safety, and proper infant clothing. You are not mentioning the absence of furniture, a full set of bottles, or a layette of clothing. You would continue with the visit to discuss the services of your agency and assess whether she feels any of them would be of interest to her. You would allow her to make decisions for her family and to use you as a resource and guide (Reutter & Ford, 1997). This encourages empowerment.

EVALUATING IMPLEMENTED FAMILY HEALTH PLANS

The final step in the nursing process is evaluation. The evaluation process leads to a reassessment of your work with the family and what is needed to be prepared for the next family visit. This reassessment will guide you to further individualize services to the family. Evaluation of the structure-process of the visit and yourself can be done informally in a reflective manner. Outcomes will be documented in the client record, and the evaluation becomes formalized. A thorough evaluation also assists you with making the most appropriate referrals and contacting key resources to meet family needs.

Types of Evaluations

Each family visit should be evaluated in three ways: structure-process, outcomes, and self-evaluation. Each gives you a different piece of information about the success of the visit. If it was not successful, what part of it made it less than successful? Most importantly, were the outcomes achieved? If not, was there something about the structure-process or your own preparedness or behavior that needs to be changed? When conducting an evauation of the home visit, you are looking for answers to these questions.

STRUCTURE-PROCESS

First, the structure-process of the visit should be analyzed. Were there aspects of the organization, timing, environment, or sequencing of the components that needed to be changed or modified to make it a more effective visit? What could you have done about these? Were you organized? Would better preparation help with your organization? Were there distractions in the home that influenced organization? Ask yourself questions such as these, and then make mental plans to avoid or reduce disorganizing distractions. For example, if you made the visit based on limited information found on a referral, you now have additional family data and can be better prepared for the next visit. If transportation schedules made the family late to the clinic, could other transportaiton be arranged? If the distractions on a home visit were school-aged chidren arriving home from school, visit earlier in the day before they get home. If the television was playing loudly, make it a point to ask the family whether they would mind turning down the volume, or visit at a time when they do not watch TV. Make the modifications that you can to assist with the visit process.

OUTCOME EVALUATION

Second, and most important, are the outcomes of the visit. Were the anticipated outcomes of the visit achieved? If not, why? If so, what made it possible? The **outcome evaluation,** or the assessment of change in the family's (client's) health status based on mutually agreed upon activities, is a formal process demonstrated in the documentation of the home visit. Visit by visit, the changes observed in the family may be small. Progress toward outcome expectation is noted. At the conclusion of the agency services to the family, the accumulated change achievement of outcomes are evaluated. This may necessitate a reevaluation of the decision to terminate services and to continue them with renegotiated additional services. Whatever the decision, the family must be included in the decision-making process.

SELF-EVALUATION

The third component of evaluation is self-evaluation. What about your performance as a community health nurse during the home visit helped toward outcome achievement? Were you prepared? Did you gather all data needed to assist the family on the next visit? What would you do differently if you could do the visit over? What went right? What went wrong? What are you going to do on the next visit to make it better? This close look at yourself is important for your own growth and effectiveness as a community health nurse.

Sometimes we cannot see our own strengths or flaws and being evaluated by others is helpful. In some agencies regular peer evaluations are conducted. An agency staff nurse makes a family visit with you and gives you feedback based on her or his observations. This is a useful technique to use even when it is not a planned evaluation time for all staff in the agency. You might ask a colleague to accompany you on a home visit to a family that is not progressing toward outcome achievement or to a family you feel you have not been able to "reach" or find difficult to work with (Cuellar & Glazer, 1996; Josten et al., 1995). For a variety of reasons, consulting with peers regarding certain visits and how to best conduct them can assist you to be better prepared or more focused or to improve your interaction with families from different cultures or in difficult situations (Spector, 2000; Walsh, 1999).

Planning for the Next Visit

Part of the evaluation of one family visit is planning for the next visit. What occured on the previous visit will guide you toward activities on subsequent visits. Goals may need to be modified, or family situations may change and specific outcomes are no longer relevant. For example, you may be planning to visit a prenatal family one last time before they give birth to reinforce when to leave for the hospital with a second pregnancy, to arrange babysitting for the older child, and to assess the pregnant woman's rising blood pressure and complaints of backache. When you arrive for the visit, the husband is home alone with the younger child, planning to leave soon to bring his wife and new baby home from the hospital; he asks you about the diaper rash that just came up on their 2-year-old and how to secure the new car seat into the car as the instructions do not seem to make sense in his make of car. Outcomes for a problem-free pregnancy and healthy birth are not relevant; there are new outcomes to be formulated and worked on with this young family.

More frequently, the planning for subsequent visits is more predictable and is done to ensure that steps toward outcome accomplishment are achieved on the visit. Being totally prepared each time is the best predictor of a successful family visit. Once you have met and gotten to know a family during a visit, the planning can be individualized and tailored to meet their unique needs. This information cannot come through clearly on a paper referral, making the planning for a first home visit important in setting the tone for your continued success with the family.

REFERRALS

A referral in written or verbal form (by agency-created form, telephone, fax, or e-mail) initiates contact with a family. In addition to responding to a referral as a community health nurse, which begins the relationship with a family, the nurse makes referrals on behalf of clients. Families often need access to services beyond the agency's scope of services, and the nurse is the difference between their receiving or not receiving these services. Therefore, nurses must have information available to them about eligibility for and availability of services provided by a bevy of official, voluntary, religious, and neighborhood organizations. If this information is not readily at hand, community health nurses need to know how to locate needed services. This is a daunting challenge as the services are many and frequently organizations change telephone numbers, services, and the populations they serve. Networking with colleagues on a regular basis helps keep nurses up to date with community services from which they can generate referrals for clients.

CONTACTING RESOURCES

At times, community health nurses implement their role as a client advocate and help families gain services in a more timely manner than they can operating on their own. Community health nurses know how to access key personnel in agencies and can eliminate some of the red tape involved in obtaining some services. They share with families specific aspects to receiving the needed services, such as arriving at the agency mid-week and early in the morning, having all forms completely filled out, bringing the last 3 months' rent and utility receipts, asking to speak with a certain worker, etc.

When nurses are seeking to obtain more informal services for families, their relationship with the director of the agency can help them gain services for the clients. For example, a family being visited is having a personal crisis and needs a donation of food and a volunteer to stay with a handicapped child for 3 days while a spouse is having surgery. The nurse telephones the religious leader of a neighborhood church and shares the family's requests, clarifying their situation, and is able to get a donation of food from the church's food pantry and the name of a member of the church to stay with the child. The family may not have been aware such services were available to them, and the nurse's linking them to the service is as important as other community health nursing functions.

SUMMARY

Making family health visits is a unique role for nurses and is one of the activities that is common to most community health nurses. In some agencies, family health visits are con- ducted for only the most high-risk families. In other agencies, a visit is the method of choice for most care.

When nurses visit families, they must use acute observation skills, good verbal and nonverbal communication, assessment skills, and a "sixth sense" to guide them safely in the community and with the families. At times, visits are conducted with families in community health settings other than their homes. Neighborhood clinics, school, and work or recreational settings may be the preferred settings or the only settings in which you can gather most of the family members for the visit. Other families may be in transition and are in homeless shelters or living with relatives or neighbors. These settings are familiar to the family and provide a unique environment for the nurse to visit with the family.

Pre-visit preparing, conducting, and documenting the visit make up the main components of the family health visit. Each step is important and has value towards the success of the next step. Being well prepared with the location and family health status information and having the needed materials for the visit is a first concern. Conducting the visit is best done in an orderly and organized fashion. Time is allowed for getting acquainted; for the body of the visit, which includes teaching and anticipatory guidance; and for any other nursing care that may be a part of the visit. Concluding with a summary of the important parts of the visit and planning for the next visit ensures an appropriate ending.

Going into the neighborhood safely is important for all people. However, community health nurses spend a great part of their day in the community, and traveling safely is of constant importance. Using a personal or agency car, public transportation, or walking to visit families each has its own set of precautions for personal safety. Even in a family's home you must think of personal safety. If family members are arguing, using drugs, or are alcohol intoxicated, the safety of the situation may deteriorate rapidly and it is best to terminate the visit.

During the implementation phase of the family health visit, the nurse establishes a verbal or written contract with the family. This permits both the family and the nurse to know personal roles and responsibilities in the relationship. Empowering family members is significant to clients. With empowerment, people can help themselves for a lifetime and become independent decision-makers for their own health.

Evaluating and preparing for the next visit completes the cycle of family health visiting. Three types of evaluation can be conducted at the end of a visit. Recalling the structure-process of the visit assists you in reflecting on the physical aspects of the visit that were positive or negative. Discovering these can help you enhance the positive and eliminate the negative. Evaluating whether the outcomes of the visit were achieved is done in a more formal way through agency documentation techniques. Since the purpose of conducting family health visits is to bring about positive changes in family behaviors, it is necessary to evaluate the achievement of mutual goals you made with the family. The hardest part of evaluation is looking at yourself and how you make home visits. Often having a peer evaluate you is a most helpful way to obtain feedback. We often minimize our strengths and may overlook our weaknesses.

Conducting family health visits involves making referrals to other agencies and services on behalf of the family. One agency cannot provide all the services a family needs. These written or verbal forms of communicating a need involve contacting resources available in the community. Community health nurses have unique skills in knowing and locating both official and voluntary services within their community that come with experience.

ACTIVITIES TO PROMOTE CRITICAL THINKING

1. Invite a peer to go on a family health visit with you, and be open to feedback regarding your strengths and weaknesses on the visit. How does it make you feel to have someone else on a family health visit with you, knowing that they are observing your skills? Offer to do the same with a peer and provide him or her with feedback. Discuss your experiences.

2. Go on several family health visits with an experienced community health nurse to observe her or his visiting techniques. Observe how he or she contacted the family, knocked on the door, greeted the family, conducted the visit, summarized and concluded the visit, and made plans for the next visit. Discuss the various techniques used, and ask questions about your observations to get a better feeling for why things were done as they were. Use some of this information on your next home visit.

3. Initiate a small group discussion among your peers about safety on your school campus and community, encouraging each to share the safety habits used. How are these techniques different from safety techniques used when making family visits in the community? If they are different, why are they? Should they be different?

4. Locate nursing websites on the internet and look for the following studies on family health: Kitzman, H., Olds, D., Henderson, C., et al. (1997); Olds, D., Eckenrode, J., Henderson, C., et al. (1997); and Olds, D. L., Henderson, C.R. Jr., Kitzman, H.J., et al. (1999). All three studies include intensive home visits to high-risk families. How does intensive family health visiting make a difference in the lives of the participants of these studies? Do you know any communities where the Olds model of home visiting to families is being replicated? If so, how do the results of visiting these families compare with the results found in this classic study?

REFERENCES

Allender, J.A. (1998). *Community and home health nursing.* Philadelphia: Lippincott-Raven.

Cuellar, I., & Glazer, M. (1996). The impact of culture on the family. In M. Harway (Ed.), *Treating the changing family: Handling normative and unusual events.* American Counseling Association. New York: John Wiley & Sons.

Farren, M. (1999). Ensuring safety for the elderly client at home. In S. Zang & J.A. Allender, *Home care of the elderly* (pp. 59–77). Philadelphia: Lippincott Williams & Wilkins.

Friedman, M.M. (1998). *Family nursing: Research, theory, and practice* (4th ed.). Stamford, CT: Appleton & Lange.

Gorin, S.S., & Arnold, J. (1998). *Health promotion handbook.* St. Louis: Mosby.

Josten, L., Mullett, S., Savik, K., et al. (1995). Client characteristics associated with not keeping appointments for public health nursing home visits. *Public Health Nursing, 12*(5), 305–311.

Karoly, L.A., Everingham, S.S., Hoube, J., et al. (1998). *Investing in our children: What we know and don't know about the costs and benefits of early childhood interventions.* MR—898, Santa Monica, CA: RAND.

Kitzman, H., Olds, D., Henderson, C., et al. (1997). Effect of prenatal and infancy home visitation by nurses on pregnancy outcomes, childhood injuries, and repeated childbearing: A randomized controlled trial. *Journal of the American Medical Association, 278*(8), 644–652.

Murry, R.B., & Zentner, J.P. (1997). *Health assessment and promotion strategies through the life span* (6th ed.). Stamford, CT: Appleton & Lange.

Olds, D., Eckenrode, J., Henderson, C., et al. (1997). Long-term effects of home visitation on maternal life course and child abuse and neglect: Fifteen-year follow-up of a randomized trial. *Journal of the American Medical Association, 278*(8), 637–643.

Olds, D. L., Henderson, C.R. Jr., Kitzman, H.J., et al. (1999). Prenatal and infancy home visitation by nurses: Recent findings. *The Future of Children. Home Visit: Recent Program Evaluations, 9*(1), 44–65.

Pender, N.J. (1996). *Health promotion in nursing practice* (3rd ed.). Stamford, CTL Appleton & Lange.

Reutter, L., & Ford, J. (1997). Enhancing client competence: Melding professional and client knowledge in public health nursing. *Public Health Nursing, 14*(3), 143–150.

Schorr, T.M. & Kennedy, M.S. (1999). *100 years of American nursing.* Philadelphia: Lippincott Williams & Wilkins.

Spector, R.E. (2000). *Cultural diversity in health and illness* (5th ed.). Upper Saddle River, NJ: Prentice-Hall Health.

Stanhope, M. & Kronmueller, R.N. (1997). *Public and community health nurse's consultant: A health promotion guide.* St. Louis: Mosby.

Tapia, J.A. (1997). The nursing process in family health. In B.W. Spradley & J.A. Allender, *Readings in community health nursing* (5th ed., pp. 343–350). Philadelphia: Lippincott-Raven.

Walsh, M. (1999). Dealing effectively with physically and verbally abusive elderly clients and families. In S. Zang & J.A. Allender (Eds.), *Home care of the elderly* (pp. 190–206). Philadelphia: Lippincott Williams & Wilkins.

Zerwekh, J.V. (1997). Making the connection during home visits: Narratives of expert nurses. *International Journal for Human Caring, 1*(1), 25–29.

SELECTED READINGS

Baltazar, V., Ibe, O.B., & Allender, J.A. (1999). Maintaining optimum nutrition among elderly clients at home. In S. Zang & J.A. Allender (Eds.), *Home care of the elderly* (pp. 98–121). Philadelphia: Lippincott Williams & Wilkins.

Barton, J. & Brown, N. (1995). Home visitation to migrant farm workers: An application of Zerwekh's family caregiving model for pubic health nursing. *Holistic Nursing Practice, 9*(4), 34–40.

Becvar, D.S. & Becvar, R. (1996). *Family therapy: A systematic integration.* Needham Heights, MA: Allyn and Bacon.

Biller, H.B. (1993). *Fathers and families: Paternal factors in child development.* Westport, CT: Auburn House.

Bomar, P.J. (Ed.) (1996). *Nurses and family health promotion: Concepts, assessment, and interventions* (2nd Ed.). Philadelphia: W.B. Saunders.

Bulechek, G.M. & McCloskey, J.C. (Eds.) (1999). *Nursing interventions: Essential nursing treatments* (3rd ed.). Philadelphia: W.B. Saunders.

Byrd, M.E. (1995). The home visiting process in the contexts of the voluntary vs. required visit: Examples from fieldwork. *Public Health Nursing, 12,* 196–202.

Cherry, B., & Giger, J.N. (1995). African-Americans. In J.N. Giger & R.E. Davidhizar, *Transcultural nursing: Assessment and intervention* (2nd ed., pp. 165–203). St. Louis: Mosby.

Cooper, W.O. (1996). Use of health care services by inner-city infants in an early discharge program. *Pediatrics, 98,* 686–691.

David, L.L. (1996). Dementia caregiving studies: A typology for family interventions. *Journal of Family Nursing, 2*(3), 30–55.

Jacobs, J. (1993). Families under siege. *Family Therapy Networker, 17*(1), 24–25.

Liepert, B.D. (1996). The value of community health nursing: A phenomenological study of the perceptions of community health nurses. *Public Health Nursing, 13,* 50–57.

Parecl, T.L., & Menaghan, E.G. (1997). Effects of low-wage emolyment on family well-being. *The Future of Children. Welfare to Work, 7*(1), 116–121.

Pearson, J.L., Hunter, A.G., Cook, J.M., et al. (1997). Grandmother involvement in child caregiving in an urban community. *Gerontologist, 37*(5), 650–657.

Rhein, L.M., Ginsburg, K.R., Schwarz, D.F., et al. (1997). Teen father participation in child rearing: Family perspectives. *Journal of Adolescent Health, 21,* 244–252.

Robinson, C.A. (1994). Nursing interventions with families: A demand or an invitation to change? *Journal of Advanced Nursing, 19*(5), 897–904.

Schwebel, A.I. & Fine, M.A. (1994). *Understanding and helping families: A cognitive-behavioral approach.* Hillsdale, NJ: Lawrence Erlbaum Associates.

Snelling, J. (1994). The effect of chronic pain on the family unit. *Journal of Advanced Nursing, 19,* 543–551.

Thompson, P. (1998). Adolescents from families of divorce: Vulnerability to physiological and psychological disturbances. *Journal of Psychosocial Nursing and Mental Health Services, 36*(3), 34–39.

Vaughn-Cole, B., Johnson, M.A., Malone, J.A., & Walker, B.L. (1998). *Family nursing practice.* Philadelphia: W.B. Saunders.

Wagner, M.M., & Clayton, S.I. (1999). The parents as teachers program: Results from two demonstrations. *The Future of Children. Home Visiting: Recent Program Evaluations, 9*(19), 91–115.

Wallace, H.M., Green, G., Jaros, K., Paine, L., & Story, M. (1999). *Health and welfare for families in the 21st century.* Boston: Jones and Bartlett.

Wright, L.M. & Leahey, M. (1994). *Nurses and families* (2nd ed.). Philadelphia: F.A. Davis.

Families in Crisis: Domestic Violence and Abuse

KEY TERMS

- Battered child syndrome
- Child abuse
- Coping
- Corporal punishment
- Crisis theory
- Cycle of violence
- Dating violence
- Developmental crisis
- Domestic violence
- Elder abuse
- Emotional abuse
- Family crisis
- Family violence
- Homicide
- Incest
- Intrafamilial sexual abuse
- Mandated reporters
- Munchausen syndrome by proxy
- Neglect
- Pedophile
- Physical abuse
- Rape
- Sexual abuse
- Sexual exploitation
- Shaken baby syndrome
- Situational crisis
- Spousal abuse
- Suicide

LEARNING OBJECTIVES

Upon mastery of this chapter, you should be able to:

- Explain the difference between developmental crises and situational crises and give several examples of each within families.
- Discuss strategies to prevent the impact of a situational crisis and a developmental crisis at each level of prevention.
- Discuss the global incidence and prevalence of family violence.
- Describe how the U.S. has historically responded to family violence.
- Describe three main categories of family violence.
- Identify characteristics of five forms of abuse against infants, children, and adolescents.
- Describe the "cycle of violence" seen in partner/spousal abuse.
- Explain the types of mistreatment common to the elderly.
- Describe the role of a community health nurse with families in crisis at each level of prevention.
- Use the steps of the nursing process to outline nursing actions in developmental and situational crises.

Family crisis is a stressful and disruptive event (or series of events) that comes with or without warning and disturbs the equilibrium of the family. A family crisis can also result when usual problem-solving methods fail. All families experience periods of crisis: a toddler is diagnosed with a serious illness; a teenager discovers she is pregnant; a father and sole breadwinner in a family loses his job; a mother's social drinking becomes habitual after her children go off to college; a family's home is destroyed in a hurricane, earthquake, flood, or fire. If you think back on your own family's history, you will likely be able to identify one or more periods of crisis that you and your family members have experienced. If so, how directly were you affected? How did the crisis resolve? As a result of the crisis, were there any permanent changes in your family's dynamics or individual behaviors?

People respond to crises differently. Some approach them as a challenge, an event to be reckoned with; others are overwhelmed and feel defeated or give up. Some seek help if needed and come through the experience unscathed or as survivors, perhaps even stronger than before. Others who are unable to cope with the crisis, or do not cope well, may suffer severe psychological damage or may inflict their feelings of rage, frustration, or powerlessness on their children, partners, or elders. In this chapter, we will focus on families that have responded to stressors with violence, neglect, and abuse.

Regardless of their responses, families in crisis need help, and community health nurses have a unique opportunity and responsibility to provide that help in a broad variety of situations. For example, in one family, an 8-year-old boy begins doing poorly in school, wets his pants during class twice in one week, and starts a small fire in the schoolyard. The school nurse is astute enough to begin an investigation into the family dynamics that may be contributing to these symptoms. In another family, a pregnant woman reschedules her appointment at a community clinic twice, then arrives with multiple faded bruises on her face and arms. The clinic nurse uses sensitivity and caring to screen her for domestic violence. In addition to assessment, community health nurses provide direct assistance during times of crisis, and they help prevent crises by teaching families parenting skills and coping strategies. This chapter examines how nurses can sharpen their knowledge and skills in the practice of crisis prevention and intervention in order to promote the health of families in the community.

DYNAMICS AND CHARACTERISTICS OF A CRISIS

Researchers have studied the nature of crises and have developed a body of knowledge called **crisis theory.** Initially limited to the field of mental health, crisis theory now influences every field of health care, helping to explain why people respond in certain ways to predict the phases that people will go through in a crisis of any kind. These are important ideas for the community health nurse to understand before crises can be prevented or managed.

How does a crisis occur? All people are dynamic systems living within a given environment under circumstances unique to us alone. Our behavior—both consciously and subconsciously—is gauged to maintain a balance within ourselves and in our relations with others. When some internal or external force disrupts our system's balance and alters its functioning, loss of equilibrium occurs. We then attempt to restore our equilibrium by using whatever resources we have available to us, in an effort to cope with the situation. **Coping** refers to those actions and ways of thinking that assist people in dealing with and surviving difficult situations. If we cannot readily cope with a stressful event—for example, if our home is destroyed by fire, or we fail all our final exams—we experience crisis.

Thus, crises are precipitated by specific identifiable events that become too much for the usual problem-solving skills of those involved. Often, a single distressing event follows a host of previous difficulties and becomes the "straw that breaks the camel's back." For example, a wife who suffers years of spousal abuse finally becomes unable to cope and shoots her husband during a violent attack. Occasionally tragic events occur suddenly without previous stressors—a father is killed in a plane crash or a child drowns in the family swimming pool.

Crises are normal in that all people feel overwhelmed occasionally. It is very possible that a person who intervenes in today's crisis will be tomorrow's crisis victim. No individual is immune from sudden overwhelming difficulties. For example, a hospice nurse assists families through crises as part of her job. Suddenly the nurse learns that her own spouse is diagnosed with cancer.

A crisis is not an event per se, but rather a person's perception of the event. Each person reacts in his or her own individual way. A situation that throws one person off course may merely create an interesting detour for another (Display 25–1). It is the individual's interpretation of the event, rather than the event itself, that is crucial.

DISPLAY 25–1. Two Families' Response to Crisis

The Redondos and the Fosters will be moving to a town in another state, 900 miles away, because of a job change. The Redondos are in crisis over the move. They have never lived in any other town. They will have to leave relatives and lifelong friends who live nearby and a community in which they have been very involved. Mrs. Redondo is the secretary at her family's house of worship. Their teenage daughter, a cheerleader, just started high school. Their son is in kindergarten; Grandma happily watches him in the mornings before school. Everyone is upset because of how the move will affect them. The family is stressed and argues each evening. They don't want to put their house up for sale or even to visit the new community to which they will be moving. Mr. Redondo is second guessing his decision to move, but his choices were limited as his company is relocating. The Redondos, in crisis, are not exploring alternatives that may allow them to stay in their present community. One possible alternative might be for Mrs. Redondo to work while Mr. Redondo looks for another job. When people perceive that they are in crisis, decision making and solving problems becomes more difficult.

The Fosters, however, are excitedly looking forward to their move. They have two young children who are not yet in school. The move will bring them only 50 miles from old college friends. They hope to realize a significant profit on their house, which they recently remodeled. They can't wait to go "house hunting" in the new town. Everyone is enjoying planing the anticipated move; their two children, aged 3 and 4, have been playing "moving day" with their favorite toys.

Both families are experiencing the same event. The difference is each person's situation and perception of the event. The Redondos' equilibrium is being disrupted. They have not developed previous coping skills and do not see the move as a positive experience. They are at a different time in their family life cycle than are the Fosters. Although the move upsets their equilibrium, too, the Fosters experienced it as an exciting event that conjures positive feelings; they are passing these feeling on to their children. They see this move as an opportunity.

Crises are resolved, either positively or negatively, within a brief period of time, usually 4 to 8 weeks (Tyra, 1996; Aguilera, 1997). People's strong need to regain homeostasis and the intense nature of crises both work to make them temporary conditions that cannot continue indefinitely. In the family of the wife who shot her abusive husband, as shocking as the event might seem, life returns to a recognizable pattern in a few weeks. Although the members will feel the change for years, the crisis will soon disappear. The husband is hospitalized and recovers from his wound; the wife's case goes to trial, and she is sentenced to 2 years in prison; the children stay with relatives and attend school.

Crisis resolution can be an adaptive process in which growth and improved health occur, or it can be maladaptive, resulting in illness or even death. The battered wife reevaluates her life, gets divorced, learns employment skills in jail, becomes more assertive with stronger self-esteem, and returns to her children able to support them financially and emotionally when she is paroled. She finds growth and health while successfully resolving the crisis. The children settle into their aunt's home with minimal difficulty, start a new school, and visit their mother and father regularly. When their mother is released, she finds an apartment near her sister's home so the children can continue in the same school district. The husband recovers from his wounds, gets counseling, relocates to another town, and sees his children frequently. This crisis situation was resolved at a higher level of wellness for all members than existed before the crisis. In this example, the members were determined to improve their situation by working with skilled health care professionals. By using the resources within the community, this family is healthier after their crisis.

Developmental Crises

Developmental crises are periods of disruption that occur at transition points during normal growth and development (Display 25–2). When developmental crises occur, people feel threatened by the demands placed on them and have difficulty making the changes necessary to fit the new stage of development.

During the process of normal biopsychosocial growth, people go through a succession of life cycle stages from birth through old age. Each stage is quite different from the previous one, and transitions from one stage to the next require changes in roles and behavior. There are periods of upset and disequilibrium. Popular authors such as Sheehy (1976, 1995) and Levinson (1978) have called these periods "passages" and "transitions." They are the times when developmental or maturational crises occur (Tyra, 1996).

Most family developmental crises have a gradual onset. The change is evolutionary rather than revolutionary. People usually anticipate and even prepare to start school, enter adolescence, leave home, marry, have a baby, retire, or die. They move into and through each transitional period knowing in

---

DISPLAY 25–2. Major Differences Between Types of Crises

Developmental Crisis
Part of normal growth and development that can upset normalcy
Precipitated by a life transition point
Gradual onset
Response to developmental demands and society's expectations

Situational Crisis
Unexpected period of upset in normalcy
Precipitated by a hazardous event
Sudden onset
Externally imposed "accident"

---

advance that some kind of change will be required. In many instances, people have already seen others experience these transitions. As a result, developmental crises have a degree of predictability. They offer the possibility of a period of time for anticipation and adjustment.

Developmental crises arise from both physical and social changes. Each new life stage confronts people with changed relationships, responsibilities, and roles. The transition to parenthood, for example, demands a change in role from caring for oneself and one's mate to include nurturing, caring for, and protecting a completely helpless infant. Relationships with adults, children, and even one's own parents also change. Parenthood is an entrance into a previously unexperienced part of the adult world. New parents may fear the unknown. Will this infant develop normally? Can I give adequate care? Parents often feel anxiety over the responsibility of shaping this new person's life and satisfying society's expectations for their child's proper education and training. They may worry about the increased financial burden and struggle with mixed feelings about giving up a large measure of freedom. These transitions put people under considerable stress, which contributes to tension, feelings of helplessness, and resultant crisis. Some people adapt quickly; others cannot cope, probably because earlier developmental crises went unresolved. When people lack a repertoire of adaptive skills, even positive and planned changes can develop into crises (Display 25–3).

Situational Crises

A **situational crisis** is a stressful disruption event arising from an external event that occurs suddenly, often without warning, to a person, group, aggregate, or community. Typically, the external events require behavioral changes and coping mechanisms beyond the abilities of the people involved.

Such events are not predicted, expected, or planned. They occur to people because of where they are in time and space.

DISPLAY 25–3. **A Developmental Crisis**

Marcia Sand is 39 years old. Married for 22 years, she has been a capable homemaker and mother of four children. Her husband, Lou, a construction worker for the past 20 years, thinks Marcia does a "super job at home." In the past, Marcia's time was filled with cooking, laundry, cleaning, shopping, and meeting the endless demands of the family. Their limited income prompted her to adopt many money-saving strategies. She made most of her own and the children's clothes, did all her own baking, and raised vegetables in her backyard garden. Now the youngest of the children, Tommy, has just left home to join the Navy. Her husband spends much of his spare time at the local bar with his friends, leaving Marcia alone. With a nearly empty house and little need for cooking, baking, and sewing, Marcia has lost her sense of usefulness. She thinks of taking a job, but knows her choices are limited because she has only a high school education. Marcia has not slept well in weeks; she wakes up tired and drags through the day barely able to manage the simplest task. She cries frequently but does not know why. Her hair, always neat and attractive in the past, looks bedraggled, and her shoulders slump. "I just can't seem to get on top of things any more," she complains.

Marcia has entered a developmental crisis that is sometimes called the "empty nest syndrome." She faces a turning point in her life, a time when parenting has seemingly ended. Leaving her satisfying homemaker role, she faces a new life stage filled with unknowns, changes, and a seeming lack of purpose. The transition came about gradually, almost imperceptibly, but now she must deal with it. Yet she feels unable to cope and wishes to turn to someone who would understand and lend her strength. She can be helped, but her crisis could also have been prevented at the pre-crisis phase. Anticipatory planning could have prevented the dilemma Marcia finds herself in now.

For instance, a baby grabs her mother's hot cup of tea and burns her chest; a college student is raped in the library parking lot; an older adult falls and fractures a hip; a mother with a van full of Little League baseball players has a crash at a busy intersection; a couple, after 25 years of marriage, gets divorced; and a hurricane devastates a town. These kinds of events, which involve loss or the threat of loss, represent life hazards to those affected. Some crisis-precipitating events can be positive, such as a significant job promotion or sudden news of acquiring great wealth; however, they still make increased demands on individuals who must make major life adjustments. Even positive events involve a modified grieving process as individuals may be losing or giving up old, familiar, and comfortable situations and facing stressful changes.

Community health nurses see an almost infinite variety of situational crises, including debilitating disease, economic misfortune, unemployment, physical abuse, divorce, unwanted pregnancy, chemical abuse, sudden death of a loved one, tragic accidents such as drownings or plane crashes, and many others. In each situation, people feel overwhelmed and need help to cope. Skilled intervention can make the difference between a healthy or an unhealthy outcome.

Multiple Crises

Different kinds of crises can overlap in actual experience, compounding the stress felt by the persons involved. For example, a couple could experience a developmental crisis (birth) and a situational crisis (birth defect) simultaneously, with the resulting stress compounded. The developmental crisis of midlife may be complicated by situational crises such as divorce and job change. With older adults the developmental crisis of retirement may be compounded by the situational crisis of a fire that destroys the family home. The transition a child faces entering school may occur at the same time the family moves to a new neighborhood and a new infant joins the family. The child must share his parents' attention and affection with a new sibling at a time when all the child's resources are needed to cope with starting school and adjusting to the new neighborhood. Classic research has shown that these accumulated stresses can lead to ill health (Holmes & Rahe, 1967). Those who might normally work through one crisis in a healthy way may find that compound events overwhelm them and cause more stress than they can handle.

HISTORY OF FAMILY VIOLENCE

Family crisis is not limited to the developmental crises that we all experience or the situational crises that come upon us suddenly, usually from forces—such as nature—that are external to the family. Unfortunately, many women and children in the world also experience the crisis of domestic violence. **Domestic violence** refers to morbidity and mortality attributable to violence within the home setting. **Family violence** involves action by a family member with the intent to cause harm to or control another family member (American Psychological Association, 1996). This is becoming more of a global burden.

Global History

Family violence is not new. For centuries, children were thought of as the property of their parents, and any treatment doled out by the parents was their prerogative. In fact, most countries had animal welfare laws long before child welfare laws were adopted. In addition, the ideology of childhood that emerged in the Western world in the late 1800s assumed that just the "abnormal" child needed protection. These were the children who were casualties of urban industrial society and were abandoned, dependent, and delinquent or products of social dislocation, such as the orphaned or refugee child.

In the early 1900s, sensitive leaders concerned with child welfare issues emerged. Several international agencies were created that were designed to positively affect the health of children. Examples include the British Children's Act of 1908 and the first White House Conference of 1909 in the United States. These were early attempts to define a role for the state. In the U.S. the conference was the forerunner of the development of the United States Children's Bureau (USCB) and a national voluntary organization, what was to be the Child Welfare League of America, which would complement any federal agency (Rooke & Schnell, 1995). The USCB became a model for other countries with well-developed programs targeting infant mortality. One innovative program, in the early 1900s, "was a heated mobile child welfare center for rural communities staffed by a female physician, a public health nurse, and an advice agent" (Rooke & Schnell, p. 179).

Other international organizations emerging in the early 1900s included the International Association for the Promotion of Child Welfare (IAPCW), Save the Children International Union (SCIU), League of Red Cross Societies (LRCS), Save the Children Fund (SCF), and Save the Children International Union (SCIU). The later two were immensely successful in raising funds for children in Germany, Austria, France, Hungary, and Serbia. As these organizations began serving the needs of children internationally, they moved from a sentimental depiction of victims to a medico-social scientific view of children at risk that expanded the concepts of victimization, exploitation and abuse (Rooke & Schnell, 1995).

By the mid-1920s the work of these agencies began to focus on children from non-European countries. The first conference on children from non-European countries focused on African children in 1931 and included such issues as infant mortality, child labor and education, and child slavery. In 1924 the League of Nations adopted the Declaration of the Rights of the Child, which would influence the League of Nation's successor, the United Nations, in years to come in the form of the Declaration of the Rights of the Child in 1959 and the Convention on the Rights of the Child in 1989.

Children are not the only victims of family morbidity and mortality from violence. Historically, women too have been treated as property, often causing physical and psychological damage. Huge numbers of women suffer from domestic and other forms of violence (between 16% and 52% of women in some parts of the world) ranging from emotional abuse to rape (1 in 5 women worldwide suffer rape or attempted rape in their lifetimes) and genital mutilation (it is estimated that 130 million girls and women alive today have been subjected to this practice) (World Health Report, 1998). As with children, the rights of women are socially, culturally, and religiously motivated, with change coming slowly.

U.S. History

The history of treatment of children, women, and elders begins with the emigration to the United States in the 1500s and has been influenced by the practices of the groups settling the country. In addition to the cultural or religious practices of the early settlers, necessity, attitudes of the time, and the stress and hardship of life in the colonies and on the frontier influenced how people were treated.

Children were born into families to help with the chores of an agricultural society. Families had many children, again out of necessity: because of high infant mortality rates, it was not uncommon for families to lose half of their children before their 2nd birthday. Older people did not retire; they contributed to the family survival until they died. There were no special considerations for children, women, or elders. The best a woman could hope for was that she would marry someone who would not abuse her emotionally, physically, sexually, or fiducially (taking advantage of a person's financial resources). Women had limited or no education, resources, and rights; children had none. If a woman married "poorly" she would have to live with the consequences. Separation and divorce were either unheard of or were a "death sentence" for her and her children, as there would be nowhere she could go and no way for her to support her family.

It took many years for the United States to establish laws that benefited women and children. Nonetheless, we did so earlier than many other countries. The Childrens's Bureau began to focus on child abuse in the 1960s and in 1962 developed a child abuse mandatory reporting law to be used by the states as a model. It stated that health professionals or child care workers must report suspected child abuse to the appropriate officials.

In 1974 the Child Abuse Prevention and Treatment Act was passed, becoming Public Law 93-247. It served to reinforce the earlier mandatory reporting law model in order to solve the growing problem of child abuse in the country. Public Law 93-247 was amended several times since 1974. Four years later the Child Abuse Prevention and Treatment and Adoption Reform Act of 1978 was passed. This was followed by the Family Violence Prevention and Services Act of 1984. All three acts were consolidated into one act entitled "The Child Abuse Prevention, Adoption, and Family Services Act of 1988" (Public Law 100-294) in 1988.

Public Law 100-294 mandates funding designed to support states in their efforts to prevent violence in families and to identify and treat the victims. Funding from this act supports the work of the National Center on Child Abuse and Neglect, a national commission on childhood deaths. This center studies the national incidence of family violence. It focuses on eliminating barriers to the adoption of older children, minority children, and children with physical and mental disabilities, in addition to supporting professional training and research (USDHHS, 1988). Each state acts on Public Law 100-294 in ways that best meet its needs. Elder abuse laws that are newer are modeled after the Family Services Act.

HEALTHY PEOPLE 2000 GOALS

Of the more than 300 national objectives of *Healthy People 2000,* 19 objectives were directed toward violent and abusive behavior. As of 1998 (United States Department of Health and Human Services [USDHHS]), three of the objectives surpassed their year 2000 targets: reduction of weapon carrying, implementation of child death review systems, and an increase in nonviolent conflict resolution programs in schools.

Six objectives progressed toward the year 2000 targets: reducing suicides; reducing firearm-related deaths; reducing physical fighting and weapon-carrying among adolescents aged 14 to 17; increasing the proportion of elementary and secondary schools that teach nonviolent conflict resolution skills, preferably as part of comprehensive school health education; and enacting laws requiring that firearms be properly stored to minimize access and the likelihood of discharge by minors. Disappointingly, eight objectives indicate movement away from the year 2000 targets: homicide; maltreatment of children younger than age 18; physical abuse directed at women by male partners; assault injuries among people aged 12 and older; rape and attempted rape of women aged 12 and older; suicide attempts among adolescents aged 14 to 17; battered women and their children turned away from emergency housing due to lack of space; and the number of states with protocols to facilitate identification and appropriate intervention for the prevention of suicides in jails.

As we look at these trends, six of the eight objectives moving away from the year 2000 goals are related to violence against women and children. This is disturbing information, and many reasons account for these results. Youth continue to be involved as both *perpetrators,* those people committing the violence, and victims of violence. Women, including their children, continue to be the targets of both physical and sexual assault perpetrated by individuals known to them, specifically the women's current and former intimate partners. Other issues, including the lack of comparable data sources, definitional issues, and the lack of resources to adequately establish consistent tracking systems, contribute to the negative data trends (USDHHS, 2000).

HEALTHY PEOPLE 2010 GOALS

The goal for *Healthy People 2010* regarding violence and abuse is to reduce injuries, disabilities, and death due to violence among all people of the United States. On an average day in America, 70 people die from homicide, 87 people commit suicide, as many as 3,000 people attempt suicide, and a minimum of 18,000 people survive interpersonal assaults. The problem is pervasive, affecting the victim directly and all the family members indirectly.

Selected violence and abuse objectives for 2010 include:

- reduce maltreatment and maltreatment fatalities of children from 13.9 victims per 1000 to 11.1 per 1000 by 2010
- reduce physical assault by current or former intimate partners from 4.5 per 1000 people to 3.6 per 1000 by 2010

- reduce the annual rate of rape or attempted rape of persons aged 12 and older to less than 0.7 per 1000 persons from 0.9 per 1000 in 1998
- reduce sexual assault other than rape to less than 0.2 per 1000 people from 0.6 in 1998
- reduce weapon carrying by adolescents on school property (by 9–12 graders) from 8.5% in 1997 to 6% by 2010 (U.S. Dept. of Health and Human Services, 2000)

Myths and Truths About Family Violence

There are many beliefs or myths about family violence that need to be dispelled as they may influence violent behavior in families. Strongly held myths by members of society, including community health nurses and other health care providers, may interfere with families in crisis getting the help they need. Table 25–1 displays some common myths and truths about family violence.

FAMILY VIOLENCE AGAINST CHILDREN

As a cause of morbidity among children, communicable diseases "are coming under control through a combination of health promotion, prevention and simplified standard treatment regimens. But at the same time, the healthy growth and development of many children is threatened by very rapid, often disruptive social, cultural and economic changes." (WHO, 1998, p. 71.) This emerging new morbidity is of a psychosocial nature, is associated with behavioral problems, and is much more difficult to prevent than diseases known for centuries.

Child abuse is the maltreatment of children, including any or all of the following: physical, emotional, medical, or educational neglect; physical punishment or battering; and emotional or sexual maltreatment and exploitation. Types can occur alone or in combination.

Child abuse and psychosocial developmental problems are taking a toll globally. It is estimated that the child abuse mortality rates for infants in most countries is 7 per 100,000 live births (WHO, 1998). This provides a rough global estimate and indicates only the "tip of the iceberg." There are abuses against children in many countries where accurate data are hard to uncover. Very young children are expected to aid the family financially. Their "chores" may include spending the whole day scrounging around city dumps for bits of food, clothing, or other useful or saleable items. Other children may be sold for sexual favors to whomever asks. Still others spend all day working in fields, home businesses, or in "sweat shops" for the equivalent of pennies a day. In some societies female children are not valued and are killed at birth, given away, or sold into slavery for a pittance.

More than 3 million children were reported because of

TABLE 25–1. Common Myths and Truths About Abuse in Families

Myth	Truth
Violence in families is rare	Family violence is common and increasing
Violence occurs most frequently among low-income families	Family violence occurs across all incomes
Violence occurs more frequently in some racial and cultural groups	Family violence occurs across all racial and cultural groups
Violence in families does not coexist with love	Love may exist but is unable to be displayed appropriately due to conflicting emotions
Men who batter women are mentally ill	The percentage of batterers who are mentally ill is the same as in the general population
Women who accept battering are mentally ill	The percentage of battered women who are mentally ill is the same as in the general population; however, they have low-esteem and a damaged spirit
Violence occurs only in heterosexual relationships	Domestic violence has no gender or sexual boundaries; it can occur among all people
Abused women instigate the battering	Quite the contrary, they go out of their way not to agitate or confront the abuser
Abuse occurs when the abuser is under the influence of drugs or alcohol	It can, but many abusers do not drink or use drugs
Children should not be taken from their parents	In some violent families, the safest place for the child is with another family member or a foster home (temporarily or permanently)
Even abusive parents are better for a child than a child living elsewhere	Children must be protected, and living away from abusive parents may save their lives
Abused children become abusive adults	Some may, but most can learn how to channel their emotions positively if the cycle of violence is broken

suspected child abuse incidents in the United States in 1995, a 20-fold increase since the 150,000 in 1963 (Besharov, 1998). This indicates we are doing a better job of protecting children from death and serious injury. In fact, the best estimate is that child abuse and neglect deaths fell from more than 3,000 (and perhaps as many as 5,000) a year in the late 1960s to about 1,200 a year in the mid-1990s (National Committee to Prevent Child Abuse, 1996).

With the release of *Healthy People 2010* goals in 2000, the nation remained without a clear baseline for child abuse cases, mainly because of evaluation and follow-up documentation issues among the states (USDHHS, 2000). However, in 1997 there were 13.9 child victims per 1000 children in the general population. The types of maltreatment were physical abuse (24.6%), general neglect (55.9%), sexual abuse (12.5%), and emotional abuse (6.1%) (USDHHS, 2000).

Child Neglect

Neglect occurs when the physical, emotional, or educational resources necessary for healthy growth and development are withheld or unavailable. It is obvious to an observer when a very young child is playing unattended outside, not dressed appropriately for the weather, or has an unkempt appearance. However, neglect is not always so obvious. A child may need eyeglasses and the parents never buy them—medical neglect. An 8-year-old gets to school only 3 days a week, usu-

ally without breakfast and no lunch money or a packed lunch—educational neglect. A family with three children lives in a sparsely furnished apartment, very little food is available, the heat works intermittently, and the children appear at school unwashed and without coats in winter weather—general neglect.

Thousands of children in the United States experience neglect each day. They are frequently "invisible" victims. At times stories of severe child neglect hit the media and we are all appalled. On the television we hear, "Twelve children are found among piles of garbage in an abandoned apartment building during a drug raid" or we might read, "Parents vacation in Florida while their two daughters aged 6 and 4 are left unattended at home." However, most children suffering from neglect do not make newspaper headlines or the television. They go to school alongside your own children or your younger brothers and sisters. If they are fortunate, their plight is uncovered by a community health nurse, teacher, or counselor. Because of the invisibility of neglect, the prevalence is hard to estimate. Often cases of neglect are brought to the attention of the proper authority only when another form of abuse is being explored (Display 25–4).

Emotional Abuse

Emotional abuse of children involves psychological mistreatment and/or neglect, such as when parents do not pro-

DISPLAY 25–4. Signs and Symptoms of Neglect

Neglect may be suspected when one or more of the following conditions exist:
- The child is lacking adequate medical or dental care.
- The child is often sleepy or hungry.
- The child is often dirty, demonstrates poor personal hygiene, or is inadequately dressed for weather conditions.
- There is evidence of poor or inadequate supervision for the child's age.
- The conditions in the home are unsafe or unsanitary.
- The child appears to be malnourished.
- The child is depressed, withdrawn, or apathetic; exhibits antisocial or destructive behavior; shows fearfulness; or suffers from substance abuse, speech, eating or habit disorders (biting, rocking, whining).

(From the Crime and Violence Prevention Center. [1996]. *Child abuse: Educator's responsibilities.* Sacramento, CA: California Attorney General's Office.)

DISPLAY 25–5. Signs and Symptoms of Emotional Abuse or Deprivation

Emotional abuse should be suspected if the child displays the following behavioral indicators:
- Is withdrawn, depressed or apathetic.
- Is clingy and forms indiscriminate attachments.
- "Acts out" and is considered a behavior problem.
- Exhibits exaggerated fearfulness.
- Is overly rigid in conforming to instructions of teachers, doctors, and other adults.
- Suffers from sleep, speech, or eating disorders.
- Displays signs of emotional turmoil that include repetitive, rhythmic movements (rocking, whining, picking at scabs).
- Pays inordinate attention to details or exhibits little or no verbal or physical communication with others.
- Suffers from enuresis and fecal soiling.
- Unwittingly makes comments such as "Mommy always tells me I'm bad."
- Experiences substance abuse problems.

Emotional deprivation should be suspected if the child:
- Refuses to eat adequate amounts of food, thus is very frail.
- Is unable to perform normal learned functions for a given age, eg, walking, talking, etc.
- Displays antisocial behavior (aggression, disruption) or obvious delinquent behavior (drug abuse, vandalism); conversely, the child may be abnormally unresponsive, sad, or withdrawn.
- Constantly "seeks out" and "pesters" other adults such as teachers or neighbors for attention and affection.
- Displays exaggerated fears.

(From the Crime and Violence Prevention Center. [1996]. *Child abuse: Educator's responsibilities.* Sacramento, CA: California Attorney General's Office.)

vide the normal experiences producing feelings of being loved, wanted, secure and worthy (Crime and Violence Prevention Center, 1996). This too can take several different forms. It may involve verbal abuse—calling the child names, belittling, or threatening. A mother may shout at the child, "You're just like your father, a real good-for-nothing lazy bum." A father may say, "You're ugly. You look just like your mother." When a child spills some juice, a parent may scream, "Everything you do you do wrong. Can't you do anything right?"

Emotional abuse may also take the form of emotional abandonment. Some parents "shun" their children as a form of punishment. They will not speak to them, they do not look at them—they behave as if their children do not exist. This may continue for a day or more whenever the children displease the parent. In some cases the shunning may last for days.

Verbal threats, although a common discipline practice among many parents, are a form of emotional abuse—for example, "Take your feet off the furniture or I'll chop your feet off" or "Do that again and you'll really know what my belt feels like." In the first instance, the child may realize the parent really won't chop her feet off, but hearing the parent say such a violent thing can be emotionally scarring. In the second instance, the parent may have beaten the child with a belt previously, so merely threatening to use it again causes emotional trauma. Emotional abuse often accompanies other forms of abuse. Emotional abuse alone is rarely reported, as it too, is a "hidden" form of abuse. However, **mandated reporters,** people who have responsibility for the welfare of children, such as nurses, doctors, teachers, counselors, and certain other professionals, are required by law (in most states) to report suspected cases of severe emotional neglect, abuse, or deprivation (Display 25–5).

Physical Abuse

Physical abuse of children is intentional harm to a child by another person that results in pain, physical injury, or death. The abuse may include striking, biting, poking, burning, shaking, or throwing the child. **Corporal punishment,** which involves violence against a child as a form of discipline, was an acceptable form of discipline earlier in our country's history and is still condoned in some subgroups. Many parents today were raised in families in which physical punishment was used as a form of discipline. Even today it is not unusual to see a parent slap the hand of a toddler to get his attention after he has been told not to do something several times or to prevent her from touching something that will hurt her more than the slap on the hand. Some families know where to draw the line. Others—especially if they were raised with "the belt" or "the switch"—see no harm in using the same disciplinary practices with their children.

Some parents cannot control the degree of physical punishment they give their child. If physical punishment is done in anger, when the parent is under the influence of mind-altering substances, or out of a parent's sense of frustration, the physical punishment may cross over to battered child syndrome (Fig. 25–1). **Battered child syndrome** is the collection of injuries sustained by a child as a result of repeated mistreatment or beatings (U.S. Department of Justice, 1996). Display 25–6 lists physical and behavioral indicators of physical abuse.

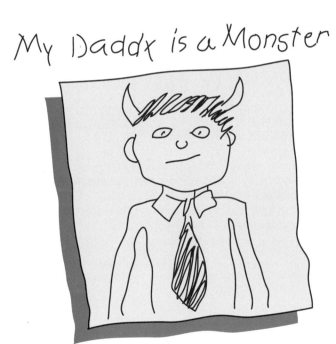

My Daddy is a Monster

He hurts my mommy
He hurts me too
Sometimes he hits
Sometimes he says things
That scare me and
make my mommy cry
after he leaves
Sometimes I wish he
won't come back ... <u>ever</u>.
I love my daddy.

National Coalition Against Domestic Violence • P.O. Box 34103 • Washington, DC 20043-4103 • 1-800-799-SAFE

FIGURE 25–1. Poster of "My Daddy is a Monster." (National Coalition Against Domestic Violence.)

DISPLAY 25-6. Physical Abuse: Types of Injuries

Bruises
Burns
Bite marks
Abrasions
Lacerations
Head injuries
Internal injuries
Fractures

Behavioral Indicators of Physical Abuse
The following behaviors are often exhibited by physically abused children:

- The child is frightened of parents/caretakers or, at the other extreme, is overprotective of parent or caretakers.
- The child is excessively passive, overly compliant, apathetic, withdrawn or fearful or, at the other extreme, excessively aggressive, destructive, or physically violent.
- The child and/or parent or caretaker attempts to hide injuries; child wears excessive layers of clothing, especially in hot weather; child is frequently absent from school or misses physical education classes if changing into gym clothes is required; child has difficulty sitting or walking.
- The child is frightened of going home.
- The child is clingy and forms indiscriminate attachments.
- The child is apprehensive when other children cry.
- The child is wary of physical contact with adults.
- The child exhibits drastic behavioral changes in and out of parental/caretaker presence.
- The child is hypervigilant.
- The child suffers from seizures or vomiting.
- The adolescent exhibits depression, self-mutilation, suicide attempts, substance abuse, or sleeping and eating disorders.

Other indicators of physical abuse may include:

- A statement by the child that the injury was caused by abuse. (Chronically abused children may deny abuse.)
- Knowledge that the child's injury is unusual for the child's specific age group (eg, any fracture in an infant).
- Knowledge of the child's history of previous or recurrent injuries.
- Unexplained injuries (eg, parent is unable to explain reason for injury; there are discrepancies in explanations; blame is placed on a third party; explanations are inconsistent with medical diagnosis).
- A parent or caretaker who delays seeking or fails to seek medical care for the child's injury.

(Adapted from the Crime and Violence Prevention Center. [1996]. *Child abuse: Educator's responsibilities.* Sacramento, CA: California Attorney General's Office.)

Sexual Abuse

Sexual abuse of children includes acts of sexual assault or sexual exploitation of a minor and may consist of many acts over a long period of time, or a single incident. Sexual assault includes rape, gang rape, incest, sodomy, lewd or lascivious acts with a child under 14 years of age, oral copulation, penetration of a genital or anal opening by a foreign object, and child molestation. **Sexual exploitation** of children includes conduct or activities related to pornography depicting minors in sexually explicit situations and promoting prostitution by minors (U.S. Department of Justice, 1997). **Incest** is sexual abuse among family members who are blood-related (parent, grandparent, older siblings, aunts and uncles) and constitutes the most hidden form of child abuse. **Intrafamilial sexual abuse** refers to sexual activity between family members not related by blood (step-parents, boyfriends, etc.).

In most reported cases, the father or male caretaker is the initiator and the victim is usually a female child; however, boys are victims more often than previously believed. It is estimated that 1 in 4 girls is sexually abused and 1 in 7 boys, a much higher percentage for boys than reported numbers indicate. The initial sexual abuse may occur at any age, from infancy through adolescence. However, the largest number of cases involves females under the age of 11 years. Regardless of how gentle, trivial, or coincidental the first approach may have seemed, sexual coercion tends to be repeated and to escalate over a period of years. The child may eventually accept the blame for tempting and provoking the abuser.

The mother in the family, who would usually be expected to protect the child, may purposely try to stay isolated from a problem of sexual abuse. Sometimes she may be distant, uncommunicative, or so disapproving of sexual matters that the child is afraid to speak up. Sometimes she may be extremely insecure, and the potential loss of her husband or boyfriend, and the economic security he provides, is so threatening that she cannot allow herself to believe or even to suspect that her child is or could be at risk. She may have been a victim herself of child abuse and may not trust her judgment or her right to challenge the man in authority in the home. Some mothers consciously acknowledge that their children are being sexually abused, but for whatever reason they "look the other way."

Until the victim is old enough to realize that incest or intrafamilial sexual abuse is not a common occurrence and/or the victim is strong enough to obtain help outside the family, there is no escape unless the abuse is reported (Crime Prevention Center, 1993).

Indicators of sexual abuse, including the history, sexual behavioral indicators of children, behavioral indicators of sexual abuse in younger children, behavioral indicators of sexual abuse in older children and adolescents, and physical symptoms, provide information to assist community health nurses in their mandated reporter role (Display 25–7). It should be noted that sexual abuse of a child may surface through a broad range of physical, behavioral, and social symptoms. Some of these indicators, taken separately, may not be symptomatic of sexual abuse. They are presented here as a guide and should be examined in the context of other behavior(s) or situational factors.

Although there are several classifications of child molesters, pedophiles present the greatest danger. A **pedophile** is an adult whose main sexual interest is a child. A pedophile tends to be well-liked by children. Pedophiles, who are most often men, frequently choose to work in professions or volunteer organizations that allow them easy access to children, where they can develop the trust and respect of children and their parents. The pedophile believes that sex with children is appropriate and often lures children into sexual relationships with love, rewards, promises, and gifts. He may be among a child's family members (grandfather, father, uncle, cousin, etc.) or a trusted community leader the child knows (next-door neighbor, teacher, scout or religious leader, etc.).

Specific Abusive Situations

Although the above information discusses the major types of violence occurring in families, two specific patterns of abuse against children should be discussed here. Shaken baby syndrome and Munchausen syndrome by proxy are fairly rare, but when they are discovered it is often too late, as the diagnosis is made during an emergency room visit or at autopsy.

SHAKEN BABY SYNDROME

Shaken baby syndrome is the intentional abusive action of violently shaking an infant or toddler, usually less than 18 months old. The type of damage that occurs to these infants very seldom occurs through play, such as the minor falls a baby at play may experience or by parents tossing a baby in the air. The classic medical symptoms associated with infant shaking include bilateral retinal hemorrhage, subdural or subarachnoid hematomas, absence of other external signs of abuse, and symptoms including breathing difficulties, seizures, dilated pupils, lethargy, and unconsciousness (U.S. Department of Justice, 1996). These injuries are caused by a violent, sustained action in which the infant's head, which lacks muscular control, is violently whipped forward and backward, hitting the chest and shoulders. Experts say that an observer watching the shaking would describe it as "as hard as the shaker was humanly capable of shaking the baby" or "hard enough that it appeared the baby's head would come off." (U.S. Department of Justice, 1996). Within minutes to hours of the injury, the baby will begin to show symptoms, such as seizures or unconsciousness. A typical explanation given by the parents or caretakers is that the baby was "fine" and then suddenly went into respiratory arrest or began having seizures—both common symptoms of shaken baby syndrome.

MUNCHAUSEN SYNDROME BY PROXY

Munchausen syndrome is a psychological disorder in which a client fabricates the symptoms of a disease in order to

DISPLAY 25–7. Indicators of Sexual Abuse

I. History of Sexual Abuse
- A child confides to a friend, classmate, teacher, a friend's mother, or other trusted adult that she/he has experienced sexual abuse.
- A child may disclose information indirectly by such statements as:
  "I know someone . . ."
  "What would you do if . . . ?"
  "I heard something about somebody . . ."
- The child has torn, stained, or bloody underclothing (among her/his clothing or is wearing it).
- Knowledge that a child's injury/disease (vaginal trauma, sexually transmitted disease) is unusual for the specific age group.
- Unexplained injuries/diseases (parent/caretaker unable to explain reason for injury/disease); there are discrepancies in explanation; blame is placed on a third party; explanations are inconsistent with medical diagnosis.
- A very young girl is pregnant or has a sexually transmitted disease. Pregnancy alone does not constitute sexual abuse, but if there are indications of coercion or significant age disparity between the minor and her partner, this may lead to reasonable suspicion of sexual abuse that must be reported.

II. Sexual Behavioral Indicators of Sexually Abused Children
- Detailed and age-inappropriate understanding of sexual behavior (especially among very young children).
- Sexually explicit language.
- Inappropriate, unusual, or aggressive sexual behavior with peers or toys.
- Compulsive indiscreet masturbation.
- Excessive curiosity about sexual matters or genitalia (self or others).
- Unusually seductive or flirtatious behavior with classmates, teachers, and other adults.
- Excessive concern about homosexuality, especially by boys.

III. Behavioral Indicators of Sexual Abuse in Younger Children
- Enuresis (wetting pants or bedwetting).
- Fecal soiling.
- Eating disturbances such as overating or undereating.
- Fears or phobias.
- Overly compulsive behavior.
- School problems or significant change in school performance (attitude and grades).
- Age-inappropriate behavior that includes pseudomaturity or regressive behavior such as bedwetting or thumb sucking.

- Inability to concentrate.
- Sleeping disturbances (nightmares, fear of falling asleep, fretful sleep pattern, sleeping long hours).
- Drastic behavior changes.
- Speech disorders.
- Frightened of parents/caretaker or of going home or being at home.

IV. Behavioral Indicators of Sexual Abuse in Older Children and Adolescents
- Withdrawal.
- Chronic fatigue.
- Clinical depression, apathy.
- Overly compliant behavior.
- Over or under reaction (hysteria or cavalier attitude) to a genital exam.
- Poor hygiene or excessive bathing.
- Poor peer relations and social skills; inability to make friends.
- Acting out, running away, aggressive, antisocial or delinquent behavior.
- Alcohol or drug abuse.
- Prostitution or excessive promiscuity.
- School problems, frequent absences, sudden drop in school performance.
- Refusal to change clothes for physical education class.
- Non-participation in sports and social activities.
- Fearful of showers or restrooms.
- Fearful of home life as demonstrated by arriving at school early and leaving late.
- Suddenly fearful of other things (going outside or participating in familiar activities).
- Extraordinary fear of males (in cases of male perpetrator and female victim).
- Self-consciousness of body beyond that expected for age.
- Sudden acquisition of money, new clothes, or gifts with no reasonable explanation.
- Suicide attempt or other self-destructive behavior.
- Crying without provocation.
- Setting fires.

IV. Physical Symptoms of Sexual Abuse
- Sexually transmitted diseases, especially in pre-pubescent girls.
- Genital discharge or infection.
- Physical trauma or irritation to the anal/genital area (pain, itching, swelling, bruising, bleeding, lacerations, abrasions), especially if injuries are unexplained or there is an inconsistent explanation.
- Pain during urination or defecation.
- Difficulty in walking or sitting due to genital or anal pain.
- Psychosomatic symptoms (stomach aches, headaches, chronic pain).

(Adapted from the Crime and Violence Prevention Center. [1996]. *Child abuse: Educator's responsibilities.* Sacramento, CA: California Attorney General's Office.)

undergo medical tests, hospitalization, or even medical or surgical treatment. Clients with this disorder may intentionally injure themselves or induce illness in themselves. In cases of **Munchausen syndrome by proxy,** a parent or caretaker suffering from Munchausen syndrome attempts to bring medical attention to himself or herself by injuring or inducing illness in his or her children. The following scenarios are typical of these cases:

- The child's parent or caretaker brings the child to the emergency room or calls the paramedics repeatedly for alleged problems that have no medical basis.
- The child only experiences "seizures" or "respiratory arrest" when the parent or caretaker is present—never in the presence of a neutral third party or when hospitalized, unless the parent or caretaker reports that the incident occurred in his or her presence.
- While the child is hospitalized, the parent or caretaker shuts off IVs or life-support equipment, causing the child distress, and then turns everything back on and summons help.
- The parent or caretaker induces illness by introducing a mild irritant or poison into the child's body; chronic ingestion may cause the child's death.

PARTNER/SPOUSAL VIOLENCE

Adult violence is rooted in childhood violence. A father hits a mother. The mother hits her son. The son hits his sister. The sister hits her little brother. The little brother sets fire to the cat, pulls wings off butterflies, and grows up to be a spouse batterer. Although abused girls may grow up to be abusing mothers, more often they grow up to be abused wives.

Partner violence often begins during adolescent dating, or dating at any age, with a push or shove that at first is overlooked by the girlfriend (Foshee et al., 1998). As these "minor" episodes of violence continue, the victim typically feels that she is doing something wrong and attempts to modify her behavior. She also assumes wrongly that once she and her boyfriend are married, these physical assaults will stop automatically or that in time she will be able to "change" him. The cycle of violence has begun.

Cycle of Violence

The **cycle of violence** is the repetitive, cyclical pattern of abuse seen in domestic violence situations. This cycle was first labeled the three-phase theory of family violence by Walker in 1979, after she studied more than 1,000 battered women, as well as a smaller group of battering men (Carden, 1994). It includes the tension-building phase, the acute battering incident, and the loving reconciliation. The psychological dynamics of these three phases help explain why women feel so guilty and ashamed of their partner's violence

toward them and why they find it so difficult to leave, even when their lives are in danger (Display 25–8).

The Domestic Abuse Intervention Project in Duluth, Minnesota has developed a wheel of violence, identifying power and control at the center, with eight categories of perpetrator behaviors. This model is a useful tool for visualizing the dimensions of abuse (Fig. 25–2).

Dating Violence

Dating violence in adolescent relationships is a serious and prevalent problem. Because of its prevalence, community health nurses should include screening for dating violence in all encounters with teens. **Dating violence** is physical, sexual, emotional, and/or verbal abuse between persons who are or have been in a casual or serious dating relationship (Furniss, 1996). Adolescent dating violence begins on average at age 15. About 50% of rape victims are between 10 and 19 years old, which indicates that teenage girls are vulnerable to the violence of sexual abuse (Goring & Arnold, 1998).

Partner/Spousal Abuse

Spousal abuse is violence against an intimate partner. Because of the nature of intimate partner violence, the problems are difficult to study. Thus, much remains unkown about the factors that increase or decrease the likelihood that men will behave violently towards women, the factors that endanger or protect women from violence, and the physical and emotional consequences of such violence for women and their children.

In the Commonwealth Fund Survey, the researchers operationalized domestic violence as pushing, grabbing, shoving, slapping, choking, kicking, biting, hitting with a fist or some other object, being beaten, or being threatened with a knife or gun by a spouse or cohabiting partner (Plichta, 1996). In this study more than 8% of the women in a married or cohabiting relationship reported partner/spousal abuse in the past year. This is consistent with studies done in the 1980s in which it was found that 8.3% to 11.3% of women experienced partner/spousal abuse in the past year. Additionally, 29% of female homicide victims in the general population were killed by a husband, ex-husband, boyfriend, or ex-boyfriend in 1993 (Federal Bureau of Investigation, 1994). Nationwide, battering exceeds rapes, muggings, and motor vehicle crashes combined as the leading cause of injury to women age 15 to 44 (*The Nation's Health,* 2000).

In Oklahoma, the number of domestic violence reports rose 42% from 1989 to 1998. Nearly 88,000 women and children sought shelter or crisis intervention from 1993 to 1997. Because of these alarming trends, through a grant from the Centers for Disease Control and Prevention, Oklahoma is conducting intimate partner violence injury surveillance in an attempt to determine the prevalence of intimate partner vio-

---

DISPLAY 25–8. The Cycle of Violence

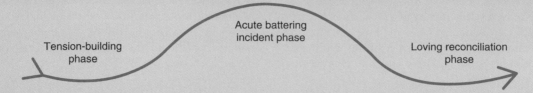

Tension-building
phase

Acute battering
incident phase

Loving reconciliation
phase

Tension-Building Phase

The woman senses her partner's increasing tension. She may or may not know what is wrong. The partner is "edgy" and lashes out in anger. He challenges her, calls her names, and tells her she is stupid, incompetent, and unconcerned about him. She "tries hard" not to make any "mistakes" that may upset him. She takes the responsibility for making him feel better, and begins to set herself up to feel guilt when he eventually explodes in spite of her best efforts to calm and please him. During the increasing tension, the woman is rarely angry even at the most outrageous demands or blame. Rather, she internalizes her appropriate anger at the partner's unfairness and, instead, experiences depression, anxiety, and a sense of helplessness. As the tension in the relationship increases, minor episodes of violence increase, such as pinching, tripping, or slapping. The batterer knows his behavior is inappropriate, and he fears the woman will leave him. This fear of rejection and loss increases his rage at the woman and his need to control her.

Acute Battering Incident

The tension-building phase ends in an explosion of violence. The incident that sets off the man's violence is often trivial or unknown, leaving the woman confused and feeling helpless. The woman may or may not fight back. She may try to escape the violence or call for help. If she cannot escape the beating, she may have a sense of unreality—as if it is a dream. Following the battering, the woman is in a state of physical and psychological shock. She may be passive and withdrawn or hysterical and incoherent. She may not be aware of the seriousness of her injuries and may resist help. The man discounts the episode and also underestimates

the woman's injuries. He may not summon medical help even when her injuries are life-threatening.

Loving Reconciliation

The loving reconciliation phase may begin a few hours to several days following the acute battering incident. Both partners have a profound sense of relief that "it's over." Although the woman is initially angry at the man, he begins an intense campaign to "win her back." Just as his tension and violence were overdone, his apologies, gifts, and gestures of love may also be excessive. Showering her with love and praise helps her repair her shattered self-esteem. It is nearly impossible for her to leave him during this phase as he is meeting her desperate need to see herself as a competent and lovable woman. The woman's feelings of power and romantic ideals are nurtured. She believes this gentle, loving person is her "real" lover. She believes that if only she can find the key, she can stop him from further violent episodes. She believes that, no matter how often it has happened before, somehow this episode seems different this time and it will never happen again.

The Increasing Spiral of Violence

One aspect of the cycle of violence of particular concern is its progressive and spiraling nature. Once violence has begun, every study indicates that it not only continues but over time increases in both frequency and severity. As the violence continues, the three-phase cycle begins to change. The tension-building phase becomes shorter and more intense, the acute battering incidents become more frequent and severe, and the loving reconciliation phase becomes shorter and less intense. After many years of battering, the man may not apologize at all.

---

lence and the extent of injuries resulting in hospital treatment (*The Nation's Health*, 2000).

Physical and/or sexual violence is used as a tactic to maintain power and control over another. Behaviors often include:

- physical violence
- sexual violence, intimidation
- coercion and threats
- emotional abuse
- isolating the victim
- using issues around children to harass or threaten
- rigid imposition of beliefs in male superiority and privilege

- economic abuse (Fitzgerald, Dienemann, & Cadorette, 1998)

Although victims may be of either sex and any sexual orientation, 95% of victims are women.

Violence During Pregnancy

Domestic violence continues through childhood and adolescence and follows a woman into long-term relationships and into pregnancy. Studies show that between 4% and 14% of adult pregnant women experience physical

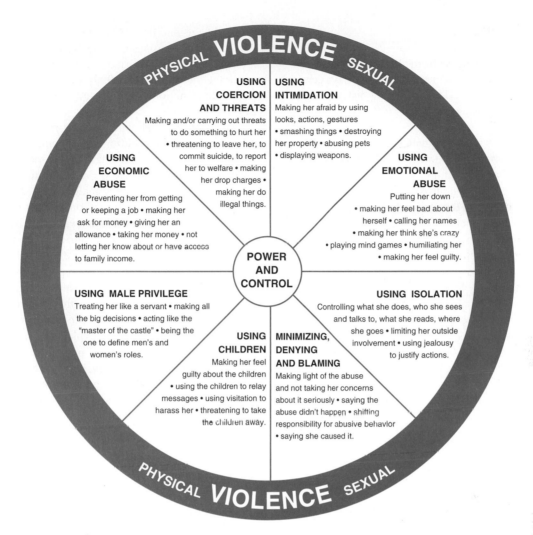

FIGURE 25–2. Wheel of violence. (Adapted from the Domestic Abuse Intervention Project, Duluth, MN.)

violence from an intimate partner (Campbell, 1999). Abuse is more likely to be reported by pregnant adolescents than pregnant adults (Parker, McFarlane, & Soeken, 1994) and by women with unplanned pregnancies (Stewart & Cecutti, 1993).

Abuse during pregnancy has been linked with maternal health problems, such as smoking, decreased weight gain, and substance use (Cokkinides & Coker, 1998). The fetus is also endangered with problems such as spontaneous abortions, pre-term deliveries, fetal distress, and lower birth weight. Curry, Doyle, & Gilhooley (1998) found that pregnant teens who were abused were more likely to be high school dropouts, smoke more, and experience more second-trimester bleeding. Once born, the infant of the abused teen or adult is at risk for child abuse.

The most serious aspect of domestic violence as a threat to a woman's safety is the link between abuse during pregnancy and homicide, called femicide. Femicide is now the leading cause of maternal mortality (rather than medical complications of pregnancy) in several cities in the United

States (Dannenberg et al., 1995). Men who abuse their partners during pregnancy are more likely to own guns and/or knives, which puts the women at greater risk, and the batterings during pregnancy are associated with increased severity (Campbell, 1998).

Studies have found that prenatal care is one of the few times when women are seen by the helping professions. It is an important opportunity to identify women who are abused and therefore at risk for homicide. It is imperative that nurses conduct an assessment for danger and lethality so that the women can be aware of their own level of risk and take safety precautions as needed. A series of questions requiring a "yes" or "no" response and inquiring about occurrences of abuse, escalation of abuse, frequency, severity, weapons, drugs or alcohol use by perpetrator, safety of other children, etc., should be incorporated into prenatal home visit assessments. This is especially important with women who have not followed through with prenatal care duiring which health care professionals can monitor the progress of their pregnancies.

Batterer Characteristics

Although men who batter come from all walks of life educationally, culturally, and socioeconomically, they have certain characteristics in common. The following list represents some characteristics of batterers:

- Low self-esteem
- Believe all myths regarding battering relationships, such as the woman "asks for it" or "if she would do what the man says it wouldn't happen" or "abuse doesn't happen in the suburbs, it happens only among low-income people in the inner city"
- Traditionalists who believe in male supremacy and stereotyped male sex role in the family
- Blame others for their actions
- Pathologically jealous
- Have severe stress reactions
- Use sex as an act of aggression to enhance self-esteem
- Do not believe their violent behavior should have negative consequences
- Low frustration threshold; poor impulse control; violent, explosive temper; external locus of control
- Presents a dual personality
- Emotionally dependent on his partner/spouse and children
- Family history of domestic violence
- Sees violence as a viable method of problem-solving
- Uses threat of violence as a control mechanism
- Physically and/or sexually abused as a child or saw mother abused
- High level of job dissatisfaction, under- or unemployment
- Unrealistic expectations of the relationship
- Preoccupation with weapons

MISTREATMENT OF ELDERS

In 1996 it was estimated that there were between 820,000 and 1,860,000 abused elders in the United States (Archstone Foundation, 1996). **Elder abuse** is the mistreatment or exploitation of older adults. Elders are abused by family members in similar ways that younger family members are abused: by abandoning or neglecting (physically or emotionally) them; by physically, sexually, or emotionally abusing them; or by exploiting them. Adult children, divided between males and females equally, are the most frequent abusers of the elderly. However, spouses who were batterers did not stop at age 65, and they committed 13.8% of the 241,000 *reported* cases of elder abuse in the United States in 1994 (Archstone Foundation, 1996). In 1994 the victims of elder abuse had a median age of 76.5 years, and 65.4% of them were white.

Abuse against elders is not new, but research on elder abuse is new. Until recently, the reasons for elder abuse were extrapolated from the literature on abuse in younger popula-

tions. By the middle 1980s more research was being conducted, and the findings indicate that elder abuse results from multiple, interrelated variables associated with the perpetrator or the victim (Miller, 1999). For example, elders can be physically, emotionally, or sexually abused, neglected, or exploited.

Forms of physical abuse include rough handling during caregiving, pinching, hitting, or slapping. Emotional abuse can take many forms, including being shouted at or threatened or having needed care withheld. More rarely, elders are sexually abused, which may include rape. Some elders are neglected by those they depend on to meet their caregiving needs. This form of abuse is often identified by the elder: being unwashed and unkempt and suffering from malnutrition, dehydration, and ultimately pressure sores. Elders dependent on the care of others often will not report such abuses for fear of being abandoned. They feel powerless and at a loss about how to change a bad situation, and they fear reprisal from the perpetrator(s) if they tell others about the abuse.

Older adults are frequently exploited in a variety of ways. They can be exploited by family members who take their Social Security retirement money, savings, or investments and use it on themselves. Criminals who approach elders with get-rich-quick schemes, sham investment opportunities, or illegitimate charities often prey on the trusting nature of older adults.

Perpetrator and Victim Characteristics

The dominant underlying factors that contribute to a family member abusing an elder are social isolation and pathology on the part of the perpetrator. Research has identified emotional or financial dependence on the victim, alcohol use, and fewer external contacts or isolation as major contributing factors. Men are more likely to exploit or physically abuse elders, whereas women are more likely to neglect elders physically or abuse them psychologically. Since women are more frequently the caretaker of elders, they are in a position to provide either appropriate or neglectful care to frail older adults (Miller, 1999). Frequently caregiver "burnout" contributes to the too-casual, neglectful, or obvious hurtful practices some family member or employed caregivers may impose on the elder.

Some characteristics of older people appear to increase their risk of abuse. They include dementia and poor health (Miller, 1999). Newly diagnosed cognitive impairment correlates with occurrences of abuse (Lachs et al., 1997). If violence or threats of violence by the elder toward the caregiver accompany dementia, this contributes to elder abuse. The failing health of an elder may contribute to self-neglect or diminished ability for self-defense or escape from maltreatment (Lachs & Pillemer, 1995). Finally, if the abuser and victim live together, the close proximity can bring up unresolved family conflict or create new conflicts when the expectations of cohabitating are not met (Miller, 1999).

Risk Factors

Regardless of the type of abuse an elder suffers or the motivation of the abuser in the family, two factors are common to all elder abuse situations. The first is the *invisibility* of elders in general and the abused elder specifically. It is estimated that less than 10% of elder abuse is reported. Pillemer and Finkelhor (1988) found that only 1 of 14 cases of elder abuse came to public attention in Massachusetts, a state with model reporting laws. Reasons for invisibility among the elderly are multifaceted. Older people usually have less contact with the community. They are no longer in the workforce and in public on a regular basis, which keeps their problems hidden longer. In addition, older adults are reticent to admit to being abused or neglected. Since the abuser is most often a family member, the elder desires to protect him or her; without this abusing family member, the elder would be entirely alone. On the other hand, the elder may fear reprisal from the abuser for coming forward with a self-report of abuse or telling another about the home situation.

The second risk factor is the *vulnerability* of older adults. Many elders who are becoming frail are dependent on others for some aspect of their day-to-day survival. At first they may need to rely on others for transportation, shopping, and housekeeping. Later they may need help with financial affairs, cooking, and laundry. In time they may need help managing their medications, bathing, and eating. The degree to which an elder needs assistance is often kept hidden from others for fear of being removed from their present living situation and placed in a more restrictive environment. This contributes to their vulnerability, and they can become easy victims for abusive family members. In addition, vulnerability in elders is increased when the following four sets of characteristics are present: (1) impairment and isolation; (2) poverty and pathologic caregivers; (3) learned helplessness and living in a violent subculture; and (4) deteriorating housing and crime-ridden neighborhoods (Anetzberger, 1990).

OTHER FORMS OF FAMILY VIOLENCE

There are three forms of family violence not previously discussed in detail. They are suicide, homicide, and rape. These three forms of violence demonstrate the ultimate extreme of violence to the victim and are the most traumatic to the surviving family members.

Suicide

Suicide is taking action that causes one's own death. Globally, 820,000 people commit suicide each year (World Health Report, 1998). In the United States, on an average day 87 people successfully commit suicide and over 3,000 people attempt suicide (USDHHS, 2000). The *Healthy People 2010* goal is to reduce sucides to no more than 6.0 per 100,000 people. White males over age 65 are at the highest risk, with 35.5 deaths per 100,000 in 1997. Suicide was the third leading killer of young persons between the ages of 15 and 24 in the U.S. in 1996 (USDHHS, 2000).

Parasuicidal acts are deliberate acts with non-fatal outcomes that attempt to cause or actually cause self-harm. The yearly prevalence of parasuicidal acts varies between 2% and 20%. The prevalence of parasuicide is estimated to be 10 to 20 times higher than that of completed suicides. Three times more women than men attempt suicide, whereas three times more men than women succeed. Cutting one's wrists is often dramatized on television but is not an effective way to die. People who attempt suicide, or commit a parasuicidal act, may use this method.

Completed suicides are carried out in a variety of ways, some more violent than others. Women usually choose less violent methods, such as overdosing on medications. Men choose more violent forms of suicide, such as hanging, use of firearms, or vehicle crashes. Deaths from suicide are under-reported because of a tendency to group them as accidental deaths or deaths from undetermined causes.

Any verbalization of suicide ideation from clients (or others) should be taken seriously and appropriate intervention steps taken immediately (Kalafat, 1991). Intervention strategies, including early recognition of depression, eliminating or treating the use of drugs and abuse of alcohol, and violence prevention programs, are available. Many more are being developed, implemented, and evaluated for effectiveness.

Homicide

Homicide is any action taken to cause non–war related death in another person. Globally, some 560,000 homicides occur each year. In many developed and developing countries, 20% to 40% of deaths in men aged 15 to 34 years are the result of homicide or suicide (World Health Report, 1998). Fifty-three people died each day in the United States from homicide in 1997. A goal for *Healthy People 2010* is to reduce homicides to less than 3.2 per 100,000 people. Our baseline was 16.2 in 1998 (USDHHS, 2000).

Many homicide casualties are victims of domestic abuse. The cycle of violence escalates and the partner is killed, most often in a violent episode, or by arrangement and committed by a third party. In 1994, of the 500,000 women who were seen in hospital emergency departments for violence-related injuries, 37% had suffered injuries inflicted by spouses, ex-spouses, or nonmarital partners (Bureau of Justice Statistics, 1997).

Rape

Rape is an act of aggression in which the perpetrator is motivated by a desire to dominate, control, and degrade the victim. It was once considered an act of sexuality. It is now believed that it is a combination of the two, with rape defined as the "sexual expression of aggression" (Congressional Caucus for Women's Issues, 1991).

In 1997 the Department of Justice reported that over 407,000 females aged 12 and over were victims of rape, attempted rape, or sexual assault in 1994. These are conservative figures, with other studies reporting that over 683,000 women experienced a forcible rape in a year and 12.1 million American women have been victims of forcible rape sometime in their lives (USDHHS, 2000).

LEVELS OF PREVENTION: CRISIS INTERVENTION AND FAMILY VIOLENCE

Family violence is a family crisis and needs interruption. Community health nurses are in a unique position to prevent, detect, and intervene during crisis situations. They encounter people in their own settings where direct observation, discussion, and intervention can occur. Because of their assessment skills, familiarity with the community, access to resources, and opportunity to go into the homes of families, community health nurses are ideally situated to help families in crisis. By implementing the three levels of prevention, the nurse can begin to put back together the lives of family members encountering violence.

Primary Prevention

The cycle of violence within the family can be interrupted. Even when partners/spouses, or parents, have been brought up in violent homes by abusive parents, they can learn to rechannel and control their emotions and behaviors to be appropriate. Primary prevention is obviously the most effective level of intervention, both in terms of promoting clients' health and in terms of cost containment. Primary prevention reflects a fundamental human concern for well-being and includes planned activities, undertaken by the nurse, to prevent an unwanted event from occurring, to protect current states of health and healthy functioning, and to promote desired states of health for the members of a particular community. For the community health nurse, any activity that fosters healthful practices and counteracts unhealthful influences can help prevent a crisis. Health promotion should take into account physical, psychological, sociocultural, and spiritual needs.

Several opportunities exist for families who want to improve relationships with their partner or spouse and children. First, social problem-solving skills for both partners and assertiveness skills for women provide a foundation on which additional programs can build. Many people have not learned positive problem-solving skills that are socially acceptable. Women have learned passivity and submissiveness, perhaps in response to their own inadequate parenting or abusive upbringing. Men and women can benefit from these two types of skill development.

Secondly, people need to have the self-esteem that improved education and occupational success can bring. If poverty is a related factor to the violence, educational preparation and a successful employee role may eliminate this stressor. As stated earlier, violence occurs across all socio-economic levels of society; however, if a family is so impoverished that their basic needs cannot be met, the stress can lead the more vulnerable family members to seek out illegal ways to solve their financial problems. This happens especially in neighborhoods where criminal activity is easily accessed.

People must take lessons or pass a test in order to drive; to get into college; to become nurses, attorneys, teachers, and other licensed professionals; and to join the military. The most important job an adult will ever have is that of parent, yet no lessons are required and there are no tests to pass. Parenting training is something all parents would benefit from, but especially those potential parents at high risk: teen parents, people with no exposure to children in their upbringing, and people raised in violent and abusive families.

Community health nurses often make home visits to families based on referrals from hospital maternity departments. During the mother's postpartum stay, a nurse may have noted some inappropriate parenting behaviors or the parents may meet high-risk parameters set by the hospital, such as being 17 years old or younger, being single, or having a history of substance abuse. On the first few visits to the family, the nurse can assess parenting skills and any need for training. If a parenting class is recommended, it should cover age-appropriate content, such as safety, breast-feeding, formula preparation, food progression, anticipatory guidance for growth and development, discipline techniques including behavior modification and time-out, well-baby care and immunizations, etc. An additional benefit for the parents is the social support they get from other attending parents.

The opportunity for home visiting has been formalized into model programs around the country that effectively prevent abuse (Olds et al., 1997). In such programs the nurse visits on a regular basis over several years, teaching and role-modeling many parenting techniques, providing needed support, and initiating necessary referrals.

The interrelatedness between families and communities cannot be overlooked or underestimated. Neighborhoods need to be enfranchised; they need to be developed; they need to be safe for all members; they need to be healthy. Empowered families can take back their neighborhoods from criminals, and they can be sources of growth for families.

Secondary Prevention

Early diagnosis and prompt treatment of the effects of family crisis or violence is the focus of the secondary level of prevention. It seeks to reduce the intensity and duration of a crisis and to promote adaptive behavior. By creating a positive relationship with family members and seeing them in their homes, the community health nurse can often uncover and intervene in a crisis or stop abusive situations.

People in crisis need help. They often desperately want help. The crisis or violence and its associated disequilibrium has a twofold effect on the individuals involved: (1) it renders them temporarily helpless, unable to cope on their own, and (2) it makes them especially receptive to outside influence. There are crisis resolution models that community health nurses can use to help clients at the secondary level. The following steps (Roberts, 1991: Aguilera, 1997) have been used successfully by people in the mental health field working on crisis hot lines, in mental health centers, and in emergency rooms: (1) establish rapport, (2) assess the individual and the problem for lethality, (3) identify major problems and intervene, (4) deal with feelings, (5) explore alternatives and coping mechanisms, (6) develop action plan, and (7) follow up, including anticipatory planning for coping with future crises. People in crisis will seek and generally receive some kind of help, but the nature of that help can rule in favor of or against a healthy outcome in which the participants can grow and evolve (Shaw & Halliday, 1992). Clients' desires for assistance give the helping professional a prime opportunity to intervene; this opportunity also presents a challenge to make that intervention as effective as possible.

One goal of crisis intervention should be to help clients reestablish a sense of safety and security while allowing them to ventilate their feelings and be validated. This will help to reestablish equilibrium at as healthy a level as possible and can result in change and growth within clients (Dean, 1994). Minimally, that goal involves resolving the immediate crisis and restoring clients to their pre-crisis levels of functioning. Ultimately, however, intervention seeks to raise that functioning to a healthier, more mature level that will enable clients to cope with and prevent future crises. As discussed earlier, crises tend to be self-limiting; intervention time lasts from 4 to 8 weeks, with resolution, one way or another, within 2 to 3 months (Roberts, 1991; Aguilera, 1997). The urgency of the situation represents a window of opportunity that invites the prompt, focused attention of clients and nurse working together to achieve intervention goals.

Special programs for children living in homes where crises and violence are chronic include Head Start programs for pre-kindergarten children meeting certain socioeconomic characteristics. These programs give children the social and academic stimulation to be on par with peers when they enter kindergarten. Other programs include those for social skills development and Special Friends Programs explicitly for children who have survived abusive situations. Survivors experience multiple developmental and psychological problems. Assessment of children experiencing learning and social failure should be an ongoing service in both elementary and high schools. Just as important is the early identification

of and intervention with conduct-disordered youth. School nurses can be an important interprofessional team member in such programs.

Intervention at the secondary level for adults who experience abuse focuses on women and their children. Shelters for women and children are available in most communities and offer a bevy of services, including counseling for the woman, classes in self-esteem building and assertiveness training, referrals to or programs for job acquisition training, even money and time management classes. Some shelters offer programs that last for up to 2 years of progressive independence and employment skill development, where the women and their children live in protective home environments with addresses being kept confidential from the abuser.

Depending on the situation that brings the woman to a shelter, the perpetrator may or may not be incarcerated or on probation. If the abuser was arrested during the most recent violent episode, he may be released, on parole, or incarcerated. Even while incarcerated, the abuser may take part in an anger-management class, psychological counseling, substance abuse treatment, Alcohol Anonymous (AA) meetings, or Narcotics Anonymous (NA) meetings. Visits with his children are supervised if they are part of a court order.

At times the nurse may be responding to a referral regarding suspected abuse; other times an abusive or neglectful situation is uncovered on a home visit being made for another reason. Regardless, the community health nurse has an important role in reporting the suspected abuse and encouraging the child, partner/spouse, or elder to go to the appropriate facility for care and documentation of the abuse.

REPORTING ABUSE

All states have reporting laws for suspected abuse. The particulars regarding the timing, who is notified, and the sequence of events may differ from state to state. The following steps are one state's guidelines for reporting suspected child abuse:

1. All mandated reporters must report known or suspected abuse. (Mandated reporters include public and private school employees, administrators and employees of a youth center, recreation program, child welfare employees, foster parents, group home and residential facility personnel, social workers, probation workers, health care workers, including nurses, doctors, and chiropractics, and animal control workers and personnel working in film development laboratories.)

2. Immediately, or as soon as reasonably possible, a local child protective agency (police department after normal working hours) must be contacted and given a verbal report. During this verbal report, mandated reporters must give their name, which is kept confidential and may only be revealed in court or when the reporter waives confidentiality (others can give information anonymously), name and age of the child, present location of the child, nature and

characteristics of the injury, and any other facts that led the reporter to suspect abuse and/or would be helpful to the investigator.

3. Within 2 working days, a written report must be completed by the mandated reporter and filed. If a mandated reporter fails to report known or suspected instances of child abuse, she or he may be subject to criminal liability, punishable by up to 6 months in jail or a fine of $1000 (Family Violence Prevention Fund, 1995).

Similar steps are required for nurses to report elder abuse. Cases of maltreatment and self-neglect among elders are reported to a local office of the area agency on aging (or police), and a screening/documentation form is used to gather and record the pertinent abuse/neglect information.

In cases of partner/spousal abuse, adults who are mentally competent cannot be removed involuntarily from the abusive situation. The community health nurse can encourage the victim to leave the perpetrator for her safety until he gets professional help and give information regarding community resources, such as going to a shelter for women and children. If the adult has a life-threatening injury or illness, medical follow-up must be encouraged; however, the victim may still be reluctant to seek help. At times another family member or neighbor witnessing the abusive event may call 911; when the police and paramedics arrive, the victim may have the support to seek the care and protection needed. A Domestic Violence Screening/Documentation Form is completed and filed by the nurse as a part of the official health records for the client.

TOOLS

Assessment of suspected abuse cannot be overemphasized. The community health nurse may be the only person entering the home of a family in crisis where abuse is occurring. Asking the right questions, being a careful observer, and following the right reporting and recording procedure may mean the difference between life and death for the victims of the cycle of violence.

Appendices A, B, and C consist of three sample tools that the community health nurse and other advocates use in their role of mandated reporter. The tools are the Suspected Child Abuse Report, a two-page medical report of suspected child abuse, and a Domestic Violence Screening/Documentation Form.

Tertiary Prevention

Tertiary prevention of family violence focuses on the rehabilitation of the family. The family may never again be the same unit of service as the partners may separate, either by choice, motivated by fear or hate; by court order, when the perpetrator is incarcerated; or by death.

If the family chooses to stay together, long-term intervention for all family members is needed to establish a climate conducive to family normalcy. Many of the services discussed during the secondary level of prevention are continued into tertiary prevention to heal, restore, and promote the growth of the family.

If incarceration is a part of tertiary prevention, the effects of one family member living in this environment must be factored into the services and support provided by the community health nurse to the family as a whole (see Chapter 36). Even if the partner/spouse has separated from the perpetrator emotionally and/or legally, the perpetrator usually has legal rights to see his children. This means that other family members, usually from the abuser's side of the family, bring the children to the prison to visit their father. Just making these arrangements can cause stress for the mother and the children. The community health nurse needs to be aware of the complicated dynamics and emotional stress such difficult situations can produce for all family members. The victim–perpetrator relationship is as complex as the forces that created the violence and abuse.

METHODS OF INTERVENTION

Crisis intervention in community health nursing may use one or both of two approaches: generic and individual. For the majority of crisis encounters, the generic approach is more appropriate. Family violence is a major situational crisis in which community health nurses intervene. However, many other situational and developmental crises affect families who are benefited by the skills of the community health nurse.

Generic Approach

The generic approach designs interventions to fit a particular type of crisis, focusing on the nature and course of the crisis rather than on the psychodynamics of each client (Aguilera, 1997). Crisis intervention using the generic approach is tailored to a specific kind of crisis, situational or developmental, and comprises four important elements: (1) encouraging use of adaptive behavior and coping strategies, (2) support, (3) preparation for the practical and emotional future, and (4) anticipatory guidance.

An example of the generic approach is used with families experiencing child abuse. The child may be in foster care while the family receives needed services and rebuilds itself. The nurse encourages the parents to discuss and analyze their feelings, teaches stress-reduction techniques and positive coping skills, and creates a supportive, caring atmosphere especially through self-help groups such as Parents Anonymous. The nurse can help individual family members strengthen self-esteem by encouraging positive interpersonal relationships. The community health nurse also teaches the parents needed parenting skills and provides anticipatory guidance so that they are prepared to raise their children by using consistent and appropriate discipline techniques that are age-appropriate.

The generic approach does not require advanced professional psychotherapy skills. More important for community health practice, it works well with families, groups, and even communities in crisis. The community health nurse may work with a group of cancer clients, abused elders, adolescents struggling with developmental crisis, or an entire community recovering from some natural or man-made disaster. The generic approach allows the nurse to intervene with any group of people who have a crisis in common. It offers a broad base of support, since such a group can offer resources for the members beyond those brought by the nurse.

Individual Approach

The individual approach is used when clients do not respond to the generic approach or when they need special therapy. Individual crisis intervention should not be confused with individual psychotherapy, which tends to focus on clients' developmental past. In contrast, crisis intervention directs treatment toward the immediate state of disequilibrium, identifying its causes and developing coping mechanisms. Family members or significant others are included during the process of crisis resolution. An entire group may need this type of intervention. When this approach is needed, clients are usually referred to a professional with specialized training.

ROLE OF THE COMMUNITY HEALTH NURSE IN CARING FOR FAMILIES IN CRISIS

Crisis intervention in community health assumes that clients have resources. If their potential for managing stressful events can be tapped, people in crisis will need minimal direct assistance. In accordance with the self-care concept, crisis intervention seeks to identify and build on client strengths. Aguilera (1997) outlines a series of four steps for intervention during crisis: assessment, planning, intervention, and resolution. Interventions to promote crisis resolution are presented using the three levels of prevention in Table 25–2.

Assessment and Nursing Diagnosis

Initially, the nurse must assess the nature of the crisis and the clients' response to it. How severe is the problem, and what risks do the clients face? Are other people also at risk? Assessment must be rapid but thorough, focusing on certain specific areas.

First, the nurse concentrates on the immediate problem during the assessment. Why have clients asked for help right now? How do they define the problem? What precipitated the crisis? When did it occur? Was it a sudden accidental or situational event, or a slower developmental one?

Next, the nurse focuses on the clients' perceptions of the event. What does the crisis mean to them, and how do they think it will affect their future? Are they viewing the situation realistically? When a crisis occurs to a family or group, some members see the situation differently from others. During intervention, all should be encouraged to express themselves, to talk about the crisis, and to share their feelings about its meaning. Acceptance of the range of feelings is important.

Determine what persons are available for support. Consider family, friends, clergy, other professionals, community members, and agencies. With whom are the clients close, and whom do they trust? One advantage of group intervention is that the members provide some of this support for one another. In subsequent sessions the quality of support should be evaluated. Sometimes a well-meaning individual may worsen the situation or deter clients from facing and coping with reality.

Finally, the nurse needs to assess the clients' coping abilities. Have they had similar kinds of experiences in the past? What techniques have they previously used to relieve tension and anxiety? Which ones have they tried in this situation, and if they have not worked, why not? Clients should be encouraged to think of other stress-relieving techniques, perhaps ones they have used in the past, and to try them.

The nurse gathers all of these data and mentally begins to form nursing diagnoses. As a plan of care is developed for the client, these nursing diagnoses are formalized in writing. Standardized nursing diagnoses are available for reference, or the agency for whom the nurse works may have a format of nursing diagnoses that it prefers. These nursing diagnoses are effective tools as the nurse begins planning intervention.

Planning Therapeutic Intervention

Several factors influence clients' reaction to crises. Nurses should try to determine what factors are affecting clients before making intervention plans. The major balancing factors—clients' perceptions of the event, situational supports, human resources, and clients' coping skills—have been assessed in the first step (Aguilera, 1997). While continuing to explore these, the nurse now also considers the clients' general health status, age, past experiences with similar types of situations, sociocultural and religious influences, and the actual assets and liabilities of the situation. This helps to clarify the situation and gives the nurse the opportunity to further encourage clients' participation in the resolution process. If clients are defensive, resistant, and rigid, they are not processing clearly and can complete only simple tasks. It will take time before clients can begin to problem-solve the ef-

TABLE 25–2. Interventions to Promote Crisis Resolution

Phase	Goals	Interventions
Precrisis	Health promotion Disease prevention Education	**PRIMARY INTERVENTION** Anticipatory guidance Reduce factors that increase vunerability Reduce hazards in some events (safety and multiplicity of stressors) Reinforce positive coping strategies Mobilize social support and other resources
Crisis	Reduction of stress load Cure or restoration of function	**SECONDARY PREVENTION** Assist with reaction to the event and functioning Allow behavior: dependence, grief Set goals with client Refer to resources
Postcrisis	Rehabilitation and maintenance	**TERTIARY PREVENTION** Promote adaptation to a changed level of wellness Promote interdependence Reinforce newly learned behaviors, lifestyle changes, coping strategies Explore application of learned behaviors to new situations Identification and use of additional resources

fects of the crisis on themselves and the loss they are experiencing, but reaching this level needs to be encouraged by the nurse.

The plan is based on the kind of crisis (situational or developmental, acute or chronically recurring), the effect the crisis is having on clients' lives (can they still work, go to school, keep house?), where they are in coming to resolution of the crisis, the ways significant others are affected and respond, and the clients' strengths and available resources.

Using the problem-solving process, nurse and clients develop a plan. They review the event that precipitated the crisis, obvious symptoms, and the disruption in the clients' lives. The plan may focus on one or several areas. For instance, clients may need to grasp intellectually the meaning of the crisis, to engage in greater expression of feelings, or both. Part of the plan may be directed toward finding appropriate and safe shelter, counseling, or physical care. Another part may focus on helping clients identify and use more effective coping techniques or locate supportive agencies and resource people (Roberts, 1991). The plan will also include the development of realistic goals for the future.

Implementation

During implementation it is important for nurse and clients to continue to communicate. They should discuss what is happening, review the plan and the rationale behind its elements, and make appropriate changes when indicated. It is helpful to assign definite activities at the end of each session so that clients can try out different solutions and evaluate various coping behaviors.

The implementation step is enhanced by use of the guidelines below (Murray & Zentner, 1993; Roberts, 1991):

1. Demonstrate acceptance of clients. A crisis will often shatter the ego. Clients need to feel the support of a positive, caring person who does not judge their feelings or behavior. Some negative expressions, such as anger, withdrawal, and denial, are normal aspects of the crisis phase. Accept them as normal.

2. Help clients confront crisis. Clients need to face and discuss the situation. Expressing their feelings reduces tension and improves reality perception. Recounting what has actually occurred may be painful, but it helps clients confront the crisis. Do not assume that once clients have told about the event, no further recounting is necessary. Each time the story is told, they come closer to dealing realistically with the crisis.

3. Help clients find facts. Distorted ideas and unknown factors of the situation create additional tension and may lead to maladaptive responses. For instance, it would help inexperienced parents to know that children under the age of 2 years cannot deliberately misbehave. Facts about childhood development and patenting training would be important for preventing crisis.

4. Help clients express feelings openly. Suppressed feelings can be harmful. For instance, a widow may feel guilty that she is glad her husband is gone. Expression of such feelings as these helps reduce tension and gives clients an opportunity to deal with them.

5. Do not offer false reassurance. Clients need to face reality, not avoid it. A statement such as "Don't worry, it will all work out" is demeaning and meaningless.

Instead, make positive statements about faith in their ability to cope: "It is a very difficult situation, but I believe you will be able to deal with it."

6. Discourage clients from blaming others. Clients often blame others as a way to avoid reality and the responsibility for problem solving. Withhold judgment when they blame others, but point out other causal factors and avenues for dealing with the situation.

7. Help clients seek out coping mechanisms. Explore and test old and new techniques to reduce stress and anxiety. Ask questions. What are all the things the client and nurse might do together to resolve the problem? What are the things that need to be done? What do clients think they can do? This assistance gives clients more adaptive energy to work toward resolution.

8. Encourage clients to accept help. Denial in the early phases of crisis cuts off help. Encouraging clients to acknowledge the problem is a first step toward acceptance of help. Often, however, clients fear the loss of their independence and the invasion of their privacy. They may say, "We ought to be able to handle this problem." At this point, the community health nurse can assure clients that people in a crisis of this sort almost always need help. Preparing people to accept help will enable them to make the best use of what others have to offer.

9. Promote development of new positive relationships. Clients who have lost significant persons through death, divorce, or incarceration should be encouraged to find new people to fill the void and provide needed supports and satisfactions.

Evaluation of Crisis Resolution and Anticipatory Planning

In the final step, clients and nurse evaluate, stabilize, and plan for the future. First, evaluate the outcome of the intervention. Are clients using effective coping skills and exhibiting appropriate behavior? Are adequate resources and support persons available? Is the diagnosed problem solved, and have the desired results been accomplished? Analysis of these outcomes gives a greater understanding for coping with future crises.

To stabilize the change, identify and reinforce all the positive coping mechanisms and behaviors. Discuss why they are effective, and explore ways to use them in future stressful situations. Summarize the crisis experience, emphasizing the clients' successes with coping in order to reconfirm progress and reinforce self-confidence. Point to evidence that they have reached their pre-crisis, or an even higher, level of functioning.

Clients' plans for the future should include setting realistic goals and a means for implementing them. Review with clients how their handling of the present crisis can help them cope with, minimize, or preferably prevent future crises.

SUMMARY

Crisis is a temporary state of severe disequilibrium for persons who face a threatening situation. It is a state that they can neither avoid nor solve with their usual coping abilities. A crisis occurs when some force disrupts normal functioning and thus causes a loss of balance or normalcy in life. A crisis creates tension; subsequently, efforts are made to solve the problem and reduce the tension. When such efforts meet with failure, people feel upset, redefine the situation, try other solutions, and, if failure continues, eventually reach the breaking point.

There are two main types of crisis: developmental and situational. Developmental crises are disruptions that occur during transitional periods in normal growth and development. They usually have a gradual onset and are often predictable. Situational crises are precipitated by an unexpected external event and occur suddenly, sometimes without warning.

Family violence constitutes a unique crisis for the victim and the entire family and is becoming disturbingly prevalent in the United States. Historically, family violence is not new. Until recently in our nation's history, there have not been laws or societal concerns about the treatment of spouses/partners or children. Although we have made human rights advances, abuses against women and children remain socially and culturally accepted in some countries in the world.

Abuse can be physical, emotional, and sexual. Neglect and sexual exploitation are additional forms of abuse. Neglect may be general or specific, such as medical or educational neglect. Child abuse occurs among children of all ages, from infancy through the teen years. There are specific forms of abuse that are identified sometimes only upon autopsy—shaken baby syndrome and Munchausen syndrome by proxy. Teen dating violence, violence during pregnancy, and violence against women in general constitute partner/spousal abuse. Finally, a most unsettling form of violence—elder abuse, neglect, and exploitation—occurs more frequently than we know.

Community health nurses use three levels of prevention when working with families. Primary prevention focuses on providing people with the skills and resources to prevent violent situations. Secondary prevention involves immediate intervention at the time of the violent episode. This involves providing different services for each family member, such as medical attention, emotional support, and police involvement. Tertiary prevention offers family rebuilding services and helps the family establish equilibrium with a structure that may be different, but healthier.

People in crisis need and often seek help. Crisis intervention builds on these two phenomena to achieve its primary goal—reestablishment of equilibrium. The two major methods of crisis intervention are the generic and individual approaches. The generic approach is used with groups of people involved in the same type of crisis, such as rape victims, mothers who have lost children from drunken driving, or a family experiencing child abuse. The individual approach is used when clients do not respond to the generic approach or need additional therapy. Crisis intervention begins with assessment of the situation; then a therapeutic intervention is planned. Next, the nurse carries out the intervention, building on the strengths and self-care ability of clients. Crisis intervention concludes with resolution and anticipatory planning to avert possible future crises.

Regardless of the method of intervention the community health nurse uses, the steps of the nursing process provide a framework in which to intervene. Assessing the family's assets and liabilities, willingness to change, and nature of the violence helps the nurse form a nursing diagnosis. With this diagnosis, the nurse can begin to plan appropriate interventions and implement the plans in concert with the family. Evaluation of the intervention techniques provides the nurse with new data that will assist with ongoing assessment of the family's progress and additional anticipatory guidance needs.

CLINICAL CORNER | **Community Health Nursing and a Potential Family in Crisis**

You are a community health nurse working for Smithville Health Department. You are following up on a referral from a community clinic's family planning clinic. The referral was made for a 19-year-old woman, Sandy, who presented in clinic and exhibited inappropriate behaviors with her 6-month-old daughter. In their referral, staff stated that they observed the mother shouting at the child, accusing her of "being spoiled rotten." They added that the mother appeared quite anxious and seemed to have difficulty waiting the 15 minutes for her examination. Although the behaviors described in this referral were insufficient to warrant a report to social services, the staff felt that this young mother would benefit from intervention on the part of the nurse.

You prepare for this home visit by reviewing the medical records of both Sandy and her child to determine whether the family has had previous involvement with social service agencies such as child protective services. You find that the maternal grandparents made a referral to Child Welfare on behalf of Sandy when she was 15. They were concerned about the relationship between Sandy and her step-father. The report cited suspected sexual involvement between the two. An investigation occurred but was inconclusive, and the charges were never pursued.

You also discuss the case with family planning and immunization clinic staff, since the family receives services at both clinics. The staff advise you that they are familiar with Sandy and her husband Nick. They state that their only interaction with Nick was during a family planning clinic 2 months ago. They report that Sandy appeared anxious and in a hurry on that day, stating, "I really need to hurry, Nick is waiting in the car and he gets impatient." Shortly after that, the staff tells you, Nick came running into the clinic shouting, "What the hell is taking you people so long?" He reportedly glared at Sandy, and the two quickly exited the clinic.

You phone the client and advise her that you are a nurse with the local health department. You inform her that nurses often visit new mothers to assist them in finding resources. You add that as a community health nurse, you will be available to talk with her about her child's growth and development.

The client expresses interest in the visit and states, "I want you to show me some things about feeding her and stuff. I need help figuring out what to do at night, she still isn't sleeping much and it's driving me crazy." You advise the client that you will be happy to discuss those issues with her, that you will bring information which you will review with her. You add that you noted in her medical record that the father of the baby is living in the home and assure her that she may involve other family members, including the father of the baby, in the home visit. You jointly decide that the visit will occur the following day at 10:30 AM and that the father of the baby will be present if his work schedule allows.

On the day of the visit, as you walk up the stairs toward the apartment, you notice someone looking at you through the curtains. As you near the apartment door the curtains close. Your repeated knocking on the door is met with no response. You call the client's name but there is no answer.

Questions
1. Would this scenario provoke anxiety for you? How would you deal with your reaction?
2. How is this different from a scenario in the acute care setting in which a supervisor would be readily available?
3. Given this scenario, what actions will you take?
4. If you had been working in the family planning clinic on the day that Nick came in, what, if anything, would you have done differently?
5. As young parents, Nick and Sandy are part of an aggregate that has unique risk factors for parenting. List as many of these risk factors as you can think of and brainstorm about possible community health nursing interventions for each.
6. What methods would you suggest the clinic staff utilize to detect signs and symptoms of physical, sexual, or emotional abuse among this aggregate?

ACTIVITIES TO PROMOTE CRITICAL THINKING

1. What are the major differences between a developmental and a situational crisis? Give examples of each from personal experiences.
2. Describe a developmental crisis experienced by a family. What was this family's response? Describe some actions a community health nurse might have taken (alone or within an interdisciplinary team) to help the family cope with the crisis.
3. Children, even the very young, are becoming violent. What preventive actions can the community health nurse take? Design actions at each level of prevention.
4. Watch a news station on television. Listen for examples of developmental or situational crises occurring to families in the world. Analyze the situations and anticipate what the role of a community health nurse would be during the crises selected.
5. Family violence is a significant public health problem. Assume that a battered wife becomes a community health nurse's client, and the nurse suspects there may be more women with this problem in the community. Describe how the nurse might provide assistance using the crisis intervention steps. Then discuss how a three-level preventive program might be instituted in the community.
6. Using the Internet, select a situational crisis, such as spousal abuse, adolescent sexual exploitation, or neglect of the elderly, and read about the most current information on this topic. Depending on your personal interests or current community health nursing experiences, develop a file of articles you have uncovered using the Internet. This file can be useful to you, to agency staff in your clinical setting, and to families you visit.

REFERENCES

Aguilera, D. C. (1997). *Crisis intervention: Theory and methodology* (8th ed.). St. Louis: Mosby.

American Psychological Association. (1996). *Violence and the family: Report of the American Psychological Association Presidential Task Force on Violence and the Family.* Washington, D.C.: American Psychological Association.

Anetzberger, G.J. (1990). Abuse, neglect and self-neglect: Issues of vulnerability. In Z. Hanel, P. Ehrlich, & R. Hubbard (Eds.), *The vulnerable aged: People, services, and policies* (pp. 140–148). New York: Springer.

Archstone Foundation. (1996). *Silent suffering: Elder abuse in America.* Long Beach, CA: Archstone Foundation.

Besharov, D.J.(1998). Four commentaries: How we can better protect children from abuse and neglect. *The Future of Children: Protecting Children from Abuse and Neglect, 8*(1), 120–123.

Bureau of Justice Statistics (August, 1997). *Violence-related injuries treated in hospital emergency departments.* Washington, D.C.: U.S. Department of Justice.

Campbell, J. (1998). *Empowering survivors of abuse: Health care, battered women and their children.* Thousand Oaks, CA: Sage.

Campbell, J. C. (1999). If I can't have you no one can: Murder linked to battery during pregnancy. *Reflections, 25*(3), 8–12.

Carden, A.D. (1994). Wife abuse and the wife abuser—Review and recommendations. *The Counseling Psychologist, 22*(4), 539–582.

Child Care Law Center. (October, 1992). *Mandatory reporting of child abuse.* San Francisco: Fresno County Department of Social Services.

Cokkinides, V.E., & Coker, A.L. (1998). Experiencing physical violence during pregnancy: Prevalence and correlates. *Family Community Health, 20*(4), 19–37.

Congressional Caucus for Women's Issues. *Effects of rape* (monograph). Washington, D.C.: Author.

Crime and Violence Prevention Center. (1996). *Child abuse: Educator's responsibilities* (3rd ed.). Sacramento, CA: California Attorney General's Office.

Crime Prevention Center. (1993). *Child abuse prevention handbook.* Sacramento, CA: Office of the Attorney General.

Curry, M.A., Doyle, B.A., & Gilhooley, J. (1998). Abuse among pregnant adolescents: Differences by developmental age. *Maternal and Child Nursing, 23*(3), 144–150.

Dannenberg, A.L., Carter, D.M., Lawson, H.W., et al. (1995). Homicide and other injuries as causes of maternal death in New York City, 1987 through 1991. *American Journal of Obstetrics and Gynecology, 172,* 1557–1564.

Dean, C. (1994). Strengthening families: From "deficit" to "empowerment." *Journal of Emotional and Behavioral Problems, 2*(4), 8–11.

Family crisis. Conflict theories and symbolic interaction theory, 1–19. Fcnote5a.htm at *www.uakron.edu* (accessed 9/12/98)

Federal Bureau of Investigation. (1994). *Uniform crime reports for the United States, 1993.* Washington, D.C.: U.S. Department of Justice, Federal Bureau of Investigation.

Fitzgerald, S., Dienemann, J., & Cadorette, M.F. (1998). Domestic violence in the workplace. *American Association of Occupational Health Nurses Journal, 46*(7), 345–353.

Foshee, V.A., Bauman, K.E., Arriaga, X.B., et al. (1998). An evaluation of safe dates, an adolescent dating violence prevention program. *American Journal of Public Health, 88*(1), 45–50.

Furniss, K. (1996). Common clinical problems and issues. In Association of Women's Health Obstetric and Neonatal Nurses (AWHONN) and National Association of Nurse Practitioners and Reproductive Health (NANPRH) (Eds.), *Current practice issues in adolescent gynecology. Contemporary studies in women's health.* Fair Lawn, NJ: MPE Communications.

Gorin, S.S., & Arnold, J. (1998). *Health promotion handbook.* St. Louis: Mosby.

Holmes, T. & Rahe, R. (1967). The social readjustment rating scale. *Journal of Psychosomatic Research, 11,* 213–217.

Kalafat, J. (1991). Suicide interventions in the schools. In A.R. Roberts (Ed.), *Contemporary perspectives on crisis intervention and prevention* (pp. 218–239). Englewood Cliffs, NJ: Prentice-Hall.

Lachs, M.S., & Pillemer, K. (1995). Abuse and neglect of elderly persons. *New England Journal of Medicine, 332*(7), 437–443.

Lachs, M.S., Williams, C., O'Brien, S., Hurst, L., & Horwitz, R. (1997). Risk factors for reported elder abuse and neglect: A nine-year observational cohort study. *The Gerontologist, 37,* 469–474.

Levinson, D. J. (1978). *The seasons of a man's life.* New York: Knopf.

Miller, C.A. (1999). *Nursing care of older adults: Theory and practice* (3rd ed.). Philadelphia: Lippincott Williams & Wilkins.

Murray, R. & Zentner, J. (1993). *Nursing assessment and health promotion strategies* (5th ed.). Englewood Cliffs, NJ: Prentice-Hall.

National Committee to Prevent Child Abuse. (1996). *Current trends in child abuse reporting and fatalities: The result of the 1995 fifty-state survey.* Chicago: Author.

Olds, D.L., Eckenrode, J., Henderson, C.R., et al. (1997). Long-term effects of home visitation on maternal life course and child abuse and neglect: Fifteen-year follow-up of a randomized trial. *Journal of the American Medical Association, 276*(8), 637–643.

Parker, B., McFarlane, J., & Soeken, K. (1994). Abuse during pregnancy: Effects on maternal complications and birth weight in adult and teenage women. *Obstetrics and Gynecology, 84,* 323–328.

Pillemer, K., & Finkelhor, A. (1988). The prevalence of elder abuse: A random sample survey. *The Gerontologist, 28,* 51–57.

Plitcha, S.B. (1996). Violence and abuse: Implications for women's health. In M.M. Falik & K.S. Collins (Eds.), *Women's health: The commonwealth fund survey* (pp. 237–270). Baltimore: The Johns Hopkins University Press.

Roberts, A. (Ed.) (1991). *Contemporary perspectives on crisis intervention and prevention.* Englewood Cliffs, NJ: Prentice-Hall.

Rooke, P.T., & Schnell, R.L. (1995). "Uncramping child life": International children's organisations, 1914–1939. In P. Weindling (Ed.), *International organisations and movements, 1918–1939* (pp. 176–202). Cambridge, UK: Cambridge University Press.

Ryan, J.M. (1997). Child abuse and the community health nurse. In B.W. Spradley & J.A. Allender (Eds.), *Readings in community health nursing* (5th ed., pp. 371–376). Philadelphia: Lippincott-Raven.

Shaw, M.C. & Halliday, P.H. (1992). The family, crisis and chronic illness: An evolutionary model. *Journal of Advanced Nursing, 17,* 537–543.

Sheehy, G. (1995). *New passages: Mapping your life across time.* New York: Random House.

———. (1976). *Passages: Predictable crises of adult life.* New York: Dutton.

Stewart, D., & Cecutti, A. (1993). Physical abuse in pregnancy. *Canadian Medical Association Journal, 149,* 1257–1263.

Oklahoma monitors intimate partner violence. (March, 2000). *The Nation's Health, 30*(2), 1, 7.

Tyra, P.A. (1996). Helping elderly women survive rape using a crisis framework. *Journal of Psychosocial Nursing and Mental Health Services, 34*(12), 20–25.

United States Department of Health and Human Services (USDHHS). (1988). *Administration for children, youth and families: Child Abuse Prevention, Adoption and Services Act of 1988.* Washington, D.C.: U.S. Government Printing Office.

———. (1998). *Healthy people 2010 objectives: Draft for public comment.* Washington, D.C.: U.S. Government Printing Office.

———. (2000). *Healthy people 2010* (conference edition in two volumes). Washington, D.C.: U.S. Government Printing Office.

U.S. Department of Justice. (1996). *Battered child syndrome: Investigating physical abuse and homicide.* Washington, D.C.: Office of Justice Programs.

———. (1997). *Understanding and investigating child sexual exploitation.* Washington, D.C.: Office of Justice Programs.

Walker, L.E. (1979). *The battered woman.* New York: Harper & Row.

World Health Organization (WHO). (1998). *Report of the Director-General. The world health report 1998: Life in the 21st century: A vision for all.* Geneva: World Health Organization.

COMMUNITY RESOURCES

Parents Anonymous. Self-help groups for potentially abusive or abusive parents. Facilitators consist of a professional and a formerly abusive parent. Usually no fee/low fee, child care and transportation provided.

Parents United. Self-help groups for sexually abusive families. Consists of groups for offenders, children, and mothers. Also have groups for Adults Molested as Children (MAC). Comprehensive child sexual abuse program.

Parental Stress Hotlines. 24-hour crisis telephone assistance for persons under stress. Telephone counseling primarily, but can also provide home visiting program and respite care. Usually offer parent rap groups and other services.

Respite Care Programs. Licensed homes that provide care for children when their parents "need a break." Not a baby-sitting service. Designed for high-risk parents. Voluntary.

Emergency Family Care. In-home based services. Workers literally "move in" with the family to provide concrete services. Frequently work with neglectful parents whose children might be removed without this service.

Parent-Infant Bonding (Perinatal Programs). Designed to help new parents with bonding skills; provide parent education regarding the child's needs. Provide early intervention services.

Child Abuse Councils. Provide information and referral; educational services including book and film library. Usually are multidisciplinary in nature, and help coordinate service delivery. Provide visibility to the problem of child abuse.

Parent Education Classes. Designed to help parents gain better understanding of child development and learn skills for disciplining their children in a safe way.

Parent Discussion Groups. Provide a forum in which parents may discuss childrearing problems, gain peer support, and minimize their isolation.

Community Mental Health Departments. Provide low-fee therapeutic services to families and children. Available in every community. Frequently serve a broad range of abusive families.

Child Care Resource Centers. Provide valuable child care information to parents who may be overwhelmed by the demands of patenting. Information and referral.

Private Mental Health Clinics/Therapist Groups. There are many private therapists who specialize in working with child abuse. Child Abuse Councils or Child Protective Agencies are usually familiar with good referral possibilities.

Family Service Agencies. Many of these agencies have taken a leadership role in child abuse prevention/treatment services. Therapeutic services are available on a sliding-fee scale.

NATIONAL RESOURCES

National Center on Child Abuse and Neglect (NCCAN) Clearinghouse
National Center on Family Violence Clearinghouse
P.O. Box 1182
Washington, D.C. 20013
1-800-FYI-3366
National Committee for the Prevention of Child Abuse (NCPCA)
332 S. Michigan Avenue, Suite 1600
Chicago, IL 60604
1-312-663-3520
The American Professional Society on the Abuse of Children (APSAC)
332 S. Michigan Avenue, Suite 1600
Chicago, IL 60604
1-312-554-0166
National Center for the Prosecution of Child Abuse
American Prosecutors Research Institute
1033 North Fairfax Street, Suite 200
Alexandria, VA 22314
1-703-739-0321

SUGGESTED READINGS

Ales, B. (1998). Community collaboration: The nursing administrator's role in implementing a child abuse prevention program. *Journal of Nursing Administration, 28*(6), 43–48.

Baron, S., & Welty, A. (1996). Elder abuse. *Journal of Gerontological Social Work, 25*(1/2), 33–57.

Blakeley, J., & Ribeiro, V. (1997). Community health and pediatric nurses' knowledge, attitudes, and behaviors regarding child sexual abuse. *Public Health Nursing, 14*(6), 339–345.

Cummings, E.M. & Davies, P. (1994). *Children and marital conflict: The impact of family dispute and resolution.* New York: Guilford Press.

Durch, J.S., Bailey, L.A., & Soto, M.A. (Eds.) (1997). *Improving health in the community: A role for performance monitoring.* Washington, D.C.: National Academy Press.

Fulmer, T.T. (1998). Mistreatment of elders: Assessment, diagnosis, and intervention. In J.A. Allender & C.L. Rector (Eds.), *Readings in gerontological nursing* (pp. 396–407). Philadelphia: Lippincott-Raven.

Fulmer, T. (1999). Our elderly—harmed, exploited, abandoned. *Reflections, 25*(3), 16–18.

Goldsmith, C. (September 21, 1998). Sheltering pets: Helping abused women by helping their pets. *NurseWeek,* 11.

Gullotta, T.P., & McElhaney, S.J. (1999). *Violence in homes and communities: Prevention, intervention, and treatment.* Thousand Oaks, CA: Sage.

Hatcher, P.A. (1997). Violence prevention begins at home—with nurses. *American Journal of Nursing, 97*(5), 80.

Karp, C.L., & Butler, T.L. (1996). *Treatment strategies for abused children: From victim to survivor.* Thousand Oaks, CA: Sage.

Karp, C.L., & Butler, T.L. (1998). *Treatment strategies for abused adolescents: From victim to survivor.* Thousand Oaks, CA: Sage.

Kübler-Ross, E. (1969). *On death and dying.* New York: Macmillan.

Lane, P.S. (1994). Critical incident stress debriefing for health care workers. *Omega: Journal of Death and Dying, 28*(4), 301–315.

Liefland, L., Caporale, E.M., Wellington, T., & Barber, L. (1997). A crisis intervention program: Staff go the extra mile for client improvement. *Journal of Psychosocial Nursing and Mental Health Services, 35*(2), 32–35.

Limbos, M.A.P., & Berkowitz, C.D. (1998). Documentation of child physical abuse: How far have we come? *Pediatrics, 102*(1), 53–58.

Long, N.J. (1992). Managing a shooting incident. *Journal of Emotional and Behavioral Problems, 1*(1), 23–26.

Mandt, A.K. (1993). The curriculum revolution in action: Nursing and crisis intervention for victims of family violence. *Journal of Nursing Education, 32*(1), 44–46.

Parnell, T.F., & Day, D.O. (1997). *Munchausen by proxy syndrome: Misunderstood child abuse.* Thousand Oaks, CA: Sage.

Pitcher, G.D. & Poland, S. (1992). *Crisis intervention in the schools.* New York: Guilford Press.

Quinn, M.J. (1998). Stopping elder abuse—new research, new strategies. Undue influence: An emotional con game. *Aging Today, 19*(6), 9, 11.

Schornstein, S.L. (19997). *Domestic violence and health care: What every professional needs to know.* Thousand Oaks, CA: Sage.

Song, L., Singer, M.I., & Anglin, T.M. (1998). Violence exposure and emotional trauma as contributors to adolescents' violent behaviors. *Archives of Pediatric and Adolescent Medicine, 152,* 531–536.

Stanhope, M., & Knollmueller, R.N. (1997). *Public and community health nurse's consultant: A health promotion guide*. St. Louis: Mosby.

Stanley, M., & Beare, P.G. (1999). *Gerontological nursing: A health promotion/protection approach* (2nd ed.). Philadelphia: F.A. Davis.

U.S. Department of Justice. (1997a). *Criminal investigation of child sexual abuse*. Washington, D.C.: Office of Justice Programs.

U.S. Department of Justice. (1997b). *Law enforcement response to child abuse*. Washington, D.C.: Office of Justice Programs.

Uphold, C.R. & Graham, M.V. (1993). Schools as centers for collaborative services for families: A vision for change. *Nursing Outlook, 41*(5), 204–211.

Van Auken, E. (1991). Crisis intervention: Elders awaiting placement in an acute care facility. *Journal of Gerontological Nursing, 17*(11), 30–33.

Veninga, R. & Spradley, J. (1981). *The work-stress connection*. Boston: Little, Brown.

Wilson, K., & James, A.(1995) *The child protection handbook*. Philadelphia: W.B. Saunders.

Wright, L.M. & Leahey, M. (1994). Calgary family intervention model: One way to think about change. *Journal of Marital and Family Therapy, 20,* 381–395.

CHAPTER

26

Maternal, Prenatal, and Newborn Populations

KEY TERMS

- Developmental disability
- Drug dependent
- Drug exposed
- Fetal alcohol effects
- Fetal alcohol syndrome
- Gestational diabetes mellitus
- Low birth weight
- Passive smoking
- Self-help groups
- Smokeless tobacco products
- Sudden infant death syndrome (SIDS)
- Very low birth weight

LEARNING OBJECTIVES

Upon mastery of this chapter, you should be able to:

- Discuss the global view of maternal and infant health.
- Identify the *Healthy People 2010* goals established for the maternal–infant population.
- Discuss major risk factors and special complications for childbearing families.
- Describe the important considerations in designing effective health promotion programs to fit the needs of diverse maternal–infant populations.
- List several features of a typical health promotion program for maternal–infant populations.
- Identify six methods of delivering services to maternal–infant populations.
- Describe various roles of a community health nurse in serving the maternal–infant population.

You will notice as you start to work in the community that the majority of your clients will be pregnant teens, women having a third, fourth, or fifth child, and subsequently, lots of infants and young children. Working with maternal and infant populations is a primary facet of community health nursing. More than 70% of nursing practice in official health agencies involves primary preventive work with mothers and infants. Why should maternal–infant populations require this amount of attention from community health nursing? Despite the existence of advanced technology and the availability of excellent perinatal services in our society, certain segments of the maternal and infant populations, such as adolescent mothers and those who are economically disadvantaged, remain at high risk for disease, disability, and even death. Although some women receive excellent prenatal care and benefit from the diagnostic capabilities of advanced technology, other women go without prenatal care and even without proper nutrition.

Historically, the health needs of pregnant women and their newborns began to receive priority status in the public health arena after we began to gain control over communicable diseases. By the mid-20th century, many health programs had been established at the local level. In the 1970s, funding from state and federal revenues enhanced existing prenatal and newborn services. The community health nurse has always had a prominent role in the planning, implementation, and evaluation of these programs.

This chapter addresses three major areas in the health of maternal–infant populations: (1) health status and needs; (2) design, implementation, and evaluation of maternal–infant health programs; and (3) availability of community resources.

HEALTH STATUS AND NEEDS OF PREGNANT WOMEN AND INFANTS

Community health nurses constitute a key group of health care workers involved in both the planning of programs and the actual delivery of services to mothers and babies. A solid understanding of vital statistics and other data regarding maternal–infant populations serves nurses as they determine both the appropriateness and the effectiveness of programs and services. Reviewing some of the global and national vital statistics of the past decade provides insight into the problem areas in maternal–infant health and gives direction for the future.

Global Overview

Almost 600,000 women die each year of pregnancy-related causes, 99% of them in developing countries (World Health Organization [WHO], 1998). In Africa, the rate is 1 death for every 16 pregnancies, compared with 1 in 65 in Asia and 1 in 1,400 in Europe. About 80% of the maternal deaths are due to direct causes, such as complications of pregnancy, labor and postpartum; to interventions, omissions, or incorrect treatment; or to the chain of events resulting from any one of these. Postpartum hemorrhage accounts for 25% of these maternal deaths.

Globally, the infant mortality rate (IMR) has been decreasing. In 1955 the IMR was 148 per 1,000 live births. Twenty years later, it had fallen to 90 per 1,000 live births and to 59 per 1,000 by 1995. Overall, the number of countries with an IMR below 50 per 1,000 live births increased to 102 countries in 1995, or 34% of global live births, from only 23 countries in 1955. It is expected that the world will continue to experience a decline, reaching a level of 32 by the year 2025. However, in 1995, there were 24 countries, 20 of them in Africa, where one in ten children dies before the first birthday.

Adolescence increases the maternal–infant mortality potential. In 1997, adolescents aged 15 to 19 gave birth to 17 million infants. Sixteen million of these births occurred in developing countries in Asia, Africa, Latin America, and the Caribbean (WHO, 1998). Other countries report only modest decreases in the number of women experiencing a pregnancy at an early age, except in Asia. All countries in Asia report a decline. Both the teenage mother and the infant are at risk. Teenage mothers have a higher rate of pregnancy-related complications, and their infants are more likely to have a low birth weight or to be premature, injured at birth, or stillborn. Mortality rates of infants born to adolescent mothers are higher than for those of women who give birth at older ages. Globally, it is expected that the 1997 figures of 17 million infants being born to adolescents aged 15 to 19 will decrease to 16 million infants by 2025 (WHO, 1998).

Perinatal transmission of human immunodeficiency virus (HIV) is an emerging global health crisis. The majority of children with acquired immunodeficiency syndrome (AIDS) are children of HIV-positive mothers who are being infected. AIDS is seen in 15% to 35% of the children with HIV-positive mothers. A significant portion of these children are born to HIV-infected adolescent mothers, especially in sub-Saharan Africa where both adolescent pregnancy and HIV rates are the highest in the world. Pediatric AIDS will increase accordingly.

National Overview

Over 4 million women in the United States give birth each year. Thirty-two percent of these women are single, and over 20% have no medical insurance (Statistical Abstract of United States, 1998). Many of these women do not have the financial or social resources to sustain minimal health levels for themselves and their infants.

In addition, a significant number of births are to adolescent women. In 1993, 36% of all U.S. births—almost 100,000—were to women in their teens with less than 12 years of schooling (Zill, 1996). Although the majority of pregnant adolescents are European Americans, the proportion of pregnant adolescents is higher in the African- and Hispanic-American populations. Additionally, there was an increasing trend throughout the last decades of the 20th century for unwed teenage mothers to keep their babies. These "children having children" with limited educational and economic advantages will affect the health of society well into the future.

Another area of concern is substance use and abuse among the childbearing population. The range of adverse consequences associated with the use of tobacco, alcohol, and illicit drugs during pregnancy is wide and includes preterm birth, low birth weight, and fetal alcohol syndrome (FAS), described shortly. Several studies have shown that many women who abuse drugs while pregnant do not receive prenatal care (Russell et al., 1996; Shah, Hoffman, Shinault & LaPoint, 1998). This puts these women and their unborn children in "double jeopardy." Not only are they at risk due to the consequences of the alcohol or drugs, but they also are not receiving the preventive prenatal care that can eliminate or reduce other obstetric complications.

Healthy People 2000 included specific goals for the maternal–infant population along with significant vital statistics and baseline information. The *Healthy People 2010* objectives for this population are based on the previous achievements in the same or similar areas (U.S. Department of Health and Human Services [USDHHS], 1991, 2000) (Table 26–1).

After years of working toward improving maternal–infant health, the United States has made very limited progress. Although the U.S. infant mortality rate (deaths for all babies up to 1 year of age) has dropped substantially from the 20.0 per 1,000 live births in 1970 to 7.2 per 1,000 live births in 1998, it remains higher than those of 24 other industrialized nations, including Japan, France, Italy, and the countries of Scandinavia (USD-

---

TABLE 26–1. Selected Maternal and Infant *Healthy People 2010* Target Objectives

Objective	Baseline
Reduce infant mortality rate from all birth defects to 1.1 per 1,000 live births.	1.6 (1998)
Reduce the sudden infant death syndrome (SIDS) mortality rate to 0.3 per 1,000 live births.	0.77 (1997)
Reduce the rate of child mortality to 25 per 100,000 children aged 1 to 4.	34.2 (1998)
Reduce the rate of child mortality to 14.3 per 100,000 children aged 5 to 9.	17.6 (1998)
Reduce the perinatal mortality rate per 1,000 live births plus fetal deaths as follows:	
Deaths of infants from 28 weeks' gestation to 7 days after birth to 4.5	7.5 (1997)
Deaths of infants from 20 weeks' gestation to 7 days after birth to 4.1	6.8 (1997)
Reduce to less than 20% the proportion of pregnant women who experience maternal complications during labor and delivery.	32.1% (1997)
Increase to at least 90% the proportion of all pregnant women who begin prenatal care in the first trimester of pregnancy.	83% (1998)
Reduce the prevalance of serious developmental disabilities arising from events in the prenatal and infant periods for:	
Mental retardation to 124 per 10,000	131 (1991–1994)
Cerebral palsy to 31.5 per 10,000	32.2 (1991–1994)
Reduce cesarean deliveries:	
Primary (first time) cesarean delivery	17.8 (1997)
Repeat cesarean deliveries to 12.5% to 63%	71% (1997)
Increase to 70% the percentage of infants who are put to sleep on their backs.	35% (1996)
Increase abstinence from alcohol use by pregnant women as follows:	
No use in the past month—increase to 94%	86% (1996–1977)
No binge drinking in the past month—increase to 100%	99% (1996–1997)
Increase abstinence from tobacco use by pregnant women to 98%.	87% (1996–1997)
Eliminate use of illicit drugs by pregnant women to 100%.	98% (1996–1997)
Reduce the incidence of spina bifida and other neural tube defects to 3 per 10,000 live births.	6 (1996)
Increase to at least 80% the proportion of women of childbearing age who take a vitamin with the recommended 0.4 mg of folic acid daily.	21 (1991–1994)
Increase breastfeeding among mothers as follows:	
To at least 75% in the early postpartum period	64% (1998)
To at least 50% until babies are 6 months old	29% (1998)
To at least 25% until babies are 1 year old	16% (1998)
(Retain *Healthy People 2000* target)	

(Adapted from U.S. Department of Health and Human Services [2000]. *Healthy people 2010* [conference edition in two volumes] Washington, DC: U.S. Government Printing Office.)

HHS, 2000). However, the rate for African-American infants remains more than twice that of white infants (USDHHS, 2000).

Low-birth-weight (LBW) babies (less than 2500 g at birth), **very-low-birth-weight** (VLBW) babies (a weight at birth of less than 1500 g), and maternal mortality are three areas in which the statistics have gotten worse. Statistics indicate a rise in the number of LBW babies for the total population from a low of 6.8% in 1985 to 7.6% in 1998 (Ventura, Martin, Curtin & Natgewsm, 1997; USDHHS, 2000). The rate of VLBW babies was 1.4% in 1998 among the total population. This rate has remained fairly stable in the country since 1990, but it has risen among African Americans while falling slightly among whites. Table 26–2 lists 1998 percentages of LBW and VLBW babies for selected populations and the goals for 2010.

In addition to infant deaths and low birth weights, the effects of pregnancy and childbirth on the woman are other important indicators of health and access to reproductive health care. The number of maternal deaths in 1997 was reported as

327, for an overall maternal mortality ratio of 8.4 per 100,000 live births. This ratio (fluctuating between 7 and 8 per 100,000 live births in the 1990s) has not declined since 1986, when it was 6.6 per 1000,000 live births, nor has the disparity between African-American and white women. The maternal mortality ratio among African-American women has consistently been three to four times that of white women (USDHHS, 2000). Ectopic pregnancy is the leading cause of maternal mortality in the first trimester, and the risk increases with age for women of all races. Other major causes of maternal morbidity include hemorrhage, pregnancy-induced hypertension, embolism, and infection (USDHHS, 2000).

There are, however, several areas in which great progress has been made toward the year 2000 goals. The neonatal mortality rate (deaths for all infants up to 28 days old) decreased from 15.1 per 1,000 live births in 1970, to 5.8 per 1,000 live births in 1990, and to 4.8 per 1,000 live births in 1998—a considerable decrease. Also, the number of all cesarean section deliveries has slowly been decreasing from a peak rate of

TABLE 26–2. LBW and VLBW Statistics in Selected Populations for 1998 and *Healthy People 2010* Goals

Healthy People 2010 target goal is to reduce the incidence of LBW babies to no more than 5% of live births and VLBW babies to no more than 0.9% of live births. (1998 baseline was 7.6% and 1.4%, respectively.)

Selected Population	1998 Statistics	
	LBW	VLBW
African American	13.0%	3.0%
American Indian/Alaska Native	6.8%	1.2%
Asian/Pacific Islander	7.2%	1.1%
Hispanic	6.4%	1.1%
White	6.5%	1.1%
Mothers under age 15	13.6%	3.1%
Mothers age 15 to 19	9.5%	1.8%
Mothers age 35 and over	8.6%	1.7%

(Adapted from U.S. Department of Health and Human Services [2000]. *Healthy people 2010* [conference edition in two volumes]. Washington, DC: U.S. Government Printing Office.)

24.7% of deliveries in 1998, with first cesarean deliveries at 17.8% in 1997 (USDHHS, 2000).

Progress in other areas has been mixed. Breastfeeding during the early postpartum period has increased. There has been progress among racial and ethnic minorities, with gains of 48% and 20% among African Americans and Hispanics, respectively. However, little progress has been shown among all women in breastfeeding at 5 and 6 months postpartum. Progress is also being made among women receiving early prenatal care, with 83% of women entering care in the first trimester in 1997.

The success in reaching the year 2000 objectives for abstinence from alcohol, tobacco, and drug use during pregnancy has been mixed. The rate of abstinence from tobacco has increased to 87%, whereas rates of abstinence from alcohol, cocaine, and marijuana have remained nearly unchanged.

Risk Factors for Pregnant Women and Infants

Most pregnant women in the United States are healthy, have normal pregnancies, and produce healthy babies. Nevertheless, many factors contribute to the health problems of those mothers and babies who figure in the statistics on infant mortality and low birth weight. The factors associated with low birth weight and infant mortality can be grouped into three categories:

1. Lifestyle—smoking, inadequate nutrition, low prepregnancy weight, high alcohol consumption, narcotic addiction, environmental toxins, prolonged standing, strenuous work, stress, and lack of social support
2. Sociodemographic—low maternal age, low educational level, poverty, and unmarried status
3. Medical and gestational history—primiparity, multiple gestation, short interpregnancy intervals, premature rupture of the membranes, uterine abnormality, febrile illness during pregnancy, abortion, genetic factors, gestation-induced hypertension, and diabetes (Basso, Olsen, Knudsen & Christensen, 1998; USDHHS, 2000).

It is in the realm of lifestyle choices that the work of community health nurses can have the most significant impact. Data related to these factors are provided below.

DRUG USE

Cities, suburbs, and rural areas are being overwhelmed with drug-related problems. Substance abuse during pregnancy is a problem of enormous scope and staggering social and medical implications as the VLBW infant is primarily associated with preterm birth, which may itself be associated with the use of illicit drugs during pregnancy (USDHHS, 2000). According to *Healthy People 2010,* two thirds of cases of LBW and 98% of cases of VLBW are attributable to preterm delivery. Preterm birth is associated with a number of modifiable risk factors, including the use of illicit drugs during pregnancy (Jacob, Harrison & Tigert, 1995; Zuckerman, 1998).

In the last three decades, when IMRs should have been decreasing, an increasing number of women were using illicit drugs during their pregnancy. This increases the proportion of women entering pregnancy at a greater risk for poor pregnancy outcomes. Many of these women have unintended pregnancies attributable to prostitution to support a drug habit or to inconsistent contraceptive protection when under the influence of drugs. In one study, researchers questioned women entering a detoxification center, and well over half (56%) reported inconsistent contraceptive use (Shah et al., 1998). Their focus on drug acquisition and use leaves everything and everyone else in their life a distant second.

Associated with drug use is limited prenatal care, inadequate nutrition, low prepregnancy weight, alcohol consumption, and smoking (Lundsberg, Bracken, & Saftlas, 1997). In addition, cocaine use during pregnancy is associated with impaired fetal growth, neonatal seizures, and congenital anomalies; neonatal withdrawal characterized by abnormalities of the gastrointestinal tract, the central nervous system, and the respiratory system; poor feeding; abnormal sleep patterns; long-term learning disabilities in the infant; and high risk of infectious diseases, including hepatitis B and HIV. Infants exposed to heroin or cocaine prenatally are also more likely to succumb to **sudden infant death syndrome (SIDS)** (American Academy of Pediatrics Committee on Substance Abuse, 1995; USDHHS, 2000).

It is difficult to determine precisely the rates of substance abuse among pregnant women. Nevertheless, current estimates of the number of women who are **drug exposed** (use drugs intermittently) and give birth to crack- or cocaine-exposed newborns range from 30,000 to 100,000 or greater annually (Novello, Degraw & Kleinman, 1997). Other illicit substances may be abused in combination, contributing to higher numbers of exposed women and infants. Another 5000 to 10,000 infants each year are born to women who are **drug dependent** (physically and psychologically require use of drugs to function). Many pregnant addicts do not receive prenatal care, and it is not until their newborns exhibit signs of withdrawal after birth that many of these women are identified (USDHHS, 2000).

All these factors contribute to LBW infants at a time when technological advancement is approaching maximum benefit from neonatal intensive care (Holzman & Paneth, 1998). There is only so much care that can be given extra utero for the VLBW infant. All of these issues contribute to a slowing of the decrease in infant mortality, leveling off in 1998 at 7.2 deaths per 1,000 live births. The year 2010 goal of 4.2 deaths per 1,000 live births is an ambitious goal to achieve.

A lifestyle choice that includes the use of drugs during pregnancy has placed millions of children at risk. These children are seen in neonatal intensive care units, the foster care system, special-education programs in the public school system, and later in the juvenile court system. Family structure patterns are altered as grandparents find themselves primary caregivers for their grandchildren. A woman who is an intravenous drug user introduces another public health problem, that of acquiring and possibly spreading the HIV virus to the fetus and possibly others (Chervenak & McCullough, 1996; USDHHS, 2000). The primary, secondary, and tertiary prevention role of the community health nurse cannot be underestimated when the results of drug use demonstrate such a high toll on all aspects of society.

ALCOHOL USE

Use and especially addiction to alcohol as the substance of choice is another problem in society. Because alcohol is a legal and socially acceptable substance, it is the most commonly abused drug by pregnant women (Shah et al., 1998). It is difficult to establish accurate statistics on the number of women who drink during pregnancy because inquiring about drinking triggers denial and minimization of intake, especially in heavy drinkers (Russell et al., 1996).

Alcohol use can cause devastating effects in the fetus, even when limited to early in the pregnancy and without addiction. For example, regular intake of alcohol during pregnancy, especially in the first trimester can cause **fetal alcohol syndrome** (FAS), which is characterized by structural abnormalities of the head and face including microcephaly, flattening of the maxillary area, intrauterine growth retardation, decreased birth weight and length, developmental delays, intellectual impairment, hyperactivity, altered sleep pattern, feeding problems, perceptual problems, impaired concentration, mood problems, and language dysfunction. It is a national health problem that was only first identified in 1973 (Lundsberg, Bracken, & Saftlas, 1997). FAS is the primary cause of mental retardation in the Western world, with an estimated incidence of 0.2 to 1.0 per 1,000 live births, yet it is 100% preventable (USDHHS, 2000). Among the Native-American population, the incidence of FAS is four times higher than in the general U.S. public (CDC, 1996); with African Americans, it has risen steeply to 5.4 cases per 1,000 live births. Worldwide, the estimated rate of FAS among pregnant women who are heavy drinkers is 43.1 cases per 1,000 live births (Abel, 1995). Shah and colleagues (1998) report that a study conducted in Colorado found that 68% of women who had children with FAS had no prenatal care during the first trimester. These statistics demonstrate the importance of primary prevention before a pregnancy is planned, or at least during the first weeks of a pregnancy.

Fetal alcohol effects (FAE) is a syndrome in which children suffer some but not all of the symptoms of fetal alcohol syndrome. It occurs in children whose mothers have used varying amounts of alcohol while pregnant, including those who engaged only in occasional binge drinking. FAE is seen three times more often than fetal alcohol syndrome (Robertson, 1993).

Alcohol use during pregnancy also increases the risk for abruptio placentae, stillbirth, spontaneous abortion, congenital anomalies, prematurity, postmaturity, and infections (Robertson, 1993). Offspring of mothers who both drank heavily and smoked during pregnancy delivered babies that weighed 500 g less than babies of nondrinking, nonsmoking mothers. The combined effects of drinking and smoking are important factors in infant mortality and impaired mental and physical development. Research studies indicate demographic markers strongly linking use of alcohol and tobacco, thus placing the woman and fetus at twice the risk (Britton, 1998).

TOBACCO USE

Tobacco use increased among women dramatically in the last third of the 20th century, inevitably affecting maternal and newborn health. The nicotine in tobacco is a major addictive substance, and smoking is an addiction that many people find difficult to stop. Although the risk factors of smoking are well documented, many pregnant women continue to smoke. Smoking during pregnancy is one of the most studied risk factors in obstetric history. It has been associated with ectopic pregnancy, spontaneous abortions, intrauterine growth retardation, preterm birth, stillbirths, higher perinatal mortality, small for gestational age birth, LBW, neonatal anomalies, and lower Apgar scores (Britton, 1998; Heinonen, Ryynanen & Kirkinen, 1999). Health problems do not end once the infant is born. Infants of women who smoked during pregnancy continue to be at higher risk for SIDS, respiratory infections, asthma, ear infections, and decreased lung function (American Lung Association, 1994; Britton, 1998; Zuckerman, 1998). As the children get older, they are at higher risk for learning disabilities, lower intelligence-quotient scores (at ages 3 and 4), and behavioral problems as preteens (Fergusson, Horwood, & Lynskey, 1993; Olds, 1994).

Passive smoking, which is exposure to tobacco smoke from other people smoking in one's environment, also puts a person at risk for smoking-related disease. It has been found that the smoke from a burning cigarette sitting on an ashtray, inhaled passively by the nonsmoker, contains a higher concentration of toxins and carcinogens than the smoke inhaled directly by the smoker (Rienzo, 1993). If a pregnant woman lives with a smoker, she and her fetus can be negatively affected by inhaling the cigarette smoke from the other person's addiction.

The use of **smokeless tobacco products,** such as snuff and chewing tobacco, has led to an increase in oral cancers related to tobacco exposure, without exposure to smoke. Any form of tobacco is extremely hazardous to health (Rienzo, 1993).

> The current trend to restrict smoking in public may induce the heavily addicted to turn to smokeless tobacco as a substitute, just as restrictions against public expectoration once contributed to the social acceptance of smoking instead of "dipping" or chewing (Rienzo, 1993, p. 26).

At this time, it is not known whether the use of smokeless tobacco has any direct adverse effects on the fetus.

Community health nurses and other health care professionals must be involved in the control of tobacco products on many levels, especially in health policy development, client assessment, planning and intervention, as a positive role model, and in research implementation (Britton, 1998). Health policy development has made important strides at the grassroots level, with 17 states receiving funding since 1992 through the American Stop Smoking Intervention Study Program supported by the CDC, the National Cancer Institute, and the American Cancer Society. A top priority of health care policy development is to reduce access of youth to tobacco products by restricting tobacco product advertising and promotion, imposing dramatic cigarette excise taxes, making public places such as malls and restaurants smoke-free, and monitoring tobacco retailers for illegal sales to minors and for keeping cigarettes in locked cases. Most smokers begin their addiction in their early teens. If fewer adolescents begin smoking, there will be fewer women of childbearing age who smoke in the future.

Initial health history taking of a pregnant woman should always include the assessment of tobacco use, smoking status, and smoke in their personal environment. The nurse must not only advise clients to quit smoking but also offer methods or interventions to help. For example, the nurse may counsel clients individually, which, in one study, resulted in a 14% cessation rate among pregnant women. This is a much more dramatic success rate than the 2% cessation rate reported in 17 studies in which family practice physicians offered unsolicited advice. Other, more effective methods were based on behavioral therapy and self-help manuals. These were effective for 16% of the pregnant women studied (Zuckerman, 1998; Law & Tang, 1995; O'Conner et al., 1992). Nicotine replacement therapy trials, including 2-mg nicotine gum and a nicotine patch, were effective among 11% and 13% of the self-referred adult nonpregnant smokers, respectively (Law & Tang, 1995). Although nicotine replacement is not recommended for pregnant smokers, it does appear to be safer for the fetus than maternal smoking of 20 cigarettes or more a day (Kilby, 1997). Other approaches, such as support groups or even a controlled use of tobacco, can be helpful. Any permanent reduction in the number of cigarettes smoked, amount of secondhand smoke inhaled, or amount of smokeless tobacco used can only improve the health of the mother and her fetus.

In addition, nurses should be positive role models for health and demonstrate health-promotion strategies to clients by their own behavior. If a nurse smokes, "this suggests passive approval of smoking behavior and the diminution of its negative effects on health" (Britton, 1998, p. 246).

Finally, there is a need for more research on the reasons why women smoke. Specific attention needs to address the effects of depression and social isolation on the initiation and continuation of smoking by women. Also, studies are needed on the effectiveness of various nursing interventions on a woman's smoking behaviors.

SEXUALLY TRANSMITTED DISEASES

The public has been lulled into a sense of false security about the presence of sexually transmitted diseases (STDs) in the community. Because the major media sources have focused on HIV and AIDs for the last two decades, information about the effects of other STDs has been essentially ignored. However, Ena and Butler (1997) indicate that STDs represent a growing threat to the nation's health and that national action is urgently needed.

Globally, the prevalence patterns of STDs in developing countries are up to 100 times those in developed countries for syphilis, 10 to 15 times higher for gonorrhea, and 3 times higher for chlamydial infection (WHO, 1998). The age of sexual initiation is between 16 and 20 for a majority of both men and women in most parts of the world. Although contraceptive use has increased in most countries in the last 25 years, many sexually active people do not protect themselves against STDs. WHO estimates that one in 20 teenagers contracts an STD each year. Teens are less likely to seek care for STDs, and this delay can contribute to permanent health effects, including sterility and death. If the teen becomes pregnant, it may mean negative health effects for the fetus or infant.

In the United States, herpes affects 20 million people every year, and there are nearly 2 million reported cases of gonorrhea. Other common STDs include syphilis, chancroid, lymphogranuloma venereum, granuloma inguinale, and human papillomavirus (HPV), the infectious agent causing venereal warts and associated with cervical cancer. In a study by Southwick and colleagues (1999), researchers followed an epidemic of congenital syphilis in Texas in 1994–1995 to determine the cause of the outbreak. They found that inadequate prenatal testing for syphilis after an outbreak in adults contributed to the epidemic. In other studies, bacterial vaginosis has been associated with spontaneous preterm birth in the United States, especially among African-American women, accounting for as many as 40% of early preterm births (Goldenberg et al., 1998; Hauth et al., 1995). Two thirds of all cases of STDs occur in persons 15 to 24 years old—the same age group in which over one third of all births occur (U.S. Census Bureau, 1999).

Women who discover that they have an STD often feel ashamed, betrayed, embarrassed, and angry. Those who are asymptomatic may deny the existence of the disease and not carry out the treatment plan. Although educating the pregnant client about the effects of STDs is critical, providing information alone is not enough. The community health nurse has a pivotal role in enhancing the empowerment of women so they can act on the information. The nurse talks with the women and helps them understand that they have control over their bodies. Usually STDs are first discovered in pregnancy during routine prenatal screening, which places the clinic nurse and the nurse who may make home visits in a position to take an affirmative approach to treatment and follow-up (Killion, 1994).

HIV AND AIDS

A positive HIV status is the tragedy of the last 20 years of the 20th century. However, being pregnant or postpartum and HIV positive calls for special nursing management of the pregnancy and of the family after the birth of the newborn. There are many teaching opportunities for the community health nurse during a high-risk pregnancy, such as helping the client identify, change, or curtail high-risk behaviors. Success in changing behaviors often requires an interdisciplinary approach of health care, social, emotional, and financial resources. What follows is a discussion of some of the pregnancy-management issues.

Antepartum Management. Evidence suggests that there is a higher rate of genitourinary tract infections and an increased incidence of STDs in HIV-positive women during pregnancy. The nurse should advise clients to see their health provider for an evaluation immediately if they develop fever, sweats, cough, or diarrhea. HIV-positive clients should also receive nutritional counseling and be encouraged to gain weight appropriately. It should not be overlooked that a woman may be HIV negative at the beginning of a pregnancy and seroconvert, especially if she is continuing high-risk behaviors, because HIV can be acquired at any time during pregnancy.

The first effective intervention to reduce the perinatal transmission of HIV was developed in the United States in AIDS Clinical Trials Group (ACTG) Study 076, in 1994 (Annas & Grodin, 1998). In that study, zidovudine was ad-

ministered orally to HIV-positive pregnant women beginning in the second trimester of pregnancy, intravenously during labor, and orally to their newborns for 6 weeks. This regimen reduced the incidence of HIV infection among the newborns by two thirds—from about 25% to 8%. Within 6 months after the study was completed, the U.S. Public Health Service recommended the ACTG 076 regimen as the standard of care in the United States (Annas & Grodin, 1998).

Postpartum Management. There is no clear evidence that an HIV-positive woman experiences increased rates of postpartum or postoperative morbidity. Some studies show other STDs coexist in HIV-positive women more frequently than in the non–HIV-positive women. Thus, the HIV-positive woman should be monitored for the development of any signs and symptoms of infections. If a community health nurse is doing a newborn assessment, a lochia check, or in some way coming into contact with maternal or infant blood, he or she should use universal precautions. The use of universal precautions is no longer the "ideal to be achieved" but the standard under which all nurses must practice.

Breastfeeding. HIV-infected women are advised not to breastfeed their infants because 8% to 18% of them will infect their infants with HIV from their breast milk (Van de Perre, 1995). The community health nurse focuses teaching on providing a safe, available form of infant formula. In developing countries, the lack of clean water still makes formula feeding dangerous and breastfeeding is overwhelmingly recommended. The infection rate for HIV from breastfeeding and the mortality rate from formula made with impure water are about the same, thus causing a dilemma for women and health care providers in developing countries. The best immediate intervention would be to put increased effort into providing clean water and sanitation (Annas & Grodin, 1998). In the long term, the nurse must focus on preventing and eliminating HIV infection. Additional information on the role of the community health nurse working with the HIV-positive client is found in Chapter 15.

POOR NUTRITION AND WEIGHT GAIN

Research has demonstrated a positive correlation between weight gain during pregnancy and normal birth weight babies. Weight gain of 25 to 35 lb during pregnancy is recommended for women at a normal weight, 28 to 40 lb. for underweight women, and 15 to 25 lb. for obese women (USDHHS, 2000). Obese women have a higher incidence of gestational hiatal hernia, diabetes, preeclampsia, primary cesarean section, gestation-induced hypertension, and perinatal mortality if there are prenatal complications (Carmichael, Abrams, & Selvin, 1997). Community health nurses who work with morbidly obese pregnant women can help them most by emphasizing good nutrition and even by encouraging them to maintain their prepregnant weight without reducing caloric intake. This can be accomplished primarily by a marked decrease in consumption of "empty calories" from junk food. Pregnancy is never a time for dieting, but eating foods from the Food Guide Pyramid established by the U.S. Department of Agriculture (1992) or Vegetarian Food Pyramid presented by The Health Connection (1994; see Chapter 1) will ensure the proper servings and proportions of foods. Nutritional counseling, however, can have an additional benefit in that it may ultimately decrease the risk of obesity or eating disorders in the client's children.

Underweight women have twice as many LBW babies as women whose weight is within normal range. There is a correlation between weight gain (excessive or low) in pregnancy and poor obstetric outcomes (Carmichael, Abrams & Selvin, 1997). Associated with excessive weight gain are maternal hypertension and diabetes. Low maternal weight gain is associated with LBW infants who have higher incidences of growth problems, developmental delays, central nervous system disorders, and mental retardation (Hickey et al., 1996).

Nutritional teaching, again, is within the community health nurse's role with pregnant woman who have difficulty gaining the recommended 25 to 35 lb during pregnancy. Finding ways to add calories to foods or increase the woman's desire to eat are effective methods to improve maternal weight gain. Insufficient caloric intake in pregnant adolescents (who themselves are still growing) is an additional concern. For women who are prone to gaining too much weight, finding nutrition-rich, low-calorie foods is recommended. After assessment, the community health nurse determines if the unwanted weight gain is in relation to the consumption of additional calories and limited activity, or fluid retention. Each must be managed differently.

TEENAGE PREGNANCY

Each year, more than 1 million American teenagers become pregnant. There is a strong association between young maternal age and high IMR, and infants born to teenagers are at increased risk for neonatal and postneonatal mortality (Alpers, 1998). Infants born to African-American adolescents are at higher risk of low birth weight than are white infants. Infants born to very young adolescents (aged 10 to 14 years) are at very high risk for neonatal mortality. Teen mothers have increased psychological risks such as isolation, powerlessness, depressive disorders, lowered self-concept, and increased somatic complaints; developmental and maturational processes that are disrupted and compromised; and diminished prospects for completing their education. Thus, the markers for successful pregnancy outcomes and future life events are more complex (Alpers, 1998). The mother's educational attainment, marital experiences, subsequent fertility behavior, labor force experience and occupational attainment, and her experiences with poverty and public assistance are all directly related to the adolescent pregnancy.

The issues of adolescent parenting are complex. They encompass many areas, including (1) emotional, (2) physical, and (3) social issues. The community health nurse has a

unique challenge when teaching teens about pregnancy-related changes, accompanying needs, and preparing for the important role of parenting the infant.

Emotional Needs. Pregnant teens deal with this change in their life in a variety of ways. Some may have such a strong denial system that they deny the pregnancy, even to themselves. It may take 3 or 4 months into the pregnancy before they can admit it and seek out a physician's diagnosis. Often, their parents are the last to know.

What is difficult about this scenario is that prenatal care is delayed into the second trimester of pregnancy. If the teen's choice is to continue with the pregnancy, the delayed prenatal care could compromise the well-being of the teen and the fetus.

What the teen needs at this time is supportive and caring parents and professionals. The teen parents have difficult choices to make. Most teens plan to continue with their pregnancy, whereas others choose abortion or adoption. These choices are difficult and fraught with emotion. Supportive parents along with their teens, in consultation with professionals, can explore all options. It may be at this time that the community health nurse first begins to work with the teen. It may begin at school as a school nurse in a school-based clinic, in a clinic or physician's office, or as the community health nurse who visits pregnant teens based on referrals from health care providers. The nurse can offer educational services, emotional support, and referrals for services as needed. Adolescent parenting programs set up in some communities have positive effects on the pregnancy. In one program, paraprofessionals indigenous to the community made intensive home visits to pregnant teens. This program, implemented by a visiting nursing service, demonstrated that mentorship and social support improved pregnancy outcomes by reducing the number of LBW babies born to the teens participating in the program to 4.6% when the national percentage for LBW infants of teens was 13.5% (Flynn, 1999).

The goal of any pregnancy is positive maternal–infant outcomes, including a positive relationship. For some teen mothers, a positive relationship is more difficult to achieve than for older mothers. One recent study found that maternal education and self-esteem, as well as the infants' fathers' involvement contributed toward positive relationships (Diehl, 1997). In another study, using the Nursing Child Assessment Teaching Scale (NCATS), mothers and infants were observed during an age-appropriate teaching situation (Barnard, 1994). The importance of positive self-esteem was demonstrated in this study because the mothers with higher self-esteem responded more positively to infant distress. Typically, older adolescents had higher self-esteem than younger mothers. This information helps to guide nurses in their work with the pregnant adolescent population.

Physical Needs. Pregnant teens have a gamut of physical needs that can be addressed by the continuity of routine prenatal care and education. Routine prenatal care is one of the most important needs, and teens may require assistance in recognizing the value of monitoring the pregnancy. Some may feel embarrassed and uncomfortable with male health care providers and refuse to keep appointments. If these feelings are shared, adjustments can be made so that the teen is seen by female professionals or is allowed to bring the baby's father or a girlfriend. Whatever it takes to get the teen to prenatal appointments should be encouraged. It may also include arranging for transportation requiring bus tokens, getting a taxi, or arranging a friend or social worker to drive the teen to her appointments.

The pregnant teen needs education regarding changes in her body, the growth and development of the fetus, dietary requirements, emotional changes, rest and relaxation needs, and anticipatory guidance for infant caregiving and parenting.

Teaching can take place as part of each prenatal appointment, in specific classes at school for pregnant teens, in the health department clinic, or during home visits. In each setting, the community health nurse can modify the teaching methods to the setting and the individual needs of the teen. Changing teen behavior during pregnancy can be challenging. The community health nurse may focus on one important and seemingly less complex issue of nutrition during pregnancy. However, it is a more difficult task to change the eating habits of teens than it is with adults. They are in a stage of development where they usually are more concerned with their body image than the growth and development of the fetus they are carrying. Fad dieting, peer pressure, and personal control are all issues with which the pregnant teen is struggling. If this teen has been raised in poverty, multiple other issues impact her motivation to make dietary changes during the pregnancy.

Social Needs. Pregnant teens are dealing with two stages of their own growth and development at the same time, which makes their social needs complex. They are struggling with the normal adolescent challenges along with the responsibilities of pregnancy and parenting of the young adulthood stage of development.

There may be changes in acceptance by previous social groups due to their parental pressure or type of activities they are involved in, such as surfboarding or mountain climbing. The group may participate in other activities that the pregnant teen should not participate in, such as smoking, drinking, or taking illicit drugs. This causes conflict for a pregnant teen who has a strong need to be accepted by her peer group and also knows that she has a responsibility to her unborn child. The community health nurse can help the teen in such a dilemma by providing a social support system among the attendees in prenatal classes and involving the teen's parents or other adults in her life to be more supportive. Often, such a developmental crisis as a teen pregnancy can help bond a mother–daughter relationship. It takes time and work on the part of the parents and the teen. The teen will need the support of her parents when the baby is born, and strengthening the relationship during pregnancy is an important start.

Another social outlet and an important resource is school.

The teen should be encouraged to continue her studies with a goal toward graduation. The health and welfare of children are related to the educational level of their parents. Higher educational levels make it more likely that children will receive adequate medical care and that their daily environments will be protected and responsive to their needs (Zill, 1996). Teen pregnancy and education are discussed more thoroughly in Chapter 28.

MATERNAL DEVELOPMENTAL DISABILITY

As important as the maternal–infant relationship between adolescent mothers and their infants, so is this relationship with mothers and/or fathers who are developmentally disabled. **Developmental disability** is the preferred term for a broad scope of limitations, which include intellectual limitations identified before age 22 and limitations in ability to perform certain activities of daily living. The disability may be mild, moderate, or severe. For couples who are developmentally disabled, having a child puts increased stress on a system already burdened. Studies have shown that child abuse, neglect, and developmental delays; intergenerational disability; and inadequate home environments accompany the parenting style of developmentally disabled parents (Keltner, 1994; Keltner, Finn & Shearer, 1995).

Much of the pediatric literature discusses the needs of developmentally disabled infants and children and role of the nurse and other health care professionals in working with the families of these children. However, these people, as adults, are rarely represented in studies of disability, giving us limited information about their success as parents. In the 1980s, several studies identified that a primary problem affecting the children of developmentally disabled mothers is the poor quality of maternal–infant or child interaction (Keltner, Finn & Shearer, 1995). The parenting style of mothers with developmental disabilities is often nonstimulating, punitive, and restrictive (Keltner, 1994). In addition, unusual and sometimes bizarre behaviors, such as locking a toddler out of the house or hitting a child for asking a question, have been documented (Keltner, Finn & Shearer, 1995).

How does the community health nurse work with developmentally disabled parents effectively? Most importantly, nursing support must enhance the natural resilience of the family. The success of family support depends on immediate and continuing health promotion visits. The goal is to establish safe parenting routines that will serve as a foundation to the parenting skills needed when the infant begins to walk and explore—a time when their safety is in greater jeopardy.

Establishing a trusting relationship between the nurse and the family is foremost. Teaching, by using demonstration and many visual aids and prompts, challenges the nurse's creativity. Role modeling appropriate parenting needs to occur on each visit. Supervision and monitoring of the family functioning must continue until the child (or children) reach adulthood. Many agencies for which community health nurses work cannot provide the intensive followup that such a family requires. It is then necessary to make referrals to organizations that can provide the support, such as the American Association of Retarded Citizens (AARC) or Exceptional Parents. The nurse may still stay involved as a consultant to the paraprofessionals or for periodic home visits at times of developmental or situational crises (see Chapter 25).

Complications of Childbearing

Although we have covered some major risk factors among pregnant women and infants, several common complications of childbearing need to be mentioned. The effects of hypertensive disease in pregnancy, gestational diabetes, postpartum depression, and grief in families who have lost their child are important areas in which the community health nurse can intervene successfully.

HYPERTENSIVE DISEASE IN PREGNANCY
Blood pressures in all people show daily variations regardless of physical and mental activities. At times, people demonstrate an elevated blood pressure during a clinic visit, due to a phenomenon know as "white coat" hypertension, that does not necessarily indicate excessive blood pressure at other times. However, for pregnant women, chronic and untreated hypertension has a negative effect on the health and safety of the fetus and the outcome of the pregnancy.

Preterm birth is a frequent and negative occurrence in a pregnancy that is associated with maternal infections, smoking, drinking, and hypertension. Additional maternal risk factors associated with hypertensive disease in pregnancy include lung disease, older age (>30), and proteinuria (Meis et al., 1998).

A variety of methods are employed to prevent and control hypertension during pregnancy, namely, a diet high in fresh fruits and vegetables, weight gain limitations, sodium restriction, rest, and regular exercise. They remain the most common preventive suggestions community health nurses can give their pregnant clients in collaboration with the client's primary health care provider. Additional assessment data may guide the nurse to focus teaching on stress reduction techniques and modifying or eliminating smoking. At times, these modifications have a very limited effect on successfully reducing blood pressure during pregnancy, and medications or even hospitalization may be necessary. The nurse can offer support and understanding while continuing to be a resource for the client as the pregnancy progresses and the infant is born.

GESTATIONAL DIABETES
Gestational diabetes mellitus (GDM) is defined as glucose intolerance of variable degree with onset or first recognition during pregnancy. For the mother with GDM, there is a higher risk of hypertension, preeclampsia, urinary tract infections, cesarean section, and future diabetes (Siccardi, 1998). The prevalence of GDM varies worldwide partly because of the different criteria and screening regimens. In the United States, the prevalence rates usually span between 1.4% and 12.3% of the pregnant population tested (Siccardi, 1998). Pathophysiologically, GDM is similar to type 2 diabetes.

Because the growth and maturation of the fetus are closely associated with the delivery of maternal nutrients, particularly glucose, maintaining appropriate glucose levels is essential to the health of the fetus. This is most crucial in the third trimester and is directly related to the duration and degree of maternal glucose elevation. Thus, the negative impact is as highly diverse as the variety of carbohydrate intolerance that women bring to pregnancy.

The community health nurse can help in the control of GDM by encouraging early prenatal care, adequate nutrition, rest and exercise, and following the particular regimen suggested by the woman's health care provider. The infants of GDM women often weigh significantly more than other full-term infants. Some infants have been born weighing 12 or more pounds. For some women, having such a large baby may encourage them to expect more of the infant, because the infant is born weighing what a 2- to 3-month-old infant weighs. Teaching and providing anticipatory guidance become particularly important for these women.

POSTPARTUM DEPRESSION
Depression is a fairly common phenomenon for women during the weeks after delivery. It occurs in primiparas as well as women with several children. In some women, it can even last for a year or more (Beck, 1996). Depressive symptoms may not indicate major clinical depression; nevertheless, symptoms may cause considerable psychological distress (see Voices From the Community) (Hall, Kotch, Browne & Rayens, 1996).

Through numerous studies over the years, researchers have been able to develop a profile of women with postpartum depression (Hall, Kotch, Browne & Rayens, 1996). Most depressed postpartum women have low self-esteem, which is reinforced by the infant's temperament: an irritable infant that demands more from the fatigued new mother who has limited support from a significant other can increase the depressive symptoms. Other mothers, who have a "good" baby, feel guilty for their apathy toward their infant. This, too, affects maternal–infant bonding. In addition, stressful life events combined with a lack of social support and everyday stress are etiologic factors in postpartum depressive symptoms—the greatest everyday stressor being interpersonal conflict. The value of a confidant to new mothers becomes evident as studies show that depressed new mothers do not perceive they have their spouses or others as confidants (Hall, Kotch, Browne & Rayens, 1996).

The critical nature of postpartum depressive symptoms and the potential negative ramifications for mothers and their

Voices From the Community

Voices of three women experiencing postpartum depression:

"I had no control of my own self-being, nothing, mind, soul, nothing. It basically controlled me. I wanted to reach out to my baby, yet I couldn't."

"Every time my baby cried when she woke up, I 'd feel a chill go up my body, and I wanted her to stay asleep because I knew it was so hard when she woke up. The fear of the baby needing you or crying for your help. . . ."

"After 4 months of suffering from postpartum depression, I do remember my very first moment of clarity and total joy in the whole depression. I was sitting with my daughter and rocking in a chair, giving her a bottle. I realized that I was feeling incredibly close to her. I remember this totally piercing sense of okay. We will be okay."

(Beck, C.T. [1996]. Postpartum depressed mothers' experiences interacting with their children. *Nursing Research, 45*[2], 98–104.)

---

children are quite evident. Community health nurses can intervene by initiating health promotion activities through primary prevention during the pregnancy and continuing into the postpartum period. Assessing the pregnant woman for factors that contribute to depression, by using standardized questionnaires or ones developed by the nursing agency, is a beginning. If women are identified with compromised mental health resources, supporting their self-esteem, optimizing the quality of their primary intimate relationship, and reducing day-to-day stressors, fosters positive mental health outcomes. At times, the nurse's efforts alone are not sufficient and a referral to community mental health services is essential for the women and their children.

FETAL OR INFANT DEATH

An infrequent role for community health nurses in maternal–infant care is that of grief counselor. A couple may experience a miscarriage, a stillbirth, or the death of an infant. In each situation, the nurse has an important and supportive role.

People respond to grief in a variety of ways. Some may express deep sadness, shock, or disbelief. Some will weep and be unable to talk, or, conversely, they may talk incessantly about regrets or guilt (Levin, 1998). Even if a miscarriage occurs early in a pregnancy, the bonding between the mother and fetus has begun and expressions of grief may be as intense as with the loss of an infant or child. The nurse should encourage the parents to express their feelings through the use of supportive statements and open-ended questions if needed. The parents may have doubts about actions or behaviors they took that they believe may have caused the miscarriage. Reassurance and clarifying any misconceptions

may alleviate the parents' feelings of guilt and help them cope with their grief in a healthy manner.

For couples who have delivered a stillborn baby, the shock is compounded by the experience of the entire length of the pregnancy, the anticipation of an imminent delivery and addition to the family, especially if all signs up to the birthing event have been positive. They may say such things to you as, "We felt him move just yesterday and now he's dead—what did I do wrong?" or "I did everything right during this pregnancy. Why did this happen?" These are questions for which there may be no answers, even for the family's health care provider. Frequently, a stillbirth is related to fetal entanglement in the umbilical cord or an infection. Mostly, the family needs reassurance that they did nothing wrong or there is nothing they could have done differently to prevent this. Tenderly encouraging the family to talk about the baby and the sadness they feel is important. Therapeutic touch, offering food, a beverage, tissues, or a blanket, and simply being there for them and listening are invaluable nursing interventions. Not allowing them to accept blame will help them through the grieving process.

When a family experiences the loss of an infant after they have brought him or her home from the hospital, their grief and guilt are compounded by the loss of an anticipated future and the continuity in their lives. An infant may die from SIDS, a congenital anomaly, an infection, or an accident. There are constant reminders of the infant's presence in the home from memories, photos, videos, and accumulated possessions. This death disrupts family homeostasis and the psychological and physiologic equilibrium of the family (Levin, 1998). In many cases, the police may be involved and an autopsy required, contributing to the anguish of the grieving family. This promotes both guilt and loss of self-esteem and can even threaten the marriage. The nurse's presence at this time is very important. Often, families are inundated with support and visits immediately after a death and during the burial ceremony. Then the parents are visited less frequently or not at all, although this is usually a very lonely and critical time for them. Providing continuity and support to the family for months after the death of an infant gives the nurse an opportunity to assess the family for signs of healthy or unhealthy grief resolution. In addition, grieving families may find comfort, support, and helpful information from support groups, such as The Compassionate Friends or the SIDS Alliance. If the grief is protracted and not resolving, referral to the appropriate support group is more than important—it is crucial.

PLANNING FOR THE HEALTH OF MATERNAL–INFANT POPULATIONS

To design programs and services for maternal–infant populations, planners need to have a sound understanding of the population they are attempting to serve. Specific aggregates of pregnant women have needs that the community health nurse should assess and incorporate into a prenatal program. Two important considerations include (1) specific needs identified through data collection and client input and (2) the developmental stage of the population being served.

Vital statistics assist planners to identify problems and pinpoint segments of the population where problems are more likely to occur, yet statistics alone cannot fully characterize the populations they represent. Society has witnessed numerous ineffective community, health care, and public works projects. Programs often have failed because the targeted populations were assessed incompletely or not involved in the planning process (see Chapter 19).

Most nurses realize that a predetermined, generalized plan may not meet the needs of any one specific client. To increase effectiveness, the nurse involves the client in designing a plan to meet individual needs and must consider the client's level of education, previous life experiences, level of motivation, culture, and developmental stage. A prenatal program would be very different when planned for a group of college-educated career women, pregnant adolescents, women in rural Appalachia, or Hispanic migrant farm workers. The needs of the women in each of these subpopulations are very different, and programs should be adjusted accordingly. The career women may want information on nurse-midwives, alternative birthing methods, and sources for literature on pregnancy, birthing, and newborn care. The pregnant teens may benefit by special teen pregnancy clinics, group classes on parenting, and assistance with selecting the supplies needed for the baby. The women living in rural Appalachia may respond best to a mobile health clinic staffed by a female nurse practitioner, a social worker to assist with completing the application process for social services, and someone to watch their other children during the appointments. The migrant workers may best be served by bilingual health care workers who offer a clinic in the evenings at a migrant camp or one that is mobile and can come to the workers in the fields. Women from each of these groups can provide valuable information to planners regarding their specific needs. As with individual clients, input from the targeted population increases the program's chances for success.

As people grow and mature, they continually experience physiologic changes, personality changes as new psychosocial issues are met (Erikson, 1968), and increasingly sophisticated thought processes (Piaget, 1950). Consequently, a person's most pressing concerns at one stage in life may seem insignificant at the next stage of development. When planning maternal–infant health programs, the community health nurse must consider the developmental stages of the women being served. For example, adolescents are in a stage of intellectual development in which their thinking processes are beginning to move from concrete thinking patterns to abstract thinking patterns (Piaget, 1950). Concrete thinking is based on what the person has actually experienced or is experiencing. Abstract thinking involves the ability to hear or read something and be able to apply it to a future problem or dilemma. Some adolescents may have difficulty comprehending the complex psychosocial issues and problems with which they will be faced when caring for an infant and young child. Nurses must use innovative and creative approaches when helping adolescents to understand the complex and demanding nature of child care. Some maternal–infant health programs and high schools involve pregnant adolescents (and those judged at risk of becoming pregnant) in child day care programs in which the adolescents participate in the day-to-day care of infants and toddlers. In some health education classes, young teens are given a lifelike doll to parent for 24 to 48 hours (Baby Think-It-Over). It comes with a computer inside, which causes the doll to cry intermittently and when not handled properly. A minute of crying with no attention is recorded as a neglectful event. Students experience firsthand the intense demands and heavy responsibility of being a parent.

The needs of pregnant women in the developmental stages of young adulthood and middle adulthood differ substantially from those of adolescents and will vary between individuals (Erikson, 1968). Women in young and middle adulthood more frequently have planned their pregnancy and make realistic decisions regarding their expanding responsibilities. The community health nurse's most valuable skills are teacher, coordinator, resource manager, counselor, and collaborator. The nurse uses these skills to design programs that meet the needs of the more mature prenatal client. Thorough understanding of the developmental tasks and the psychosocial issues confronting each population should be the cornerstone of solid, well-developed programs. Such programs can be adapted to the developmental needs of clients in adolescence, young adulthood, or middle adulthood (see Levels of Prevention).

HEALTH PROGRAMS FOR MATERNAL–INFANT POPULATIONS

For over a half century, the federal government has been granting money to states for the promotion of maternal and child health. Through the Maternal and Child Health Block Grant Program, millions of dollars come to individual states each year. This money supplements the state's own funds to meet the maternal and child health care needs for people at the local level. With this money, each state provides basic services to its maternal–child population. An additional companion program provides services to special needs children. Community health nurses need to become familiar with their

A HEALTHY PREGNANCY OUTCOME

GOAL
A healthy, full-term infant comes into the world.

PRIMARY PREVENTION
(Planning a pregnancy) The parents plan the pregnancy at a time in life when it's "right." Pregnancies are spaced 2 years (or more) apart. Mother has a positive attitude going into the pregnancy. A health care provider is selected. The parents do not use alcohol, tobacco, or other mood-altering substances when planning to conceive. The mother begins a vitamin regimen containing folic acid and attempts to have weight as close to ideal as possible, before conception. Family and significant others are supportive. There are financial resources to meet the expanding family's needs.

SECONDARY PREVENTION
(The pregnancy) The mother starts prenatal care early in the first trimester, and it is continuous. She does not use alcohol, tobacco, or other mood-altering substances. She takes a daily prenatal vitamin. Parents avoid exposure to people with infectious diseases. Mother has adequate nutrition, rest, and exercise. Mother begins support services if eligible (AFDC, WIC). Family and significant others continue to be supportive. The parents attend labor preparation, infant care, and parenting classes. Name(s) are selected for the infant. Delivery method and location are selected. The home is prepared for the infant—adequate infant furnishings and supplies are acquired within the parents' budget. Preparations and plans are made regarding breast or bottle feeding. A pediatrician or pediatric nurse practitioner is selected. An infant car seat is acquired. Plan(s) are made to get to the health care facility when in labor.

TERTIARY PREVENTION
(After delivery) The parents and significant others begin to bond with the newborn. Parents get to know the newborn and establish breast or bottle feeding routine. Infant returns home in an age-appropriate infant car seat, which is used whenever traveling in a car. Exposure to people with infectious diseases is avoided. Infant's birth is celebrated according to cultural and religious preferences. Appointments are made and kept for postpartum and newborn visits to health care provider. Parents resume sexual intercourse using a family planning method of their choice. Infant immunization schedule begins on time. The parents enjoy the new life they created!

(Display 26–1). Through teaching, nurses help mothers adapt to the physiologic and emotional changes they are experiencing and help them anticipate and plan for the impact their infants will have on their daily lives.

During the comprehensive, ongoing client assessments, in addition to considering their clients' physiologic and emotional status, nurses must assess the clients' social support systems, access to medical care, financial status, housing needs, and ability to provide for their babies. If clients need assistance in any or all of these areas, nurses must intervene and refer them to other appropriate community resources. Nurses often must serve as advocate for the client in the referral process and should continue to work collaboratively with other professionals during follow-up services to meet clients' needs.

Types of Health Programs

Methods of delivering services will vary based on the population and its specific needs. The geographic distribution of clients and the size of the nursing staff available to deliver the services also play significant roles. For example, in rural areas where clients are scattered over a large area, it may be appropriate to deliver services to the population on a one-to-one basis through nurse-run clinics (stationary or mobile) or home visits.

CLINIC PROGRAMS
In the clinic setting, each client receives an individualized examination, immunizations, and health teaching. Unfortunately, there are time constraints placed on the nurse; thus, the actual time spent in teaching clients is relatively short. Clinics may be effective on Native-American reservations where the population is centrally located and on sites where migrant farm workers and their families are temporarily located.

A motorhome, bus, or van converted to serve as a mobile clinic may be the resource needed in some rural or isolated areas that are populated by groups experiencing physical barriers to health care services. Often, the community health nurse working in a mobile health clinic provides routine prenatal, postpartum, and newborn care including teaching and administering scheduled immunizations. These are much-needed services in some areas, and ones that cannot be provided as cost-effectively by other methods. The recommended immunization schedule for children, which is started in infancy, is discussed in detail in Chapter 27.

HOME VISITS
Home visits provide clients with a one-to-one opportunity for teaching with the community health nurse. There are two major benefits to home visits. First, the client is in the comfortable, familiar surroundings of her own home. Second, the nurse's assessment is enhanced by observations in the home setting of such things as family interactions, values, and

state's Maternal and Child Health Program and the services provided by the program.

Program plans for maternal–infant populations across the country include many typical features. For example, there are concerted efforts to educate clients during the antepartum and postpartum periods and assess their specific needs. A major focus of community health nurses is teaching. Nurses introduce new information or reinforce existing knowledge of pregnancy, delivery, and postpartum health considerations

DISPLAY 26–1. Typical Features of Maternal–Infant Health Programs

I. Antepartum teaching
  A. Significance of prenatal care
  B. Self-responsibility
  C. Physiologic changes during pregnancy
  D. Fetal growth and development
  E. Nutrition
  F. Proper exercise
  G. Hazards of substance use: Drugs/alcohol/tobacco
  H. Breastfeeding techniques and problem solving
  I. Stages of labor
  J. Delivery—Process and options available
  K. Future birth control
II. Introduction to community resources for prenatal care
  A. Childbirth classes
  B. Self-help groups (pregnant teens, parents of twins, and so forth)
  C. WIC
  D. Department of Social Services
  E. Family planning services
  F. School-based clinics
  G. High-risk clinics
III. Postpartum teaching
  A. Newborn assessments
  B. Care of the newborn
  C. Growth and development of the infant
  D. Infant immunization schedule/health care followup
  E. Mother–infant bonding
  F. Postpartum physiologic changes in the mother
  G. Breast/bottle feeding techniques
  H. Postpartum health care followup
  I. Exercise to regain muscle tone
  J. Family planning
  K. Returning to work (balancing home, family, and work)
  L. Child care
IV. Delivery of services for prenatal/postnatal care
  A. Clinic/private health care provider visits
  B. Home visits
  C. Formal classes
  D. Self-help groups
  E. Community education
V. Client advocacy and coordination with other community resources
  A. Physicians/nurse practitioners/nurse midwives
  B. Clinics
  C. Hospitals
  D. High schools
  E. Industries
  F. WIC
  G. Department of Social Services

priorities. Chapter 24 has detailed information about how to make home visits.

However, home visiting to any client is costly for an agency. One-to-one delivery of service is becoming a luxury for some agencies with limited finances. In such agencies, the nurses provide most of the routine care in clinic or group settings. Home visits are made to the most serious of cases only. If clients are not at home at scheduled visit times and must be rescheduled, this increases an already strained agency budget.

In metropolitan areas where community health nurses and clients are located near one another, nurse-run clinics and home visits may still be appropriate mechanisms for the delivery of services. In these cases, clients can visit the clinic frequently, and nurses can make more home visits with less distance to travel between clients. In addition, metropolitan areas afford community health nurses an opportunity to use a group approach with clients. This may include small, informal group discussions or larger, more formal classes. Whether small or large, groups can provide a vehicle for teaching by the nurse as well as a means for clients to teach and learn from one another. Group discussions can complement clinic and home visits and be ongoing at both neighborhood clinics and Special Supplemental Food Program for Women, Infants, and Children (WIC) clinics (see The Global Community).

SELF-HELP GROUPS

Self-help groups are usually formed by peers who have come together for mutual assistance to satisfy a common need, such as overcoming a handicap or life-disrupting problem. The group goal is to bring about specific desired behavior changes. Although many groups are formed by peers, the community health nurse can often facilitate the formation, function, and direction of the group. The nurse's role is that of facilitator.

Community health nurses should be familiar with the concept of self-help groups, because it is a concept that needs to be integrated consistently into community health nursing practice. The role of the nurse will vary depending on the size, interests, and level of sophistication of the group. For example, with a group of well-educated women who are effective problem solvers, the nurse may initiate the group and then serve primarily as a resource person. With a group of adolescents, on the other hand, the nurse may need to be present at each meeting to facilitate group process as well as to clarify information shared within the group. In Chapter 8, group work is described in greater detail.

Self-help groups provide many benefits to participants. Within the present health care system, clients often express feelings of insignificance and loss of control. However, in a self-help group environment, individuals regain their sense of identity and control. Acceptance of responsibility for health-promoting behaviors is a key concept supported by the majority of self-help groups. Members who lose sight of their responsibility are readily confronted by the group. Individuals reach out to help other members and, in the process,

THE GLOBAL COMMUNITY

The Community Mothers' Program, Dublin, Ireland

Lloyd, K. (1993). Mothering instinct. *Nursing Times, 89*(26), 42–44.

In Dublin, Ireland, there is a large urban housing development rented by people who are largely unemployed and have problems with low self-esteem, alcoholism, depression, and anxiety. The incidence of violence against women and children and burglary is also high in the development. Against this background, the community mothers' program was developed. It is a support program for first- and second-time parents with infants in the first year of life and occasionally up to the age of 2.

The model is one of parent enablement and empowerment. The program aims to recruit and train experienced mothers within the local community to give support and encouragement to parents in rearing their children. Emphasis of the program is on health care, nutrition, language, and social and cognitive development. Community mothers are expected to use patience, skill, and sensitivity to develop trust, empathy, and mutual respect with the parents taking part in the program. The community mothers are recruited, trained, and visited monthly by public health nurses, to provide support and discuss visits. Each "family development nurse" is responsible for up to 20 community mothers.

The program has contributed to the social and mental well-being of the community. An evaluation of the program revealed, in the families visited compared to a control group, more children completed immunizations, formula was used longer before switching to cow's milk or more mothers breast-fed their infants, 98% of the parents read to their children, and the parents reported greater feelings of self-esteem. By 1991, 1100 families were in the program with 150 community mothers visiting. A shift in emphasis toward client involvement requires the families' acceptance that lay people can understand and implement activities previously carried out by professionals. The program also demonstrates how nurses can use their expertise and expand their scope of influence, which reaches a widening circle of clients.

help themselves to become better informed and stronger in their own beliefs.

Self-help groups have been successfully developed for the prenatal population to address common concerns such as prenatal changes, adapting to pregnancy, fetal growth and development, and labor and delivery. For postpartum women, groups have been established for breastfeeding mothers, mothers of infants, mothers of toddlers, and mothers of twins. In each instance, members of healthy populations help one another to remain healthy and prevent potential problems.

The term *peer counseling* is used in some settings for the self-help group process. For instance, in a high school, an informed and respected group of peers are identified and trained and then work with their classmates in small groups to discuss safe sex, saying no to drugs, self-esteem, conflict resolution, or teen parenting. The topics vary to meet the needs of the peers. The concept of peer counselor and self-help groups can be initiated by the innovative and creative community health nurse.

SCHOOL-BASED PROGRAMS

Delivering maternal and child health care programs in the school setting has been growing over the last two decades. Many high schools offer special courses for pregnant teens and at home study programs after delivery, followed by on-site day care for the infants and toddlers of the postnatal teens. All of these services may be part of school-based programs. Some schools have initiated innovative programs that include additional health care services to their pregnant teens. This type of care may include family planning services, immunizations, and primary health care for illness and injury. Each community and school district needs to decide, in consultation with community health nurses, school nurses, community leaders, parents, teens, and the board of education, what services the community desires and/or needs.

HIGH-RISK CLINICS

High-risk clinics are established especially to meet the needs of women whose pregnancy is considered at high risk. The risk may be due to a multiple pregnancy, a very young primipara client (under 15 years old), an older primipara client (over 40 years old), a grand multipara client, hypertension, or GDM. The high-risk clinic is staffed by health care providers with special maternal–child health skills and advanced diagnostic equipment. They see clients experiencing a variety of conditions that might lead to fetal distress and so require special monitoring. In some communities, health care facilities have several types of high-risk clinics. Some just see teens or substance abusers. In smaller communities, there may be one high-risk clinic meeting the needs of all those experiencing a special pregnancy. A community health nurse often becomes involved in the referral to such clinics, or may work in one as part of the job description in a small health department. The nurse needs to be knowledgeable about the clinic's services so potential clients can be referred if necessary.

INFORMATION SERVICES

Providing safe and cost-effective prenatal and postpartum care is more and more a focus of the health care delivery system. Shortened hospital stays for childbirth and limited community health agency budgets impact services available for new mothers and their families. Routine home visits are becoming rare and are reserved for high-risk families. Such conditions make a telephone service or health education centers viable options.

A phone line that is staffed by community health nurses can link parents and professionals with information and community resources (Valaitis, Tuff & Swanson, 1996). An information line can help parents adjust to the postpartum period, address concerns regarding infant care and nutrition, make referrals for home visits, provide information regarding services available within the larger system, and refer to other community agencies. Telephone lines can be specialized by using a bank of numbers on a touch-tone phone, and parents can get recorded information on such topics as breastfeeding or other postpartum concerns. Other telephone lines can be answered by specialists in contact through a paging system, such as a lactation specialist, or an on-call community health nurse who could make a home visit if needed. Parents often find these types of services reassuring, and health care practitioners find they reduce the number of office visits for minor problems that can be handled over the telephone, thus keeping costs down.

The Kaiser Permanente Health Maintenance Organization system, the largest HMO in the country, uses such a method to assist clients to solve their health concerns. In addition to this service, they provide their members with a comprehensive *Healthwise Handbook,* and in each regional center they have a health education center where members can obtain written materials, videos, and information about classes and other programs (Kaiser Permanente, 1996).

Both types of services, phone lines and handbooks, rely on the client's self-care capacity. Clients takes the initiative to seek the information they need to optimize their health. Community health nurses can link clients to such services if they are available in their community. If not available, the community health nurse can help to establish such services in collaboration with public or private health care agencies. They can prove to be beneficial for all involved—client as well as health care provider.

Another form of information services was part of a 4-year project in Detroit. The program, called INREACH, was designed to meet the needs of maternal walk-ins (women who do not receive prenatal care from the hospital systems in which they deliver their infants or who received five or fewer prenatal visits) and their newborns, to provide them with a comprehensive needs assessment, and to link them with community-based agencies, such as substance abuse treatment programs or mental health treatment. INREACH nurses remained in contact with both the mother and the agency to which they were referred for 12 weeks to monitor effectiveness. Over 80% were linked to an agency, and one third of these women remained with the agency for 12 weeks. Benefits of the program were many. The program was influential in the development of health and social service policies at the local and state levels; agencies demonstrated more willingness to coordinate services and became open to adopting new approaches to client care; participants, who had previously had negative experiences with the health care system, appreciated the caring interventions (McComish, Lawlor & Laken, 1996).

The Community Health Nurse and Maternal–Infant Health

The maternal–child population makes up a major portion of a community health nurse's caseload. There is a need for commitment to excellence in service for this special aggregate within the community. The reality is that the future health of the nation lies within each woman who is pregnant. The challenges are great for the nurses who work with this vulnerable group. Three areas/roles are the special focus with the maternal–child population: (1) special professional qualities, (2) the role of educator, and (3) the role of client advocate and liaison with community resources. In addition, the community health nurse has an important role in the evaluation of maternal–infant health programs and as a facilitator to influence government policies for the maternal–infant population.

SPECIAL PROFESSIONAL QUALITIES
Nurses working with maternal–infant health populations require special qualities and education. It is recommended that nurses have the following qualifications:

1. A sound educational background, with the minimum of a baccalaureate degree in nursing
2. A solid understanding of nursing process and ability to use it in working with individuals, families, and groups
3. A knowledge of and willingness to work with other community resources
4. Effective communication skills
5. Effective organizational and leadership skills
6. A sincere, nonjudgmental approach to clients (see Voices From the Community)

ROLE OF EDUCATOR
Because teaching is such an integral part of any maternal–infant program, nurses working in this area must possess good communication skills and teaching skills. For the teaching to be effective, however, the content and methods must vary depending on the needs, characteristics, and developmental stage of each population. For example, when teaching nutrition to pregnant women, the nurse must alter the recommended calorie intake according to the woman's height and weight, age group, culture, and lifestyle. Nutrition information would be presented differently to groups who were college graduates and already familiar with the basics of the Food Guide Pyramid, whereas information presented to pregnant teens may need to include basic nutritional information.

In addition to tailoring subject matter to fit the client population, community health nurses should select teaching methodologies appropriate to clients. Some groups, such as couples attending childbirth education classes, may respond positively to structured classes; others, such as teens, may prefer a less formal discussion format. Peer-group counseling and self-help support groups may be appropriate formats

Voices From the Community

I thought I knew what hands-on nursing was all about because I had been working in a high acuity hospital 5 years previous to public health. Frustration—what could be more frustrating than a CODE at the end of your shift!

Upon entering my young pregnant client's home, armed with my college degree and prepared to teach her everything she needed to know in a very short time, I soon became frustrated and angry when not only were her blood sugars not coming down but she was not following my perfect 2400 calorie diabetic diet plan. She was frustrated too, thinking she was doing the right things for her baby. I conferred with her MD, and, after much deliberation, we came up with a diet plan to 'squeeze' out the fat in her current diet.

My next visit was to behold. I drove up to her home, left my starched, bleached nurse's jacket, stethoscope, charts, etc. in the car, rolled up my sleeves, sat my client on a stool in her kitchen, and began cooking class 101. I showed her how to cook her favorite foods in as healthy a manner as possible, including removing fat by washing the Mexican sausage under warm water after thoroughly cooking it and using a spray oil instead of lard when she made tortillas. I also kept my fingers crossed when I lifted the lid to a pot of steamed rice that I would not encounter any steamed bugs! Environmental health and safety principles were included in the cooking classes as well.

After several visits of cooking instruction, reinforcement of positive health changes, and encouragement, we noticed, together, a decrease in her blood sugars to the 150s from 200+. Needless to say, we were both highly pleased. The visits continued and focused on her gestational diabetes along with preparation for delivery and infant care. Her pregnancy proceeded without complications, and she delivered a healthy 8-lb baby at 38 weeks' gestation. She is early in a second pregnancy and maintaining good blood sugar levels using the techniques taught the year before. The foci of the visits with this pregnancy are broader because we have developed rapport, and because she had a healthy outcome with her first pregnancy, she is very interested in making changes to ensure success again.

Until I was a public health nurse, I had no clue what hands-on nursing and frustration were all about.

Barbara, RN, BSN, PHN
Public Health Nurse

for small groups who respond to the structure and support this format provides.

Teaching aids used should be appropriate for each audience. It is important to remember that many of the available teaching aids are in English and depict white, middle-class women and infants. Although these will be appropriate for some populations, not all people will be able to identify with the mothers and babies portrayed. When possible, teaching aids should be congruent with the language, race, and culture of the population being served so that clients can understand and identify with them. For example, pamphlets on infant care need to be made available in appropriate languages, with pictures portraying people from that cultural group and using supplies and equipment available in all homes. For instance, pamphlets that show infant room monitors, expensive educational toys, or fancy cribs with canopies may not depict the environment of the audience the nurse is trying to reach.

Teaching and motivating women to promote their own health and the health of their babies are major challenges, and there is no single correct way to approach the task. Community health nurses need to be innovative and creative in their approach to teaching, and also to be aware that not all women are interested in their pregnancy. In Chapter 9, further information and resources, including appropriate teaching methods and materials for community health settings, are presented in more detail. In Chapter 8, the client with whom it is difficult to communicate is discussed.

ROLE OF CLIENT ADVOCATE AND LIAISON WITH COMMUNITY RESOURCES

The maternal–infant population has complex needs. It is not unusual for community health nurses to see multiple personal and family problems in this group, and, because community health nurses clearly cannot meet all these needs, it is essential that they act as client advocates in referring clients to other community resources. The nurse must have a working knowledge of available community resources for maternal–infant health, which include family planning services, community childbirth education classes, those resources available through the Department of Social Services (state level), as well as WIC, a federal program administered by the states. A clear understanding of the services available and a positive working relationship between agency personnel will facilitate effective provision of services to this population group.

Department of Social Services. The Department of Social Services assigns each family a trained social worker. After interviewing the family, the social worker determines whether the family or individual members of the family meet eligibility criteria for programs administered by the Department of Social Services such as the Medicaid program (health insurance for low-income families), the Food Stamp program (a program to increase low-income families' buying power of most foods), and the Aid to Families with Dependent Children program (financial grants to low-income and unemployed families with dependent children for a combined lifetime limit of 5 years). If the social worker establishes family or individual eligibility, she or he starts the process of applying for benefits. These benefits are essential for the basic survival of many families, and it may be the community health nurse who first

Bridging Financial Gaps

Long, S.H. & Marquis, M.S. (1998). The effect of Florida's Medicaid eligibility expansion for pregnant women. *American Journal of Public Health, 88* (3), 371–376.

In July 1989, Florida expanded the Medicaid income eligibility threshold for pregnant women to 150% of the poverty level. This increased the number of women eligible for Medicaid by removing a financial barrier. In Florida, there are about 200,000 births a year, and, with this expanded eligibility, the researchers wanted to study whether newly eligible women received more or earlier prenatal care and whether their birth outcomes were improved.

Medicaid eligibility records, and records from county health departments for women giving birth from July 1988 to June 1989 with the old Medicaid eligibility requirements (56,000 clients) and from calendar year 1991 with the expanded Medicaid eligibility requirements (78,000 clients) were compared. Measures included amount and timing of prenatal care, rates of low birth weight, and infant deaths.

The number of deliveries covered by Medicaid increased by 47% insuring women who would have been otherwise unin-sured. Outcomes included access to prenatal care improved significantly, more prenatal visits were made, the number of LBW babies decreased from 67.9 per 1,000 to 61.8 per 1,000, and the number of infant deaths decreased from 7.3 per 1,000 to 5.9 per 1,000.

An interesting finding is that the additional prenatal care financed by Medicaid was provided largely by county health departments. This may have been an important factor in the better outcomes for the expansion population. The rate of LBW infants per 1,000 among the mothers in the Medicaid expansion group who used the county health departments was 49.9 vs 70.4 for the other mothers in the expansion group. The incidence of VLBW babies and infant deaths was also significantly lower among women in these same groups. The county health department expansion was an important feature of the Florida intervention. The results suggest the importance of the coordinated care and expanded nonclinical services that the public system offers (educational classes, social work, home visits). Direct examination of the role of these services in birth outcomes for low-income women is an area for further research.

---

identifies a family in need of such social services and makes the initial referral (see Bridging Financial Gaps).

Supplemental Food Program for Women, Infants, and Children (WIC). The Special Supplemental Food Program for Women, Infants, and Children (WIC) is a federal program that provides nutrition education for low-income women and children and vouchers for the purchase of specific supplemental foods and infant formula. Pregnant, breastfeeding, and postpartum women, infants, and children up to age 5 who are at medical or nutritional risk are eligible. The food provided by the program helps pregnant women to produce healthy, normal-birth-weight babies. WIC also refers participants to prenatal care, well-child care, and other services. Established in 1972 as a pilot program, WIC receives its funding from the Food and Nutrition Service of the U.S. Department of Agriculture.

Eligibility for WIC is based on income level, geographic area, and nutritional risk. Determining income eligibility is relatively uncomplicated, because guidelines are clearly defined by each state. Geographic eligibility varies, because many states offer services in all areas whereas others do not. Clients must live in an area that has been designated to receive funding. Nutritional risk is determined by the nurse or nutritionist through interviews with individual clients and review of their previous medical and nutritional history. Eligibility factors for pregnant or postpartum women include age (ie, adolescents or over 40); poor obstetric history, such as previous LBW infants, miscarriages, short periods between pregnancies, and gestational diabetes; anemia; inappropriate weight gain (low or high); and inadequate consumption of food. Risk factors for infants and children include poor growth, anemia, obesity, chronic illnesses, or nutrition-related diseases.

Based on these risk factors, the health professional identi-fies areas of strength and areas for change. The program then offers supplemental food to clients. The food offered contains high-quality protein, iron, calcium, and vitamins A and C. The specific foods offered tend to be combinations of fruit juice fortified with vitamin C, eggs, milk (low-fat or whole), cheese, beans, fortified cereals, and fortified infant formula. Distribution of food varies within states. In some states, local dairies deliver the food to the home; in other states, clients receive vouchers and exchange them for food at local grocery stores. The WIC program reevaluates clients at predetermined intervals. It reassesses needs, continues nutrition education, and recertifies food distribution if appropriate.

Family Planning Services. Family planning services may be an integral part of the comprehensive services of a local health department or community clinic. However, in some communities, these specialized services are provided by separate organizations, such as Planned Parenthood. Depending on the prevailing attitudes and needs in the community, the family planning services may include teen counseling, abortions, and long-term family planning methods such as administering Depo-Provera injections or inserting devices such as Norplant. Family planning service agencies provide counseling, gynecologic examinations that include Pap smears, breast examinations, and mammograms. Some agencies may provide a broader range of services for which there is a need, such as genetic counseling, infertility counseling, and diagnosis and treatment of problems related to male and female sexual dysfunction.

Childbirth Education Classes. Most community clinics or health departments that provide maternal–child health care services also hold childbirth education classes. However, many community groups develop and provide their own classes; possible sources include religious centers, YW-

CAs, and hospitals. If the agency for which the nurse is working does not provide such a service, it is the nurse's responsibility to know the community resources and refer interested women, and their significant others, to childbirth education classes. Women find these classes very helpful in preparing them for the birthing experience in addition to preparing them for the demands of parenthood. The group support effect from being in a class with other pregnant women is also rewarding. For childbirth education classes to be used, they must be accessible; this means they must be held at convenient times and locations. For example, for some clients, the availability of public transportation may be a factor in accessing classes (Serafine & Broom, 1998).

EVALUATION OF MATERNAL–INFANT HEALTH PROGRAMS

Evaluation is a critical aspect of maternal–infant health program planning as it is with any health planning. Four questions, in particular, should be addressed. (1) Did the program meet the identified needs of this particular population? (2) Did the program meet its goals and objectives? (3) Was the program cost-effective? Did the outcomes justify the resources used? (4) What was the program's long-term impact on the health of this population?

Community health nurses find the answers to the above questions through a carefully designed, systematic evaluation plan. Program evaluation is discussed in detail in Chapter 19. For the purposes of this chapter, three useful methods for obtaining evaluation data are examined.

Vital statistics provide an important database for evaluating maternal–infant programs. Local, state, or national figures can help agency personnel determine whether their own statistics are improving, remaining constant, or worsening. Using vital statistics, nurses can make comparisons between or within population groups. For instance, they might compare the incidence of LBW babies born to their clients with rates reported by similar agencies in other urban areas or in their agency the previous year. One disadvantage of using vital statistics is that the time required to compile these data can make it difficult to have the most current figures.

A second mechanism for evaluation within individual maternal–infant programs is measuring quality through performance improvement programs. They are used by health care agencies to monitor service and care of clients in order to maintain or improve delivery of care. The quality management and improvement process looks at maternal–infant program goals and raises questions such as the following:

How soon after receiving the referral were clients seen?
Was the database complete?
Was the plan of care appropriate?
Were the established outcomes reasonable and
 achievable?
Were clients involved in the planning process?
Were appropriate referrals made?
Was there follow-up on the referrals?
Was discharge of the client appropriate?

Quality management systems use various methods to gather this type of information, such as feedback from clients through periodic questionnaires and personal interviews or telephone surveys. Disadvantages of these methods may be the time consumed, the expense for the agency, and the questionable reliability of self-reported feedback rather than using more objective data obtained from client records and health outcomes. Chapter 12 discusses quality management and improvement and the role of the nurse in more detail.

A cost-effective mechanism for assessing a program and the client care delivered is by auditing client records. It is not feasible for an agency to review every client record, but random samplings can be done at predetermined times each year. If clearly defined criteria are established, then those conducting the audit can easily review a record and determine, in their professional judgment, whether the criteria have been met. Auditing client records can be a positive learning experience, and agency staff should be encouraged to participate in the process. Reading through another nurse's documentation can be a positive reminder of the impact that the community health nurse can have on the effectiveness of services delivered.

ROLE AS FACILITATOR TO INFLUENCE GOVERNMENT POLICIES

Another responsibility of the nurse in maternal–infant health programs is in the role of client advocate. This is done with clients at the local level on a daily basis; however, changes are often needed at the state or federal level. The community health nurse can influence the legislation and policies that affect the services provided at the local level. Funding of maternal–child programs occurs through the state legislature. So, by giving testimony on behalf of the maternal–infant population, the community health nurse can attest to the needs of this population and promote the funding of additional programs at the local level. However, this takes time, and, in the meantime, funding may begin to dwindle. Other sources for funding must be found (see Bridging Financial Gaps).

The role of facilitator may include writing grants to obtain the funding for new projects or even to maintain existing programs. Writing grants and getting them funded is becoming a more important skill of the nurses in agencies that are experiencing fiscal constraints. Public and private grants, both large and small, can supplement the shrinking state funding. Limited funding and increasing client needs will continue into the 21st century, and the programs provided through local agencies may depend on grant monies generated by proposals written by community health nurses.

SUMMARY

Global and national vital statistics indicate that the status of maternal–infant health in the world has been improving but is still of major concern. Significant numbers of pregnancies are unplanned, and children are born into unwanted situations or into families already burdened by multiple socioeconomic stressors. The vital statistics for the maternal–infant population in the United States can be improved greatly when compared with that of other industrialized nations. Both the knowledge and the resources to improve the quality of life for mothers and babies are available in this country. However, the issues and importance of maternal–infant well-being extend beyond the borders of any single country.

Factors influencing the health of pregnant women and infants may be related to obstetric history, genetics, socioeconomics, or lifestyle choices. The latter category is a prime target for community health nursing intervention. Lifestyle-related factors influencing the health status of pregnant women and infants include illicit drug, alcohol, and tobacco use; presence of STDs, HIV/AIDS, and other infectious diseases during pregnancy; and weight gain during pregnancy. Pregnancy during adolescence, especially early adolescence, adds additional risk. Emotional, physical, and social needs of pregnant teens need special consideration. In addition, the special circumstances caused by hypertensive disease in pregnancy, gestational diabetes, developmental disability, postpartum depression, and fetal or infant death can be addressed through community health nursing intervention.

In planning effective maternal–infant programs, community health nurses must consider needs identified by the populations themselves as well as vital statistics. Maternal–infant programs across the country have certain features in common, including perinatal followup and teaching, client assessment, service delivery, coordination with other community resources, and client advocacy. These common features assist community health nurses in designing maternal–infant programs. Two other planning considerations include specific needs identified through data and client input and the developmental stage of the population being served.

Creative and innovative methods of implementation such as discussion and self-help groups should be used more widely for teaching and working with maternal–infant populations. Effective implementation of health programs also depends on appropriately qualified staff members. The nature of the maternal–infant population is complex and diverse; thus, appropriate preparation of the community health nurse with highly developed professional skills and the knowledge and use of community resources provide important adjuncts to community health nursing services.

To evaluate the effectiveness of maternal–infant health programs, the community health nurse needs to ask the following questions: (1) Was the program relevant? (2) Did it meet identified goals and objectives? (3) Was the program cost-effective? (4) What was the program's long-term impact on the health of the population of mothers and infants? Three methods for obtaining evaluation data are collection of vital statistics, use of quality management processes, and use of the auditing process.

There is an increasing need for the community health nurse to influence government policies and funding to the lo-

cal level. More often, the nurse will be called on to acquire grant funding to maintain or promote needed programs that were once automatically funded or for the development of programs for a more complex client need now being experienced (see Clinical Corner).

ACTIVITIES TO PROMOTE CRITICAL THINKING

1. What specific objectives has your local health department developed for mothers and infants to help achieve the objectives listed in the U.S. *Healthy People 2010* document? How do your county's statistics compare with those of others in your state on (1) infant death rates (collectively and by specific ethnic groups [eg, Asian, African-American, white, Hispanic]), (2) incidence of LBW and VLBW infants, and (3) incidence of birth defects?

2. Describe three different maternal–infant populations in your county. What are their most pressing health needs? Do any existing services target these populations? How well, in your judgment, are clients' needs being met? Interview a city or county community health nurse as well as other public health professionals to help you find your answers.

3. Select one lifestyle-related factor that affects pregnant women and infants (such as drug, alcohol, tobacco use, or nutritional status) and design a health program to deal with it. Be sure to include the main factors, discussed in this chapter, for planning and evaluating a maternal–infant program.

4. Sonia, an 18-year-old woman, is single and 14 weeks pregnant. Her first prenatal visit was made at the urging of her aunt who uses the clinic. Sonia reluctantly admitted to the clinic nurse that the pregnancy was unplanned; she consumes alcohol two to three times a week, frequently amounting to six 12-oz cans of beer and 16 oz of wine; she smokes one pack of cigarettes a day; and she has tried a variety of street drugs in the last 3 months, but does not use any regularly.

    The clinic nurse believed that the client might not return for regular prenatal care and made a referral to the community health nurse to make follow-up home visits to assess Sonia's home environment and teach prenatal care and preparation for the infant. You were given the case. Design a plan of care to address Sonia's needs. What specific services and programs might you recommend? What barriers might exist? How would the prenatal and postpartum teaching delivered to Sonia differ from care needed by other single teens?

5. Use the Internet to locate international maternal–infant vital statistics. In which countries are the statistics the worst? In which countries are the statistics the best? What do you think accounts for these dramatic differences? What do you know about each group of countries that may account for the differences, such as economic level, type of government, overall physical environment? What activities could a community health nurse become involved within the countries with the worst statistics to help to improve them?

CLINICAL CORNER | **Maternal, Perinatal and Newborn Clients**

Scenario 1

You are a public health nurse working in the high-risk infant follow-up program in Capitol City. You are responsible for home visits to families whose infants have been exposed, in utero, to illicit drugs. The determination of perinatal substance abuse may be made prenatally but is primarily identified in routine postpartum toxicology screening. Both of your clients today tested positive for methamphetamines while in the immediate postpartum period.

Mrs. Boyle is your first client of the day. She is a 35-year-old Anglo woman. She lives in an exclusive gated community north of Capitol City. She has private insurance and is employed by a local software company. Her husband is an architect. This is the couple's first child. Prenatal records indicate that this child was the result of artificial insemination. The pregnancy was without complications. There was no toxicology screen performed prenatally. When you phoned Mrs. Boyle to arrange for the visit, she seemed surprised and initially reluctant to agree to the visit. She stated, "I know they said there was something wrong with my tests, but I don't do drugs and I'm very upset about their accusations." She agreed to the visit after your assurances that you had information for her about infant development and parenting classes in her community.

Next, you will visit *Ms. Craig.* She is a 21-year-old Anglo woman who lives in a low-income housing complex downtown. Ms. Craig is single, and prenatal records indicate involvement by the father of the baby. Ms. Craig's medical costs were covered by Medicaid for this pregnancy. Ms. Craig is gravida three, para one. She has had two therapeutic abortions. Prenatal records document a toxicology screen performed at 7 months' gestation, which was also positive for methamphetamines. At that time, Ms. Craig stated that her boyfriend was a "dealer" and that she was cutting down and would eventually attempt to discontinue drug usage. When you telephoned to schedule an appointment for the visit, she stated, "I know why you're coming . . . it's okay with me but we have to do it when my boyfriend is at work or he'll get mad."

Questions:

1. What considerations must be made for safety in preparation for these visits?

- Mrs. Boyle
- Ms. Craig

Discuss the following issues as they relate to the initial visit with each client:

2. "Getting in the door"
- Mrs. Boyle
- Ms. Craig
3. Establishing a trusting relationship, empathy, and rapport
- Mrs. Boyle
- Ms. Craig
4. Assessing for drug usage
- Mrs. Boyle
- Ms. Craig
5. Involving significant family members
- Mrs. Boyle
- Ms. Craig
6. Making appropriate referrals
- Mrs. Boyle
- Ms. Craig

After you complete your visits with Mrs. Boyle and Ms. Craig, your supervisor asks you to develop a postpartum visitation protocol for women who have tested "toxicology positive" and their children. You will be allowed four to six visits postpartum. Your aggregate will consist of all women testing positive who deliver at any of the three Capitol City hospitals. An average of eight to twelve women each month fit this category. Your aggregate's average age is 23. Most are single women with limited involvement by the father of the baby or the woman's extended family. The ethnicity breakdown for this aggregate is 12% African-American, 38% Anglo, 18% Asian, 30% Hispanic, and 2% other. Most of your aggregate falls at or below poverty level for income, and most have completed high school.

Questions:

1. What additional information do you need to plan an effective program? How will you go about obtaining this information?
2. Identify the components of a program that will lead to effective home visits with this aggregate.
3. How will you accommodate for individual variances within your aggregate?

REFERENCES

Abel, E. L. (1995). An update on incidence of FAS: FAS is not an equal opportunity birth defect. *Neurology, Toxicology, and Teratology, 17*, 437–443.

Alpers, R. R. (1998). The importance of the health education program environment for pregnant and parenting teens. *Public Health Nursing, 15*(2), 91–103.

American Academy of Pediatrics Committee on Substance Abuse (1995). Drug exposed infants. *Pediatrics, 96*(2), 364–367.

American Lung Association. (1994). *Fact sheet, women and smoking*. New York: Author.

Annas, G. J., & Grodin, M. A. (1998). Human rights and maternal–fetal HIV transmission prevention trials in Africa. *American Journal of Public Health, 88*(4), 560–563.

Barnard, K. E. (1994). *NCATS teaching manual*. Seattle, WA: NCATS Publication.

Basso, O., Olsen, J., Knudsen, L. B., & Christensen, K. (1998). Low birth weight and preterm birth after short interpregnancy intervals. *American Journal of Obstetrics and Gynecology, 178*(2), 259–263.

Beck, C. T. (1996). Postpartum depressed mothers' experiences interacting with their children. *Nursing Research, 45*(2), 98–104.

Britton, G. A. (1998). A review of women and tobacco: Have we come such a long way? *Journal of Obstetric, Gynecologic, and Neonatal Nursing, 27*, 241–249.

Carmichael, S., Abrams, S. B., & Selvin, S. (1997). The pattern of maternal weight gain in women with good pregnancy outcomes. *American Journal of Public Health, 87*(12), 1984–1988.

Centers for Disease Control and Prevention (CDC). (1996). Alcohol and other drug-related birth defects awareness week, May 12–18. *Morbidity and Mortality Weekly Report, 45*, 378–379.

Chervenak, F. A., & McCullough, L. B. (1996). Common ethical dilemmas encountered in the management of HIV-infected women and newborns. *Clinical Obstetrics and Gynecology, 39*(2), 411–419.

Diehl, K. (1997). Adolescent mothers: What produces positive mother–infant interaction? *MCN: American Journal of Maternal Child Nursing, 22*, 89–95.

Eng, T. R., & Butler, W. T. (Eds.) (1997). *The hidden epidemic: Confronting sexually transmitted diseases*. Washington, DC: National Academy Press.

Erikson, E. H. (1968). *Identity, youth, and crisis*. New York: Norton.

Fergusson, D. M., Horwood, J., & Lynskey, M. T. (1993). Maternal smoking before and after pregnancy: Effects on behavioral outcomes in middle childhood. *Pediatrics, 92*(6), 815–822.

Flynn, L. (1999), The adolescent parenting program: Improving outcomes through mentorship. *Public Health Nursing, 16*(3), 182–189.

Goldenberg, R. L., Iams, J. D., Mercer, B. M., et al. (1998). The preterm prediction study: The value of new vs standard risk factors in predicting early and all spontaneous preterm births. *American Journal of Public Health, 88*(2), 233–238.

Hall, L. A., Kotch, J. B., Browne, D., & Rayens, M. K. (1996). Self-esteem as a mediator of the effects of stressors and social resources on depressive symptoms in postpartum mothers. *Nursing Research, 45*(4), 231–238.

Hauth, J. C., Goldenberg, R. L., Andrews, W. W., et al. (1995). Treatment with metronidazole and erythromycin reduces preterm delivery in women with bacterial vaginosis. *New England Journal of Medicine, 333*, 1732–1736.

Health Connection (1994). *The vegetarian food pyramid*. Hagerston, MD: Author.

Heinonen, S., Ryynanen, M., & Kirkinen, P. (1999). The effects on fetal development of high fetoprotein and maternal smoking. *American Journal of Public Health, 89*(4), 561–563.

Hickey, C. A., Cliver, S. P., McNeal, S. F., et al. (1996). Prenatal weight gain patterns and birth weight among nonobese black and white women. *Obstetrics and Gynecology, 88*(4), 490–496.

Holzman, C., & Paneth, N. (1998). Preterm birth: From prediction to prevention. *American Journal of Public Health, 88*(2), 183–184.

Jacob, J., Harrison, H., Jr., & Tigert, A. T. (1995). Prevalence of alcohol and illicit drug use by expectant mothers. *Alaska Medicine, 37*, 83–87.

Kaiser Permanente. (1996). *Partners in prevention*. Kaiser Permanente Northern California Region Department of Quality and Utilization and Department of Regional Health Education: Kaiser Foundation Health Plan, Inc. Boise, ID: Healthwise, Inc.

Keltner, B. (1994). Home environments of mothers with mental retardation. *Mental Retardation, 32*, 123–127.

Keltner, B., Finn, D., & Shearer, D. (1995). Effects of family intervention of maternal–child interaction for mothers with developmental disabilities. *Family Community Health, 17*(4), 35–49.

Kilby, J. W. (1997). A smoking cessation plan for pregnant women. *Journal of Obstetric, Gynecologic, and Neonatal Nursing, 26*, 397–403.

Law, M. D., & Tang, J. L. (1995). An analysis of the effectiveness of interventions intended to help people stop smoking. *Archives of Internal Medicine, 155*, 1933–1941.

Levin, B. (1998). Grief counseling. *American Journal of Nursing, 98*(5), 69–72.

Lloyd, K. (1993). Mothering instinct. *Nursing Times, 89*(26), 42–44.

Long, S. H., & Marquis, M. S. (1998). The effects of Florida's Medicaid eligibility expansion for pregnant women. *American Journal of Public Health, 88*(3), 371–376.

Lundsberg, L. S., Bracken, M. B., & Saftlas, A. F. (1997). Low-to-moderate gestational alcohol use and intrauterine growth retardation, low birthweight, and preterm delivery. *Annals of Epidemiology, 7*(7), 498–508.

McComish, J. F., Lawlor, L. A., & Laken, M. P. (1996). INREACH: Linking walk-ins and their infants to community-based care. *MCN: American Journal of Maternal Child Nursing, 21*, 132–136.

Meis, P. J., Goldenberg, R. L., Mercer, B. M., et al. (1998). The preterm prediction study: Risk factors for indicated preterm births. *American Journal of Obstetrics and Gynecology, 178*(3), 562–567.

Novello, A. C., Degraw, C., & Kleinman, D. V. (1997). Healthy children ready to learn: An essential collaboration between health and education. In B. W. Spradley & J. A. Allender (Eds.), *Readings in community health nursing* (pp. 391–409). Philadelphia: Lippincott-Raven.

O'Conner, A. M., Davies, B. L., Dulberg, C., et al. (1992). Effectiveness of a pregnancy smoking cessation program. *Journal of Obstetric, Gynecologic, and Neonatal Nursing, 21,* 385–392.

Olds, D. L. (1994). Intellectual impairment in children of women who smoke cigarettes during pregnancy. *Pediatrics, 93*(2), 221–227.

Piaget, J. (1950). *The psychology of intelligence.* London: Routledge and Kegan Paul, Ltd.

Rienzo, P. G. (1993). *Nursing care of the person who smokes.* New York: Springer.

Robertson, B. E. (1993). *Alcohol disabilities primer: A guide to psychosocial disabilities caused by alcohol use.* Boca Raton, Fl.: CRC Press.

Russell, M., Martier, S. S., Solok, R. J., Mudar, P., Jacobson, S., & Jacobson, J. (1996). Detecting risk drinking during pregnancy: A comparison of four screening questionnaires. *American Journal of Public Health, 86*(10), 1435–1439.

Serafine, M., & Broom, B. L. (1998). Predicting low-risk pregnant women's attendance at a preterm birth prevention class. *Journal of Obstetric, Gynecologic, and Neonatal Nursing, 27*(3), 279–287.

Shah, S., Hoffman, R., Shinault, R., & LaPoint, S. (1998). Screening for pregnancy and contraceptive use among women admitted to a Denver detoxification center. *Public Health Reports, 113,* 336–340.

Siccardi, D. C. (1998, September 27). Gestational diabetes. Available: http://www.medstudents.com.br/ginob/ginob4.htm.

Southwick, K. L., Guidry, H. M., Weldon, M. M., et al. (1999). An epidemic of congenital syphilis in Jefferson County, Texas, 1994–1995; Inadequate prenatal syphilis testing after an outbreak in adults. *American Journal of Public Health, 89*(4), 557–560.

U.S. Census Bureau (1999). *Statistical abstract of the United States, 1999* (119th ed.). Washington, DC: Author.

U.S. Department of Agriculture. (1992). *The food guide pyramid.* Washington, DC: Author.

U.S. Department of Health and Human Services. (2000). *Healthy people 2010* (conference edition in two volumes). Washington, DC: U.S. Government Printing Office.

———. (1991). *Healthy people 2000: National health promotion and disease prevention objectives* (S/N 017-001-00474-0). Washington, DC: U.S. Government Printing Office.

Valaitis, R., Tuff, K., & Swanson, L. (1996). Meeting parents' postpartal needs with a telephone information line. *MCN: Maternal and Child Nursing, 21,* 90–95.

Van de Perre, P. (1995). Postnatal transmission of human immunodeficiency virus type 1: The breast-feeding dilemma. *American Journal of Obstetrics and Gynecology, 173,* 483–487.

Ventura, S. J., Martin, J. A., Curtin, S. C., & Natgewsm, T. H. (1997). *Report of final natality statistics, 1995. Monthly Vital Statistics Report, 45*(11, S2). Hyattsville, MD: National Centers for Health Statistics.

World Health Organization. (1998). *The world health report, 1998: Life in the 21st century, a vision for all.* Geneva, Switzerland: Author.

Zill, N. (1996). Parental schooling and children's health. *Public Health Reports, 3*(1), 34–43.

Zuckerman, B. (1998). Marijuana and cigarette smoking during pregnancy: Neonatal effects. In F. I. Chasnoff (Ed.). *Drugs, alcohol, pregnancy, and parenting.* Boston: Kluwer Academic.

SELECTED READINGS

Beck, C. T. (1996). A meta-analysis of the relationship between postpartum depression and infant temperament. *Nursing Research, 45*(4), 225–230.

Bedics, B. C. (1994). Nonuse of prenatal care: Implications for social work involvement. *Health and Social Work, 19*(2), 84–92.

Bennett, T. R. (1997). "Racial" and ethnic classification: Two steps forward and one step back? *Public Health Reports, 112,* 477–480.

Burton, J. (1999). When your patient is postpartum: Are you confident in your skills? *American Journal of Nursing, 99*(2), 64–70.

Choudhry, U. K. (1997). Traditional practices of women from India: Pregnancy, childbirth, and newborn care. *Journal of Obstetric, Gynecologic, and Neonatal Nursing, 26*(5), 533–539.

Fein, S. B., & Roe, B. (1998). The effect of work status on initiation and duration of breast-feeding. *American Journal of Public Health, 88*(7), 1042–1046.

Freeman, E. W., & Rickles, K. (1993). *Early childbearing: Perspectives of black adolescents on pregnancy, abortion, and contraception.* Newbury Park, CA: Sage.

High-Laukaran, V., Rutstein, S. O., Peterson, A. E., & Labbok, M. H. (1996). The use of breast milk substitutes in developing countries: The impact of women's employment. *American Journal of Public Health, 86*(9), 1235–1240.

Horns, P. N., Ratcliffe, L. P., Leggett, J. C., & Swanson, M. S. (1996). Pregnancy outcomes among active and sedentary primiparous women. *Journal of Obstetric, Gynecologic, and Neonatal Nursing, 25,* 49–54.

Julnes, G., Konefal, M., Pindur, W., & Kim, P. (1994). Community-based perinatal care for disadvantaged adolescents: Evaluation of the resources mothers program. *Journal of Community Health, 19*(1), 41–53.

Kardel, K., & Kase, T. (1998). Training in pregnant women: Effects on fetal development and birth. *American Journal of Obstetrics and Gynecology, 178*(2), 280–286.

Koenig, M. A., Roy, N. C., McElrath, T., et al. (1998). Duration of protective immunity conferred by maternal tetanus toxoid immunization: Further evidence from Matlab, Bangladesh. *American Journal of Public Health, 88*(6), 903–907.

Lutenbacher, M., & Hall, L. A. (1998). The effects of maternal psychosocial factors on parenting attitudes of low-income, single mothers with young children. *Nursing Research, 47*(1), 25–34.

McFarlane, J., & Parker, B. (1994). Preventing abuse during pregnancy: An assessment and intervention protocol. *Journal of Obstetric, Gynecologic, and Neonatal Nursing, 18,* 245–246.

Miranda, J., Azocar, F., Komaromy, M., & Golding, J. M. (1998). Unmet mental health needs of women in public-sector gynecologic clinics. *American Journal of Obstetrics and Gynecology, 178*(2), 212–217.

Nag, M. (1994). Beliefs and practices about food during pregnancy: Implications for maternal nutrition. *Economic and Political Weekly, 29*(37), 2427–2428.

Nesbitt, T. S., Latson, E. H., Rosenblatt, R. A., & Hart, L. G. (1997). Rural Washington: Its effect on neonatal outcomes and resource use. *American Journal of Public Health, 87*(19), 85–90.

Olds, D. L., Henderson, C. R., & Kitzman, H. (1994). Does prenatal and infancy nurse home visitation have enduring effects on qualities of parental caregiving and child health at 25 to 50 months of life? *Pediatrics, 93*(1), 89–98.

Pearson, M. A., Hoyme, E., Seaver, L. H., & Rimsza, M. E. (1994). Toluene embryopathy: Delineation of the phenotype and comparison with fetal alcohol syndrome. *Pediatrics, 93*(2), 211–215.

Petrini, J., Damus, K., Roy, S., et al. (1998). The effect of using "race of child" instead of "race of mother" on the black–white gap in infant mortality due to birth defects. *Public Health Reports, 113,* 263–267.

Rossiter, J. C. (1998). Promoting breast feeding: The perceptions of Vietnamese mothers in Sydney, Australia. *Journal of Advanced Nursing, 28*(3), 598–605.

Tharaux-Deneux, C., Bouyer, J., Job-Spira, N., et al. (1998). Risk of ectopic pregnancy and previous induced abortion. *American Journal of Public Health, 88*(3), 401–405.

Promoting and Protecting the Health of Infant, Toddler, and Preschool Populations

KEY TERMS

- Attention deficit disorder (without hyperactivity; ADD)
- Attention deficit hyperactivity disorder (ADHD)
- Developmental disabilities
- Head Start
- High-risk families
- Infant
- Oppositional defiant disorder (ODD)
- Preschooler
- Toddler

LEARNING OBJECTIVES

Upon mastery of this chapter, you should be able to:

- Identify the changing demographics found in the infant, toddler, and preschool populations.
- Identify major health problems and concerns for infant, toddler, and preschool populations globally and in the United States.
- Describe a variety of programs that promote and protect health and prevent illness and injury of infant, toddler, and preschool populations.
- State the recommended immunization schedule for infants and children, and give the rationale for the timing of each immunization.
- Give examples of methods the community health nurse might use in working with infants, toddlers, and preschool populations to help promote their health.

Healthy children are a vital resource to ensure the future well-being of a nation. They are the parents, workers, leaders, and decision makers of tomorrow, and their health and safety depend on today's decisions and actions. Their future lies in the hands of those people responsible for their well-being, including the community health nurse.

The well-being of children has been a subject of great concern globally and in this country for many years. In the United States, we have emphasized its importance through development of numerous laws and services, yet the needs of millions of children continue to go unmet. Many young children go to bed hungry. All infants and toddlers do not receive even the most basic of immunizations until reaching school age. Accidents and injury are a leading cause of death. Preventable communicable diseases increase the mortality among the very young. In a world-leading country in many areas, including technology, business, agriculture, and education, the failure to protect and promote the health of our youngest is a blemish we must not ignore. Globally, in many nations, infant health and well-being are in even greater jeopardy.

In this chapter, we will explore the global needs of and related services available for the youngest and most vulnerable of society's members. We examine infant, toddler, and preschool population health services commonly available in the United States, and explore the role of the community health nurse in providing those services.

GLOBAL VIEW OF INFANT, TODDLER, AND PRESCHOOL HEALTH

The health of children in one country will affect the health of children in other countries, including the United States. Infants and young children travel internationally with their parents. Refugee populations cross the borders of other countries in an attempt to escape intolerable political changes in their country. Major natural disasters create an environment that places whole populations at risk, especially the very young and very old, such as the nationwide flooding in Mozambique during the winter and spring of 2000. It behooves each country to consider this and do what is necessary to promote and protect the health of children worldwide. A review of the changing demographics and current health status of the world's infants, toddlers, and preschool-aged children will provide you with a more complete picture of where we came from, where we are, and what more we have to do.

Global History of Children's Health Care

Only recently in the history of the world have children been considered valuable assets. This is true in many countries where there are well-developed programs of infant health promotion and protection, infant and child day care services, and strict educational expectations for all children. However, in some countries, female infants and children are not valued. They may be sold to another family or prevented from going to school to get an education. Some countries, such as China, limit population growth, and couples are allowed to raise only one child. Subsequent pregnancies are forbidden and termination encouraged. Among some cultures, a child born with a congenital anomaly is not treated. Some birth and growth and developmental rituals are harsh and considered illegal when judged by Western beliefs. Cultural practices that are fostered by political forces prevent many countries from improving the health of infants and young children.

For many developing countries, the health care system is a system of superstition and faith, as it was in colonial America (Spector, 2000). Presently in the United States, the system is "predicated on strong scientific beliefs; the epidemiological model of disease; highly developed technology; and strong values of individuality, competition, and free enterprise" (Spector, 2000, p. 51). Many other countries follow a similar pattern in their approach to health care.

Countries burdened with political unrest, poverty, and a lack of, or political misuse of, natural resources have elevated numbers of low-birth-weight infants. Low birth weight is associated with an elevated risk of infant mortality, congenital malformations, and other physical and neurologic impairments (Valanis, 1999). The most developed countries have the lowest infant mortality rates (Display 27–1). Yet even in these countries, infants and young children are not always provided with all the services they need.

DISPLAY 27–1. Countries With the Lowest Infant Mortality Rates—1999

Country	Rate (per 1,000 live births)
Iceland	2.6
Sweden	3.6
Norway	4.1
Finland	4.2
Luxembourg	4.2
Austria	4.8
Switzerland	4.8
France	5.0
Netherlands	5.1
Hong Kong	5.1
Denmark	5.2
Australia	5.3
Italy	5.5
Spain	5.5
Canada	5.6
Israel	5.8
United Kingdom	5.9
Belgium	6.0
Germany	6.0
Canada	6.1
Ireland	6.2
Greece	6.3
United States	7.0

(From Population Reference Bureau. [1999]. World population data sheet. Available: http://www.prb.org.)

Demographics

Spectacular global improvements in infant and child health have occurred in the past 50 years. This is likely to continue into the new millennium (World Health Organization [WHO], 1998). For example, just 45 years ago, one in five children died before their fifth birthday—a total of 20.6 million deaths in 1955. By 1995, the death rate had fallen to less than one in ten children. This should decline further to 3.7 children per 100 by 2025 (WHO, 1998).

When measuring the infant through preschool population's morbidity and mortality trends globally over the past 50 years, three dimensions of health development need to be taken into account. These include:

- Each country's epidemiologic patterns of disease and deficiencies
- Social, economic, and health infrastructure of the country
- Priority strategies and adequacy of the actions taken to address the preventable and treatable causes of death and illness in infants and children

Globally, the quality of family living conditions, the prevalence and modes of transmission of infectious disease agents, and the nutritional status of the child are among the strongest immediate determinants that set the different levels of mortality rates in children younger than age 5. Significant improvement in at least one, but more desirably all three of these factors is required to effect a substantial overall decline in the rates. For example, the decline in deaths among the population under 5 years of age in developed countries since the late 1940s is largely attributed to improved sanitation, safe water supply, secure housing, adequate food supply and distribution, and general hygiene. Various childhood diseases such as diphtheria, scarlet fever, and rheumatic heart disease were in steady decline long before immunizations and antibiotics became widely available.

Today, in most developing countries, general improvement in sanitation, water, education, and access to preventive and curative health care has led to declines in childhood mortality similar to those seen in the West 50 to 80 years ago. However, progress in developing countries has been more rapid because of the historic lessons learned along with improved technologies for disease prevention and treatment, nutrition, and fertility management.

Unfortunately, progress is not rapid in all countries. Among the least developed countries, progress either has not been made, or it has not been sustained over the years. In a few countries, child mortality levels are as high as 15% among live births, such as in the Western Sahara, almost 50 years behind other countries.

Health Status

In the poorest of countries, infants and young children are most vulnerable. They often die of diarrhea, acute lower respiratory infections, measles, tuberculosis, or pertussis (Fig. 27–1). In the morbidity associated with these diseases, malnutrition is a significant factor.

Although childhood mortality rates have markedly decreased in most countries since the early 1900s, morbidity rates remain high. The most common types of acute conditions seen in the United States are respiratory illnesses (which account for the largest group), infectious and parasitic diseases, injuries, and digestive diseases (U.S. Department of Health and Human Services [USDHHS], 1998).

Other childhood health problems, less easy to detect and measure but often as debilitating, are those of emotional, behavioral, and intellectual development. Although these problems are not new, awareness and concern for them have increased as the rates of occurrence for infectious diseases such as measles, mumps, rubella, and polio have diminished. Emotional disorders are quite prevalent, and "it is estimated that 20% of children and adolescents may have a diagnosable mental, emotional, or behavioral problem that can lead to school failure, alcohol or other drug use, violence, or

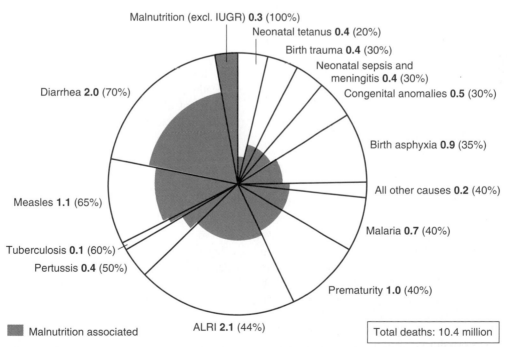

Disease clusters

Neonatal and perinatal causes. Neonatal tetanus, birth trauma, neonatal sepsis and meningitis, congenital anomalies, birth asphyxia, prematurity.
Integrated management of childhood illness. Malaria, acute lower respiratory infection (ALRI), measles, diarrhea, malnutrition.

FIGURE 27–1. Main cause of death among children under age 5, developing world, 1995. (World Health Organization [1998]. *The world health report 1998: Life in the 21st century.* Geneva: World Health Organization.)

suicide" (USDHHS, 1998). The roots of these problems are often traced to the toddler and preschool years. For example, studies have found an association between learning disorders in children and violent behavior in adolescents and adults (Foley, Carlton & Howell, 1996).

Causes of learning disorders and emotional behavioral problems appear to have genetic and environmental influences. Increased use of illicit drugs by pregnant women is producing a generation of children with developmental delays and learning disabilities (Butz, Lears, O'Neil & Lukk, 1998; Haack, 1997). The number of children affected by parental drug use has surpassed childhood disabilities caused by lead poisoning, which has, itself, been a major contributor to developmental problems in children.

In the United States, 21% of children live below the poverty level, compared with the adult poverty rate of 11% (U.S. Census Bureau, 1999). Because many poor adults have more than two children, the total number of children who are poor is greater than the number of poor adults. Single parents contribute to this number as well, because there is just one parent and often two or more children in the family. Cultural factors may also contribute. For example, it is traditional in the Southeast Asian, Northern Laotian, and Hmong cultures for teenage girls to marry as young as 15 or 16 to young men in their late teens. Family planning measures are not widely practiced, and it is not unusual that from this union the partners will have 6 to 10 children. Such early marriages and large families limit educational and employment opportunities and promote poverty. Additionally, there are millions of children worldwide in moderate-income families who have inadequate child care, poor housing, limited health insurance, and limited access to higher education.

HEALTH PROBLEMS OF INFANTS, TODDLERS, AND PRESCHOOLERS

The **infant** (birth to 1 year), **toddler** (ages 1 and 2 years), and **preschooler** population (ages 3 and 4 years) has a low mortality rate in the United States that is becoming lower every year. Currently, the infant mortality rate, often considered to be a fairly sensitive indicator of the general health status in a population, is 7.2 per 1,000 live births (USDHHS, 2000). This has steadily declined since infant mortality rates were first recorded in 1915, when it was at 99.9; it had fallen to 47 by 1940 (Kovner & Jonas, 1999). This dramatic change can be credited to improved maternal health, the spacing of children, infant immunizations, and infant safety. The major cause of death among the birth-to-4-year-old population is unintentional injuries (motor vehicle accidents, falls, drownings, fires and burns), followed by malignant neoplasms, birth defects, and heart disease (USDHHS, 2000).

Accidents and Injuries

Toddlers and preschoolers are vulnerable to many types of accidents or unintentional injuries such as those from unsafe toys, falls, burns, drownings, automobile crashes, and poisonings, especially for children under age 4. Injury from many sources may result in death.

The loss of children's lives resulting from all injuries combined suggests a staggering number of years of productive life lost to society. Unintentional injuries are the leading cause of death for people aged 1 to 34 and are the fifth leading cause of death in the United States (USDHHS, 2000). Motor vehicle crashes account for approximately half the deaths from unintentional injuries. Greater efforts are being made to reduce play and recreational injuries for young children through better monitoring of toy safety and improved playground construction and maintenance. Product safety is monitored by the Federal Consumer Product Safety Commission.

Infants are at risk of falling when they are not supervised adequately. Falls from a bed or other furniture item when not properly secured or supervised can cause permanent injury or death. Infants should never be left unattended when not in a crib or play yard. Even a safely made crib placed near a window with a dangling cord from window blinds is an infant injury or death waiting to happen. Many children are killed each year by getting entangled in these cords. As the infant grows and begins to learn to walk, frequent falls are common and continuous supervision and "childproofing" of the home are essential. Young children are curious, and their exploring can lead to additional forms of injury, such as burns, drowning, or poisoning.

Injury from burns can happen to children of all ages. Child deaths and injuries from burns result primarily from house fires but also from electrical burns, cigarette lighters and matches, and scalds. Cigarette lighters and matches are fascinating to young children. Toddlers or preschoolers may be able to start a flame, injuring or killing themselves and others. Infants are often burned by touching a parent's cigarette or by reaching for a cup of hot coffee or the handle of a pot on the stove. Being placed into bath water that is too hot can cause a scalding injury. A crawling or toddling child can pull an iron cord, causing the iron to topple on him or her, resulting in a burn or injury. By inserting a finger or toy into an electrical outlet, the child is at risk of electrocution.

Preventing all possible sources of injury or death from burns can be accomplished by eliminating opportunity and source. Through child supervision, safe storage of matches and lighters, and keeping children away from the stove and electrical outlets, burning can be prevented. Adults can protect children by keeping pot handles turned toward the center of the stove, by not using the stove burners or ovens to heat their homes, by modifying water temperatures in water heaters, by always testing bath water with an elbow before placing a child in the bath, and by keeping electrical outlets covered with inexpensive plastic inserts. Many local fire departments and public health programs offer safety education in this area, emphasizing the use of heat- and smoke-detecting systems; fire drills and home evacuation plans; less flammable structural materials, furnishings, and clothing; and careful smoking—or better yet, no smoking.

Drownings among young children occur wherever water occurs in depths exceeding only a few inches, such as in toilet bowls, bathtubs, buckets or cans left outside that have filled with rainwater, puddles, ponds, and swimming pools. Infants, toddlers, and preschool-aged children are especially vulnerable because they are not aware of water dangers and will explore unafraid. Parents need to provide a "drown-free" environment by:

- Bathing young children in shallow water
- Never leaving young children unattended during a bath
- Keeping the lid down on toilets and the bathroom door closed—preferably secured with a childproof safety handle
- Eliminating water collection sites around the home by turning over or removing empty buckets, containers, empty flower pots, and so forth, from collecting rainwater
- Having a swimming pool fenced with a childproof lock or alarm device that sounds when the water is disturbed
- Promoting water safety measures, including teaching young children to swim
- Vigilantly observing young children at play to protect them from wandering off toward neighborhood water sources

Injury and death from automobile crashes continue to be a major safety problem in the United States. Some families do not use infant restraint seats consistently even though they have been required by law for decades. Other families have them and use them regularly, but they are not installed properly and the child is at as much risk as not being restrained. There is much opportunity in this area for the community health nurse to educate the public and ensure that parents have the information and skills to properly secure their children whenever traveling by car.

Poisoning is a constant safety concern for young children. Sources of poisoning include household plants, prescription medications and over-the-counter drugs, unintentional medication overdoses, household cleaning products, other chemicals stored within a child's reach, and lead.

Childproofing the home to eliminate major sources of poisoning is the best method of keeping children safe. This includes keeping plants out of a child's reach or eliminating them from the home until the child is older, locking up household chemicals and storing them out of a child's reach, using childproof medication containers and storing all medicines in a locked box with a key that is kept out of reach, and eliminating sources of lead.

A major cause of poisoning comes from lead. The primary sources of lead exposure in preschool-aged children continue to be lead-based paint, lead-contaminated soil and dust, and drinking water from lead-soldered pipes (Manheimer & Silbergeld, 1998; USDHHS, 1998). Children living and playing in substandard housing areas remain at risk for being directly exposed to significant sources of lead. Community health nurses should include opportunities for blood screening for lead levels when it is suspected that a children in certain homes, apartments, or neighborhoods are at risk for lead poisoning.

Safety programs seek to protect children from the hazards of poisonings, ingestion of toxic substances, prescription medications, and over-the-counter drugs. Poison control centers in many localities offer information and emergency assistance. Toxic household substances, such as cleaning supplies, must be clearly labeled, and harmful drugs must be packaged with special seals and safety caps. Generally, the community health nurse can educate families to recognize potentially hazardous situations and encourage efforts to eliminate them.

Homicide is the most frequent cause of death for infants—8.3 per 100,000 in 1997. The 2010 target is 3.2 per 100,000, with a 1998 baseline of 6.2 (USDHHS, 2000). Homicides of children under the age of 3 most often result from family violence.

A child's culture influences the level of violence to which the child is exposed. Increased aggressive behavior among children has been attributed to violence in the child's home (spousal and child abuse) and community, as well as violent scenes on television and in movies.

Communicable Diseases

Toddlers and preschool-aged children experience a high frequency of acute illnesses, more than any other age group. These account for a large number of days of restricted activity and disability requiring bed rest. Respiratory illness makes up over one half of acute conditions in toddlers and preschoolers (USDHHS, 2000). Morbidity from communicable diseases among young children is high. Respiratory illnesses, followed by infectious and parasitic diseases, injuries, and digestive conditions, are the most common. The incidence of measles, rubella (German measles), and infectious parotitis (mumps) has dropped considerably because of widespread immunization efforts. Yet cases of communicable diseases still occur. Some have potentially serious complications, such as pertussis. Pertussis had a *Healthy People 2000* goal of 1,000 cases and has remained high, with 3417 cases in 1998 (USDHHS, 1998, 2000). The *Healthy People 2010* goal is revised to 2,000 cases.

Vigorous campaigns have been undertaken by health departments to get children immunized. For example, in 1991 routine infant hepatitis B vaccination was first recommended, and in 5 years the proportion of 19- to 35-month-old children who received three doses of the vaccine increased from less than 10% to 82% (USDHHS, 1998). With the introduction of *Haemophilus influenzae* type b (Hib) conjugate vaccine in 1990, the incidence of Hib meningitis among infants declined by 94% from 1986 to 1995 (Centers for Disease Control and Prevention [CDC], 1996). An immunization for mumps, measles, and rubella (MMR) has been available for almost 30 years and for varicella (chickenpox) since 1995. In 1998, immunization coverage levels for children aged 19 to 35 months were at record high levels (CDC, 1999c).

Guidelines for polio immunization have recently undergone change. Experts recommend giving most infants inactivated polio virus (IPV) for the first two doses, and then oral polio virus (OPV)—made from live, attenuated virus—for the second two doses, rather than giving all IPV or OPV. This new schedule is intended to decrease the incidence of vaccine-associated paralytic polio. Approximately nine such cases occur each year after administration of OPV (Forshner & Garza, 1999).

The financing of immunizations for infants and children has been significantly improved as a result of two major initiatives. The Vaccines for Children Program and the Child Health Insurance Program cover children on Medicaid, uninsured children, and American Indian and Alaska Native children. In addition, underinsured children who receive immunizations at federally qualified health centers and rural health clinics are covered. Also, additional state programs and funds help provide free vaccines for children not covered by the other programs. There are several ways for community health nurses to help all families obtain free immunizations.

Even if financial barriers are removed, there are other barriers. Transportation is a significant problem for some parents, especially in rural areas, and for families in urban areas who have several children and need to take public transportation. Even with public health announcements in the media, there are mothers who are unaware of the disabling consequences of diseases such as polio and do not realize the importance of a fully vaccinated child (Fig. 27–2).

There are no immunizations against human immunodeficiency virus/acquired immunodeficiency syndrome (HIV/AIDS). In 1996, there were 830,000 HIV-positive children (Pediatric AIDS, 2000). In 1999 over 10,000 children in the United States were HIV positive. AIDS is the seventh leading cause of death in children between ages 1 and 4 in the United States. These children acquire the virus while in utero and are infected at birth. Pediatric AIDS is declining due to the antiretroviral agents that HIV-positive pregnant women now have access to. There were 947 new cases in 1992 and 225 in 1998 (CDC, 1999c). Many young children become orphaned at an early age because their mothers may have been living with AIDS for several years. The children may enter foster care because of the mother's declining health and an inability or reluctance by other family members to care for an HIV-infected child. Also, because HIV-infected children are infrequently adopted, they often remain in foster care throughout their short lives.

Chronic Diseases

Many young children are afflicted with chronic diseases that affect quality of life. Asthma is the most common chronic illness among children in the United States, affecting 4.8 million children and adolescents (Walsh, Kelly & Morrow, 1999). Many of that number begin to show signs and symptoms of asthma as infants and toddlers. It is a leading cause of hospitalization in children. Inner city low-income and minority children are affected disproportionately. Head Start, a federally funded program that provides early childhood education to low-income children between 3 and 5 years of age, is an ideal setting for community health nurses to address asthma awareness, education, and prevention.

The incidence of food allergies is increasing in the population. Fortunately, once allergies are diagnosed, they can be managed through dietary changes and by avoiding allergy-producing foods. Discovering food allergies early in an infant's life can be accomplished by parents offering one new food at a time, with a 3-day interval between new foods. This helps to identify which foods the infant or child may be allergic to. Parents need to be educated to read food labels consistently and to alert family members about the child's allergy so foods are not given to the child inappropriately.

Other chronic illnesses have a more profound effect on child and family. Muscular dystrophy (MD) and cystic fibrosis (CF) are two diseases that not only affect quality of life but also severely shorten the child's life.

MD is a familial disease characterized by progressive atrophy and wasting of muscles. Onset is usually at an early age, and it occurs more frequently in males than females. Its cause is thought to be a genetic defect in muscle metabolism. A child with MD is often confined to a wheelchair and needs assistance with activities of daily living, especially as the disease progresses.

CF usually begins in infancy and is characterized by chronic respiratory infection, pancreatic insufficiency, and increased electrolytes in sweat. It is the major cause of severe chronic lung disease in children. CF occurs in 1 in 2,000 white and 1 in 17,000 African-American live births. Parents must be taught positioning, clapping, and vibration followed by deep breathing and coughing to help mobilize secretions. Community health nurses reinforce these techniques and teach the family to avoid respiratory infections and to initiate prescribed antibiotic prophylaxis promptly. The young child should be involved in his or her own care, offering valid choices and encouraging decision-making. The family needs emotional support as they work through feelings of anticipatory grief.

Behavior and Learning Problems

Behavioral disorders and developmental disabilities are problems first recognized in children in this age group, which often become exacerbated when the child enters school. The

Birth	1 m	2 m	4 m	6 m	12 m	15 m	18 m	24 m	4-6 y	11-12 y	14-16 y
Hepatitis B	Hepatitis B										
		Hepatitis B			Hepatitis B					#	
		DTaP	DTaP	DTaP		DTaP			DTaP	Td	
		Hib	Hib	Hib		Hib					
		IPV	IPV			IPV			IPV		
						MMR			MMR	##	
						Var				###	
									Hep A in Certain Areas		

General Notes on Immunizations

- **Remember:** these guidelines are for **HEALTHY CHILDREN**, modifications may need to be made if certain illnesses exist or if immunocompromised
- age is post-partum age, therefore, be careful in premies
- by law, DT-Pertussis + MMR must be given before going to school
- in Canada, pentavalent vaccine (DTaP/IPV + Hib; Pentavax®) is licensed for use, but not in the United States; therefore, in U.S. don't mix DTaP and Hib (unless it's Hib powder)
- in multivalent vaccines, be careful if CI to single agent, whole multimodal vaccine CI, need individual components
- # means reassess and give vaccine if necessary, DOES NOT mean a fourth dose
- ## means reassess and give vaccine if necessary, DOES NOT mean a third dose
- ### means susceptible children may be given this vaccine at this time, but for > 13 yoa, 2 doses must be given at least one month apart

FIGURE 27-2. Recommended childhood immunization schedule—United States, January 2000. (Centers for Disease Control and Prevention [1999a]. General recommendations on immunizations: Recommendations of the Advisory Committee Practices [ACIP], American Academy of Pediatrics and American Academy of Family Physicians. *Morbidity and Mortality Weekly Report.*)

prevalence of these problems is difficult to measure epidemiologically, but as many as 20% of school-aged children have learning disabilities and behavioral problems first recognized in preschool years. The cause is multifaceted and often difficult to identify. The child's future mental health as an adult will be influenced by how well emotional needs are met during the early childhood phase of development.

Attention deficit hyperactivity disorder (ADHD) is a cluster of problems related to hyperactivity and impulsivity. **Attention deficit disorder (without hyperactivity; ADD)** is a cluster of problems related mainly to inattention, poor motivation, and disorganization. Both are seen in children and adults. It is estimated to affect 2% to 5% of American children, with boys more commonly affected than girls (Bussing et al., 1998; Marks, 1998). These disorders are being diagnosed with increasing frequency in children, adolescents, and adults; however, frequently, the signs are recognized in the preschool years. Descriptions of ADHD and ADD are displayed in Table 27–1 (Aust, 1994; Marks, 1998). A detailed discussion of ADHD occurs in Chapter 28.

Oppositional defiant disorder (ODD) is a set of "externalizing" behavior problems including noncompliance,

temper tantrums, and other socially provocative behaviors first diagnosed in the preschool years (Speltz, McClellan, DeKlyen & Jones, 1999). ODD is often considered to be a "gateway" for diverse psychopathologies in later life, and preschool-aged children (predominantly boys) with confirmed diagnoses of ODD or ODD/ADHD have these clear indicators for ongoing risk (Speltz, McClellan, DeKlyen, & Jones, 1999). Children diagnosed with ODD have lower verbal IQ scores, higher probability of insecure attachments to parents, and conflicted family interactions (DeKlyen, Speltz & Greenberg, 1998; Stormschak, Speltz, DeKlyen & Greenberg, 1997).

There is much controversy about using medications to modify and control behavior. The use of mood-modifying drugs begins for some children during preschool years with even more children being medicated by school age. Drugs used in combination with behavior modification practices and tapered off when behavior improves is a productive approach to out-of-control behavior.

Developmental disabilities are severe, chronic disabilities that manifest before the person attains age 22. They share the following characteristics:

1. They are accompanied by a mental or physical impairment or a combination of mental and physical impairments.
2. They are likely to continue indefinitely.
3. Impairments result in substantial functional limitations in three or more of the following areas:
   a. Self-care
   b. Receptive and expressive language
   c. Learning
   d. Mobility
   e. Self-direction
   f. Capacity for independent living
   g. Economic sufficiency

There are several categories of causes for such developmental disability: birth defects, prematurity, birth trauma, injury from falls, auto crashes, poisonings, or near drowning. Other disabling chronic conditions that limit activities and self-care are speech, hearing, and visual defects; seizure disorders; asthma; cancer; and AIDS. Together, disabilities affect approximately 12% of children through school age. The percentage is smaller among the infant, toddler, and preschool population because developmental and other chronic conditions may not occur until the child is older. Children with special needs, however, affect the health of families, educational and support services in communities, as well as the role of the community health nurse.

Poor Nutrition and Dental Hygiene

Other health problems found in this age group are nutritional problems (under- or overfeeding, overeating, and inappropriate food choices) and poor dental health. Nutritional and dental health needs are great during this period of rapid growth. Many factors contribute to early nutrition and dental problems.

A healthy start in life is foundational to well-being later in life. Nutrition is basic to the strength of this foundation. Bonding between mother and infant and overall maternal health are predictors of infant weight gain. Both nutrition and bonding can be accomplished by breastfeeding. Some of the benefits of breastfeeding include (Olds, London, & Ladewig, 1999):

- Convenience: The milk is always the perfect temperature and no preparation is needed
- Cost: A healthy diet for the mother, breast pads, nursing bras, and (possibly) a breast pump
- Nutrition: Breast milk is species specific, the proteins are easily digested, and fats are well absorbed
- Anti-infective and antiallergic properties: Breast milk contains immunoglobulins, enzymes, and leukocytes that protect against pathogens; breast milk decreases the incidence of allergy by eliminating exposure to potential antigens

Overfeeding an infant can lead to childhood obesity and becomes a risk factor for heart disease, hypertension, and diabetes. Eleven percent of school-age children are overweight, with the foundation begun in the preschool years (USDHHS, 2000; Tropiano & Flegal, 1998). The propensity for obesity begins as early as infancy and by childhood for most people. Obese children are three times more likely to become obese adults (Karp, 1993).

Young children's diets, often unreasonably high in sugar, increase the incidence of dental caries in this population group. The practice of allowing infants to continue to bottle feed beyond 15 to 16 months, or to fall asleep with a bottle, can lead to "nursing bottle syndrome." This causes the decay of the front teeth and, eventually, the molars, requiring extraction of the affected teeth (Reisine & Douglass, 1998). Parents of infants over 6 months of age should be instructed to rub the infant's gums with a damp clean cloth and begin toothbrushing, without toothpaste, using a soft pediatric toothbrush when several teeth have erupted. Liquid vitamins with added fluoride should be used if formula is premixed and not made from local fluoridated water supplies or if local water is not fluori-

TABLE 27–1. **ADHD and ADD: The Differences**	
Attention Deficit Disorder With Hyperactivity (ADHD)	**Attention Deficit Disorder Without Hyperactivity (ADD)**
A CHILD WITH THIS DIAGNOSIS OFTEN:	
Is impulsive	Has difficulty following through on instructions
Distracts easily	Has difficulty sustaining attention
Is inattentive when spoken to	Seems not to listen
Has difficulty waiting turn in group situations	Loses things necessary for tasks
Interrupts or intrudes on others	Fails to give close attention to details
Blurts out answers to questions	Is disorganized
Has difficulty playing quietly	Makes careless mistakes in schoolwork or work
Doesn't stay seated	Is forgetful
Runs about or climbs excessively	Daydreams when should be attending
Fidgets or squirms	Is unmotivated to complete tasks
Talks excessively	
Acts as if "driven by a motor" and cannot remain still	

dated. As children reach the toddler years, they are able to brush their own teeth with enthusiasm. Toothpaste should be used sparingly, and toothbrushing should be supervised by an adult because children this age can get overzealous with the amount of toothpaste they use, which should not be ingested. At age 3 or earlier, a first visit to a dentist should be planned and biannual visits should commence. American children begin a lifetime history of dental caries as preschoolers. Dental caries is a preventable condition that, if left unaddressed, can lead to self-esteem issues and body image disorders when children live with teeth that are discolored, misshapen, or missing. Chronic health conditions such as heart disease and nutritional problems from bacteria forming in the rotted teeth or food not being masticated properly occur when the teeth are missing. Dental caries increases with age and is more prevalent in Native-American populations (68% of children 2 to 4 years old with dental decay go untreated), in groups underserved by dentists, and in areas where there is no fluoridated water (USDHHS, 2000).

The Effects of Poverty

Poverty steals childhood from over one in five American children. It robs them of the resources needed to build a strong foundation for a healthy life. Urban and rural poverty are issues addressed in detail in Chapters 31 and 32 and are problems affecting greater numbers of children each year.

Contributing to the growing numbers of children living in poverty is the increasing number of single-mother households. In addition, there are higher rates of mortality, morbidity, and disability in families with lower income, less education, lower occupational level, and racial or ethnic minority status (Montgomery, Kiely & Pappas, 1996).

Children living in poverty have parents who are more unlikely to seek preventive family care, who underuse existing health care services, who lack general or systematic communication with health professionals, and who suffer from more acute and chronic health problems (Hatton, 1997). These problems are exacerbated when the poverty is severe and the family is homeless.

Being homeless brings with it additional problems that affect the health of young children. Exposure to the elements places children at risk for illness and injury. Sleeping in the street, parks, or occasional shelters interrupts a child's sleep patterns. The lack of a stable physical home environment can contribute to self-esteem, emotional, and mental health disturbances.

Community health nurses can make a big difference in the well-being of families with young children living in poverty. Assisting the family to apply for financial resources they are eligible for and helping them locate permanent, low-cost, and safe housing are priorities. Helping the parents locate employment, health care, and educational resources will promote wellness and give them the skills to help themselves and their children. Community health nurses can provide on-going contact to teach preventive health practices and to provide anticipatory guidance for young families.

HEALTH SERVICES FOR INFANTS, TODDLERS, AND PRESCHOOLERS

There are many ways in which the health of a child can be influenced. The goal is for health to be influenced positively. A variety of programs now exist that directly or indirectly serve the health needs of children. Community health nurses play a major and vital role in delivering these services. In community health, they fall into three categories approximating the three practice priorities of community health nursing practice: Health prevention, protection, and promotion.

Preventive Health Programs

Neighborhood community centers found in urban and rural settings provide families with parenting education, health and safety education, immunizations, various screening programs, and family planning services. Community health nurses, in collaboration with an interdisciplinary team, are usually the primary care providers in these programs. Their major goals are to keep communities well by focusing on primary and secondary prevention services.

Two examples of preventive health programs for infants and young children include immunization programs and quality day care services. In addition, parenting classes and other parental support services yield long-term benefits to children.

IMMUNIZATION PROGRAMS
Health departments and the private sector continue to offer immunization against the major childhood infectious diseases—measles, mumps, rubella, chickenpox, polio, diphtheria, tetanus, pertussis, and *Haemophilus influenzae*—some of which can cause permanent disability and sometimes even death. Although the threat of these diseases has been substantially reduced, vigilance cannot be relaxed. Low immunization levels in many areas, particularly among the poor, and increased disease rates signal the need for constant surveillance, outreach programs, and educational efforts. Community health nurses are deeply involved in each of these preventive activities. Health departments and schools often work collaboratively to provide immunization services (see Fig. 27–2). A compulsory immunization law, varying in its application from state to state, has enabled public health personnel to carry out these preventive services.

QUALITY DAY CARE PROGRAMS
Quality child care provides a significant avenue for preventing illness and injury among young children. In 1975, 39%

of women with children under the age of 6 were in the labor force; by 1994, more than 60% were employed (Gormley, 1995). Today, those figures are even higher as a result of economic necessity, changes in family structure, or personal career and lifestyle choice, making the two-wage-earner family the single largest employee group in the United States (Carabin et al., 1999). With these changes comes the demand for accessible and quality child care and, for some parents, the desire to provide children with educational experiences to prepare them for school (Hernandez, 1995).

Children in day care tend to contract a significantly higher number of illnesses than children cared for at home (Carabin et al., 1999). Carabin and colleagues found that there was an incidence rate of 6.1 upper respiratory tract infections (URTI) per toddler in day care studied throughout a 6-month period and compared this with children cared for at home in an earlier study of 3.8 URTI, for an incidence rate difference of 2.3 episodes per child-year, or a 38% increase among toddlers in day care. Many day care disease occurrences can be prevented through improved policies and adherence to those policies regarding sick children. Adhering to requirements for completed immunizations for all children and staff should be part of the community health nurse's role in services provided to aggregates in the community. Further preventive measures are needed to ensure cleanliness, good nutrition, proper ventilation, lighting, exercise, and a safe, emotionally secure environment (Helburn & Howes, 1996; Howes & Smith, 1995). Many children suffer injuries and even death due to lack of safe child care; one important preventive measure is to ensure lower child-to-caregiver ratios (Table 27–2).

Availability and accessibility of affordable, quality, licensed day care are recognized as one long-term solution for the prevention of child abuse. When young children can be safely cared for, it allows two parents or a single parent to work and provide more resources for the family, thus decreasing the stress that often precipitates abuse. However, the quality of day care and preschool programs varies considerably. Licensing laws can regulate only minimum safety and health standards. In addition, numerous child care operations are too small to require licensing, which leaves their quality open to individual discretion. Community health nurses can influence the quality of day care and preschool programs through active educational efforts, through monitoring of health and safety standards, and working to improve the state's role in passing stronger licensing laws.

PARENTAL SUPPORT SERVICES

Parental support services, available through many public and private agencies, including religious communities, have long-range effects on children's health. Emotionally healthy parents and stable families offer a healthful environment and support system for growing children. In most states, community health nurses provide teaching and counseling services to parents in their homes and in groups. Discussing parenting concerns and increasing parents' understanding of normal child growth and development allay fears and prevent problems. Through such efforts, family violence and abuse can be reduced or averted.

Health Protection Programs

Health protection programs for infants and young children are designed to protect them from illness and injury. Ultimately, these programs may even protect their lives.

SAFETY AND INJURY PROTECTION

Accidents and injury control programs serve a critical role in protecting the lives of children. Efforts to prevent motor vehicle crashes, a major cause of death, include driver education programs, better highway construction, improved motor vehicle design and safety features, and continuing research into the causes of various types of crashes. Injury prevention and reduction have been addressed through strategies such as state laws requiring the use of safety restraints, front and side driver and passenger airbags, substituting other modes of travel (air, rail, or bus), lower speed limits, stricter enforcement of drunk driving laws, safer automobile design, and helmets for motorcyclists, bicycle riders, and skaters.

For infants, toddlers, and preschool-aged children to be the most safe when traveling in vehicles, they must be restrained in an approved infant carrier, child restraint seat, or booster seat. These must be positioned and secured as described by the manufacturer; used at all times, even for the shortest of distances; placed in the vehicle in the back seat, never in the front seat; and installed in the appropriate position (facing rear or front) based on the weight/age of the infant or toddler. Children under the age of 12 should never sit in the front passenger seat. The force of the erupting airbag

---

> ### TABLE 27–2. The National Association for the Education of Young Children (NAEYC) Guidelines
>
> Developed in 1984, the NAEYC criteria for accreditation were based on research and professional consensus. The criteria include guidelines for staff–child interactions, curriculum content, parental involvements, staff qualifications and training, administration, staffing patterns, physical environment, health and safety, and nutrition and food service. One example is the NAEYC standards for group size and adult–child ratio:
>
> | Age of Child | Number of Children per Group | Adult–Child Ratio |
> | --- | --- | --- |
> | 0 to 12 months | 6 to 8 | 1:3 to 1:4 |
> | 12 to 24 months | 6 to 12 | 1:3 to 1:4 |
> | 2 years | 8 to 12 | 1:4 to 1:6 |
> | 3 years | 14 to 20 | 1:7 to 1:10 |
> | 4 to 5 years | 16 to 20 | 1:8 to 1:10 |

during a vehicle crash may be forceful enough to seriously injure or kill a small child.

Falls, a major killer of infants, toddlers, and preschool-aged children and the cause of injuries for millions of children each year, occur mostly in the home. Here, the community health nurse plays a major role in observing potential hazards, teaching safety measures, and reinforcing positive practices. Preventive and protective measures may be achieved through simple and inexpensive changes in the home. They include guards on windows and across stairways; removal, securing, or shortening of window blind cords; safer walking surfaces; and elimination of sharp objects or modification of surfaces that a child might fall against. Clearly, close supervision of infants and young children is primary to their safety and survival.

Programs to reduce environmental hazards for all people, not just infants, toddlers, and preschoolers, begin at the federal level, where the government sets and enforces pollution standards and regulates environmental contamination that poses health risks. At the state and municipal government levels, enforcement of regulations occurs. Measures include monitoring air and drinking water safety; installing carbon monoxide detection devices in housing units; providing proper sewage disposal; controlling ionizing radiation, asbestos, lead, and radon contamination and removing barrier provisions installed; enforcing auto safety and emission standards; and controlling use of agricultural chemicals and pesticides. Locally, protective measures include educational programs warning against toxic agents in the environment, community surveillance, and enforcement of environmental health standards. At all levels, epidemiologic research probes the causes and seeks answers to provide better protection for the public. Community health nurses need to be alert to environmental hazards and to work collaboratively with other members of the public health team to report problems and educate parents so their children are safe. Improved environmental control protects today's children against disease and disability and tomorrow's children against birth defects and the long-range hazards of environmental contamination. Chapter 16 explores environmental health and safety.

PROTECTION FROM COMMUNICABLE DISEASE

It has been demonstrated in community health that infectious diseases can be controlled and, in some cases, eliminated. Witness the successful worldwide eradication of smallpox, the dramatic decline in paralytic polio, and the decreasing incidence of the other communicable diseases of childhood, especially measles and chickenpox. Control of infectious diseases comes largely through immunization programs, discussed earlier, and surveillance of communicable disease incidence.

Programs protecting children against infectious diseases encompass efforts such as closing swimming pools with unsafe bacteria counts, conducting immunization campaigns in conjunction with influenza or measles outbreaks, and working with hospital pediatric units to reduce the incidence and threat of iatrogenic disease.

PROTECTION FROM DENTAL CARIES

Dental caries is the single most common chronic disease of children in the United States, occurring five to eight times more frequently than asthma (USDHHS, 2000). Eighteen percent of children aged 2 to 4 have been affected by dental caries. The average number of decayed and filled teeth among 2- to 4-year-olds has remained unchanged over the past 25 years. Children whose parents or caregivers have less than a high school education or whose parents and caregivers are Hispanic, American Indians, or Alaska Natives appear to be at markedly increased risk for developing early childhood caries (ECC) (USDHHS, 2000).

Fluoridation of community water supplies is the single most effective, safe, and low-cost means of protecting children's and adults' dental health, regardless of education or income level. Fluoride makes teeth less susceptible to decay by increasing resistance to the bacteria-produced acid in the mouth. Public acceptance of community water fluoridation has been slow, despite 40 years of research indicating its safety and effectiveness. Since 1980, just 62% of persons served by community water systems in the United States received optimally fluoridated water (USDHHS, 2000). The goal for 2010 is to increase this to at least 75% of the population (USDHHS, 2000). For those without this passive protection, supplemental fluorides, both systemic and topical, are available. In addition to regular dental care, good nutrition, and proper oral hygiene, community health nurses can safely promote public water fluoridation as an important program for protecting children's dental health.

However, there remains the need to focus on good dental health care. Professional dental health care has not changed dramatically in recent years, yet there are new products such as fluoride-releasing sealants, antibacterial rinses, plaque and tartar control dentifrices, and slow-release, intraoral drug delivery systems. Nevertheless, none of these products or treatments takes the place of personal oral health care supplemented with regular professional care. *Healthy People 2010* has a goal of reducing untreated cavities in the primary and permanent teeth so the proportion of children with decayed teeth not filled is no more than 9% among children ages 2 to 4, down from a baseline of 16% in 1988 to 1994 within this age group (USDHHS, 2000).

Some barriers to children's dental health are more prevalent among minority populations and the poor. Financial barriers and lack of education lead to poor dental health values, and adversely affect use of dentists and conscientious personal oral health care. Only about 40% of the population are covered by dental insurance, which accounts for 48% of dental reimbursement. The greater costs of dental care is assumed directly "out of pocket" by the consumer. Furthermore, dental insurance often is with limited coverage and high copayments and available only to children through employed parents or guardians with dental insurance (USDHHS, 1998). Medicaid pays for less than 4% of dental expenditures. The disparities in oral health care need to be reduced and, ideally, eliminated (Display 27–2).

DISPLAY 27-2. Disparities in Oral Health Care Among Young Children

Health Status
The level of untreated dental caries among members of racial and ethnic minority groups is greater than the national average.

Access
Poor children and members of racial and ethnic minority groups have less private dental insurance than the average for all children.

Poor children have 37% fewer dental visits than nonpoor children.

Smaller proportions of members of racial and ethnic minority groups have dental insurance than the national average.

Smaller proportions of members of racial and ethnic minority groups had a dental visit in the preceding year.

Preventive Services
Smaller proportions of minority and poor children have dental sealants.

(From U.S. Department of Health and Human Services [2000]. *Healthy people 2010* [conference edition in two volumes]. Washington, D.C.: Author.)

PROTECTION FROM CHILD ABUSE AND NEGLECT

Child abuse and neglect are major concerns for the United States. In 1994, over 3 million reports of possible abuse or neglect were made to authorities across the country with over 1 million children found to be victims of maltreatment (English, 1998). Child abuse is the maltreatment of children, including any or all of the following: physical abuse, emotional abuse, neglect (physical, medical, or educational), and sexual abuse (including sexual exploitation and child pornography). Exposing infants to drugs while in utero is a form of abuse (see Research: Bridge to Practice).

It is believed many more children also suffer from forms of abuse and neglect, but thousands of cases are not reported and not reflected in the statistics. The problem is often difficult to detect and often under-reported (Browne, 1995). In recent years, there has been an alarming increase in reported cases of physical and sexual abuse in day care centers, nursery schools, children's organizations, and churches. It is alarming to note that, regardless of race, culture, or socioeconomic origin, today's children run a high risk of suffering violence by their own caregivers.

Risk factors for abusive behavior include immaturity, stress, poverty, alcoholism, unstable employment, and physical and social isolation (English, 1998). Child abuse is seldom the result of any single factor, but rather a combination of stressful situations and parents who are unable to cope with problems and stress in a normal manner. Abusive adults often were abused, molested, or neglected themselves as children, carry low self-images into their adult lives, and are unable to cope with the demands of parenting (see Chapter 25). Other characteristics of abusive parents include immaturity, dependency, inability to handle responsibility, and low self-esteem. They often believe in the value of physical punishment, misunderstand their children's ability to understand and perform certain tasks, and frequently make unreasonable demands beyond their child's capability. During times of crisis, these parents often direct their anger and frustration at their children. These negative life patterns can continue for generations if intervention does not occur (McCroskey & Meezan, 1998).

Families at high risk for child abuse may be those that are chronically troubled or temporarily stressed. Teenage mothers and families with closely spaced children may also be more likely to engage in abusive behavior. Although poverty and lack of education are often linked with child abuse and neglect, no socioeconomic level is immune.

Services to protect children from abuse are not as well developed or effective as safety and injury protection programs. A variety of factors account for this. Most child abuse occurs in the home; thus, only the most blatant situations become evident to outsiders. Community health nurses and physicians who see injured children may find parents' explanations plausible and not suspect or want to believe that abuse might be responsible. Avoidance of legal involvement keeps others from reporting suspected cases. Fortunately, this attitude is changing among professionals who work with children and other community members.

For many years, states have had mandatory reporting laws. The first reporting law was passed in 1963 and required mandatory reporting of suspicious cases of child abuse, only by physicians. By 1966, all states had a reporting law. Over the years, numerous amendments have expanded the definition of child abuse and the persons required to report. People mandated to report suspected child abuse include all people who work with children—day care providers, teachers, social workers, nurses, doctors, clergy, coaches, and so forth. In addition, animal humane workers and commercial photograph developers are mandated reporters. Procedures for reporting categories of child abuse have also been clarified. Today, professionals and the public are more aware of the problem, and there is an increase in reporting. Nonetheless, it is estimated that less than 10% of abused child cases are actually reported. In 1974, the National Center for Child Abuse and Neglect was established as a result of the Child Abuse Prevention and Treatment Act. The center collects and analyzes information on child abuse and neglect, serves as an information clearinghouse, publishes educational materials on the subject, offers technical assistance, and conducts research into the problem. In addition, this act spurred all of the states to pass mandatory reporting laws and set up procedures for investigating suspected cases of child abuse and neglect. The government entity know as Child Protective Services was born (Larner, Stevenson & Behrman, 1998).

RESEARCH Bridge to Practice

Butz, A. M., Lears, M. K., O'Neil, S., & Lukk, P. (1998). Home intervention for in utero drug-exposed infants. *Public Health Nursing, 15*(5), 307–318.

Researchers from Johns Hopkins University conducted a study in 1997, which included 204 mother–infant dyads, to determine whether intensive early intervention, including home-based intervention, is an effective method to improve cognitive development, parent–child interaction, and health-related problems in high-risk children. There is a paucity of home intervention studies specifically examining in utero drug-exposed (IUDE) infants. This study is part of a larger clinical trial examining the effectiveness of home nurse interventions for the little-studied IUDE infants.

Each infant in this study received a total of 16 home visits during the first 18 months of life. Home visits were conducted by community health nurses adept in home visits to inner-city populations, specializing in pediatrics, and trained in basic pediatric assessment for IUDE infants.

On each home visit, the nurse assessed for signs and symptoms of in utero drug exposure, developmental problems, and common infant conditions. At 3, 6, 12, and 18 months of age, each infant received the Denver Developmental Screening Test (DDST-II) in the home to screen for developmental delays. Parenting information was provided, and selected skills were taught to the mother/caregiver to enhance maternal–infant interaction. In addition, role modeling was used by the community health nurse to promote positive maternal–infant interaction.

An analysis of home visit data for the first 20 enrolled mother–infant dyads is based on 229 visits to these 20 pairs of study participants. Health problems were encountered during approximately one third of the home visits and social problems during 80% of the visits. Basic parenting and personal skills were the primary educational information shared with the mother/caregiver. Basic parenting skills were important teaching topics in addition to well-child care. One third of the mothers continued drug use during the infant's first year of life. Infectious disease symptoms and preventable dermatologic problems were common, suggesting that basic personal hygiene is a necessary component of parent education before discharge of high-risk infants. Most mothers were unable to receive support from an identified support person and tended to be socially isolated, which can contribute to depression and continued drug use.

The implications for nursing practice indicate the need for vigilant monitoring through frequent home nurse visits for the first 12 months of life. These mothers experience a myriad of social, economic, and health problems during the first 12 months after birth. It is suggested that home visiting should be incorporated into the discharge planning of any IUDE infant to monitor the safety of these infants and maintain them in the health care delivery system.

prevent the stress and problems that might lead to dysfunction and abuse or neglect. Prevention should focus on parent preparation during the prenatal period; practices that encourage parent–child bonding during labor, delivery, the postpartum period, and early infancy; and provision of information regarding support services for families with newborns.

Provide parents of children of all ages with information regarding child-rearing and community resources.

Secondary Prevention. Services are designed to identify and assist high-risk families to prevent abuse or neglect. **High-risk families** are those families exhibiting the symptoms of potentially abusive or neglectful behavior or are under the types of stress associated with abuse or neglect.

Tertiary Prevention. Intervention and treatment services are designed to assist a family in which abuse or neglect has already occurred, to prevent further abuse or neglect. Intervention ranges from "early" intervention in the initial stages of abuse or neglect to "late stage" intervention in severe cases or after services have failed to stop the abusive or neglectful behavior.

The community health nurse has a major role in primary prevention of child abuse. In addition, the nurse is in a unique position to detect early signs of neglect and abuse; establish rapport with abusing parents, family members, or others; and assist with appropriate interventions and referrals at the secondary and tertiary levels of prevention in an interdisciplinary manner with teachers, the department of social services, foster families, and other health care providers (Chernoff, Combs-Orme, Risley-Curtiss & Heisler, 1994) (Display 27–3). The effectiveness of local programs depends, in large measure, on the willingness of community health professionals to increase their awareness and work as a team to detect, report, and develop interventions for abusers and abused children. Ongoing education of health care providers is recommended to increase their awareness of changing child abuse patterns, new reporting laws, and resources available to families (see Levels of Prevention).

Health Promotion Programs

Early childhood programs are designed to have positive effects on the outcomes of children's cognitive and social development. Some have considered children's physical health, and fewer have focused on parent–child interaction and parenting skills. All are considered health promotion programs.

EARLY CHILDHOOD DEVELOPMENT PROGRAMS

Early childhood development programs serve an increasingly important function for the escalating number of children enrolled in day care centers and preschools. More than half of all children today have mothers who work, and that figure keeps rising. Economic pressures eat into family time together and often diminish the quality of children's physical and psychosocial nourishment. Childhood development programs,

Most professionals adopt the "levels of prevention" model to define child abuse and neglect prevention efforts.

Primary Prevention. Establish community education to enhance the general well-being of children and their families.

Provide educational services designed to enrich the lives of families, to improve the skills of family functioning, and to

---

DISPLAY 27–3. Reports of an Emergency Foster Home

The following are examples of the various situations from which abused and neglected children come, as reported by a couple who had an emergency foster home for the county department of social services. The examples represent children placed with them over a 2-year period in which they cared for 256 children.

- Two-week-old Jose was brought to their home because the parents (under the influence of drugs) were found swinging Jose upside down in circles in an infant carrier as they walked along a downtown street at 3 AM. After being returned to his parents, he returned to foster care 1 month later after being found abandoned in an infant carrier at the county fair.
- Andre, Otis, and Selma, ages 8, 5, and 4, were brought to the foster home when social services discovered they had been living with their father in an abandoned car for 2 years. They stayed for 3 weeks while the social worker found suitable housing for this family and counseling for the father.
- Victoria, 5 years old, a loving and passive child, arrived wearing a diaper and appeared developmentally delayed. She had a history of being physically and sexually abused. Her family was very dysfunctional, and it took the social worker several weeks to sort out relatives and their intentions before placing Victoria in a long-term foster home.
- Ronald and Randall, 6-year-old twin boys who were forced to "sexually please their mother" for several years, came to the emergency foster home before being placed with relatives while their mother underwent psychiatric treatment. The boys began counseling during their stay in the emergency foster home.
- Antoinette, age 7, had severe asthma and was very withdrawn. She came to the emergency foster home because her mother (and the mother's boyfriend) refused to care for her. The child came with every photograph of herself and personal mementos because the mother wanted no reminders of the child. The social worker located a grandmother who would be the child's guardian.
- Thirteen-year-old Robert came home from school one day and found his mother and all their furniture gone. After a few weeks of living in the basement of the apartment building, someone alerted social services and Robert was placed in the emergency foster home for 2 months. His mother finally called social services after 6 weeks, saying Robert was too difficult for her to handle, but she may want to see him again someday. Robert was eventually placed in a group home for boys.
- Quyn, a 17-year-old Laotian girl, came into foster care after being referred by the school nurse because of wounds observed on her wrists and ankles. Quyn reported being strapped to a chair for 12 or more hours at a time by her father because she was not following the old ways and was shaming the family by being seen in public, unchaperoned, with a boy. Several meetings were held between the parents, a Southeast Asian community leader, and the social worker to resolve this situation so Quyn could go home safely.

---

such as **Head Start** (federally funded preschool programs for 3- to 5-year-old children from families in disadvantaged communities), provide physical, emotional, intellectual, and social stimulation. This is provided during a critical period in children's growth when impressions are being made and patterns are formed that will influence what kind of adults these children will be in the future. Comprehensive preschool programs promote good physical health, proper nutrition, a positive self-concept, and cognitive and social skill development. Many such programs exist, but more are needed.

In 1990, the president and the state governors set six national education goals to be reached by the year 2000; the first is "By the year 2000, all children in America will start school ready to learn" (U.S. Department of Education, 1990). We have not achieved that goal. Children are entering school without being ready to learn—for many, major emotional, physical, financial, and social barriers still exist. A physically and emotionally healthy child will be able to start school ready to learn. Where and how they achieve that health is the challenge to society. The stresses some parents feel are compounded when affordable and accessible licensed child care is not available; these stressed parents are more likely to abuse their children or place their children at risk of abuse, neglect, or exploitation.

NUTRITIONAL PROGRAMS

Adequate nutrition must begin at birth. However, some low-income children in the United States (8% in 1997) were growth retarded (USDHHS, 2000), which is defined as height-for-age below the fifth percentile. One of the most productive health outcome programs is the Special Supplemental Food Program for Women, Infants, and Children (WIC) program. Besides supporting women and young children with nutritious foods, in some cases, it makes a difference between life and death. Moss and Carver (1998) found that participation in the WIC program during pregnancy and infancy was associated with a reduced risk of infant deaths.

Nutrition and weight control programs form an additional important set of health-focused promotion services. Children need to learn sound dietary habits early in life to establish

LEVELS OF PREVENTION

PRIMARY, SECONDARY, AND TERTIARY LEVELS OF PREVENTION: A CONTINUUM OF FAMILY AND CHILDREN'S SERVICES

Family Type	Examples of Possible Services Used
PRIMARY PREVENTION	
All families and healthy families	Advocacy
	Income support
	Housing
	Health care services
	Accessible child care
	Family-centered policies at work
	Parenting education
	Recreation resources
	Family-planning services
	Information and referral services
Families needing additional support/facing minor challenges	Family support centers and programs
	Home visiting programs
	Family counseling
	Support groups at times of developmental and situational crisis
	Services for single parents
SECONDARY PREVENTION	
At-risk families—those with serious challenges and having special needs	Substance abuse treatment
	Respite child care
	Special health and educational services
	Teen pregnancy/parenting services
	Mental health services
TERTIARY PREVENTION	
Families in crisis, at risk of dissolution, or who place children at risk	Child protective services
	Intensive family preservation services
	Services for chronically neglectful families
	Domestic violence shelters and counseling
Families in which children cannot be protected within the home and needing restorative services	Diagnostic services
	Foster care and therapeutic foster care
	Group homes and therapeutic group homes
	Residential treatment centers
	Reunification services
Families who cannot be reunified	Adoption services

(Adapted from McCroskey, J., & Meezan, W. [1998]. Family-centered services: Approaches and effectiveness. *The Future of Children, 8*[1], 54–71.)

healthy lifelong patterns. Some preschool programs teach, as well as provide, good nutrition and encourage the kinds of eating patterns that prevent obesity and encourage the importance of a healthy breakfast and lunch. Weight control programs are available for overweight young children through health departments, community health centers, health maintenance organizations, and private groups.

Parents are becoming more aware of the need to reduce their consumption of saturated fat, salt, sugar, and overprocessed foods in order to feel better and look better and pass these beliefs along to their children. The community health nurse, through nutrition education and reinforcement of positive practices, plays a significant role in promoting the health of infants and young children (see Levels of Prevention).

PHYSICAL FITNESS PROGRAMS

The value of developing a lifetime pattern of exercise and physical fitness programs for children has been recognized for some time. Organized groups, such as the YMCA, YWCA, Boy and Girl Scouts, and Campfire Girls, have offered sports and character development programs for many years. Good day care and preschool programs provide equipment and opportunities for large-muscle activity as well as fine-motor development. Schools, parks, and recreation centers encourage exercise through use of playground

LEVELS OF PREVENTION

OBESITY IN YOUNG CHILDREN

PRIMARY PREVENTION

Foster good eating habits from infancy. Introduce foods according to health care provider's recommendations. Reserve empty calories for special occasions only. Reward good behavior with items/activities rather than food. Family dietary practices should model the recommendations in the Food Guide Pyramid (see Chapter 1). Encourage an active lifestyle with physical activity being a more important and time-consuming part of early childhood than TV and video games.

SECONDARY PREVENTION

Increase age-appropriate physical activity. Have fruits and vegetables available for snacks. Limit purchasing empty calorie foods. Don't focus on the child dieting; the entire family should eat appropriately. A child should not lose weight, especially if the increased weight is mild to moderate, but weight should stabilize as the child grows.

TERTIARY PREVENTION

Assist the family to recognize the need for the young child to lose weight. Have a physical examination by a health care provider before any major dietary changes. Initiate other actions according to those listed in primary and secondary prevention. If child is morbidly obese, additional medical intervention may be necessary, including psychiatric intervention.

equipment and organized sports activities. In addition, many programs are available for the very youngest children and their mothers, through "Mommy and Me" programs that offer simple play and exercises that mother and baby can participate in together and swimming classes for infants and toddlers where a parent accompanies the child. Despite these opportunities, many children do not exercise often enough or vigorously enough. Even team sports such as soccer and baseball that begin for children as young as age 4 or 5 keep players inactive much of the time and are not activities that most children continue in their adult lives. More comprehensive physical education programs that encourage and focus on vigorous individual exercise and self-discipline as lifetime habits would better serve the health needs of even the youngest in this population. Community health nurses can promote the development of and participation in such programs in their contacts with children of all ages.

PROGRAMS FOR CHILDREN WITH SPECIAL NEEDS

Many children have special needs. They may have been born with or acquired a developmental disability or may have an emotional, mental health, or physical chronic disease. Children as young as infants, toddlers, and preschoolers are diagnosed with asthma, diabetes, cerebral palsy, cystic fibrosis, muscular dystrophy, autism, ODD, ADHD, or ADD. Educational, health, and social or recreational services should be available for all children.

Public schools have been mandated by federal law since the 1970s to provide a full and equal educational program for all children, regardless of their ability level. Children as young as 3 months of age can receive infant stimulation services at home or in some schools especially designed to meet the needs of such young children. These programs are offered on a part-time basis for 1 to 2 hours, two to three times a week. By preschool age, they advance to half-day programs. Additional services are provided to assist the families in getting their children to the programs. Door-to-door bus service in specially equipped small buses or vans safely transports young children who arrive in school in wheelchairs or with other assistive devices.

Head Start programs serve 3- to 5-year-old children from low-income families to give them a "head start" on being successful in school. Head Start programs seek to prepare children for the challenges of a structured school environment.

Availability of health services for children with special needs vary with the size of the community. In small, rural communities, children and their parents may have long distances to go to receive the specialized services the child needs. In inner-city neighborhoods, a lack of finances for transportation to nearby services makes the services just as inaccessible. Accessibility is also influenced by lack of knowledge, attitudes, and prejudices. Community health nurses must recognize the power of these immobilizing factors and be able to deal with them effectively in order to make positive changes.

Most communities offer additional social and recreational programs for children with special needs. Children as young as age 3 to 4 can participate in special camping programs established by voluntary organizations that are usually "disease specific." For example, the American Lung Association affiliate offices sponsor camping programs for children with asthma or other lung diseases. Often, these are weeklong sleep-away camps for the school-aged child, but they also may be day camps with parents in attendance for the preschooler. Similar services are offered by other voluntary organizations.

Nationwide programs such as the Special Olympics offer recreational competition for children with special needs of all ages in a variety of sports, such as bowling, track and field events, skiing, and swimming.

The community health nurse best serves families as a resource for such programs. Some parents are not aware of the rights or services available to their children with special needs. Nurses can advocate for parents and help establish services in communities where the services are needed and are lacking.

ROLE OF THE COMMUNITY HEALTH NURSE

Community health nurses face the challenge of continually assessing each population's current health problems as well as determining available and needed services. Some gaps can be filled by nursing interventions. Others must be referred to various members of the community health team with whom the nurse may sometimes collaboratively develop services.

Community health nursing interventions with infant, toddler, and preschool populations are focused on education, engineering, and enforcement. The nurse uses educational interventions when teaching family planning, nutrition and exercise, safety precautions, or child care. Each of these involves providing information and encouraging client groups—parents and young children—to participate in their own health care. Engineering interventions are those strategies in which the nurse uses a greater degree of persuasion or positive manipulation, such as conducting voluntary immunization programs, encouraging enrolling in nutrition programs, preventing communicable diseases, or encouraging appropriate use of child safety devices, such as car seats. Finally, the nurse uses enforcement interventions in which the nurse must use coercion to make people comply with the law, such as requiring certain immunizations, reporting suspected child abuse, or reporting environmental health standards violations, such as sanitation issues.

The community health nurse acts as an advocate and a resource for families of young children. The nurse is aware of federal, state, and local laws that preserve and protect the rights of children. Availability of the educational, medical, social, and recreational services needed by young families is a necessity. The nurse helps to secure these services in the community she or he serves. Ensuring that families have the resources to provide for a safe and healthy environment for their children can take many forms, from lobbying to change existing laws, to initiating the effort needed to establish programs and services in the community, to teaching families infant safety or the importance of immunizations, during a home visit.

SUMMARY

Young children are an important population group to community health nurses because their physical and emotional health is vital to the future of society and because the very youngest are unable to help themselves.

Mortality rates for children in the United States have decreased dramatically since the early 1900s, but morbidity rates among young children remain high. Children are still vulnerable to many illnesses and injuries, often as a result of our complex and stressful environment. In many other countries, child health has improved. However, in countries with long histories of political unrest and a lack of natural resources, the welfare of young children still remains bleak.

Worldwide, toddlers and preschoolers are at risk for accidents (falls, drownings, burns, and poisonings); acute illnesses, particularly respiratory illnesses; and nutritional, dental, and emotional ailments. Violence against children and deaths due to homicide have an alarming occurrence in the United States. These problems create major challenges to the community health nurse who seeks to prevent illness and injury among children and promote their health.

Health services for children span three categories: preventive, health protecting, and health promoting. The community health nurse plays a vital role in each. Preventive services include quality child care, immunization programs, parental support services, and family planning programs. Health protection services include accident and injury control, programs to reduce environmental hazards, control of infectious diseases, services to protect children from child abuse, and fluoridation of community water supplies to protect children's dental health. Health promotion services include health outcome programs in early childhood development, nutrition and weight control, and exercise and physical fitness.

The role of community health nurses includes three basic interventions while serving young children's health needs. With educational interventions for the young child, such as nutrition teaching, nurses provide information and encourage parents to act responsibly on behalf of their children to assist in healthy habit formation for a lifetime. With engineering interventions, such as encouraging age-appropriate immunizations, nurses employ persuasive tactics to move clients toward more positive health behaviors. With enforcement interventions, such as reporting and intervening in child abuse, nurses practice some form of coercion to protect children from threats to their health.

ACTIVITIES TO PROMOTE CRITICAL THINKING

1. What is the major cause of death among infants, toddlers, and preschool-aged children? What community-wide interventions could be initiated to prevent these deaths? Select one intervention for each age group, and describe how you and a group of community health professionals might develop this preventive measure.
2. Describe one health promotion program you, as a community health nurse, could initiate and carry out to improve the health of children in a day care center or preschool program.
3. How can environmental health protection programs affect the future health of infants? Why is control of environmental hazards important for children of any age? List three things a nurse can do to protect children from environmental hazards.
4. A 1-year-old girl from a middle-class family and a 4-year-old girl from a poor family both come to the office you use when working with one preschool program in your community. The girls have similar symptoms that possibly indicate pediculosis capitis (head lice). Would your assessment and interventions be the same or different for the two girls? What are your values and attitudes toward people with "nuisance" diseases such as pediculosis capitis? Does social class, race, age, or sex make any difference in how you feel about them? What is one action the community health nurse can take to prevent such diseases in this population group?
5. Using the Internet, locate national websites that give you the current information about our progress toward meeting some of the *Healthy People 2010* goals with infants, toddlers, and preschool-aged children. Are we making progress? Will we meet the 2010 goal with these populations? If so or if not, what can a community health nurse do locally to promote the positive trend or turn around a negative trend in your community? What needs to be done on the regional, state, or national level?

REFERENCES

Aust, P. H. (1994). When the problem is not the problem: Understanding attention deficit disorder with and without hyperactivity. *Child Welfare, 73*(3), 215–227.

Browne, K. (1995). Preventing child maltreatment through community nursing. *Journal of Advanced Nursing, 21,* 57–63.

Bussing, R., Zima, B. T., Perwien, A. R., et al. (1998). Children in special education programs: Attention deficit hyperactivity disorder, use of services, and unmet needs. *American Journal of Public Health, 88*(6), 880–886.

Butz, A. M., Lears, M. K., O'Neil, S., & Lukk, P. (1998). Home intervention for in utero drug-exposed infants. *Public Health Nursing, 15*(5), 307–318.

Carabin, H., Gyorkos, T. W., Soto, J. C., et al. (1999). Estimation of direct and indirect costs because of common infections in toddlers attending day care centers. *Pediatrics, 103*(3), 556–564.

Centers for Disease Control and Prevention. (1996). Progress towards elimination of *Haemophilus influenzae* type b disease among infants and children—United States, 1987–1995. *Morbidity and Mortality Weekly Report, 45,* 901–906.

———. (1999a). General recommendations on immunizations: Recommendations of the Advisory Committee on Immunization Practices (ACIP), American Academy of Pediatrics and American Academy of Family Physicians. *Morbidity and Mortality Weekly Report, 49*(2), 35–38.

———. (1999b). *HIV/AIDS Surveillance Report,* Year end 1998, *10*(2).

———. (1999c). Notice to readers: National vaccination coverage levels among children aged 19 to 35 months—United States, 1998. *Morbidity and Mortality Weekly Report, 48*(32), 829–830.

Chernoff, R., Combs-Orme, T., Risley-Curtiss, C., & Heisler, A. (1994). Assessing the health status of children entering foster care. *Pediatrics, 93*(4), 594–601.

DeKlyen, M., Speltz, M., & Greenberg, M. (1998). Attachment of disruptive preschool boys to their fathers. *Clinical Child and Family Psychology Review, 1,* 3–21.

English, D. J. (1998). The extent and consequences of child maltreatment. *The Future of Children, 8*(1), 39–53.

Foley, H. A., Carlton, C. O., & Howell, R. J. (1996). The relationship of attention deficit hyperactivity disorder and conduct disorders to juvenile delinquency: Legal implications. *Bulletin of the American Academy of Psychiatry Law, 24,* 333–345.

Forshner, L., & Garza, A. (1999). Childhood vaccines: An update. *RN, 62*(4), 32–37.

Gormley, W. T. (1995). *Everybody's children: Child care as a public problem.* Washington, DC: The Brookings Institution.

Haack, M. R. (1997). *Drug dependent mothers and their children: Issues in public policy and public health.* New York: Springer.

Hatton, D. C. (1997). Managing health problems among homeless women with children in a transitional shelter. *Image: Journal of Nursing Scholarship, 29*(1), 33–37.

Helburn, S. W., & Howes, C. (1996). Child care cost and quality. *The Future of Children, 6*(2), 62–82.

Hernandez, D. J. (1995). Changing demographics: Past and future demands for early childhood programs. *The Future of Children, 5*(3), 145–160.

Howes, C., & Smith, E. W. (1995). Relations among child-care quality, teacher-behavior, children's play activities, emotional security, and cognitive activity in child care. *Early Childhood Research Quarterly, 10*(4), 381–404.

Karp, R. J. (Ed.). (1993). *Malnourished children in the United States: Caught in the cycle of poverty.* New York: Springer.

Kovner, A. R., & Jonas, S. (Eds.). (1999). *Jonas & Kovner's Health care delivery in the United States.* New York: Springer.

Larner, M. B., Stevenson, C. S., & Behrman, R. E. (1998, Spring). Protecting children from abuse and neglect: Analysis and recommendations. *The Future of Children, 8*(1), 4–22.

Manheimer, E., & Silbergeld, E. (1998). Critique of CDC's retreat from recommending universal lead screening. *Public Health Reports, 113,* 36–46.

Marks, M. G. (1998). *Broadribb's introductory pediatric nursing* (5th ed.). Philadelphia: Lippincott-Raven.

McCroskey, J., & Meezan, W. (1998). Family-centered services: Approaches and effectiveness. *The Future of Children, 8*(1), 54–71.

Montgomery, L. E., Kiely, J. L., & Pappas, G. (1996). The effects of poverty, race, and family structure on US children's health: Data from the NHIS, 1978 through 1980 and 1989 through 1991. *American Journal of Public Health, 86*(10), 1401–1405.

Moss, M. E., & Carver, K. (1998). The effect of WIC and Medicaid on infant mortality in the United States. *American Journal of Public Health, 88*(9), 1354–1361.

Olds, S. B., London, M. L., & Ladewig, P. A. W. (1999). *Maternal–newborn nursing: A family and community-based approach* (6th ed.). Upper Saddle River, NJ: Prentice Hall Health.

Pediatric AIDS. Available: http://www.caring4babieswithaids.org.

Reisine, S., & Douglass, J. M. (1998). Psychosocial and behavioral issues in early childhood caries. *Community Dentistry and Oral Epidemiology, 26*(Suppl.), 32–34.

Spector, R. E. (2000). *Cultural diversity in health & illness* (5th ed.). Upper Saddle River, NJ: Prentice-Hall Health.

Speltz, M. L., McClellan, J., DeKlyen, M., & Jones, K. (1999). Preschool boys with oppositional defiant disorder: Clinical presentation and diagnostic change. *Journal of the American Academy of Child and Adolescent Psychiatry, 38*(7), 838–845.

Stormschak, E., Speltz, M., DeKlyen, M., & Greenberg, M. (1997). Family interactions during clinical intake: A comparison of families containing normal or disruptive boys. *Journal of Abnormal Child Psychology, 25,* 345–357.

Tropiano, R. P., & Flegal, H. M. (1998). Overweight children and adolescents: Description, epidemiology, and demographics. *Pediatrics, 101,* 497–504.

U.S. Census Bureau (1999). *Statistical abstract of the United States, 1999* (119th ed.). Washington, DC: Author.

U.S. Department of Education. (1990). *America 2000: An education strategy sourcebook.* Washington, DC: Author.

U.S. Department of Health and Human Services. (1998). *Healthy people 2010 objectives: Draft for public comment.* Washington, DC: U.S. Government Printing Office.

———. (2000). *Healthy people 2010* (conference edition in two volumes). Washington, DC: U.S. Government Printing Office.

Valanis, B. (1999). *Epidemiology in health care* (3rd ed.). Stamford, CT: Appleton & Lange.

Walsh, K. M., Kelly, C. S., & Morrow, A. L. (1999). Head start: A setting for asthma outreach and prevention. *Family Community Health, 22*(1), 28–37.

World Health Organization. (1998). *The world health report, 1998: Life in the 21st century, a vision for all.* Geneva, Switzerland: Author.

SELECTED READINGS

Baker, A. J. L., Piotrkowski, C. S., & Brooks-Gunn, J. (1999). The home instruction program for preschool youngsters (HIPPY). *The Future of Children, 9*(1), 116–133.

Ball, J., & Bindler, R. (1999). *Pediatric nursing: Caring for children* (2nd ed.). Stamford, CT: Appleton & Lange.

Currie, J. M. (1997). Choosing among alternative programs for poor children. *The Future of Children, 7*(2), 113–131.

Duckitt, J., Wall, C., & Pokroy, B. (1999). Color bias and racial preference in white South African preschool children. *Journal of Genetic Psychology, 160*(2), 143.

Friedman, M. M. (1998). *Family nursing: Research, theory, and practice* (4th ed.). Stamford, CT: Appleton & Lange.

Gullotta, T. P. (Ed.). (1999). *Children's health care: Issues for 2000 and beyond.* Thousand Oaks, CA: Sage.

Hediger, M. L., Oberpeck, M. D., McGlynn, A., et al. (1999). Growth and fatness at three to six years of age of children born small- or large-for-gestational age. *Pediatrics, 104*(3)1–6. Available: http://www.pediatrics.org/cgi/content/full/104/3/e33.

Hott, J. R. (1998). Sexual awareness. In S. S. Gorin & J. Arnold (Eds.), *Health promotion handbook.* St. Louis: Mosby.

Kitzman, H., Olds, D. L., Henderson, C. R., et al. (1997). Effect of prenatal and infancy home visitation by nurses on pregnancy outcomes, childhood injuries, and repeated childbearing: A randomized controlled trial. *Journal of the American Medical Association, 278*(8), 644–652.

Mitchell, L. M. (1999). Reporting abuse and neglect of children with disabilities: Early childhood service providers' views. *Infants and Young Children, 11*(3), 19–26.

Nix, S. T., Ibanez, C. D., Strobino, B. A., & Williams, C. L. (1999). Developing a computer-assisted health knowledge quiz for preschool children. *Journal of School Health, 69*(1), 9.

Parnell, T. F., & Day, D. O. (1997). *Munchausen by proxy syndrome: Misunderstood child abuse.* Thousand Oaks, CA: Sage.

Silver, J., DiLorenzo. P., Zukoski, M., et al. (1999). Starting young: Improving the health and developmental outcomes of infants and toddlers in the child welfare system. *Child Welfare, 78*(1), 148–165.

Stein, R. E. K. (Ed.). (1997). *Health care for children: What's right, what's wrong, what's next.* New York: Springer.

CHAPTER

28

Promoting and Protecting the Health of School-Aged and Adolescent Populations

KEY TERMS

- Anorexia nervosa
- Attention deficit hyperactivity disorder (ADHD)
- Bulimia
- Learning disability
- Pediculosis
- School nurse
- School nurse practitioner
- School-based health center (SBHC)

LEARNING OBJECTIVES

Upon mastery of this chapter, you should be able to:

- Identify major health problems and concerns for school-aged and adolescent populations in the United States.
- Describe types of programs and services that promote health and prevent illness and injury of school-aged and adolescent populations.
- State the recommended immunization schedule for school-aged children and give the rationale for the timing of each immunization.
- Describe the three main functions of school nursing practice (health services, health education, and improvement of the school environment).
- Evaluate the potential benefits of school-based health centers, and discuss possible parental or community objections.

There are over 46 million school-aged children and adolescents in this country. Every school day, they attend over 100,000 schools. These children are the parents, workers, leaders, and decision-makers of tomorrow, and their future depends in good measure on their achieving their educational goals today (U.S. Department of Health and Human Services [USDHHS], 1995). Their successful schooling, in turn, depends on their health.

Think back to your own elementary and secondary schooling. Did you have access to a school nurse? If so, how did that person influence your health and the health of your peers? If not, how do you think a school nurse might have improved your school environment or experience? In this chapter, we explore the health needs of school children and adolescents. We then describe various services to address those needs, and describe the role of the school nurse as a key provider of these services. We hope this chapter will increase your understanding of the vital role of the school nurse in promoting the health of school-aged and adolescent populations. Perhaps it will also lead you to investigate a career in school nursing for yourself.

HEALTH PROBLEMS OF SCHOOL-AGED CHILDREN

The well-being of children has been a subject of great concern in this country for many years. International organizations, including the World Health Organization (WHO) and the United Nations Children's Fund (formerly, United Nations International Children's Education Fund [UNICEF]) as well as U.S. governmental organizations, nonprofit groups, and charitable foundations have focused their resources on improving the health and well-being of children, but the needs of millions of children worldwide continue to go unmet. Even in the wealthiest nations, many children face complex and often chronic health problems that cause them to miss school days or participate only marginally in the classroom. The chronic health problems of children under age 18 are ranked in Display 28–1; we will explore many of these here.

Problems Associated With Economic Status

The dramatic increase in single-parent (usually mother-only) families and economic trends that keep less well-educated populations from entering all but the most menial jobs combine to produce a powerful synergistic effect (Brooks-Gunn & Duncan, 1997). Poor children and adolescents are more likely to experience poor health, score lower on standardized tests, be held back a grade, drop out of school, have out-of-wedlock births, experience violent crime, and end up as poor adults (Lewit, Terman & Behrman, 1997). According to the Children's Defense Fund, low-income children are 2.7 times more likely to have stunted growth, 2 to 3 times more likely to have fatal accidental injuries, and 1.5 to 3 times more likely to die in childhood when compared to children in upper-income or never-poor families (Sherman, 1997). Noting that "everyone pays the costs of child poverty," the Chil-

dren's Defense Fund purports that schools, businesses, consumers, and society in general pay for poor children who must repeat a grade or require special education, and for the subsequently less educated and less productive workers whose lower productivity leads to higher prices and a greater tax burden (Sherman, 1997). It is clearly in society's best interest to care for its children.

Furthermore, the many needs of America's 14.5 million poor children are only part of the picture. There are millions more children in moderate-income families who have inadequate child care, limited health insurance, limited access to higher education, and poor housing. In fact, Vissing and Diament (1997) surveyed over 3,600 high school students in New Hampshire and Maine and found that between 5% and 10% had been homeless during the past year. Almost 20% lived in distressing situations and were at risk of being homeless. Currently, over 11 million children age 18 and under lack health insurance (U.S. Bureau of Census, 1997). This is the largest number ever reported, even though over 90% of uninsured children have one or more parents who work and more than 66% have family incomes above the poverty level.

There are specific physical health problems related to poverty (eg, lead poisoning, iron deficiency anemia, an increased susceptibility to illness). Many school-aged children suffer from the effects of poverty-related hunger. It is difficult to concentrate and to learn properly when meals are often skipped or when food is consistently less nutritious. Benjamin (1996) notes that children living in poverty demonstrate poor academic achievement, developmental and cognitive delays, and suffer from chronically poor nutrition. Even with programs like food stamps and Special Supplemental Food Program for Women, Infants, and Children (WIC), children go hungry because less than 64% of eligible families and about half of eligible women use these worthwhile services. Those children who participate in school lunch and breakfast programs suffer less of the side effects of hunger that affect their learning. However, only about 50% of schools participate in these programs (Food Research and Action Center, 1998).

DISPLAY 28–1. Chronic Health Problems of School-Aged Children and Adolescents

Chronic Conditions Under Age 18	Rank (by condition prevalence)
Hay fever or allergic rhinitis without asthma	1
Chronic sinusitis	2
Asthma	3
Chronic bronchitis	4
Dermatitis	5
Deformities/orthopedic impairments	6
Acne	7
Chronic disease of tonsils/adenoids	8
Heart disease	9
Deafness/hearing impairments/speech impairments	10

(From Collins, J. [1997]. *Prevalence of selected chronic conditions: United States, 1990–1992.* Washington, DC: National Center for Health Statistics.)

Accidents and Injuries

The loss of children's lives resulting from all injuries combined suggests a staggering number of years of productive life lost to society. Accidental trauma is the leading cause of death for children ages 5 to 14 years (Centers for Disease Control and Prevention [CDC], 1998a). Motor vehicle accidents lead all other types of accidental death for this age group.

Communicable Diseases

The mortality rates of school-aged children (5 to 14 years old) are low and decreasing; they have dropped from 4.0 per

1,000 in 1900 to less than 0.22 per 1,000 currently (CDC, 1998a). Again, this reduction can be credited to effective prevention and control of the acute infectious diseases of childhood.

Although mortality rates may be low, morbidity in schoolchildren is high. Children of this age group are most often affected by respiratory illness, followed by infectious and parasitic diseases, injuries, and digestive conditions. Among schoolchildren, the incidence of measles, rubella (German measles), pertussis (whooping cough), infectious parotitis (mumps), and varicella (chickenpox) has dropped considerably because of widespread immunization efforts. Yet, cases of communicable diseases still occur, some with potentially serious complications, such as birth defects from rubella and nerve deafness from mumps. Reported cases of pertussis have increased from 1980 to 1996 (U.S. Bureau of Census, 1998a). Vigorous campaigns have been undertaken by health departments to get children immunized. An immunization for mumps, measles, and rubella (MMR) has been available for over 20 years, and newer vaccines for *Haemophilus influenzae* type b (Hib) and varicella have been developed and are now part of the childhood immunization schedule. As increasing numbers of school-aged children must show proof of required vaccinations before entry to school, the numbers of children in this age group immunized against specific diseases will continue to rise.

Chronic Diseases

The numbers of school-aged children afflicted with chronic diseases are rising. Commonly seen problems include hay fever, sinusitis, dermatitis, tonsillitis, asthma, diabetes, seizure disorders, and hearing difficulties. Stomachaches, headaches, and colds and flu are frequent complaints of school-aged children.

Asthma is the most common chronic disease of childhood. It is estimated that over 5 million children under age 18 have asthma, with inner-city children suffering the highest asthma-associated hospitalizations and the highest prevalence rates ("Are State Health Departments Concerned With Asthma," 1998). Although reasons for the increased cases of asthma are somewhat unclear, experts speculate that better recognition and diagnosis of the disease, along with overcrowded conditions and exposure to allergens and irritants in the environment are probable culprits.

Children with asthma may have attacks triggered by exposure to cigarette smoke, stress, strenuous exercise, weather changes (eg, cold, windy, rainy weather), allergens, and air pollutants (indoor or outdoor). Commonly used medications include inhaled corticosteroids and chromolyn or sustained-release theophyllines (Skoner & Adelson, 1999).

Asthma may also result in mortality and growth retardation. Many children, especially the poor, have inadequate access to regular medical care. They may suffer from poorly controlled asthma and an ongoing inflammatory process that leads to permanent scarring and damage to their airway structures (Skoner & Adelson, 1999).

School nurses often work with students, their families, and the child's doctor to develop an asthma action plan to keep the child in good control and prevent or minimize untoward effects of acute asthma episodes. Peak flowmeters can be used frequently to determine early signs of asthma problems. Monitoring asthma medications and teaching the proper methods of using inhalers are also vital school nursing functions.

Diabetes is also a common chronic illness in children. Experts now conclude that both type 1 and type 2 diabetes mellitus are found in school-aged children. Type 2 diabetes is rising almost exponentially in this age group, largely due to obesity, sedentary lifestyle, and the predisposition of certain ethnic groups. Almost one third of new cases of diabetes in children under age 18 have type 2 diabetes (Kaplowitz, 1999). A recent study by Hale and Gomez (1999) on a middle-school–aged sample of Mexican-American youth found that 8% had impaired fasting glucose tests and 54% had a family history of diabetes. They also found a marked increase in obesity, insulin resistance, and hypertension in this sample.

Prevention of type 2 diabetes, through education and improvement in exercise, nutrition, and lifestyle, can be one of the most important areas of focus for health professionals working with the school-aged population. Diabetic children and adolescents may be reluctant to comply with medical regimens. Testing blood sugar and taking insulin at school can be frustrating and cause children to feel singled out. It is important for school nurses to understand each child's unique concerns and to alert teachers and school personnel to the signs and symptoms (as well as treatment) of hypoglycemia. Besides the obvious emergency, health-related concerns for diabetic children, studies have shown that diabetes-related severe hypoglycemia can affect memory tasks (Hershey, Bhargava, Sadler, White & Craft, 1999). Over a period of time, memory deficits can affect learning and progress in school.

Juvenile rheumatoid arthritis is an often painful immune disorder that is generally treated with nonsteroidal anti-inflammatory drugs and occasionally steroid injections (Cron, Sharma & Sherry, 1999). Exercise is often an important component of therapy, and an adapted physical education program may be developed.

Seizure disorders are not uncommon in the school-aged population. It is important to monitor medication compliance and teach school staff about first aid measures related to seizures. Treatment of epilepsy has been greatly enhanced by the use of newer antiepilepsy drugs (AEDs) specific to the pediatric population (Shields & Koh, 2000).

The second leading cause of death in the 5- to 14-year-old group is malignant neoplasms (CDC, 1998a). Childhood cancers (eg, leukemia) now have better outcomes than ever before. From 1960 to 1993, there has been a 60% to 70% decrease in all childhood cancer deaths in North America

(American Cancer Society, 1999). Many children return to school after initial hospitalization and treatment. School nurses can be helpful in making this transition by educating classmates about cancer facts (eg, it is not contagious) and by being vigilant in protecting any immunocompromised students from communicable diseases.

Behavioral Problems and Learning Disabilities

Other child health problems, less easy to detect and measure but often as debilitating, are those of emotional, behavioral, and intellectual development. Although these problems are not new, awareness and concern for them have increased as the rates of occurrence for other life-threatening childhood diseases (measles, mumps, rubella, and polio) have diminished. Emotional or behavior problems and learning disabilities are prevalent in childhood; it is estimated that between 2% and 15% of school-aged children have conduct or oppositional defiant disorders, 3% to 10% have attention deficit hyperactivity disorder (ADHD), 2.5% are mentally retarded, less than 1% have autism or cerebral palsy, and 2% to 10% have some type of **learning disability** (Kurtz, Dowrick, Levy & Batshaw, 1996). Children or adults with average or above-average intelligence who demonstrate significant difficulties in one or more areas of learning (eg, reading, writing, mathematics) may have a learning disability. Causes of learning disabilities and emotional behavioral problems appear to have genetic, environmental, and cultural influences. Increased use of illicit drugs by pregnant women is producing a generation of children with developmental delays and learning disabilities. Immature, stressed, and dysfunctional families have high incidence of child abuse (physical and sexual) and neglect. The numbers of children affected by parental drug use has surpassed childhood disabilities caused by lead poisoning, which has, itself, been a major contributor to developmental problems in children.

Behavioral and emotional problems of school-aged children may stem from many causes. About 26% of all children and adolescents under the age of 18 live with a divorced or separated parent or a stepparent (Behrman & Quinn, 1994). Research validates that, overall, children of divorce are more likely to exhibit conduct problems, have lower academic achievement and more symptoms of psychological maladjustment, and have more social problems and poorer self-concepts, as well as a lower standard of living, than children raised in intact families (Amato, 1994; Teachman & Paasch, 1994). Those children who are products of highly contentious divorces are most at risk (Johnston, 1994). The results of this maladjustment can also be found in later adult life (Amato, 1994). Community health nurses can be alert to early symptoms and refer parents to marital counseling or suggest family therapists.

Attention deficit hyperactivity disorder (ADHD) is a cluster of problems related to hyperactivity, impulsivity, and inattention (Display 28–2). It is estimated to affect 3% to 5%

of all school-aged children (Kwasman, Tinsley & Lepper, 1995) but is being diagnosed with increasing frequency. Interestingly, girls are at increased risk for not receiving appropriate services because they are not often recognized as having the condition. This may be because they often do not exhibit the hyperactivity component (Bussing, Zima, Perwien, Belin & Widawski, 1998).

There seem to be multiple reasons for ADHD, with research into inherited tendencies for decreased action of several neurotransmitters and decreased blood flow to prefrontal regions of the brain or generalized resistance to thyroid hormone supporting a neurobiologic basis for the condition (Aust, 1994). Although some health professionals believe that many of the symptoms found in people with ADHD are part of the spectrum of human behavior, others note that those people with ADHD have functional impairment in academic, social, or occupational areas resulting from their problem behaviors (Cara, 1999).

ADHD is sometimes found with associated disorders, such as communication or language disorders. It is estimated that close to 28% of children with ADHD have more than one co-existing condition. School-aged children with ADHD may also have learning disabilities (12%) and other problems such as poor social skills, aggression, depression (18%), anxiety (25%), oppositional defiant disorders (35%), and conduct disorders (26%; Cara, 1999; Hinshaw, 1994). They may also be more accident prone and have more school-related problems, such as grade retention and suspension or expulsion.

There is a need for collaboration between the child's family, the school, and the child's physician to diagnose ADHD and to plan appropriate interventions and educational accommodations (Wender, 1996). Teacher confirmation of ADHD-related behaviors is very important (Cara, 1999). Community health nurses and school nurses can assist parents in recognizing the symptoms of ADHD and obtaining appropriate treatment. A multimodal treatment approach is recognized as most effective. This includes medication, usually methylphenidate (Ritalin) or dextroamphetamine and amphetamine (Adderall); school accommodations for learning problems; and social skills training for the child with ADHD (Pelham, Aronoff & Midlam, 1999). Family and individual counseling, parent support groups and training in behavior management techniques, as well as family education about the condition, are also essential features of this method of treatment. Not all children and adolescents respond to medication, and medication dosage must be carefully monitored and titrated. The main goal of medication for school-aged children is academic improvement. If this does not occur, medication may need to be changed or discontinued. School nurses and community health nurses can work closely with school staff, parents, and physicians in determining the efficacy of treatment regimens.

Parents often voice concern about giving their child a stimulant medication to treat ADHD. Resistance to treatment may stem from fears about later abuse of substances. As adolescents, people with ADHD may begin experimenting with

DISPLAY 28–2. Attention-Deficit/Hyperactivity Disorder (*DSM-IV*)

A. Either 1 or 2:
  1. **6** (or more) of the following symptoms of **inattention** have persisted for at least 6 months to a degree that is maladaptive and inconsistent with developmental level:
    a. Often fails to give close attention to details or makes careless mistakes in schoolwork, work, or other activities
    b. Often has difficulty sustaining attention in tasks or play activities
    c. Often does not seem to listen when spoken to directly
    d. Often does not follow through on instructions and fails to finish schoolwork, chores, or duties in the workplace (not due to oppositional behavior or failure to understand instructions)
    e. Often has difficulty organizing tasks and activities
    f. Often avoids, dislikes, or is reluctant to engage in tasks that require sustained mental effort (eg, homework)
    g. Often loses things necessary for tasks or activities (eg, toys, books, tools)
    h. Is often easily distracted by extraneous stimuli
    i. Is often forgetful in daily activities
  2. **6** (or more) of the following symptoms of **hyperactivity-impulsivity** have persisted for at least 6 months to a degree that is maladaptive and inconsistent with developmental level:
    Hyperactivity
    a. Often fidgets with hands or feet or squirms in seat
    b. Often leaves seat in classroom or in other situations in which remaining seated is expected
    c. Often runs about or climbs excessively in situations in which it is inappropriate (in adolescents or adults, may be limited to subjective feelings of restlessness)
    d. Often has difficulty playing or engaging in leisure activities quietly
    Impulsivity
    a. Often blurts out answers before questions have been completed
    b. Often has difficulty waiting turns
    c. Often interrupts or intrudes on others (eg, butts into conversations or games)
B. Some hyperactive-impulsive or inattentive symptoms that caused impairment were present before age 7 years.
C. Some impairment from the symptoms is present in two or more settings (eg, school and home).
D. There must be clear evidence of clinically significant impairment in social, academic, or occupational functioning.
E. The symptoms do not occur exclusively during the course of a pervasive developmental disorder, schizophrenia, or other psychotic disorder and are not better accounted for by another mental disorder (eg, mood disorder).
  ■ Attention-Deficit/Hyperactivity Disorder, Combined Type
  ■ Attention-Deficit/Hyperactivity Disorder, Predominately Inattentive Type
  ■ Attention-Deficit/Hyperactivity Disorder, Predominately Hyperactive-Impulsive Type

(From American Psychiatric Association. [1994]. *Diagnostic and statistical manual of mental disorders* [4th ed.]. Washington, DC: Author.)

---

alcohol and other substances at an earlier age than non-ADHD teens; however, new research indicates that those treated with medication for ADHD in childhood are less likely to abuse substances later (Stocker, 1999).

Children with disabilities make up over 10% of the total school-aged population. In descending order, the most common disabilities include learning disorders, speech or language impairment, mental retardation, serious emotional disturbances and other disabilities such as autism, deaf-blindness, orthopedic problems, traumatic brain injury, and other health impairments such as asthma and epilepsy (Reschly, 1996). One study found that 5% of children under age 18 have two or more chronic conditions and less than 1% have three or more (Newacheck & Stoddard, 1994).

Many children with perceived disabilities or problems are referred for assessment and possible placement in special education programs each year. Teachers and other school personnel refer between 3% to 5% of the school-aged population each year, and 92% of children referred are tested, with 74% of those tested placed in special education (Hocutt, 1996). However, most children are given special services in a regular classroom through "full inclusion" or "mainstreaming," with fewer children being segregated into special classes or separate schools.

Head Lice

Pediculosis (head lice) is a frustrating and common problem for many school-aged children. It is estimated that close to 10 million people in this country get head lice every year; one in four elementary school-aged children had an occurrence in 1998 (Price, Burkhart, Burkhart & Islam, 1999). An infestation of *Pediculus humanus capitis,* the parasite that lives and feeds on the human scalp, can be an embarrassing nuisance to many families. These very tiny, wingless insects need blood to survive and can cause itching and skin irritation (Miller, 1999). They are most often found toward the nape of the neck where hair is generally the thickest, but their pearly white eggs (nits) are usually distributed all over the head. They are attached to the hair shaft with a gluelike substance and are easily detected with careful examination. Because nits open within 10 days and the immature louse can reach reproductive maturity within 8 to 9 days, recurring cycles of infection are common. To completely eradicate the problem, all nits must be removed along with lice.

Head lice are transmitted by direct contact or through shared items, such as combs and brushes, hats and scarves, as well as sheets and towels. Contrary to some popular myths, they do not fly or jump, and they cannot be contracted from animals (Price, Burkhart, Burkhart & Islam, 1999).

Many schools have recurring outbreaks of head lice that can be traced back to particular families who have had difficulty in successfully treating head lice cases and removing all nits. Some schools resort to "no nits" policies and establish routine head lice examinations with a goal of early detection and treatment.

Treatment of head lice commonly includes over-the-counter insecticide shampoos and rinses such as RID or Nix along with Kwell, a prescription shampoo (Price, Burkhart, Burkhart & Islam, 1999). School nurses also need to educate families about the need to reduce reinfestation by careful cleaning and treatment of any fomites (eg, combs, hats, towels, sheets, clothing) and scrupulous nit removal. In some larger cities, entrepreneurs have started nit removal businesses (eg, Nit Pickers) to assist parents with this tedious task.

Poor Nutrition and Dental Health

Other health problems found in this age group are nutritional problems (primarily overeating and inappropriate food choices) and poor dental health. Obesity often begins in childhood and becomes a risk factor for cardiovascular disease and diabetes. Of children ages 6 to 11, 11% are characterized as having excess body fat (defined as 25% or greater percent weight as fat for boys and 30% for girls). For 12 to 17 year olds, that percentage increases to 14% ("Guidelines for School Health Programs," 1997). Obese children are generally more likely to become obese adults. School children's diets are high in fat, saturated fat, and sodium ("Guidelines for School Health Programs," 1997). Results of a recent Youth Risk Behavior Survey indicate that 72% of those surveyed ate fewer than five servings of fruits and vegetables the day before (CDC, 1999c). An analysis of dietary sources of nutrients for children ages 2 to 18 revealed that foods such as milk, yeast bread, cake/cookies/doughnuts, beef, and cheese were among the top 10 sources of energy, protein, and fat (Subar, Krebs-Smith, Cook & Kahle, 1998). The poor eating habits that develop during childhood are generally thought to persist into

adulthood, contributing to the leading causes of death and disability—cardiovascular disease, cancer, and diabetes. In fact, evidence of early coronary atherosclerosis has been found in autopsy studies of children and adolescents (Harrell et al., 1998). Education and multicomponent school-based programs have been shown to be effective in changing children's food choices (Perry et al., 1998; Tershakovec et al., 1998).

Undernutrition can also have serious consequences, including lasting effects on the cognitive development and academic performance of children ("Guidelines for School Health Programs," 1997). Irritability, lack of energy, and difficulty concentrating are only part of the problem of skipped meals or consistently inadequate nutrition. Risk of infection and illness, leading to loss of school days, can affect academic progress and interfere with the acquisition of basic skills such as reading and mathematics. Undernutrition is frequently associated with poverty and hunger, but social pressure to be thin can also spark purposeful undernutrition. In an English study by Roberts, McGuiness, Bilton & Maxwell (1999), girls as young as 8 years old reported that they were actively dieting.

INACTIVITY

An association between poor eating habits and physical inactivity has been found in several studies of school-aged children and adolescents (Pate, Heath, Dowda & Trost, 1996). In a study of 2,200 third and fourth grade children, 33% of boys reported that they most often played video games when asked to report their leisure activities (Harrell, Gansky, Bradley & McMurray, 1997). Girls in the study most often reported homework as their most frequent activity (39%). Girls were generally more sedentary than boys, but both genders reported that watching television was a common activity (28% for boys, 30% for girls). The 1995 Youth Risk Behavior Survey revealed that 40% of those surveyed were not enrolled in physical education classes; of those who were enrolled, 75% admitted that they did not attend class daily (CDC, 1999c). Also, only 27% of time in these classes is typically spent in physical activity (Fleming, 1996).

Dental caries affect over half of school-aged children. School days are lost to dental problems and dental visits ("Guidelines for School Health Programs," 1997). Although there has been a downturn in the rate of dental caries in school-aged children over the past two decades (Brown, Wall & Lazar, 2000), the prevalence of dental caries remains high in this country and the cost for dental services in 2000 is estimated to be around $60 billion (CDC, 2000). The peak incidence of dental caries is found among school-aged children and adolescents, although the effects of decay can be felt throughout adulthood as various restorations fracture or wear out and must be replaced, or as caries activity recurs.

Dental trauma can occur in playground injuries, motor vehicle accidents, and during sports-related activities. In studies of emergency room visits for dental trauma (Lombardi, Sheller & Williams, 1998; Wilson, Smith, Preisch & Casamassimo, 1997), researchers found that 87% of primary tooth injuries were to maxillary incisors (front teeth) and that the most common injuries were lacerations (32%) and tooth fractures (33%).

Barriers to care are more prevalent among the poor and those who are institutionalized. Financial barriers and lack of education lead to poor dental health values and adversely affect use of dentists and conscientious personal oral health care. Lack of access to dental insurance or a local dentist can deter many people from caring for their oral health.

HEALTH PROBLEMS OF ADOLESCENTS

A growing number of youth suffer from spiritual poverty and disengagement from home and school. Plagued with boredom, low self-esteem, and lack of motivation, children in wealthy homes are often insulated from challenge and risk. Many of the same problems exist for children of the rich as for those of the poor, with a number of young people turning to drugs, alcohol, and indiscriminate sexual activity. School violence, an increasingly common phenomenon, is often carried out by "quiet loners" who attract little attention and feel socially and emotionally alienated (Gorski, 1999; Kachur et al., 1996). Clearly, there is a need for improvement in the nation's efforts to prepare young people adequately for the future.

Adolescents, during the period roughly encompassing the teen years, encounter many complex changes—physically, emotionally, cognitively, and socially. Rapid and major developmental adjustments create a variety of stresses, with concomitant problems, that have an impact on their health. Mortality and morbidity rates for adolescents are low overall and demonstrate considerable improvement over the early 1900s. However, the death rate for ages 15 to 24 years is 89.6 per 100,000 residents, which is much higher than the rate of 21.7 for 5- to 14-year-olds (National Center for Health Statistics [NCHS], 1998).

Unintentional injuries, homicide and legal intervention, and suicide are the top three causes of death in the 15- to 24-year-old age group (NCHS, 1998). Death rates from motor vehicle-related injuries for this age group peaked during the 1970s and 1980s, but have declined through the 1990s to a rate of 29.4 (NCHS, 1998). A gender difference is apparent, though, with the rate for males more than double that of females. Death rates from homicides have increased over the past three decades, to an overall rate of 20.3, with males thirty times more likely to die from homicides than females (NCHS, 1998). Death rates from firearm-related injuries have almost doubled since 1970 (NCHS, 1998).

Emotional Problems and Teenage Suicide

The adolescent years are a time of rapid growth and change. Hormonal influences can cause a teen to be emotional and, at times, unpredictable. Peer pressure becomes more important than parental concerns. Teens test family rules and generally search for their own identity and individuality apart from the family. Most parents and teens ride out this period with love and understanding and no long-term negative effects. However, for some teens, there is a real or perceived lack of emotional support, which can lead to temporary or permanent emotional problems.

Depression, anxiety, behavioral problems, or eating disorders may first appear during adolescence. Approximately 1 in 5 children and adolescents may have emotional, behavioral, or mental health problems, and at least 1 in 10 may have "a serious emotional disturbance that disrupts his or her ability to function" (USDHHS, 1996). Many adolescents are reluctant to seek help for emotional problems, or help may not be readily available to them.

Suicide is the third leading cause of death in 15- to 24-year-olds (CDC, 1998a). The death rate from suicide in this age range has shown a gradual increase, from 5.2 in 1960 to 15.2 in 1996 (NCHS, 1998). As youth move toward adulthood, they become more likely to take their life. Females generally attempt suicide more frequently than males, but male suicide rates are higher than female rates (Fleming, 1996). The suicide rate among American Indians is highest, and the rate among African Americans is lowest. Gay and lesbian youth are more likely to attempt suicide than heterosexual youth (Foote, 1997).

Although teachers come into contact with troubled youth on a more direct and daily basis, they do not always feel comfortable in assessing suicide risk. A recent study of high school health teachers found that only 1 in 10 thought that they could effectively recognize a student at risk for suicide, and less than half believed they would be effective at offering support or even asking for further information to determine suicide intent (King, Price, Telljohann & Wahl, 1999). Suicide prevention programs and direct interventions by counselors or schools nurses to determine an adolescent's suicide intentions are the most effective school-based approaches. Community health nurses and community mental health counselors may serve as consultants to schools in the development of sound prevention programs.

Violence

A study by the American Academy of Pediatrics (1999) found that over half a million children and adolescents under the age of 17 had emergency room visits for assault-related injuries in 1995. Children are assaulting and killing other children at school, as well as on the streets. Recent reminders include Columbine High School and other chilling incidents in middle schools and elementary schools across this country. A recent incident involved a child as young as 6 years old killing a classmate of the same age with a .32 caliber semiautomatic weapon brought from home ("List of Recent School Shootings," 2000).

Many parents are frightened and concerned about the issue of violence at school. In a *Los Angeles Times* poll, a majority of parents reported that they think, overall, California public schools are unsafe (53% to 44%), although 70% of parents of school-aged children said they still believe their children are safe at their own neighborhood schools—an interesting case of "it always happens to the other guy" (Helfand, 1999).

The U.S. Department of Education (1999) reports that school violence has actually declined from a rate of 155 school-related crimes per 1,000 students to 102 crimes per 1,000 over the 4-year period ending in 1997. However, the number of homicides involving multiple victims increased from one incident in 1994–1995 to a total of five in 1997–1998. Comprehensive school safety plans are advocated, and grants as well as technical assistance are available to local school districts through the federal government (U.S. Department of Education, 1998).

Cultural and environmental influences include the violence to which children and adolescents are exposed. Increased aggressive behavior among children and teens has been attributed to violence in the environment, violence in the home (spousal and child abuse), and what the child sees in the community, on television, and in the movies. Violence is an increasing threat for teenagers. According to recent research, the percentage of young adolescents who do not feel safe at school is increasing dramatically (Kandakai, Price, Telljohann & Wilson, 1999), and recent crime statistics lend credence to their fears. According to the most recent Youth Risk Behavior Survey, 20% of adolescents reported carrying a weapon to school during the past month, and 39% were in a physical fight in the last year (CDC, 1990). Schools have developed zero-tolerance policies to counteract and prevent violence (Weiler, Dorman & Pealer, 1999). Many schools now have metal detectors and security guards, and some schools conduct random searches of students' lockers in an effort to prevent violence. Physical fighting at school is more prevalent among ninth and tenth graders, and the number of females reporting that they were involved in a physical fight increased from 1993 to 1995, while the number for males decreased slightly, according to a recent study (Hill & Drolet, 1999). The researchers also noted that white teens were less likely to be involved in school violence than black, Hispanic, or Asian adolescents.

Violence (either homicide or suicide) accounts for 40% of all adolescent deaths (CDC, 1999a). Homicide is the second highest cause of death for the 15- to 24-year-old age group, with suicide the third. Homicide is the leading cause of death for African-American males. Adolescents between the ages of 12 and 24 comprise only 22% of the population, but they represent 35% of murder victims (U.S. Department of Justice, 1997). Almost 90% of 15- to 19-year-old homicide victims were killed with a firearm in 1994 (CDC, 1999b). One in four deaths among 15- to 19-year-olds is caused by a firearm, and the risk of death from firearm injury has jumped by 77% since 1985 (CDC, 1999a).

Substance Abuse

Substance abuse among young people was almost unknown before 1950 and rare before 1960. Now, adolescent drug ex-

perimentation and use pose serious physical and psychological threats. Almost 55% of high school seniors reported that they had used an illicit drug, and almost 82% had used alcohol (National Clearinghouse on Alcohol and Drug Information, 1997).

Using data from the Youth Risk Behavior Survey, researchers examined the age of initiation of substance abuse among high school students (Warren et al., 1997). The median age for first use of alcohol was 14 years. Students reported beginning to smoke cigarettes between the ages of 15 and 16 years. Overall, they noted that males initiated cigarette smoking and alcohol use earlier than females. However, by age 15, females accelerated their pace of behavior initiation so that the proportion of male and female risk behaviors was similar. Females appear to be initiating cigarette smoking and marijuana use at earlier ages, indicating a need for additional education and public health interventions. Marijuana use has fluctuated between 14% in 1979 to a low of 3% in 1992, with a surge upward again to 7% in 1996 (NCHS, 1998) (see Research: Bridge to Practice).

Inhalant abuse is another very real problem. Around 17% of adolescents report that they have sniffed inhalants (eg, glue, lighter fluid, spray paint) at least once, and over 5% of eighth graders reported sniffing within the past 30 days. The level of use is similar to stimulant use, and inhalant abuse can result in severe nervous system damage, according to the National Institute for Drug Abuse (National Clearinghouse on Alcohol and Drug Information, 1999b). Control of such legal products as spray paint, lighter fluid, and glue is difficult, making the scope of this problem almost impossible to adequately monitor.

RESEARCH Bridge to Practice

Neumark-Sztainer, D., Story, M., French, S., Cassuto, N., Jacobs, D., & Resick, M. (1996). Patterns of health-compromising behaviors among Minnesota adolescents: sociodemographic variations. *American Journal of Public Health, 86*(11), 1599–1606.

Unfortunately, adolescents who abuse substances are also more likely to engage in other health risk behaviors such as unprotected sexual intercourse, suicide attempts, and delinquent behaviors. A study comparing the prevalence rates of these behaviors among adolescents from different ethnic groups in Minnesota found very high prevalence rates consistent with other national studies. There was also a trend toward higher prevalence among older adolescents, and the greatest difference was found between sixth and ninth graders.

Girls more often reported unhealthy weight loss behaviors and suicidal attempts, and boys reported higher alcohol and marijuana use.

Variation between ethnic groups was noted, with very high rates of health risk behaviors found in American-Indian youth and a low prevalence of tobacco use among African-American youth. The strongest association noted in this study, among all ethnic groups, was between delinquency and substance abuse.

The illicit use of anabolic steroids is also difficult to monitor; however, over 325,000 teenage males and over 175,000 teenage females have reported taking them despite close to 70% of teens stating that they are fully aware of the dangers of steroid use (National Clearinghouse on Alcohol and Drug Information, 1999c).

Other drugs popular with adolescents and young adults include Ecstasy, a synthetic drug with amphetamine and hallucinogenic properties; Rohypnol, the "date rape" drug that is often mixed with alcohol to produce sedative hypnotic effects; and GHB, a drug touted as a synthetic steroid in fitness clubs and associated with sexual assaults across the country.

Since 1979, the percentage of 12 to 17 year olds reporting cocaine use has dropped from 1.5% to 0.6%. The National Institute of Drug Abuse reports that, whereas cocaine use seems to have leveled off, the use of marijuana, methamphetamine, and heroin is rising (National Clearinghouse on Alcohol and Drug Information, 1999a). Smoking or snorting heroin, popular among adolescents and young adults because they mistakenly believe it precludes the strong physical addictiveness of this drug, frequently leads to intravenous abuse. Methamphetamine may also be smoked, along with marijuana, but the most popular method of use is injection.

Teenage Pregnancy

Teenage pregnancies, sexually transmitted diseases (STDs), and human immunodeficiency virus/acquired immunodeficiency syndrome (HIV/AIDS) are public health concerns associated with the sexual activity of adolescents. The United States leads most developed nations in rates of teenage pregnancy, abortion, and childbearing. There was a 24% rise in teen births from 1986 to 1991. The trend over the past few years, though, has been a decline in the teen birth rate (US-DHHS, 1998b). Between 1991 and 1996, teen birth rates for all ethnic groups and in all states declined by 12%.

The fall in teen birth rates is encouraging because of the public health concerns related to teen pregnancy and birth. Young mothers are at high risk of bearing infants with low birth weight and are more likely to smoke. They are also less likely to receive adequate prenatal care or to gain the recommended weight during pregnancy (USDHHS, 1998b). They are also at risk for a greater number of physical, psychological, and social problems, including dropping out of high school, continued limited earning potential, social isolation, unstable relationships with child's father, and child abuse and neglect (NCHS, 1998). Those who choose to end their pregnancies with abortion may encounter other physical and psychosocial complications (see Research: Bridge to Practice).

Sexually Transmitted Diseases and HIV

About 12 million cases of STDs other than HIV are reported annually in the United States, and almost 66% of those cases

RESEARCH Bridge to Practice

Clifford, C., & Brykczynski, K. (1999). Giving voice to childbearing teens: Views on sexuality and the reality of being a young parent. *Journal of School Nursing, 15*(1), 4–15.

Teenage pregnancy has long been viewed as a moral problem, but, recently, the focus has shifted toward studying the underlying psychosocial aspects. Researchers have found that adolescent sexual experiences are often attempts at dealing with loneliness, bolstering self-esteem, confirming masculinity or feminity, and finding affection rather than satisfying libido.

A school nurse and a university professor used a qualitative research approach, interpretive phenomenology, to examine the "meanings embedded in situations" of the lived experiences of nine pregnant African-American students (ages 15 to 16) in a large urban high school in Texas. They conducted hour-long interviews over the period of a school year to gain a better understanding of the experience of development, sexuality, decision-making, relationships, and future hopes of the study participants.

They began by asking the girls about their experiences at menarche, how they felt about their first sexual experiences and their subsequent pregnancies and deliveries, as well as their relationships with their families and the fathers of their babies throughout their pregnancies and afterward. Several major themes emerged. Their first sexual experiences were frightening and uncomfortable; they viewed menarche as a rite of passage into adulthood and saw abortion as undesirable; they knew about birth control but did not conscientiously use it; and they were aware of the threat of sexually transmitted diseases but did not perceive STDs as an imminent threat.

The authors stated that early adolescents need to be aware of normal growth and development and recognize their own unique patterns as different from their peers. Parent support groups were also noted as helpful to mothers of young adolescents, as are counseling services for teens. Supervised after-school experiences—because most of the sexual encounters of teens in this study occurred between the hours of school dismissal and parents' return home from work—are essential. Case management for teen mothers to access medical care, housing, babysitting, and other services is also vital. When sexual choice is no longer based on submission or rebellion but on self-discovery and a planned future, we may begin to see real changes in the rate of teen births.

affected young people under the age of 25 (CDC, 1999e). These diseases include syphilis, gonorrhea, chlamydia, human papillomavirus, and herpes simplex virus. It is estimated that one in ten adolescent females is infected with chlamydia, and teenage girls ages 15 to 19 have the highest rates of gonorrhea. Syphilis rates are two times higher for adolescent females than adolescent males (CDC, 1997c).

Of the 33 million new cases of gonorrhea, chlamydia, syphilis, and trichomoniasis reported each year worldwide, over 3 million cases occur in the 13- to 19-year-old age range (CDC, 1998d). This is further global evidence of this public health concern. Serious complications from STDs include pelvic inflammatory disease (PID), sterility, an increased risk of cancers of the reproductive system, and blindness, mental illness, and death (with syphilis). There are also complications for unborn children of those infected with STDs (WebMD, 1999).

Even though death rates from HIV infection have dramatically fallen, new HIV infections reported annually do not reflect the same decline. New medications are thought to be the cause of the declining death rate (USDHHS, 1998a). However, as cohorts enter their late teens and early twenties, the rate of infection for HIV increases substantially (CDC, 1997b). In 1998, almost 1800 Americans 13 to 24 years old were reported to have AIDS. Most AIDS cases in males of this age group were among young men reporting sexual experiences with other men (50.1%), whereas the majority of cases in young females were reported to have been heterosexually related (47%). There is a much greater proportion of HIV than AIDS reported in this age group (CDC, 1999e).

Effective methods of preventing STDs and HIV/AIDS include decreasing sexual activity among adolescents, either by promoting abstinence or delaying sexual initiation, as well as by fostering safer sex messages, which promote the use of condoms (CDC, 1997b). Sex education has been shown to be effective at both delaying the onset of sexual activity and decreasing sexual activity in those adolescents who are already sexually active. It has also been shown to be effective in increasing safer sex practices, as has early mother–adolescent communication about condoms and sexually transmitted diseases (CDC, 1998c). There has been some indication that sexual activity among adolescents is reflecting more concern for risks. In a study examining HIV-related sexual risk behaviors among high school students in several large U.S. cities, there was a reported decrease in the proportion of sexually experienced students in most cities, a decrease in the numbers of students reporting four or more sex partners, and an increase in condom use (CDC, 1999d).

Acne

Acne is now recognized as a genetic disease; three out of four children of a mother or father who had acne as a teenager will usually follow in their footsteps (Fulton, 1999). Acne begins during puberty (10 to 12 years of age) with the increase in circulating male hormones that stimulate sebaceous glands in the skin. The excess sebum (oil) leads to irritation in the pores of sensitive adolescents and results in a buildup of cells leading to whiteheads. Open pores are known as blackheads. A red and inflamed pustule can develop or, in serious cases of acne, cysts or nodules can form. This can lead to pitting and scarring if not treated.

It is now known that greasy foods or chocolate do not cause acne but can contribute as aggravating factors (along with stress and certain cosmetics) in susceptible adolescents. Common treatment regimens include skin cleansers, peelers, and medication to decrease sebaceous gland activity. Benzoyl peroxide is used to kill the bacteria on the skin and in the pores. Retin A (a topical vitamin A ointment), glycolic acid, and alpha hydroxy acids help to peel the impacted cells from the pores. Accutane (isotretinoin) reduces the size and activity of sebaceous glands but can cause liver or kidney dysfunction. Because of an extremely high risk of birth defects, female adolescents taking Accutane are prescribed oral contraceptives (Fulton, 1999).

The best preventive measures include keeping the skin clean, eating a balanced diet that includes fresh fruits and vegetables, drinking lots of water, and getting adequate sleep. Adolescents with severe acne may need to be referred to dermatologists who specialize in this skin disorder.

Poor Nutrition and Eating Disorders

Poor nutrition and obesity are both common among adolescents, whose diets often consist of snacks with limited nutritional value interspersed among unhealthful meals. Adolescent females are more at risk for problems with nutrition for several reasons: they are known for more inappropriate dieting, have more finicky eating habits, and are less physically active than teen males. Adolescent males eat large quantities of food, which increases their chances for obtaining adequate nutrients, and they are also noted to be more physically active (CDC, 1999c).

Issues with body image and control are at the heart of anorexia nervosa and bulimia nervosa, common problems for adolescent girls.

Anorexia nervosa is an eating disorder of emotional etiology characterized by a body image disturbance (ie, seeing themselves as fat although they may be extremely thin), an intense fear of becoming fat or gaining weight, and a refusal to maintain an adequate body weight (ie, body mass index of 18 or above). **Bulimia** is an eating disorder characterized by recurrent episodes of binge eating with repeated compensatory mechanisms to prevent weight gain (eg, purging type—vomiting, or nonpurging type—fasting or exercise). These diseases have emotional etiologies that pose a complex challenge to treatment, which generally includes techniques such as nutrition education, psychological counseling and cognitive-behavioral techniques to control stimuli, substitute alternative behaviors, positive visualization, and a support network (Muscari, 1998). Self-concept is often distorted, and self-esteem is generally low; therefore, activities are initiated to improve the adolescents' feelings about themselves and to bolster their coping mechanisms (Pesa, 1999).

HEALTH SERVICES FOR SCHOOL-AGED CHILDREN AND ADOLESCENTS

A variety of programs directly or indirectly serve the health needs of school-aged children and adolescents. Community health nurses play a major and vital role in delivering these services. In community health, they fall into three categories approximating the three practice priorities of community health nursing practice: illness prevention, health protection, and health promotion.

Preventive Health Programs

IMMUNIZATIONS

Low immunization levels in many areas, particularly among the poor, and increased disease rates signal the need for constant surveillance, outreach programs, and educational efforts. Community health nurses are deeply involved in each of these preventive activities. Health departments and schools often work collaboratively to provide immunization services (see schedule in Chapter 27, Fig. 27–2). Compulsory immunization laws, varying from state to state, have enabled public health personnel to carry out these preventive services. Most adolescents are now required to be immunized against hepatitis B, and school nurses are working with community health nurses to provide immunization clinics at elementary and middle school sites to accomplish that goal by making them convenient to adolescents and their parents (Krahn, Guasparini, Sherman & Detsky, 1998). Researchers from the National Immunization Program at the CDC recommend that 11- to 12-year-old adolescents be scheduled for a routine visit to their physician so immunizations can be checked and updated. They recommend that a second dose of MMR be given (if not already done), along with a tetanus-diphtheria booster and the first dose of hepatitis B vaccine. Adolescents who have not had chickenpox and not received prior vaccination should be given the varicella virus vaccine. Influenza vaccine, pneumococcal polysaccharide vaccine, and hepatitis A vaccine should also be given to adolescents who have specific chronic health conditions or who routinely come in close contact with persons at risk from influenza or who are at risk of exposure to hepatitis A (Averhoff, Williams & Hadler, 1997).

In addition to immunizations required for school entry, many states or local school districts now require tuberculosis (TB) skin testing for school-aged children and adolescents. Close to 40% of TB cases in this country occur in foreign-born people, and children have a much higher risk of disease progression than adults (Steele, 1999). Children should be screened for TB if they meet the following criteria:

- Family history of infection (back two to three generations)
- Foreign birth, foreign travel, or contact with foreign visitor
- Contact with HIV-infected persons or inmates
- Foster children (due to poor history)
- Local epidemiology (health department recommendation)

EDUCATION AND SOCIAL SERVICES

Education of school-aged children and adolescents includes a wide variety of approaches and can range from the basics of handwashing for early elementary students (Early et al., 1998) to hearing conservation for high school students who like to listen to loud music (Lukes & Johnson, 1998).

Parental support services, available through many public and private agencies including churches, are also commonly found, and they can have long-range effects on school-aged children's health. Emotionally healthy parents and stable families offer a healthful environment and support system for children and facilitate their progress in school. In most states, community health nurses provide teaching and counseling services to parents in their homes and in groups. School nurses, school mental health counselors, and school psychologists also organize parent support groups in local schools. This is particularly important during periods of transition (eg, from elementary school to middle school and from middle school to high school). Discussing parenting concerns and increasing parents' understanding of normal child growth and development help to allay fears and prevent problems. Through such efforts, family violence and abuse can be averted. There is also research that indicates that by strengthening family resilience, alcohol and other drug use can be prevented or reduced (Johnson et al., 1998). Reduction in rates of divorce, and its attendant consequences, may also be a sequelae of strengthening family resilience.

Family planning programs, often stationed strategically in inner cities, near schools, and in school-based clinics, provide birth control information and counseling to young people. In some communities, the school-based clinic dispenses condoms. Community health nurses, in collaboration with an interdisciplinary team, are usually the primary care providers in these programs. Their major goals are to prevent teenage pregnancy, educate teenagers about reproduction and contraception, and encourage responsible sexual behavior.

Providing STD services and HIV/AIDS education can be a daunting task. Young people with STDs are often afraid or embarrassed to seek help. Others, exposed to the HIV virus, may not know they have been infected. Furthermore, community health professionals receive very little training in these areas and may be uncomfortable and judgmental in their approach. Quality services that are easily accessible, provide anonymity for clients, and are staffed with health care providers who exhibit nonjudgmental attitudes are better able to attract young people who need help.

Vulnerable groups, particularly minority youths, inner-city residents, and homosexuals, are being reached through STD clinics, HIV testing sites in clinics and health departments, family planning clinics, private health care providers, schools, and employers. Community health nurses, available in most of these settings, are generally the professionals who deal most directly with these clients (Lane et al., 1999). Improved public awareness and education, screening of high-risk groups, appropriate treatment of infected people, and identification and treatment of sexual contacts can reduce the threat of STDs.

Physicians are also concerned about the health risks common to adolescents. Pediatricians, especially, are instituting better history taking, more consistent monitoring, and anticipatory guidance for risks from unintentional and intentional injury, substance abuse, and sexually related risks (Jenkins & Saxena, 1995). Community health nurses need to work with local physicians and other community care providers to ensure that adequate education and social services are available to school-aged children and adolescents.

Educational efforts to prevent risk-taking behaviors that can lead to adverse health conditions have been shown to be effective. A preliminary examination of the effects of a school-based program to prevent pregnancy, HIV, and other STDs demonstrated that, after only 1 year, participants decreased unprotected sexual intercourse by one half, increased the use of condoms, and reduced the number of sexual partners (Coyle et al., 1999). A multilevel, multiyear, community-wide education program to prevent or reduce alcohol use among early adolescents was successful in delaying onset and in decreasing prevalence of alcohol use in program participants when compared with nonparticipants (Perry et al., 1996). Besides school-based education, peer leadership, parental education and involvement, and community-wide task forces were developed to lobby for local legislation and strengthen community–school ties.

Other social-influence–based intervention programs have been shown to be successful in reducing cigarette and alcohol use (Chou et al., 1998), and those with peer-led education were more effective than teacher-led, noninteractive programs in reducing alcohol, tobacco, and other drug use among adolescents (Black, Tobler & Sciacca, 1998). Enforcement of laws that restrict tobacco sales to minors is another very effective method of prevention and has been shown to reduce the rates of adolescent smoking (Gemson et al., 1998). Community health nurses often work in conjunction with law enforcement officials, school district administrators, and other community agencies to ensure compliance with local regulations and prevent or delay tobacco use (Forster et al., 1998).

Health Protection Programs

SAFETY AND INJURY PREVENTION

Accident and injury control programs serve a critical role in protecting the lives of school-aged children and adolescents. Efforts to prevent motor vehicle accidents, a major cause of death, include driver education programs, better highway construction, improved motor vehicle design and safety features, and continuing research into the causes of various types of crashes. Injury prevention and reduction have been addressed through strategies such as state laws requiring the use of safety restraints, driver and front passenger airbags, substituting other modes of travel (air, rail, or bus), lower speed limits, stricter enforcement of drunk driving laws, safer automobile design, and helmets for motorcyclists, bicycle riders, and skaters. Students Against Drunk Driving (SADD) and Friday Night Live activities can promote more

responsible driving habits among teens. Communities can also work with law enforcement to ensure compliance with mandatory seat belt laws and to promote safe speeds and appropriate driving behaviors around schools.

Child deaths and injuries from burns result primarily from house fires, but also from electrical burns, cigarette lighters, and scalds. Many local fire departments and public health programs offer safety education in this area, emphasizing the use of heat- and smoke-detecting systems, fire drills, and home evacuation plans; less flammable structural materials, furnishings, and clothing; and careful smoking or, better yet, no smoking.

Safety programs also seek to protect school-aged children from the hazards of poisonings, ingestion of prescription and over-the-counter drugs, product-related accidents (unsafe toys, bicycles, skateboards, skates, playground equipment, and furniture), and recreational accidents, including drownings and sports injuries. Safety services assume various forms. Poison control centers in many localities offer information and emergency assistance. Product safety is monitored by the Federal Consumer Product Safety Commission. Education programs in schools or through local fire or police departments teach school-aged children about bicycle and water safety, fire danger, and hazards related to poisoning.

Generally, the community health nurse can educate families to recognize potentially hazardous situations and encourage efforts to eliminate them. Working with school nurses and school district officials to reduce playground hazards can contribute to the reduction of school-related injuries.

Environmental hazards and other dangers await school-aged children and adolescents in the workforce. It is estimated that over 4 million children and adolescents are legally employed, with another 1 to 2 million employed illegally, and that over 64,000 annual emergency room visits by children and adolescents are work related (Landrigan & McCammon, 1997). Deaths due to exposure to toxic vapors, electrocution, and work-related motor vehicle accidents are not uncommon. Community health nurses can join with occupational health nurses and school nurses to teach parents and children about the dangers and risks inherent in the workplace, and they can work with local employers to ensure safer working conditions and more reasonable hours of employment that do not interfere with school.

INFECTIOUS DISEASES

Programs protecting school-aged children and adolescents against infectious diseases encompass efforts such as closing swimming pools with unsafe bacteria counts, conducting immunization campaigns in conjunction with influenza or measles outbreaks, and working with hospital pediatric units to reduce the incidence and threat of iatrogenic disease.

CHILD PROTECTIVE SERVICES

Services to protect children from abuse are generally not as well developed or effective as safety and injury protection programs. A variety of factors account for this. Most child abuse occurs in the home; thus, only the most blatant situations become evident to outsiders. Avoidance of legal involvement keeps others from reporting suspected cases. Fortunately, this attitude is changing among professionals who work with children and other community members. In some areas, community health nurses are working together with social workers, mental health workers, and substance abuse counselors as part of a team providing services to families. Improved training of mandated reporters, such as teachers and physicians, has led to better reporting of abuse. Today, professionals and the public are more aware of the problem, and there is an increase in reporting. In 1974, the National Center for Child Abuse and Neglect was established as a result of the Child Abuse Prevention and Treatment Act. The center collects and analyzes information on child abuse and neglect, serves as an information clearinghouse, publishes educational materials on the subject, offers technical assistance, and conducts research into the problem.

ORAL HYGIENE AND DENTAL CARE

School-based programs that provide fluoride rinses and promote toothbrushing, along with nutrition education to promote dental health, can be found across the country.

Fluoridation of community water supplies is promoted as the most effective, safe, and low-cost means of protecting children's dental health. Fluoride makes teeth less susceptible to decay by increasing resistance to the bacteria-produced acid in the mouth. Since 1945, public water supplies have been fluoridated, at an average cost of less than $1 per child per year (CDC, 1995b).

Some individuals and groups oppose fluoridation because of possible adverse effects (including fluorosis, which can cause mottling of tooth enamel). Research results have sometimes been mixed; however, most have supported the low risk of water fluoridation versus the benefits of decreased caries. For instance, a British study examined the risk of hip fracture in adults over the age of 50 who lived in areas with fluoridated water supplies; they found a very low risk of hip fracture with lifetime exposure to drinking water concentrations of fluoride at 1 ppm (Hillier, 2000). A study conducted in Finland sought to determine whether selected symptoms of fluorosis were related to actual exposure to fluoridated water (Lamberg, Hausen & Vartiainen, 1997). Although fluoridation of the community water system ended in November, respondents to a survey had similar rates of symptoms for both November and December (45%), and fewer reported symptoms in March (32%). Researchers concluded that fluoridation may have had some psychological effects that were perceived as symptoms of fluorosis. In the U.S., however, some researchers have concluded that because of children's potential for multiple exposure to fluoride through drinking water, processed foods and beverages, toothpaste, gels, and rinses, lower doses (or no) fluoride supplements are now required (Burt, 1999; Horowitz, 1999).

In addition to regular dental care, good nutrition, and proper oral hygiene, community health nurses can safely promote public water fluoridation as an important program for protecting children's dental health.

Dental researchers are continuing to work to fight dental caries by developing new products and methods. In addition to the now more commonly used protective sealants and advanced restorative treatments, new studies are examining the feasibility of laser light, polymeric coatings, and remineralization agents to strengthen and protect teeth (American Dental Association, 1996). Extending the natural protection of saliva, discovering foods that may have protective components to fight dental caries, and increasing tooth resistance by the use of more effective toothpastes and mouth rinses are also being studied. Perhaps the most promising areas, though, include the development of an antibacterial agent that interferes with plaque buildup, or a replacement therapy that trades acid-producing bacteria for harmless counterparts through the use of gene therapy, as well as the recently tested caries vaccine (American Dental Association, 1998).

SCHOOL HEALTH SCREENING PROGRAMS

Most local school districts provide some type of health screening services, usually through the school nurse or local health care providers. Common examples are routine vision screenings, done at periodic intervals, for early detection of vision problems, which can interfere with learning (eg, near- or farsightedness, strabismus, amblyopia). Lions Clubs may be involved in paying for local optometrists to assist in or direct these screenings.

Hearing screenings are also commonly done to detect any serious hearing deficits that may be related to recurrent ear infections or some type of sensorineural hearing loss. Height, weight, and sometimes cholesterol screenings are done on a regular basis to monitor normal growth and development, and allow for early intervention with populations who are especially susceptible to hypertension and heart disease.

In some areas, scoliosis screening is also done, frequently during middle school years, to permit early detection and referral for medical intervention (eg, bracing or surgery). Dental screenings or clinics may be conducted to determine the incidence of dental caries, especially in elementary school children, and to encourage followup with local dentists for necessary restorations.

The goal of all screening is to promote early intervention. Referral information is generally given to parents, and school nurses may contact parents to encourage follow through.

Children who are not present in school may not receive the benefits of these screenings, as well as the socialization experiences that are part of school attendance. A growing number of children in this country are being home-schooled by their parents, and are not present at school for most or all of the day. Approximately 1% to 2% of the total school-aged population is being home-schooled; the number of home-schooled children doubled or tripled over the 5-year period ending in 1996 (Lines, 1999). Montana and South Dakota report the largest percentage of home-schooled children (2.1%), and Arkansas, Georgia, North Carolina, and Maryland have the lowest (about 1.3%). Because many parents do not continue to home-school their children throughout their entire school-aged years, the total number of children having some home-schooling experience by age 18 may be closer to 6% to 12%. Parents may try home-schooling and find that it is very time consuming; consequently, their children generally return to public schools within about 2 years. At some point, those children will participate in health screenings. However, it may be necessary to work with those children and parents who do not, to better ensure their health.

Health Promotion Programs

NUTRITION AND EXERCISE PROGRAMS

Nutrition and weight control programs form another important set of health promotion services. Children need to learn sound dietary habits early in life to establish healthy lifelong patterns ("Guidelines for School Health Programs," 1997). Overweight acquired during childhood or adolescence may persist into adulthood and increase the risk for some chronic diseases later in life (NCHS, 1998). Some school programs teach, as well as provide, good nutrition and encourage the kinds of eating patterns that prevent obesity (Story & Neumark-Sztainer, 1996). A number of weight control programs for overweight children and adolescents are available through schools, health departments, community health centers, health maintenance organizations (HMOs), and private groups.

Adolescents are particularly vulnerable to media and peer pressures for nonnutritious snacks, including diet sodas, based on a desire to be accepted and to look trim. Fad diets can also be harmful if they are not nutritionally balanced. Programs aimed at more nutritionally sound advertising are having a positive effect. Parents and children are becoming more aware of the need to cut down their consumption of saturated fat, salt, sugar, and overprocessed foods in order to feel and look better. Acceptance of the U.S. Department of Agriculture's Food Guide Pyramid as a guide to daily food choices is an approach to sensible eating that assists people in limiting consumption of the foods shown to affect health negatively. The nurse, through nutrition education and reinforcement of positive practices, plays a significant role in promoting the health of children.

The value of exercise and physical fitness programs for young people has been recognized for some time. Organized groups, such as the YMCA, YWCA, Boy Scouts and Girl Scouts, as well as Campfire Girls, have offered sports and character development programs for many years. Schools, parks, and recreation centers encourage exercise through use of playground equipment and organized sports activities. Despite these opportunities, many young people do not exercise often enough or vigorously enough. Poor female children are the most sedentary, with poor males the most sedentary among male groups distinguished by income level (NCHS, 1998). Even team sports keep players inactive much of the time and are not activities that young people continue in their adult lives. More comprehensive physical education programs that encourage and focus on vigorous individual exercise and self-discipline as lifelong habits would better serve the health needs of this population group. Community health nurses can promote such programs through the schools as well as encourage these activities in their contacts with students of all ages.

EDUCATION TO PREVENT SUBSTANCE ABUSE

The demonstrated hazards of cigarette smoking, alcohol, use of inhalants, and drug abuse have prompted the development of substance abuse programs particularly targeting school-aged children and adolescents. Health education efforts involving school nurses, teachers, and counselors have been a major source of influence encouraging students to make responsible decisions about smoking, drinking, and other behaviors affecting their health (Black, Tobler & Sciacca, 1998; Chou et al., 1998; Perry et al., 1996).

Health departments, community health nursing agencies, and private groups such as the American Cancer Society and the National Lung Association also provide educational materials and promote antismoking and drug use prevention campaigns. The more successful programs emphasize how the human body works and how behaviors affect it. They also help young people resist social pressures to smoke and take drugs by pointing out that those who do are in the minority and by showing the deleterious effects of these practices. These groups can also work as advocates for changes in the schools that allow for broader health education (Smith, Zhang & Colwell, 1998). Using students themselves as health educators is a positive use of peer pressure and has proved to be a successful means of influencing attitudes (Black, Tobler & Sciacca, 1998).

Other groups, such as 4-H clubs, churches, the Catholic Youth Organization, and Scouts, use peer counseling to influence young people to assume responsibility for healthy lifestyles. Decision-making skills that lead to healthy lifestyle choices, enhanced in adolescence and remaining through adulthood, are the goals. The community health nurse participates in and supports existing programs in addition to counseling and referring young people who need help.

COUNSELING AND CRISIS INTERVENTION

Stress control programs for children and adolescents do not exist in any great number, yet they are very much needed. Many of the health problems discussed in this chapter relate to the emotional health of young people. Reckless driving, suicide, homicide, unplanned pregnancy, smoking, alcoholism, illicit drug use, obesity, anorexia nervosa, and bulimia, as well as other problems, all signal the presence of stress and the absence of coping skills sufficient to handle it.

Crisis intervention programs and services that treat a problem after it occurs are helpful and can prevent problems from worsening, but it is estimated that 17% of youth have unmet needs for mental health services (Bickham, Pizarro, Warner, Rosenthal & Weist, 1998).

More needed, however, for this population group are programs that build coping skills early, including conflict resolution, self-help, peer counseling, peer intervention, and mutual support activities. Support groups for children of divorce or children with chronic health problems (eg, asthma, diabetes), as well as groups to promote proper nutrition and weight management, and those focused on preventing teenage pregnancies have been instituted in diverse areas with varying degrees of success. Many of these activities are occurring in some of our nation's schools; however, they may often be discontinued when grant funding dries up or budget cuts must be made (Girard, 1995).

Programs offered in a group context have proved most effective. For the nurse, recognition of young people at risk, counseling, and early referral to sources of help can prevent crisis situations. Reduction of stresses in the family and community environments can further enhance this group's health.

School-Based Health Clinics

Because of the complex and intertwined emotional, physical, and educational needs of school-aged children and adolescents, a more comprehensive, interdisciplinary approach to services is needed than the piecemeal approaches that have been previously attempted. On a national level, experts are recognizing the link between learning and health and calling for an integrated, coordinated approach (Kolbe, 1994; Maix, Wooley & Northrop, 1998). The goal is to keep children and adolescents healthy and in school so they will have a greater chance of graduating and succeeding as citizens.

Adolescents are notorious for low utilization of health care services, lower rates of health insurance than other age groups, and engaging in high-risk behaviors (CDC, 1997a). With adolescents, emotional and physical problems are frequently entwined and can only be discerned by a well-trained, caring, and consistent practitioner. Also, by 2010 the cohort of school-aged children (ages 6 to 17) is expected to duplicate the baby-boom level of 1970, one of the largest groups ever (U.S. Bureau of Census, 1998b). In addition, more parents are working and less available to take care of their children's health care needs during the day. **School-based health centers (SBHC)** provide ready access to health care for large numbers of children and adolescents during school hours, making absences from school due to health care appointments unnecessary. SBHCs provide a variety of services in a user-friendly manner at a convenient location.

There are currently more than 1100 SBHCs in the United States, up from only 200 in 1990 (National Survey of School-Based Health Centers, 1997–1998). Some clinics provide services only to school children, whereas others extend services to the families of those children and other families in the neighborhood with preschool-aged children.

The most commonly reported diagnoses are mental health/substance abuse (eg, crisis intervention, counseling) and health supervision/acute disease (eg, immunizations, physical examinations, risk behavior screenings).

SBHCs are staffed by an interdisciplinary team of helping professionals, paraprofessionals, and staff. Many hospitals, HMOs, and health departments are sponsors of these school clinics because it is a cost-effective way to decrease emergency room visits and promote health, especially to underserved groups like adolescents (Kaplan, Calonge, Guernsey & Hanrahan, 1998). Third-party billing, especially to access Medicaid funding, is increasingly more common among SBHCs, and private foundations have also been instrumental in providing financial and technical support.

Evaluation research has demonstrated that SBHCs are effective in increasing student access to health care and improving student health knowledge (Kisker & Brown, 1996), improving rates of mental health, reducing substance abuse visits (Kaplan, Calonge, Guernsey & Hanrahan, 1998), and delaying sexual activity (Kirby et al., 1994).

ROLE OF THE SCHOOL NURSE

Historical Background

At the end of the last century, immigrants flooded the northeastern cities of the United States, and mandatory education was instituted. Poor, foreign-born children enrolled in schools, and as early as 1870 New York City was immunizing children in public schools (Lear, 1996). Sanitation and identification of sources of contagion were the focus, and many children were excluded from school with no follow-up. Some schools reported that 10% to 20% of their students were absent. Lillian Wald sent one of her Henry Street Settlement visiting nurses to four schools in New York City with high numbers of exclusions, and the numbers of absentee children dropped significantly within 1 year from 10,567 to 1,101 (Hawkins, Hayes & Corliss, 1994; Woodfill & Beyrer, 1991). Not only were medical inspections of school children conducted, but medical clinics also were established in schools. Home visiting and health education were also provided. Over the years school health services dwindled, and medical care was shifted to private practitioners, largely at the insistence of the American Medical Association. By the 1920s school health services consisted mainly of health education and minimal health services (eg, emergency care, periodic health assessments, documentation of state or district health requirement compliance). During the 1960s and 1970s, however, federal legislation providing Early Periodic Screening Diagnosis and Treatment (EPSDT) examinations for children and education for disabled students (Education for the Handicapped, Americans with Disabilities Act) expanded services to children and adolescents in public schools (Hawkins, Hayes & Corliss, 1994; Woodfill & Beyrer, 1991). During this time the first nurse practitioner programs began at the University of Colorado (Igoe, 1994). Nurse practitioners continue to work in conjunction with school nurses, especially in SBHCs. The school nurse role in these clinics is one of triage, referral, and follow-up—especially in the role of case manager for children and their families (National Association of School Nurses [NASN], 1996b).

School nurses began working in public schools at the turn of the 19th century, and they continue as a specialty branch of professional nursing that serves the school-aged population. It is estimated that there are over 40,000 nurses working in 82,000 public schools in the United States (Beverly Farquahr, Executive director of the National Association of School Nurses, personal communication, April 24, 1996). "School nursing delivers services to students of all ages from birth through age 21 and serves students, families, and the school community in regular education, in special education, and in other educational arenas" (Hass, 1993, p. 11). A school nurse, depending on the state of residence, can be a licensed practical nurse or a registered nurse (frequently with additional educational preparation beyond the bachelor's degree in nursing, including a master's degree) who has primary responsibility for the health care of school-aged children and school personnel in an educational setting. The National Association of School Nurses (NASN) is a professional organization of school nurses that has been incorporated since 1979. There are chapters in each state, and members meet nationally every summer to address the professional needs of school nurses. It is the position of NASN that school nurses, at minimum, possess a bachelor's degree (see Voices From the Community).

Responsibilities of the School Nurse

The primary responsibilities of the school nurse are to prevent illness and to promote and maintain the health of the school community (Display 28–3). The school nurse not only serves individuals, families, and groups within the context of school health, but also the school as an organization and its membership (students and staff) as aggregates.

The school nurse identifies health-related barriers to learning, serves as a health advocate for children and families, and promotes health while preventing illness and disability (NASN, 1996a). Further, the role of the school nurse includes that of care provider, change agent, teacher, manager, and educator. Health services include programs such as vision and hearing screening; scoliosis screening; monitoring of height, weight and blood pressure; oral health; tuberculosis screening; immunization monitoring; health examinations (especially for athletics or school entry); emergency care; and referrals (Lordi & Schneider, 1996). School health services also include health appraisal, health counseling, and services for school personnel to promote employee wellness.

Functions of School Nursing Practice

The three main functions of school nursing practice are health services, health education, and promotion of a healthy school environment (Hass, 1993). Health services have been

Voices From the Community

I have a new job that I love and that I have been shooting for since I graduated from nursing school. I now work for a school district as a school nurse. I have three year-round elementary schools in the central area of town, and it was exactly the assignment that I wanted because I wanted to expand my Spanish. It doesn't pay as much as I would get if I were still working at a hospital, but I have a life, good pay and benefits and, out of 365 days a year, I work 183 days. This job allows me to continue with other work interests and do the traveling and mission work I've always wanted to do. I do love working with kids. I feel like I'm able to make a positive impact on the kids' health and their future. I have to admit that the job is very different than I had expected. Some people, especially other nurses, think that school nurses aren't "real nurses." Boy, they could not be more wrong. In the hospital, you have all these backups. If someone stops breathing, you call the code blue team. If a patient has some family problems, you call the social worker. If a patient's symptoms are puzzling, you grab another nurse or the doctor. As a school nurse, you are the code blue team, the other nurse, the social worker, and often, although you are not the doctor, you become a diagnostician (enough so that you send people into the ER or the doctor's office). You go from putting Band-Aids on knees, to running out to the playground hoping the kid on the ground is breathing and hasn't broken his neck (oh, yes, we've been there, done that one). Then, there is the paper work. You know the wave that can roll over us? This is more like a tsunami. I manage the cases of 3,400 kids, give or take a hundred. They are actually being nice to the new school nurses. Most of us only have three schools. The more experienced nurses may have five or more schools. I have to admit, my boss is great to work for. She is very encouraging and gives us a lot of support, both in orientation and mentoring and kindness. It is a very challenging job, and I love it. I head back to school in the fall to get my school nurse certification, and am also working toward my nurse practitioner license.

Kate, new school nurse,
in a letter to a friend.

discussed above. The health education function of school nursing practice involves planned and incidental teaching of health concepts; curriculum development, which includes classes in health science and healthful living; and use of educational media, library resources, and community facilities. These activities aim to integrate health information with students' daily living experiences, to build positive attitudes toward health, and to establish sound health practices that will carry forward into adulthood.

The third function of school nursing practice is the promotion of healthful school living. Emphasis on a healthful physical environment includes proper selection, design, organization, operation, and maintenance of the physical plant. Consideration should be shown for areas such as adaptability to student needs; safety; visual, thermal, and acoustic factors; aesthetic values; sanitation; and safety of the school bus system and food services. Healthful school living also emphasizes planning a daily schedule that monitors healthful classroom experiences, extra class activities, school breakfasts and/or lunches, emotional climate, program of discipline, teaching methods, and reporting illegal drug use, suspected child abuse, or reporting violations of environmental health standards. It also seeks to promote the physical, mental, and emotional health of school personnel by being accessible as a resource to teachers and staff regarding their own health and safety.

DISPLAY 28–3. Professional School Nurse Roles and Responsibilities: Education, Certification, and Licensure

Functions: The practice of professional nursing by school nurses occurs within the complex and unpredictable setting of the school agency. The school nurse acts as a care provider, advocate, change agent, teacher, manager, and educator. The school nurse collaborates with other education and health care professionals to provide optimal school nursing care to the school community.

The functions of the specialized school nurse include, but are not limited to, the following:

1. Promotes and protects the optimal health status of children.
2. Provides health assessments.
   a. Obtains a health and developmental history.
   b. Screens and evaluates findings of deficit in vision, hearing, scoliosis, growth, and so forth.
   c. Observes the child for development and health patterns in making nursing assessment and nursing diagnosis.
   d. Identifies deviant health findings.
3. Develops and implements a health plan.
   a. Interprets the health status of pupils to parents and school personnel.
   b. Initiates referrals to parents, school personnel and community health resources for intervention, remediation, and follow-through.
   c. Provides ongoing health counseling with pupils, parents, school personnel, and health agencies.
   d. Recommends and helps to implement modification of school programs to meet students' health needs.
   e. Utilizes existing health resources to provide appropriate care of students.
4. Maintains, evaluates, and interprets cumulative health data to accommodate individual needs of students.
5. Participates as the health team specialist on the child education evaluation team to develop the Individual Education Plan (IEP).
6. Plans and implements school health management protocols for the child with special health needs, including the administration of medication.
7. Participates in home visits to assess the family's needs as related to the child's health.
8. Develops procedures and provides for crisis intervention for acute illness, injury, and emotional disturbances.
9. Promotes and assists in the control of communicable diseases through preventive immunization programs, early detection, surveillance, and reporting and followup of contagious diseases.
10. Recommends provisions for a school environment conducive to learning.
11. Provides health education.
    a. Participates in health education directly and indirectly for the improvement of health by teaching persons to become more assertive health consumers and to assume greater responsibility for their own health.
    b. Counsels with students concerning chronic health conditions, mental health issues, problems such as pregnancy, sexually transmitted diseases, and substance abuse, in order to facilitate responsible decision-making practices.
    c. Serves as a resource person to the classroom teacher and administrator in health instruction and as a member of the health curriculum development committees.
12. Coordinates school and community health activities and serves as a liaison person between the home, school, and community.
13. Acts as a resource person in promoting health careers.
14. Provides health counseling for staff.
15. Provides leadership and/or support for staff wellness programs.
16. Engages in research and evaluation of school health services to act as a change agent for school health programs and school nursing practices.
17. Assists in the formation of health policies, goals, and objectives for the school district.

(From National Association of School Nurses [1996a]. *Position statement. Professional school nurse roles and responsibilities: Education, certification, and licensure.* Scarborough, ME: Author.)

Liaison With the Interdisciplinary School Health Team

School health, like all health programs in the community, requires an interdisciplinary team effort (Lordi & Schneider, 1996; NASN, 1999). Although the school nurse plays a central role, collaboration with many other individuals is important. The coordinated school health program includes eight components and involves a variety of professionals and other people ranging from teachers, administrators, and school staff to families. The components are:

- School health services (preventive services, referral)
- Health education (K–12 curriculum)
- Health promotion for faculty and staff (employee health)
- Counseling, psychological and social services
- School nutrition services
- Physical education programs
- Healthy school environment
- Family and community involvement (partnership between school, families, community groups)

The school principal influences all phases of the school health program by promoting good school health through actively supporting all the school's health services, participating in the setting of policies, and tapping community resources. The principal can reinforce positive efforts within the school ranging from health teaching to cleaning activities of the custodian. Because of the principal's influential position, it is absolutely essential for the nurse and principal to maintain a positive and cooperative working relationship.

Teachers, whether they are involved in regular instruction, physical education, or special education classes, play a major role in school health. Because they spend so much time with students, their observations, health teaching, and personal health habits have a profound effect on student health and the quality of school health services. The school nurse and teachers must collaborate constantly.

Other health team members, such as health educators, health coordinators, psychologists, audiologists, speech therapists, occupational therapists, physical therapists, counselors, health care providers, dentists, dental hygienists, social workers, security personnel, health aides, and volunteers, may be present depending on the size and financial resources of the school. All team members, including students, parents, bus drivers, and custodians, have a specialized role complementary to that of the school nurse. Consultation and referral between team members are crucial to the successful implementation of the school health program.

If the school system desires the services, a physician may work part-time or be available on a consultation basis only. This role focuses largely on advising and consulting in policy and medical–legal matters. A community physician may serve on a school advisory panel and serve as a liaison with the community, other health agencies, and the school. The physician or a nurse practitioner may become involved in student health appraisal, rescreening, health problem intervention, sports physicals, or be in attendance at sporting events.

Special Training and Skills of the School Nurse

School nurses operate from one of two administrative bases, the school system or the health department. There is controversy over which system best serves the population's needs. In most localities, school nurses are hired through the public or private school system and maintain a specialized, school-based service. An advantage of this specialized school nurse's role is that the nurse can concentrate all the time and effort on the school health program and thus develop specialized skills in school health assessment and intervention. Today, with emphasis on delivering health care at community sites where clients spend most of their time (eg, schools for children, the workplace for adults), the nurse specializing in school health care seems better prepared to meet the complex needs of the school-aged population.

In contrast, the more generalized role of the community health nurse who operates under the board of health's jurisdiction provides services to schools as one part of generalized services provided to the community. The community health nurse working through the health department devotes only a portion of the workday in the school and has other responsibilities such as clinic nursing and making home visits. Many argue that such generalized school nurses are at a disadvantage with not enough time spent on meeting school health needs. The advantage is that this broader base allows contact with preschoolers and families, strengthened knowledge of the community and its resources, and integration of in-school and out-of-school care.

School nurse practitioners are registered nurses with advanced academic and clinical preparation (certification or a master's degree in nursing) with experience in physical assessment, diagnosis, and treatment, so that primary care can be provided to school-aged children. Many school districts see the advantage of having school nurse practitioners on staff rather than having the limited services of a physician. Assessments, diagnosis, treatment, and referral of injuries, communicable diseases, or other health problems can be managed more efficiently by a nurse practitioner who is educationally prepared to work holistically with the school-aged population and is part of the educational setting. If this is impractical, one school nurse practitioner available to school nurses for consultation or employed on a part-time basis can be the start of the development of more comprehensive school health services.

Some states are requiring even more specialized training for school nurses as the needs of school-aged populations become increasingly complex. In California, school nurses are expected to hold a school health services credential. This credential is obtained through a post-baccalaureate program that includes a minimum of 24 semester units of coursework in audiology, guidance and counseling, exceptional children, school health principles and practice, a practicum in school nursing, child psychology, and health curriculum development in addition to other courses.

As the population continues to become more diverse and the problems of children and families grow in complexity, the school nurse with specialized training in school health, the education system, case management, and advanced practice nursing (eg, nurse practitioner, clinical nurse specialist) becomes even more essential.

SUMMARY

Children and adolescents are important population groups to community health nurses because their physical and emotional health is vital to the future of society and because they are unable to help themselves without guidance and direction.

Mortality rates for children and adolescents have decreased dramatically since the early 1900s, but morbidity rates remain high. Children and adolescents are still vulnerable to many illnesses, injuries, and emotional problems, often as a result of our complex and stressful environment.

Violence against children and deaths due to homicide have an alarming rate of occurrence in the United States. Violent deaths, suicides, injuries, and HIV/AIDS are the leading threats to life and health for adolescents. Other health problems include alcohol and drug abuse, unplanned pregnancies, STDs, and poor nutrition. All these problems create major challenges to the community health nurse who seeks to prevent illness and injury among children and promote their health. Chronic illnesses such as asthma and diabetes are important to monitor. Commonly seen irritating problems, such as head lice and acne, can respond to treatment and education.

Health services for children and adolescents span three categories: preventive, health protection, and health promotion. The community health nurse plays a vital role in each. Preventive services include immunization programs, parental support services, family planning programs, services for those with STDs, and alcohol and drug abuse prevention programs. Health protection services include accident and injury control, programs to reduce environmental hazards, control of infectious diseases, and services to protect children and adolescents from child abuse and neglect. Health promotion services include programs in nutrition and weight control; exercise and physical fitness; smoking, alcohol, and drug abuse education; and stress control. School-based health centers provide a convenient place for the provision of primary health care as well as health education and mental health counseling.

The role of school nurses includes three basic interventions while serving children's and adolescent's health needs. With educational interventions, such as nutrition teaching, nurses provide information and encourage clients to act responsibly on behalf of their own health. With engineering interventions, such as encouraging use of contraceptives, nurses employ persuasive tactics to move clients toward more positive health behaviors. With enforcement interventions, such as reporting and intervening in child abuse, nurses practice some form of coercion to protect children from threats to their health.

Nursing of the school-aged population involves providing health services and health education and ensuring a healthful school environment. School nurses may provide these services as part of their role within a health department or be hired by the school district full time. The increasingly complex needs of the school-aged population and the collective accessibility to children in schools as a site to provide primary health care services are prompting schools to hire nurses with advanced preparation as nurse practitioners and credentialed school nurses to expand their services to this aggregate (see Clinical Corner).

ACTIVITIES TO PROMOTE CRITICAL THINKING

1. You are a community health nurse assigned to work at a school. You learn that over 20% of the students in this school district are being treated with Ritalin, Cylert, Adderall, or some other medication for attention deficit hyperactivity disorder (ADHD). What things should you consider in determining if these medications are being appropriately prescribed?

2. What is the major cause of death among school-aged children? What community-wide interventions could be initiated to prevent these deaths? Select one intervention, and describe how you and a group of community health professionals might develop this preventive measure.

3. A 14-year-old girl from a middle-class family and a 14-year-old girl from a poor family both come to the office where you work as a school nurse. The girls have similar symptoms that possibly indicate gonorrhea. Would your assessment and interventions be the same or different for the two girls? What are your values and attitudes toward people with diseases that are sexually transmitted? Does social class, race, age, or sex make any difference in how you feel about them? What is one action the community health nurse can take to prevent such diseases in this population group?

4. Discuss possible methods of doing nutritional assessments in school-aged children. What programs could be instituted to encourage healthier diets? What other factors might need to be considered? How could you, as a community health nurse, work with schools and parents to increase physical activity and improve nutrition for school-aged children and adolescents?

CLINICAL CORNER | Veronica Williams Gets Head Lice

Scenario

Your client is Veronica Williams, a 9-year-old girl with recurring episodes of pediculosis capitis (head lice). This is her fifth episode this school year. You are the school nurse for Brownsville Elementary School, where Veronica is in the fourth grade. You are responsible for coordination of health services for two elementary and one junior high school. You spend one day each week at Brownsville Elementary School.

You have gone into the classrooms and talked to the children about head lice prevention (not sharing combs, barrettes, hats, and so forth), but head lice continue to be a problem in the elementary schools. Protocol for head lice in Brownsville Elementary School includes prevention, treatment, and followup as follows:

1. At the beginning of each school year, head lice prevention packets of information are sent home to all families.
2. First episode—An informational notice is sent home.
3. Second episode—A personal notice is sent and a phone call to the parents is made.
4. Three or more episodes—The school nurse makes a home visit.

This procedure has been followed in Veronica's case.

Veronica lives with her mother, Ms. Williams, a 5-year-old brother, and 3-year-old sister in an apartment complex in Brownsville. Your health clerk spoke with Ms. Williams 3 months ago when Veronica experienced the second episode of head lice. She also lives near, and has personal knowledge of, the family. Based on information obtained from Veronica's teacher, you know that Veronica is a bright child who has frequent absences from class. She often comes to school with no lunch and wearing inappropriate cloth-

ing for the weather. She reportedly informed her teacher that her mother works "a lot" and that she does not know where her father is. She stated that she must stay home to care for her siblings when they are ill "since they can't go to day care and my mom has to go to work."

The school health clerk, who has information about this family based on her telephone call as well as second-hand knowledge of them as members of her neighborhood, informs you that Ms. Williams is a single mother. She tells you that she heard the father was addicted to heroin and that he left town shortly after the birth of the youngest child. Ms. Williams works two jobs to support her family—as a security guard for a local company during the daytime and three evenings a week in a convenience store.

Questions

1. Based on the above information, what are realistic goals for your initial home visit with Ms. Williams and her family?
2. What preparation might assist you in maximizing the effects of your home visit?
3. How will you work with this family to identify mutual goals?
4. What are your professional goals for this family based on the above information?
5. What issues does this situation elicit for you regarding:
    Fears and anxiety in dealing with this family?
    Knowledge of community resources available to this family?
    Social justice?
    Building partnerships with families, schools, and communities?

5. Describe possible benefits of school-based health centers (SBHCs). What are the most common misperceptions about them? What are common barriers to starting SBHCs? What steps can community health nurses take to promote community awareness and facilitate development of SBHCs in local schools?

6. A new elementary school to which you have been assigned has repeated outbreaks of head lice and very limited access to health care. Using the Internet, research causes for recurrent head lice infestations and effective over-the-counter treatments. Are head lice most often found seasonally? Discuss possible education programs you might implement or other innovative methods of treatment and control you might be able to institute.

REFERENCES

Amato, P. R. (1994). Life-span adjustment of children to their parents' divorce. *The Future of Children, 4*(1), 1 43–164.

American Academy of Pediatrics. (1999). New AAP policy addresses violence in children. Available: http://www.aap.org/advocacy/archives/janviol.htm.

American Cancer Society. (1999, January 8). Researchers say outlook good for childhood cancer patients. *ACS NewsToday*. Available: http://www.cancer.org.

American Dental Association. (1998). *Scientists develop vaccine against tooth decay*. Available: www.ada.org/prac/position/vaccine.html.

———. (1996). *Dental researchers developing new ways to fight tooth decay*. Available: www.ada.org/newsrel/9611/ur-05.html.

Are state health departments concerned with asthma? (1998). *BioMedicina, 1*(6), 205–206.

Armbruster, P., Gerstein, H., & Fallon, T. (1997). Bridging the gap between service need and service utilization: A school-based mental health program. *Community Mental Health Journal, 33,* 199–211.

Aust, P. H. (1994). When the problem is not the problem: Understanding attention deficit disorder with and without hyperactivity. *Child Welfare, 73*(3), 215–227.

Averhoff, F., Williams, W., & Hadler, S. (1997). Immunization of adolescents. *American Family Physician, 55*(1), 159–167.

Behrman, R. & Quinn, L. (1994). Children and divorce: Overview and analysis. *The Future of Children, 4*(1), 4–14.

Benjamin, R. (1996). The troubling verdict on poverty and health care in America. *National Forum, 76*(3), 39–42.

Bickham, N., Pizarro, J., Warner, B., Rosenthal, B., & Weist, M. (1998). Family involvement in expanded school mental health. *Journal of School Health, 68*(10), 425–428.

Black, D., Tobler, N., & Sciacca, J. (1998). Peer helping/involvement: An efficacious way to meet the challenge of reducing alcohol, tobacco, and other drug use among youth? *Journal of School Health, 68*(3), 87–93.

Brooks-Gunn, J., & Duncan, G. J. (1997). The effects of poverty on children. *The Future of Children, 7*(2), 55–71.

Brown, L., Wall, T., & Lazar, V. (2000). Trends in untreated caries in primary teeth of children 2 to 10 years old. *Journal of the American Dental Association, 131*(1), 93–100.

Burt, B. (1999). The case for eliminating the use of dietary fluoride supplements for young children. *Journal of Public Health Dentistry, 59*(4), 269–274.

Bussing, R., Zima, B. T., Perwien, A. R., Belin, T. R., & Widawski, M. (1998). Children in special education programs: Attention deficit hyperactivity disorder, use of services, and unmet needs. *American Journal of Public Health, 88*(6), 880–886.

Cara, J. (1999). Attention deficit/hyperactivity disorder: Guidelines and practice. Presented at the American Academy of Pediatrics Annual Meeting. Available: http://www.medscape.com/Medscape/CNO/1999/AAP/AAP-15.html.

Centers for Disease Control and Prevention. (2000). Improving oral health: Preventing unnecessary disease among all Americans. Available: http://www.cdc.gov/nccdphp/oh/ataglanc.htm#top.

———. (1999a). *Facts on adolescent injury.* National Center for Injury Prevention and Control. Washington, DC: Author.

———. (1999b). *Firearm injuries and fatalities.* National Center for Injury Prevention and Control. Washington, DC: Author.

———. (1999c). 1995 United States Youth Risk Behavior Data. Available: www.cdc.gov/needphp/dash/yrbs/index.htm

———. (1999d). Trends in HIV-related sexual risk behaviors among high school students: Selected U.S. cities, 1991–1997. *Journal of School Health, 69*(7), 255–257.

———. (1999e, August). *Young people at risk: HIV/AIDS among America's youth.* Washington, DC: Author.

———. (1998a). Deaths and death rates for the 10 leading causes of death in specified age groups, by race and sex: United States, 1996. *National Vital Statistics Report, 47*(9), 26.

———. (1998b, September). *National data on HIV prevalence among disadvantaged youth in the 1990s.* National Center for HIV, STD and TB Prevention. Washington, DC: Author.

———. (1998c, October). *Patterns of condom use among adolescents: The impact of mother–adolescent communication.* National Center for HIV, STD and TB Prevention. Washington, DC: Author.

———. (1998d, June). *Prevention and treatment of sexually transmitted diseases as an HIV prevention strategy.* National Center for HIV, STD and TB Prevention. Washington, DC: Author.

———. (1997a). *Access to health care, part 1: Children.* National Center for Health Statistics. Washington, DC: Author.

———. (1997b, January). *Comprehensive HIV prevention messages for young people.* National Center for HIV, STD and TB Prevention. Washington, DC: Author.

———. (1997c, November). *Sexually transmitted diseases.* Office of Women's Health. Washington, DC: Author.

———. (1995a, January 6). General recommendations on immunizations: Recommendations of the Advisory Committee on Immunization Practices (ACIP), American Academy of Pediatrics and American Academy of Family Physicians. U.S. Public Health Service. *Morbidity and Mortality Weekly Report, 44,* RR05,01.

———. (1995b, December 14). *Surgeon General's statement on community water fluoridation.* Washington, DC: Author.

Chou, C., Montgomery, S., Pentz, M., Rohrbach, L., Johnson, C., Flay, B. & MacKinnon, D. (1998). Effects of a community-based prevention program on decreasing drug use in high-risk adolescents. *American Journal of Public Health, 88*(6), 944–948.

Clifford, J., & Brykczynski, K. (1999). Giving voice to childbearing teens: Views on sexuality and the reality of being a young parent. *Journal of School Nursing, 15*(1), 4–15.

Coyle, K., Basen-Engquist, K., Kirby, D., Parcel, G., Banspach, S., Harrist, R., Baumler, E., & Weil, M. (1999). Short-term impact of safer choices: A multicomponent, school-based HIV, other STD, and pregnancy prevention program. *Journal of School Health, 69*(5), 181–188.

Cron, R., Sharma, S., & Sherry, D. (1999). Current treatment by United States and Canadian pediatric rheumatologists. *Journal of Rheumatology, 26*(9), 2036–2038.

Early, E., Battle, K., Cantwell, E., English, J., Lavin, J., & Larson, E. (1998). Effect of several interventions on the frequency of handwashing among elementary public school children. *American Journal of Infection Control, 26*(3), 263–269.

Fleming, M. (1996). *Healthy youth 2000: A mid-decade review.* Chicago, IL: American Medical Association.

Food Research and Action Center. (1998). *Fact sheet on hunger in the United States.* Washington, DC: Author.

Foote, J. (1997). Teenage suicide attempts. *Nursing Times, 93*(22), 46–48.

Forster, J., Murray, D., Wolfson, M., Blaine, T., Wagenaar, A., & Hennrikus, D. (1998). The effects of community policies to reduce youth access to tobacco. *American Journal of Public Health, 88*(6), 1193–1198.

Fulton, J. (1999). Prevention and treatment of teen acne. Available: http://my.webmd.com/content/article/l707.50068.

Gemson, D., Moats, H., Watkins, B., Ganz, M., Robinson, S., & Healton, E. (1998). Laying down the law: Reducing illegal tobacco sales to minors in central Harlem. *American Journal of Public Health, 88*(6), 936–939.

Girard, K. L. (1995, September). Preparing teachers for conflict resolution in the schools. *ERIC Digest, 94,* 4.

Gorski, E. (1999, April 22). Colorado school massacre: Schools have few resources for spotting troubled kids. *The Fresno Bee,* p. A1.

Guidelines for school health programs to promote lifelong healthy eating. (1997). *Journal of School Health, 67*(1), 9–26.

Hale, D. & Gomez, J. (1999). *Prevalence of glucose abnormalities in Mexican-American youth* [Abstract 0121]. 59th Annual Scientific Sessions of American Diabetic Association, San Diego, CA.

Harrell, J. S., Gansky, S. A., Bradley, C. B., & McMurray, R. G. (1997). Leisure time activities of elementary school children. *Nursing Research, 46*(5), 246–253.

Harrell, J. S., Gansky, S. A., McMurray, R. G., Bangdiwala, S. I., Frauman, A. C., & Bradley, C. B. (1998). School-based interventions improve heart health in children with multiple cardiovascular disease risk factors. *Pediatrics, 102*(2), 371–380.

Hass, M. B. (Ed.). (1993). *The school nurse's source book of individualized healthcare plans* (Vol. 1). North Branch, MN: Sunrise River Press.

Hawkins, J., Hayes, E., & Corliss, C. (1994). School nursing in America—1902 to 1994: A return to public health nursing. *Public Health Nursing, 11*(6), 416–425.

Helfand, D. (1999, June 17). Most parents say their local schools are safe. *Los Angeles Times* poll. Available: http://www.latimes.com/poll-99.

Hershey, T., Bhargava, N., Sadler, M., White, N., & Craft, S. (1999). *Diabetes Care, 22*(8), 1318–1324.

Hill, S. C., & Drolet, J. C. (1999). School-related violence among high school students in the United States, 1993–1995. *Journal of School Health, 69*(7), 264–272.

Hillier, S. (2000). Fluoride in drinking water and risk of hip fracture in the UK: A case-control study. *Lancet, 355*(9200), 265–269.

Hinshaw, S. P. (1994). *Attention deficits and hyperactivity in children.* Thousand Oaks, CA: Sage.

Hocutt, A.M. (1996). Effectiveness of special education: Is placement the critical factor? *The Future of Children, 6*(1), 77–102.

Horowitz, H. (1999). The role of dietary fluoride supplements in caries prevention. *Journal of Public Health Dentistry, 59*(4), 205–210.

Igoe, J. (1994). School nursing. *Nursing Clinics of North America, 29*(3), 443–420.

Jenkins, R., & Saxena, S. (1995). Keeping adolescents healthy. *Contemporary Pediatrics, 12*(6), 76–89.

Johnson, K., Bryant, D., Collins, D., Noe, T., Strader, T., & Bernbaum, M. (1998). Preventing and reducing alcohol and other drug use among high-risk youths by increasing family resilience. *Social Work, 43*(4), 297–308.

Johnston, J. R. (1994). High-conflict divorce. *The Future of Children, 4*(1), 165–182.

Kachur, S. P., Stennies, G. M., Powell, K. E., Modzeleski, W., Stephens, R., Murphy, R., Kresnow, M., Sleet, D., & Lowry, R. (1996). School-associated violent deaths in the United States, 1992 to 1994. *Journal of the American Medical Association, 275*(22), 1729–1733.

Kandakai, T., Price, J., Tolljohann, S., & Wilson, C. (1999). Mothers' perceptions of factors influencing violence in schools. *Journal of School Health, 69*(5), 189–195.

Kaplan, D., Calonge, N., Guernsey, B., & Hanrahan, M. (1998). Managed care and school-based health centers. *Archives of Pediatric and Adolescent Medicine, 152*, 25–33.

Kaplowitz, P. (1999). Type 2 diabetes in children: Concerns about a growing threat. Presented at the American Academy of Pediatrics Annual Meeting. Available: http://www.medscape.com/Medscape/CNO/1999AAP/AAP-11.html.

King, K. A., Price, J. H., Telljohann, S. K., & Wahl, J. (1999). High school health teachers' perceived self-efficacy in identifying students at risk for suicide. *Journal of School Health, 69*(5), 202–207.

Kirby, D., Short, L., Collins, J., Rugg, D., Kolbe, L., Howard, M., Miller, B., Sonenstein, F., & Zabin, L. (1994). School-based programs to reduce sexual risk behaviors: A review of effectiveness. *Public Health Reports, 109*, 339–360.

Kisker, E., & Brown, R. (1996). Do school-based health centers improve adolescents' access to health care, health status, and risk taking behavior? *Journal of Adolescent Health, 18*, 335–343.

Kolbe, L. (1994). Our children's future. *Healthcare Trends and Transitions, 6*(1), 14–17.

Krahn, M., Guasparini, R., Sherman, M., & Detsky, A. (1998). Costs and cost-effectiveness of a universal, school-based hepatitis B vaccination program. *American Journal of Public Health, 88*(11), 1638–1644.

Kurtz, L. A., Dowrick, P. W., Levy, S. E., & Batshaw, M. L. (Eds.). (1996). *Handbook of developmental disabilities: Resources for interdisciplinary care.* Gaithersburg, MD: Aspen.

Kwasman, A., Tinsley, B. J., & Lepper, H. S. (1995). Pediatricians' knowledge and attitudes concerning diagnosis and treatment of attention deficit and hyperactivity disorders: A national survey approach. *Archives of Pediatric and Adolescent Medicine, 149*, 1211–1216.

Lamberg, M., Hausen, H., & Vartiainen, T. (1997). Symptoms experienced during periods of actual and supposed water fluoridation. *Community Dentistry and Oral Epidemiology, 25*(4), 291–295.

Landrigan, P. & McCammon, J. (1997). Child labor: Still with us after all these years. *Public Health Reports, 112*, 446–473.

Lane, M., McCright, J., Garrett, K., Millstein, S., Bolan, G., & Ellen, J. (1999). Features of sexually transmitted disease services important to African American adolescents. *Archives of Pediatric and Adolescent Medicine, 153*(8), 829–833.

Lear, J. (1996). School-based services and adolescent health: Past, present and future. In L. Juszczak & M. Fisher (Eds.), *Adolescent medicine: Health care in schools* (pp. 163–180). Philadelphia: Hanley & Belfus.

Lewit, E. M., Terman, D. L., & Behrman, R. E. (1997). Children and poverty: Analysis and recommendations. *The Future of Children, 7*(2), 4–24.

Lines, P. (1999). *Home-schoolers: Estimating numbers and growth.* National Institute on Student Achievement, Curriculum, and Assessment. Washington, DC: US Department of Education.

List of recent U.S. school shootings (2000). *Yahoo-News.* Available: http://dailynews.yahoo.com/hlap/20000926/US/school_shootings_list.1.html.

Lombardi, S., Sheller, B., & Williams, B. (1998). Diagnosis and treatment of dental trauma in a children's hospital. *Pediatric Dentistry, 20*(2), 112–120.

Lordi, S., & Schneider, M. (1996). Roles and responsibilities of school nurses and physicians in adolescent school health programs. In L. Juszczak & M. Fisher (Eds.), *Adolescent medicine: Health care in schools* (pp. 273–286). Philadelphia: Hanley & Belfus.

Lukes, E., & Johnson, J. (1998). Hearing conservation: Community outreach program for high school students. *American Association of Occupational Health Nurses Journal, 46*(7), 340–343.

Maix, B., Wooley, S., & Northrop, D. (Eds.). (1998). *Health is academic: A guide to coordinated school health programs.* New York: Teachers College Press.

Miller, D. (1999). Dealing with a "lousy" situation. Available: http://my.webmd.com/content/dmk/dmk_article5962913.

Muscari, M. E. (1998). Walking a thin line: Managing care for adolescents with anorexia and bulimia. *Maternal Child Nursing, 23*(3), 130–141.

National Assembly on School-Based Health Care. (1998). *Census.* Washington, DC: Author.

National Association of School Nurses. (1999). *Coordinated school health program.* Scarborough, ME: Author.

———. (1996a). *Professional school nurse roles and responsibilities: Education, certification and licensure.* Scarborough, ME: Author.

———. (1996b). *School-based/school-liked health centers.* Scarborough, ME: Author.

National Center for Health Statistics. (1998). *Health, United States.* Washington, DC: Author.

National Clearinghouse on Alcohol and Drug Information. (1999a). *Heroin, marijuana, methamphetamine use on the rise.* NIDA/NIH Report. Rockville, MD: Author.

———. (1999b). Inhalants. *NIDA Notes, 13*(5).

———. (1999c). *Steroids (anabolic).* Publication #13557. Rockville, MD: Author.

———. (1997). *High school and youth trends: Monitoring the future study.* Publication #13565. Rockville, MD: Author.

National Clearinghouse on Child Abuse and Neglect Information. (1999). *Prevention fundamentals.* Washington, DC: Author.

———. (1997). *Child abuse and neglect national statistics.* Washington, DC: Author.

National Heart, Lung, and Blood Institute. (1994). *Strategy development workshop for public education on weight and obesity: Summary report.* Bethesda, MD: Author.

National Survey of School-Based Health Centers. (1997–1998). *Making the grade.* Washington, DC: The George Washington University.

Neumark-Sztainer, D., Story, M., French, S., Cassuto, N., Jacobs, D., & Resnick, M. (1996). Patterns of health-compromising behaviors among Minnesota adolescents: Sociodemographic variations. *American Journal of Public Health, 86*(11), 1599–1606.

Newacheck, P. W., & Stoddard, J. J. (1994). Prevalence and impact of multiple childhood chronic illnesses. *Journal of Pediatrics, 124*(1), 40–48.

Pate, R., Heath, G., Dowda, M., & Trost, S. (1996). Associations between physical activity and other health behaviors in a representative sample of US adolescents. *American Journal of Public Health, 86*(11), 1577–1581.

Pelham, W., Aronoff, H., & Midlam, J. (1999). A comparison of Ritalin and Adderall: Efficacy and time-course in children with attention-deficit hyperactivity disorder. *Pediatrics, 103*(4), 43.

Perry, C., Bishop, D., Taylor, G., Murray, D., Mays, R., Dudovitz, B., Smyth, M., & Story, M. (1998). Changing fruit and vegetable consumption among children: The 5-a-day power plus program in St. Paul, Minnesota. *American Journal of Public Health, 88*(4), 603–609.

Perry, C., Williams, C., Veblen-Mortenson, S., Toomey, T., Komro, K., Anstine, P., McGovern, P., Fiknnegan, J., Forster, J., Wagenaar, A., & Wolfson, M. (1996). Project Northland: Outcomes of a communitywide alcohol use prevention program during early adolescence. *American Journal of Public Health, 86*(7), 956–965.

Pesa, J. (1999). Psychosocial factors associated with dieting behaviors among female adolescents. *Journal of School Health, 69*(5), 196–201.

Price, J., Burkhart, C., Burkhart, C., & Islam, R. (1999). School nurses' perceptions of and experiences with head lice. *Journal of School Health, 69*(4), 153–158.

Reschly, D. (1996). Identification and assessment of students with disabilities. *The Future of Children, 6*(1), 40–53.

Roberts, S., McGuiness, P., Bilton, R., & Maxwell, S. (1999). Dieting behavior among 11–15 year-old girls in Merseyside and the Northwest of England. *Journal of Adolescent Health, 25*(1), 62–67.

Sherman, A. (1997). *Poverty matters: The cost of child poverty in America.* Washington, DC: Children's Defense Fund.

Shields, W., & Koh, S. (2000). The role of newer antiepileptic drugs in children with epilepsy. Neurology Treatment Updates. Available: http://www.medscape.com/medscape/neurology/TreatmentUpdate/2000/tu03/public/toc-tu03.html.

Skoner, D., & Adelson, J. (1999). New developments in corticosteroid therapy for children with asthma. Presented at the American Academy of Pediatrics Annual Meeting. Available: http://www.medscape.com/Medscape/CNO/1999/AAP/AAP-07.html.

Smith, D., Zhang, J., & Colwell, B. (1998). Roles of community organizations in improving cancer prevention instruction in schools. *Journal of Community Health Nursing, 23*(1), 45–57.

Steele, R. (1999). A new look at TB skin testing in children. Available: http://www.medscape.com/Medscape/cno/1999/AAP/AAP-05.html.

Stocker, S. (1999). Medications reduce incidence of substance abuse among ADHD patients. *NIDA Notes, 14*(4), 6–8.

Story, M., & Neumark-Sztainer, D. (1996). School-based nutrition education programs and services for adolescents. In L. Juszczak & M. Fisher (Eds.), *Adolescent medicine: Health care in schools* (pp. 287–302). Philadelphia: Hanley & Belfus.

Subar, A. F., Krebs-Smith, S. M., Cook, A., & Kahle, L. L. (1998). Dietary sources of nutrients among US children, 1989–1991. *Pediatrics, 102*(4), 913–923.

Teachman, J. D., & Paasch, K. M. (1994). Financial impact of divorce on children and their families. *The Future of Children, 4*(1), 63–83.

Tershakovec, A., Shannon, B., Achterberg, C., McKenzie, J., Martel, J., Smiciklas-Wright, H., Pammer, S., & Cortner, J. (1998). One-year follow-up of nutrition education for hypercholesterolemic children. *American Journal of Public Health, 88*(2), 258–261.

U.S. Bureau of Census. (1998a). *Acute conditions by type, 1980–1995.* Washington, DC: Author.

———. (1998b). *Current population reports.* Series P-25, No. 311, No. 519, No. 917, No. 1130. Washington, DC: Author.

———. (1997). *Current population survey.* Washington, DC: Author.

U.S. Department of Education. (1999). School violence continues to decline: Multiple homicides in schools rise. Available: http://www.ed.gov/PressReleases/10–1999/violence.html.

————. (1998). Annual report on school safety. Available: http://www.ed.gov/pubs/AnnSchoolRept98/exesum.html.

U.S. Department of Health and Human Services. (1998a, October 7). AIDS falls from top ten causes of death. *HHS News, 47*(4), 42.

————. (1998b, April 30). Teen birth rates down in all states. *HHS News.*

————. (1996). *Mental health, United States.* Center for Mental Health Services, Substance Abuse and Mental Health Services Administration. Washington, DC: Author.

————. (1995). *School health programs: An investment in our future.* Washington, DC: Author.

U.S. Department of Justice. (1997). *Special report: Age patterns of victims of serious violent crime.* Bureau of Justice Statistics. Washington, DC: Author.

Vissing, Y. M., & Diament, J. (1997). Housing distress among high school students. *Social Work, 42*(1), 31–41.

Warren, C., Kann, L., Small, M., Santelli, J., Collins, J., & Kolbe, L. (1997). Age of initiating selected health-risk behaviors among high school students in the United States. *Journal of Adolescent Health, 21*(4), 225–231.

WebMD. (1999). Sexually transmitted diseases. Available: http://my.webmd.com/content/dmk/dmk-article-6462879.

Weiler, R., Dorman, S., & Pealer, L. (1999). The Florida school violence policies and programs study. *Journal of School Health, 69*(7), 273–279.

Wender, E. (1996). Evaluation and management of learning difficulties. In L. Juszezak & M. Fisher (Eds.), *Adolescent medicine: Health care in schools* (pp. 239–247). Philadelphia: Hanley & Belfus.

Wilson, S., Smith, G., Preisch, J., & Casamassimo, P. (1997). Epidemiology of dental trauma treated in an urban pediatric emergency department. *Pediatric Emergency Care, 13*(1), 12–15.

Woodfill, M., & Beyrer, M. (1991). *The role of the nurse in the school setting: A historical perspective.* Kent, OH: American School Health Association.

SELECTED READINGS

Allen, K., Ball, J., & Helfer, B. (1998). Preventing and managing childhood emergencies in schools. *Journal of School Nursing, 14*(1), 20–24.

Altman, D., Levine, D., Coeytaux, R., Slade, J., & Jaffe, R. (1996). Tobacco promotion and susceptibility to tobacco use among adolescents aged 12 through 17 years in a nationally representative sample. *American Journal of Public Health, 86,* 1590–1593.

Armstrong, M., Ekmark, E., & Brooks, B. (1998). Adolescent body piercing. *The Prevention Researcher, 5*(3), 7–10.

Armstrong, M., & Pace Murphy, K. (1998). Adolescent tattooing. *The Prevention Researcher, 5*(3), 1–4.

Bachman, J., Johnston, L., & O'Malley, P. (1998). Marijuana use: Impacts of perceived risks and disapproval, 1976 through 1996. *American Journal of Public Health, 88,* 887–892.

Bainbridge, C., Klein, G., Neibart, S., Hassman, H., Ellis, K., Manring, D., Goodyear, R., Newman, J., Micik, S., Hoehler, F., & Walicke, P. (1998). Comparative study of the clinical effectiveness of a pyrethrin-based pediculicide with combing versus a permethrin-based pediculicide with combing. *Clinical Pediatrics, 37,* 17–22.

Brindis, C. (1997). Adolescent pregnancy prevention for Hispanic youth. *The Prevention Researcher, 4*(1), 8–10.

Copeland, L., Shope, J., & Waller, P. (1996). Factors in adolescent drinking/driving: Binge drinking, cigarette smoking, and gender. *Journal of School Health, 66*(7), 254–260.

Coyle, K., Kirby, D., Parcel, G., Basen-Engquist, K., Banspach, S., Rugg, D., & Weil, M. (1996). Safer choices: A multicomponent school-based HIV/STD and pregnancy prevention program for adolescents. *Journal of School Health, 66*(3), 89–94.

Cull, V. (1996). Exposure to violence and self-care practices of adolescents. *Family and Community Health, 19*(1), 31–41.

Driscoll, D., & Tronic, B. (1996). Images in clinical medicine: Pediculosis capitis. *New England Journal of Medicine, 336*(10), 790.

Dryfoos, J., Brindis, C., & Kaplan, D. (1996). Research and evaluation in school-based health care. In L. Juszczak & M. Fisher (Eds.), *Adolescent medicine: Health care in schools* (pp. 207–220). Philadelphia: Hanley & Belfus.

Foshee, V., Bauman, K., Arriaga, X., Helms, R., Koch, G., & Fletcher Linder, G. (1998). An evaluation of Safe Dates, an adolescent dating violence prevention program. *American Journal of Public Health, 88,* 45–50.

Friman, P., Hauwerk, M., Swerer, S., McGinnis, J., & Warzak, W. (1998). Do children with primary nocturnal enuresis have clinically significant behavior problems? *Archives of Pediatric and Adolescent Medicine, 152,* 537–539.

Goodson, P., Evans, A., & Edmundson, E. (1997). Female adolescents and onset of sexual intercourse: A theory-based review of research from 1984 to 1994. *Journal of Adolescent Health, 21,* 147–156.

Gould, J., Blackwell, T., Heilig, C., & Axley, M. (1998). Utility of percentage of births to teenagers as a surrogate for the teen birth rate. *American Journal of Public Health, 88,* 908–912.

Hu, T., Lin, Z., & Keeler, T. (1998). Teenage smoking, attempts to quit, and school performance. *American Journal of Public Health, 88,* 940–943.

Jenson, J., & Howard, M. (1998). Youth crime, public policy and practice in the juvenile justice system: Recent trends and needed reforms. *Social Work, 43*(4), 324–334.

Koh, H. (1997). Kids, cancer, and the Joe Camel connection. *Journal of Clinical Oncology, 15*(6), 2181–2182.

MacFarlane, R. (1997). Summary of adolescent pregnancy research: Implications for prevention. *The Prevention Researcher, 4*(1), 5–7.

Martin, A. (1998). On teenagers and tattoos. *The Prevention Researcher, 5*(3), 10–12.

McDermott, S., Scott, K., & Frintner, M. (1998). Accessibility of cigarettes to minors in suburban Cook County, Illinois. *Journal of Community Health, 23*(2), 153–159.

McKeown, R., Jackson, K., & Valois, R. (1998). The frequency and correlates of violent behaviors in a statewide sample of high school students. *Family and Community Health, 29*(4), 38–53.

Meijer, B., Branski, D., Knol, K., & Kerem, E. (1996). Cigarette smoking habits among schoolchildren. *Chest, 110*(4), 921–926.

Montealcgre, F. (1998). Do you know how asthma affects Hispanics? *BioMedicina, 1*(6), 197.

Montessoro, A., & Blixen, C. (1996). Public policy and adolescent pregnancy: A reexamination of the issues. *Nursing Outlook, 44,* 31–36.

Murphy, A., Youatt, J., Hoerr, S., Sawyer, C., & Andrews, S. (1995). Kindergarten students' food preferences are not consistent with their knowledge of the dietary guidelines. *Journal of the American Dietetic Association, 95,* 219–223.

Schachner, L. (1997). Treatment resistant head lice: Alternative therapeutic approaches. *Pediatric Dermatology, 14*(5), 409–410.

Schrier, L., Emans, S., Woods, E., & DuRant, R. (1996). The association of sexual risk behaviors and problem drug behaviors in high school students. *Journal of Adolescent Health, 20,* 377–383.

Schuster, M., Bell, R., & Kanouse, D. (1996). The sexual practices of adolescent virgins: Genital sexual activities of high school students who have never had vaginal intercourse. *American Journal of Public Health, 86,* 1570–1576.

Shearer, C. A. (1995). *Where the kids are: How to work with schools to create elementary school-based health centers.*

Washington, DC: National Health and Education Consortium.

Sonenstein, F., Ku, L., Duberstein Lindberg, L., Turner, C., & Pleck, J. (1998). Changes in sexual behavior and condom use among teenaged males: 1988 to 1995. *American Journal of Public Health, 88,* 956–959.

U.S. Department of Transportation. (1997). *Traffic safety facts. Alcohol.* National Highway Traffic Safety Administration. Washington, DC: Author.

———. (1997). *Traffic safety facts. Young drivers.* National Highway Traffic Safety Administration. Washington, DC: Author.

Weissbourd, R. (1996). The feel-good trap: Self-esteem movement in education. *The New Republic, 215*(8), 12–13.

Widom, C., & Kuhns, J. (1996). Childhood victimization and subsequent risk for promiscuity, prostitution, and teenage pregnancy: A prospective study. *American Journal of Public Health, 86,* 1607–1612.

Yawn, B., & Yawn, R. (1997). Adolescent pregnancy: A preventable consequence? *The Prevention Researcher, 4*(1), 1–4.

Promoting and Protecting the Health of Adults and the Working Population

KEY TERMS

- Adult
- Disabling injury
- Employee assistance program
- Ergonomics
- Life expectancy
- Occupational disease
- Occupational health
- Occupational health nurse
- Unintentional injury
- Unsafe condition

LEARNING OBJECTIVES

Upon mastery of this chapter, you should be able to:

- Identify key national and global demographic characteristics of adult men and women.
- Provide a health profile of adult men and women in the United States.
- Identify potential physical, chemical, biologic, ergonomic, and psychosocial stressors in a variety of work environments.
- Describe the history of state and federal legislation relative to occupational health.
- Discuss a variety of health problems related to occupation, including disorders related to ergonomics and workplace violence.
- Compare and contrast three main types of occupational health programs.
- Describe the role of the occupational health nurse and other members of the occupational health team in protecting and promoting workers' health and safety.

The term *adult* has many different meanings in our society. When we are children, an adult is anyone in authority, including a 14-year-old babysitter. As we age, we tend to redefine the term upward: It is not unusual, for example, to hear an elderly person describe a couple in their mid-thirties as "kids." Our criminal justice system distinguishes between adults and juveniles for purposes of delimiting both types of crimes and possibilities for punishment, and labor legislation provides different protections for children than for adult workers. Even hospitals and health care systems vary somewhat in the age at which they distinguish pediatric and geriatric clients from middle adults.

How would you characterize an adult? Does your definition rest solely on age, or is it influenced by other factors, such as marital status, employment status, financial independence, amount of responsibility for self and others, and so on? For the purposes of this chapter, we will define an **adult** as anyone between the ages of 18 and 64. Obviously, within this range are tremendous differences in health profiles and health care needs. We begin this chapter, therefore, with a discussion of the characteristics of adult clients.

This chapter also examines adult clients as workers. **Occupational health** is a specialty health practice that focuses on the health and well-being of the working population, including both paid and unpaid laborers, and thus covers most of the country's well adults. We will look at the environmental factors that affect workers' health, as well as the evolution of the role of occupational health nurse in meeting those needs.

ADULT CLIENTS

Young adults, whom we can describe as between the ages of 18 and 40, and middle adults, age 40 to 64, have characteristics, developmental tasks, and health problems different from those of adolescents or older adults. An awareness of the normal physical profile and developmental tasks of the adult helps the community health nurse assess for deviations from that norm. Similarly, an awareness of the health problems most common to this age group is essential for planning health promotion programs appropriate to this population.

Who Are Adult Clients?

Typically, adult clients have few interactions with health care providers in any given year. It is often assumed that this age range is not necessarily associated with physical or psychological disease. Single mental conditions or disease are not related to the passage of time. However, the adult should be assessed for signs of illness.

There are several normal physical changes associated with this age group. Because different body parts age at varying rates, a physical profile of middle-aged adults is organized by body system (Display 29–1).

DEMOGRAPHICS

It is difficult to identify the transition from wellness to poor health. Therefore, mortality statistics are considered the most reliable indicator of the health status of a population. In addition, they can be used to calculate other important measures such as life expectancy.

According to the National Center for Health Statistics (1997), in 1996 there were 529,300 registered deaths for adults in the United States. The mortality rate for that year was 177.8 per 100,000 for 25- to 44-year-old adults and 708.0 per 100,000 for adults in the 45- to 65-year-old range. Causes of death vary by age. The leading causes presented in this chapter reflect the adult population (Table 29–1).

The 20th century has seen a shift in the mortality statistics. At the turn of the century, communicable diseases such as tuberculosis and pneumonia were the leading causes of death. However, the impact of significant advances in biomedical research and public health is such that noncommunicable diseases are now the leading causes of death. At present, 70% of all deaths in the United States are attributed to heart disease, cancer, cerebrovascular disease, and unintentional injuries (Table 29–1).

LIFE EXPECTANCY

Life expectancy is another standard measurement that is used to compare the health status of various populations. **Life expectancy** is defined as the average number of years that an individual member of a specific cohort (usually of a single

DISPLAY 29–1. Physical Profile of Middle-Aged Adults by Body System

Body System	Physical Characteristic
Skeletal system	Intervertebral disks flatten over time
Integumentary system	Decreased secretions by sebaceous glands leads to drier skin
	Sweat glands diminish in size and number
	Skin loses elasticity and is more prone to wrinkles
	Hair bulbs lose melanin usually resulting in gray hair by age 50
Muscular system	Muscle fibers decrease by approximately 10%
	Lean body mass is replaced by adipose tissue
	Decreased grip strength occurs at this age
Endocrine and reproductive system	Menses stops
	Synthesis of estrogen decreases
	Tissues of the reproductive system (eg, cervix and uterus) gradually atrophy
	Uterine changes make pregnancy less likely
	Intercourse may be more painful due to diminishing natural lubrications
Neurologic system	Nerve impulses are conducted 5% slower
	Cognition is unaffected, although there is a gradual loss of neurons
	Eyesight is poorer due to loss of elasticity in the lens
	Auditory discrimination of certain tones and consonants gradually decreases
Cardiovascular system	By age 50, the heart's efficiency may be only 80%
	Elasticity of heart and blood vessels decreases
	Cardiac output decreases
Respiratory system	Elasticity of lungs decreases
	Breathing capacity decreases to 75% due to diminished strength of chest wall muscles
Urinary system	Decreased glomerular filtration rate appears in women
	Loss of bladder tone and tissue atrophy may lead to incontinence or possibly prolapse
	In men, an enlarged prostate may result in nocturia or dribbling

TABLE 29-1. Deaths and Rates for the 10 Leading Causes of Death for 25 to 44 and 45 to 64 Year Olds: United States, 1996

Cause of Death	Number	Rate (per 100,000)
25 TO 44 YEAR OLDS		
All causes	148,904	177.8
Accident and adverse effects	26,554	31.7
Motor vehicle accidents	14,528	17.3
All other accidents	12,026	14.4
HIV infection	22,795	27.2
Malignant neoplasms (cancer)	22,147	26.4
Diseases of the heart	16,261	19.4
Suicide	12,536	15.0
Homicide and legal intervention	9,261	11.1
Chronic liver disease/cirrhosis	4,230	5.1
Cerebrovascular diseases	3,418	4.1
Diabetes mellitus	2,520	3.0
Pneumonia and influenza	1,972	2.4
All other causes	27,210	32.5
45 TO 65 YEAR OLDS		
All causes	380,396	708.0
Malignant neoplasms (cancer)	132,805	247.2
Diseases of the heart	102,510	190.8
Accidents and adverse effects	16,332	30.4
Motor vehicle accidents	7,659	14.3
All other accidents	8,673	16.1
Cerebrovascular diseases	15,526	28.9
Chronic obstructive pulmonary diseases	12,849	23.9
Diabetes mellitus	12,678	23.6
Chronic liver disease/cirrhosis	10,718	19.9
HIV infection	8,443	15.7
Suicide	7,717	14.4
Pneumonia and influenza	5,646	10.5
All other causes	55,172	102.7

(From Ventura, S. J., Peters, K. D., Martin, J. A. & Maurer, J. D. [1997]. Annual summary of births, marriages, divorces, and deaths: United States, 1996. *Monthly Vital Statistics Reports, 46* [1, Supp. 2], p. 33.)

birth year) is projected to live. Health statistics generally report life expectancy figures for birth and 65 years of age (Table 29–2). In the United States, life expectancy has increased consistently over time. When compared with other countries, the United States compares favorably with the exception of countries with upper-middle income and high income economies (Table 29–3). Japan reports the highest life expectancy figures whereas countries with poorly developed economies have the lowest life expectancy predictions.

Developmental Tasks of Adult Clients

Developmental tasks vary depending on the age of the adult. The developmental stages and corresponding tasks are incremental. A young adult enters the stage of "becoming adult" between the ages of 23 and 28. Associated tasks include starting their career, becoming a parent, and becoming a homeowner. Between the ages of 29 and 34, adults reassess relationships and develop better problem-solving skills. These attributes contribute to the likelihood that, in this stage, greater career success can be achieved.

The term of "midlife" is applied to the age of 35 to 43 years. Developmental tasks focus on reappraisal of values, priorities, and personal relationships, especially marriage. In addition, they may be faced with issues related to aging parents and teenagers. As the term "midlife crisis" implies, this is one of the more difficult stages and tends to challenge adult ability to problem solve. Successful navigation of this stage can be very fulfilling but may require enhanced coping skills.

The developmental stage between 44 and 55 years of age can be considered as "rehabilitation." Most adults will face issues of parents that demand more attention both physically and economically because extended care needs may arise. Simultaneously, these adults are faced with the economic crunch of putting their children through college. Meanwhile, they are adjusting to the reality that their career path is now set.

TABLE 29-2. Life Expectancy at Birth and 65 Years of Age According to Sex: United States, Selected Years, 1900–1995

Year	At Birth			At 65 Years		
	Both Sexes	Male	Female	Both Sexes	Male	Female
1900	47.3	46.3	48.3	11.9	11.5	12.2
1950	68.2	65.6	71.1	13.9	12.8	15.0
1960	69.7	66.6	73.1	14.3	12.8	15.8
1970	70.8	67.1	74.7	15.2	13.1	17.0
1980	73.7	70.7	77.4	16.4	14.1	18.3
1990	75.4	71.8	78.8	17.2	15.1	18.9
1995	75.8	72.5	78.9	17.4	15.6	18.9

(Adapted from National Center for Health Statistics (1997). *Health, United States 1996–97 and injury chartbook* [DHHS pub. no. PHS 97-12232]. Hyattsville, MD: Public Health Service, p. 108.)

TABLE 29–3. Life Expectancy at Birth for Selected Countries by Sex

	Male	Female
Nicaragua	64	68
Poland	67	75
United Kingdom	72	79
United States	72	79
Greece	75	80
Sweden	75	81
Japan	76	82

(From *World development report 1993: Investing in health.* [1993]. New York: Oxford University Press [for the World Bank].)

TABLE 29–4. Adult Deaths due to Unintentional Injuries, 1998

Causes	Age		
	15–24	25–44	45–64
Motor vehicle accidents	9,300	13,200	8,000
Falls	240	1,000	1,700
Poisoning by solids and liquids	600	5,000	2,150
Drowning	650	1,300	700
Fires/burns	230	850	800
Suffocation by ingested object	60	240	400
Firearms	310	250	130
Poisoning by gases and vapors	60	200	120
All other types*	1,150	2,850	3,200

*Most important types included are medical and surgical complications and misadventures, machinery, air transport, water transport (except drownings), mechanical suffocation, and excessive cold.
(From National Safety Council. [1999]. *Injury facts: Report on injuries in America.* Itasca, IL: National Safety Council.)

The final stage, 56 to 64 years, involves preparation for retirement. Health problems may have emerged for these adults, and they begin to adjust to the potential loss of loved ones, particularly a spouse. In anticipation of retirement, this stage is marked by expanded social relationships and pursuit of new hobbies to fill leisure time.

Health Problems of Adult Clients

ACCIDENTS

Accidents are unforeseen and unfortunate happenings. In health care, accidents are usually referred to as **unintentional injuries,** a more precise term that refers to any injury that results from unintended exposure to physical agents, including heat, mechanical energy, chemicals, or electricity (Table 29–4). Thus, a motor vehicle collision could result in unintentional injuries, as could exposure to pesticides. When we think about injuries, what usually comes to mind are mechanical injuries of the musculoskeletal system. However, chemical injuries commonly affect the skin, eyes, lungs, and gastrointestinal organs, and both heat and electricity typically injure the skin. The Centers for Disease Control and Prevention (CDC) (1999) estimates that 42,000 people die each year in unintentional motor vehicle crashes.

In 1995, 29 million persons visited emergency departments as a result of unintentional injuries (Shappert, 1997). Injuries cost more than $224 billion annually in the late 1990s, an increase of 42% over the 1980s (U.S. Dept. of Health and Human Services [USDHHS], 2000).

Injuries are the result of an acute exposure to physical agents, including heat, mechanical energy, chemicals, or electricity. As the name implies, unintentional injuries are the result of unintended harm such as falls or motor vehicle accidents. Injury prevention or injury control refers to any effort to prevent injuries, or lessen their severity.

Disabling injuries occur disproportionately among the young and the elderly. Child safety seats, bicycle helmets, smoke detectors, and poison control centers save billions of dollars in direct and indirect medical costs. Primary preven-

tion saves lives and money. A **disabling injury** is one that results in restriction of normal activities of daily living beyond the day on which the injury occurred.

An **unsafe condition** is any environmental factor, either social or physical, that increases the likelihood of an unintentional injury. An icy walkway is an example of an unsafe condition: although it poses a hazard, it does not cause an injury, but only makes it more likely that an injury will occur.

Injury prevention and *injury control* refer to any effort to prevent injuries or lessen their severity. These efforts often focus on assessment of the environment for unsafe conditions, such as loaded guns in the home, or asbestos in school buildings.

CANCER

Chronic disease poses a significant threat to the health of American adults. Cancer is the major chronic illness in the United States. It affects more people over the age of 15 than any other disease and remains the leading cause of death for these people. Major preventable risk factors that contribute to cancer include smoking, alcohol abuse, diet, exposure to radiation and sunlight, water and air pollution. There is a proven link between exposure to cigarette smoke and lung cancer, and, until legislation curtailed it, many workers were exposed to secondhand smoke in the workplace.

Chemicals and other potential cancer-causing materials are produced and used every year. In addition, known carcinogens, such as asbestos and vinyl chloride, continue to threaten the health of workers who, without adequate protection, develop malignancies not commonly found in the general population. In fact, mesothelioma, a lung cancer related to asbestos exposure, has been documented among people whose only known exposure was from the contaminants carried home on the shoes and clothing of a worker. Because asbestos was once a common construction material, it is being removed from older buildings to protect people from asbestos exposure. Asbestos removal experts are at risk of exposure and, therefore, must follow elaborate procedures to protect themselves.

CARDIOVASCULAR DISEASE

More than one fourth of all deaths of adults aged 25 to 64 are due to cardiovascular diseases, primarily coronary artery disease and cerebral vascular accidents (CVAs). Heart disease has been the leading cause of death for men older than 40. Women have only one third the heart disease rate of men before menopause, although the incidence among women increases after menopause. But men still have twice the incidence rate up to age 75. By age 85, the rates are nearly the same (U.S. Bureau of the Census, 1997).

Heart disease is also the largest contributor to permanent disability claims for workers younger than 65 and accounts for more days of hospitalization than any other single disorder. It is the principal cause of limited activity for some 5 million to 6 million Americans under age 65 (Burt et al., 1995).

Approximately 600,000 Americans suffer strokes each year, resulting in 158,000 deaths (USDHHS, 2000). African Americans between the ages of 25 and 64 are almost twice as susceptible to stroke as whites, largely because of the high incidence of hypertension among the black population. In the southeastern United States (the "Stroke Belt"), stroke death rates for both blacks and whites are higher than in any other part of the country.

Risk factors contributing to coronary artery disease can be separated into three categories: Personal, hereditary, and environmental. Personal risk factors include gender, age, race, cholesterol level (specifically low-density lipoprotein to high-density lipoprotein ratio), blood pressure, and cigarette smoking. The most preventable of these include cholesterol, high blood pressure, and cigarette smoking. Heredity obviously cannot be changed. The understanding of environmental risk factors, especially as they relate to occupational exposures, is limited (Office of Disease Prevention and Health Promotion, 1997). The likelihood of heart disease or CVA multiplies with the increasing number of risk factors present.

ADULT SUICIDE

Suicide is the fourth leading cause of death overall for young adults in the United States. Although biomedical advances in science continue to improve survival rates for most physical diseases, our present lifestyle has caused increased emotional and mental stress for individuals. Because accidental deaths are not always closely investigated for clues that they were suicides, it may be that our current statistics do not reflect the actual number of suicides that take place.

The majority of unsuccessful attempts at suicide are made by women. The method selected also seems to reveal a gender bias. Men tend to use more lethal methods such as hanging or gunshots to the head. Women more often take an overdose of pills or cut their wrists. Usually, the person is not trying to kill himself but is trying to escape what they perceive as a hopeless and desperate situation.

How do you know when to pay attention to the signs of depression that may lead to suicide? Signs of depression must be reported to others such as a physician, or friends and relatives. It is important to note that the individual is more likely to commit suicide when their depression lifts slightly because they will have increased energy at that point to act out their suicidal thoughts.

Demonstrate understanding and mutual respect for the person at risk. As a nurse, your responsibility is to listen to the person and make an effort to connect them with available resources.

HIV/AIDS

Acquired immunodeficiency syndrome (AIDS) is a progressive disease that is caused by human immunodeficiency virus (HIV) infection. Adults are usually infected with the virus through intravenous drug use or through sexual activity with an infected partner. By the year 2000, it is estimated that over 40 million people in the world will be living with HIV/AIDS (World Health Report, 1998). Over 1 million people in the United States are infected with HIV, and 670,000 have been diagnosed with AIDS since 1981 (CDC, 1998; UNAIDS, 1998). Unfortunately, the greatest increase in the incidence of HIV/AIDS is in the age group of 25- to 44-year-olds (see Chapter 15).

Our best hope for better control of this public health problem rests with education of the public. Safer sex practices, including abstinence, need to be encouraged. Several cities are implementing needle exchange policies to limit transmission by way of contaminated needles. Use of condoms needs to be taught at a variety of settings ranging from schools to gay bars. Educational programs that instill hope and not just fear have proven to be more successful.

OTHER PROBLEMS

Other problems that threaten the health of American adults are kidney disease, substance abuse, and alcohol abuse. Each has taken a tremendous toll in lives lost, quality of life, and on health and productivity. The National Health Promotion and Disease Prevention Objectives, outlined in *Healthy People 2010,* provides a compelling case for the preventability of substance abuse and alcohol abuse especially (USDHHS, 2000).

Drug abuse is increasing in young adults. Although alcoholism and drug dependence are more common in males, the number of addicted females is increasing. Treatment for drug abuse and addiction requires acceptance of individuals as sick people and deserving of your support (see Research: Bridge to Practice).

Health Promotion of Adult Clients

Several measures can be instituted for adults to promote enhanced health status. Primary prevention strategies such as providing health and safety education and encouraging adults

RESEARCH Bridge to Practice

Bass, E. B., Jenckes, M. W., & Fink, N. E. (1999). Dialysis patients' quality-of-life concerns deserve greater attention from providers. *Medical Decision Making, 19,* 287–295.

Patients with chronic kidney failure have multiple concerns about the impact of dialysis treatments on their quality of life. A study supported by the Agency for Health Care Policy and Research (HS08365) shows that medical providers do not fully appreciate these concerns. Both hemodialysis (HD) and peritoneal dialysis (PD) patients participated in the focus groups in this qualitative study.

Because these patients have end-stage renal disease (ESRD), dialysis treatment substitutes for the kidney by removing waste products from the body and regulating the water and chemical balance. CHOICE (Choices for Health Outcomes in Caring for ESRD) researchers from the following institutions enrolled clients: New England Medical Center, Johns Hopkins University, Tufts University, and the Independent Dialysis Foundation in Baltimore, MD. They conducted focus groups with adult patients receiving either HD or PD at four Baltimore dialysis centers. Separate focus groups were then conducted with nurses, nephrologists, dietitians, medical technicians, and social workers from the dialysis centers. Focus groups were audiotaped while discussing quality-of-life issues for dialysis patients. The tapes were then analyzed to compare group comments.

Dialysis patients identified ten different areas of quality of life that were affected by their dialysis treatment and ESRD, whereas providers usually focused on only five of these areas of concern. Providers consistently mentioned the issue of loss of freedom and loss of control owing to these patients' circumstances but neglected issues such as anxiety, body image, cognitive function, and sleep. Specifically, some patients mentioned that they were anxious about the possibility of getting an infection (from PD), became depressed, felt weak and tired, often had to take cat naps to get through the day, and believed they did not think clearly or easily forgot things.

Findings of this study have implications for health care providers' approach to dialysis patients. It may be that patients would be less likely to suffer anticipatory grief about possible complications if they were encouraged to discuss their fears and concerns. In addition, perhaps these patients should be screened for depression and treated for the condition when indicated.

1. Does this study change your view of dialysis for ESRD patients? If so, in what way?
2. What recommendations would you make to screen dialysis patients for the variety of concerns they raised in the study?

to keep their immunizations up to date are a healthy start. In addition, adults should be encouraged to learn moderate eating habits and gradually increase their exercise. Using safety guidelines to move oneself and lift people or materials at work and in day-to-day activities is an important health promotion activity.

Other measures that promote health include regular physical examinations, moderation in smoking and drinking, and learning relaxation techniques. Adults often sacrifice their need to enjoy leisure activity to their work schedule, but they need an emotional release to avoid frustration. If adults do not have a hobby or a favorite pastime, encourage them to develop an avocation.

ENVIRONMENTAL WORK FACTORS

Healthy adult workers, whether in urban or rural settings, have similar issues in their work environment. Five environmental factors are common to every work setting: (1) physical factors, (2) chemical factors, (3) biologic factors, (4) ergonomic factors, and (5) psychosocial factors.

Physical Factors

Physical factors are structural elements of the workplace that influence worker health and productivity. The various features that make up the physical work environment include work space, temperature, lighting, noise, vibration, color, radiation, pressure, and the soundness of the building and the equipment. The effects of such elements can influence worker health. Excessive noise, for example, may disrupt concentration, prevent verbal communication, impair job performance and safety, and, over time, cause hearing loss. Exposure to the sun is another problem. Those who work outdoors, including migrant farm workers, construction workers, and groundskeepers, are especially at risk for skin cancer, dust, chemical pollutants, and so forth. These workers are also exposed to temperature extremes that put them at risk for frostbite in the winter and heatstroke in the summer.

Exposure to blood-borne pathogens, such as hepatitis B and C and HIV, can have serious or deadly effects on health care workers. Extremes in pressure, such as those experienced by deep-sea divers or by persons working at high altitudes or in tunnels, may cause improper gas exchange and tissue damage affecting ears, sinuses, and teeth.

Some employees work in confined spaces in mines, chemical plants, oil refineries, cargo ships, and airplanes. These workers typically breathe recycled air and may also suffer from insufficient exposure to sunlight. They may be exposed to additional hazards from sudden events such as fires or explosions. Many physical factors in confined work areas can threaten safety, such as lack of protection against sparks from an acetylene torch, insufficient lighting, or weak scaffolding. Despite awareness of these hazards, incidences of occupational injury leading to death continue to remain high.

Each day, an average of 137 persons die from work-related disease, and an additional 17 die from injuries on the job (USDHHS, 2000). There were 4.3 fatal injuries per 100,000 from 1990 through 1995 with motor vehicle-related fatalities at work accounting for the single largest percentage (23%) of deaths since 1980. Industries with the highest traumatic occupational fatality rates per 100,000 workers are mining, agriculture, forestry and fishing, and construction (USDHHS, 2000).

Chemical Factors

Chemical factors are the chemical agents present in the work environment that may threaten worker health and safety. Numerous chemicals are found in the raw materials, production processes, and daily operations of industries and businesses such as dry cleaners, painters, food companies, photographers, automobile manufacturers, plastics factories, farms, pharmaceutical companies, and hospitals. In addition, the petroleum and chemical industries have introduced substances at an alarming rate, subjecting workers to unknown hazards (McKinney & Schoch, 1998). Although chemicals are frequently associated with gases, they are also present in solvents, mists, vapors, dusts, and solids.

Depending on their form and structure, chemicals can enter the human body through the lungs, gastrointestinal tract, and/or skin. Therefore, understanding the toxicology of chemicals is essential for identifying (1) the amount of chemical exposure that produces toxicity, (2) the routes by which chemicals enter the body, and (3) the appropriate personal protection for workers (Institute of Medicine, 1995). For example, lead enters the body through all three routes—lungs, gastrointestinal tract, and skin. Workers exposed to toxic levels of lead must wear protective clothing, maintain good handwashing practices, avoid eating or smoking on the job to prevent ingestion, and employ appropriate respiratory protection to prevent inhalation.

Many toxic chemicals, such as insecticides, are taken for granted in daily use, and their toxicity is frequently ignored. But careless handling and needless exposure can cause serious burns, poisoning, asphyxia, tissue damage, or even cancer. Some inert, nontoxic industrial materials, such as resins and polymers, may decompose and form toxic byproducts when heated. Workers need to be warned of and protected from the hazards associated with the materials they use on the job (Tiedje & Wood, 1995). With proper handling and protection, toxicity can be prevented. Ideally, all toxic substances should be eliminated through substitution of nontoxic agents, when such chemicals exist.

Biologic Factors

Biologic factors are living organisms found in the work environment. These include bacteria, viruses, rickettsiae, molds, fungi, parasites of various types, insects, animals, and even toxic plants. Potential hazards, such as infectious or parasitic diseases, may derive from exposure to contaminated water or to insects. Other vehicles include improper waste or sewage disposal, unsanitary work environments, improper food handling, and unsanitary personal practices.

Workers in every setting have a unique set of potential bi-

ologic hazards. Agricultural workers, for instance, are subject to a condition called "farmer's lung," which comes from inhaling fungi-contaminated grain dust. *Staphylococcus aureus,* hepatitis B virus, HIV, and other infectious agents threaten health care workers. Brucellosis (undulant fever) and Q fever from infected cattle are threats to slaughterhouse workers. Outdoor workers, such as builders, forest rangers, or environmental specialists, face the hazards of insect and animal attack as well as exposure to toxic plants, such as poison oak and ivy.

Ergonomic Factors

Ergonomic factors include all the interactions between the worker, the demands of the job, the work setting, and the overall environment. **Ergonomics** (sometimes called human engineering) has become a field of study in occupational health concerned with "the design of workplaces, tools, and tasks to match the physiological, anatomical, and psychological characteristics and capabilities of the worker" (Ross, 1994).

For our purposes, ergonomic factors are the customs, laws, design, and expectations of the work itself. They include all the physiologic and psychological demands on the job as well as other workplace stressors that can cause anxiety. These can include physical conditions in a work space (called engineering stressors), such as the design of necessary tools, equipment, lighting, or ventilation; physical positions workers must assume; motions they must make to do the job; or bad habits associated with carrying out the work, such as improper lifting habits. Increasing diversity in the workforce underscores the need for changes in the work environment (Travers & McDougall, 1997).

Migrant farm workers in some southwestern states as recently as 1984 were required to use short-handled hoes to speed production and maximize crop yield and were required to spend hours stooping over plants in this doubled-up position. This caused serious skeletal and internal injuries, some of which were permanent. Farm workers often suffer from a lack of toilet facilities or drinking water in the fields. Stooping or squatting for hours can cause bladder and uterine problems in females (Lambert, 1995; see Chapter 33).

There can be organizational stressors in the company or industry itself involving the chain of command, policies, or procedures. Sometimes, an employer's expectations or unrealistic job demands can provoke stress as well. In such situations, the organization becomes the target of treatment, not the individual. When these factors begin to have an impact on individuals' health, job stress results. Long periods of job stress, which is manifested in feelings of anxiety, frustration, and fatigue, can lead to job strain. Job strain can cause workers to lose interest in the job; it can also undermine the morale of others and may even be unsafe. Some extreme cases of job burnout result in former employees using violence or sabotage against the company or its employees.

Psychosocial Factors

Psychosocial factors include the responses and behaviors that workers exhibit on the job. These behaviors come from the attitudes and values learned from their culture, life experiences, and work-site norms. They are the workers' responses to the work and the work milieu. Similar work conditions can evoke different responses. Within the same work setting, some people may seem fatigued, tense, bored, angry, depressed, or agitated, whereas others may seem enthusiastic and energized. Repetitive work may bore some people, whereas others may see it as an opportunity for reflection. Certain types of work may challenge some, but threaten others.

The nature of the work as much as the working conditions can evoke certain responses. Work that is time sensitive or that conflicts with personal values may create tremendous stress for some employees. Ethical dilemmas, such as selling or promoting a product or service that might be injurious to the public (e.g, unreliable used cars), can cause emotional conflict for people. Peer pressure can also add stress, for instance, when one employee is forced to agree with the majority, such as during strikes or labor disputes. Unrealistic personal expectations and unattainable aspirations can lead to chronic stress and fatigue. Psychological stress can result from personal problems such as a terminally ill spouse, a painful divorce or child custody battle, or other family difficulties or crises. Such problems can result in depression or even despair. These types of personal dilemmas influence the quality and quantity of work produced and, in many professions, can compromise worker safety if a worker is preoccupied and functioning inadequately.

Obviously, these five factors will vary in intensity and potential for threat to worker health, depending on the individual and the work environment. They present a core of critical data for occupational health assessment and planning (see Levels of Prevention). The nurse is required to assess not only the environment but also the worker's response to the factors discussed (American Nurses Association, 1995).

EVOLUTION OF OCCUPATIONAL HEALTH

Modern occupational health is an outgrowth of the 19th-century Industrial Revolution in England. Deplorable work conditions and worker exploitation created a growing public concern and spawned the development of many protective laws. This influence was felt in the United States, which was rapidly becoming an industrialized nation. Between 1890 and 1914, more than 16.5 million immigrants from all over the world poured into the United States. As industrial growth escalated, these new citizens worked in the plants, factories, railroads, and mines, creating a new market for manufactured goods. Workers, children as well as adults, commonly worked 12- to 14-hour shifts, 7 days a week, under unspeakable conditions of grime, dust, physical hazards, smoke, heat,

---

LEVELS OF PREVENTION

BACK INJURIES AMONG HOME HEALTH WORKERS

GOAL

To prevent work-related back injuries among nurses, home health aides, and physical therapists employed in one home health agency.

PRIMARY PREVENTION

In-service training is required of all staff who provide direct client care that includes positioning, transferring, and lifting clients. On home visits, supervisors should observe appropriate safety techniques used with clients. They should also observe appropriate use of lifting devices, back supporters, and other appropriate working attire, such as wearing sturdy shoes.

SECONDARY PREVENTION

The injured employee should report the injury immediately and take appropriate actions, including rest, medical follow-up, drug therapy, exercise, heat, or hydrotherapy. On return to work, the employee should gradually work up to full potential and use all safety precautions mentioned above.

TERTIARY PREVENTION

For a long-term back injury, seek alternative treatment including transcutaneous electric nerve stimulation (TENS) units, acupressure, acupuncture, biofeedback, surgery, or other treatment modalities offered at reputable pain clinics. If those treatments provide no relief, consider a change of occupation, part-time work, or, as a last resort, disability and the consequences of living on a limited income.

---

cold, and noxious fumes. People accepted work-related illnesses and injuries as part of the job and lived shorter lives, frequently dying in their forties and fifties, with workers in some trades dying in their thirties (Lee, 1978).

No connection was made between work conditions and health. Employers attributed employees' poor health and early deaths to the workers' personal habits on the job or their living conditions at home. Physicians, uneducated in the relationship between work and health, blamed industrial-related diseases, such as silicosis, lead poisoning, and tuberculosis, on other causes.

Early Research in Occupational Health

Public awareness and understanding were necessary before changes could be made to improve working conditions. That understanding is based on continuing research into occupational health.

In 1700, Bernardino Ramazzini, an Italian physician known as the "father of occupational medicine," conducted the earliest systematic study of occupational disease. His treatise was entitled *Discourse on the Disease of Workers*. Ramazzini had the foresight, when attempting a diagnosis, to ask about his patient's occupation. Despite his influence, interest in and information concerning worker health evolved slowly.

It was not until the early 1900s that the Public Health Service conducted one of the first scientific studies on occupational hazards by investigating dust conditions in mining, cement manufacturing, and stone cutting. Other studies followed. Lead poisoning was as high as 22% among the pottery workers studied. A 1914 study of garment workers showed a high incidence of tuberculosis related to poor ventilation, overcrowding, and unsanitary work conditions. Other investigations revealed phosphorus poisoning among workers in the match industry (1912), radium poisoning among watchmakers (1920s), and mercury poisoning in those who manufactured felt hats (1930s) (Lee, 1978). The public was awakening to the effect of work conditions on people's health.

The birth of the labor movement increased the demand for healthful and safe working conditions. Workers' compensation laws provided for occupational injury and disease coverage, and other efforts were made to protect workers against health hazards in the workplace. Unfortunately, it took such disastrous events as the Triangle Shirtwaist Factory fire to create the impetus for further legislation. This notorious fire, which occurred in New York City in 1911, took the lives of 154 workers, most of whom were young women. Investigations after the incident revealed nonexistent fire escapes and locked exit doors. This tragic event resulted in establishment of the first serious safety laws to protect working people (Morris, 1976).

Current Legislation

Today, a growing body of legislation exists to protect the health and safety of workers. The following is a list of current laws that employers must follow to meet health and safety codes.

The Workmen's Compensation Act of 1910 was initially enacted in New Jersey before it became national law in 1948. This law requires employers to carry employee insurance that provides compensation for lost wages and medical and rehabilitative costs associated with work-related disease and injury. Application of the law varies from state to state. All states, however, emphasize early intervention and rehabilitation.

The Social Security Act of 1935 was enacted to provide financial resources to the "aged, blind, and disabled" as well as state and federal unemployment insurance programs. Amendments to the act in 1965 and 1972 created benefits for high-risk mothers and children and additional benefits for the elderly.

The Federal Coal Mine Health and Safety Act of 1967 is the only federal program that deals with a specific occupational disease. The act originally established health standards in coal mines and provided medical examinations for actively employed underground coal miners. Through the Social Security Administration, it also provided benefits for black lung (pneumoconiosis) disease. Specifically, it required all exposed

workers to have radiographic examinations and made available federal funds to compensate victims and their families. The subsequent *Federal Mine Safety and Health Amendments Act of 1977* retains most of the original provisions.

The Occupational Safety and Health Act of 1970 generally provides workers with protection against personal injury and illness resulting from hazardous working conditions. More specifically, its purpose and functions are "to ensure safe and healthful working conditions for working men and women by authorizing enforcement of the standards developed under the act; by assisting and encouraging the states in efforts to ensure safe and healthful working conditions; by providing for research, information, education, and training in the field of occupational safety and health; and for other purposes" (Lee, 1978, p. 50).

The act created two federal agencies: the Occupational Safety and Health Administration (OSHA) and the National Institute for Occupational Safety and Health (NIOSH).

OSHA, housed in the Department of Labor, became the regulatory branch of the Occupational Safety and Health Act in 1970. OSHA brought about several changes in the workplace. One of the most critical changes is that, for the first time, an employee could request an OSHA inspection for any suspected violation of work standards. And the employee could remain anonymous if he wished to do so. In addition, OSHA provided grants to states to assist in compliance with the act, and some states regained local authority over occupational safety and health.

NIOSH, based in the Public Health Service (under the Department of Health and Human Services), is responsible for research. NIOSH responsibilities include the following (NIOSH, 1986):

- Research on occupational safety and health problems
- Hazard evaluation
- Toxicity determinations
- Workforce development and training
- Industry-wide studies of chronic or low-level exposures to hazardous substances
- Research on psychological, motivational, and behavioral factors as they relate to occupational safety and health
- Training of occupational safety and health professionals

The Toxic Substances Control Act of 1976 ensures that the risk of using chemical substances in the workplace does not present an undue hardship for either the employee or the environment. The act requires that certain chemical substances and mixtures be tested and their use restricted. It is also concerned with the manufacture, processing, commercial distribution, and disposal of such substances. The Environmental Protection Agency enforces this act.

The Hazard Communication Act of 1986, known as the worker right-to-know legislation, ensures that workers are adequately educated regarding hazards in their places of work through a hazards communication program. This is especially important because all hazards and toxic substances cannot be removed from workplaces because of the nature of the product being developed or service provided by a company. This standard was extended in 1988 to all employers covered by OSHA. One of the most frequently cited OSHA violations has been noncompliance with this standard.

The Americans with Disabilities Act (ADA) was passed by Congress in 1990 as a civil rights law to prevent discrimination against qualified workers with disabilities. For employers with 25 or more employees, the law went into effect in 1992. Employers with 15 to 24 employees were obligated to comply with its provisions by 1994 (McKenna, 1994). A disabled person is someone with a physical or mental impairment that substantially limits an aspect or aspects of daily living and work activity. Employees must identify themselves as disabled. The employer and employee then begin a process of defining the essential characteristics of the job and the accommodations that need to be made to allow the employee to work. This is usually done through a job description or a collective-bargaining contract.

The OSHA Blood-Borne Pathogens Standard was enacted in 1992. Guidelines published since the early 1970s addressed infection-control compliance for the protection of health care workers against the transmission of blood-borne diseases. This new standard requires employers to do two things: Offer the hepatitis B vaccine free of charge to all employees and practice general infection control, as recommended by the CDC. The universal precautions recommended by the CDC instruct health care workers to consider any direct contact with blood or body fluids as potentially infectious and provide guidelines on ways of handling such materials. This requires employers to provide such personal protective equipment as gloves, masks, gowns, and eye protectors, and to establish education, training, and some form of record keeping.

Annual compliance costs to employers are considerable, and noncompliance with this new standard puts employers at risk of costly citations. However, the responsibility for adhering to universal precautions remains literally in the hands of the employees. With HIV infection—the most significant public health crisis of this century—compliance with standards for blood-borne pathogens becomes the responsibility of every health care employer and employee.

The Family and Medical Leave Act of 1993 was enacted as a labor standards act. It requires employers of 50 or more people to provide unpaid leave of up to 12 weeks to their employees to care for family members with serious health conditions, their own serious medical condition, or newborn or newly adopted children. The employer must also continue providing medical benefits and ensure that the employee can return to the same or comparable job (McKenna, 1994).

WORK-RELATED HEALTH PROBLEMS

What are the health problems of the working population specifically? As previously mentioned, Americans are ex-

posed to numerous safety and health hazards in the workplace. *Healthy People 2010* focuses on the following eleven occupational health areas:

> *Goal:* **Promote the health and safety of people at work through prevention and early intervention.**

OBJECTIVE AREAS

1. Reduce deaths from work-related injuries
2. Reduce work-related injuries resulting in medical treatment, lost time from work, or restricted work activity
3. Reduce the rate of injury and illness cases involving days away from work due to overexertion or repetitive motion
4. Reduce pneumoconiosis deaths
5. Reduce deaths from work-related homicides
6. Reduce work-related assault
7. Reduce the number of persons who have elevated blood lead level concentrations from work exposures
8. Reduce occupational skin diseases or disorders among full-time workers
9. Increase the proportion of worksites employing 50 or more persons that provide programs to prevent or reduce employee stress
10. Reduce occupational needlestick injuries among health care workers.
11. Reduce new cases of work-related, noise-induced hearing loss (USDHHS, 2000)

Occupational Disease

Occupational disease is any condition or disorder that results from an exposure that resulted from employment. Collecting data on occupational diseases has been difficult because the lag time is so great between exposure and onset of the disease and actual clinical evidence. Silicosis, for example, takes 15 years to develop. Some cases of mesothelioma have not become evident until 25 years after the worker was last exposed to asbestos. Lung disease in workers occurs gradually over time. Most often, exposures do not result in acute symptoms, and, once the symptoms do occur, little can be done. It is for this reason that respiratory disease prevention is so important. Many workers who have changed jobs or retired are only now discovering disease that may be connected to previous employment. Documenting this connection poses problems. Nonetheless, more sophisticated epidemiologic methods and an improved database are enabling public health and industrial researchers to demonstrate linkages and make more accurate predictions.

Occupational settings give rise to a number of environmental health hazards. Workers exposed to heavy metals, such as lead, mercury, and arsenic, will likely develop related diseases. Although miners are often exposed to high levels of radon, sawmill workers are at greater risk for lymphomas (Hertzman et al., 1997). Researchers have also demonstrated the relationship between cotton mill dust and byssinosis, a lung disease formerly thought not to exist in the United States. Epidemiologists are also studying the connection between skin diseases and materials used on the job, a problem of considerable magnitude because dermatologic problems are among the most common occupational diseases.

It is estimated that 30 million workers are exposed to noise levels that can cause impaired hearing, and more than 9 million workers in the United States have some degree of noise-induced hearing loss (NIOSH, 1996). As many as 28% of all reported occupational conditions relate to noise-induced hearing loss (Dembe, 1996). Nurses will be better equipped to design more effective protective and preventive measures as knowledge of occupational illnesses increases.

Health Problems Related to Ergonomics

Another set of health problems affecting workers stems from the ergonomic stressors. With increasing technology and changing work environments, new concerns over such things as lack of natural light and air, poor lighting, loud noise, isolation, and temperature extremes have surfaced. Also, an increasing amount of research is being devoted to the study of video display terminal exposure, which may result in visual problems, and to musculoskeletal problems such as carpal tunnel syndrome resulting from inappropriate positioning at workstations.

Work-Related Emotional Disturbances

There is some evidence that up to 30% of absenteeism from work is due to emotional disturbances (North, Syme, Feeney, Shipley & Marmot, 1996). Pressures at work to increase productivity or a physically stressful work environment (eg, excessive noise, heat, or vibration), coupled with a perception of an inability to control the demands, can result in job strain (Curtis, James, Raghunathan & Alcser, 1997). Personal problems, such as those dealing with finances or relationships, can also adversely affect the worker's job performance. Either source of stress creates a vicious circle, perpetuating and escalating the problems in both settings with the potential for unsafe practices at work and harmful behavior at home.

Workplace Violence

A related stressor is violence in the workplace stemming from "disgruntled employee syndrome," or from interpersonal relationship problems that escalate into violent acts against an employed spouse or significant other. Each year between 1992 and 1996, more than 2 million persons were victims of a violent crime while they were at work (USDHHS, 2000). Homicide is the second-leading cause of death at work. Workers in retail establishments, taxi drivers, and people working at night are the most vulnerable when robbery is the motive. More than three fourths of workplace homicides involve a firearm.

Prevention strategies for violence in the workplace fall into three separate categories: administrative controls, behavior strategies, and environmental designs. Administrative controls include procedures for handling money, unlocking and opening up for business each day, and staffing policies. Behavior strategies include training all employees in conflict resolution and implementation of a nonviolence policy. Environmental designs may include such factors as lighting, security alarm systems, and protective equipment.

OCCUPATIONAL HEALTH PROGRAMS

Because the working population is primarily composed of healthy adults, the goal of occupational health is to maintain that healthy, productive workforce by providing a safe and healthy work environment and promoting healthful personal behavior. Thus, occupational health programs encompass the entire spectrum of health care, including the practice of disease prevention, health protection, and health promotion (Pender, 1996).

Occupational health programs have grown tremendously since World War II. Many manufacturing plants, service organizations, and commercial establishments, including department stores, have instituted some kind of health program for employees. Some programs still concentrate on providing emergency care, but most are beginning to recognize the importance of prevention and health promotion. For example, in 1981 the Adolph Coors Company opened the nation's first comprehensive wellness facility. Mesa Petroleum estimates annual savings of $1.6 million in health care costs for its 650 employees as a result of its wellness program. Other major companies, such as General Electric Aircraft, Tenneco, AT&T Communications, and Johnson & Johnson, have lowered absenteeism and health care costs by initiating health promotion programs.

The variety of work in the United States, as well as the number and type of workers employed, creates a wide range of potential hazards and the need for various on-site health programs. For example, construction and mine workers are a high-risk group for certain types of injuries and illnesses. Workers require an aggressive surveillance program that focuses on prevention and personal protection. In contrast, professionals such as lawyers and accountants are generally at low risk for encountering hazardous physical conditions at work but may experience psychological stress and, therefore, may benefit from a health promotion program that emphasizes stress management and physical fitness.

Disease Prevention Programs

To determine the priorities for intervention and the appropriate health goals and objectives for an aggregate of workers, it is essential to conduct an assessment of both workers and the workplace environment. Knowledge of workers' job classifications and the types of materials they handle and are exposed to will provide clues to potential hazardous substances and working conditions. This information, together with data on the characteristics of the aggregate in terms of age, gender, race, and existing health conditions, should be compiled. In addition, workers' compensation claims and occupational safety and health reports should be examined to identify subpopulations at risk for occupational illness and injury.

The practice of making prevention a priority holds primary importance in occupational health because work-related injuries and illnesses are frequently irreversible. Development of a mesothelioma from asbestos exposure and loss of a limb are conditions for which there are no cures. Interventions, therefore, are aimed at eliminating the hazards by such methods as redesigning equipment to provide safeguards and substituting materials that are as effective but less toxic. *Healthy People 2000* promotes health and disease prevention objectives in the area of occupational health and safety.

The reduction of leading work-related injuries and illnesses and the prevention of new problems require that accrediting bodies of all scientific disciplines understand the role of their professions in recognizing or preventing occupational and environmental problems. Progress in this area also depends greatly on improvements in surveillance to identify high-risk groups and to assist in developing appropriate prevention strategies (USDHHS, 1997).

Healthy People 2010 objectives add the goal of eliminating health disparities to the framework (USDHHS, 2000) (Fig. 29–1).

Once occupational hazards are identified, they can be controlled by substituting safer materials and/or safer practices. In addition, manufacturing processes can be changed and hazardous materials can be isolated. Exhaust methods and other engineering techniques can be used to control the source of occupational hazards. Special clothing and other protective devices can be used. Efforts must be made to educate and motivate employees and employers to comply with safety procedures that focus on prevention.

Health Protection Programs

Making protection a priority becomes essential when hazardous exposures cannot be eliminated. Construction workers, for example, wear hard hats and steel-toed safety shoes to protect themselves from falling objects. Health care work-

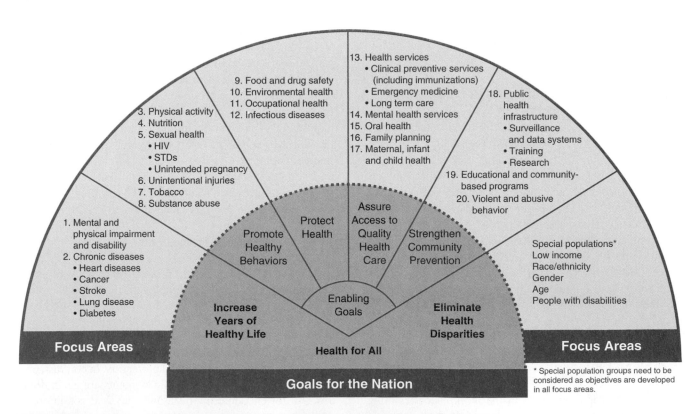

FIGURE 29–1. Vision of 2010: Healthy people in healthy communities. (U.S. Department of Health and Human Services, Office of Disease Prevention and Health Promotion [1997]. *Developing Objectives for Healthy People 2010.* Washington, DC: U.S. Printing Office, p. 14.)

ers who may be exposed to bodily fluids wear gloves, gowns, masks, and/or eye protectors. The protection of workers is frequently achieved through legislation and regulation. The Occupational Safety and Health Act of 1970 provided the impetus for worker protection. More recently, employee right-to-know legislation has been passed, focusing on safety training for employees who are working with potentially hazardous agents. Some of the changes made in the workplace environment include the use of international symbols to warn employees of potentially hazardous materials (electrical hazard is red on white background, biohazard is black on red background, radiation hazard is black on yellow background). Other OSHA-prompted changes include the use of Material Safety Data Sheets (MSDS) and implementation of OSHA's new standards regarding exposure to blood-borne pathogens. The enforcement of such regulations will continue to be the key intervention for ensuring that workers are adequately protected on their jobs.

Occupational safety programs are available in most industries, especially those employing larger numbers of workers. These programs include plant surveillance, safety violation reporting, and worker safety education. All have the goal of protecting the employee.

Health Promotion Programs

A health promotion program is designed to promote healthier lifestyles by encouraging necessary behavioral change. The practice of making health promotion a priority has appropriately received much attention and activity in the workplace over the past decade. The workplace is ideal for conducting health promotion efforts for two important reasons: (1) the majority of the healthy population can be reached at work and (2) employers view wellness programs as legitimate, worthwhile employee benefits to promote and support.

Employee assistance programs are offered in federal and state governmental agencies and many private industries. These programs are cooperatively sponsored by employers and bargaining agencies. The intent is to promote the mental health of the employee by providing an outlet for employee concerns.

It is significant for community health that health promotion activities in the workplace can involve long-term interventions. This allows for the use of various educational and motivational strategies as well as a systematic plan for monitoring and evaluating the programs.

The work environment can serve as a model for a healthy community. Such health policies as creating a smoke-free environment, offering low-fat meals in the company cafeteria, discouraging alcohol abuse, and encouraging injury prevention including seat belt use will establish health norms for company personnel. Many of these healthy behaviors can also have a positive impact on employees' homes and families (Pender, 1996).

Typical health promotion programs include exercise, weight loss, smoking cessation, and nutrition education. There is growing evidence that wellness efforts are effective. Some research indicates that as a result of wellness promotion, employees have increased self-esteem, improved job performance and job satisfaction, decreased absenteeism, and use company health services less frequently (Vail, 1997).

Health promotion programs in the workplace have the potential to provide a significant contribution to adult health as well as to research and development in this new arena of wellness. Cost and production incentives increase employers' acceptance of methods that enhance employee wellness. More research is needed to demonstrate the correlation between healthy employees and increased productivity on the job. Health promotion will continue to be a vital area of emphasis for the working community as the nation enters the 21st century.

Additional Workplace Health Services

Although employers are not presently required to provide treatment for nonoccupational injuries and illnesses (ie, injury and illness not incurred at work), many companies do provide such services. One reason is that it is difficult to determine where health problems such as muscle strain, influenza, and minor rashes are acquired. Therefore, it is simpler to provide care for the problem regardless of its source. The on-site treatment of minor acute injury and illness as well as employee counseling depends on the philosophy of the company, the employment of an occupational health nurse, and the company's prior experience with offering these services as an employee benefit.

From the nurse's perspective, the advantages of offering nonoccupational health services are the following:

1. The occupational health nurse develops rapport with employees and can detect health problems early.
2. Loss of employee productivity is minimized when treatment is given on site.
3. The occupational health nurse, through triage, can decide which cases require medical attention as opposed to those that can safely be managed by the nurse.
4. The occupational health nurse can provide needed, ongoing, personal health education and counseling in the context of a more holistic view of the worker.
5. On-site chronic disease management, such as hypertension monitoring, increases compliance, thereby saving costs of physician visits and complications associated with noncompliance.
6. The occupational health nurse provides employees with personal contact—a valued commodity in our high-technology work environments.

A number of occupational health nurses have expressed concern that spending too much time on nonoccupational illnesses could keep them from pursuing an aggressive occupational health surveillance program. As occupational health nurses learn more about environmental factors that threaten workers' health, they will likely spend less time with illness management and move more aggressively toward primary prevention, protection, and health promotion efforts. The direction of health care programs in the future is covered later in this chapter.

ROLE OF THE OCCUPATIONAL HEALTH NURSE

Community health nurses have a long history of involvement in occupational health. In 1895, the Vermont Marble Company hired the first industrial nurse in the United States to care for its employees and their families. At the time, it was an unusual demonstration of interest in employee welfare. The nursing service, which consisted mostly of home visiting and care of the sick, was free to employees and their families. Gradually that role changed. World War II showed a marked increase in employment of industrial public health nurses who practiced illness prevention and health education among employees at work.

In addition to emergency care and nursing of ill employees, the activities of many industrial nurses involved safety education, hygiene, nutrition, and improvement of working conditions. Yet a significantly high number of industrial injuries and sick employees kept many nurses too busy to do anything but care for the ill. They might see more than 75 patients a day in the plant dispensary, where they provided first aid and medications. Employee health programs have improved as socioeconomic and political pressures have created improved safety and health standards for the work environment. Similarly, these developments have changed and expanded the nurse's role. The role of an **occupational health nurse** is to ensure that the workforce is healthy and productive, as evidenced by the nursing practice standards developed by the professional organization known as the Association of Occupational Health Nurses (Display 29–2).

Special Skills and Demands

The nurse's role in occupational health, as previously mentioned, has traditionally focused on illness and injury care. This directly resulted from the knowledge and skills obtained in basic nursing education. During the last decade, a number of nursing education programs (primarily on the graduate level) have developed a specialty focus in occupational health. In addition, many continuing education programs provide occupational health nurses with updated information and skill training for identifying and assisting in the management of the physical, chemical, biologic, ergonomic, and psychosocial factors in the work environment that can affect worker health and safety. As a result, the occupational health nurse's role is not universal; it depends on the type and philosophy of the company, type and number of workers, the health professionals involved, exposures and potential haz-

---

DISPLAY 29–2. Standards of Occupational Health Nursing Practice

Standards of Clinical Nursing Practice

Standard I. Assessment: The occupational health nurse systematically assesses the health status of the client.

Standard II. Diagnosis: The occupational health nurse analyzes data to formulate a nursing diagnosis.

Standard III. Outcome Identification: The occupational health nurse identifies expected outcomes specific to the client.

Standard IV. Planning: The occupational health nurse develops a plan of care that is comprehensive and formulates interventions for each level of prevention and for therapeutic modalities to achieve expected outcomes.

Standard V. Implementation: The occupational health nurse implements interventions to promote health, prevent illness and injury, and facilitate rehabilitation, guided by the plan of care.

Standard VI. Evaluation: The occupational health nurse systematically and continuously evaluates the client's responses to interventions and evaluates progress toward the achievement of expected outcomes.

Professional Practice Standards

Standard I. Professional Development/Evaluation: The occupational health nurse assumes responsibility for professional development and continuing education and evaluates personal professional performance in relation to practice standards.

Standard II. Quality Improvement/Quality Assurance: The occupational health nurse monitors and evaluates the quality and effectiveness of occupational health practice.

Standard III. Collaboration: The occupational health nurse collaborates with employees, management, other health care providers, professionals and community representatives in assessing, planning, implementing, and evaluating care and occupational health services.

Standard IV. Research: The occupational health nurse contributes to the scientific base in occupational health nursing through research, as appropriate, and uses research findings in practice.

Standard V. Ethics: The occupational health nurse uses an ethical framework as a guide for decision-making in practice.

Standard VI. Resource Management: The occupational health nurse collaborates with management to provide resources that support an occupational health program that meets the needs of the worker population.

(Adapted from American Association of Occupational Health Nurses. [1994]. *Standards of occupational health nursing practice.* Atlanta, GA: Author.)

ards in the work environment, and the knowledge and skills of the nurse.

Nurses who select the field of occupational health and safety will encounter experiences that differ significantly from those found in an acute care setting. To make the adjustment, the nurse should be aware of the factors that make occupational health unique.

Unlike hospitals or ambulatory care centers, the workplace is a non-health care institution in which production or service (not health care) is the primary goal of the organization. The occupational health nurse participates in the organization's goals through activities that will contribute to the productivity of the workforce.

An occupational health nurse in the organization is in a staff position, taking on the role of a consultant, educator, or role model in the workplace, but has no supervisory responsibilities or power to hire or fire workers. The nurse is generally responsible for the management of the occupational health unit, serving the needs of employees and management personnel.

The occupational health nurse, especially in many smaller organizations, may be the only nurse in the company. As a result, he or she has no on-site consultation and direction that is needed for comfortable, competent, and independent decision-making. Nurses who use critical thinking skills to develop a framework for independent problem solving will enhance their efficiency (Kuhar, 1998). A nurse who works alone may feel isolated and need to collaborate with the occupational health and safety team members.

There are various causes of job stress for the occupational health nurse, and there may be related personal, professional, and employer factors. The nurse may experience role ambiguity due to a lack of professional preparation or inadequate orientation and continuing education. The corporate culture and leadership may foster work overload, be nonsupportive, and have limited career opportunities for the nurse. Occupational health nurses need to apply strategies to reduce job stress and potential job strain by modeling health-affirming choices, networking with other nurses and professional organizations in the community, and setting appropriate occupational health standards.

The client base served in occupational health is a well-adult population with whom long-term contact is possible. Occupational health nurses, therefore, have the chance to know their clients well and have opportunities to work with them through various stages of personal as well as health service-related incidents. Such continuity of health care can challenge occupational health nurses to use all the community health nursing model interventions—education, engineering, and enforcement.

Finally, the practice focus is oriented to the aggregate; the nurse serves a worker population. Environmental factors significantly influence the health and safety of workers. Therefore, occupational health nurses need to constantly monitor the work environment and assess the health needs of

the entire worker population to identify those at risk, particularly workers in hazardous lines of work, and develop prevention, promotion, and protection programs.

Community-Based Occupational Health Nursing

Agencies external to business and industry also provide occupational health nursing services. Historically, public health nurses from visiting nurse associations made home visits to sick employees and their families. In subsequent years, public health agencies provided part-time nursing services to small companies. These services included supervising the work environment, conducting health examinations, keeping records, teaching about and counseling on health issues, providing first aid, giving immunizations, and referring workers to community resources. More recently, community health nursing services have offered health screening and health promotion programs. Furthermore, occupational health nurse consultants based in state departments of health provide consultation and continuing education programs to nurses employed in occupational health settings.

Hospital-based occupational health programs, large medical-industrial health clinics, and insurance companies also provide occupational health nursing services. These services may be in the form of direct care (rehabilitation of an injured worker) or indirect care (consultation on implementing regulations regarding record keeping or compiling health statistics).

A continuing unmet need is attending to the health of workers in smaller companies. These companies have more hazards because equipment and controls are often inadequate. They seldom, if ever, have a health professional on site. Attempts have been made by some communities to provide needed health protection services, but no sustained efforts exist. Community health nurses are in a position to accept this challenge and develop a system that will ensure ongoing service to this high-risk population.

Members of the Occupational Health Team

Today, the two professionals who generally provide on-site occupational health services are the occupational health nurse and the safety engineer. Other members of the interdisciplinary team may include an industrial hygienist, epidemiologist, toxicologist, and occupational physician. However, only large corporations usually employ these specialists, or they provide only selected part-time services on a contractual basis. Therefore, the position of occupational health nurse in a large company or the community health nurse who serves smaller companies is the cornerstone of occupational health.

Collaboration may take time but will be worth the investment. The occupational health nurse must gain the respect and trust of management and establish open communication to influence company policies regarding the nature and scope of health programs.

Depending on the size of the company and its products or services, the occupational health nurse may also collaborate with any or all of the following people: insurance carriers, union representatives, employee assistance counselors, industrial hygienists, safety engineers, company and/or outside lawyers, toxicologists, human resources personnel, and the community (Slayle, Sun, & Mathis, 1998). Any comprehensive assessment of employee health and safety problems, as well as any health promotion program, requires cooperation and assistance from many people working in various departments within the organization.

Finally, the occupational health team is not complete without the workers themselves. Employees can help identify problems and needs and contribute to decision-making about health programs. Their cooperation in implementing and evaluating programs is essential for an effective health protection and promotion effort.

Future Trends

A broad goal for occupational health is to promote and maintain the highest level of physical, social, and emotional health for all workers. In practice, this goal is only beginning to be realized in selected instances. Nevertheless, it is a worthy and, more important, an essential objective in the realization of an energized and productive working community.

However, the rapid and fundamental changes in U.S. businesses in the 1990s have added three critical issues that affect the practice of occupational health nursing. First, increasing worldwide competition requires business to remain competitive by reducing and/or controlling operating costs at the lowest level possible. Second, there has been an increase in technological hazards that require sophisticated approaches as well as a knowledge of toxicology, epidemiology, ergonomics, and public health principles. Third, health care costs continue to escalate at faster rates than most company profits (Vail, 1997) (see The Global Community).

Current occupational health nurse practices will continue to evolve to meet future needs. The focus will shift from one-on-one health services to a new role involving broader business and research skills.

Current occupational health nurse activities include:
1. Supervising care for emergencies and minor illnesses
2. Counseling employees about health risks
3. Following up with employees' workers' compensation claims
4. Performing periodic health assessments
5. Evaluating the health status of employees returning to work

Future occupational health nurse activities will involve:
1. Analyzing trends (health promotion, risk reduction, and health expenditures)

THE GLOBAL COMMUNITY

Impact of a National Health Care System on Canadian Nurses

Shamian, J. (2000). On the heels of Florence Nightingale: Re-energizing hospital care. *Reflections on Nursing Leadership, 26*(1), 24–26.

Health Canada's new executive director of nursing, Dr. Judith Shamian, notes that Canada enjoys a first rate, publicly funded health care system. As a result, Canadian citizens view health as a right, not a privilege. Although most Canadian nurses share this perspective, they also acknowledge a dissonance between educational preparation of nurses and the demands that the current health care environment makes on their clinical practice. In 1998, Dr. Shamian was a co-investigator in a study of 8,000 hospital nurses in Ontario, Canada. It was part of a comprehensive, multinational examination whose purpose was to determine which characteristics of the nurses are most likely to produce the best clinical outcomes and result in job satisfaction. Results from the Ontario study showed the following:
- When compared to other employee groups, nurses suffer greater emotional exhaustion.
- Nurses trust peers but are less trusting of their managers.
- The health condition of the nurse is described as being poor when compared to other employee groups.

Implications of the study are that nurses deserve greater respect for the important service they provide. Canadian nurses bear a tremendous social obligation to deliver health services in a system that does not appear to value them. Politicians and decision-makers need to be informed of nurses' contributions to both the physical and economic well-being of a country. Health and nursing knowledge should address the impact of public policy. Continued research and resultant evidence-based practice have the potential to influence decisions regarding allocation of health care resources. The primary motivation for this paradigm shift is to enhance the health of the people served by any type of health care program.

2. Developing programs suited to corporate needs
3. Recommending more efficient and cost-effective in-house health services
4. Determining cost-effective alternatives to health programs and services
5. Collaborating with others to identify problems and propose solutions

As we move into the 21st century, occupational health nurses and management will share the goal of developing a healthy, productive, and profitable company. A healthy company consists of healthy and productive employees, and healthy employees mean lower health care costs. Lower costs result in an increased competitive edge and higher profits. Higher profits can make more resources available to support more programs and to improve employee health.

The occupational health nurse will particularly need skills in effective communication, leadership, change management, research, business acumen, and assertiveness. These tools will be crucial for effectively interpreting the occupational health nurse's role and promoting ideas. Success of programs developed by the occupational health nurse depends on establishment of positive working relationships with the other team members. Nurses involved in occupational health have a unique opportunity to help shape the health profile of the working population. The degree of that influence depends on how the nurse defines the occupational health nurse role. Also, the nurse must be able to overcome the many obstacles found in the occupational setting, including restrictive company policy, misunderstanding of the nurse's role, and lack of time for innovative program development. The nurse's role in occupational health, therefore, varies considerably. It ranges from only providing emergency care for on-the-job injuries or illness to establishing comprehensive policies and programs covering health promotion, accident and disease prevention, and innovative care for disease and disability.

Occupational health nursing demands a great deal from the nurse. Individual needs in the workplace will always compete for the nurse's time and take attention away from aggregate needs, often to the detriment of the latter. To maintain a proper focus on aggregate needs requires discipline and commitment—commitment based on a different mindset and the realization that the health and productivity of workers are interrelated with the health of the community.

SUMMARY

The 20th century has seen a shift in the three leading causes of death from communicable diseases to noncommunicable diseases. Currently, the leading causes of death in adults are accidents, cancer, cardiovascular disease, suicide, and HIV/AIDS.

The working population in the United States, numbering 127 million, makes up the majority of the American people. The profile of this aggregate is changing from an industrialized labor force to one of more white-collar workers and professionals. The environment of the workplace is changing as well.

Five types of environmental factors, common to all work settings, can influence worker health or safety. Physical or structural elements include such things as temperature and noise extremes. Chemical factors refer to the presence of potentially hazardous chemical agents. Biologic organisms, such as viruses, bacteria, and fungi, may contaminate the work environment and cause disease. Ergonomic factors include the customs, design, and expectations of the job that influence the way people interact with their work environment. Psychosocial factors are the workers' feelings and behavior at work. Assessment of all of these is critical in determining appropriate occupational health interventions.

Historically, workers' health has been of little importance to the government. As a result, many have suffered unhealthy, dangerous working conditions and have contracted debilitating, often fatal, diseases and injuries. More recently, however, worker health has become a target for health intervention. The government has become more involved and passed major legislation to ensure workers' rights to a safe and healthy work environment. Three of the most significant pieces of legislation are the Occupational Safety and Health Act of 1970, the Hazard Communication Act of 1986, and the Americans with Disabilities Act of 1990.

Leading work-related health problems include occupational lung disease, injuries, and occupational cancers. New health concerns have arisen in this population that reflect our changing society, work patterns, and environment. They include job stress, ergonomic issues that relate to the computer age, emotional disturbances, and workplace violence.

The number and type of workplace injuries vary by place, time, and type of industry. Homicide is currently the second leading cause of deaths in the workplace. A variety of prevention strategies can be implemented to control workplace injuries.

Programs designed to serve the health needs of the working population should be based on an assessment of the unique needs of each setting. Occupational health services encompass the three public health practice priorities—prevention, protection, and health promotion. Preventive programs seek to eliminate potential hazards to worker health and safety. Protective services shield workers from remaining hazards. Health promotion or wellness programs seek to maintain and improve workers' health. Health services for workers may also cover nonoccupational illnesses.

Occupational health nursing applies the philosophy and skills of nursing and community health to protecting and promoting the health of people in their work environment. The occupational health nurse's role is evolving as business becomes more competitive and health care costs escalate at a frightening rate. That expanded role will include analyzing current trends, recommending more cost-effective and innovative in-house health services, and collaborating with other members of the multidisciplinary occupational health team, including management, to develop appropriate programs.

ACTIVITIES TO PROMOTE CRITICAL THINKING

1. Using a local newspaper, select three articles that relate to workplace violence. For each article, (a) summarize the content, (b) identify the likely cause of the violence, and (c) describe how the violence might have been prevented.
2. You are asked to offer a weight-control program for a local milk-processing plant that has 100

employees. What steps would you take to develop a successful program?

3. Using the Internet and the school library, research an injury and a disease often associated with your future profession. Write a two-page paper in which you identify the selected concerns and discuss both the employee's and employer's responsibility regarding management of these problems.

4. Survey your living quarters and make a room-by-room environmental assessment of potentially unsafe conditions. Describe a strategy for improving each condition.

REFERENCES

American Nurses Association. (1995). *Nursing: A social policy statement.* Washington, DC: Author.

Burt, V. L., Colter, J. A., Higgins, M., et al. (1995). Trends in the prevalence, awareness, treatment, and control of hypertension in the adult U.S. population. *Hypertension, 26,* 60–69.

Centers for Disease Control and Prevention (CDC), National Center for Health Statistics (NCHS) (1999). Deaths: Final data for 1997. *National Vital Statistics Reports, 47*(19).

————. (1998). 1998 guidelines for treatment of sexually transmitted diseases. *Morbidity and Mortality Weekly Report, 47*(RR-I).

Curtis, A. B., James, S. A., Raghunathan, T. E., & Alcser, K. H. (1997). Job strain and blood pressure in African Americans: The Pitt County Study. *American Journal of Public Health, 87,* 1297–1302.

Dembe, A. E. (1996). *Occupation and disease: How social factors affect the conception of work-related disorders.* New Haven, CT: Yale University Press.

Hertzman, C., Teschke, K., Ostry, A., et al. (1997). Mortality and cancer incidence among sawmill workers exposed to chlorophenate wood preservatives. *American Journal of Public Health, 87,* 71–79.

Institute of Medicine. (1995). *Nursing, health and the environment.* Washington, DC: National Academy Press.

Kuhar, M. B. (1998). Critical thinking: A framework for problem solving in the occupational setting. *AAOHN Journal, 46*(2), 80–81.

Lambert, M. (1995). Migrant and seasonal farmworker women. *Journal of Obstetric, Gynecologic, and Neonatal Nursing, 24*(3), 265–268.

Lee, J. (1978). *The new nurse in industry: A guide for the newly employed occupational health nurse* (DHEW [NIOSH] Pub. No. 78–143). Cincinnati, OH: U.S. Government Printing Office.

McKenna, B. (1994). *The Americans With Disabilities Act and the health care worker.* Healthwire. Washington, DC: Federation of Nurses and Health Professionals.

McKinney, M. L., & Schoch, R. M. (1998). *Environmental science: Systems and solutions.* Sudbury, MA: Jones and Bartlett.

Morris, R. B. (Ed.) (1976). *The United States Department of Labor bicentennial history of the American worker.* Washington, DC: U.S. Government Printing Office.

National Center for Health Statistics. (1997). *Health, United States 1996–97 and injury chartbook.* DHHS pub. no. PHS-9712232. Hyattsville, MD: Public Health Service.

National Institute for Occupational Safety and Health. (1996). *National occupational research agenda.* Cincinnati: Author.

————. (1986). *NIOSH recommendations for occupational safety and health standards.* Atlanta: Centers for Disease Control.

North, F. M., Syme, S. L., Feeney, A., Shipley, M., & Marmot, M. (1996). Psychosocial work environment and sickness absence among British civil servants: The Whitehall II Study. *American Journal of Public Health, 86,* 332–340.

Office of Disease Prevention and Health Promotion. (1997). Progress review: Environmental health. *Prevention Report, 12*(2), 1–13.

Pender, N. J. (1996). *Health promotion in nursing practice* (3rd ed.). Stanford, CT: Appleton & Lange.

Ross, P. (1994). Ergonomic hazards in the workplace: Assessment and prevention. *American Association of Occupational Nurses Journal, 42*(4), 171–176.

Schappert, S. M. (1997). Ambulatory care visits to physician offices, hospital outpatient department and emergency departments: U.S., 1995, NCHS. *Vital and Health Statistics, 13*(29), 1–38.

Slagle, M. W., Sun, S. M., & Mathis, M. G. (1998). A conceptional model of occupational health nursing: The resource model. *AAOHN Journal, 46*(3), 121–126.

Tiedje, L., & Wood, J. (1995). Sensitizing nurses for a changing environmental health role. *Public Health Nursing, 12*(6), 359–365.

Travers, P. H., & McDougall, C. E. (1997). The occupational health nurse: Roles and responsibilities, current and future trends. In J. M. Swanson & M. Nies (Eds.), *Community health nursing: Promoting the health of aggregates* (pp. 767–795). Philadelphia: W. B. Saunders.

USAIDS (1998). *Report on the global HIV/AIDS epidemic.* Geneva: UNAIDS/World Health Organization.

U.S. Bureau of the Census. (1997). *Statistical abstract of the United States, 1997* (117th ed.). Washington, DC: U.S. Government Printing Office.

U.S. Department of Health and Human Services. (2000, January). *Healthy People 2010* (conference edition, in two volumes). Washington, DC: U.S. Government Printing Office.

————. Office of Disease Prevention and Health Promotion. (1997). *Developing objectives for Healthy People 2000.* Washington, DC: U.S. Government Printing Office.

Vail, S. (1997). A question of values. *Canadian Nurse, 93*(10), 59–60.

Ventura, S. J., Peters, K. D., Martin, J. A., & Maurer, J. D. (1997). Annual summary of births, marriages, divorces, and deaths: United States, 1996. *Monthly Vital Statistics Report, 46*(1, Suppl. 2), 33.

World Health Report (1998). *Report of the director-general.* Geneva: World Health Organization.

INTERNET RESOURCES

American Lung Association: http://www.alaw.org

American Public Health Association (APHA): http://www.apha.org

American Red Cross: http://www.redcross.org

Centers for Disease Control and Prevention (CDC): http://www.cdc.gov

MSU Radiation, Chemical and Biological Safety: http://www.orcbs.msu.edu

National Institute for Occupational Safety and Health (NIOSH): http://cdc.gov/niosh/homepage.html

National Institutes of Health: http://www.nih.gov

National Safety Council: http://www.nsc.org

U.S. Department of Health and Human Services: http://os.dhhs.gov

World Health Organization: http://www.who.ch

SELECTED READINGS

Abusabha, R., Peacock, J., & Achterberg, C. (1999). How to make nutrition education more meaningful through facilitated group discussions. *Journal of the American Dietetic Association, 99*(1), 72–76.

Andrews, J. (1998). Optimizing smoking cessation strategies. *The Nurse Practitioner, 23*(8), 47–65.

Bishop, C. E. (1998). Health cost containment: What it will mean for workers and local economies. *Public Health Reports, 113,* 204–213.

Burton, W. N., & Connerty, C. M. (1998). Evaluation of a worksite-based patient education intervention targeted at employees with diabetes mellitus. *Journal of Emergency Medicine, 40*(8), 702–706.

Cerrelli, E. C. (1998). *Traffic crashes, injuries and fatalities—preliminary report.* National Highway Traffic Safety Administration Technical Report, DOT HS 909 695. Available from the National Technical Information Service, Springfield, VA 22161.

Cookfair, J. M. (1996). *Nursing care in the community* (2nd ed.). St. Louis, MO: Mosby–Year Book.

Freedman, R. I., Krauss, M. W., & Seltzer, M. M. (1999). Patterns of respite use by aging mothers of adults with mental retardation. *Mental Retardation, 37*(2), 93–103.

Grisso, G. A., Schwartz, D. F., Miles, C. G., & Holmes, J. J. (1996). Injuries among inner-city minority women: A population-based longitudinal study. *American Journal of Public Health, 86*(1), 67–70.

Halm, M. A. & Penque, S. (1999). Heart disease in women. *American Journal of Nursing, 99*(4), 26–32.

Haws, J. M., Butta, P. G., & Girvin, S. (1997). A comprehensive and efficient process for counseling patients desiring sterilization. *The Nurse Practitioner, 22*(6), 52–67.

Henderson, A. K., Payne, M. M., Ossiander, E., et al. (1998). Surveillance of occupational diseases in the United States. *Journal of Emergency Medicine, 40*(8), 714–719.

Hipkins, K. L., Materna, B. L., Kosnett, M. J., et al. (1998). Medical surveillance of the lead-exposed worker: Current guidelines. *American Association of Occupational Health Nurses Journal, 46*(7), 330–339.

Jeffery, R. W., & French, S. A. (1998). Epidemic obesity in the United States: Are fast foods and television viewing contributing? *American Journal of Public Health, 88*(2), 277–280.

Johnson, K. M., Taylor, V. M., Lessler, D., et al. (1998). Inner city primary care providers' breast cancer screening knowledge: Implications for intervention. *Journal of Community Health, 23*(1), 1–13.

Korrick, S. A., Hunter, D. J., Rotnitsky, A., et al. (1999). Lead and hypertension in a sample of middle-aged women. *American Journal of Public Health, 89*(3), 330–335.

Kotecki, J. E. (1996). Interpersonal violence among youth: A priority issue for public health. *The Health Education Monograph Series, 14*(3), 21–25.

Lai, S. C., & Cohen, M. N. (1999). Promoting lifestyle change. *American Journal of Nursing, 99*(4), 63–67.

Mas, F. S., Papenfus, R. L., & Guerrero, J. J. (1997). Hispanics and worksite health promotion: Review of the past, demands for the future. *Journal of Community Health, 22*(5), 361–371.

Middleton, A. D. (1997). Managing asthma: It takes teamwork. *American Journal of Nursing, 97*(1), 39–43.

Murray, C. J., & Lopez, A. D. (Eds.). (1996). *The global burden of disease: A comprehensive assessment of mortality and disability from diseases, injuries, and risk factors in 1990 and projected in 2020.* Geneva, Switzerland: World Health Organization.

Mustard, C. A., Kaufert, P., Kozyrskyj, A., & Mayer, T. (1998). Sex differences in the use of health care services. *New England Journal of Medicine, 338*(23), 1678–1683.

National Institute for Occupational Safety and Health. (1991). *Environmental tobacco smoke in the workplace: Lung cancer and other health effects.* DHHS (NIOSH) pub. no. 91-108. Cincinnati: Author.

Nies, M. A., Buffington, C., Cowan, G., & Hepworth, J. T. (1998). Comparison of lifestyles among obese and nonobese African American and European American women in the community. *Nursing Research, 47*(4), 251–257.

Nusselder, W. J., van der Velden, K., van Sonsbeek, J. L. A., et al. (1996). The elimination of selected chronic diseases in a population: The compression and expansion of morbidity. *American Journal of Public Health, 86*(2), 187–194.

Rogers, B., & Cos, A. R. (1998). Integrating environmental health in occupational health nursing. *American Association of Occupational Health Nurses Journal, 46*(1), 9–13.

U.S. Bureau of the Census. (1998). *United States population estimates by age, sex, race, and Hispanic origin, 1990–1997.* Population Division, PPL-91. Washington, DC: U.S. Government Printing Office.

Wilby, M. L. (1998). Improving the health profile: Decreasing risk for cancer through primary prevention. *Holistic Nursing Practice, 12*(2), 52–61.

Wold, J. L., & Williams, A. M. (1996). Student/faculty practice and research in occupational health: Health promotion and outcome evaluation. *Journal of Nursing Education, 35*(6), 252–257.

Zandee, G. L. (1996). Effectiveness of contingency contracting: Component of a worksite weight loss program. *American Association of Occupational Health Nurses Journal, 44*(4), 183–188.

Zerwic, J. J., & Prasun, M. A. (1998). Acute myocardial infarction in the workplace. *American Association of Occupational Health Nurses Journal, 46*(4), 195–202.

Promoting and Protecting the Health of the Older Adult Population

KEY TERMS

- Ageism
- Alzheimer's disease
- Assisted living
- Baby boomers
- Board and care homes
- Case management
- Confidant
- Continuing care center
- Custodial care
- Elite-old
- Frail elderly
- Geriatrics
- Gerontology
- Group home
- Hearty elderly
- Hospice care
- Intermediate care
- Long-term care
- Osteoporosis
- Personal care homes
- Respite care
- Senility
- Skilled nursing facility

LEARNING OBJECTIVES

Upon mastery of this chapter, you should be able to:

- Describe the global and national health status of older adults.
- Identify and refute at least four common misconceptions about older adults.
- Describe characteristics of healthy older adults.
- Provide an example of primary, secondary, and tertiary prevention practices among the older population.
- Discuss four primary criteria for effective programs for older adults.
- Describe various living arrangements and care options for older adults.
- Describe the future of an aging America and the role of the community health nurse.

Older Americans constitute a large and growing population group. You will be part of it in the future. Perhaps your parents and grandparents are in that group now. In fact, people aged 65 and older make up the fastest-growing segment of the American population (American Association of Retired Persons [AARP] & Administration on Aging, 1997). This trend is expected to continue, with the most rapid increase expected between the years 2010 and 2030 when the "baby boom" generation reaches 65 (AARP & Administration on Aging, 1997). Older adults make up a group whose health needs are not fully understood, and the nation has yet to offer the full complement of services they require and deserve.

For community health nursing, this population group poses a special challenge. The increasing number of seniors in the community increases the need for health-promoting and preventive services. These services help maximize an older person's ability to remain an independent, contributing member of society and maintain a high quality of life. With this group's potential for longevity comes the myriad problems brought on by these extended numbers of years, including dwindling finances that may not be keeping up with inflation; increasing chronic disease and disability; diminishing functional capacity; dealing with ongoing losses regarding work, home, family members and other loved ones. Significant economic, environmental, and social changes create a demand for greater protective and preventive services for older adults in addition to requiring adjustments in health care provision patterns. The challenge is clear. Nursing must study the needs of this group and respond with appropriate, effective, and cost-effective interventions.

This chapter focuses on population-based nursing for the elderly. There are four fundamental requirements for effective nursing of any population:

1. Know the characteristics of the population.
2. Set aside stereotypes based on misconceptions about the population.

3. Know the health needs of the population as a basis for nursing intervention.
4. View the population from an aggregate, public health perspective that emphasizes health protection, health promotion, and disease prevention.

This chapter first examines the global challenge of an aging society and the characteristics of the aging population in the United States. We look at some myths and misconceptions about the elderly and discuss ageism. Next, the primary, secondary, and tertiary health needs of older adults are explored. Finally, population-based health services and nursing interventions applied to the health of the aging population are discussed in light of cost containment and comprehensive care as we enter a new millennium.

HEALTH STATUS OF OLDER ADULTS

Never before has the population of older adults been so large, and its numbers are on the increase. This progressive aging of populations in the 20th century will continue into the 21st century and is hailed as a triumph for the human species. People are living longer as a result of improved health care, eradication and control of many communicable diseases, use of antibiotics and other medicines, healthier dietary practices, regular exercise, and accessibility to a better quality of life. This is especially true for people in developed countries, particularly for residents of the United States.

Global Demographics

It is estimated that more than 420 million people worldwide are over age 65. This is about 7% of the world's population. In the United States, more than 33 million people (13% of the population) are older than 65, and by 2030 that number is expected to increase to 20% of the population (World Health Organization [WHO], 1998). In 1996, 11.8% of the U.S. population were among the oldest of older adults, those over 75 years old. This compares with 17.9% of those in China, 8.2% of the Indian population, and 5.7% of the Japanese. In some African and Asian countries, the population age 75 and older constitutes less than 1% of the total population (WHO, 1998). Display 30–1 lists the world's oldest countries, where 13% or more of the population are over age 65. In Africa, 3% of the population is over 65; in India, 4%, and Mexico 5% (Population Reference Bureau, 1999).

Women outnumber men in the older population because they have an advantage in life expectancy that averages 8 years. In fact, older women outnumber older men in most countries. However, the advantage is partially offset by disability. There is no advantage to a longer life if the quality of that life is poor. In fact, extending the healthy years of life is a goal of the U.S. Department of Health and Human Services *Healthy People 2010* objectives (U.S. Department of Health

and Human Services [USDHHS], 2000). It will be a focus of public health practices in the United States for the next decade. According to data from selected European countries, women in Switzerland can expect 15 years of disability-free years of life after age 65 and 5 years of disability, compared to a low of 8 years of disability-free years of life after age 65 for women in the Netherlands, with 12 years of disability. In the United States, disability-free years after age 65 are slightly above 10 years, followed by 7 years of disability (National Institute on Aging, 1996). More than half of the women in the United States older than 65 are widowed (Eliopoulos, 1997).

National Demographics

The average life expectancy has increased to 76.5 years for white Americans (72.5 for men, 78.9 for women). This compares with 69.6 for nonwhite males and females (USDHHS, 1998). Although life expectancies have been increasing, a variety of factors have caused those figures to level off in recent years. These include unhealthy lifestyles; societal problems, such as deaths caused by firearms, substance abuse,

---

DISPLAY 30–1. The World's "Oldest" Countries—1999

	Percentage of population age 65 and over (%)
Italy	17
Sweden	17
Norway	16
Greece	16
Belgium	16
Spain	16
Bulgaria	16
Japan	16
Germany	16
United Kingdom	16
France	16
Portugal	15
Denmark	15
Austria	15
Hungary	15
Switzerland	15
Finland	15
Luxembourg	14
Czech Republic	14
Ukraine	14
Belarus	13
Netherlands	13
Russia	13
United States*	**13**

*Twenty-two countries have a greater percentage of people over 65 than does the United States.
(From World Population Data Sheet. [1999]. Population Reference Bureau. Available: www.prb.org.)

and human immunodeficiency virus/acquired immunodeficiency syndrome (HIV/AIDS); and the rise of Alzheimer's disease among the elderly.

However, older people are healthier than ever before. Although statistics indicate people in the United States aged 65 years have 14.8 (men) to 19.5 (women) years of life remaining, it is estimated that only 9.5 of those years will be disability free (Burke & Walsh, 1997; National Institute on Aging, 1996). Increasing numbers of capable elderly people older than 65 are living independently, and **hearty elderly**—people older than 65 who maintain a high level of wellness and activity well above present expectations for that age—are increasing in number. Not only can many people older than 65 maintain independent living, but they can and do contribute to society and become involved in community programs and activities. Some have become valuable volunteers, helping others in such community activities as foster grandparents and literacy programs for adults, working in libraries and homeless shelters, or providing services such as Meals on Wheels.

Not only are more people living into old age, but also, once they get there, they are living longer. Specifically, the number of people living into "older" old age (75 years and older) is increasing. Forty percent of elderly people in the United States are among the "oldest old," over age 85, with a projected number of 4.2 million in the year 2000. More than 200,000 claim to be among the **elite-old,** or centenarians. Until the year 2030, the 85-and-older age group is projected to be the most rapidly growing segment of the entire U.S. population (Eliopoulos, 1997). During the early decades of the 21st century, the large cohort of **baby boomers,** those people born between 1945 and 1964, after World War II, will be the major influence on these numbers. As the number of "old-old" people increases, so, too, will the need for assistance with activities of daily living (ADL). Many will be among the **frail elderly,** those older than 85 who need assistance in attending to activities of daily living, such as dressing, eating, toileting, and bathing. Even now, about half of those over age 85 need some help with daily activities.

Other statistics on older adults may also help community health nurses anticipate the psychosocial needs of the older population. Most older men (76%) live out their years with their spouse and thus have someone for companionship, whereas almost 60% of older women are widowed, single, or divorced (Staab & Hodges, 1996). In fact, there are five times as many widows (8 million) as widowers (1.5 million) in the United States, and the incidence of widowhood increases with advancing age. Community health nurses should anticipate the needs of many older adults (particularly women) who will face the loss of a spouse, helpmate, and companion and may experience loneliness, social isolation, and depression.

Only 6% of all older adults live in institutions, with the overwhelming majority of older people living in family settings (Atchley, 1997). Two thirds (66%) of older adults live within 30 minutes of an adult child. Approximately 80% of older adults have seen one of their children within the previous week. These figures contradict the popular notion of abandoned elderly who have been forgotten or neglected by their families (Atchley, 1997).

In the total U.S. population, almost twice as many women (16%) as men (8%) live below the poverty level, and this trend continues into old age (Miller, 1999). More than one eighth (12.9%) of older Americans are poor, and many live in profound poverty. They are unable to afford clothing, recreation, transportation, or other items that most people consider necessary for mental health, social status, and continued personal growth. The differences among various ethnic groups experiencing poverty in old age are broad. Among white older adults, approximately 10% live below the poverty level, whereas in the African-American community, 30% of elders live in poverty, as do 23% of Hispanic elders (Miller, 1999). In no other age group is there such a variance of assets, with 20% of the nation's elderly holding 50% of all assets held by this age group.

The education level of the older population is increasing. The percentage of older adults who have completed high school or a higher level of education is 66.7% (whites), 37% (African-American), and 30% (Hispanic) (Miller, 1999). These figures are predicted to change as the United States witnesses a trend toward a more educated senior population because of the significant numbers of baby boomers who completed high school and entered college during and since the 1960s.

DISPELLING AGEISM

Stereotyping older adults and perpetuating false information and negative images and characteristics regarding older adults is called **ageism.** These stereotypes often arise from negative personal experience, myths shared throughout the ages, and a general lack of current information. Ageism can interfere with effective practice and prevent the kind of comprehensive and interdisciplinary service aging persons need and deserve.

Misconceptions About Older Adults

Community health nurses must guard against ageism in their practice by dispelling common misconceptions.

MISCONCEPTION: MOST OLDER ADULTS CANNOT LIVE INDEPENDENTLY

On the contrary, 94% of the elderly live in the community, outside formal facilities or institutions. Some live alone or with friends, and others may live in the homes of nonrelatives where room and board are provided. In some homes, assistance in activities of daily living is provided. There are also alternative-housing arrangements—group-living situations for older adults in which many types of housing arrangements and care possibilities are offered. This concept is not new, but these centers are being built now in greater numbers to meet the needs of a growing segment of the older adult population. These situations are well suited to those who desire such comprehensive living choices and have the financial means for the housing and care arrangements provided.

Most elders who are vigorous and functioning independently live in their own homes. Only 6% live in institutions, such as skilled nursing facilities, extended care facilities, supervised living facilities, and Alzheimer's disease centers, and not all of these are permanent residents. Many are recovering from illnesses or rehabilitating from injuries and/or surgeries and will return to their living situation in the community within weeks.

MISCONCEPTION: CHRONOLOGICAL AGE DETERMINES OLDNESS

Older people are quite distinct from one another in the aging process, and they age at widely disparate rates (Bortz, 1996). Some people at age 85 still play golf, drive a car, and participate in social and community activities; others are frail and cannot move about well. Physical, social, and mental health parameters, life experiences, and genetic traits all combine to make aging an individualized process (see Levels of Prevention).

MISCONCEPTION: MOST ELDERLY HAVE DIMINISHED INTELLECTUAL CAPACITY OR ARE SENILE

Studies show that intelligence, learning ability, and other intellectual and cognitive skills do not decline with age.

LEVELS OF PREVENTION

SUCCESSFUL RETIREMENT

GOAL
Client will have a healthy transition into a satisfying retirement.

PRIMARY PREVENTION
Early preparation—emotional, financial. Avocation planning (preretirement workshops, support groups, financial planning).

SECONDARY PREVENTION
Celebration activity, reflect on contributions to the workforce, organization of new free time; allow time for adaptation to this life transition.

TERTIARY PREVENTION
Adaptation to changed roles with spouse and significant others, maintenance of health, participation in avocational activities, assess increasing dependency needs including alternative housing, modifications in transportation, and changing health care needs. Periodically review and update will, insurances, and other important documents as needed; keep beneficiaries or executors aware of changes in and location of documents and personal wishes regarding funeral and burial arrangements.

Cognitive deficits are caused by certain risk factors. Nutritional status has been singled out as a physical health variable that influences cognitive functioning, particularly memory performance, regardless of a person's age. Anticholinergic ingredients that are present in many medications can interfere with memory and cognitive functioning. In healthy, mentally stimulated, older adults, deficits are generally minimal and probably not even noticed. Speed of reaction tends to decrease with age, but basic intelligence does not. In fact, some abilities are viewed collectively as crystallized intelligence. Wisdom, judgment, vocabulary, creativity, common sense, coordination of facts and ideas, and breadth of knowledge and experience actually improve with age (Miller, 1999). Most older people are largely capable of making their own decisions; they want and need the freedom to make choices and to be as independent as their limitations will allow.

Senility, although not a legitimate medical diagnosis, is a term widely used by health professionals and lay people alike to denote deteriorating mental faculties associated with old age. Yet fewer than 1% of people aged 65 years, and only 18% of people older than 75 years, are affected by cognitive impairment, dementia, or Alzheimer's disease (AD). In addition, these are all physiologic consequences of disease processes (Hewett & Chang, 1998). Alzheimer's disease as a growing community health problem is discussed in more detail later in this chapter. Although most cases of cognitive impairment are not treatable, 10% to 20% of them may be reversible. These include problems caused by drug toxicity, metabolic disorders, depression, or hyperthyroidism (Miller, 1999).

Certainly, Alzheimer's disease and arteriosclerosis cause memory loss and altered behavior in the elderly, but many older adults may have similar symptoms because of anxiety, losses, grief, or just from changes in their routine. These reactions need to be diagnosed by health care providers and differentiated from disease processes.

MISCONCEPTION: ALL OLDER PEOPLE ARE CONTENT AND SERENE

The picture of Grandma sitting serenely in her rocker with her hands folded in her lap is misleading. It is true that many older people have learned to accept rather than fight the hardships and vicissitudes of life. Yet, for most people, advancing age brings increasing physical, social, and financial problems to harass and worry them. Depression, which may be a problem among the elderly, may sometimes be confused with dementia because of such symptoms as disorientation, failing memory, and eccentric behavior. However, one must not forget that, to attain the status of senior citizen (meaning one who has survived 65 years or more of living), one has had a great deal of strength, tenacity, adaptation, and a sense of humor about many of the trials, tribulations, and absurdities in life. These people are survivors, and survivors do not always sit contentedly in a rocking chair on the sidelines of life.

MISCONCEPTION: OLDER ADULTS CANNOT BE PRODUCTIVE OR ACTIVE

More than two thirds (between 65% and 68% since the mid-1980s) of the male work force retire before age 65. In contrast, the participation rate for women between 45 and 64 continually rose through 1997 (Fronstin, 1999). Some reasons for early retirement include health, availability of private pension benefits, social expectations, and long-held plans to do something else with their time (Staab & Hodges, 1996). These additional years give older adults time for travel, volunteering, and hobbies. This "third phase of life" is a gift of the 20th century available for people to pursue these and other interests. Many older retired adults care for grandchildren, great-grandchildren, or even their very old surviving parent. One fifth of women older than 65 have a living parent who is 85 or older and needs some degree of assistance.

More than 4 million Americans older than 65 work full or part time, and many others, not included in labor statistics, work but do not report their earnings. One example includes the grandmother who chooses to give up full-time employment in an unsatisfying job to babysit for three preschool grandchildren and is paid in cash by her two children. The grandmother gets to spend time with growing grandchildren and not lose all income potential, the parents feel comfortable that their children are being cared for by a loving family member, and the grandchildren are experiencing the joy of being with their grandparents. In another situation, active retired older adults assist with their two children's businesses. The mother types legal documents for the son's law practice during busy times, and the father helps out on Saturdays in the daughter's pool supply store. Everyone wins in these situations.

Healthy older people generally do not disengage or withdraw and isolate themselves from society; rather, they are active and involved. Remaining active, through a daily routine, organized purposeful behavior, and a positive view of life, produces the best psychological climate for the elderly (Bortz, 1996).

MISCONCEPTION: ALL OLDER ADULTS ARE RESISTANT TO CHANGE

People at any age can learn new information and skills. Research indicates that older people can learn new skills and improve old ones, including how to use a computer (Finn, 1997). The elderly have spent a lifetime adapting to change, with varying measures of success. People over 65 years old grew up in an age when having an automobile was a luxury and many did not have a television, microwave oven, or VCR until they were in middle adulthood. Elders learned to adapt to these changes, and they are becoming increasingly computer literate today. The ability to change does not depend on age but rather on personality traits acquired throughout life or, sometimes, on socioeconomic difficulties. For example, an elder on a fixed income may be faced with inflationary costs. This may cause the elder to vote against a school levy

that would increase taxes, when he or she would support schools if finances were different.

MISCONCEPTION: SOCIAL SECURITY WON'T BE THERE WHEN I RETIRE

The Social Security fund is healthy! Although the government has borrowed from it, the amount the fund has accumulated is huge—over $566 billion at the end of 1996—and still growing (Quinn, 1997). Money still pours into it from payrolls, and not until 2019 will Social Security have to start tapping the trust fund to meet obligations. Around 2029, the fund will be exhausted, but even at that point, payroll tax revenues will be enough to pay 75% of everyone's benefits for the next 75 years.

Even with this system secure, most people who reach retirement age in the next few decades have experienced a lifestyle well beyond what Social Security benefits are scheduled to pay to retirees. This necessitates that people plan for retirement early and contribute to retirement plans at work or establish their own retirement fund if self-employed, invest, and save regularly. This would guarantee multiple sources of income at the time of retirement and provide the resources necessary so decisions about when to start or how to spend one's retirement can be based on personal preference, not on a restricted and fixed Social Security check.

Characteristics of Healthy Older Adults

No one knows conclusively all of the variables that influence healthy aging, but it is known that a lifetime of healthy habits and circumstances, a strong social support system, and a positive emotional outlook all significantly influence the resources people bring to their later years. Most people recognize a healthy older person when they meet one.

What is healthy old age? As we said earlier, the vast majority (94%) of the elderly, even those with chronic diseases and other disabilities, are living outside institutions and are relatively independent. Their ability to function is a key indicator of health and wellness and is an important factor in understanding healthy aging. Good health in the elderly means maintaining the maximum degree possible of physical, mental, and social vigor. It means being able to adapt, to continue to handle stress, and to be active and involved in life and living. In short, healthy aging means being able to function, even when disabled, with a minimum of ordinary help from others (USDHHS, 1991, 2000).

Wellness among the older population varies considerably. It is influenced by many factors, including personality traits, life experiences, current physical health, and current societal supports. Some elderly people demonstrate maximum adaptability, resourcefulness, optimism, and activity (Display 30–2). Others, often those from whom we tend to draw our stereotypes, have disengaged and present a picture of dependence and resignation. Most of the elderly population fall somewhere in between those two extremes. Although the level of wellness varies among the elderly, that level can be raised. The challenge in community health nursing is to maximize the wellness potential of the elderly. Nurses must analyze and capitalize on an older person's strengths rather than focus on the difficulties. The goal is to enable older people to thrive, not merely survive (Eliopoulos, 1997; Miller, 1999).

HEALTH NEEDS OF OLDER ADULTS

Effective nursing in any population requires familiarity with that group's health problems and needs. Aging in and of itself is not a health problem. Rather, aging is a normal, irreversible physiologic process. Its pace, however, can sometimes be delayed, as researchers are discovering (Bortz, 1996), and many of the problems associated with aging can be prevented (Staab & Hodges, 1996). The aging process is subtle, gradual, and lifelong. One can see remarkable differences among different individuals' rates of aging. Even in a single individual, various systems of the body age differently (Bortz, 1996; Eliopoulos, 1997). Thus, chronologic age cannot serve as an indicator of health needs, however, the proportion of people with health problems increases with age, and as a group older adults are more likely than younger ones to suffer from multiple, chronic, and often disabling conditions.

The elderly, like any age group, have certain basic needs: physiologic and safety needs as well as the need for love and belonging, self-esteem, and self-actualization. Their physi-

cal, emotional, and social needs are complex and interrelated. Here, we discuss them according to primary, secondary, and tertiary prevention activities.

Primary Prevention

As discussed earlier in this text, primary prevention activities involve those actions that keep one healthy. Health education, follow-through of sound personal health practices, and maintaining an immunization schedule will ensure that older adults are doing all that they can to maintain their health. The National Institute on Aging (1997) has identified "10 Tips for Healthy Aging," which focus on primary prevention, and Bortz (1996) identifies several strategies for aging successfully (Display 30–3).

NUTRITION NEEDS

People who have maintained sound dietary habits throughout life have little need to change in old age. Many have not established such habits but may wish to. It is generally believed

---

DISPLAY 30–2. Profile of a Healthy Older Adult

Minerva Blackstone, affectionately called Minnie by her friends, is a lively 87-year-old woman who enjoys life. Every day, except in bad weather, she walks a half mile to visit her granddaughter, Karen. There she works on the quilt, which is stretched on a frame, that she is making for Karen. In addition, twice a week Minnie takes the city bus to the senior citizens' center to join her friends in an exercise class. Although her eyesight has somewhat diminished, Minnie enjoys reading in the evening or crocheting while she watches television. Mysteries and comedies are her favorite kinds of stories.

She is not content, however, unless she is up on the latest political developments. She always has opinions on current events and expresses them with vigorous shakes of her curly white hair at her monthly group meeting on women and politics. She has a good appetite and generally sleeps well. Minor arthritis does not hamper her activities, nor does the hypertension that she controls by taking her medication with conscientious regularity. Minnie is enjoying a healthy, successful old age.

DISPLAY 30–3. Strategies for Successful Aging

1. Do at least 30 minutes of sustained, rhythmic, vigorous exercise four times a week.
2. Eat "like a bushman" (a healthy diet of fruits, whole grains, vegetables, and lean meat).
3. Get as much sleep and rest as needed.
4. Maintain a sense of humor and deflect anger.
5. Set goals and accept challenges that force you to be as alive and creative as possible.
6. Don't depend on anyone else for your well-being.
7. Be necessary and responsible; live outside yourself (give to others, become involved).
8. Don't slow down. Stick with the mainstream. Avoid the shadows. Stay together. Maintain energy flow in a purposeful direction; aging need not be characterized by losses. Maintain contacts with family and friends, and stay active through work, recreation, and community.
9. Get regular check-ups.
10. Don't smoke—it's never too late to quit.
11. Practice safety habits at home to prevent falls and fractures—always wear seat belts when traveling by car.
12. Avoid overexposure to the sun and the cold.
13. If you drink, moderation is the key—when you drink, let someone else drive.
14. Keep personal and financial records in order to simplify budgeting and investing—plan long-term housing and financial needs.
15. Keep a positive attitude toward life—do things that make you happy.

that older people need to maintain their optimal weight by eating a diet that contains low fats, moderate carbohydrates, and high protein. Foods with "empty calories" such as salty snacks, candy, fatty foods, and alcohol should be limited because they meet a hunger need by satisfying appetite while providing little nutrition. However, John E. Morley (1994) of the division of geriatric medicine at St. Louis University states that as people age (70 and older), the need for calories increases. He states, "Over age 70 there is no need to be on a diet except to eat anything you can. [In fact,] older fat women [among skilled nursing home inhabitants he has studied] live longer than older thin women."

Most people can keep their teeth for a lifetime with optimal personal, professional, and population-based preventive practices. Yet in 1997, 26% of adults 65 to 74 years old had all their teeth extracted. The *Healthy People 2010* target is to reduce this number to 20% (USDHHS, 2000). Since the 1960s, water supplies and toothpastes have been fluoridated and regular dental care has become more accessible and acceptable to most people, all of which has helped prevent periodontal disease, a major component of tooth loss in adults. Oral health and hygiene needs do not decrease with age. Eating, chewing, and swallowing should be an uncomplicated and natural process (Meadows, 1999). Frequently, older adults are on medications that cause dry mouth, taste alterations, and loss of appetite that limit the desire for food. Eating should remain a pleasurable social experience, preferably taking place in the company of others. Community health nurses can assist older adults with meal management by following the suggestions outlined in Display 30–4.

In addition to maintaining a healthy diet, older adults should avoid habitual use of laxatives, adding instead more fiber and bulk to their diet. Inadequate fluid intake often contributes to bowel and bladder problems. Consuming a diet that includes six to eight 8-oz glasses of water a day will assist the gastrointestinal and genitourinary system in their functions. Also, more exercise will help keep an older adult's bowel patterns regular.

EXERCISE NEEDS

Older adults need to exercise; in fact, they thrive when exercise is incorporated into their daily routine. Research shows that exercise can slow the loss of bone density and increase the size and strength of muscles, including the heart (Mayo Clinic, 1999). Aging does not and should not involve passivity; instead, physical activity and movement contribute to the quality of intellectual and physical performance in old age. Exercise, such as a daily walk, can keep muscles in good tone, enhance circulation, and promote mental health. Exercise may occur in connection with such activities as homemaking chores, gardening, hobbies, or recreation and sports. Often, such physical outlets are done in the company of other people, which meets social and emotional needs as well. Preparing for exercise by warming up helps to keep muscles free from injury and helps to prevent falls (Schoenfelder & Van Why, 1997; Tibbits, 1996). Even among the very old, an

---

DISPLAY 30–4. Meal Management Considerations

- Complete a safety check with the older adult to assess the ability to operate stoves and microwave ovens. Include the elder's ability to reach, and put things on and off stove burners.
- Arrange cupboards so commonly used items can be reached from an easy standing level. Suggest use of turntables and long-handled "grabbers" while discouraging use of stepstools or ladders.
- Assess the elder's typical meal for quality and availability.
- To ensure that elders eat an appropriate number of times a day, suggest that they "eat by the clock" or with a certain TV show.
- Help older adults build support system for sharing grocery shopping, cooking, and meals. Suggest they bake once a week for an activity.
- Suggest buying convenience foods, making sure they have nutritional value, such as frozen vegetables or dinners.
- Consider community resources to assist with shopping, transportation, or meal preparation as needed. Keeping a continuous shopping list helps elders remember needed grocery items and provides a reference if someone offers to assist with shopping.
- Help elders consider increasing socialization by eating out with friends, selecting restaurants that are physically and financially accessible.

(Adapted from Bonnel, W.B. [January, 1999]. Meal management strategies of older adult women. *Journal of Gerontological Nursing, 25,* 41–47.)

---

exercise routine that includes activities that improve strength, flexibility, and coordination may also indirectly, but effectively, decrease the incidence of osteoporotic fractures by lessening the likelihood of falling (American College of Sports Medicine, 1995; Burghardt, 1999).

ECONOMIC SECURITY NEEDS

Economic security is another major need for older adults. Worrying about finances is often one of the most debilitating factors in old age. Fearing the potential costs of major illness and not wanting to be a burden on family or friends, many older people will conserve their limited finances by establishing frugal eating patterns, using health resources sparingly, taking medications in partial doses, and spending little on themselves. Too often, the fear, let alone the reality, of financial difficulties prevents older adults from leading full and active lives.

For older adults today, living many years past retirement and perhaps not planning for financial security to maintain them throughout these additional, unexpected, years, the fears are not unfounded. Putting older people in touch with appropriate community resources can do much to relieve the source of that stress and anxiety. The community health nurse can also help the younger, working adult plan for a physically and emotionally, as well as financially, vigorous old age (Fronstin, 1999).

PSYCHOSOCIAL NEEDS

All human beings have psychosocial needs that must be met in order for lives to be rich and fulfilling. Without other people and healthy relationships with them, life can be very lonely and lacking quality for many elderly. With advancing age, the psychosocial issues are many. A major issue is coping with multiple losses, discussed below. In addition, maintaining independence, social interaction, companionship, and purpose is necessary for a healthy old age. Older adults who have maintained good health and have developed a supportive system of family and friends have a more fulfilled life.

Coping With Multiple Losses

Elders experience multiple losses—loss of income and prestige from a career once practiced or the economic stability of an enjoyable job; space needs change and larger residences are often replaced by much smaller homes or apartments; and health and vitality may change and limited movement or pain may be a daily concern, which may necessitate another move to a more dependent setting. Repetitive losses occur as significant others, relatives, friends, and acquaintances die.

Inadequate coping with the compounding losses can make an older person believe that life holds no meaning (Moore et al., 1999). Depression may be a difficult problem for older adults. Social and emotional withdrawal can often occur, as can suicide. Although older populations have a much lower rate of suicide attempts than younger age groups, the rate of completed suicide is high. It is the highest among elderly men, who account for about 80% of suicides age 65 and older. Moreover, elderly white males have a suicide rate six times the national average (Moscicki et al., 1998). Concern for the increased suicide rates among older white men led to a key health objective in *Healthy People 2000:* By the year 2000, the goal was to reduce the suicide rate to 38.9 per 100,000 from 46.1, which was the rate in 1987 (USDHHS, 1991). In 1997, for white males aged 65+, the rate was 35.5 per 100,000, exceeding the 2000 goal 3 years early. Suicide continues to be of concern and is included in the *Healthy People 2010* objectives (USDHHS, 2000). Because most elderly have visited their primary care provider in the month before their suicides, recognition and treatment of depression in health care settings is a promising way to prevent elderly suicide.

Mortality after bereavement is high and can be prevented through nursing intervention. Loss and the mourning process among elders have been examined in many studies. It has been found that crucial to successful aging is the ability to mourn prior states of one's self and the past. This can be liberating and can give energy for current living, including planning for the future (Pollock, 1987). Although men and women experienced similar levels of depression during early

bereavement, it was more difficult for widowers to seek and receive social support. Higher levels of perceived social support were associated with lower levels of depression in widows and widowers (Kanacki, Jones & Galbraith, 1996). In addition, Bowling and Windsor (1995) followed widowed older adults for up to 13 years and found more men died closer to the death of their spouses than women. Women had stronger social support systems throughout their lives, sustaining them during losses in old age.

In addition to preventing early deaths after the loss of a spouse, the greater goal for the nurse in promoting successful aging can be accomplished when the nurse recognizes the significance of accepting all the losses of aging. The loss of a spouse is much more frequent for women than for men (Eliopoulos, 1997). With this knowledge, a woman can age successfully by planning for the future through anticipatory guidance, with the help of a community health nurse. Actually, many women can expect to live alone up to 20 years at the end of their life. This is due to a longer life expectancy compounded with the fact that women in most cultures marry men older than themselves. The nurse can help to make these years meaningful and as healthy as possible.

Maintaining Independence

Older people need independence, and those who stay independent are happier ("Full-Life Counselors," 1998). As much as possible, the elderly need to make their own decisions and manage their own lives. Even those with activity limitations because of disability can still exercise decision-making options about many, if not most, aspects of their daily living. The need for autonomy—to be able to assert ourselves as separate individuals—is great for all of us. With life's restrictions ever increasing for the elderly person, this need is all the greater (Eliopoulos, 1997). Independence helps to meet the need for self-respect and dignity. The elderly need to have their ideas and suggestions heard and acted on and to be addressed by their preferred names in a respectful tone of voice. Respect for the older adult is not a strong value in the American culture, but it is highly valued in Asians, Italians, Hispanics, and Native Americans. Older people represent a rich resource of wisdom, experience, and patience that is generally wasted in the United States.

Social Interaction, Companionship, and Purpose

Older people need companionship and social interaction, particularly when they live alone. The company of other people as well as the companionship of a household pet offers avenues for expression and response and adds meaning to life (Jorgenson, 1997). Many studies of mortality patterns demonstrate that older adults living together have a greater survival rate and retain their independence longer than those who live alone (Miller, 1999). The problem is of greatest significance for women, who outnumber men considerably in the later years and who live alone more frequently.

It is also important for older adults without companions to discover and develop a friendship with someone who can be considered a **confidant,** someone in whom the older adult can confide, reflect on the past, and trust. It could be a close friend, a sibling, a son or daughter, or an acquaintance. This person is usually seen daily or talked with on the telephone each week. In particular, mothers and daughters form confidant bonds (Martin Matthews, 1991). In one study, many women considered a sibling a confidant, especially if that person lived close by; this was especially true for childless and single women (Connidis & Davies, 1992).

Meaningful activity is another need of the elderly that adds purpose to life. Some kind of active role in community life is essential for mental health, satisfaction, and self-esteem. These activities can range from involvement in hobbies, such as gardening or crafts, to volunteer work or even full-time employment. One current example is the federally supported Foster Grandparents and Senior Companions programs that engage the help of more than 20,000 seniors. These older adults work part-time offering companionship and guidance to handicapped children, the terminally ill, and other people in need. Senior Partners is another program that keeps older adults involved. Volunteers earn service credits by providing support services so persons aged 60 or older can remain independent and active in their own homes. Each hour of volunteer service earns one service credit. Credits may be "spent" in several ways. They can be used to obtain services, should the volunteer need them, or they can be donated to another person in need or donated back to Senior Partners to help others.

Additional volunteering opportunities abound. Internationally, many older professionals join the Peace Corps. Initially started in the early 1960s, people of all ages have worked for 2-year periods in global communities in need of services to improve their personal health, education, environment, and the larger community. On the national level, the newer AmeriCorps*VISTA (Volunteers in Service to America) programs are similar, but with a 1-year commitment; the volunteer lives among and at the economic level of the low-income people in the United States served by its projects. Retired people can volunteer, donating their skills, to help others at a time in their lives when they transition from employment to retirement or to fill active retirement years. The RSVP (Retired and Senior Volunteer Program) engages seniors in a bevy of activities designed to improve people's lives and the environment. EASI (Environmental Alliance for Senior Involvement) sponsors various environment-focused programs, such as assisting the Hawk Mountain Sanctuary, protecting birds of prey or monitoring streams and other waterways for cleanliness.

Many older adults choose not to engage in long-term volunteering, and other programs are more appropriate for them. Elderhostel, Inc., is a nonprofit organization with 25 years of experience providing high-quality, affordable, educational adventures for adults who are 55 and older. They offer short-term educational programs that are fun and exciting for seniors to share new ideas, explore new places, and make new friends. In 1998, 175,000 adults took advantage of the unique experiences that Elderhostel has to offer (Elderhostel, 1999). The success of this program is based on the fact that learning is a lifelong process that is rewarding at any age. Elderhostel is inspired by the youth hostels and folk schools of Europe, but guided by the needs of older citizens.

SAFETY NEEDS

People of all ages have safety needs, and this concept has been threaded throughout the five chapters in this unit on developmental needs of clients. Likewise, safety issues are a major concern among older adults and the community health nurses who work with them. Several areas of safety focus are discussed here: personal health and safety, home safety, and community safety.

Personal health and safety include three major areas: immunizations, fall prevention, and drug safety. Immunizations are not just for children. Older adults are at risk for not only the diseases of influenza and pneumonia but dying from them. Pneumococcal disease, influenza, and hepatitis B account for more than 45,000 deaths annually, mostly among older adults. Ninety percent of influenza-related deaths occur in people aged 65 and over (Thurm, 1998). In September 1997 the U.S. Department of Health and Human Services approved an agency-wide plan to improve adult immunization rates and reduce disparities among racial and ethnic minorities (USDHHS, 2000). Immunizations protect more than the at-risk population—they protect society as a whole (Thurm, 1998). People with chronic illnesses, such as diabetes and asthma, at any age and people over 65 should be encouraged to receive a yearly flu vaccine and the pneumonia vaccine, which is recommended every 5 years.

Approximately 30% to 40% of people over age 65 who are independent and living on their own fall each year (Schoenfelder & Van Why, 1997; Tibbits, 1996). Falls in this age group account for 250,000 hip fractures each year (see Research: Bridge to Practice). Causative factors involve both environmental hazards and host issues. Fall prevention, which involves education, strengthening and balance exercises, medication evaluation, and environmental improvements, is an important part of the role of the community health nurse. Using a home safety checklist can give the nurse a baseline of information from which to begin teaching (Display 30–5).

A significant safety issue for the older adult arises from adverse drug effects. Older people may need to take several medications to control the effects of chronic conditions, and their bodies may react differently from those of younger people (on whom most new drugs are tested). It is not unusual for older people to be taking four to six medications daily and filling 13 prescriptions each year (Hobson, 1992). It is estimated that 25% to 40% of all U.S. prescriptions are written for older adults (Walker & Foreman, 1999). Thus, multiple medications or complicated drug regimens for many older people can lead to unexpected and dangerous drug interactions. The elderly need education about the drugs they take and their possible effects. They also need proper supervision of their overall medication intake. This is an area in which

RESEARCH Bridge to Practice

Older Adults: Preventing Disability and Falls

Wagner, E. H., LaCroix, A. Z., Grothaus, L., Leveille, S. G., Hecht, J. A., Artz, K., Odle, K., & Buchner, D. M. (1994). Preventing disability and falls in older adults in Los Angeles population-based randomized trial. *American Journal of Public Health, 84,* 1800–1806.

The purpose of this CDC grant-supported study was to test a multicomponent intervention program to prevent disability and falls in ambulatory older adults. Morbidity associated with advanced age can be delayed or compressed by interventions to prevent disability; this is a national priority.

More than 1550 ambulatory adults 65 years and older were randomly selected from health maintenance organization (HMO) enrollees. They were randomly placed in one of three groups: group one (N = 635) received a nurse assessment visit and followup interventions targeting risk factors for disability and falls; group two (N = 317) received a general health promotion nurse visit; and group three (N = 607) received the usual care (the control group). The average age of the subjects was 73, 59% were female, 93% were white, and 25% held college degrees. Data collection consisted of a baseline and two annual followup surveys.

The findings indicated that after 1 year, group one subjects reported a significantly lower incidence of declining functional status and a significantly lower incidence of falls than group three subjects. Group two subjects had intermediate levels of most outcomes. However, after 2 years of follow-up the differences narrowed.

The results of this study suggest that a modest, one-time prevention program appeared to confer short-term health benefits on ambulatory HMO clients, although the benefits diminished by the second year of follow-up if the intervention was not sustained over time. The recommendations are to intensify and sustain a disability and fall prevention/intervention without making costs prohibitively expensive for community health application.

---

the community health nurse can intervene very effectively and with much success.

Safety in the community is an additional concern. Safety involves pedestrian and driving issues, fear of and crime against elders, and environmental factors such as sun exposure, pollution, heat, and cold.

Because of age-related changes in vision, hearing, mobility, and the effects of polypharmacy, elders are at risk in the community as pedestrians and drivers. Automobile crashes and pedestrian injuries can be life-threatening events when elders are involved. As pedestrians, elders must be increasingly vigilant of traffic patterns, sidewalk irregularities, and the possibility of being a victim of street crime. Often out of necessity and pride, elders drive longer than their ability permits. In 1997, older adults made up 10% of the licensed driving population but accounted for 14% of all traffic fatalities and 17% of all pedestrian fatalities. On the basis of estimated annual travel, the fatality rate for drivers aged 85 and over is nine

times as high as the rate for drivers 25 through 69 years of age (U.S. Department of Transportation, 1998). To stop driving is usually a difficult and painful decision for the elder to make. At times, the keys may have to be taken from the elder for the safety of the elder and others, especially elders with dementia, Alzheimer's disease, uncorrectable vision problems, or stroke-related physical or cognitive after-effects.

Actual crime against elders in the community is 50% lower than among other segments of the population (Vander Zanden, 1993). However, the fear of crime among elders is perceived as a major issue by 74% of the general public, and about 25% of elders consider the fear of crime a major concern (Benson, 1997). Display 30–6 lists client-centered nursing interventions designed to reduce fear among older adults and empower them to feel safer in their communities.

Environmental factors can have an effect on the health and safety of elders when they are outside. Sun exposure, pollution, and exposure to heat and cold can have negative effects on older adults. They are just as vulnerable as infants and children to climatic changes and should take a variety of preventive measures, including using sun block when gardening, reading, or walking outside for more than 10 minutes, even on days with an overcast sky; staying indoors on days when the air quality is poor or there is an air safety alert; drinking additional fluids, wearing protective covering, and limiting outdoor activities and exposure on days with elevated temperatures; and, conversely, limiting outdoor exposure and wearing appropriate winter clothing, especially layers of clothes, on cold, snowy, or icy days. Teaching geographically and seasonally appropriate safety precautions is the responsibility of the community health nurse providing services to groups of elders in the community.

SPIRITUALITY, ADVANCE DIRECTIVES, AND PREPARING FOR DEATH

A final need of the elderly, and one that is receiving increasing attention, is that of preparing for a dignified death. Elisabeth Kübler-Ross (1975) describes death as the final stage of growth and one that deserves the same measure of quality as other stages of life. Many older people fear death as an experience of pain, humiliation, discomfort, or financial concerns for their loved ones. Planning for a dignified death is an important issue for many older people. For most, this includes choosing, if possible, where and under what circumstances death will occur, being free of financial worries, knowing that their affairs and their family members are taken care of, having the opportunity to receive spiritual counseling, and dying in peaceful surroundings, preferably at home with the support of loved ones.

Some elders make arrangements with a funeral home of their choice, selecting interment or cremation, memorial service or celebration of life gathering, music selections, and other personal details rather than leaving these choices to their family. Other older adults place less emphasis on the rituals, as demonstrated by one elder who left these choices to her children by telling them, "Surprise me!"

DISPLAY 30–5. Guidelines for Assessing the Safety of the Environment

Illumination and Color Contrast
- Is the lighting adequate but not glare producing?
- Are the light switches easy to reach and manipulate?
- Can lights be turned on before entering rooms?
- Are nightlights used in appropriate places?
- Is color contrast adequate between objects such as a chair and floor?

Hazards
- Are there throw rugs, highly polished floors, or other hazardous floor coverings?
- If area rugs are used, do they have a nonslip backing and are the edges tacked to the floor?
- Are there cords, clutter, or other obstacles in pathways?
- Is there a pet that is likely to be running underfoot?

Furniture
- Are chairs the right height and depth for the person?
- Do the chairs have arm rests?
- Are tables stable and of the appropriate height?
- Is small furniture placed well away from pathways?

Stairways
- Is lighting adequate?
- Are there light switches at the top and bottom of the stairs?
- Are there securely fastened handrails on both sides of the stairway?
- Are all the steps even?
- Are the treads nonskid?
- Should colored tape be used to mark the edges of the steps, particularly the top and bottom steps?

Bathroom
- Are grab bars placed appropriately for the tub and toilet?
- Does the tub have skidproof strips or a rubber mat in the bottom?
- Has the person considered using a tub seat?
- Is the height of the toilet seat appropriate?
- Has the person considered using an elevated toilet seat?
- Does the color of the toilet seat contrast with surrounding colors?
- Is toilet paper within easy reach?

Temperature
- Is the temperature of the room(s) comfortable?
- Can the person read the markings on the thermostat and adjust it appropriately?
- During cold months, is the room temperature high enough to prevent hypothermia?

- During hot weather, is the room temperature cool enough to prevent hyperthermia?

Overall Safety
- How does the person obtain objects from hard-to-reach places?
- How does the person change overhead light bulbs?
- Are doorways wide enough to accommodate assistive devices?
- Do door thresholds create hazardous conditions?
- Are telephones accessible, especially for emergency calls?
- Would it be helpful to use a cordless portable phone?
- Would it be helpful to have some emergency call system available?
- Does the person wear sturdy shoes with non-skid soles?
- Are smoke alarms present and operational?
- Is there a carbon monoxide detector (if the house has gas appliances)?
- Does the person keep a list of emergency numbers by the phone?
- Does the person have an emergency exit plan in the event of fire?

Bedroom
- Is the height of the bed appropriate?
- Is the mattress firm at the edges to provide enough support for sitting?
- If the bed has wheels, are they locked securely?
- Would side rails be a help or a hazard?
- When side rails are in the down position, are they completely out of the way?
- Is the pathway between the bedroom and bathroom clear of objects and adequately illuminated, particularly at night?
- Would a bedside commode be useful, especially at night?
- Does the person have sufficient physical and cognitive ability to turn on a light before getting out of bed?
- Is furniture positioned to allow safe use of assistive devices for ambulation?
- Is a telephone situated near the bed?

Kitchen
- Are storage areas used to the best advantage (eg, are objects that are frequently used in the most accessible places)?
- Are appliance cords kept out of the way?
- Are nonslip mats used in front of the sink?
- Are the markings on stoves and other appliances clearly visible?
- Does the person know how to use the microwave oven safely?

(continued)

DISPLAY 30–5. Guidelines for Assessing the Safety of the Environment (Continued)

Assistive Devices
- Is a call light available, and does the person know how to use it?
- What assistive devices are used?

- Would the person benefit from any assistive devices that are not being used?
- Are assistive devices being used safely and properly, or do they present additional hazards?

(Miller, C.A. [1999]. *Nursing care of older adults: Theory and practice* [3rd ed.]. Philadelphia: Lippincott Williams & Wilkins.)

Living wills and medical directives are legal documents whose purpose is to give people legal power over the medical treatment they would want if they became incapacitated or terminally ill. Living wills are legal in all states and the District of Columbia (Miller, 1999). Having such documents prepared and made known among significant others can ensure that the older adult's wishes will be honored.

Secondary Prevention

Secondary prevention focuses on early detection of disease and prompt intervention (see Chapter 1). Much of the community health nurse's time is spent in encouraging individuals to obtain routine screening for diseases such as hypertension or cancer, which, when identified early, are able to be treated successfully. Many nurses are in positions to establish screening programs based on the desires and demographics of the community and agency focus, making them accessible to the population being served.

Older adults need to be encouraged to follow the routine health screening schedule prescribed by their clinic or health care provider. The health screening schedule described in Table 30–1 is based on the recommendations of Kaiser Permanente (1994, 1998), serving millions of clients, and is presented here as a guide. A more comprehensive view of interventions and recommendations for the periodic health examination of people over age 65 has been proposed by the United States Preventive Services Task Force (USPSTF). They have identified age-specific, evidenced-based preventive services guidelines for people age 65 and older, which are outlined in Display 30–7 (U.S. Preventive Services Task Force, 1996).

Tertiary Prevention

Tertiary prevention involves follow-up and rehabilitation as needed after a disease or condition has occurred or been diagnosed and initial treatment has begun. Chronic diseases that are common among older adults, such as congestive heart failure, emphysema, and arthritis, often cannot be prevented but frequently can be postponed into the later years of life through a lifetime of healthy living. However, when they occur, the de-

bilitating symptoms and damaging effects can be controlled through healthy choices encouraged by the community health nurse and recommended by the primary care practitioner.

Although most of the elderly population is healthy, 80% have at least one chronic condition, causing nearly half of the elderly to experience some kind of limitations in activity (Miller, 1999). A small portion suffer more disabling forms of disease, such as chronic obstructive pulmonary disease (COPD), cerebral vascular accidents (CVAs), or cancer or diabetes mellitus (DM), both of which can require more extensive care. The most frequent health problems of older people

---

DISPLAY 30–6. Reducing the Fear of Crime

1. Allow them time to discuss their fears of crime.
2. Facilitate a realistic self-assessment of their ability to avoid crime and to defend themselves.
3. Teach basic safety and security techniques.
4. Correct the elder's sensory losses when possible, such as by getting a hearing aid or glasses.
5. Correct a physical disability when possible, such as treating the pain of arthritis or obtaining physical therapy.
6. Facilitate access to safe, reliable, and affordable transportation.
7. Identify family members, friends, neighbors, or caregivers who can support efforts to leave the home on a more regular basis.
8. Encourage an elder to make a daily telephone or e-mail contact with at least one supportive person.
9. Encourage the elder to get to know his or her neighbors.
10. Encourage elders to travel and conduct community activities and errands together.
11. Encourage participation in local senior centers and other community-based programs.
12. Refer to alternative housing options available for older adults.
13. Provide information on local services that assist and support crime victims.

(Adapted from Benson, S. [1997]. The older adult and fear of crime. *Journal of Gerontological Nursing, 23*[10], 24–31.)

TABLE 30-1. Recommended Health Screening Schedule for Older Adults

Test	Age 50–64	Age 65+	Comments
MEN AND WOMEN			
Blood pressure	1–3 years	Yearly	More often if elevated
Total cholesterol	5 years	5 years	More often if elevated
Flexible sigmoidoscopy	10 years	10 years	
Vision	4 years	2 years	
Hearing	Not recommended	Once	Evaluate at regular health care practitioner visits
WOMEN			
Breast self-examination	Monthly	Monthly	
Pap test	1–3 years	1–3 years*	*May discontinue if prior examinations were normal
Clinical breast examination	1–2 years	1–2 years	
Mammogram	1–2 years	1–2 years	Frequency decided on an individual basis

(Adapted from Kaiser Permanente, 1998, 1994.)

in the community are arthritis, reduced vision, hearing loss, heart disease, peripheral vascular disease, and hypertension. In those older than 65, 40% have blood pressure recordings that are high enough to be considered hypertensive.

ALZHEIMER'S DISEASE

Alzheimer's disease (AD) has been recognized in the medical literature since it was first described by Dr. Alois Alzheimer in a German medical journal in 1907. It is the same illness that produces the majority of cases of progressive dementia in the elderly today (Hewett & Chang, 1998). At age 65, one's risk is about 5% for developing the disease;

by age 75, the risk has increased to about 18%; and by age 85, the risk is substantial and may be as high as 47% (Hewett & Chang, 1998). It is seen as the fourth leading cause of death among the very old in the United States (Margolin, 1994). This disease robs its victims of everything learned in life so they are unable to fall back on preserved intelligence. A simple way to describe the difference between the normal forgetfulness of aging and Alzheimer's disease is seen in the behavior described below.

With advancing age or with increased stress, an individual may say, "Where are my keys? Where did I place them? I can't find them anywhere." After several stressful moments, the

DISPLAY 30-7. Health Maintenance Programs and Services for Older Adults

Resources for Community Health Nurses to Utilize With Clients

- Communication services (phones, emergency access to health care)
- Dental care services
- Dietary guidance and food services (such as Meals on Wheels, commodity programs, or group meal services)
- Escort and protective services
- Exercise and fitness programs
- Financial aid and counseling
- Friendly visiting and companions
- Health education
- Hearing tests and hearing-aid assistance
- Home health services (including skilled nursing and home health aide services)
- Home maintenance assistance (housekeeping, chores, and repairs)
- Legal aid and counseling
- Library services (including tapes and large-print books)
- Medical supplies or equipment
- Medication supervision
- Podiatry services
- Recreational and education programs (community centers, Elderhostel)
- Routine care from selected health care practitioners
- Safe, affordable, and ability-appropriate housing
- Senior citizens' discounts (food, drugs, transportation, banks, retail stores, and recreation)
- Social assistance services offered in conjunction with health maintenance
- Speech or physical therapy
- Spiritual ministries
- Transportation services
- Vision care (prescribing and providing eye glasses; diagnosis and treatment of glaucoma and cataracts)
- Volunteer and employment opportunities (Vista, RSVP)

(Adapted from U.S. Preventive Services Task Force [USPSTF] [1996]. *Guide to clinical preventive services* [2nd ed.]. Baltimore: Williams & Wilkins.)

keys are usually found and the event is over. However, if a person with Alzheimer's disease is handed a set of keys, he or she looks at them blankly, handles them awkwardly, and has no idea what they are for or what to do with them.

Onset is gradual, and verbal memory is often affected first. AD clients lose judgment and reasoning, and safety becomes an issue early in the disease process. Victims of AD may wander away from home and cannot tell anyone exactly where they live, or they may not know that a stove can get hot and may burn themselves when trying to cook. They neglect their health and are even unaware if they are experiencing major health problems.

Probable causes are many. "Promising leads involve the role of neurotransmitters, proteins, genes, metabolism, and environmental suspects" (Hewett & Chang, 1998, p. 486). Discovering the cause and preventing the disease will be a significant achievement that it is hoped will be realized in this century. However, there are currently 16 agents under study, as compared with 90 for cardiovascular disease. The medical community is not putting the amount of effort into research for Alzheimer's as it does into other diseases. This lack of research interest today affects what will be available for those in need tomorrow.

How does this disease affect the role of the community health nurse? Often, until very late in the disease the person is cared for at home. The intense caregiving these clients require drains the reserve of their families. The client demonstrates depression, agitation, sleeplessness, and anxiety, which upset the family's normal routine. In many situations, the main caregiver is an aged spouse. The stress of caregiving puts the caregiver's health at risk as well. The intensity of caregiving is aptly described in a book written for Alzheimer's disease family members, called *The 36 Hour Day* (Mace & Rabins, 1999). Medications may be prescribed but have limited effectiveness. At best, available medications may "turn back the clock by 6 months" and the disease worsens at a slower rate (Margolin, 1994).

The community health nurse is in a position to assess the level of stress on the family, provide them with methods and means to cope and adapt as needed, and make referrals when appropriate. Most communities have resources for clients and their families. They may provide family and caregiver support groups, respite care (see discussion about respite care later in this chapter), counseling, and/or legal and financial consultation. These services are available through local agencies, but there are also government-sponsored national resources that offer information, referral services, and educational materials, all of which can be accessed by the community health nurse and/or families in need. The nurse needs to know that resources are available in order to guide families to them.

ARTHRITIS

Osteoarthritis is the deterioration and abrasion of joint cartilage. It is increasingly seen with advanced age, affecting women more than men. Classic symptoms include aching, stiffness, and limited motion of the involved joint. Discomfort increases with overuse and during damp weather. It is the leading cause of physical disability in older adults (Eliopoulos, 1997). Acetaminophen is the first drug of choice; however, clients often find a combination of medications and daily routines that helps them the most. The nurse can best help these clients by assessing the safety of using a particular regimen and being able to suggest changing treatments as they are developed, including new medications, surgical options for joint replacement, and dietary changes, including vitamins and foods high in essential fatty acids.

Rheumatoid arthritis begins in young adulthood and becomes disabling as the disease continues, causing systemic damage in the later years. This form of arthritis causes inflammation, deformity, and crippling. Rheumatoid arthritis is treated with anti-inflammatory agents, corticosteroids, antimalarial agents, gold salts, and immunosuppressive drugs. Joint discomfort is often relieved by gentle massage, heat, and range-of-motion exercises.

The community health nurse must be aware of the major differences in these two prevalent forms of arthritis. Recommended treatments, including physical therapy, diet, and medications, change as more is discovered about arthritis. The community health nurse must keep current because these conditions are treated in the community and affect a large portion of the older population.

CANCER

Cancers, characterized by the uncontrolled growth and spread of abnormal cells, steadily increase in incidence in aging adults (Staab & Hodges, 1996). "One theory is that as the body ages the immune system deteriorates, losing its ability to serve as a buffer against the abnormal cancer cells that form in the body throughout life" (Staab & Hodges, 1996, p. 414).

It is particularly important for the community health nurse to be aware of the increased incidence of cancer in older clients because they often under-report symptoms that may be early signs of cancer. Thorough assessments in the clinic or on home visits, the participation in screening programs, and encouraging reporting untoward symptoms can help to detect a cancer early, which will give the client the best chance of survival. Following the health care practitioner's recommended schedule for health screening (see Table 30–1) should be encouraged. In addition, being aware of and sharing the American Cancer Society's seven warning signals of cancer with clients can possibly save their life (Display 30–8).

DEPRESSION

Depression in older adults is a major problem. It is frequently related to experiencing major multiple losses, such as the loss related to retirement, a health change, or the death of a significant other. Depression is reported to be higher in women than in men (Kanacki, Jones & Galbraith, 1996). However, as mentioned earlier in this chapter, depression in men is more severe, resulting in suicide at a higher rate than among women. Higher levels of perceived social support are related to lower instances

DISPLAY 30-8. CAUTION

The seven warning signals can be remembered through the use of the mnemonic device, CAUTION, as follows:
1. **C**hange in bowel or bladder habits
2. **A** sore throat that does not heal
3. **U**nusual bleeding or discharge
4. **T**hickening or lump in breast or elsewhere
5. **I**ndigestion or difficulty in swallowing
6. **O**bvious change in wart or mole
7. **N**agging cough or hoarseness

of depression among all people, especially the elderly, and women seem to make these supportive connections throughout life more effectively than men do. The nurturance, reassurance, and support women get from intimate relationships with other women is not highly developed in men; thus, they display more symptoms of depression after a loss.

Community health nurses can help elders prevent the overwhelming signs and symptoms of depression related to losses by working with aggregates of elders in the community. Through senior centers, adult housing units, senior day care centers, or men's and women's groups at religious centers, the community health nurse can meet with groups of seniors to offer support, teach ways to improve the quality and quantity of support systems, invite mental health speakers on the topic of depression prevention, and generally assess the holistic health status of the elders in that setting. The increased years added to our lives in the last century should be healthy and happy ones, filled with activities that bring joy and contentment. Years lost to depression are a wasted resource that could be prevented through early intervention.

DIABETES

Diabetes mellitus (DM) is a chronic disease affecting 16 million people in the United States. Each year, an additional 800,000 people are diagnosed with diabetes. The number of people with diabetes has increased sixfold since 1958, presently involving 18.4% of the people over age 65; nearly one in five older adults (Oxendine, 1999). About 50% of all elders have some problems with glucose intolerance (Eliopoulos, 1997). More Americans than ever suffer from various forms of DM, and the resulting rates of death and serious complications, such as adult blindness, kidney disease, and foot or leg amputations, are especially high for elders and racial and ethnic minority populations (West, 1999). In the past, DM was not always managed effectively, and for elders today, the fear and misinformation about the disease may hinder them from getting an early diagnosis and the effectiveness of the teaching–learning process if diagnosed with DM.

Being diagnosed with DM can cause depression or anger, and the community health nurse must tailor educational programs to meet individual client needs. The plan needs to be thorough, with special emphasis placed where each client needs the information. For example, a spouse may be concerned about preparing meals that meet her husband's needs, whereas he may be more concerned with how this will affect his long days on the golf course; or a single older woman worries if she can see well enough to draw up her insulin and afford to pay for diabetic supplies and buy special foods. All newly diagnosed diabetics need a comprehensive overview of the disease process followed by an individualized approach.

Community health nurses are ideally situated to meet group and individual needs. They have the resources and skills to plan and implement diabetic education classes for groups of elders, in addition to making home visits to individual clients based on their specific concerns. The group setting allows elders to share their experiences, learn from each other, and benefit from the group support. Home visits permit the nurse to focus on an assessment of the client, home, family support, diabetic supplies and technique, and overall health management.

CARDIOVASCULAR DISEASE

Hypertension increases with age and generally affects men more than women. It appears at an earlier age and is more severe, with higher rates of morbidity and mortality, in African-Americans than in whites (Miller, 1999). Older adults do, however, need to have a blood pressure high enough to have sufficient cerebral circulation to avoid light-headedness and dizziness. Thus, slightly higher blood pressure readings for older adults than for younger people are within normal ranges. Elders have difficulty managing activities of daily living if antihypertension medications lower the blood pressure too dramatically. Hypotension leads to problems of safety, including being at a higher risk of falling. This point is mentioned to alert the community health nurse to the negative effects of a blood pressure that is too low. Both hypertension and hypotension can have significant detrimental effects on the health of older adults.

OSTEOPOROSIS

Osteoporosis is defined by a World Health Organization Study Group (1994) as "a systemic skeletal disease characterized by low bone mass and microarchitectural deterioration of bone tissue, leading to increased bone fragility and a consequent increase in fracture risk." It starts much earlier than old age, thus making recognition essential for preventing its progression (Kushner, 1998). Osteoporosis is a generalized, persistent, and disabling disease that can influence every facet of a person's life. Osteoporosis causes acute and chronic pain, subsequent fractures, decreased physical activity, changes in body image, role changes, a reduction in the activities of daily living, and chronic depression (Kessenich, 1998). It has become an increasingly prevalent problem that will only grow in magnitude as society ages. Community health nurses can focus their teaching on primary prevention and ensure that people eat diets rich in calcium and include calcium supplements as needed. People should be encouraged to engage in weight-bearing activities, such as walking and weight lifting. Also, people should not smoke; women who smoke have greater incidences of osteoporosis.

APPROACHES TO OLDER ADULT CARE

In general, we can divide nursing service to seniors into two approaches: geriatrics and gerontology. In addition, healthy older adults can be effectively cared for in the community through case management approaches.

Geriatrics and Gerontology

Geriatrics is the medical specialty that deals with the physiology of aging and with the diagnosis and treatment of diseases affecting the aged. Geriatrics focuses on abnormal conditions and the treatment of those conditions, and geriatric nursing in the past has focused primarily on the sick aged.

Gerontology refers to the study of all aspects of the aging process, including economic, social, clinical, and psychological, and their effect on the older adult and society. Gerontology is a broad, multidisciplinary practice, and gerontologic nursing concentrates on promoting the health and maximum functioning of older adults (Eliopoulos, 1997).

Community health nurses work with many older people. In one instance, the nurse may promote and maintain the health of a vigorous 80-year old man who lives alone in his home. As another example, the nurse may give postsurgical care at home to a 69-year-old woman, teach her husband how to care for her, and help them contact community resources for shopping, meals, housekeeping, and transportation services. Perhaps nursing intervention focuses on teaching nutrition and maintaining a healthful lifestyle in an extended family that includes the 73-year-old grandmother. The nurse may also lead a bereavement support group for senior citizens whose spouses have recently died.

A community health nurse's work with older adults is at the individual, family, and group levels. However, a community health perspective must also concern itself with the group of older adults as a whole. There are many groups composed of seniors, for example, those attending an adult day care center, belonging to a retirement community, living in a nursing home, or using Meals on Wheels. Others include residents of a senior citizens' apartment building, retired business and professional women, older postcataract-surgery patients at risk for glaucoma, the older poor, Alzheimer's disease sufferers, and the homeless elderly.

Case Management and Needs Assessment

The **case management** concept involves assessing needs, planning and organizing services, and monitoring responses to care throughout the length of the caregiving process, condition, or illness. This concept, which has been practiced by community health nurses for many years, focuses primarily on the health needs of clients. Social workers use case management to address their clients' social needs, including their financial problems. Some health maintenance organizations provide a coordinated system of services for their enrolled clients. Unfortunately, many communities provide no such advocate for their older residents. Therefore, a more comprehensive, community-wide system is needed to serve the entire older population. Such a system might be based on an agency specifically designed to serve as case manager, or "agent," to assess clients' needs and assemble existing agencies and services to meet those needs.

Various techniques are available to assess the needs of older adults:

- The Older Americans Resources and Services Information System (OARS), developed by Duke University, has two tools—Mental Health Screening Questions and the OARS Social Resource Scale. They establish baseline data on clients' well-being, available economic and social resources, physical and mental health status, and clients' capacity for self-care (Stanley & Beare, 1999).
- Clients' capacity for self-care is assessed by the Capacity for Self-Care Index, which ascertains clients' ability to go outdoors, climb stairs, move about their homes, bathe, dress, and cut their toenails (Shanas, 1980).
- The Barthel Index assesses functional independence.
- The Katz Index of ADL is based on an evaluation of the functional independence or dependence of clients with respect to bathing, dressing, toileting, and related tasks (Stanley & Beare, 1999).
- The Instrumental Activities of Daily Living Scale looks at an older adult's ability to perform such activities as using the telephone, shopping, doing laundry, and handling finances (Burke & Walsh, 1997).
- Other techniques, like the Ability to Perform Work-Related Activities survey (Kovar & LaCroix, 1987), determine an elderly person's physical, psychological, and social needs.

A frequently overlooked area of assessment is an elderly client's spiritual needs. Religious dedication and spiritual concern often increase in later years. Limited ability or lack of transportation may prevent older people from attending religious services or engaging in spiritually enhancing activities. Self-health rating, including clients' reporting on their spiritual needs, is another useful assessment technique. A tool to assess a client's self-care practices is included in Chapter 23.

HEALTH SERVICES FOR OLDER ADULT POPULATIONS

How well are the needs of older adults being met? To answer this question, other questions must be raised. Do health programs for the elderly encompass the full range of needed services? Are programs both physically and financially accessible? Do they encourage elderly clients to function independently? Do they treat senior citizens with respect and preserve their dignity? Do they recognize older adults' needs for companionship, economic security, and social status? When appropriate, do they promote meaningful activities instead of overworked games or activities like bingo, shuffleboard, and ceramics? Games can be useful diversions but must be balanced with opportunities for creative outlets, continued learning, and community service through volunteerism.

Criteria for Effective Service

Several criteria help define the characteristics of an effective community health service delivery system for the elderly. Four, in particular, deserve attention.

For a delivery system of a community health service to be effective, it should be *comprehensive*. Many communities provide some programs, such as limited health screening or selected activities, but do not offer a full range of services to more adequately meet the needs of their senior citizens. Gaps and duplication in programs most often result from poor or nonexistent community-wide planning. Furthermore, such planning should be based on thorough assessment of elderly people's needs in that community. A comprehensive set of services should provide the following:

Adequate financial support

Adult day care programs

Health care services (prevention, early diagnosis and
  treatment, rehabilitation)

Health education (including preparation for retirement)

In-home services

Recreation and activity programs

Specialized transportation services

A second criterion for a community service delivery system is *coordination*. Often, older people go from one agency to the next. After visiting one place for food stamps, they may go to another for answers to Medicaid questions, another for congregate dining, and still another for health screening. Such a potpourri of services reflects a system organized for the convenience of providers rather than consumers. It encourages misuse and discourages use. Instead, there should be coordinated, community-wide assessment and planning. Communities must consider alternatives, such as multiservice agencies, that can meet many needs in one location.

A coordinated information and referral system provides another link. Most communities need this type of information network that contains a directory of all resources and services for the elderly and includes the name and telephone number of a contact person with each listing. Such a network is available in some communities and should be developed in those without one. A simplified information and referral system that includes one number, such as an 800 number, to call to find out what resources and services are available and how to get them is particularly helpful to older people.

Unfortunately, in most communities this is not done at all, or it is not done with any regularity or thoroughness. Many

agencies in a given community do not coordinate services, but instead deliver their own services to the elderly in a patchwork and uncoordinated fashion. Collaboration among those who provide services to seniors can provide vital information for planning and implementing needed programs. This has been documented in a seven-county area in central California through the services of the San Joaquin Valley Health Consortium (Allender, Fitzgerald, Guarnera & Hewett, 1993).

A third criterion is *accessibility*. Too often, services for the elderly are not conveniently located or are prohibitively expensive. Some communities are considering multiservice community centers to bring programs and services for the elderly closer to home. More convenient and perhaps specialized transportation services and more in-home services, such as home health aides, homemakers, and Meals on Wheels, may further solve accessibility problems for many older adults. Federal, state, and private funding sources can be tapped to ease the burden on the economically pressured elderly population.

Finally, an effective community service system for older people should *promote quality programs*. This means services that truly address the needs and concerns of a community's senior citizens. Evaluation of the quality of a community's services for the elderly is closely tied to their assessed needs. What are the needs of this specific population group in terms of nutrition, exercise, economic security, independence, social interaction, meaningful activities, and preparation for death? Planning for quality community services depends on having adequate, accurate, and current data. Periodic needs assessment is a necessity to ensure updated information and to initiate and promote quality services.

Services for Healthy Older Adults

Maintaining functional independence should be the primary goal of services for the older population. Assessing needs and the ability to function and using techniques such as OARS, Instrumental Activities of Daily Living Scale, or other previously mentioned tools, form the basis for determining appropriate services. Although many of the well elderly can assess their own health status, some are reluctant to seek needed help. Thus, outreach programs serve an important function in many communities. They locate elderly people in need of health or social assistance and refer them to appropriate resources.

Health screening is another important program for early detection and treatment of health problems among older adults. Conditions to screen for include hypertension, glaucoma, hearing disorders, cancers, diabetes, anemias, depression, and nutritional deficiencies (Eliopoulos, 1997). At the same time, assessment of elderly clients' socialization, housing, and economic needs, along with proper referrals, can prevent further problems from developing that would compromise their health status.

Health maintenance programs may be offered through a single agency, such as a health maintenance organization (HMO), or they may be coordinated by a case management agency with referrals to other providers. These programs should cover a wide range of services needed by the elderly, such as those given in Display 30–7.

Living Arrangements and Care Options

Three types of living arrangements and care options are available for elders. Some living arrangements are based on levels of care, from independent to skilled nursing care, and all levels of assistance in between. At times, while seniors remain in their own homes or apartment, they need home care services brought to them. Other seniors may live with family members and go to an adult day care center during the day. The third category of living arrangements is those that are short term. It may be for respite care, to give the usual caregiver a much-needed rest from 24-hour-a-day caregiving and to prevent "burnout." Families of terminally ill clients cared for at home often use respite services. Finally, hospices provide comfort-focused care in a homelike atmosphere for people with less than 6 months to live.

To meet the multiple housing and caregiving needs of today's elders and in anticipation of the larger numbers to come, many options are becoming available. A range of housing types, from luxurious retirement communities with all amenities for the active and healthier senior to secure and more modestly priced or low-income apartments for independent senior living, are being built in most communities.

DAY CARE AND HOME CARE SERVICES
Most older adults want to remain in their own homes for the remainder of their lives and be as independent and in control of their lives as possible. Some struggle to appear to be doing well in maintaining their independence. Often, they fear that their children or others will make decisions for them that include leaving their homes. Home, whatever form it takes, is where these people believe they are the happiest. There is increased emphasis on providing needed services for elders at home. The trend started several years ago when it became evident that people improved more quickly and at lower costs when they were cared for as outpatients in their own homes.

Today's heightened emphasis on health care cost control gives added support for providing services at home. Given the increase in longevity, the potential for cost savings appears great if dependent older people can be maintained at home. This encourages functional independence as well as emotional well-being (see Bridging Financial Gaps).

Home care provides services such as skilled nursing care, psychiatric nursing, physical and speech therapies, homemaker services, social work services, and dietetic counseling (see Chapter 37). Day care services offer a place where older adults can go during the day for social activities, nutrition, nursing care, and physical and speech therapies. Both services are useful for families caring for an elderly person when the caregivers work and no one is at home or available during the day.

One disadvantage to those remaining at home is that services for the dependent elderly in the community are often fragmented, inadequate, and inaccessible, and at times they operate with little or no maintenance of standards or quality control.

Thus, the dependent elderly need someone in the community to assess their particular needs; assemble, coordinate, and monitor the appropriate resources and services; and serve as their advocate. Such case management roles are most appropriately filled by the community health nurse. This case management approach tailors services to the long-term needs of clients and enables them to function longer outside of institutions (Bower, 1992).

Bridging Financial Gaps

Rock, A. (February, 1999). You can remake your life. *Reader's Digest, 154*(922), 106–111.

Lynn Peluso from Wethersfield, Connecticut, worked as an emergency room nurse. She earned an MBA and left the emergency room to work as an assistant director of a nursing home. Something about this setting bothered Lynn. She said, "I saw many people who could have stayed in their own homes if only they'd had assistance."

Lynn decided to make a dramatic change and open a center where elderly people would be able to spend the day and enjoy recreational and social programs and medical support while continuing to live at home. She conducted market research and selected Wethersfield as a site where there was more demand than facilities for such services. She also sought out free help from the Small Business Administration's SCORE program, which pairs retired executives with entrepreneurs. Lynn says her "SCORE mentor was invaluable in reviewing the business plan that I needed to get financing."

Lynn Peluso and her husband opened Golden Care in January 1994, using savings and a loan secured by a lien on their house. By the end of the first year, the couple had 15 clients. By 1997, they had 100 and a staff of 26. Her husband earns $60,000 a year and she earns $112,000—both having doubled their salaries from previous jobs.

Lynn loves what she does, and her clients love her. The services the Pelusos provide allow many older adults to avoid going into nursing homes. Remaining at home is what elders want, and it saves the elders, family members, and the state money.

LIVING ARRANGEMENTS BASED ON LEVELS OF CARE

Although only 6% of the elderly population live in **skilled-nursing facilities,** such organizations remain the most visible type of health service for older adults. These facilities provide skilled nursing care along with personal care that is considered nonskilled or **custodial care,** such as bathing, dressing, feeding, and assisting with mobility and recreation. Currently, approximately 2 million elderly people are receiving nursing home care.

However, **long-term care** services "include all those services designed to provide care for people at different stages of dependence for an extended period of time" (Miller, 1999, p. 662). New choices are now available and are housing larger numbers of elders than nursing homes alone.

Nursing home reform was passed in 1987 with the Omnibus Budget Reconciliation Act (OBRA), which put increased demands on facilities to provide competent resident assessment, timely care plans, quality improvement, and protection of resident rights starting in 1990 (Miller, 1999). However, this increased complexity of services has caused costs in these facilities to rise. Staffing needs increase as care becomes more complex and the resident population grows. This requires licensed personnel to be knowledgeable decision-makers, managers of unskilled staff, staff educators and role models, and efficient and effective administrators in an essentially autonomous practice setting.

In the past, nursing homes had stigmas attached to them. Many people saw them as places that enforced dehumanizing and impersonal regulations, such as segregation of sexes, strict social policies, and sometimes overuse of chemical and physical restraints. Media attention to such conditions as well as the current licensing regulations should make these types of practices the rare exception. Gradually, the fear and despair associated with such facilities will begin to dissipate. In addition, as competition comes from facilities offering lower levels of care, such as assisted living centers, residents in nursing homes receiving more minimal care may be attracted to move to the new assisted living centers.

Even in institutions in which the quality of care is outstanding, costs are so high that family resources are soon depleted if not planned for long in advance of the need. Although Medicaid pays for skilled nursing costs if the client meets low income and asset requirements and Medicare pays for a limited period of time, clients and families pay more than half (Eliopoulos, 1997). Life savings that older parents had hoped to leave to their children may be quickly consumed, forcing them into indigence. In 2000, it was not unusual for a skilled nursing facility to cost over $4500 a month.

Intermediate care facilities are less costly and still provide health care, but the amount and type of skilled care given are decreased. Frequently, older adults need **assisted living,** which, according to the mission statement of the Assisted Living Federation of America, is "a special combination of housing, supportive services, personalized assistance, and health care designed to respond to the individual needs of those who need help with activities of daily living (ADLs) and instrumental activities of daily living (IADLs)" (Barton, 1997). This is a less intense level of care than intermediate care units or facilities provide. Medicare generally pays only for care in skilled nursing facilities, and Medicaid pays for care in intermediate care facilities but only after the client meets income and asset tests, leaving them essentially indigent. Costs in 2000 for assisted living choices averaged $3000 a month.

Personal care homes offer basic custodial care, such as bathing, grooming, and social support, but provide no skilled nursing services. Payment may also come from private funds, Title XIX or XX (Social Security Act) funds, or Supplemental Security Income (aid to the aged, disabled, or blind). Boarding homes, board and care homes, or residential care facilities house elderly people who only need meals and housekeeping and can manage most of their own personal care. Government funds are not available to support these institutions. Costs average $2000 a month in a shared room in 2000. **Group homes** are an alternative for specific elderly populations, such as the mentally ill, alcoholics, or developmentally disabled, and are often subsidized by concerned community organizations. Homes focusing on care of people with Alzheimer's disease are physically designed with the client's safety and individual needs considered and are staffed with para-professionals trained to meet each person's needs.

The concept of the **continuing care center** (sometimes called total life centers), in which all levels of living, from total independence to the most dependent are designed to meet the continuous living needs of older aging adults (Display 30–9). This choice is usually expensive; however, it is a very attractive alternative to wealthier segments of the aging population. Others may choose to remain in their own home because they do not desire the consolidated living arrangements in which only older adults reside or they may not be able to afford this comprehensive living arrangement. Nevertheless, demand is increasing for this type of housing option. For adults today nearing retirement, this concept is being looked into as a viable choice as they actively plan for a long old age. Many of these centers have a 5- to 10-year waiting list, so older adults need to seek them out long before they intend to live there.

HOSPICE AND RESPITE CARE SERVICES

Respite care is a service receiving increasing attention and is aimed primarily at caregivers' needs. Many older people at home are cared for by a spouse or other family member. The demands of such care can be exhausting unless the caregiver can get some relief, or respite—thus the name of this service. Respite care may be available through an agency that provides volunteers to relieve caregivers, giving them time off regularly or permitting a periodic vacation. Some skilled nursing facilities or **board and care homes** provide an extra room to give temporary institutional housing for the elderly while caregivers take a break. Elderly clients may also need a change from the constant interaction with their caregivers.

DISPLAY 30–9. Continuing Care Centers—Wave of the Future?

The Otterbein-Lebanon Retirement Community is a model continuing care center and is one of five Otterbein Homes located in Ohio. With housing options for 785 residents on a 1500-acre campus in rural southeastern Ohio, older adults can choose housing options that include freestanding two- and three-bedroom homes, one-bedroom cottages, or apartment-style one- or two-bedroom or one-room studio units, where they live independently.

Three hundred and eleven licensed beds include assisted living options from one-room studio apartments (with limited facilities for meal preparation) to semiprivate rooms in which nurses oversee medication and staff is available to assist with personal care. If caregiving needs become greater, additional services are available. Both skilled nursing services and a freestanding 30-bed Alzheimer's living unit exist for the frailest older adults.

Regardless of the living arrangement, the residents are free to come and go as they wish and all have access to congregate dining in their large and attractive restaurant-style dining room.

The retirement community is expanding. Sixty-six patio homes were built in 1999, with 44 more planned in 2000. The goal is to house 1,200 resident by the year 2006.

The Otterbein-Lebanon Retirement Community also provides home health care services, adult day care, and the other usual services found in a community—a bank, post office, ice cream parlor, hairdresser, library, and a church (the choir has 70 members, a bell choir, and men's and women's clubs). Because of the popularity of this Otterbein-Lebanon location, there is a waiting list of 1 to 4 years for the independent living area.

Many of the assisted living and skilled nursing beds are occupied by residents who moved into the independent living areas 10 to 15 years ago while they were in their seventies or eighties. Their ages now range from the late eighties to older than 100, and their caregiving needs have increased. In this type of setting, frail elderly people do not have to leave their community to get the care they need, and longtime friends are nearby to care for them or to provide companionship. It is not unusual to see many of the independent seniors volunteering to help feed frail elderly in the skilled nursing care units. In fact, they volunteer more than 80,000 hours a years to the Otterbein-Lebanon Retirement Community. They know that when they need the care, a senior friend will be there for them.

(Otterbein-Lebanon Retirement Community Admissions Director, personal communication, September 16, 1999.)

Hospice care may be offered through an institution, such as a hospital or a home health agency, or may be a freestanding facility existing solely as an inpatient hospice. Hospices and other agencies providing hospice care offer services that enable dying people to stay at home with the support and services needed. The purpose of **hospice care** is to make the dying process as dignified, free from discomfort, and emotionally, spiritually, and socially supportive as possible. Some community health nursing agencies offer hospice programs staffed by their nurses. For the elderly, it is a service that has been well received, meets important needs, and is growing in use. Hospice and respite care are two services most needed and used by the families of Alzheimer's victims.

THE COMMUNITY HEALTH NURSE IN AN AGING AMERICA

Community health nurses can make a significant contribution to the health of older adults. Because these nurses are in the community and already have contact with many seniors, they are in a prime position to begin needs assessments and mutual planning for the health of this group. Case management is often a critical aspect of the nurse's role because the community health nurse must know what resources are available and when and how to make referrals for these older clients.

The health care scene in terms of the availability of services for the elderly is changing dramatically. The numbers and types of home care services, for example, are mushrooming. Many entrepreneurs, including nurses, who recognize the potential of this growing market have begun offering goods and services targeted for older adults. Community health nurses must keep abreast of new developments, programs, regulations, and social and economic forces and their potential impact on the provision of health services.

More importantly, community health nurses need to be proactive, designing interventions that maximize nursing's resources and provide the greatest benefit to elderly clients. For example, community health nurses might develop a case management program for older adults as a community-wide assessment, information, and referral service. Such a program might contract with existing agencies to serve as a clearinghouse for the elderly and to channel clients to appropriate services. Financing of such a program might be based on tax dollars (if a public agency), grants, or some innovative fee-for-service reimbursement system.

Many of the older population's health problems can be prevented and their health promoted. Changing to a healthier lifestyle is one of the most important preventive measures the nurse can emphasize.

The role of community health nurse as a teacher is an important one. Educating the elderly about their health conditions, safety, and use of their medications is another important way to prevent problems. Influenza and pneumonia can be prevented through regular health maintenance, which includes immunizations. Other problems associated with environmental conditions and the aging process, such as arthritis, diabetes, and some cancers, can be diagnosed and treated early, thereby minimizing their effect on functional independence.

Many types of accidents that frequently happen to older adults are 100% preventable. Community health nurses can make a difference through their work with individuals, families, and aggregates in teaching safety measures to avoid such accidents. As discussed earlier, falls are a leading cause of injury and death and are caused by a combination of internal (diseases, effects of medicines) and external (lighting, scatter rugs) factors that are preventable or controllable. Nurses can make a difference in the lives of older clients by using available materials and their own resources when teaching safety.

With a growing and aging elderly population, community health nurses face a serious challenge in addressing their needs. At the same time, nursing can be on the forefront of developing innovative health services for that group and rising to meet the opportunity and the challenge.

SUMMARY

The number of older adults (aged 65 and older) is increasing. That age group is also becoming a larger percentage of the overall population. It is common that women outlive men by many years, making women a larger part of this older population. With improved medicines and medical technology, many people are now living into their eighties and nineties in relatively good health. They are able to enjoy these later years and still make contributions to their families and society. This extended life expectancy is, of course, good news; however, it has also created a myriad of new health needs and concerns, not only for the older population, but also for health care facilities and professionals who deliver services to older adults.

Healthy longevity is the goal for the aging population and is a focus of *Healthy People 2010*. That means being able to function as independently as possible; to maintain as much physical, mental and social vigor as possible; and to adapt to life's changes and cope with the stresses and losses while still being able to engage in meaningful activity.

The most frequent health problems of older adults are chronic and often progressive conditions such as arthritis, vision and hearing loss, heart conditions, hypertension, and diabetes, all of which can become disabling conditions. Other major causes of death or disability are cancer, cerebral vascular accidents, Alzheimer's disease, and accidents and injuries from falls, fire, or automobile crashes. Older adults also often suffer adverse side effects from taking multiple medications prescribed for various chronic conditions. Many of these health problems associated with old age are preventable to some extent, such that early diagnosis and treatment of some conditions can minimize the condition's adverse effects. Many accidents and injuries that render older adults unable to live independently are preventable.

Many older adults also suffer from the emotional side effects of aging, such as feelings of distress and anxiety regarding their future, loneliness, and social isolation when loved ones or friends die, and even depression—feeling that life is over and they have no purpose or meaningful function in life. But older people can also enter this phase of life determined to keep physically and mentally healthy, interacting with others and making viable contributions to others and society.

To promote and maintain health and prevent illness, older people need to be educated about their own health care needs. In particular, they should understand potential hazards of drug interactions if they are taking multiple medications. They also need good nutrition and adequate exercise; they need to be as independent and self-reliant as possible; they need coping skills to face the possibility of financial insecurity and the loss of a spouse and other loved ones; they need social interaction, companionship, and meaningful activities; and they need to resolve anxieties regarding their own disability and death.

Many programs are available to older adults, both for those who are healthy, hearty, and active and for those who need some level of dependent or semidependent care. Programs for hearty older people include health maintenance programs that cover a wide range of health services, wellness programs, health screening, outreach programs, social assistance programs, and information about volunteering and educational opportunities in the community. A variety of living arrangements and care options are available from which to choose according to the older person's desires and needs. These include the newest concepts of continuing-care centers that offer a full range of living arrangements from totally independent living to skilled nursing services, all within one community. There are also facilities that provide skilled nursing and custodial care, home care, day care, respite care, and hospice care.

The community health perspective includes a case management approach that offers a centralized system for assessing the needs of older people and then matching those needs with the appropriate services. The community health nurse should also seek to serve the entire older population by assessing the needs of the population, examining the available services, and analyzing their effectiveness. The effectiveness of programs can be measured according to four important criteria—comprehensiveness, effective coordination, accessibility, and quality (targeted to the specific needs of the population).

The community health nurse can make significant contributions to the health of the older population as a whole by being aware of new developments and programs that are available, new regulations, and new social and economic forces and their impact on the provision of health services. But more importantly, the community health nurse can design interventions that maximize nursing resources and provide the greatest benefit to the older adult population.

ACTIVITIES TO PROMOTE CRITICAL THINKING

1. Picture an elderly person whom you know well or know a great deal about. Make a list of characteristics that describe this person. How many of these characteristics fit your picture of most senior citizens? What are your biases (ageisms) about the elderly?
2. If you were Minnie Blackstone's community health nurse (see Display 30–2), what interventions would you consider using to maintain and promote her health? Why?
3. As part of your regular community health nursing workload, you visit a senior day care center an afternoon a week. You take the blood pressures of several people who are on antihypertensive medications and do some nutrition counseling. The center accommodates 60 senior clients, and you would like to serve the health needs of the aggregate population. What are some potential health needs of this group? What actions might you consider taking at an aggregate level? With whom would you consult as you plan programs at the center?
4. Assume you have been asked by your local health department to determine the needs of the elderly population in your community. How would you begin conducting such a needs assessment? What data might you want to collect? How would you find out what services are already being offered and whether they are adequate?
5. Visit a continuing care center in your community. Assess the housing options, services, and health care provisions. Would you live here when you are older? Why or why not? What would you change?
6. Using the Internet, locate innovative programs for elders in the community at the primary, secondary, and tertiary levels of care. Determine if such programs could work in your community.

REFERENCES

Allender, J., Fitzgerald, G., Guarnera, J., & Hewett, L. (1993). *Train the trainer: A program for elder care providers.* Fresno, CA: San Joaquin Valley Health Consortium.

Alzheimer, A. (1907). A unique illness involving the cerebral

cortex. In D. A. Rottenberg & F. H. Hochberg (Eds.). *Neurological classics in modern translation.* New York: Hafner Press. (Original work published 1907.)

American Association of Retired Persons. (1990). *Health risks and preventive care among older blacks.* Washington, DC: Author.

American Association of Retired Persons (AARP) & Administration on Aging, U.S. Department of Health and Human Services. (1997). *A profile of older Americans.* Washington, DC: AARP.

American College of Sports Medicine (ACSM). (1995). ACSM position stand on osteoporosis and exercise. *Medical Science and Sports Exercise, 27*(4), i–vii.

Atchley, R. C. (1997). *Social forces and aging* (8th ed.). Belmont, CA: Wadsworth.

Barton, L. J. (1997). *A shoulder to lean on: Assisted living in the U.S.* Ithaca, NY: American Demographics/Marketing Tools, Cowles Business Media.

Benson, S. (1997). The older adult and fear of crime. *Journal of Gerontological Nursing, 23*(10), 24–31.

Bonnel, W. B. (1999, January). Meal management strategies of older adult women. *Journal of Gerontological Nursing, 25,* 41–47.

Bortz, W. M. II. (1996). *Dare to be 100.* New York: Simon & Schuster.

Bower, K. A. (1992). *Case management by nurses.* Washington, DC: American Nurses Association.

Bowling, A., & Windsor, J. (1995). Death after widow(er)hood: An analysis of mortality rates up to 13 years after bereavement. *Omega, 31,* 35–49.

Burghardt, M. (1999). Exercise at menopause: A critical difference. *Medscape Women's Health, 4*(1), 1–13. Available: http://www.medscape.com/Medscape/WomensHealth/journal/1999/v04.n01/wh3078.burg/wh3078.burg-.

Burke, M. M., & Walsh, M. B. (1997). *Gerontologic nursing: Holistic care of the older adult.* St. Louis: Mosby.

Connidis, I. A., & Davies, L. (1992). Confidants and companions: Choices in later life. *The Journal of Gerontology, 47*(3), S115–122.

Elderhostel, Inc. (1999, August 13). *Elderhostel United States catalog: Winter 2000.* Issue #1.

Eliopoulos, C. (1997). *Gerontological nursing* (4th ed.). Philadelphia: Lippincott-Raven.

Finn, J. S. (1997). Aging and information technology: The promise and the challenge. *Generations, 21*(3), 5–6.

Fronstin, P. (1999). Retirement patterns and employee benefits: Do benefits matter? *The Gerontologist, 39*(1), 37–47.

"Full-life" counselors help frail seniors stay independent. (1998). *Senior Care Management, 1*(7), 97–100.

Hewett, L. J., & Chang, F. (1998). Alzheimer's disease, a hopeful note for the closing of a century: Challenges for the new millennium. In J. A. Allender & C. L. Rector (Eds.), *Readings in gerontological nursing* (pp. 484–499). Philadelphia: Lippincott-Raven.

Hobson, M. (1992). Medications in older patients. *Western Journal of Medicine, 157,* 539–543.

Jorgenson, J. (1997). Therapeutic use of companion animals in health care. *Image: Journal of Nursing Scholarship, 29*(3), 249–254.

Kaiser Permanente. (1998). *Breast cancer screening.* Author.

Kaiser Permanente healthwise handbook (11th ed.). (1994). Boise, ID: Healthwise Incorporated.

Kanacki, L. S., Jones, P. S., & Galbraith, M. E. (1996). Social support and depression in widows and widowers. *Journal of Gerontological Nursing, 22*(2), 39–45.

Kessenich, C. R. (1998). *Health-related quality of life in osteoporosis.* Available: http://www.medscape.com? HumanaPres/JCD/1. . . . n01/jed0101.06.kess/ jcd0101.06.kess.html.

Kovar, M. G., & LaCroix, A. Z. (1987). Aging in the eighties, ability to perform work-related activities. (Data from the supplement on aging). National Health Interview Survey: United States. (1984). National Center for Health Statistics Advance Data Number 136 (8, May), DHHS Pub. No. (PHS)87–1250. Hyattsville, MD: U.S. Public Health Service.

Kübler-Ross, E. (1975). *Death: The final stage of growth.* Englewood Cliffs, NJ: Prentice-Hall.

Kushner, P. R. (1998). Osteoporosis: Unmasking the silent epidemic. *Hospital Medicine, 34*(5), 25–26, 32–34, 37–39.

Mace, N. L., & Rabins, P. V. (1999). *The 36-hour day* (3rd ed.). New York: Warner.

Margolin, D. I. (1994, March 19). *Alzheimer's disease: Update on diagnosis and treatment.* Paper presented at the Seventh Annual Walter A. Rohlfing Medical Lectureship in Geriatrics and Long-Term Care, Fresno, CA.

Martin Matthews, A. (1991). *Widowhood in later life.* Toronto, Ontario, Canada: Butterworth.

Mayo Clinic. (1999). *Exercise as you age: How to get off the sidelines and back in the game.* Available: http://www.mayohealth.org/mayo/9703/htm/me9702.htm.

Meadows, M. (1999, July). Making oral health a priority. *Closing the Gap,* 1–2 [a newsletter of the Office of Minority Health, U.S. Department of Health and Human Services].

Miller, C. A. (1999). *Nursing care of older adults: Theory and practice* (3rd ed.). Philadelphia: Lippincott Williams & Wilkins.

Moore, K. H., Babyak, M. A., Wood, C. E., et al. (1999). The association between physical activity and depression in older depressed adults. *Journal of Aging and Physical Activity, 7,* 55–61.

Morley, J. E. (1994, March 19). *Malnutrition in the nursing home: A common life-threatening problem.* Paper presented at the Seventh Annual Walter A. Rohlfing Medical Lectureship in Geriatrics and Long-Term Care, Fresno, CA.

Moscicki, E. K., O'Carroll, P., Rae, D. S., et al. (1998). Suicide attempts in the epidemiologic catchment area study. *The Yale Journal of Biology and Medicine, 61,* 259–268.

National Institute on Aging (NIA). (1997). *10 tips for healthy aging.* Bethesda, MD: National Institutes of Health.

———. (1996, December). *Global aging into the 21st century.* Bethesda, MD: Office of the Demography of Aging, Behavioral and Social Research Program (NIA).

Oxendine, J. (1999, February/March). Who has diabetes? *Closing the Gap,* 5 [a newsletter of the Office of Minority Health, U.S. Department of Health and Human Services].

Pollock, G. (1987). The mourning-liberation process: Ideas on the inner life of the older adult. In J. Sadavoy and M. Leszcz (Eds.), *Treating the elderly with psychotherapy: The scope for change in later life* (pp. 3–30). Madison, CT: International Universities Press.

Population Reference Bureau (1999). World population data sheet. Available: www.prb.org.

Quinn, J. B. (1997, April). Money watch: Retirement myths. *Good Housekeeping,* 76.

Rock, A. (1999). You can remake your life. *Reader's Digest, 154*(922), 106–111.

Schoenfelder, D. P., & Van Why, K. (1997). A fall prevention educational program for community dwelling seniors. *Public Health Nursing, 14*(6), 383–390.

Shanas, E. (1980). Self-assessment of physical function: White and black elderly in the United States. In S. Haynes and M. Feinleib (Eds.), *Epidemiology of aging* (NIH Pub. No. 80-969). Washington, DC: U.S. Department of Health and Human Services.

Staab, A. S., & Hodges, L. C. (1996). *Essentials of gerontological nursing: Adaptation to the aging process.* Philadelphia: Lippincott.

Stanley, M., & Beare, P. G. (1999). *Gerontological nursing.* Philadelphia: F.A. Davis.

Thurm, K. (1998). Adult immunizations save lives. *Closing the Gap, 1,* 3 [a newsletter of the Office of Minority Health, U.S. Department of Health and Human Services].

Tibbits, G. M. (1996). Patients who fall: How to predict and prevent injuries. *Geriatrics, 51*(9), 24–32.

U.S. Department of Health and Human Services (2000). *Healthy people 2010* (conference edition in two volumes). Washington, DC: U.S. Government Printing Office.

———. (1998). *Healthy people 2010 objectives: Draft for public comment.* Washington, DC: U.S. Government Printing Office.

———. (1991). *Healthy people 2000: National health promotion and disease prevention objectives* (S/N 017-001-00474-0). Washington, DC: U.S. Government Printing Office.

U.S. Department of Transportation. (1998). *Traffic safety facts 1997–older population.* Washington, DC: National Center for Statistics & Analysis, Research & Development.

U.S. Preventive Services Task Force. (1996). *Guide to clinical preventive services* (2nd ed.). Baltimore: Williams & Wilkins.

Vander Zanden, J. W. (1993). Later adulthood. In *Human development* (5th ed., pp. 537–586). New York, NY: McGraw-Hill.

Walker, M. K., & Foreman, M. D. (1999). Medication safety: A protocol for nursing action. *Geriatric Nursing, 20*(1), 34–39.

West, J. (1999, February/March). National diabetes education program. *Closing the Gap,* 1–3 [a newsletter of the Office of Minority Health, U.S. Department of Health and Human Services].

World Health Organization (1998). *The world health report, 1998: Life in the 21st century, a vision for all.* Geneva, Switzerland: Author.

World Health Organization (WHO) Study Group. (1994). *Assessment of fracture risk and its application to screening for postmenopausal osteoporosis.* WHO Technical Report Series 843. Geneva, Switzerland: Author.

INTERNET RESOURCES

Administration on Aging: http://www.aoa.dhhs.gov

Alzheimer's Association: http://www.alzheimers.org

American Association of Retired Persons: http://www.aarp.org

Andrus Foundation: http://www.andrus.org

Association of Late Deafened Adults: http://www.alda.org

Elderhostel: http://www.elderhostel.org

Generations United: http://www.gu.org

Gerontological Society of America: http://wwwgeron@geron.org

GriefNet: http://www.rivendell.org

National Aging Information Center: http://www.aoa.dhhs.gov/naic

National Institute on Aging: http://www.nih.gov/nia

Parkinson Association: http://www.Parkinson.org

SPRY Foundation: http://www.spry.org

Statistical Abstract of U.S.: http://www.census.gov/statab/www/

The Geezer Brigade: http://www.thegeezerbrigade.com

SELECTED READINGS

Anderson, G. (1995). *Caring for people with Alzheimer's disease*. Baltimore: Health Professions Press.

Baltes, M. M., & Carstensen, L. L. (1996). The process of successful ageing. *Ageing and Society, 16,* 397–422.

Chambre, S. M. (1993). Volunteerism by elders: Past trends and future prospects. *The Gerontologist, 33*(2), 221–228.

Collins, C. E., et al. (1997). Models for community-based long-term care for the elderly in a changing health system. *Nursing Outlook, 45,* 59–63.

Fillenbaum, G. G., & Smyer, M. A. (1981). The development, validity, and reliability of the OARS multidimensional functional assessment questionnaire. *Journal of Gerontology, 36*(4), 428.

Fisher, P. P. (1995). *More than movement for fit to frail older adults*. Baltimore: Health Professions Press.

Gregory, S. (1996). Memory maintenance groups in the community. *British Journal of Occupational Therapy, 59*(1), 25–26.

Haber, D. (1994). *Health promotion and aging* (2nd ed.). New York: Springer.

Institute of Medicine. (1990). *The second fifty years: Promoting health and preventing disability*. Washington, DC: National Academy Press.

Logan, J. R., & Spitze, G. (1994). Informal support and the use of formal services by older Americans. *Journal of Gerontology: Social Sciences, 49*(2), S25–S34.

Mace, N. L., & Rabins, P. V., (1991). *The 36 hour-day* (2nd ed.). Baltimore: Johns Hopkins University Press.

Matteson, M. A., McConnell, E. S., & Linton, A. D. (1997). *Gerontological nursing: Concepts and practice*. Philadelphia: W.B. Saunders.

Maxted, G. (1998). Functional assessment in the elderly. *The IHS Primary Care Provider, 23*(11), 149–152.

Molony, S. L., Waszynski, C. M., & Lyder, C. (1999). *Gerontological nursing: A primary care clinical guide*. Stamford, CT: Appleton & Lange.

O'Neill, D. P., & Kenny, E. K. (1998). Spirituality and chronic illness. *Image: Journal of Nursing Scholarship, 30*(3), 275–280.

Palmore, E. B. (1987). Centenarians. In G. L. Maddox (Ed.). *The encyclopedia of aging* (pp. 107–108). New York: Springer.

Peters-Davis, N. D., Moss, M. S., & Pruchno, R. A. (1999). Children-in-law in caregiving families. *The Gerontologist, 39*(1), 68–75.

Pfeiffer, E. (Ed.). (1978). *Multidimensional functional assessment: The OARS Methodology* (2nd ed.). Durham, NC: Duke University Center for Study of Aging and Human Development.

Stone, J. T., Wyman, J. F., & Salisbury, S. A. (1999). *Clinical gerontological nursing: A guide to advanced practice* (2nd ed.). Philadelphia: W.B. Saunders.

Swonger, A. K., & Burbank, P. M. (1995). *Drug therapy and the elderly*. Sudbury, MA: Jones and Bartlett.

Tout, K. (1993). *Elderly care: A world perspective*. London, England: Chapman & Hall.

Wiley, D., & Bortz, W. M. II. (1996). Sexuality and aging—usual and successful. *Journal of Gerontology: Medical Sciences, 51*A(3), M142–M146.

Yale, R. (1995). *Developing support groups for individuals with early-stage Alzheimer's disease*. Baltimore: Health Professions Press.

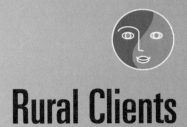

Rural Clients

KEY TERMS

- Circle of continuity of care
- Circle of family and community support
- Frontier area
- Health professional shortage area (HPSA)
- Key informant
- Metropolitan
- Nonmetropolitan
- Out-migration
- Rural
- Telehealth
- Urban area (UA)

LEARNING OBJECTIVES

Upon mastery of this chapter, you should be able to:
- Define the term *rural*.
- Discuss population characteristics of rural residents.
- Identify at-risk populations in rural communities.
- Describe five barriers to health care access for rural clients.
- Relate the broad objectives of *Healthy People 2010* to the concept of "social justice" in rural communities.
- Discuss activities to assist in the orientation of a new community health nurse to a rural community.
- Compare and contrast the "circle of continuity of care" and the "circle of family and community support" themes apparent in rural communities.
- Discuss the challenges and opportunities related to rural community health nursing practice.

Think about the last time you were in a rural community. What do you recall about it? Was there a hospital, nursing home, clinic, and/or public health department in the community? Were there schools and playgrounds? What types of small businesses lined the main street? What eating establishments were there? How many traffic signals were present? How would you describe the population living in the area, in terms of their age, income, occupation, faith, culture, and ethnicity? If you live in the rural community you describe, these questions are probably easy to answer, and you have likely at least considered a career in rural nursing. If you live in an urban community, you probably have little familiarity with rural communities, and have never considered this specialty practice.

Rural nursing practice offers many opportunities for you. Nurses are respected community members—your judgment and opinions count. Rural nurses are key members of the health care team. You can make a difference in the lives of your neighbors, friends, and community. The challenges are many, and the rewards are great! This chapter addresses the special health needs and concerns of rural clients, and how the community health nurse can address those needs. It is our hope that after reading it, you will come to appreciate the many advantages that rural nurses enjoy, and consider rural nursing as a practice choice.

DEFINITIONS AND DEMOGRAPHICS

Definitions of Rural

There are different definitions of the term *rural*. The community health nurse needs to be aware of the precise meaning of the term as it is used in a particular agency, community, or piece of legislation, because differences in semantics can affect public policy regarding rural communities. For example, federal dollars are often distributed to communities according to their rural or urban status (Johnson-Webb, Baer, & Gesler, 1997).

The U.S. Government provides three definitions of rural. The Bureau of the Census (1994) definition distinguishes between rural communities and **urban areas (UAs).** UAs have *a population of 150,000 or more residents and a population density of 1,000 or more inhabitants per square mile* (U.S. Department of Health and Human Services [USDHHS], Office of Rural Health Policy, 1998). The Census Bureau also considers as "urban" communities outside of UAs that are incorporated and have 2,500 or more residents. Rural areas, therefore, have fewer than 2,500 residents and population density below 1,000 inhabitants per square mile.

The U.S. Office of Management and Budget (OMB) classifies U.S. counties as either metropolitan or nonmetropolitan (Office of Management and Budget, 1995).

Metropolitan counties *include one or more cities of 50,000 or more residents or a Bureau of Census defined UA and a total metropolitan area population of 100,000 or greater* (Lee, 1991). **Nonmetropolitan** counties *do not have a city of 50,000 residents within their borders*. With such a broad definition, nonmetropolitan counties can be inclusive of both rural and urban areas.

The U.S. Department of Agriculture's (USDA) rural–urban continuum codes further break down the OMB definition of metropolitan area into four codes, and nonmetropolitan counties into six codes based on population density as well as proximity to metropolitan areas (Butler & Beale, 1995) (Display 31–1). Both code 8, "Adjacent to Metropolitan Area," and code 9, "Non-Adjacent to Metropolitan Area,"

have fewer than 2,500 residents and are classified as "completely rural."

For the purposes of this chapter, **rural** is defined as *communities with fewer than 10,000 residents and a county population density of fewer than 1,000 persons per square mile* (Table 31–1). In reality, this definition of rural is arbitrary, because rural clients do not consider only population density or size of their community when defining their "ruralness."

DISPLAY 31–1. U.S. Department of Agriculture Economic Research Service Rural–Urban Continuum Codes

Code	Metropolitan Counties
0	Central counties of metropolitan areas of 1 million population or more
1	Fringe counties of metropolitan areas of 1 million population or more
2	Counties in metropolitan areas of 250,000–1 million population
3	Counties in nonmetropolitan areas of fewer than 250,000 population

Code	Nonmetropolitan Counties
4	Urban population of 20,000 or more, adjacent to a metropolitan area
5	Urban population of 20,000 or more, not adjacent to a metropolitan area
6	Urban population of 2,500 to 19,999, adjacent to a metropolitan area
7	Urban population of 2,500 to 19,999, not adjacent to a metropolitan area
8	Completely rural or less than 2,500 urban population, adjacent to metro area
9	Completely rural or less than 2,500 urban population, not adjacent to metro area

(From Butler, M. A., & Beale, C. A. [1994]. *Rural-urban continuum codes for metropolitan counties,* 1993. Washington, DC: Agriculture and Rural Economy Division, Economic Research Service, U.S. Department of Agriculture.)

TABLE 31–1. Definitions of Rural

Source	Nomenclature	Definitions
U.S. Bureau of the Census	Rural	Communities with less than 25,000 residents *and* population density below 1,000 people per square mile
U.S. Office of Management and Budget	Nonmetropolitan	Counties without a city of 50,000 residents
U.S.D.A.—Rural–Urban Continuum Codes	Completely rural	Completely rural or less than 2,500 urban population either adjacent to *or* not adjacent to metro area
U.S. Government	Frontier area	Less than six people per square mile
Author	Rural	Communities with less than 10,000 residents *and* county population of less than 1,000 people per square mile

Instead, they have a multitude of reasons for defining their community as rural, such as distance from a large city, major occupations in the area, or numbers of students in the local schools. If you have access to a small community, ask some of the residents why they consider their community to be urban or rural. You will get a variety of comments based on their individual experiences. These stories will only add to the richness to be found in rural communities.

You also need to be familiar with the term **frontier area,** which is used to designate *sparsely populated places with six or fewer persons per square mile* (USDHHS, 1998). Rural health issues of concern to rural areas may be of even greater concern to frontier areas. Another term critical to rural health is **health professional shortage areas (HPSAs),** which are *federally designated areas with too few physicians and, therefore, eligible for a wide variety of governmental assistance* (Rosenblatt & Hart, 1999). HPSAs included 802 whole counties and 641 partial counties in 1997 (Fig. 31–1).

Population Statistics

The number of persons living in rural areas in the United States has tripled since the mid-1800s from 20,000,000 persons in 1850 to over 60,000,000 rural residents in 1990. During the same time period, the proportion of persons living in rural U.S. communities decreased from about 85% to 25% (USDHHS, 1998; Ricketts, Johnson-Webb, & Randolph, 1999). The highest proportion of rural populations in the United States is located in the South, in Appalachia, and in the Great Plains; the Northeast region has the smallest proportion (Ricketts, Johnson-Webb, & Randolph, 1999).

Rural populations are generally older than their urban counterparts. In 1996, the median age of nonmetropolitan residents was 35.6 years, whereas the metropolitan median age was 33.8 years (Ricketts, Johnson-Webb, & Randolph, 1999). The older age of rural residents has health care implications.

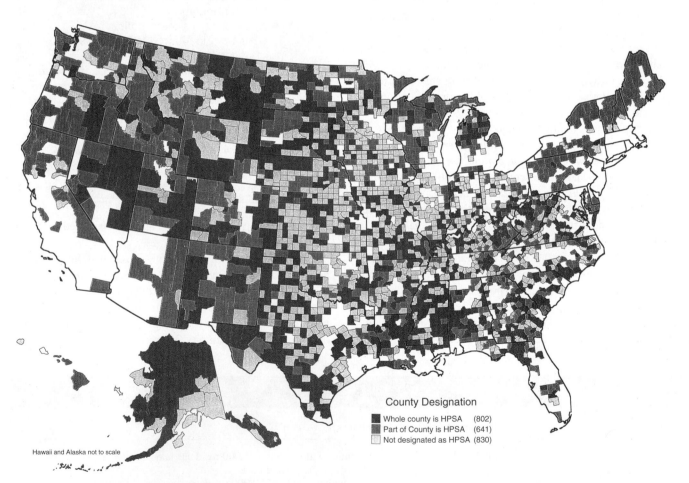

County Designation

■ Whole county is HPSA (802)
▨ Part of County is HPSA (641)
□ Not designated as HPSA (830)

Hawaii and Alaska not to scale

Note: Metropolitan counties are aggregated into white areas on the map.
Source: Division of Shortage Designation, BPHC, HRSA, DHHS, 1997.
Produced by: North Carolina Rural Health Research and Policy Analysis Center, Cecil G. Sheps Center for Health Services Research, University of North Carolina at Chapel Hill, with support from the Federal Office of Rural Health Policy, HRSA, US DHHS.

FIGURE 31–1. Primary care health professional shortage areas (HPSAs), 1997. (Ricketts, T. [Ed.] [1998]. *Mapping rural health: The geography of health care in rural America* [p. 17]. Bethesda, MD: Office of Rural Health Policy, Health Resources, and Services Administration.)

It is also important to note the concentration of rural population from age 25 to 44 years. This group is responsible for most of the childbearing in rural communities. This growth in population related to births is called "natural increase." In 1990, the Northeast and the West regions of the United States had the largest proportion of 25- to 44-year-old residents (Ricketts, Johnson-Webb, & Randolph, 1999).

Changing Patterns of Migration

Population changes in nonmetropolitan areas have generally been related to natural increase, by way of births or **out-migration** by *residents moving out of rural communities and into urban places* (Ricketts, Johnson-Webb, & Randolph, 1999). Johnson and Beale (as cited in Ricketts et al., 1999) noted that there was more natural increase than out-migration of population during the 1800s in the United States, causing a growth in rural population. In the 1970s the proportion of births decreased, but many people moved into rural communities, with, again, an increase in population. During the 1980s the population trends shifted as nonmetropolitan areas lost population to out-migration. Most rural communities lost population, and any gains were due to increased births. Trends since the early 1990s have shown a gradual increase in nonmetropolitan population (Ricketts, Johnson-Webb, & Randolph, 1999). Population trends as noted have many implications for the health services needed by rural communities. The patterns of rural migration appear to be "shifting sands," which adds to the challenge of planning health resources for rural communities.

POPULATION CHARACTERISTICS

The following information is meant to describe, not stereotype rural clients. Each rural community is unique, as are its residents. You, the community health nurse, must determine whether the population characteristics discussed "fit" the selected rural community. Keep in mind, too, that many rural clients reside in countries outside of the United States. The nursing student planning to practice in the international arena will need to seek out relevant information about the rural population to be served.

Age and Gender

The elderly, 65 years and older, are the fastest growing population group in the United States in all communities, including rural America. From 1980 to 1990 there was a 20% growth in the number of nonmetropolitan people 65 years and older, as compared with a total metropolitan growth of 4% (Fugitt, 1995). Sigler (1995) notes that of the over 10 million rural elderly in the United States in 1990, more than 3 million were age 75 or older. Older women outnumbered older rural men by more than 1 million.

When compared with metropolitan counties, nonmetropolitan counties have a slightly increased proportion of residents under age 15 (Fugitt, 1995). Population trends have a direct relationship to the kinds of health services that are needed in rural communities. Growing families with young children need maternity, pediatric, and family health medical services. They can also benefit from health promotion and disease prevention services.

The elderly, on the other hand, need health care to manage their increased numbers of chronic health conditions. Rural communities need to provide access to nursing homes and other rehabilitative services, as well as hospitals, clinics, and health promotion programs that serve the elderly and the entire community.

Race and Ethnicity

Rural areas have less racial diversity than urban areas. In 1990, 88% of nonmetropolitan area residents were Caucasian; 8% African American; 2% American Indian, Eskimo, or Aleut; and 0.5% Asian or Pacific Islander. The number of rural residents classified as Hispanic/Latino is unclear because people who identify themselves as "Hispanic" may be counted under any of the racial categories (U.S. Bureau of Census, 1990).

Some rural areas of the country have much greater racial diversity. Nonmetropolitan Hispanics generally live in the Western United States and the state of Texas, whereas the majority of nonmetropolitan Asian Americans live in Hawaii. Two thirds of nonmetropolitan Native Americans live in the Western United States, or in the state of Oklahoma. Most African-American nonmetropolitan residents live in the Southern states (Fugitt, 1995).

Level of Education

Rural clients in the United States generally have lower educational attainment than urban clients. Nonmetropolitan adults (25+ years), as reported in the 1990 census, had fewer college degrees and more were high school dropouts, as compared with adults (25+ years) living in metropolitan areas (Table 31–2). This may be due to the fact that rural clients have little access to higher education, such as community colleges and universities close to home. Teixeira (1995) concludes that the majority of rural residents have the education they need to work in their communities.

Income and Occupations

There are rural communities with a moderate number of very wealthy residents. On average, however, the income of people

TABLE 31-2. Educational Level of Adults—1990

	Metropolitan	Nonmetropolitan
Associate degree, bachelor's degree, or advanced degree	28.9%	18.4%
High school diploma, some college	48.1%	50.8%
High school dropout	23%	30.8%

Adapted from Teixeira, 1995, and 1990 census.

in rural communities is lower than that of persons living in urban communities. Mills (1995) notes that wages are higher in nearly every metropolitan area as compared with nonmetropolitan areas.

There are a number of economic advantages to living in a rural area. The cost of land is lower than in urban areas; therefore, housing costs are also lower. Taxes are lower and restrictions on land use are less stringent (Mills, 1995). Lower cost land is advantageous to business such as manufacturing, which may need large parcels of land.

Although many people equate farming with rural life, as of 1990 only 1.9% to 2.4% of the total U.S. population were rural farmers (Mills, 1995; USDHHS, 1998). Only 1 in 16 people in 1990 lived on farms (Hart, 1995). The United States is unique in that it feeds its population with such a small percentage of its workers and still exports food products to the rest of the world.

Other typically rural work, such as mining and forestry, varies by locale. Rural areas have manufacturing, business, education, and service occupations just like more urban communities. The use of the telephone and Internet for commerce is now becoming common in rural areas (Mills, 1995). You may never know that a business is located in a rural community the next time you order a product from an Internet website or by telephone.

RURAL POPULATIONS AT RISK

Homeless Families

The homeless are a population at risk in many rural communities. Although fewer in number, rural homeless families are similar to their urban counterparts. They are often headed by a female (Wagner, Menke, & Ciccone, 1995). They have frequently suffered a series of personal crises—illness, loss of work, loss of housing, or others that have led to their homelessness. Finally, although they usually consider themselves to have few major health needs, studies frequently report heavy smoking, alcohol use, and illegal drug use with some in this population (Wagner, Menke, & Ciccone, 1995).

Homeless children are at risk for developmental delays, nutritional deficits, and other health problems.

In rural settings the problems of homelessness may be compounded by lack of transportation, inadequate shelters, few employment opportunities, limited access to health and social services, and a lack of cheap housing. Community health nurses need to attempt to address the multiple needs of this population. They should (1) seek out homeless families, (2) assess their health needs, (3) connect the families with available resources—health, financial, housing, and others, and (4) remain connected with the families until they have stabilized (see Research: Bridge to Practice).

Perinatal Clients

Historically, the best outcomes for obstetric clients have been with white urban women (Lishner, Larson, Rosenblatt & Clark, 1999). The question is, do rural women have adequate access to prenatal care to ensure the births of healthy infants? Perinatal clients are *pregnant women in the last half of their pregnancy and their newborn infants until 1 month of age.*

Local access to obstetric care is basic to positive birth outcomes. The Council on Medical Education (as cited in Lishner et al., 1999) states that 20% of the U.S. population lives in rural areas, yet only 9% of physicians practice in these communities. It is understandable that many pregnant women either receive care from primary care physicians in their own community or need to travel distances into an urban center for care by an obstetrician. Babies born to these women enter into the rural system of health care as soon as they are born.

Larson, Hart, and Rosenblatt (1997) report their analysis of single births in the United States during 1985 to 1987. Over 11 million infant births were analyzed about a number of factors, including metropolitan versus nonmetropolitan residence. In this national group, residence in an nonmetropolitan county was not associated with low birth weight or increased neonatal mortality. However, the study also found that nonmetropolitan women often sought prenatal care later than urban women, suggesting that access to early obstetric care remains a problem for rural women. Obviously, the initiation of early prenatal care is an issue of concern for rural community health nurses seeking to optimize birth outcomes in their community.

Omar, Schiffman, & Bauer (1998) identified four barriers to care—economics, transportation, attitudes, and organizational barriers—from a convenience sample of 61 Midwest rural pregnant women and their providers. In this study, *economic* barriers were paramount. Rural women were concerned about paying for care, and Medicaid was the number one problem. Pregnant women did not know that they could seek care with Medicaid approval pending. *Transportation* was not identified as a barrier to seeking prenatal care for 80% of respondents. Providers, however, viewed transporta-

RESEARCH Bridge to Practice

Hornberger, C. A. & Cobb, A. K. (1998). A rural vision of a healthy community. *Public Health Nursing, 15*(5), 363–369.

Nurses can assist rural clients to identify their vision of a healthy community. Delivery of primary health care in a rural community requires that nurses understand the rural communities' perceptions of health and health care. The purpose of the part of the ethnographic study reported in this article was to determine "What is your vision of a healthy community?" Horton, Kansas, a town of 2,000 residents, was the site for this study.

Seven nurses participated on the research team. They first looked at secondary data such as town history, census information, and county health statistics. Then they held key informant interviews with the town leaders. Before contacting the other residents, the Horton community was told about the study by radio announcements and an interview with research team members.

One hundred and fifty residents of Horton were involved in the next part of this study. Eight focus group sessions and 56 individual interviews were conducted by the research team over a 5-day period. The nurses kept field notes that were clarified after each session, and all researchers met daily to discuss and share their findings, and plan for the next day. It is interesting to note that the research team initially identified the entire county where Horton is located as the focus of the study. However, during the interviews it became clear that the residents saw their "community" as a smaller area encompassing Horton, the surrounding 5 miles of farms and farmland, and a Native American reservation a short distance away.

To determine "what is the people's vision of a healthy community," Leininger's (1985) theoretical framework was used. Data were collected in each of the following areas: (1) economics, (2) social-kinship, (3) cultural, (4) religion, (5) political–legal, (6) technology, and (7) education. An eighth category of *environment* emerged from the data and was also used.

The selected findings shared here indicate that the residents of Horton shared a vision of a healthy community. For example, regarding *economics,* they valued the hospital and nursing home in their community. They liked local, affordable, accessible health care services. They wanted a good downtown, more jobs, and new industry. The residents also wanted their town to be a place "where children want to return and raise their families." Regarding the *social-kinship* dimension, the residents emphasized the need for people in their community to care for each other. They spoke about a safe community for their children, a community with good schools and recreational activities. Considering the *environment,* residents shared their concerns about both the physical environment and the social environment. The people of Horton wanted a community with clean water and less air pollution and a social environment with healthy people, pride in their community, and recreational opportunities.

In Horton, no specific recommendations for a healthier community were made by the research team nurses. Instead, the community members were asked to develop their own recommendations. Indeed, the residents of Horton had their vision of a healthy Horton community. It was up to the town's residents to make that vision happen.

Directions: Answer these questions related to the research abstract above
1. Share how the term *empowerment* applies to this research study.
2. What was the value of gathering some data about the community before the nurses began their interviews of community members?
3. How would you respond to nurses doing a similar study in your neighborhood/community?

tion as a barrier to care. There was also disagreement among patients and providers about *attitudinal* barriers, with all patients viewing early prenatal care as important. Providers thought that women did not value early prenatal care and that was their reason for not seeking it. *Organizational* barriers relating to access to perinatal care, as reported by the women, included issues with scheduling of physician appointments and needing to take time off work. Physicians did not perceive their office hours as an access issue. These findings cannot be generalized to the larger population but provide some context about perinatal care issues.

Birth in rural communities also is an area of concern. High-risk infants born in rural hospitals are at risk for many potential complications. Alexia, Nichols, Heverly, and Garzon (1997), in a study of nearly 800 pregnant urban and rural women, report that rural women had a higher incidence of low-birth-weight babies. The rural group was younger, but the incidence of poor Apgar scores, congenital anomalies, and neonatal mortality was not significantly different between the urban and rural sample.

Rural community health nurses need to be advocates for the improvement of care for perinatal clients in their communities. Pregnant women, new parents, and their infants are a special population that need the skills and talents of rural community health nurses. These nurses are familiar with the rural community's resources, programs, and needs and are in a position to influence policy changes. Rural community health nurses can optimize the outcomes for perinatal clients through their assessment of the strengths and weaknesses of the system of perinatal care for rural consumers.

The Elderly

The elderly are a population of special concern for rural community health nurses. Some elderly are well and live independently throughout their lives. As an aggregate, however, the elderly have increased chronic disease, disabilities, and functional impairments (U.S. Congress, 1990). Himes and Rutrough (1994) found that the elderly in nonmetropolitan counties had fewer physician visits annually than elders in metropolitan areas. Rural elders in their study sought out doctors most often when they were in poor health, had difficulty with walking or bathing, or lived alone. Findings from the National Health Interview Survey (1990 to 1994) indicate that 35% of rural elders between 65 and 69 years of age rate their own health status as poor (Coburn & Bolda, 1999).

Rural elders rarely have close access to the sophisticated health care that they need. Oncologists, cardiologists, neurologists, and other specialists do not typically practice in rural communities. Extended travel to these specialists can be a severe barrier to obtaining needed care.

Older adults tend to stay in their own homes, even when ill. They do not want to move to a dependent living situation. Rural elders in poor health often have limited alternative housing arrangements when they can no longer live by themselves (Griffin, 1999). Many of the community services required to maintain ill elders in their homes may not be available in rural communities. They may need to move to a nursing home when in-home or assisted living placements are not available.

The Mentally Ill

Rural residents experience mental illness as do people in urban communities. The mental health resources available to rural residents, however, may be limited to primary care physicians, community mental health centers (CMHC), state hospitals, and clergy (Bane, 1997). CMHCs may be restricted to treating only individuals with severe mental illness (Hartley, Korsen & Marc, 1998). Less severely ill people may be placed on long waiting lists and never receive needed services. These individuals may lack health insurance that could enable them to seek private mental health services.

There is a stigma associated with having a mental illness. Rural residents may be unwilling to use mental health specialists' services because of the stigma and their concerns about confidentiality. Rural practitioners need to consider ways to reduce the stigma of mental illness, ensure confidentiality, and connect rural residents with the mental health services that they need.

Primary care providers may be in the best position to make these connections. These physicians, physician assistants, and nurse practitioners should be alert to the signs and symptoms of depression and other mental health disorders. They need to note that depression in women is often an indicator of domestic violence. Two studies on rural women seeking services through a clinic reported that 19% to 20% of the women had experienced abuse in the past year (Kershner, Long & Anderson, 1998; Van Hightower & Gorton, 1998). All women should be questioned about violence in their lives. Rural women who present to primary care providers with physical problems may be depressed and/or living in a violent situation and need to have their situation exposed and services offered.

Another overlooked group is the elderly in rural communities with mental health problems. Outpatient services for elders with mental illness may not be available. These elders may be unable to care for themselves any more without in-

tensive home health and other support services, which may be limited or nonexistent in their area. Rural residents may be admitted to nursing homes for long-term custodial care (Bane, 1997).

Ideally, there should be an integration of primary care and mental health services so that people who need mental health services receive them. Integration can be accomplished through (1) diversification—coordinating primary care and mental health services in one organization, (2) linkages—having mental health providers at the same site, (3) referrals—primary care providers to mental health specialists, or (4) enhancement—training primary care providers to give the necessary mental health services themselves (Lambert, Bird, Hartley & Genova, 1996).

Community health nurses need to be aware of the mental health resources available in the rural community and to assist rural residents to access those services appropriately. Rural community health nurses can work with other professionals to "get the word out" about mental health and illness issues to churches, service clubs, businesses, and the community at large. Only then can the stigma associated with mental illness be lessened and rural residents receive the mental health services that are needed.

Native Americans

Nearly 2 million Native Americans live in rural America, most often on or near tribal reservations in 28 states (Joho & Ormsby, 2000) (Fig. 31–2).

> **A unique feature of a federally recognized tribe is that the tribe has signed a treaty with the U.S. government providing eligibility of the tribe to participate in federal programs such as the Indian Health Service (IHS) while at the same time placing the land once occupied by the American Indian in trust to the U.S. government, thus the term reservation (Joho & Ormsby, 2000, p. 210).**

Takeuchi and Jehara (as cited in Hartley, Bird & Dempsey, 1999) note that Native Americans may move back and forth between their rural homes and nearby urban cities because of unemployment and poverty. Native Americans who leave the reservation may be ineligible for health care services by the IHS. This can be problematic because Native Americans are at risk for numerous health problems.

American Indians have an infant mortality rate twice that of whites. They also have some of the highest rates of diabetes, obesity, alcoholism, and smoking (USDHHS, 2000). Stubben (as cited in Hartley, Bird & Dempsey, 1999) states that Native American adolescents drink more alcohol and use more marijuana and inhalants than other American adolescents. Native American adolescents also have higher suicide levels.

Nurses and other professionals working with Native Americans should attempt to identify the traditions and beliefs of their patients. They can ask their Native American patients about their traditions related to healing and attempt to incor-

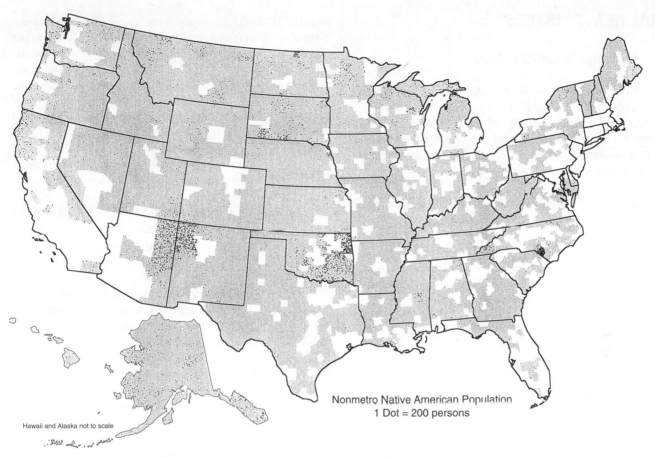

Nonmetro Native American Population
1 Dot = 200 persons

Hawaii and Alaska not to scale

Note: Metropolitan counties are aggregated into white areas on the map.
Source: US Bureau of the Census, 1990.
Produced by: North Carolina Rural Health Research and Policy Analysis Center, Cecil G. Sheps Center for Health Services Research,
University of North Carolina at Chapel Hill, with support from the Federal Office of Rural Health Policy, HRSA, US DHHS.

FIGURE 31–2. Distribution of nonmetropolitan Native American population, 1990.
(Ricketts, T. [Ed.] [1998]. *Mapping rural health: The geography of health care in rural America* [p. 10]. Bethesda, MD: Office of Rural Health Policy, Health Resources, and Services Administration.)

porate those into the health services delivered. Nurses working with this population should encourage health promotion activities such as exercise, no smoking, and reduced alcohol consumption to minimize health consequences related to these behaviors.

Farm Workers

Agricultural workers operating family farms are another population at risk. There are many potential health and safety issues associated with farming. Agricultural workers are exposed to hazards every day, yet they generally receive little injury prevention education. For example, farming today is a high-technology industry with much potentially hazardous equipment. Heavy machinery such as tractors, forklifts, and combine harvesters can cause serious injuries, especially when operated by unskilled workers. Toxic pesticides and

other chemicals are commonplace on farms. Power tools, ladders, and discarded farm equipment account for many electrical shocks, falls, and other injuries.

Farms are also places where people live and play. Farm families are exposed to potential dangers daily. More than 24,000 farm children are injured each year from falls, drownings, electrical shocks, suffocations, and other causes (Hammett & Mock, 1997). Some children die from their injuries.

The community health nurse can intervene with farm workers by using tools that identify farm hazards. A walk-through of a farm can assist the nurse in the process. Farm safety checklists and a risk-mapping tool are available through the National Institute for Occupational Safety and Health (NIOSH). The community health nurse can obtain additional assessment tools through the local Department of Agriculture extension agent. Community health nurses can include injury prevention in all interactions with farm workers and their families. A multifaceted approach works best with this population.

RURAL HEALTH ISSUES

Self, Home, and Community Care

Historically, self-management of health care problems has been the most common way for rural people to cope with illness. This may be a strength. Rural clients are resourceful and often have a supportive network to get their health needs met. Because cost, travel, weather, and distance are barriers to obtaining health services from formal health care providers, rural clients will often employ a variety of folk treatments and home remedies before consulting a nurse or physician. Thus, they tend to visit providers at a much later stage than people in urban areas. Magilvy, Congdon, and Martinez (1994) found that home health care (HHC) fits well with the culture of rural life. HHC allows people to stay at home, supports their hardiness, and compensates for the long distance between home and formal health care.

In the same ethnographic study of rural older adults, the researchers discovered two "circles of care" themes apparent in rural communities. These are (1) a circle of continuity of care and (2) a circle of family and community support.

The **circle of continuity of care** relates to the formal plan of care integral to health care delivery. For example, when a person is hospitalized, discharge planning is critical to the "circle." A continuum of formal providers give support; physicians, community health nurses, pharmacists, social workers, and others are essential to the client doing well after discharge.

The **circle of family and community support** forms another informal circle around many rural clients. This supportive network may provide meals, transportation, errands, household tasks, personal care, shopping, and other services. Sometimes, family members just need to identify what they cannot provide, and the supportive network of neighbors and community agencies responds.

Major Health Problems

CARDIOVASCULAR DISEASE

Pearson and Lewis (1998) found that heart disease, diabetes, and cancer rates in 44,406 rural New York residents exceeded the mean rates for urban dwellers. Their study also found that, often, rural residents do not focus on prevention early enough to make significant differences in health outcomes. Another study on rural Appalachian adults (Ramsey & Glenn, 1998) showed that the subjects had significant risk factors for heart disease, including excessive smoking, lack of exercise, and high-fat diets.

There are clear differences in cardiovascular mortality rates when comparing metropolitan and nonmetropolitan rural residents. Data compiled by the National Center for Health Statistics (1991 to 1995; as cited in Ricketts, Johnson-Webb, & Randolph, 1999) showed that rural residents were at greater risk in every instance when compared with the urban popula-

tion. The 1995 age–sex-adjusted cardiovascular death rate was highest for the African-American rural population (2,800 per 100,000), followed by the urban African-American population (2,600 per 100,000). The rate for nonmetropolitan Caucasian population (1,800 per 100,000) exceeded that for the urban Caucasian group (1,700 per 100,000). Other rural populations together had cardiovascular mortality rates of 1,450 per 100,000, whereas their urban counterparts had fewer heart-related deaths (1,000 per 100,000).

There may be many reasons for these data. Rural residents may ignore their early cardiovascular symptoms and give little heed to preventive interventions such as exercise and low-fat diets. They also live in areas that usually have less high-tech equipment available, which may affect patient outcomes for rural patients with cardiovascular emergencies.

HIV/AIDS

Almost 700,000 cases of acquired immunodeficiency syndrome (AIDS) have been reported in the United States since 1981. There are estimates that nearly a million people are infected with the human immunodeficiency virus (HIV), many of whom do not know of their infection (USDHHS, 2000). HIV/AIDS was first identified in the United States in urban populations. Brownlea and colleagues and the CDC (as cited in Ricketts, Johnson-Webb, & Randolph, 1999) report that, although the numbers of HIV/AIDS cases in rural areas are small, the numbers are increasing, especially in the rural regions of the South and Midwest. Residents of Southern states have a higher proportion of black residents who are particularly affected by this disease.

The early diagnosis and treatment of HIV/AIDS are issues that must be faced by all rural communities. Physicians, nurses, and other health practitioners need to be educated about the changing face of this disease. Because of the relatively few numbers of HIV/AIDS-affected people in any one community, it can be a challenge to stay up to date with the newest treatment protocols. Sowell and Opava (1995) reported on the "Rural-Based Nurse Model" implemented in Georgia to provide extensive education to public health nurses, correctional nurses, and home health/hospice nurses across the state. They propose that their model of educational classes and clinical practice has the potential for improving the quality of care for those with HIV/AIDS in rural areas and that the model can be easily adapted for other settings.

It may be difficult for a person to seek diagnosis or treatment from a rural health practitioner. Confidentiality is an issue of concern, as is the lack of anonymity. People with HIV/AIDS may fear for their jobs or "place in the community" if their diagnosis is learned. Rural people may, instead, choose to seek out HIV/AIDS testing through an urban health facility where they know no one. Returning to their community can be devastating without the support services in place that they may need and because of fearing to share their diagnosis with others.

Another issue that is becoming all too common is that of urban residents with "rural roots" returning to their home rural communities as their illness worsens. These people seek family support and can overwhelm their caregivers, especially if the caregivers do not seek support for themselves. Community health nurses are in a good position to assist families with any health issues.

The impact of HIV/AIDS on other rural areas of the world is devastating. Large populations of countries in Africa and elsewhere are being engulfed by this disease. Often, people with HIV/AIDS have no access to treatment modalities and little understanding about the epidemiology of the disease. Certainly, the key to this disease lies in its prevention. Nurses worldwide are in a position to provide education and advocate for policies that provide for humane treatment for people with HIV/AIDS.

Access to Health Care

INSURANCE AND MANAGED CARE

Health insurance in today's market is costly, especially for individual purchasers. Some people, therefore, forego health insurance for themselves and their families. Depending on their income, these people may or may not be eligible for Medicaid. The 1996 American Nurses Association (ANA) Rural/Frontier Health Care Task Force document states that the proportion of low-income people eligible for Medicaid is lower in nonmetropolitan areas because of more stringent Medicaid rules in rural areas. Even people eligible for government health assistance may not apply because of their belief that it is a sign of weakness to "accept a handout."

Historically, health care in rural and urban communities was delivered by a traditional fee-for-service model. The managed care model, attempting to control costs and improve health care delivery, has diffused into rural communities slowly. By the end of 1995, fewer than 11% of rural Medicaid recipients were enrolled in managed care organizations (MCOs) ("How Do We Make Managed Care," 1998).

Building provider networks in rural communities is more time- and effort-intensive because rural providers are often inexperienced with MCOs (Felt-Lisk, Silberman, Hoag & Slifkin, 1999). These providers are geographically dispersed in solo and small group practices. Amundson (as cited in "How Do We Make Manage Care," 1998) sees three major choices for rural communities related to MCOs. The community's providers can join an existing health maintenance organization (HMO), they can form a local or regional network for managed care, or they can operate their own health plan with its inherent costs. Amundson believes that rural communities should explore the formation of community health plans (CHP). The CHPs are composed of local or regional organizations that pull together the providers with a financing system, often an existing MCO. This model supports the local providers, maintains local control, and attempts to retain local dollars. The costs of MCOs, however, are high and their future development in rural areas is uncertain (see Bridging Financial Gaps).

BARRIERS TO ACCESS

Access to health care for rural clients has numerous barriers. The physical distance between place of residence and place for health care can be considerable. Rural clients may be referred to a distant urban medical center for cancer therapy or other sophisticated health care. This population may be frustrated when they travel to a faraway site for care and do not have their problem solved. Rural clients need to be advised before they travel "into town" to check and make sure that their health care provider is not behind schedule or unable to see them.

Transportation can also be an issue, especially for people who do not drive or lack dependable transportation. Unpredictable weather adds to potential barriers for rural clients.

Bridging Financial Gaps

Rural community health nurses often serve as school nurses for the local schools. One fall day, a 15-year-old student was referred to the nurse because he didn't have the required physical examination form signed by a physician so that he might play basketball. The nurse met with the student, John, that day and inquired about the needed physical examination. John explained that his father had recently lost his job and now the family didn't have health insurance. He would have to wait until he could earn the money to pay for the doctor examination. John said that he understood that he would not be able to start the basketball season with his classmates. Mrs. J., the community health nurse, asked if she could meet with John's parents; he agreed.

The next afternoon, Mrs. J. visited John's parents at their home and confirmed that John had their permission to play basketball. They discussed the family's loss of health insurance and limited income to purchase private insurance. Mrs. J. told the family that she would attempt to help John get a free or low-cost physical, if that was acceptable to them.

Mrs. J. made a few telephone calls that afternoon and was able to get John an appointment to see Dr. Z., the "Team Doctor," at his office the next afternoon. Dr. Z. was pleased to give John the necessary examination. Mrs. J. also let John and his parents know about the appointment; they were pleased. Mrs. J. then shared that she had an application for a new state subsidized health insurance plan for families that was available at minimal cost. She encouraged John's parents to apply for the reduced premium insurance.

Weeks later, at a basketball game, John's mother approached Mrs. J. and thanked her for helping their family to get enrolled in the subsidized insurance plan. The family now had the basic health insurance for their family's health care needs and John was enjoying playing basketball on the school team.

Snow, ice, wind, and rain may make travel dangerous, even for short distances. Parents may decide not to risk driving on poorly maintained roads to get their children immunized or have their own hypertension evaluated. Travel in emergency situations can be life threatening not only because of the emergency situation itself but also because of the distance involved to get the ill or injured person to the nearest health facility.

Limited choice of health providers may be a barrier for some rural residents. There are fewer physicians, nurses, dentists, and other providers. Sometimes client concerns about confidentiality or provider expertise may cause people to seek care services from even more distant providers.

NEW APPROACHES TO IMPROVE ACCESS

The *Healthy People 2010* objectives (2000) mandate improvements in health education, health screening, immunizations, and disease morbidity for the United States. Creative ways of delivering these and other services to rural clients need to be explored. Access to care is a social justice issue; clients who live in rural areas should receive quality health care.

One approach that has been successful in numerous rural areas is the use of mobile clinics (Lee & O'Neal, 1994). These clinics bring health care providers to remote places for health screenings, immunizations, and other service delivery. Mobile health clinics are frequently staffed by nurse practitioners and can improve access to health care for low-income residents.

School-based clinics are another approach to improve access. These clinics in schools provide available, community-based, affordable, and culturally acceptable care to well and sick children (Terwilliger, 1994). Often, grant-supported, school-based clinics facilitate the receipt of health education and primary care by children who are otherwise without easy access to health services.

Telehealth is the newest approach for increasing access to care. **Telehealth** provides electronically transmitted clinician consultation between the client and the health care provider. Burtt (1997) describes a pilot program for this new technology. A home health nurse monitored a patient with congestive heart failure effectively using two-way audiovisual transmission over telephone lines. The patient controlled the process by turning his home monitor on and off himself. Clients can be assessed quickly by way of this interactive communication from physician offices and other sites. Telehealth technology may decrease emergency room visits and hospitalizations. The U.S. Department of Health and Human Services now provides Medicare reimbursement to health care providers for telehealth services (Burtt, 1997) in designated health professional shortage areas.

Healthy People 2010 Goals

The two broad objectives of *Healthy People 2010* are (1) increase quality and years of health life and (2) eliminate health disparities. The report notes that injury-related death rates are 40% higher in rural communities and that 20% of the rural population is uninsured as compared with 16% of urban residents (USDHHS, 2000). Model standards are being written by communities with community-specific objectives to reduce morbidity and mortality and determine the preventive services to emphasize in their locale. It may be useful for rural communities to consider focusing on these health indicators:

- Access to health care
- Mental health
- Tobacco use
- Injury and violence
- Overweight and obesity
- Environmental health

Rural community health nurses need to consider the *Healthy People 2010* objectives as guides for improving the health status of rural communities throughout the next decade.

RURAL COMMUNITY HEALTH NURSING

Working in a Rural Community

Rural community health nurses are most often women who either grew up in rural areas or lived for a time in small communities. They frequently have extended family there (Bushy, 1994). Rural nurses are active members of their community and are highly respected professionals. Display 31–2 lists characteristics of rural nurses (ANA Rural/Frontier Health Care Task Force, 1996). The ANA also states in its "Statement on Rural Nursing" (1990) that the organization is concerned about the availability and quality of rural health services. The ANA recommends recruitment of rural residents into nursing and rural nurses into leadership roles.

Rural community health nurses will utilize the levels of primary, secondary, and tertiary prevention in their practice. Primary prevention may be used as the community health nurse provides immunizations to children at a well-child clinic or influenza vaccine to elders at the local community center. The nurse may engage in secondary screening while doing blood pressure checks with adults or while screening school children for scoliosis. Rural community health nurses will have opportunities to practice tertiary prevention as they work with a child with special health care needs or when they visit a recently hospitalized rural resident needing home health care. It is important that the rural community health nurse emphasize each of the levels of prevention.

How do you begin to learn about a rural community? If you are going to have a rural clinical experience in community health nursing, these simple steps are for you (Display 31–3). Your community assessment skills (see Chapter 18) will come in handy. It is helpful to (1) approach the community without preconceived ideas, as a stranger, and (2) observe and describe the people, places, and activities of the community at different times of day. You should (3) use your

DISPLAY 31–2. Rural Nurse Characteristics

- They have close community ties.
- They are expected to be all things to all people.
- Confidentiality is a concern because of blurring of social and professional roles.
- Autonomy is important in retaining and satisfying rural nurses.
- Rural nursing staffs are generally cohesive; there is less burnout than urban nurses.
- Rural nurses are seen as positive assets to their community.

(Adapted from American Nurses Association [ANA] Rural/Frontier Health Care Task Force [1996]. *Rural/frontier nursing: The challenge to grow.* Washington, DC: American Nurses Publishing.)

DISPLAY 31–3. Working as a Community Health Nurse in a Rural Community

- Approach the community without preconceived ideas.
- Observe/describe the people, places, and activities.
- Use all of your senses.
- Talk with key informants.
- Review available demographic, morbidity, and mortality data.
- Determine potential community strengths and problems.
- Verify your impressions.
- Enjoy your learning!

senses—your eyes, ears, and nose to learn about the neighborhood and (4) identify key informants and talk with them about their community. **Key informants** are people who know much about their community and are willing to share their information with you. You need to (5) review the demographic, morbidity, and mortality data that are available about the locale and (6) determine potential strengths and potential problems for the community. Lastly, you must (7) verify your impressions with community members—including the health providers you will be working with—and (8) enjoy your learning experience!

Roles of the Nurse

There are many roles for the rural community health nurse. They include:

1. Advocate—for rural clients and families, assisting them to obtain the best possible health care
2. Coordinator/case manager—connecting rural clients with the health and social services they need
3. Health teacher—providing education to individuals, families, or groups on health promotion or other health-related topics (rural community health nurses frequently teach Lamaze, parenting, and other classes)
4. Referral agent—making appropriate connections between rural clients and urban providers of services
5. Mentor—to new community health nurses, nursing students, and other nurses new to the rural community
6. Change agent/researcher—suggesting new approaches to solving patient care or community health problems based on research, professional literature, and community assessment
7. Activist—willing to take appropriate risks to improve the community's health

It may be helpful to see how all these roles come into play during a typical day for a rural community health nurse. Carol M. arrives at the Stevens County Public Health Department in rural America. She reviews her caseload for the

day and begins her work. First, she telephones the principal of the local high school to let him know that she is able to speak next week to the Parent-Teacher Association about raising healthy adolescents (*health teacher*). Then, Carol calls the family of a hospitalized patient (*coordinator/case manager*) to begin the plans related to discharge of their family member. At 10 AM Carol makes a home visit to the Wesley family. They explain that they have been unable to enroll for needed food stamps because they do not understand the process. Carol encourages the family to contact the appropriate agency (*referral agent*) and even calls her neighbor who works at that office to inform her of the referral (*advocate*). After lunch, the nurse returns to her office for a staff meeting and discusses a new charting system that she is recommending (*change agent/researcher*) that the department consider implementing. At the same meeting, Carol is asked if she will work with a visiting community health nursing student during his rural practicum (*mentor*). Carol agrees. That evening, Carol, as a concerned citizen, participates in a meeting at the town hall about concerns related to local water quality. Carol addresses the group (*activist*) and volunteers to lead others concerned about this issue. As you can see, community health nurses like Carol M. often play many roles during their day. As a nursing student working in a rural community, you may have the opportunity to "try on" many of these roles (see Voices From the Community).

Challenges and Opportunities

AUTONOMY

Rural community health nurses have the opportunity to use autonomy in daily practice. Nurses must rapidly assume independent and interdependent decision-making roles, due to the small workforce and the large workload. Rural community health nurses learn to prioritize tasks quickly and work effectively with others to "get the job done." Referrals to other rural providers are facilitated because providers frequently know one another. The rural community health nurse

Voices From the Community

I knew where this road would end. After a mile or so, I would have to stop, open, drive through, and then close the cattle gate before arriving at a complex of old buildings. There would be two houses, a trailer home, plus all the other assorted ranch buildings. The end house was the home of an elderly lady that I had visited monthly for an injection. She was the mother of the two men who ran this rural ranch, and the visits that accompanied the treatment to the elderly lady were delightful. As a rural public health nurse, I now had been called to visit the home of the hired man. His wife had given birth to a new baby the month before. The new mom, Ellen, invited me into her cluttered kitchen. She was somewhat quiet and only 17 years old. She stated that her delivery had gone well, and that this was her fist baby. Her husband had three other children living with his first wife. He was quite a bit older than Ellen and wasn't particularly interested in another child. Ellen's family was in another state, and I got the indication that marriage was a good reason for her to leave home. When I asked to see the baby, I was led into another small room in the trailer. The 1-month-old infant was lying on his back, awake, staring at the ceiling. Ellen stated that her son was a good baby, who rarely cried and spent most of his time in the crib. She made no effort to talk with him or pick him up. I told her what a beautiful baby he was, and that I would like to visit her several times to help answer her questions about child care, or any other matters. Before I left that day, she began asking questions about mixing formula and feeding her infant, and I felt that she truly wanted to be a good mom. As I drove back to town, I contemplated where to start with my next visit. Basic infant care needed to be addressed, as well as how Ellen and her son would get to their medical appointments, when her husband and the beat-up pickup truck were her only means of transportation. The ranch owners were neighborly but didn't appear interested in supporting Ellen in the mothering of her son. Isolation certainly was a potential problem for Ellen. I also was very concerned about the brain development of an infant with such little stimulation. Unfortunately, before I could put any more interventions into place, I learned that the family had moved without leaving a forwarding address. To this day, I still wonder about the life of that child, and whether Ellen was able to find the resources to parent effectively.

Deborah, a public health nurse

has an advantage over urban nurses in that the rural health care system is smaller and easier to influence and change.

"ALWAYS A NURSE"
Anonymity is not easy for the rural community health nurse. These nurses are always "on duty." A trip to the grocery store on a Saturday morning may include interactions with rural clients and their families about pressing health concerns.

Rural community health nurses may have confidentiality and personal/professional boundary issues that need to be addressed. However, rural community health nurses are often respected, known, and trusted by the population they serve.

FUNDING YOUR EDUCATION
Some of the educational loans available to you at the undergraduate and graduate levels may be reduced or forgiven if you practice nursing in a rural community after graduation. You should inquire through your nursing program about that possibility. It is also possible to contact a specific rural community to see if the community will offer some monetary support in return for your working in the host community for several years.

ISOLATION
Rural community health nurses may experience the challenge of physical isolation from personal and professional opportunities associated with urban areas. Travel to cities for basic and continuing education can be a barrier. Rural nurses may also feel isolated in their clinical practice because of the scarcity of professional colleagues. Many rural community health nurses can overcome these barriers and learn to appreciate the benefits of clinical practice in a rural setting by discussing their concerns with peers and seeking ways to combat isolation.

"DOLLARS AND SENSE"
The rural community health nurse will often receive a salary less than urban nurses in comparable positions. However, there are other benefits to rural nursing. Housing costs are usually cheaper than larger cities, and long commutes to and from work on congested highways are avoided. Rural communities are a great place to live and raise a family. The slower pace of life, open spaces, clean air, and friendly atmosphere may make more "sense."

MANY POSSIBILITIES
The smaller system of health care in a rural community may be an advantage to the community health nurse. It may be easier to "understand the system" and initiate planned change. For example, if a rural nurse wanted to continue his or her education, a college of nursing could be contacted to offer the needed classes. There are many possibilities to enhance rural nursing practice, including continuing education by way of satellite or Internet, partnerships with larger medical centers, and invitations to clinical experts to provide on-site workshops. Grants can be written to facilitate these endeavors.

An Innovative Nursing Model

In 1993, the University of North Dakota's (UND) nursing program developed a nursing center to assist rural residents to meet many of their health needs. The UND Nursing Center also provides clinical education for nursing students and a practice site for faculty. The UND Nursing Center is "population specific, family-focused, community based . . . and directed toward primary prevention and care during chronic illness" (Henly, Tyree, Lindsey, Lambeth & Burd, 1998, p. 22). The Center adopted the World Health Organization model of Primary Health Care that "emphasizes the five principles of:

- Equitable distribution
- Community involvement
- Appropriate technology
- Focus on prevention
- Multisectoral approach" (Henly et al., 1998, p. 24)

The nursing students provide care and collaborate with other community agencies and providers. Emphasis at the Nursing Center is on care rather than cure, and on chronic illness rather than acute illness. Much emphasis is placed on primary prevention. Junior-level students provide community-based, family-centered prenatal nursing care to expectant parents; a child health program delivers care to families with children having chronic illnesses or special needs. Senior nursing students deliver community health services to high-risk populations (eg, those with diabetes or other chronic illnesses).

The UND Center also provides health education in public and private schools, and health screening (Henly et al., 1998). This innovative program serves as a model to other educational institutions. Rural residents are the real "winners" when they are the recipients of increased options for care.

SUMMARY

Rural clients are a unique aggregate. Community health nurses are key to ensuring the delivery of appropriate health services to this population. There are numerous definitions of the term *rural*. In this chapter, rural is defined as communities with fewer than 10,000 residents and a county population density of fewer than 1,000 people per square mile. The numbers of people living in rural communities have increased over the last century. During the same time span the proportion of rural residents decreased, whereas the proportion of urban residents increased. The elderly are a rapidly growing population in rural communities. Rural areas have less diversity than urban places. Rural clients generally have lower educational attainment than urban clients. This may be due to less access to higher education. Income levels and housing costs are frequently lower than in larger cities.

Healthy People 2010 identifies national health goals applicable to rural communities. There are many at-risk populations in these communities. Homeless families often face inadequate shelters, few employment opportunities, lack of inexpensive housing, and limited access to health and social services. Rural elders may have limited alternatives for housing when they can no longer live alone. Perinatal clients may not have the health services they need close to home. Mental health services are limited. Health care providers need to ensure confidentiality and attempt to reduce the stigma of mental illness for these clients. There are numerous risks associated with farming. The community health nurse must help

this population to identify possible hazards and practice injury prevention. Native American clients are at great risk for diabetes, obesity, alcoholism, and smoking.

Community health nurses need to engage in a community assessment of their rural area as part of their orientation. It is helpful to identify the strengths of the community. Rural clients are frequently resourceful and have a supportive network of people to meet their needs.

Access to care is an important issue in rural communities. Health insurance is expensive, and some rural residents choose not to purchase it. Others may be too proud to apply for government assistance. Managed care organizations are diffusing into rural communities, and their long-term impact is uncertain. Barriers to access include distance, weather, transportation, limited choice of providers, and others. Some ways to improve access in these communities are school-based clinics, mobile health vans, and use of the latest technology. University-sponsored nursing centers serving rural populations should be explored.

Rural community health nurses are key members of the professional community. Their roles include advocate, coordinator, case manager, health teacher, referral agent, mentor, change agent/researcher, and activist. Community health nurses have both challenges and opportunities related to their clinical practice. They may have confidentiality and personal/professional boundary issues. Their salaries may be lower than nurses in urban areas. Rural community health nurses are highly respected individuals who make a difference for the community they serve. Maybe you should consider a career as a rural community health nurse.

ACTIVITIES TO PROMOTE CRITICAL THINKING

1. Interview a peer who grew up in a rural community about his or her family and school life. Determine what he or she considers to be his or her best experiences growing up. Compare the peer's best experiences with your own.

2. Complete a community assessment of a rural community with a small group of peers. Compare your assessment findings with an assessment done in an urban neighborhood. Discuss the similarities and differences of the community assessments with your peers.

3. Assume you are a community health nurse in a rural community. Describe your approach to solve the problem of overuse of the emergency room for minor childhood illnesses by community residents.

4. Go on the Internet to locate rural health programs in various states. In addition, see whether the Internet has rural job opportunities for community health nurses.

REFERENCES

Alexy, B., Nichols, B., Heverly, M. A., & Garzon, L. (1997). Perinatal factors and birth outcomes in the public health service: A rural/urban comparison. *Research in Nursing & Health, 20*(1), 61–70.

American Nurses Association. (1990). Statement on rural nursing. *The Kansas Nurse, 65*(5), 6–7.

American Nurses Association (ANA) Rural/Frontier Health Care Task Force. (1996). *Rural/frontier nursing: The challenge to grow*. Washington, DC: American Nurses Publishing.

Bane, S. D. (1997). Rural mental health and aging: Implications for case management. *Journal of Case Management, 6*(4), 158–161.

Bushy, A. (1994). When your client lives in a rural area, part II: Rural professional practice-considerations for nurses providing mental health care. *Issues in Mental Health Nursing, 15*(3), 267–276.

Burtt, K. (1997). Nurses use telehealth to address rural health care needs, prevent hospitalization. *The American Nurse, 29*(6), 21.

Butler, M. A., & Beale, C. A. (1994). *Rural–urban continuum codes for metropolitan counties, 1993*. Washington, DC: Agriculture and Rural Economy Division, Economic Research Service, U.S. Department of Agriculture.

Coburn, A. F., & Bolda, E. J. (1999). Rural elderly and long-term care. In T. C. Ricketts (Ed.), *Rural health in the United States* (pp. 179–189). New York: Oxford University Press.

Felt-Lisk, S., Silberman, P., Hoag, S., & Slifkin, R. (1999). Medicaid managed care in rural areas: A ten-state follow-up study. *Health Affairs, 18*(2), 238–245.

Fugitt, G. V. (1995). Population change in nonmetropolitan America. In E. N. Castle (Ed.), *The changing American countryside* (pp. 77–100). Lawrence, KS: University of Kansas Press.

Griffin, J. (1999). Parish nursing in rural communities. In P. A. Solari-Twadell & M. A. McDermott (Eds.), *Parish nursing: Promoting whole person health within faith communities* (pp. 75–82). Thousand Oaks, CA: Sage.

Hammett, W. S., & Mock, J.E. (1997). Safety on the farmstead. In R. Longley, R. McLymore, W. Meggs & G. Robertson (Eds.), *Safety and health in agriculture, forestry, and fisheries* (pp. 397–418). Rockville, MD: Government Institutes.

Hartley, D., Bird, D., & Dempsey, P. (1999). Rural mental health and substance abuse. In T. C. Ricketts (Ed.), *Rural health in the United States* (pp. 38–51). New York: Oxford University Press.

Hartley, D., Korsen, N., & Marc, D. (1998). Management of patients with depression by rural primary care practitioners. *Archives of Family Medicine, 7*(2), 139–145.

Henly, S. J., Tyree, E. A., Lindsey, D. L., Lambeth, S. O., & Burd, C. M. (1998). Innovative perspectives on health services for vulnerable rural populations. *Family & Community Health, 21*(1), 22–31.

Himes, C. L., & Rutrough, T. S. (1994). Differences in the use of health services by metropolitan and nonmetropolitan elderly. *The Journal of Rural Health, 10*(2), 80–88.

Hornberger, C. A., & Cobb, A. K. (1998). A rural vision of a healthy community. *Public Health Nursing, 15*(5), 363–369.

How do we make managed care work for us? (1998, Fall). *State Rural Health Watch, 5*(1), 2–3, 8–9, 10.

Joho, K. A., & Ormsby, A. (2000). A walk in beauty: Strategies for providing culturally competent care to Native Americans. In M. L. Kelley & V. M. Fitzsimons (Eds.), *Understanding cultural diversity* (pp. 209–218). Sudbury, MA: Jones & Bartlett.

Johnson, K. M. & Beale, C. L. (1993). Demographic change in nonmetropolitan America, 1980–1990. *Rural Sociology, 58*(3), 347–365.

Johnson-Webb, K. D., Baer, M. A., & Gesler, W. M. (1997). What is rural? Issues and considerations. *Journal of Rural Health, 13*(3), 253–256.

Kershner, M., Long, D., & Anderson, J. (1998). Abuse against women in rural Minnesota. *Public Health Nursing, 15*(6), 422–431.

Lambert, D., Bird, D. C., Hartley, D., & Genova, M. (1996). *Integrating primary care and mental health services*. Kansas City, MO: National Rural Health Association.

Larson, E. H., Hart, L. G., & Rosenblatt, R. A. (1997). Is non-metropolitan residence a risk factor for poor birth outcome in the U.S.? *Social Science and Medicine, 45*(2), 171–188.

Lee, E. J., & O'Neal, S. (1994). A mobile clinic experience: Nurse practitioners providing care to a rural population. *Journal of Pediatric Health Care, 8*(1), 12–17.

Lee, H. J. (1991). Definitions of rural: A review of the literature, In A. Bushy (Ed.), *Rural nursing* (Vol. 1). Newbury Park, CA: Sage.

Leininger, M. (1985). Transcultural care diversity and university: A theory of nursing. *Nursing and Health Care, 6*(4), 209–214.

Lishner, D. M., Larson, E. H., Rosenblatt, R. A., & Clark, S. J. (1999). In T. C. Ricketts (Ed.), *Rural health in the United States* (pp. 134–149). New York: Oxford University Press.

Magilvy, J. K., Congdon, J. G., & Martinez, R. (1994). Circles of care: Home care and community support for rural older adults. *Advances in Nursing Science, 16*(3), 22–33.

Mills, E. S. (1995). The location of economic activity in rural and nonmetropolitan United States. In E. N. Castle (Ed.), *The changing American countryside* (pp. 103–133). Lawrence, KS: University Press of Kansas.

Office of Management and Budget (1995). *Revised statistical definitions of metropolitan areas (MAs) and guidance on uses of MA definitions* (OMB Bulletin No. 95–04). Washington, DC: Author.

Omar, M. A., Schiffman, R. F., & Bauer, P. (1998). Barriers to rural prenatal care. *Journal of Community Health Nursing, 15*(4), 237–249.

Pearson, T. A., & Lewis, C. (1998). Rural epidemiology: Insights from a rural population laboratory. *American Journal of Epidemiology, 148*(10), 949–957.

Ramsey, P. W., & Glenn, L. L. (1998). Risk factors for heart disease in rural Appalachia. *Family and Community Health, 20*(4), 71–82.

Ricketts, T. (Ed.). (1998). *Mapping rural health: The geography of health care and health resources in rural America*. Bethesda, MD: Office of Rural Health Policy, Health Resources and Services Administration.

Ricketts, T. C., Johnson-Webb, K. D., & Randolph, R. K. (1999). Populations and places in rural America. In T. C. Ricketts (Ed.), *Rural health in the United States* (pp. 7–24). New York: Oxford University Press.

Rosenblatt, R. A., & Hart, L. G. (1999). Physicians and rural America. In T. C. Ricketts (Ed.), *Rural health in the United States* (pp. 38–51). New York: Oxford University Press.

Sigler, J. E. (1995). *Profile of rural older Americans*. Washington, DC: National Council on Aging.

Sowell, R. L., & Opava, W. D. (1995). The Georgia rural-based nurse model: Primary care for person with HIV/AIDS. *Public Health Nursing, 12*(4), 228–234.

Teixeira, R. A. (1995). Rural education and training: Myths and misconceptions dispelled. In E. N. Castle (Ed.), *The changing American countryside* (pp. 419–435). Lawrence, KS: University of Kansas Press.

Terwilliger, S. H. (1994). Early access to health care services through a rural school-based health center. *Journal of School Health, 64*(7), 284–289.

U.S. Bureau of the Census. (1994). *Geographic areas reference manual*. Washington, DC: Economics and Statistics Administration, Bureau of the Census.

_____. (1990). *1990 census of the population and housing*. Washington, DC: U.S. Government Printing Office.

U.S. Congress. (1990). *Health care in rural America* (OTA Publication No. OTA-H-434). Washington, DC: U.S. Government Printing Office.

U.S. Department of Health and Human Services. (2000, January). *Healthy people 2010* (conference edition, in two volumes). Washington, DC: U.S. Government Printing Office.

U.S. Department of Health and Human Services, Office of Rural Health Policy. (1998). *Definitions of rural: A handbook for health policy makers and researchers* (Tech. Issues Paper) Bethesda, MD: Equal Three Communications.

Van Hightower, N. R., & Gorton, J. (1998). Domestic violence among patients at two rural health clinics: Prevalence and social correlates. *Public Health Nursing, 15*(5), 355–362.

Wagner, J. D., Menke, E. M., & Ciccone, J. K. (1995). What is known about the health of rural homeless families? *Public Health Nursing, 12*(6), 400–408.

SELECTED READINGS

Alexy, B. B., & Elnitsky, C. (1998). Rural mobile health unit: Outcomes. *Public Health Nursing, 15*(1), 3–11.

Bosch, D., & Bushy, A. (1997). The five a's of rural home care. *Caring, 16*(1), 20–25.

Bushy, A. (1997). Case management: Considerations for coordinating quality services in rural communities. *Journal of Nursing Care Quality, 12*(1), 26–35.

_____. (1994). When your client lives in a rural area, part I: Rural health care delivery issues. *Issues in Mental Health Nursing, 15*(3), 253–266.

_____. (1994). Women in rural environments: Considerations for holistic nurses. *Holistic Nursing Practice, 8*(4), 67–73.

Bushy, A. (Ed.). (1991). *Rural nursing*, Vol. 1. Newbury Park, CA: Sage.

Congdon, J. G., & Magilvy, J. K. (1995). The changing spirit of rural community nursing: Documentation burden. *Public Health Nursing, 12*(1), 18–24.

Council on Graduate Medical Education. (1997). *Ninth Report: Graduate Medical Education Consortia: Changing the governance of graduate medical education to achieve physician workforce objectives*. Washington, DC: U.S. Government Printing Office.

Cromartie, J. B., & Swanson, L. L. (1996). Census tracts more precisely define rural populations and areas. *Rural Development Perspectives, 11*(3), 31–39.

Dansky, K. H. (1995). The impact of healthcare reform on rural home health agencies. *Journal of Nursing Administration, 25*(3), 27–33.

Elnitsky, C., & Alexy, B. (1998). Identifying health status and health risks of older rural residents. *Journal of Community Health Nursing, 15*(2), 61–75.

Felton, G. M., Parsons, M. A., Pate, R. R., Ward, D., Saunders, R., Valois, R., Dowda, M., & Trost, S. (1996). Predictors of alcohol use among rural adolescents. *The Journal of Rural Health, 12*(5), 378–385.

Garrett, D. K. (1995). Mobile access: Opening health care doors. *Nursing Management, 26*(10), 30–33.

Hart, J. F. (1995). "Rural" and "farm" no longer mean the same. In E. N. Castle (Ed.), *The changing American countryside* (pp. 63–76). Lawrence, KS: University of Kansas Press.

Hulme, P. A., & Blegen, M. A. (1999). Residential status and birth outcomes: Is the rural/urban distinction adequate? *Public Health Nursing, 16*(3), 176–181.

Irwin, R. (1998). The work of clinical nurse specialists (HIV/AIDS) in areas with a low prevalence of HIV infection. *Journal of Advanced Nursing, 27*, 649–656.

Johnsen, M. C., Morrissey, J. P., Calloway, M. O., Fried, B. J., Blank, M., & Starrett, B. E. (1997). Rural mental health leaders' perceptions of stigma and community issues. *Journal of Rural Health, 13*(1), 59–70.

Knight, D. W. (1997). The challenges of hard-to-reach patients. *Caring, 16*(1), 26–27.

Knollmueller, R. N. (1994). Rural health care and health care reform. *Public Health Nursing, 11*(3), 143–144.

Lee, P. R., & Estes, C. L. (Eds.). (1997). *The nation's health* (5th ed.). Sudbury, MA: Jones & Bartlett.

Lishner, D. M., Richardson, M., Levine, P., & Patrick, D. (1996). Access to primary health care among persons in rural areas: A summary of the literature. *The Journal of Rural Health, 12*(1), 45–52.

May, K. M., Mendelson, C., & Ferketich, S. (1995). Community empowerment in rural healthcare. *Publish Health Nursing, 12*(1), 25–30.

National Rural Health Association. (1995). *Community development applied to rural health care*. Kansas City, MO: Author.

Nesbitt, T. S., Larson, E. H., Rosenblatt, R. A., & Hart, L. G. (1997). Access to maternity care in rural Washington: Its effect on neonatal outcomes and resource use. *American Journal of Public Health, 87*(1), 85–90.

Olds, S. (1997). Designing a care pathway for a maternity support service program in a rural health department. *Public Health Nursing, 14*(6), 332–338.

Pierce, S. F., & Luikart, C. (1996). Managed care: Will the healthcare needs of rural citizens be met? *Journal of Nursing Administration, 26*(4), 28–32.

Ramsbottom-Lucier, M., Emmett, K., Rich, E. C., & Wilson, J. F. (1996). Hills, ridges, mountains, and roads: Geographical factors and access to care in rural Kentucky. *The Journal of Rural Health, 12*(5), 386–394.

Ricketts, T. C. (Ed.). (1999). *Rural health in the United States*. New York: Oxford University Press.

Sachs, B., & Hall, L. A. (1998). Developing community partnerships to enhance care for rural families with low birth weight children. *The Journal of Rural Health, 14*(1), 51–58.

Shaw, J. K. (1997). An assessment of two upstate New York rural counties to determine unmet health needs of the Medicaid population. *Journal of the New York Nurses' Association, 28*(1), 12–15.

Shreffler, M. J. (1996). An ecological view of the rural environment: Levels of influence on access to health care. *Advances in Nursing Science, 18*(4), 48–59.

Slifkin, R. T., Hoag, S. D., Silberman, P., Felt-Lisk, S., & Popkin, B. (1998). Medicaid managed care programs in rural areas: A fifty-state overview. *Health Affairs, 17*(6), 217–227.

U.S. Department of Agriculture, Economic Research Service. (1990). *What is rural?* Available: http://www.econ.ag.gov/briefing/rural/ruralecn/ruralnm.htm.

Van Hook, M. P. (1996). Challenges to identifying and treating women with depression in rural primary care. *Social Work in Health Care, 23*(1), 73–92.

Vrabec, N. J. (1995). Implications of U.S. health care reform on the rural elderly. *Nursing Outlook, 43*(6), 260–265.

Weinert, C., & Burman, M. E. (1994). Rural health and health-seeking behaviors. *Annual Review of Nursing Research, 12,* 65–92.

Wellever, A. (1998). Future rural managed care issues. *The Journal of Rural Health, 14*(3), 274–277.

_____. (1998). Implications of HMOs for rural providers and consumers. *The Journal of Rural Health, 14*(3), 268–273.

White, R. (1997). Rural home care: Social work intervention in social isolation and safety concerns. *Caring, 16*(1), 28–34.

Whitener, L. (Ed.). (1995). Families and family life in rural areas. *Journal of Rural Health, 11*(3), 217–220.

Winstead-Fry, P., Tiffany, J. C., & Shippee-Rice, R. V. (Eds.). (1992). *Rural health nursing.* New York: National League for Nursing Press.

Clients Living in Poverty

KEY TERMS

- Disenfranchised
- Distributive justice
- Feminization of poverty
- Homelessness
- Indigent
- Marginalized
- Poverty threshold
- Social status
- Social support
- Temporary Aid to Needy Families (TANF)

LEARNING OBJECTIVES

Upon mastery of this chapter, you should be able to:
- Identify common characteristics of people living in poverty.
- Analyze political and ethical dimensions of American poverty.
- Identify common health effects of poverty.
- Analyze causes of homelessness and the effect on health.
- Explain the forces determining global poverty and strategies for its elimination.
- Propose intervention strategies at the community, agency, and individual level.
- Assess own attitude toward poverty and identify self-caring strategies when working with impoverished people.

What is your experience with poverty or the poor? Have you or your family lived in poverty? Do you give money to charities for the poor? Why or why not? What are your opinions of the needs of impoverished people? Poverty is of great concern to nurses because of the resulting human hardship and association with poor emotional and physical health.

This chapter provides some general characteristics of the poor in America. We then examine the politics and ethics of poverty, the health effects of poverty, and homelessness in America. We will also look briefly at global poverty. Finally, we will explore the role of the community health nurse in caring for clients living in poverty.

WHO ARE THE POOR?

Poverty Defined

To be poor is to have few or no material possessions as well as inadequate access to family and community resources. Low socioeconomic position in society is determined by social and economic deprivation that includes poor income, no accumulated assets, no access to power, poor education, and low status occupation. People are said to be **indigent** when they are impoverished and deprived of basic comforts.

The U.S. government has an official poverty line or **poverty threshold;** people living below this income line are defined as poor. In 1998, the poverty threshold for a reference family of two adults and two related children was a cash income of $16,588. It was $13,133 for a single mother with two children (U.S. Bureau of the Census, 1998). This number is updated every year with changes in the federal consumer price index. Many government programs, such as Medicaid, Head Start, and food stamps, determine eligibility based on the poverty threshold.

How is the poverty threshold determined? It is assumed that a family spends one third of its budget on food. Therefore, subsistence living costs are calculated by taking a meager food budget and multiplying by three to identify the lowest amount of income needed for all other expenditures such as utilities, clothing, and shelter. This method of defining poverty is under government evaluation because it does not take into account many factors. It might underestimate poverty by not considering escalating housing costs, medical expenses, or day care. Likewise, it might overestimate poverty by ignoring noncash government benefits like housing assistance and food stamps.

Absolute poverty is defined as not having enough money for shelter, clothing, and food. However, many more people live in relative poverty; this means that they cannot afford goods and services that the rest of us consider necessities. They are isolated from consumer America and must "make do" without safe child care or health care, reliable transportation, heat, telephone service, or electricity for months or years at a stretch. They survive by trading, bartering, and sharing among friends and relatives. Consider how your family would live with a cash income at the poverty line.

Demographics

The demographics of poverty can be examined in terms of how many people are poor in any given year and how many people experience poverty during their lifetime. About 36 million Americans, or 13% of the population, were poor in 1998. This number is based on a U.S. Bureau of the Census household survey and does not include people who are homeless and living in shelters (U.S. Bureau of the Census, 1998).

The number of extreme poor—those trying to survive on less than half the official poverty line—is increasing. In 1997, 14.6 million Americans were classified as extremely poor.

Most impoverished Americans are white. However, compared with their numbers in the population, a disproportionate number of people of color are poor. For example, 27% of Hispanics and 27% of blacks are poor, in contrast with 9% of non-Hispanic whites. Native Americans are disproportionately poor; for instance, unemployment is 85% on the Pine Ridge reservation of South Dakota, and the median yearly income is $3,400 (Sink, 1999).

Children represent 40% of the poor population, with 20% of American people under age 18 living in poverty. Fifty-nine percent of children under age 6 living with single mothers heading the household were poor in 1997 (U.S. Bureau of the Census, 1998). Poverty also affects the aged; 10% of people over age 65 live below the poverty threshold. In addition, 17% of elders are considered "near poor" with incomes less than 125% of the poverty line.

Poverty also has its own geographics. Sixteen percent of people in rural areas are poor, as are 19% in central cities. New Mexico and Washington, DC, have the highest rates of poverty in the nation.

Chronic illness and disability increase the chances of living in poverty. One third of adults with disabilities live in households with annual incomes less than $15,000 (Kilborn, 1999). Growing numbers of disabled people live without income, health insurance, or family support.

More striking than the actual proportion of people who are poor at any given time is the likelihood of living in poverty sometime during one's lifetime. It is projected that by age 40, slightly over one third of all Americans will have lived in poverty (Rank & Hirschl, 1999). By age 75, over one half of adult Americans will have experienced poverty. This includes 91% of African Americans and 53% of European Americans. When viewed across the lifespan, poverty is a prevalent experience of mainstream Americans, not one afflicting a small marginal population! The typical spell of poverty is relatively brief; it often occurs when people living just above the poverty threshold lose their job or a couple breaks up. Long-standing poverty, lasting longer than 10 years, affects around 15% of the poor. Because poverty is so prevalent, many students of nursing have been touched personally by its hardships.

Social Characteristics

The wealthiest Americans have vast resources at their disposal. The net worth of the top 1% of American households is nearly equivalent to the combined wealth of the bottom 95% of Americans (Sklar, 1995). This discrepancy is deeply troubling to those who believe in equal opportunity for all. Most impoverished Americans have few resources with which to escape from poverty or to live with dignity despite poverty. In particular, the marginalization of the poor, their social status, social support, and neighborhood resources all influence their ability to escape persistent poverty (Aday, 1993).

MARGINALIZATION
Despite their numbers, the poor in America remain invisible, easily denied by mainstream America. This is, in part, because the poor are often **marginalized,** meaning that they live on the margins, or edges, of society rather than in the mainstream. Another term used is **disenfranchised;** enfranchisement refers to having full privileges and rights as a citizen. People who live in persistent poverty are especially likely to be isolated in inner-city neighborhoods through which the middle-class person never travels. The most vulnerable, the elderly, the disabled, and the young, seldom leave their own neighborhoods (Display 32–1).

DISPLAY 32–1. The Human Face of Poverty: Tommy

Four generations of Cora's impoverished African-American family live in the shadows of Chicago's loop surrounded by outstanding medical centers. The family narrative by Laurie Abraham (1993) reveals the failure of the health care system. Cora is 69 years old and suffers from diabetes and hypertension. She lives with her granddaughter, Jackie, who is caring for Cora, her three children, and her husband Robert, whose kidneys failed when he was 27 years old. Tommy is Cora's son and Jackie's father; he lives with his girlfriend, who works full time. Tommy had a stroke at age 48, when he was employed as a bartender. He has been hardened by a lifetime on the rough inner-city streets and does not trust outsiders. Tommy believes that his high blood pressure was due to stress, and he suspects that his stroke was caused by a relative's curse; he believes he was vulnerable because he had not led a virtuous life. Before the stroke, he was a drinker and smoker; he stopped taking his antihypertensive medication because it made him impotent. Now, his left arm remains partially paralyzed; he has trouble with most activities of daily living. He has stopped drinking but continues to smoke and eat a high-fat diet; he rarely exercises. Tommy leaves home primarily to cash his disability check, buy lottery tickets, and visit the doctor. He worries that he is losing strength, but he has no insurance coverage for physical therapy. Counseled by his physician to walk regularly, Tommy responds, "I do not want to be no prey" (p. 140). He is afraid of being assaulted in his crime-ridden neighborhood. Likewise, dietary advice is hard to follow, with the ingredients of a healthy diet too expensive and not available at neighborhood convenience stores. Tommy appears to agree when his doctor lectures him on smoking, but he continues his habit. The doctor concludes that Tommy is morally responsible for his persistent unhealthy choices; he is the cause of his own suffering. What do you think about Tommy's choices?

DISPLAY 32–2. The Human Face of Poverty: Mary

Mary is a poor mother in a foreign country she cannot understand. She is Haitian American, pregnant with an infant on her arm, hungry, and living on the streets of a small agricultural community in central Florida. The public health nurse received a referral from the OB clinic nurse, asking her to call on this woman because she was considered "peculiar in the head." Mary lost her welfare benefits and, therefore, her single room because the baby's father was living with her. The father was HIV positive and took any money she had. She had a single room, but the father had taken over the entire space with stored items he planned to sell overseas. There was no room to sleep. People tell the public health nurse just to leave this crazy woman alone. She does appear to have a personality disorder, but most of the difficulty is that she cannot articulate what is going on in her life because she speaks Creole and little English. Her mental illness estranges her from the local Haitian community, and she does not know how to access community resources in the broader community. Mary lives apart from mainstream society, and it will be the nurse's role to connect her to the community. What nursing priorities are evident in this situation?

Rural poverty is also "off the beaten path." Diminished opportunities to earn a decent living in mining, farming, and forestry have left many rural people living in grinding poverty. They reside in picturesque regions that mainstream America hurries through on the way to tourist destinations.

Both the inner-city and the rural poor are also politically invisible. They are less likely to vote; they are seldom organized to have a voice. They are not property owners; they are not represented by policy makers.

The poor are also rendered invisible by our difficulty in understanding and identifying with them. Perhaps they lack the language skills and education to explain their circumstances, to provide an adequate health history (Display 32–2). Perhaps our social circumstances are so different that we have trouble identifying with their problems. Unable to empathize with their circumstances, we may fail to see them as persons.

SOCIAL STATUS

Social status is a person's ranking or standing in society. Social status is affected by gender, age, and race. In the United States, women have a lower social status than men. Children and the elderly also have low social status, as do people of color. Therefore, a very young or very old female of a minority race has the lowest status and least opportunity in American society. Middle-aged Caucasian men have the highest status. It is not surprising, then, that rates of poverty are highest among females of color and lowest among white males.

SOCIAL SUPPORT

Social support involves the quality of interpersonal ties between individuals; the strength and extent of these personal ties determine the individual's abilities to cope with adversity. A single, adolescent mother living apart from family and friends has little social support and is, therefore, most vulnerable to an array of social, physical, and emotional problems.

NEIGHBORHOOD RESOURCES

Neighborhood resources can be valuable in helping people reach their potential. Such community assets include religious organizations, safe housing, crime-watch programs, good schools, libraries, safe and affordable day care centers, recreational facilities, public health care clinics, and other social services.

Consider the likelihood of persistent poverty for a Native American woman living with paraplegia. She lives on a reservation, marginalized from mainstream society. She is of low social status as a disabled woman of color. The quality of her life and health and the opportunity to move beyond poverty will, therefore, be determined by the strength of social support available from her family and friends and by the resources available in her community. If vocational rehabilitation, wheelchair-accessible housing, transportation, and employment opportunities are lacking, she will be unlikely to escape poverty.

Gender and Age

Two out of three poor adults are women (Sidel, 1992). In a process that has been called the **feminization of poverty,** growing numbers of women have fallen into poverty due to weakening of the nuclear family, women heading households alone, low-wage jobs for unskilled work, and the dismantling of social programs for women. Society expects women to care for others. Women's lives are woven into a web of caring for children, the elderly, grandchildren, men, and other relatives and friends. They are also responsible for managing households—cooking, cleaning, and organizing. How can women in poverty sustain these roles and survive economically?

As we mentioned earlier, 40% of the American poor are children. Indeed, among Western industrialized nations, the United States has the highest rate of child poverty. This means children are going to school hungry and unable to learn. Lacking preventive dentistry, they suffer from dental caries. Sometimes they are poisoned by lead from the old lead-based paint peeling off the wall of deteriorating housing. Perhaps they cannot breathe because of asthma caused by roach droppings in their infested housing. Due to poor access to preventive health care, they have more, and more severe, health problems.

Employment Status

In 1998, 42% of Americans classified as poor were employed. However, only 10% had full-time jobs year round. Others had part-time employment, often in low-paying retail service industries. Others worked seasonally as migrant farmworkers or sporadically as "temps" or day laborers. Much American poverty is a consequence of work that has disappeared (Wilson, 1996) or no longer pays a living wage.

America has shifted from an industrial economy to a postindustrial economy based on service industries such as retail trade, banking, and health care. Manufacturing plants have closed or moved overseas. The remaining manufacturing industries are becoming more and more technological, with jobs requiring advanced training. These jobs are generally located in the suburbs and are, therefore, inaccessible to inner-city and rural residents. Whereas low-skilled fathers worked in manufacturing trades, low-skilled sons can now get only the lowest-wage part-time retail or service jobs. Similarly, undereducated women are also likely to be working in low-wage, dead-end positions.

Consider just some of the challenges of obtaining and maintaining a higher wage position: completing high school and vocational training, money for the bus or to maintain a car, child care, and money for presentable clothing. These factors often have forced poor Americans—especially single mothers—to rely on public assistance at least until their children reach school age.

Persistent joblessness perpetuates self-doubt and feelings of hopelessness and powerlessness that can infect whole neighborhoods. The lack of economic opportunities for millions of American men can consign them to a lifetime at the bottom of the class structure and to estrangement from community and family commitments. They become resigned to their inability to play the traditional "breadwinner" role and walk away from fatherhood (Sidel, 1992).

Even for those employed full-time year-round, low wages perpetuate poverty. In 2000, the minimum wage in the United States was $5.15. This does not permit a decent standard of living even for an individual, let alone a family with one or more children. Conspiring to keep the minimum wage down are the increased political power of American industry, the decline of union representation of workers, the exporting of manufacturing operations overseas, and the increased reliance on part-time and temporary workers.

Lifestyle

In 1959, anthropologist Oscar Lewis first described common beliefs and coping mechanisms when poverty is persistent (Carney, 1992). These patterns are seen when wage earners are continuously unemployed or employed with low wages in unskilled work. Cash is chronically short. Possessions are pawned and money is borrowed at inflated interest rates. Food is purchased in small amounts daily. Living quarters are crowded, with no privacy. Attitudes and behaviors can include fatalism, cynicism about government, marginal connection to mainstream organizations, present-time orientation with little postponement of immediate gratification, early sexual initiation, abandonment of women and children, high frequency of alcoholism, and violence toward women and children. The external environment may be hostile, crowded, polluted, and violent. Over time, they have "internalized their poverty. . . . Many simply do not believe that they can influence the course of their lives" (Hilfiker, 1994, p. 158).

A public health nurse explains the attitude of sexually active, drug-using teen women whose families live in persistent poverty with no economic opportunities in their local community:

> **Over the years, it took me a while to figure out why the drugs and the sex and the babies. They're so poor, and the older men will come along and say, "I'm going to show you a better life. Be with me and be my girlfriend and I'll give you all the stuff you never had." Now, delayed gratification is not in their mind. They can't envision 5 years from now. I tell them, "Five years from now, you finish high school, go the vocational school or community college, and you'll be able to buy as many pairs of shoes once you're working." Instead, they can't see beyond 6 months of high living with him. It's the poverty and hopelessness causing them to take all of these risks. Then comes the babies and the HIV.**

Communication patterns can be very different from those used within the middle class (Martin & Henry, 1989). Verbalization may be minimal; silence might be valued over exploring feelings or ideas. Indirect communication of feelings is likely. Poor people are often skilled at picking up nonverbal communication of acceptance or apparent rejection. If the nurse shares some details of her or his own personal life, the disclosure is more likely to break down social barriers, which then encourages client disclosure of self.

POLITICS AND ETHICS OF POVERTY

The existence and alleviation of poverty in America are best understood in the context of American political and ethical forces.

Tensions Between Community and Self-Interest

Mainstream American values emphasize materialism and the work ethic. Individualism, focusing on individual self-interest and self-determination, has fashioned our social conscience. As a society, we believe that people do well by having strong wills and working hard. When people fall into hard times, the dominant assumption is that they are weak and failed to work hard enough. In other words, we blame the poor for their impoverished state. This has tragic effects on children. When *The Boston Globe* ran a story about high infant mortality among black and Latina mothers living in poverty, the majority of letters and phone calls were heartless. Mothers were described as irresponsible and immoral and babies as undeserving of help—"Trash begets trash" (Sklar, 1995, p. 76).

Because American social conscience denies that society is responsible to help them, we resist paying taxes to support community services. In contrast, Canada and Western Europe have emphasized sustenance rights for the population, ensuring basic social protections such as food, housing, and health care for all. European programs include housing subsidies, medical care, child care, and unemployment insurance that benefit all levels of society. The European public believes in the social origins of poverty and that society as a whole benefits when poverty is prevented or relieved (Wilson, 1996).

Cycles of Government Involvement

English and American history reveals cycles of political focus on the poor (Carney, 1992). The English Poor Law of 1601 first established government responsibility for relieving poverty (Sidel, 1992). In the American colonies, the first Poor Law was established in Plymouth in 1642. Helping people in their own homes was neglected in favor of removing them to workhouses, almshouses, and indentured servitude. The Protestant ethic emphasized individual hard work and explained poverty as individual failure. In the 1800s, counties took responsibility for public assistance, primarily in the form of almshouses. Orphanages were established; most of the children had living parents who were too poor to care for them. Not until the early 1900s was there public support for aiding needy families and reversing the policy of taking children from their own homes (Sidel, 1992).

In the United States, as a consequence of the Great Depression, President Roosevelt enacted the New Deal in 1935. It included Social Security and Aid to Dependent Children, which added a grant for the mother's expenses and was renamed Aid to Families with Dependent Children (AFDC) in 1950 (Sidel, 1992). Receiving AFDC came to be equated with "receiving welfare." AFDC was administered at the state level with federal grants; payments provided varied dramatically from state to state. The cash benefit was supposed to be enough to provide basic needs for food, clothing, shelter, and basic necessities.

In 1964, a War on Poverty was declared, ushering in Medicare and Medicaid and the Equal Opportunity Employment Act. Then, in the 1980s, many programs to assist the poor were cut in the belief that such assistance was fostering irresponsibility. The American dream continued to be that anyone can make it to the middle class through hard work. The sentiment against the poor became so strong that, in 1996, the United States abolished welfare as it had been known. In contrast, most of the industrialized, developed world continues to support women and men in their dual responsibilities as workers and parents. Cash benefits are given to supplement wages considered inadequate to nurture children. Mothers receive maternity leave and leave to care for sick children; day care is government sponsored.

Temporary Aid to Needy Families

In 1996, the Personal Responsibility and Work Opportunity Reconciliation Act restructured AFDC into **Temporary Aid**

to Needy Families (TANF). Financing is through federal funding to individual states, which have great latitude in setting up programs. The government limits the duration of family support to 5 years; this is a lifetime limit. Most states have reduced eligibility duration even further. TANF also mandates that states require that the recipient find work within 2 years. Secondary school or post-secondary education does not postpone the work requirement (Gault, Hartmann & Yi, 1998), although it is well known that education is a significant factor predicting whether welfare recipients work and eventually can earn enough to escape poverty. Federal law does not require child care provisions, although it is also known that subsidizing child care enables that about a third of families living in poverty to eventually escape. Individual states impose requirements for keeping benefits, such as up-to-date immunizations or limits on child absenteeism from school or identification of fathers and requiring their child support cooperation (Chavkin, 1999). Therefore, mothers are required to work outside the home and be highly responsible for their children, but they are given little assistance to accomplish these ends.

Income eligibility requirements are now stricter than Medicaid requirements, which causes administrative complications by creating two separate sets of criteria (Keepnews, 1998). The Act also cut back Medicaid benefits for mentally impaired children and for many noncitizen immigrants. Now, many immigrants have no recourse except the emergency room when their conditions become life-threatening. As had been feared by health advocates, many people have lost Medicaid coverage and become uninsured as a result of the TANF reforms (Pear, 1999). Even when they have found employment, their low-wage jobs do not have health benefits.

The effects of welfare-to-work programs are continuing to be evaluated. A key element of their success will be the strength of accompanying health insurance and child care provisions. Tough long-range issues will be the lack of employment opportunities, low wages, and unaffordable housing. Other challenges to maintaining steady employment include mental health issues, drug or alcohol abuse, jealous or violent male partners, unreliable babysitters, sick children, broken-down cars, and neighborhood dangers. For the most emotionally and socially impoverished, the cutoff of welfare benefits mandated by the Welfare Reform Act of 1996 could result in an enlarged group of people living in extreme hardship with no financial safety net.

TANF has been called successful because it has dramatically reduced the number of people receiving assistance. However, true success will be measured by a long-standing reduction of the number of families living in poverty. Low-wage jobs generally allow no paid leave or flexibility to meet children's health needs. Current policy forces mothers to choose between meeting their children's basic health needs and keeping a job to ensure family survival (Heymann & Earle, 1999). Many children are left alone to care for even younger children, sick and well. Whom will we blame for the resulting tragedies? In contrast, interventions that support work success include education and skill development, child care, work flexibility and family leave, and programs to respond to domestic violence and chronic disabilities, particularly those related to substance abuse (Gault, Hartmann & Yi, 1998).

Human Service Programs

Contrary to a mythology that nothing can be done and that helping the poor just weakens them, many human service programs have proved their effectiveness in alleviating hardship and improving well-being of impoverished people (Schorr & Schorr, 1988). Effective programs are interdisciplinary and comprehensive; they combine intensive social, educational, and health interventions. The programs consider people in the context of family and community, not in isolation. Successful programs include professionals who establish trusting relationships and respond to the needs of people they serve rather than the demands of bureaucracies. Such programs deliberately reduce barriers of access, money, and fragmented services. They do not wait for people to make it through the overwhelming service maze. They go where people live and work and go to school, often at nontraditional hours. Pregnancy prevention and prenatal care programs that meet these criteria have excellent outcomes. Perinatal nurse home visiting with these characteristics has been demonstrated to have dramatic effects to reduce maternal smoking, newborn low birth weight, emergency department visits, and child abuse and to improve mothers' return to school and work and postponement of further pregnancies (Olds & Kitzman, 1990) (see Levels of Prevention).

There is strong evidence that federally funded public assistance programs intended to alleviate the effects of poverty on children and families are effective (Devaney, Ellwood, & Love, 1997). Food stamps provide nationwide food assistance to all households based on financial need. They are considered central to the food assistance safety net for children. The Special Supplemental Food Program for Women, Infants, and Children (WIC) has increased intake of essential nutrients for pregnant mothers and children. School nutrition programs offer free or low-cost breakfasts and lunches to qualifying children. Head Start is a model of comprehensive services that was launched in 1965 as a preschool educational program for the disadvantaged providing educational, social, health, and nutritional intervention. Short-term benefits include improved physical, social, and cognitive development.

Distributive Justice

Justice is concerned with treating people fairly. **Distributive justice** refers to the justified distribution of burdens and benefits throughout society. Just distribution is challenging when

LEVELS OF PREVENTION

POOR SINGLE MOTHERS

GOAL

To prevent illness and diminish poverty among poor single mothers and their children. To effectively detect and treat health problems of marginalized young families.

PRIMARY PREVENTION

Support social policy that fosters income-earning opportunities so that women can make enough to move out of poverty. This requires a secondary education and jobs that pay living wages with benefits and child care. It requires elimination of racial and gender discrimination. Develop accessible health education programs with priorities on compelling issues such as family planning, strengthening parental bonds, violence prevention, smoking prevention, drug and alcohol abuse, mental health, and injury prevention. Ensure availability of client-friendly preventive measures such as nutrition and immunization. Advocate for economic opportunities for all and public assistance for those whose personal and social circumstances prevent employment for a living wage.

SECONDARY PREVENTION

Develop comprehensive humanized health services focusing on women's health and well-child screening. Develop outreach screening programs in the neighborhoods, schools, and workplaces. Encourage local community development to strengthen the capacity of women to help one another. Develop trusting partnerships with women to diagnose and manage health problems. Encourage support systems.

TERTIARY PREVENTION

Ensure effective case management of chronic conditions. Work with agencies and individuals to support women living with domestic violence, alcohol, and substance abuse. Advocate for expansion of counseling and rehabilitative services in the community.

resources are considered scarce; the paradox of growing American wealth is that resources are hoarded rather than distributed. Philosophies of economic justice are contradictory. Some believe that resources should be distributed according to merit, determined by factors such as social status and work contribution. Whom does this leave out? Some believe that resources should be distributed to ensure that basic human needs (food, shelter, education, health) are met. Do you believe that there are some human beings so unworthy that they do not get to eat or to have a roof over their head?

In the United States, the distribution of goods and services is largely determined by the marketplace. Although we claim equality as a social ideal, we accept dramatic inequities as determined by the law of the marketplace. In contrast, community health nursing is grounded in commitment to a just distribution of primary goods for all members of society. The founder of American public health nursing, Lillian Wald, was in the forefront of social reform movements emphasiz-

ing just allocation of resources for the immigrant and poor laborer (Chafey, 1997). Public health nurses inherit her legacy in the beginning of the 21st century.

HEALTH EFFECTS OF POVERTY

Increased Morbidity and Mortality

Public health professionals are committed to reducing the greater risk of illness and death that is due to poverty. Complex mechanisms related to socioeconomic disadvantage result in disadvantaged health status. As socioeconomic position improves, health improves. Just how causal variables relate to each other and result in poor health requires further investigation; however, it is clear that poverty and race are entwined as determinants of health. The greater relative risks for racial minorities are particularly striking in infant and maternal mortality, cardiovascular disease, diabetes, HIV infection, cancer, and immunization rates. African Americans have a shorter life expectancy, and twice as many African-American newborns die in the first month of life as European-American newborns. Even when adequately insured, minorities are less likely to receive advanced therapies. Institutional racism is a major reason. A recent study presented 720 physicians with videotaped actors posing in identical clothing with identical occupations, health insurance, and health histories (Schulman et al., 1999). The physicians chose to refer significantly fewer women and African Americans for cardiac catheterization. Prior studies also identified gender and race as factors affecting how aggressively heart disease is managed.

Other variables known to interact with poverty in promoting poor health include lack of education, low occupational status, jobs with high demands and low control, selected cultural health beliefs, social isolation, poor nutrition, and poor housing (Blane, 1995; Pappas, 1994). Inadequate housing may lack heat or cooling, proper ventilation, access to bathing, adequate refrigeration and cooking facilities, and security from violence. It may also be plagued with rats, fleas, roaches, and other vermin. Environmental hazards outside the home include toxic wastes in the neighborhood and toxic materials at work.

The chronic stressors of poverty, including racism, classism, self-doubt, and learned helplessness, contribute to poor health. Similarly, morbidity and mortality are greater where social bonds and the level of social trust have eroded (Kawachi, Kennedy, Lochner & Prothrow-Stith, 1997). Residents in high-trust neighborhoods are more willing to help one another and share resources; they are healthier, despite poverty. Any intervention that strengthens human connections within a community can be predicted to improve individual health.

Individual health behaviors such as inactivity, tobacco and alcohol abuse, and obesity are clearly correlated with poor health and must be understood in their social context.

Persons with the least education and the lowest income are more likely to be smokers, overweight, and physically inactive (Lantz, House, Lepkowski, Williams, Mero, & Chen, 1998). However, it is unwise to focus public health policies solely on reduction of individual risk behaviors because they explain only some of the health disadvantage.

Reduced Access to Health Care

Low-income people are less likely to have access to preventive and therapeutic health services. In addition to lack of transportation and inability to leave low-wage jobs to keep medical appointments, access to care is impeded by lack of health insurance and inability to pay out-of-pocket charges. Places where the poor have traditionally received care have been called "safety net providers." Lacking an insurance card in their pocket or purse, they have, in the past, been able to receive care in emergency rooms, public health departments, community free clinics, public and teaching hospitals, some not-for-profit hospitals, and from physicians and practitioners who have voluntarily provided uncompensated care. Now, although the demands for uncompensated care are increasing with 44 million uninsured Americans, subsidies for indigent care have been cut at all levels of government. As managed care aggressively seeks to control costs, there is no longer a way to subsidize care for the indigent ("Managed care cost pressures threaten access for the uninsured," 1999).

Those receiving Medicaid often receive unequal care. For instance, mothers covered by Medicaid in some South Florida hospitals must pay $500 or more out of their pockets if they want epidural anesthesia during childbirth; they must pay anesthesiologists up front before labor begins or endure the pain. Many Medicaid recipients are unable to access medical specialists because these physicians consider Medicaid reimbursement to be inadequate.

When they do access care, impoverished clients of the health care system are unlikely to receive health-promoting advice and unlikely to have their chronic conditions carefully managed. Instead, they are likely to be treated for the most obvious symptoms of a single illness episode. This may often be attributed to the negative attitudes of agencies and care providers. Often, agencies founded to serve the poor have developed so many regulations and obstacles for clients that they are essentially inaccessible. For instance, a nurse practitioner recently sought to immunize a population of 300 adolescents in a drop-out prevention program against hepatitis B and measles, but the nursing supervisor interpreted the regulations of the local health department to preclude both delivering the vaccine to the practitioner and authorizing transportation of the youth to the department. Additionally, the resources of institutions mandated to serve the poor may be stretched so thin that essentially no adequate services are provided. Finally, service providers may be so numbed or "burned out" by their exposures to human hardship that they decide clients are beyond help. "It is precisely in those institutions charged with serving the poor that one finds the highest proportion of workers who are no longer responsive to the real needs of clients" (Hilfiker, 1994, p. 100).

Lack of access to prevention and treatment of alcohol and drug dependency is an immense burden on the poor. The national failure to ensure access to substance abuse treatment has been estimated to cost the nation up to $276 billion annually. The cost of untreated chemical abuse includes law enforcement, motor vehicle crashes, lost work productivity, medical expenses, and incarceration (Amaro, 1999). Treatment has been proved to be more effective than law enforcement and incarceration in reducing demand, yet the federal government spends nearly double the amount on reducing supply (interdiction) than on prevention and treatment. Every dollar spent on treatment generates $7 in future costs saved. Demonstrated to save money over time, publicly funded treatment, as well as expansion of private insurance benefits, is essential to provide comprehensive and effective treatment.

HOMELESSNESS IN AMERICA

Poverty results in **homelessness** when limited resources make housing unaffordable. Homeless people lack a regular address. It is estimated that 14% of Americans become homeless sometime during their lifetime (Link et al., 1994). Finding, interviewing, and counting the homeless are challenging to officials; their numbers are always likely to be underestimated. If they have not yet exhausted the resources and good will of friends or relatives, people without their own home stay overnight in other people's homes. This condition is called "doubling-up." When unable to do this, the most deprived homeless people sleep in parks, in abandoned buildings, in cars, on benches in bus stations, on roofs, under viaducts, or in homeless shelters.

For most people, being homeless is temporary or cyclic as they struggle to keep a roof over their heads. Homeless people on the doorsteps and streets of America have become familiar sights since the 1980s. We have come to accept and even to ignore this profound hardship, although being without a home was once common only in impoverished nations, not in the United States.

Why Are People Homeless?

The absence of low-cost housing is a tremendous burden on the poor, who must pay an expanding percentage of their paycheck for housing. Over the last 25 years, low-rent apartments have disappeared quietly due to urban renewal and the process of upgrading urban housing that is called "gentrification" (National Coalition for the Homeless, 1996). At the same time, the federal government has reduced its commitment to build and maintain inexpensive housing. The resultant widening gap between affordable housing units and people needing them has created a housing crisis. Many impoverished people are forced to live in overcrowded and substandard housing. The most severe housing needs are among the elderly, families with children, and low-income disabled people. Government housing assistance programs are unable to keep up with the demand. Waiting lists are 3 to 4 years long for government programs such as Section 8 housing.

In addition to poverty and the unavailability of affordable housing, several other factors can lead to homelessness in America. Battered women without resources are often forced to choose between enduring abuse at home or becoming homeless (National Coalition for the Homeless, 1996). In addition, many uninsured or underinsured people who suffer severe physical or emotional illness will eventually become homeless. Approximately one quarter of the adult homeless population is mentally ill. The lack of community mental health support services such as case management, treatment, and supportive housing options often forces patients onto the streets, under the bridges, or into the woods. Likewise, people who are poor and addicted to drugs and/or alcohol are at high risk of homelessness. Uninsured homeless people face long waits to get into treatment programs, and then are still likely to be discharged after treatment back onto the streets or into shelters. In 1996, new federal legislation denied Social Security Income and Social Security Disability Insurance, including Medicaid, to people whose disability was due to addictions. Therefore, many chemically dependent people are unable to afford even the worst sort of housing.

Living as a Homeless Person

The poor are continually faced with multiple stressors. Mothers living in shelters report minimal social support and alienation from human relationships (Berne, Dato, Mason & Rafferty, 1990). One third suffered physical abuse as children, and one fourth were battered in adult relationships. Women and children described what it is like to be homeless in a qualitative study by Baumann (1994). Having no place of their own makes mothers feel angry, controlled by rules they do not make. They dislike the absence of privacy. They are surrounded by the hardships of others. In a life involving frequent moves, mothers worry about where they will sleep next. They are concerned that children's schooling is interrupted and inferior. Children feel imprisoned, miss school, and do not like their new schools. Relationships are impaired by shelter rules that prohibit visitors. Living so publicly causes tensions between everyone. Homeless people yearn for a stable family life, and their children dream of houses.

Health of the Homeless

Consider how living environment contributes to health. Living outside results in exposure to assault and the weather. Hypothermia or the effects of sun and heat are constantly threatening. Trauma and impaired skin integrity are common. Living in shelters results in exposure to violence and communicable diseases ranging from scabies to tuberculosis, readily transmitted due to overcrowding. What basic activities of daily living would be difficult if you were homeless? You would face sleep deprivation, fear, hunger and thirst, inadequate bathing and oral hygiene, inadequate laundry facilities, nowhere to store medicines, no privacy, no control, and perhaps no hope. If you or your children were persistently hungry, would you consider begging, stealing, selling drugs, or engaging in prostitution? A whole new set of problems would result.

Homelessness and health are interrelated in three ways: homelessness precipitates ill health, homelessness complicates treatment of ill health, and ill health causes homelessness (Reichenbach, McNamee & Seibel, 1998). Infant mortality and low birth weight are disproportionate among infants born to homeless women. Homeless children experience chronic physical disorders at double the rate of the general population (Berne et al., 1990). Most common are malnutrition, anemia, and asthma. Acute illnesses such as upper respiratory and ear infections, gastrointestinal problems, and skin disorders are especially frequent. Children's mental health is profoundly affected, with half of preschool children experiencing developmental delays and half of school-aged children manifesting anxiety and depression, including suicidal ideation. Post-traumatic stress disorder is commonly diagnosed in children.

Homeless adults suffer disproportionately from most physical and mental illnesses. Tuberculosis and AIDS can be prevalent, depending on the region. Homeless shelter residents in New York City die at an extraordinary four times the rate of the general population of the same age (Barrow, Herman, Cordova & Struening, 1999). Homeless adults suffer disproportionately from permanent physical disabilities and have a life expectancy of 20 years less than middle-class adults (Hilfiker, 1994) (see Research: Bridge to Practice).

Programs to Help the Homeless

The Interagency Council on the Homeless coordinates federal homeless resources and is made up of the leaders of 16 federal agencies that have programs for the homeless. However, health care programs for the homeless are limited and fragmented (Acquaviva & Lancaster, 1996).

Like most people living in poverty, homeless people receive their health care in emergency rooms after their health problems have reached crisis proportions. Typically, there is no plan for continuity of care. Some homeless people receive health care in community clinics, often experiencing long waits and insensitive care from health care providers who find them noncompliant with medical regimens.

Frequent barriers to health care for the homeless include the following: lack of health insurance, insensitivity of health care providers, stereotyping on the part of providers, cultural

RESEARCH Bridge to Practice

Reichenbach, E. M., McNamee, M. J., & Seibel, L. (1998). The community health nursing implications of the self-reported health status of a local homeless population. *Public Health Nursing, 15*(6), 398–405.

This descriptive study sought to better describe characteristics of homeless people, their perceived biopsychosocial concerns, reported barriers to health care, and history of disruptions in their family of origin. One hundred and thirty-two homeless people agreed to complete a semistructured questionnaire, which was administered orally to avoid possible literacy problems.

Demographic characteristics were similar to homeless populations nationally. Men were over-represented, average age was mid-thirties, they had a high rate of unemployment, and most lacked health insurance. Those living in shelters were more transient in the community. Longer-term community residents were less likely to use shelters.

One third of the subjects rated their health as fair or poor. Most frequently mentioned health problems were problems with feet, as well as musculoskeletal, cardiovascular, and pulmonary problems. About one third rated their mental health as fair or poor. One fourth stated that they had received a mental health diagnosis. Few acknowledged alcohol or substance abuse problems. This may be due to their denial, the attached social stigma, or the drinking prohibition at the shelter where they were interviewed. Loneliness was the most frequently reported fear.

Barriers to health care were financial and related to lack of health insurance. Other barriers mentioned were transportation, language, and racism.

Only half of the informants reported regular contact with the family that raised them, and only half of those with family contact reported that their family provided emotional support. Material support was even less available from families.

1. How will the self-reported physical and emotional problems eventually affect the mobility and self-sufficiency of the homeless population interviewed?
2. What are the nursing implications of the reported barriers to health care for the homeless?
3. What are the nursing implications of the reported loneliness and estrangement from family?
4. What community-level interventions would be useful for this population?

barriers regarding health beliefs and behavior, the homeless person's first priority of food and shelter instead of health, breakdown in communication with the client and between providers, bureaucratic paperwork to obtain services, transportation to those services, and homeless people's fear of "the system" (Jezewski, 1995).

The best services for the homeless provide social, educational, and health interventions. For instance, the Henry Street Settlement in New York City, originally established by the founder of American public health nursing, Lillian Wald, has offered model supportive services (Berne et al., 1990). Mental health and children's school involvement im-

prove markedly with a safe shelter, around-the-clock staff available, day care, tutoring after school, job training, assistance with obtaining government assistance, and assistance with locating homes. It is fruitless to treat symptoms in the absence of broad-based interventions that address underlying problems.

Primary prevention of homelessness requires affirmation of shelter as a basic human right. Primary prevention involves changes in social policy, including affordable housing, accessible education and job training, work at a living wage, accessible child care, timely drug treatment, health education that includes pregnancy prevention, and public assistance that guarantees shelter for all (Berne et al., 1990).

GLOBAL POVERTY: THE DEVELOPING NATIONS

The right to a life free from poverty is proclaimed by the United Nations Charter. Internationally, poverty thresholds are defined in terms of the cost of a basic diet. One common definition of poverty is daily subsistence on 1 U.S. dollar or less; one third of people in developing countries meet this definition. For example, one third of India's 1 billion people live on less than $1 a day (Crossette, 1999).

The concept of human poverty goes beyond income to identify deprivations such as lack of political freedom, lack of personal security, and inability to participate in the life of the community (United Nations Development Programmes, 1998). The Human Poverty Index measures illiteracy, child malnutrition, early death, poor health care, and inadequate access to safe water (see The Global Community). It reveals environmental and population characteristics that lead to health risks that are strikingly similar across the globe. Poverty, overpopulation, urbanization, and environmental deterioration are strongly interrelated.

Overpopulation

Poverty leads to population growth, and population growth leads to poverty (United Nations Children's Fund, 1994). High child mortality leads parents to have more children. Lack of resources increases the need for children to help in home and field and to ensure help during infirmity and aging. Poverty engenders helplessness and hopelessness, which does not lead to planning ahead to limit children. Likewise, low education and low status of women means less knowledge of family planning and less personal power over fertility.

Migration and Urbanization

As population expands, growing numbers of people are exhausting the soil and then moving to cultivate environmentally

THE GLOBAL COMMUNITY

Cancun, Mexico, is famous as a luxury destination resort. However, 15 minutes away is a community of 110,000 people, many of whom are Mayan Indians. For several years, Ms. Jackie Adames, a nursing student at Florida Atlantic University, has been visiting these people as a member of a medical mission team. Her community assessment, presented in class, provided the information that follows regarding the environment, the people, and their health risks.

There are significant environmental hazards. The climate is persistently warm and humid. The air is thick with dust; most streets are not paved. Pesticides are used weekly to prevent yellow fever and dengue fever transmission by mosquitoes. Air is polluted from the exhaust of numerous buses and cabs. There is constant migration to and from the area. Although some houses are sturdy, others are made of cardboard or bamboo with thatched roofs and dirt floors. There are no child labor laws and no mandatory school laws. The cost of living has doubled in the last 5 years. Health services are available for employed people.

There are 110,000 people living in this community, which is experiencing 21% annual population growth. Most are under 45 years of age; they live in extended families with many children. They speak Spanish and Mayan at home. Most are impoverished, with no employment or low-wage employment. The diet is tortillas, pork, rice, cheese, animal fat, and few vegetables. Newborn babies are not named for 3 months to reduce attachment if they die. Prenatal care is inadequate. Mothers work, and children babysit younger children. Water is available from an outside pipeline at set times of the day. Electricity is inconsistent. Development of neighborhood infrastructure and government services cannot keep up with the explosive community growth.

Health risks are extensive with a particularly high incidence of respiratory infections, asthma, gastroenteritis, and premature or low-birth-weight infants. Infectious diseases and diseases of malnutrition are of great concern. Dental problems include gum disease and tooth decay. Physical injuries from manual labor and domestic violence are prevalent.

vulnerable areas, where they denude the hillsides and deforest the tropics. Short-term survival takes precedence over preservation of natural resources. When rural life becomes unsustainable, the poor migrate into cities and towns. Nearly half of the world's people now live in cities, creating an unprecedented density of people. Their concentrated numbers have resulted in dramatic environmental degradation and urban sprawl that makes water a scarce commodity and causes incredible problems with waste disposal (Cohen, 1993). Increased motorization results in gridlock and air pollution. Public spending cannot keep up with the needs for food, transportation, water, sewer, garbage collection, public health protection, communication, and education. Urban crowding is strongly linked to respiratory infections. Dirty

air and water are causing serious health problems worldwide. Seventy percent of the health problems in Ghana, on the southern coast of West Africa, are environmentally related diseases. Whether poor people are urban or rural dwellers, the immediacy of making a living overshadows preservation of the forest, land, water, or air. Poverty is destroying the ecosystem, and environmental degradation disproportionately impacts the lives of the poor.

Underemployment and Industrialization

The poor are often underemployed in the "informal sector" in activities such as domestic service or street vending. Those who are formally employed are often temporary and underpaid. Industries in the underdeveloped world are under great pressure to be competitive internationally. They push production costs down by keeping wages down and hiring part-time, temporary workers. Increasingly, children, the elderly, and women are pressed into manufacturing, with all the attendant occupational hazards and none of the safety requirements of the United States. The greed of the developed world commercial interests is felt in the everyday struggles of the working poor in developing countries.

Eradicating Global Poverty

The poorest countries are so heavily burdened with debt to industrialized nations that they are falling behind in meeting the basic needs of their people (Display 32–3). Eradication of poverty requires honest central governments working in partnerships with local governments and the private sector. Vital to antipoverty programs are the organization and activation of impoverished communities themselves. Because

---

DISPLAY 32–3. Eradicating Global Poverty

Six policies are proposed by the United Nations to eradicate extreme poverty in the underdeveloped global community.
1. Empowerment of women
2. Programs to promote economic growth of developing countries where growth has been failing
3. Fair trade policies that allow poor countries to enter the world market
4. Support for poor communities to organize and act collectively
5. Promotion of accountable, open governments with active citizen participation
6. Debt reduction and peace-building for nations in particularly difficult circumstances

(From United Nations Development Programmes, 1998.)

poverty causes illness and illness causes poverty, community development is central to international public health nursing.

ROLE OF THE COMMUNITY HEALTH NURSE IN CARING FOR CLIENTS IN POVERTY

Self-Assessment

Confronting poverty and caring for people who are poor require reflective assessment of one's own assumptions and beliefs. Because poverty is prevalent over a lifetime, many students of nursing will actually have personal or family experience of living in poverty. However, because the stigma is so great and fault finding is so pervasive in our society, acknowledging and reflecting on this experience may well be painful for you. In contrast, because poverty is so hidden and frequently denied, many students of nursing may have lived apart from any knowledge of the human experience of poverty. You may have come to believe many of the negative stereotypes about poor people. How have your judgments been shaped? How can you open yourself to caring for those from whom most of society turns away?

We learn from one another's stories. First, learn from your classmates, friends, and neighbors who are courageous enough to tell you their own experiences of living with poverty. Ask them and listen well. Then let your patients teach you. One honor we have as nurses is the opportunity to work with people from all walks of life. You are particularly likely in clinical experiences in community health to meet impoverished individuals and families living outside the mainstream. Many years ago, the author had a one-to-one postclinical conference with a student at a small Roman Catholic college. She made many visits to an African-American teen mother of two thriving children. The young mother lived in a dangerous housing project, and, although she locked him out of her second-floor apartment, her abusive boyfriend had been known to climb up the drainage pipe and over the porch roof. Sometimes, he forced open a window and beat her up. Mom worked every day at a fast food establishment; her grandmother took care of the children. After a couple of months of weekly visits, the student exclaimed, "When I read her chart, I saw her as a immoral girl—a slut— and I expected her to be a loser. Now I can't believe what I've learned about how strong she is. She just keeps fighting for herself and the kids to survive! She's a great mom and I told her so!"

Improving Access

Even when government-sponsored health insurance and services are available, as we have seen, extensive barriers pre-

vent poor people from accessing services. The community health nurse serves as an advocate and bridge for families who need to gain access. Barriers to access associated with the clients themselves include reluctance to seek coverage because of feelings of pride or independence or mistrust; feeling powerless; being unaware that such services exist or are worthwhile; lacking resources such as a telephone or transportation; being illiterate; and preoccupation with meeting survival needs instead of health needs (DeChiara & Wolff, 1998). Barriers associated with applying for health insurance include a system that is unfriendly and complicated. Paperwork is overwhelming and may be returned for correction. Informative materials may be too difficult to understand; programs may seek to restrict enrollments by restricting information. The process may require a car, a phone, and appointments at inconvenient times. The nurse can intervene as a coach and guide, interpreting the system to the client and the client to the system. Likewise, the nurse can act as change agent to improve the system whenever possible.

Strengthening Communities

We are all connected. All of us as citizens have a stake in preventing the adverse hardships of poverty.

> **We all pay to support the unproductive and incarcerate the violent. We are all weakened by lost productivity. We all live with fear of crime in our homes and on the streets. We are all diminished when large numbers of parents are incapable of nurturing their dependent young, and when pervasive alienation erodes the national sense of community (Schorr & Schorr, 1988, xix).**

The common good is enhanced by strengthening community resources, including investing in people of historically low status, developing and strengthening ties within the families and among people involved in neighborhood mutual support, and redeveloping neighborhood resources (Aday, 1993). Recognizing that the foundational causes of poverty are economic, the community health nurse realizes that the alleviation of poverty can only come with major changes in American economic and social policy. Whenever possible, the nurse voices support of economic redevelopment of neighborhoods to enhance schools, housing, and employment. The community health nurse can also work to promote subsidized carpools, school-to-work transition programs, universal health insurance, and inner-city economic development programs.

McKnight (1995) cautions well-intentioned professionals to beware seeking solutions to poverty in service programs alone. First of all, a whole population of people can become defined in terms of their problems instead of their strengths. In addition, citizens acting to help themselves within their community can be weakened when they are seen as "clients" requiring professional services. Finally, McKnight worries about the disabling effect of being dependent on multiple human services, which reduces self-worth and leads to feelings of powerlessness. If you doubt this, go sit in the waiting room of your nearest public clinic. Notice how people are addressed as they wait, are processed through various clerks, and are finally seen. If you are really courageous, try seeking help for one of your own health problems in such an environment, so often dehumanized and even designed to discourage people from seeking help. Because human service interventions can have negative as well as positive effects, it is important to consider whether more community agencies are the answer to resolving community hardship. Community health planning should take seriously an organizing process that builds community, focusing on developing neighborhood competence to problem-solve and create solutions for itself. See the discussion of community development in Chapter 19.

Strengthening Individuals

Poverty nursing requires careful attention to how medical regimens can be made workable despite poverty (Display 32–4). The nurse needs to ask many questions to translate mainstream health care to what is feasible, given the person's living circumstances. For every treatment prescribed, the nurse must question how it will be accomplished. Can the client afford medications? Can the client obtain the dressings? Is it possible for the client to rest or exercise or eat as prescribed? Are caregivers available among family and friends? What compromises are necessary? What is practical? What agencies or services can be mobilized to help and for how long?

DISPLAY 32–4. **Strengthening Individuals**

A nurse with extensive experience in working with an impoverished Washington, DC, neighborhood provides the following guidelines for every encounter with the poor:

- Create trust.
- Show respect and concern.
- Don't make assumptions regarding underlying need.
- Remember the basics like food and hygiene.
- Accept that patients will miss appointments because of more pressing priorities.
- Coordinate a network of services.
- Advocate for accessible health services.
- Focus on prevention.
- Know when to take initiative on behalf of the patient and when to back off and let them take it.
- Develop a support network for oneself.

(Acquaviva, T. & Lancaster, J. [1996]. Poverty and homelessness. In Stanhope, & Lancaster, J. *Community health nursing: Promoting health of aggregates, families, and individuals.* St. Louis: Mosby.)

The author interviewed seven nurses well respected for their compassionate work with disenfranchised people. Their clients are people from whom many others withdraw and walk away. These exemplary nurses described their clients as fellow human beings who frighten many of us and are themselves afraid. Their poverty, accompanied by mental illness, HIV infection, end-stage illness, alcoholism, or status as an unwanted immigrant, has "pushed them out of the human family." They are disconnected and fearful. It seems like there is a wall between them and the rest of the community (see Voices From the Community).

David Hilfiker, who describes himself as practicing "poverty medicine," portrays this abandonment of the poor and the tragic consequences that he discovered after extensive practice experience. "What caught me completely off guard was my patients' internalization of their abandonment. Children who had not been adequately loved now saw themselves as unlovable. . . . Pushed down too many times, they now saw failure as inevitable" (Hilfiker, 1994, p. 19).

Similarly, the nurses interviewed said that compassionate caring for patients who are disenfranchised and apart from the mainstream requires a different kind of nursing. Analysis of their reflections and stories reveals three practice categories: the Human Connection, the Community Connection, and Making Self-Care Possible (Zerwekh, 2000).

The Human Connection involves deliberately honoring the human dignity of the poor, coming to know them well, and sharing one's own humanity rather than maintaining professional distance. The nurses remind other professionals who have forgotten about their clients' humanity. Clients know they are held in regard. One nurse explained, "They call me because I respect them." They are proud of knowing the clients well, drawing them out through authentic listening and paying attention. They discover their past. With discretion, they share their own life struggles and stories and insist that other nurses should do the same. One expert asserts, "They have to perceive you as real."

The Community Connection involves connecting the disconnected to other community members and services, mediating between client and those services, and persisting with the

---

Voices From the Community

A nurse who has practiced with many disenfranchised patients living with mental illness or infected with HIV describes *breaking the fear* as essential to caring:

"All of us at some level have a fear of the disenfranchised, whether it's because we could be in that place or because there may be potential harm to us. But I seek to break that fear and see someone as human. The more I work with her, the more I see her as human" (Zerwekh, 2000, p. 47).

case. The nurse has to find a way around the wall separating clients from community. One nurse said this might require "tunneling through the wall. There's always another way around."

In many cases, this means making exceptions to bureaucratic rules. Although others get tired and give up, expert nurses keep trying to pull in and coordinate resources. One nurse calls this kind of persistence "haunting the case." Another researcher interviewing nurses who work with the homeless found that staying connected is the very core of their work to facilitate health care for homeless people (Jezewski, 1995). They sought to develop rapport with each person, developing and maintaining a trusting connection. In addition, the nurses established and maintained a provider network to get the client into the health delivery system. This requires excellent working relationships and personal influence. Finally, they actively linked the homeless person to the health care system. The goal was continuity of care that addresses underlying problems, instead of a Band-Aid approach.

Making Self-Care Possible has to do with strengthening people to care for themselves. Nurses listen at length. They "help them get the anger out" and do not take it personally. One nurse explains, "I help them get through the rough spots." They teach understanding of body and emotions. Another nurse tells her clients, "You should know more about the illness than I do. You have to walk it, wash it, live it, breathe it." Another nurse who works with indigent mentally ill clients teaches them how to separate from "the voices that tell them all day long that they are no good and ugly." Nurses encourage impoverished clients to take control of their life, and they develop practical health care plans with clients in charge. "Always, always let them know that they are in control." And, as we have seen, poverty nursing involves working at the community level, to pull the entire wall down and help change underlying circumstances.

Care for Oneself as Caregiver

Sustained work with the poor requires significant self-awareness and deliberate self-caring. Work with the truly broken, "physically unappealing, disturbed, abusive, confused, unreachable, and often visibly 'ungrateful'" can exhaust the emotional and spiritual reservoirs of even the most highly motivated caregivers (Hilfiker, 1994, p. 200). Some clients are deeply damaged and degraded by poverty and feel powerless. When they fail to make the changes that we as professionals repeatedly recommend, our caring intentions can turn to fault finding and blame. Hilfiker considers the caregivers' descent into senseless blaming: "Life in our neighborhood thwarts all efforts to blame. Everyone is caught in an ugly web. . . . On whom can I vent my frustrations when their shortcomings enrage me?" (pp. 140–143).

As we experience inevitable frustration and failure, self-protection results in growing detachment, less willingness to feel the pain, anger, and cynicism. We retreat behind the wall. In contrast, sustained engagement requires ongoing, conscious exploration of one's own motivations and behaviors. Sustained caring requires ongoing, conscious care of self: nurturing through spiritual practices, rest, retreat, celebration, friendship, art, music, exercise, therapy, self-reflection, and group support with colleagues.

Many community health nurses find meaning in working with the disenfranchised through a sense of personal calling: "These are the people I am meant to help." To work effectively with the poor, nurses hold a strong conviction of their common humanity and right to sustenance and respect. Many nurses are invigorated by the ongoing challenges of helping the neediest of the needy: "They are the sickest people and I am putting an end to them falling through the cracks." Might this be your mission also?

SUMMARY

To integrate and apply your understanding of the poor and role of the community health nursing in caring for clients in poverty, consider the following ten guidelines for practice:

1. Vote for candidates and laws that diminish poverty and diminish suffering of the poor.
2. Advocate for the poor in all community groups where you are a member.
3. Listen and keep listening to people living in poverty.
4. Consciously develop trusting, respectful relationships with poor people.
5. Based on your search to understand their life circumstances, develop preventive and treatment approaches that are workable.
6. Link poor people with each other and helping resources.
7. Translate medical and psychiatric information in practical ways that assist the poor to understand themselves and take charge of their lives.
8. Maintain your own hope and well-being through deliberate self-care.
9. Always consider how you could contribute to community level or organizational changes that diminish poverty or diminish its hardships.
10. Find meaning that sustains your compassion and nursing effectiveness with every impoverished person you encounter (see Clinical Corner).

CLINICAL CORNER | Nuisance Diseases in a Homeless Shelter

Scenario

As a public health nurse working for the Capitol City health department, you are assigned to rotate through three homeless shelters once each week. Your role is assessment of physical and metal health issues, health education, basic first aid, and appropriate referrals. In recent weeks, you have noticed that individuals staying in a particular homeless shelter have complained of an increased incidence of pediculosis capitis and pubis.

The shelter is operated by an interfaith religious organization. Twelve religious groups are members of this organization (churches, synagogues, mosques, and so forth). Each agency assumes responsibility for operating the shelter three to four times per month. The hours of operation for the shelter are from 5:00 PM until 10:00 AM. Clients are provided an evening meal, a cot and blankets, and a morning meal. Hot showers are available in the morning, with clients rotating through the two showers in the shelter.

Funding and oversight of this program are provided by a volunteer organization working with officials in city government.

Available assessment data related to the problems include:

- Inclement weather has led to an increase in clients requesting shelter.
- Many of these clients would otherwise camp in the wilderness or sleep on the streets.

Questions

1. Discuss additional assessment data needed to address the issue of pediculosis in the shelter. How you will go about gathering these data?
2. Based on data presented in this scenario, present host, agent, and environmental factors that may be contributing to the problems.
   - Host
   - Agent
   - Environment
3. Discuss interventions your program will perform at the following levels of prevention:
   - Primary
   - Secondary
   - Tertiary
4. Analyze issues related to social justice for this aggregate.

ACTIVITIES TO PROMOTE CRITICAL THINKING

1. Check the web for the current year U.S. Census Bureau poverty threshold (http//www.census.gov/hhes/www/poverty.html). Now, check the costs in your community for the simplest nutritional diet, shelter, clothing, and basic necessities. Create a budget for a subsistence living in your community and compare it with the most recent poverty threshold established by the government.
2. What is your own family history of poverty? Because poverty is so stigmatized, such background in your own family may be difficult to acknowledge. Family encounters with poverty may be family secrets.
3. Drive through your own community. Are there places where the tourist books advise visitors never to venture? Are there neighborhoods with unpaved streets and homes slowly falling down on top of the residents, who live in escalating fear of the drug selling of youth on the street? How many children grow up in these places? How many finish high school? How many find work that pays a living wage?
4. Drive through two local communities, one affluent and one impoverished, to evaluate local resources.

5. What do you believe about the worth of individual human beings?
6. Are the poor to blame for their poverty?
7. See Display 32–1. What sorts of social, educational, and economic assistance programs would make it possible for Tommy to become employed at a living wage? Are there limits to his potential for self-sufficiency? What is society's responsibility?
8. Why do you think our nation emphasizes policing and punishment of drug traffic instead of prevention and treatment of drug use? What do you believe, and how does this affect your nursing care?
9. Do you believe that shelter and food are basic human rights?
10. Go sit in the waiting room of your nearest public clinic. Notice how people are addressed as they wait, are processed through various clerks, and are finally seen. Try seeking help for one of your own health problems in such an environment. What have you learned?
11. You may have come to believe many of the negative stereotypes about poor people. How have your judgments been shaped? How can you open yourself to caring for those from whom most of society turns away?

REFERENCES

Abraham, L. K. (1993). *Mama might be better off dead: The failure of health care in urban America.* Chicago: University of Chicago.

Acquaviva, T., & Lancaster, J. (1996). Poverty and homelessness. In Stanhope, M., & J. Lancaster (Eds.), *Community health nursing: Promoting health of aggregates, families, and individuals.* St. Louis: Mosby.

Aday, L. (1993). *At risk in America: The health and health care needs of vulnerable populations in the United States.* San Francisco: Jossey-Bass.

Amaro, H. (1999). An expensive policy: The impact of inadequate funding for substance abuse treatment. *American Journal of Public Health, 89*(5), 657–659.

Barrow, S., Herman, D., Cordova, P., & Struening, E. (1999). Mortality among homeless shelter residents in New York City. *American Journal of Public Health, 89*(4), 529–533.

Baumann, S. (1994). No place of their own: An exploratory study. *Nursing Science Quarterly, 7*(4), 162–169.

Berne, A., Dato, C., Mason, D., & Rafferty, M. (1990). A nursing model for addressing the health needs of homeless families. *Image: Journal of Nursing Scholarship, 22*(1), 33.

Blane, D. (1995). Editorial: Social determinants of health-socioeconomic status, social class, and ethnicity. *American Journal of Public Health, 85*(7), 903–905.

Carney, P. (1992). The concept of poverty. *Public Health Nursing, 9*(2), 74–80.

Chafey, K. (1997). Caring is not enough: Ethical paradigms for community-based care. In B. Spradley & J. Allender (Eds.), *Readings in community health nursing* (pp. 211–220). Philadelphia: Lippincott.

Chavkin, W. (1999). What's a mother to do? Welfare, work, and family. *American Journal of Public Health, 89*(4), 477–478.

Cohen, M. (1993). Megacities and the environment. *Finance and Development, 30,* 44–47.

Crossette, B. (1999, August 5). In days, India, chasing China, will have a billion people. *New York Times,* p. A10.

Devaney, B., Ellwood, M., & Love, J. (1997). Programs that mitigate the effects of poverty on children. *Future Child, 7*(92), 88–112.

DeChiara, M., & Wolff, T. (1998). Topics for our times: If we have the money, why is it so hard? *American Journal of Public Health, 89*(9), 1300–1302.

Gault, B., Hartmann, H., & Yi, H. (1998). Prospects for low-income mothers' economic survival under welfare reform. *Publius: The Journal of Federalism, 28*(3), 175–193.

Heymann, S., & Earle, A. (1999). The impact of welfare reform on parents' abylity to care for their children's health. *American Journal of Public Health, 89*(4), 502–505.

Hilfiker, D. (1994). *Not all of us are saints: A doctor's journey with the poor.* New York: Ballantine Books.

Jezewski, M. (1995). Staying connected: The core of facilitating health care for homeless persons. *Public Health Nursing, 12*(3), 203–210.

Kawachi, I., Kennedy, B., Lochner, K., & Prothrow-Stith, D. (1997). Social capital, income inequality, and mortality. *American Journal of Public Health, 87*(9), 1491–1498.

Keepnews, D. (1998). Welfare reform and health care. *American Journal of Nursing, 98*(3), 55–56.

Kilborn, P. (1999, May 31). Disabled spouses increasingly face a life alone and loss of income. *new York Times,* p. A8.

Lantz, P., House, J., Lepkowski, J., Williams, D., Mero, R., & Chen, J. (1998). Socioeconomic factors, health behaviors, and mortality. *Journal of the American Medical Association, 279*(21), 1703–1708.

Link, B., Susser, E., Stueve, A., Phelan, J., Moore, R., & Struening, E. (1994). Lifetime and five-year prevalence of homelessness in the United States. *American Journal of Public Health, 84*(12), 1907–1912.

Managed care cost pressures threaten access for the uninsured. (1999, March). *Findings from Health System Change, 19,* 1–6.

Martin, M., & Henry, M. (1989). Cultural relativity and poverty. *Public Health Nursing, 6*(1), 28–34.

McKnight, J. (1995). *The careless society: Community and its counterfeits.* New York: Basic Books.

National COalition for the Homeless. (1996). *Why are people homeless?* Fact Sheet #1.

Olds, D., & Kitzman, H. (1990). Can home visitation improve the health of women and children at environmental risk? *Pediatrics, 86*(1), 108–116.

Pappas, G. (1994). Elucidating the relationships between race, socioeconomic status, and health. *American Journal of Public Health, 84*(6), 892–893.

Pear, R. (1999, May 14). Study links Medicaid drop to welfare changes. *New York times,* p. A18.

Rank, M., & Hirschl, T. (1999). The likelihood of poverty across the American adult life span. *Social Work, 44*(3), 201–214.

Reichenbach, E., McNamee, M., & Seibel, L. (1998). The community health nursing implications of the self-reported health status of a local homeless population. *Public Health Nursing, 15*(6), 398–405.

Schorr, L., & Schorr, D. (1988). *Within our reach: Breaking the cycle of disadvantage.* New York: Doubleday.

Schulman, K., Berlin, J., Harless, W., Kerner, J., Sistrunk, S., Gersh, B., Dube, R., Taleghani, C., Burke, J., Williams, S., Eisenberg, J., & Escarce, J. (1999). The effect of race and sex on physicians' recommendations for cardiac catheterization. *The New England Journal of Medicine, 340*(8), 618–626.

Sidel, R. (1992). Women and children last: The plight of poor women in affluent America. New York: Penguin.

Sink, M. (1999, July 5). Faraway friends "adopt" a reservati n's elderly. *New York Times,* p. A8.

Sklar, H. (1995). *Chaos or community: Seeking solutions, not scapegoats for bad economics.* boston: South End Press.

United Nations Children's Fund. (1994). *The state of the world's children.* New York, NY: UNICEF.

United Nations Development Programmes. (1998). *UNDP poverty report 1998: Overcoming human poverty.* New York: United Nations.

U.S. Bureau of the Census. (1998). *Current population reports: Poverty in the United States: 1997* (Series P60–201). Washington, DC: U.S. Wovernment Printing Office.

Wilson, W. J. (1996). *When work disappears: The world of the new urban poor.* New York: Vantage Books.

Zerwekh, J. V. (2000). Caring on the ragged edge: Nursing persons who are disenfranchised. *Advances in Nursing Science, 22*(4), 47–61.

SELECTED READINGS

Chalich, T., & White, J. P. (1997). Providing primary care to poor urban women. *Nursing Forum, 32*(2), 23–28.

Douglass, R. L., Torres, R. E., Surfus, P., et al. (1999). Health care needs and services utilization among sheltered and unsheltered Michigan homeless. *Journal of Health Care for the P   or and Unsheltered, 10*(1), 5–18.

Ensign, J., & Santelli, J. (1997). Shelter-based homeless youth. *Archives of Pediatric and Adolescent Medicine, 151,* 817–823.

Gaze, H. (1997). Hitting the streets. *Nursing Times, 93*(34), 36–37.

Gelberg, L., Gallagher, T. C., Anderson, R. M., & Koegel, P. (1997). Competing priorities as a barrier to medical care among homeless adults in Los Angeles. *American Journal of Public Health, 87*(2), 217–220.

Gillis, L. M., & Singer, J. (1997). Breaking through the barriers: Healthcare for the homeless. *Journal of Nursing Administration, 27*(6), 30–34.

Harrington, M. (1962). *The other America: Poverty in the United States.* Baltimore: Penguin.

Hatton, D. C. (1997). Managing health problems among homeless women with children in a transitional shelter. *Image: Journal of Nursing Scholarship, 29*(1), 33–37.

Herman, D. B., Susser, E. S., Struening, E. L., & Link, B. L. (1997). Adverse childhood experiences: Are they risk factors for adult homelessness? *American Journal of Public Health, 87*(2), 249–255.

Hunter, J. K., Ventura, M. R., & Kearns, P. A. (1999). Cost analysis of a nursing center for the homeless. *Nursing Economics, 17*(1), 20–28.

Luttenbacher, M., & Hall, L. A. (1998). The effects of maternal psychosocial factors on parenting attitudes of low-income, single mothers with young children. *Nursing Research, 47*(1), 25–34.

Lynch, J. W., Everson, S. A., Kaplan, G. A., et al. (1998). Does low socioeconomic status potentiate the effects of heightened cardiovascular responses to stress on the progression of carotid atherosclerosis? *American Journal of Public Health, 88*(3), 389–394.

Northam, S. (1996). Access to health promotion, protection, and disease prevention among impoverished individuals. *Public Health Nursing, 13*(5), 353–364.

Phee, A. (1998). Nursing in the streets. *Nursing Times, 94*(21), 32.

Plumb, J. D., McManus, P., & Carson, L. (1996). A collaborative community approach to homeless care. *Primary Care, 23*(1), 17–30.

Power, R., French, R., Connelly, J., et al. (1999). Health, health promotion, and homelessness. *British Medical Journal, 318,* 590–592.

Randolph, F., Blasinsky, M., Leginski, W., et al. (1997). Creating integrated service systems for homeless persons with mental illness: The ACCuSS program. *Psychiatric Services, 48*(3), 369–373.

Rosenheck, R., & Lam, J. A. (1997). Homeless mentally ill clients and providers' perceptions of service needs and clients' use of services. *Psychiatric Services, 48*(3), 381–386.

Salit, S. A., Kuhn, E. M., Hartz, A. J., et al. (1998). Hospitalization costs associated with homelessness in New York City. *The New England Journal of Medicine, 338*(24), 1734–1740.

Weich, S., & Lewis, G. (1998). Material standard of living, social class and the prevalence of the common mental disorders in Great Britain. *Journal of Epidemiology and Community Health, 52,* 8–14.

_____. (1998). Poverty, unemployment, and common mental disorders: Population based cohort study. *British Medical Journal, 317,* 115–119.

Wojtusik, L., & White, M. C. (1998). Health status, needs, and health care barriers among the homeless. *Journal of Health Care for the Poor and Underserved, 9*(2), 140–152.

Zlotnick, C., Kronstadt, D., & Klee, L. (1998). Foster care children and family homelessness. *American Journal of Public Health, 88*(9), 1368–1370.

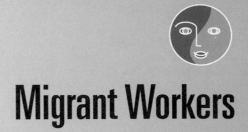

Migrant Workers

KEY TERMS

- Camp health aide
- Crew leader
- Cultural brokering
- Cultural sensitivity
- Curanderas
- Familialism
- Homebase
- Lay workers
- Machismo
- Migrant farmworker
- Migrant health program
- Migrant streams
- Outreach
- Patterns of migration
- Personalismo
- Seasonal farmworker
- Simpatica

LEARNING OBJECTIVES

Upon mastery of this chapter, you should be able to:

- Discuss the historical background of migrant workers and their demographics and patterns.
- Describe the migrant lifestyle.
- Explain how hazardous living and working conditions contribute to migrant workers' increased risk for health problems.
- Identify at least three health problems common to migrant workers and their families.
- Describe social issues resulting from the migrant lifestyle.
- Discuss barriers and challenges to migrant health care.
- Identify methods for effective health care delivery to migrant populations.
- Discuss goals and implications for effective health care delivery to migrant populations.

You may never have seen migrant workers, yet you are a direct beneficiary of their labor. Have you ever thought about the people who harvest the fruits and vegetables that you eat? Have you ever thought about exactly who these people are, where they come from, where they live, or what their health is like? This chapter addresses these questions, but you will probably come away with many new questions and concerns as you explore migrant health issues in community health nursing.

Migrant farmworkers are an integral part of the farming community in the United States. Our agricultural industry relies heavily on migrant workers to harvest the almost endless array of fresh, frozen, and canned fruits and vegetables that mark the United States as a country of plentiful harvests. Nearly 5 million migrant farmworkers are employed in the United States, and they harvest over half the produce in many communities.

Despite their importance to American agriculture, migrant workers are rarely visible beyond the fringes of the camps and farms to which they travel to pursue their livelihood. Most come to the United States from Mexico and other underdeveloped countries in hopes of improving their impoverished lives. Some are legal residents, whereas others are undocumented and live in fear of deportation. All endure backbreaking, menial labor for low wages and are often deprived of basic rights to safe working conditions, adequate sanitation, decent housing, and health care.

Because they are concerned with the health needs of underserved populations at risk, community health nurses are the prime implementers of health care to migrant workers and their families. Primarily, nurses who work with migrant communities try to simultaneously reduce their high incidence of disease and increase their low access to health care. By creating options for this vulnerable aggregate and helping them reach beyond their often abysmal conditions, community health nurses also promote social justice.

MIGRANT FARMWORKERS: PROFILE OF A NOMADIC AGGREGATE

Maintaining a low public profile, migrant workers are, for the most part, marginalized from mainstream society. They remain unseen, unheard, poorly understood, and excluded from many programs that provide health care assistance for low-income people. The migrant worker is a kind of disenfranchised citizen, an orphan within our country for whom no one wants to take responsibility (National Advisory Council on Migrant Health, 1995). Yet their needs are great. They are plagued with different and more complex health problems that occur more frequently than in the general population (Dever, 1991). In addition, their demographics, socioeconomic conditions, and lifestyle resemble those of a Third World country despite the fact that they live and work in one of the most prosperous countries on earth. Some of their most common problems include poverty, malnutrition, infectious and parasitic diseases, limited education, hazardous working conditions, and unsafe housing. Although migrant families are in dire need of health resources, economic, cultural, and language barriers prevent this aggregate from accessing available health services. According to the National Advisory Council on Migrant Health, fewer than 20% of migrant farmworkers use available health services. This astounding fact makes it essential to understand the history, demographics, environment, culture, and health care needs of the migrant worker.

Historical Background

Both historically and internationally, farmers have rarely been able to employ permanently the large workforces needed to harvest their crops. Through the 19th century, however, the small, family-owned farms typical in the United States got through the harvest by using school children, neighbors, and local day laborers. However, during the Great Depression many of these small, independently run farms went bankrupt. Within a few years, the outbreak of World War II caused an increased need for food production. To keep abreast of the demand for produce, the surviving, larger farms turned to migrant labor for help. The Bracero Agreement of 1942 enabled Mexicans to enter the United States for up to 6 months to provide agricultural assistance to farmers. The goals of the Bracero Agreement were to contract for Mexicans who would leave as soon as the harvesting season was over, prevent Mexican workers from displacing American workers, and provide for transportation and living expenses (Piniero, 1994). Between 1951 and 1964, more than 400,000 Mexicans were

brought to the United States annually (Siantz, 1994). The Bracero Agreement lasted more than 20 years and established a large core of Mexican migrant workers. Despite the Bracero Agreement, however, many employers, wanting to save time and expenses, started importing immigrants across the border illegally. Living apart from society, the plight of migrant farmworkers was largely ignored until exposure on a television documentary created a national outcry. This led to the passage of the Migrant Health Act of 1962, which addressed the health needs of migrant workers for the first time in U.S. history. The Migrant Health Act authorized delivery of primary and supplementary health services to migrant farmworkers. Federally funded migrant health clinics serve areas in the United States where there are significant numbers of migrant farmworkers. Staffing usually includes doctors, nurses, outreach workers, social workers, and health educators. An important source of health care for migrant workers, the federally funded clinics also receive monetary help from more than a hundred organizations. They provide health care services throughout more than 400 clinic sites (Fig. 33–1). However, funding is often insufficient, and many clinics are not sufficiently staffed or operated to meet the health needs of migrant farmworkers and their dependents. Additionally, although these clinics exist throughout the United States, there are large geographic regions that are not being served. Migrant workers in these areas must rely on local health departments and emergency rooms or go without health care at all. These factors may explain why migrant health clinics have struggled to provide care for over 40 years, yet statistics reveal that they serve less than 20% of the migrant population (Dever, 1991). A law passed in 1997 under the Clinton administration, the Children's Health Insurance Program (CHIP), Title XXI of the Social Security Act, insures the nation's 10.6 million uninsured children. Hopefully, CHIP will improve health care access for the nearly 1 million migrant children who move from field to field and state to state with their parents to harvest the crops (Health Resources and Services Administration, 1998).

Migrant Hero

An outstanding migrant hero, Cesar Chavez was born in Yuma, Arizona, on March 21, 1927 and died on April 23, 1993. Chavez founded the United Farm Workers (UFW), the first union in agricultural labor history to successfully organize migrant farmworkers. He spent his life fighting for social justice, "La Causa," and his tireless commitment inspired people to join the movement for social change. He traveled with his family to harvest crops, but they rarely had enough food to eat and lived in shacks. Work was often scarce, wages were low, and labor contractors cheated the family out of the money they earned (Furomoto, 1993). Moving to follow the crops, Chavez attended as many as 65 different schools, and after completing eighth grade, he dropped out of school to help support his family by working full time in the fields. His experiences as a migrant worker deeply

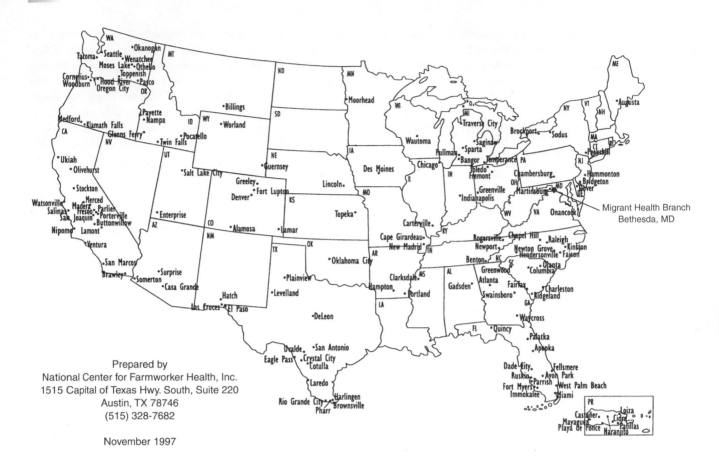

Prepared by
National Center for Farmworker Health, Inc.
1515 Capital of Texas Hwy. South, Suite 220
Austin, TX 78746
(515) 328-7682

November 1997

FIGURE 33–1. Health centers serving migrant and seasonal farmworkers.

affected him and later motivated him to devote his life to organizing farmworkers.

In early 1972, Chavez successfully organized the UFW union, whose membership now numbers 100,000, to campaign against antilabor legislation in California, Oregon, Arizona, and Florida. In 1975, the Agricultural Labor Relations Act was passed, guaranteeing farmworkers secret ballots in union elections. Chavez organized many successful strikes and boycotts, the most famous being the boycott of California grapes against the indiscriminate use of pesticides by growers. In 1988, he fasted for 36 days to protest the use of agricultural pesticides. His efforts united people who, as individuals, had no significance in the power structure. His legacy is an example of how people build power together. The persistent commitment that Chavez had for the cause of social change serves as an example to all people. Throughout his life, he ignored personal hardships to struggle with union victories and losses. As Cesar Chavez so eloquently expressed, "Fighting for social justice . . . is one of the profoundest ways to say yes to human dignity. . . . " (Furomoto, 1993).

Demographics

Comprehensive, national studies on the migrant population need to be done. Much of the research from 40 years ago is

out of date, and there is a general agreement that census figures are not reliable indicators of the actual numbers (National Advisory Council on Migrant Health, 1995). Because migrant farmworkers constitute a mobile population with shifting composition, it is difficult to know their numbers precisely or determine their origins. Estimates of the number of migrant workers vary also because of the influx of illegal and undocumented workers. Most of the estimated 5 million migrant farmworkers tend to be either newly arrived immigrants with few connections or established legal residents with limited opportunities and skills who rely on farm labor for survival. Most of the migrant workers are young. Sixty percent are under 25 years old, and 25% are less than 6 years of age (Siantz, 1994). Some are U.S. citizens, and, although predominantly Hispanic Mexicans, many are African American, Haitian, Creole, Native American, or Asian. No one can accurately count immigrants who cross the Mexican border every day, yet as many as one quarter of the migrant population may be unauthorized to work in the United States (Piniero, 1994).

Farmworkers are defined as having income derived primarily from work in the agricultural industry. **Seasonal farmworkers** live in one geographic location and labor in the fields of that particular area, whereas **migrant farmworkers** travel to find agricultural work throughout the year, usually from state to state. Some live apart from their families, forming groups of single men, whereas others travel with their entire families.

The average migrant farmworker spends from June to September doing seasonal harvesting, about 8 weeks on the road traveling from farm to farm to work, and is then unemployed unless nonagricultural work such as hauling and canning is found (Sandhaus, 1998). Agricultural labor requirements vary greatly between the different phases of planting, cultivating, harvesting, and processing. This labor is crucial to the production of a large variety of crops in almost every state of our nation, yet migrant farmworkers are among the poorest of the working poor (Siantz, 1994). Income for migrant workers is well below the poverty level, and half earn about $5,500 per year, less than half the U.S. poverty threshold (Migrant Clinicians Network, 1997).

Migrant Streams and Patterns

Migrant farmworkers usually have their permanent residence, or **homebase,** in California, Texas, Florida, Mexico, or Puerto Rico. From their homebase, they mobilize as each new crop is ready for harvest. Following the harvest seasons of agricultural crops, migrant farmworkers move from place to place, usually along predetermined routes called **migrant streams** (Fig. 33–2). Most migrant farmworkers are multigenerational; that is, their families have been farmworkers for several generations, traveling the same streams for many years.

Three principal streams formulate the agricultural routes that migrant laborers follow. The *eastern stream* originates in Texas, Puerto Rico, and Florida and extends up the East Coast to states east of the Mississippi as far as northern New York. Although predominantly Mexican, this stream is ethnically diverse, including African Americans, Anglos, Haitians, and Jamaicans. The *midwestern stream* begins in Texas and reaches across the southwestern and midwestern states, going north to the states bordering Canada and both east and west of Mississippi. The *western stream* is the largest and originates in California and Arizona and moves up the West Coast to all western states. Mexicans, Native Americans, and Southeast Asians follow the midwestern and western streams.

Weather conditions and employment opportunities affect movement and patterns of migration. Because of the unpredictable nature of farm work, the three streams are not clearly

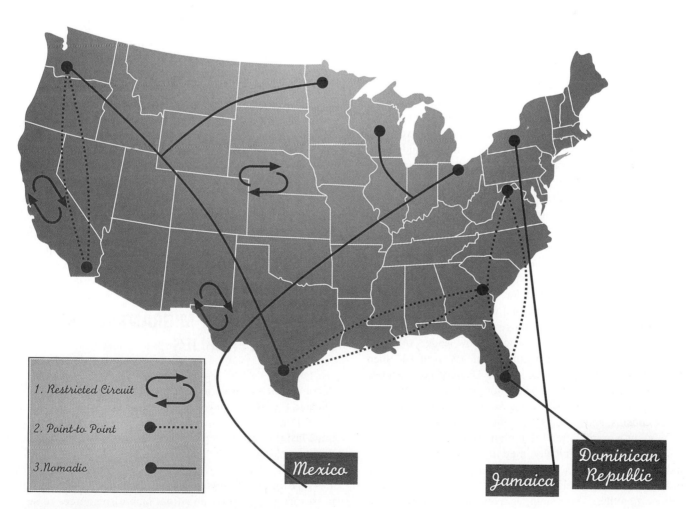

FIGURE 33–2. Migration patterns. (From the Migrant Clinicians Network Monograph Series. [1998]. The TB Net System.)

delineated, pointing to more complex patterns of movement. In addition to the migrant streams, **patterns of migration** exist with varying lengths of stay. In the *restricted circuit,* many people travel throughout a season within a small geographic area. *Point-to-point migration* entails leaving a homebase for part of the year to travel to the same place or series of places along a route during the agricultural season. *Nomadic* migrant workers travel away from home for several years, working from farm to farm and crop to crop, relying on word of mouth about job opportunities. Some of these workers eventually settle in the areas to which they have migrated, whereas others return to their homebase. An ethnic group will usually follow its own particular stream and pattern of migration.

Migrant Lifestyle

To understand the health needs of migrant farmworkers and their families, it is important to understand their lifestyle. Migrant workers and their families endure a transient and uncertain life with long hours, stressful working conditions, low wages, and poor health care. Substandard housing, unsafe work conditions, and language difficulties make life even more difficult.

Migrant workers must confront the vagaries of an unpredictable world. At any given time, migrants remain in an area for only 6 to 8 weeks to work the fields 6 days a week from sunrise to sunset. Depending on weather and crop conditions, work may be plentiful one week and virtually gone the next. Because yearly income must be earned during the harvest season, all family members contribute to harvesting. Children are essential to the core group's economy and must help in the fields and at home. Migrant laborers learn about employment opportunities from recruiters and crew leaders and from other migrants. Interestingly, there are towns in Mexico where the majority of the people migrate each year (Piniero, 1994). Migrant laborers who travel in crews, or groups, use a **crew leader** who acts as the mediator between themselves and the farmer. The farmer usually pays the crew leader who, in turn, pays the workers. An unscrupulous crew leader could withhold payment and keep the migrant workers in constant debt.

Entry into the migrant camps is contingent on the approval of the farmer and crew leader. Crew leaders often organize their crews at the beginning of a season and then transport them throughout the stream. Usually, crew leaders and crews remain the same year after year. It is not uncommon for an entire crew to be composed of a family of uncles, aunts, cousins, and siblings traveling together.

Migrant workers often drive night and day as they move from crop to crop. Typically, they travel with their children and only their most essential possessions in aging cars, vans, and trucks. Occasionally, van loads of "solos," or single men, migrate together. Their status is even more precarious because they lack family support systems (Bechtel, Shepherd & Rogers, 1995).

An average migrant farmworker usually earns about 40 cents per 5-gallon bushel of harvested crops (Bechtel et al., 1995). On a good day a worker can earn up to $100, but rain, poor harvest, injury, and disease make the average earnings only $30 to $60 (Bechtel et al., 1995), causing annual income to fall below the poverty level (Migrant Clinicians Network, 1997). Men, women, and older children all work in the fields. Because inexpensive child care is often unavailable, mothers often leave very young children alone playing in fields exposed to sun, chemicals, and dangerous machinery. Sometimes children are brought to the fields and left in cars or cardboard boxes. Often a teenage girl or the mother of an infant remains in the camps to babysit all the children and is usually stranded there because available cars are used to take workers to the fields.

Recent Population Changes

Although there is little evidence that suggests that the total number of migrant farmworkers has changed significantly in recent years, two important changes have occurred in this population. The first major change is the declining number of migrant workers traveling independently in organized work crews. Instead, family units now predominate. As a result, the number of women, young children, and infants exposed to the stress of migrant life has increased.

A second major change is in the increased number of Hispanics, particularly Mexicans in the midwestern and western states. This change reflects the shift toward family working units, with Mexican farmworkers showing a preference for traveling in family units (Siantz, 1994). Migrant farmworkers from Mexico typically have low rates of literacy and will accept employment regardless of personal cost to health. Although most Mexicans tend to resettle in the Southwest, many are now settling in areas where they were not found in previous years, such as Pennsylvania, North Carolina, and Minnesota. Work crews composed mostly of African-Americans still dominate the eastern stream.

HEALTH RISKS OF MIGRANT WORKERS AND THEIR FAMILIES

A community with varied and profound health needs complicated by disease and social isolation, migrant farmworkers and their families are at risk. Because seasonal earnings must last the entire year, the migrant farmworker avoids or delays seeking health care until the illness becomes debilitating. When work is primary, health is eclipsed (Sandhaus, 1998). Migrant farmworkers and their families suffer illnesses caused by poor nutrition, lack of resources to seek care early in the disease process, and infectious diseases from overcrowding and poor sanitation (Migrant Clinicians

Network, 1997). Keep in mind these shocking health statistics:

- Migrant life expectancy is 49 years as compared with 73 years for the general population.
- Migrant infant mortality rate is 125% higher than the national average.
- The death rate from flu and pneumonia is 20% higher than the national average.
- The rate of parasitic infection is estimated to be 11 to 59 times higher than that of the general population.
- The death rate from tuberculosis and other communicable diseases is 25 times higher than the national average.
- The hospitalization rate of migrant families is 50% higher than the national average.
- Poor nutrition often results in infant deaths, anemia, extreme dental problems, vision problems, and poor mental and physical development of children (Migrant Clinicians Network, 1997).

Occupational Hazards

The hazards of agricultural employment coupled with limited legal protection jeopardize the health of the migrant farmworker. Working in agriculture surpasses mining and construction as the most hazardous occupation in the United States, with more deaths occurring among agricultural workers than in other occupations (Gwyther & Jenkins, 1998). Frequent falls, cuts, muscle strains, and repetitive motion injuries such as carpal tunnel afflict migrant laborers. Agricultural work often requires stooping, working long hours in wet clothes, working with the soil, climbing, carrying heavy loads, and touching plants. Failure to perform these activities on a rigid timetable dictated by seasons and weather can result in crop loss. This urgency compels farmworkers to work in all weather conditions, including extreme heat, cold, rain, bright sun, and damp. Some plants such as tobacco and strawberries emit toxic chemicals that cause severe allergic reactions. Extreme cold causes frostbite; overexposure to the sun creates heat stroke, which occurs nearly four times as often as in the general population (Health Resources and Services Administration, 1998).

Farmworkers spend much of their time on their feet, picking crops, irrigating and clearing fields. Footwear is usually not adequate, and foot problems are often ignored until walking becomes painful because the migrant worker cannot afford the time off from work or treatment expenses. Minor injuries usually receive superficial treatment in the field from coworkers or the crew chief. In the fields, nonemergent and chronic health conditions merit minimal attention. Leaving work means loss of pay because farmers are not required to pay health insurance or Workers' Compensation, although migrant workers are entitled to these benefits.

Few states impose the minimum age of 16 years for field labor outside of school hours. Because migrant workers are paid on a piecework basis, the contribution of each member, including young children, is significant income (Piniero, 1994). Taken out of school to work in the fields, children are at great risk for accidents and pesticide and sun exposure. Beyond physical injury, children are at risk for school failure that is compounded by mobility and poverty.

Pesticide Exposure

Migrant farmworkers are at greater risk for pesticide poisoning when fields are sprayed or at initial reentry into the field. Many migrant camps are located within large open fields or on the periphery. Overhead pesticide sprayings then endanger not only those at work in the fields but also those in the camp. One study of migrant children found that 48% worked in fields still wet with pesticides, 36% were sprayed with chemicals directly or indirectly, and 34% were sprayed in the process of spraying nearby fields (Health Resources and Services Administration, 1998).

Pesticide exposure produces higher rates of miscarriages, birth defects, upper respiratory infections, visual problems, excessive thirst, sweating, and tremors. Skin reactions include rashes, welts, excoriated arms, facial swelling, and intense itching. Severe cases can result in blindness or death. Pesticide burns and rashes often go untreated because of lack of education about the dangers of pesticide and available services. Migrant workers are often unaware of the hazards of pesticides. A study of 460 migrant farmworkers in Washington state found that 89% did not know the name of a single pesticide to which they had been exposed, and 76% never received information on appropriate protection measures (Migrant Clinicians Network, 1997). Farmers do not always comply with the law to post Environmental Protection Agency (EPA) warnings of pesticide safety and dangers in the migrant camps and in the fields. Gloves and long-sleeved shirts are not always supplied or used. The Department of Labor cannot keep abreast of the reports of violations in safety standards. When a farm is reported, it often only closes down for a few days, and although farmers may be assessed large fines, they are seldom collected.

Contaminated water sources in the field enhance the absorption and spread of pesticides. EPA standards that require not entering a field for at least 24 hours after a spraying are often ignored. Pesticides can drift from the fields to contaminate food or children playing nearby. Children are at greater risk for pesticide-induced illnesses because of their higher metabolism rate, greater surface absorption, and chronic long-term exposure. The EPA estimates that 300,000 farmworkers suffer pesticide poisoning each year (National Advisory Council on Migrant Health, 1995). Many cases are unreported because the workers do not seek treatment and are often misdiagnosed because symptoms of pesticide poisoning can mimic those of viral infections.

Although the impact of acute pesticide poisoning is widely recognized, little is understood about the long-term effects of repeated low-level exposure to which migrant farmworkers are constantly subjected. Some farmworkers report long-term allergies and colds that last 2 or 3 years (National Advisory Council on Migrant Health, 1995). Although there are no studies on the long-term effects of pesticide poisoning, some studies reveal multigenerational effects of pesticide exposure among farmworkers and their families. Of significance are the clusters of cancer and birth defects that have been documented in areas of California (National Advisory Council on Migrant Health, 1995). Figure 33–3 shows an Assessment of Farmworker Pesticide Exposure form developed by the Migrant Clinicians Network.

Substandard Housing and Poor Sanitation

Agricultural fields are usually in isolated areas on the outskirts of rural communities. While in these isolated fields, migrant workers often are not provided with sanitation facilities or fresh drinking water. The Occupational Safety and Health Administration (OSHA) mandates field sanitation and fresh drinking water for farms with 11 workers together in a 1-mile stretch of field. Large corporate farms can, however, simply space workers and legally avoid this regulation.

When housing is available, several families live in one structure. Often 15 or more people share one or two rooms (National Advisory Council on Migrant Health, 1995). Typical living quarters include dilapidated housing units, overcrowded barracks, trailers, buses, and sheds. Most have inadequate or absent heating and cooling, poor plumbing, and little privacy. Trailers used as living quarters are often in disrepair, lacking doors, screens, and even windowpanes (Perilla, Wilson, Wold, & Spencer, 1998). Numerous pests such as roaches, fleas, snakes, rats, and scorpions invade the trailers and pose health threats to the workers and their families. Moreover, broken beer bottles, cans, IV drug needles and paraphernalia, and other trash often litter the living and outdoor spaces. Babies cannot be put down for fear of pests, toddlers are at risk as they explore their environments, and young children are at risk if they play outside (Perilla et al., 1998). When housing is unavailable, workers and their families live in boxes, cars, garages, or in the fields and orchards where they work. Some migrant workers live at least temporarily without any shelter at all. For example, southern Arizona is a first stop area for Mexicans coming into the United States. While looking for work or awaiting transportation to another state, many single men and families live under trees in orange groves. They sleep outside on the ground with no protection from cold, heat, or rain. They drink water from irrigation canals in the field and depend on food that is provided by charitable organizations (Stein, 1993). Lacking stoves, they often cook meals outside over open fires. Without proper refrigeration, their food spoils quickly. Available housing often does not meet even minimal standards of adequacy. Many migrant quarters have neither sinks nor toilets. In one migrant camp in Alabama, workers were living in a converted chicken house (Cole & Crawford,

1991). An upper portion of the wall had been removed for ventilation, creating easy access for insects and birds. A dirt floor, a single light bulb, and two portable toilets located a distance away were some of the other features. Two sinks in a common living area provided the only water for the nearly 60 people who lived in the chicken house. Many did not have mattresses, and because the workers were harvesting potatoes, potato baskets conveniently served as the only furniture.

Licensed and unlicensed field housing is especially likely to have a polluted water source contaminated by pesticides, chemical fertilizers, and organic wastes. Bathing or drinking in this water exposes the migrant worker to harmful chemicals and parasites. Migrant workers are sometimes ignorant of their hazardous conditions, but often they are fearful that if they complain to farmers they will lose their jobs.

COMMON HEALTH PROBLEMS

Health problems among migrant families are largely correlated with poverty, mobility, poor nutrition, neglect, crowded housing, and occupational hazards. Migrant community life is threatened by common denominators that threaten health, such as inaccessibility to medical care, lack of basic hygiene, and ignorance of exposure to environmental hazards. Furthermore, problems with drug, alcohol, and prostitution are eroding health and family values. The growing numbers of women and children with different and specific health care needs pose even greater health challenges for community health nurses. The migrant lifestyle also places families at risk for chronic and communicable diseases. A survey conducted in a Georgia migrant camp revealed that the health problems most often encountered were nutritional deficiencies, urinary tract infection, diabetes, dental caries, skin infections, and head lice (Bechtel et al., 1995). The hazards of agricultural work and crowded unsanitary living conditions with frequent migration to new camps expose migrant farmworkers and their families to many sources of infection and create the opportunity for disease to spread rapidly (Gwyther & Jenkins, 1998). Stressors of living a life in which work is sporadic, with no guarantee of income, affects the entire migrant family when life is physically and emotionally demanding. Unfortunately, the lack of access to health care services results in a high incidence of preventable and almost unheard-of diseases in the migrant population.

Migrant Family Health

Inadequate nutrition affects the health of the entire family. Because migrant farmworkers often cannot afford the fruits and vegetables that they harvest, they buy foods that are cheaper but higher in fat, salt, and processed sugar. These foods exacerbate the hypertension and diabetes already prevalent in Mexican groups. Poor nutrition results in ane-

PATIENT ID	Name: _____ DOB: _____ SS#: _____ Farm: _____ Address: _____
EXPOSURE INFORMATION	Date of exposure: _____ Last time field sprayed: _____ Name of pesticide: _____ Crop: _____ Method of pesticide application: ☐ Aerial ☐ Hand spray ☐ Spray rig Type of work: ☐ Mixing ☐ Loading ☐ Picking/thinning/pruning crops Exposure: ☐ Aerial ☐ Hand spray ☐ Spray rig ☐ Sprayed directly ☐ Drift Other workers involved? ☐ Yes ☐ No ☐ Who? _____ Had patient received training under the Worker Protection Standard? ☐ Yes ☐ No

SYMPTOMS

☐ Weakness	☐ Drooling	☐ Blurred vision	☐ Chest pain
☐ Skin rash	☐ Tiredness	☐ Excessive sweating	☐ Red eyes
☐ Headaches	☐ Nausea	☐ Loss of consciousness	☐ Convulsions
☐ Shortness of breath	☐ Dizziness	☐ Vomiting	☐ Abdominal pain
☐ Muscle twitches	☐ Productive cough	☐ Confusion	☐ Other: _____

How long after exposure did symptoms occur? _____

Other workers exposed who developed symptoms?   ☐ Yes   ☐ No

PHYSICAL SIGNS

☐ Hypotension	☐ Bradycardia	☐ Dermatitis	☐ ↓ DTRs
☐ Confusion	☐ Convulsions	☐ Ataxia	☐ Muscle weakness
☐ Paralysis	☐ Fasciculations	☐ Constricted pupils	☐ Other: _____
☐ ↓ Visual accommodation	☐ Sweating	☐ Drooling	
☐ Bronchospasm	☐ Bronchial exudation	☐ Red eyes	

Cholinesterase testing: Date: _____   Results: _____

Follow-up test ordered: ☐ Yes   ☐ No   Date: _____   Results: _____

TREATMENT

Atropine?   ☐ Yes   ☐ No   Dose: _____   Response: _____

2-PAM?   ☐ Yes   ☐ No   Dose: _____   Response: _____

PROVIDER ID

Provider Signature: _____   Date: _____

Address: _____   Phone: _____

ABOUT THIS REPORT

The original "Evaluation of Farmworker Pesticide Exposure" was developed by Mark Lyons, MPH, PAC, for the New Jersey Department of Health. This form was adapted by the Migrant Clinicians Network for use in a migrant health center setting and used with permission. This form may be duplicated as needed. For more information, contact MCN at 2512 South IH35, Suite 220, Austin, TX 78704, (512) 447-0770.

FIGURE 33–3. Migrant Clinicians Network evaluation of farmworker pesticide exposure.

mia, greater infant mortality and morbidity, and poor physical and mental development in children. Preschool children from Hispanic farmworker families represent a nutritionally vulnerable subset of our pediatric population. Health care providers must be aware of the nutritional risks these children face as well as the fact that many are not participating in public health supplemental food programs because of the family's migratory status and program funding limitations. In one study, one third to one half of migrant preschoolers showed clinical signs of vitamin A deficiency, largely attributed to a diet lacking in fruits and vegetables (Morrison, Rienzo & Frazee, 1995). Vitamin A is essential for maintaining the integrity of the gastrointestinal, pulmonary, immune, and integumentary systems. Deficiencies can lead to conjunctival dryness, blindness, and increased susceptibility to infection (Gargas & Sherrey, 1998). Unhealthy diets also cause other vitamin deficiencies and obesity in migrant children. Obesity is particularly harmful for the Mexican migrant children who are susceptible to developing hypertension and diabetes. In addition, anemia and upper respiratory congestion resulting from a largely milk-based diet are common in migrant children. Sometimes, infants get only milk well beyond the age when solids should be given. Many migrant infants with milk allergies have chronic diarrhea and congestion because medical interventions are not sought and allergies are not recognized (Castiglia, 1997).

Because of frequent moves, children of migrant farmworkers receive only fragmented health care. Minor health problems of migrant children are similar to the general population and include rashes, sprains, upper respiratory infections, earaches, diarrhea, urinary tract infections, anemia, headaches, and dizziness (Health Resources and Services Administration, 1998). Lack of awareness that a minor symptom such as diarrhea or fever may indicate a more serious underlying problem can cause delays in seeking medical attention. An earache is minor but can lead to a major problem such as deafness if untreated. Deafness is a frequently mentioned major health problem in the migrant population (Migrant Clinicians Network, 1997).

Although parents in migrant families may seek help for acute viral or bacterial infection, the parents may stop giving prescribed antibiotics after the child appears better or may have siblings share the medicine. As a result, infections often recur or develop into chronic subacute conditions (Castiglia, 1997). Because head lice is not considered a serious health threat among migrant families, spending money on treatment is deferred (Bechtel et al., 1995).

Mexican women tend to marry young and bear children in their teens. Higher birth rates necessitate health care and teaching in preconception, prenatal, pediatric, and family planning areas. All are sorely lacking at this time. Ironically, Hispanic women are more likely to have several children but are less likely to receive prenatal and postnatal care (Caudle, 1993). Often anemic and with little or no prenatal care because of the constant moving, young mothers bear babies who are also anemic and often underweight. In addition, exposure to pesticides causes birth defects and contamination of breast milk.

Women report frequent urinary tract infections, almost two to three times higher than the national average, because of the demanding work conditions, dehydration from the hot sun, and lack of toilet facilities in the fields (Bechtel et al., 1995). Running water and working toilets are sparsely located in the fields. The toilets are often broken and repairs delayed (Perilla et al., 1998). Because migrant farmworkers are paid by the amount of produce harvested, they do not even take out time to walk the distances to usable bathrooms. Thus, workers, especially women, either reduce their water intake or wait up to 14 hours before using a toilet (Perilla et al., 1998). Frequent complaints of bladder and kidney problems are the consequences. Overcrowding in the migrant camps further hinders personal hygiene and access to toilets.

Money for treating chronic diseases is limited, and migrant families lack knowledge of and access to helpful health measures. Besides the poor diets, the high levels of stressful living and working conditions exacerbate chronic diseases such as diabetes and hypertension that are common among Hispanic populations. Upper respiratory infections, eye problems, depression, anemia, and arthritis are commonly reported illnesses (Migrant Clinicians Network, 1997). Knowledge of appropriate skin and foot care is minimal. Spending much of their time on their feet with inadequate shoes picking crops, irrigating, and clearing fields, farmworkers develop painful foot problems. Although suffering skin rashes from exposure to pesticides and plants, migrant workers spend such a limited time in a state that it becomes difficult for health care providers to identify the relationship between dermatitis and working conditions. Long-term effects of eye irritations and systemic pesticide poisoning include cancer and neuropsychological problems.

Dental Problems

Dental problems are epidemic in the migrant population, yet dental care has very low priority among migrant families. Dental problems are often not assessed or treated. Obtaining oral health care is very difficult in migrant clinics, with waiting periods of up to 6 months for an appointment. Many migrant children are never even screened for dental problems. Many studies cite oral disease as the most frequent migrant health problem because many adults have missing and decayed teeth and gingivitis (Migrant Clinicians Network, 1997). Migrant families seek to have teeth extracted when they become painful; little consideration is given to dental repair or restoration.

"Baby-bottle" syndrome, in which toddler's teeth are rotted to the gum lines, frequently occurs when they are allowed to sleep with sweetened liquids in their bottles. Although refined sugars and soft drinks are not part of the traditional Mexican diet, migrant families frequently resort to these cheap convenience foods in the migratory lifestyle (Bechtel et al., 1995).

Many migrant families do not even own a toothbrush, and most have limited knowledge of dental care. Specifically, they have a poor understanding of the relationship between a sweet diet and caries, the connection between oral hygiene and periodontal health, and the role of fluoride in caries prevention. Oral health problems are caused by lack of early professional treatment, inadequate fluoride intake, and poor diets that, when combined with inadequate oral hygiene, lead to tooth decay.

Infectious Diseases

Although many diseases in migrant aggregates are also common in the general population, it is not unusual to find diseases that would be seen once in a lifetime, if ever, in other groups in the United States. Migrants not only live in Third World conditions but also suffer from Third World diseases. To understand why infectious diseases are so prevalent among migrant workers, you must consider their extreme poverty, their need to travel great distances to find work, their overcrowded living conditions, their lack of proper sanitation, and their limited access to health care (Poss, 1998). Diseases that have been almost eradicated in the United States are sometimes seen in migrant workers. These include typhus, encephalitis, yellow fever, malaria, and leprosy. The largest outbreak of typhoid in recent history occurred in a Florida migrant laborers' camp and was traced to contaminated water (Sandhaus, 1998). Many of the cases of polio in the United States in recent times have been found in the migrant farmworker population (Migrant Clinicians Network, 1997). A significant percentage of migrant farmworkers come from Mexico, Central America, Haiti, and the Dominican Republic, where malaria is endemic. Migrant workers frequently travel back to these countries, placing themselves at risk of acquiring and spreading malaria (Barat, 1999).

Cold and damp living quarters produce ear and respiratory infections that occur more frequently in the migrant population than in the general population (Migrant Clinicians Network, 1997). Toilets located in sleeping areas are associated with a higher incidence of anorexia and gastrointestinal diseases. Parasitic diseases, hepatitis, and gastroenteritis spread rapidly in the crowded living conditions, with no indoor plumbing or sewage disposal and open barrels used for garbage. For example, *Giardia lamblia,* the most commonly found parasite infection in the United States, had a 34% prevalence among migrant children as compared with a national incidence of 4% (Gwyther & Jenkins, 1998). Although many cases of parasite infestations go unreported, estimates of parasites in the migrant aggregate are from 11 to 59 times higher than in the general population (Bechtel, 1998).

TUBERCULOSIS AND AIDS
Tuberculosis is again emerging as a serious public health problem; the deplorable conditions of migrant life favor the spread of tuberculosis among migrant farmworkers. It has been estimated that the migrant farm population is six times more likely to develop tuberculosis than the general population (Snyder, 1998). With unsanitary, cramped, and poorly ventilated living conditions, respiratory infections and the transmission of tuberculosis become inevitable. In a Georgia migrant camp, many study participants reported a great number of coworkers with coughs, weakness, and trouble breathing who refused to go to a clinic because of loss of work hours, money, and possibly jobs. Although tuberculosis screening reveals a high prevalence of the disease, essential follow-up procedures are lacking (Bechtel et al., 1995). A 1993 study by the Centers for Disease Control showed that 44% of migrant farmworkers screened had positive tuberculosis tests. In one study, inaccessibility to a mobile chest x-ray van delayed the confirmation of active tuberculosis cases and financial constraints further precluded treatment. Those with positive tuberculin skin tests often relocated before treatment could be initiated. Others were only supplied with a 1-month supply of medication. Although court-ordered compliance is required for active tuberculosis cases, the migratory lifestyle, the absence of a nationwide tracking system, and large state financial burdens render this impossible. The Advisory Council for the Elimination of Tuberculosis has set screening for tuberculosis and preventive treatment for migrant workers, especially children, as a national priority (Centers for Disease Control and Prevention, 1992).

Acquired immunodeficiency syndrome (AIDS) is a growing problem in the migrant community. The incidence of prostitution and intravenous drug use, both risk factors for AIDS, is especially high in the East Coast stream where single migrant workers interact with day workers from large cities where drug use is frequent. Not surprisingly, research points to increases in human immunodeficiency virus (HIV) infection in the East Coast migrant community that far exceed the general population. In a 1992 study among farmworkers in North Carolina, the rate of positive HIV was eight times the national rate. Migrant families are particularly at risk for both transmission of the virus and development of HIV infection into AIDS because of their lack of access to counseling, prevention, and treatment (Lambert, 1995). Studies reveal that migrant families do not know about the transmission of HIV and that, before going to a doctor, migrant workers will attempt to self-treat with herbal compounds and other folk remedies (Perilla et al., 1998). Thus, the HIV infection may not be diagnosed until AIDS-related symptoms are manifested, and HIV may be spread unknowingly.

IMMUNIZATION
Because of the nomadic life, absence of adequate medical tracking and continuity of care are problems. Poor medical record keeping makes tracking of immunizations difficult, yet many of the diseases in the migrant population are preventable by proper immunization. Probably no other population in the United States has simultaneous high incidences of both overimmunization and underimmunization of children,

as do migrant families (Migrant Clinicians Network, 1997). Many migrant children have been immunized four or five times in the same season because of poor tracking records, whereas others have been missed completely for the same reason. The vast majority of migrant adults also do not have available or up-to-date health or immunization records. Acknowledgment of immunization is also a problem. When tetanus booster shots were offered free of charge to migrant workers in Georgia fields, some refused, stating they did not want to risk a sore arm that would interfere with crop harvesting (Bechtel et al., 1995). The irony is that many foreign-born migrant workers probably never even received primary tetanus vaccines, rendering boosters inadequate for protection.

RISKS TO COMMUNITIES

No information is available on which illnesses migrant farmworkers and their families have when they enter a state or which illnesses they take along with them when they leave. We do know that the migrant lifestyle leads to the creation and perpetuation of disease and illness, which then becomes a community health issue. Migrant workers live in close quarters with others and may send their children to local schools for brief periods of time. They and their children may remain untreated for the duration of the time they spend in a community. They, thus, may act as vehicles for disease transmission and incubators for diseases that develop into drug-resistant strains.

Many migrant workers eventually settle in the predominantly rural areas where they work. Then the need for decent health care and housing becomes more pressing not only for their safety and comfort, but also for the good of the community at large. Host communities faced with people markedly different from themselves and with threatening health problems may become polarized and hostile to the migrant workers.

Social Issues

Migrant workers work and live in places and ways apart from the mainstream population. For example, in Georgia more than 100,000 migrant workers and their families harvest approximately 90% of the crops, which generate more than $300 million in sales for the farmers. Yet it is not rare to meet native Georgians who have never met a migrant farmworker or even know of their existence (Perilla et al., 1998). Living apart from established local communities, migrant workers are especially vulnerable to isolation and neglect. Fear of deportation, poverty, and limited education intensify social isolation, which sometimes results in chronic emotional problems such as depression. Display 33–1 lists some stressors in the Hispanic Stress Inventory evaluation tool.

Lack of recreational facilities and the stressors associated with migrancy also contribute to increased rates of substance abuse. Leisure time in the camps is sometimes spent drinking, smoking marijuana, or injecting illegal drugs. In one

DISPLAY 33–1. Hispanic Stress Inventory— Brief Version

Item	Yes	No
My spouse and I disagree about who controls the money.	☐	☐
My spouse expects me to be more traditional in relationships.	☐	☐
My spouse and I disagree on how to bring up our children.	☐	☐
I've questioned the idea that "marriage is forever."	☐	☐
There have been cultural conflicts in my marriage.	☐	☐
I've felt my spouse and I haven't communicated.	☐	☐
My spouse and I disagree on the language spoken at home.	☐	☐
Both my spouse and I have had to work.	☐	☐
My spouse hasn't adapted to American life.	☐	☐
I watch my work quality so others don't think I'm lazy.	☐	☐
My income is insufficient to support family or myself.	☐	☐
Since I'm Latino I'm expected to work harder.	☐	☐
Since I'm Latino it's hard to get promotions/raises.	☐	☐
I've been criticized about my work.	☐	☐
I think my children used illegal drugs.	☐	☐
My children have been drinking alcohol.	☐	☐
My children received bad school reports/grades.	☐	☐
My children haven't respected my authority as they should.	☐	☐
My children's ideas about sexuality are too liberal.	☐	☐
My children have talked about leaving home.	☐	☐
There's been physical violence among my family members.	☐	☐
My personal goals conflict with family goals.	☐	☐
I've had serious arguments with family members.	☐	☐
Since I'm Latino it is difficult to find the work I want.	☐	☐
I thought I could be deported if I went to social/government agency.	☐	☐
Due to poor English, people treat me bad.	☐	☐
Due to poor English, it's hard dealing with daily situations.	☐	☐

(From Garcia, D. [1997]. Assessing stress among migrant and seasonal farmworkers. *Streamline: The Migrant Health News Source, 3* [5], 1–5.)

study, women in a Georgia migrant camp cited drug and alcohol abuse as the most significant health problem in their community (Perilla et al., 1998).

The children of these workers suffer homelessness, hunger, long hours of work, lack of friends, frequent relocation, poverty, and school interruption, which all pose psychosocial and developmental risks. A study that investigated children's exposure to violence found large numbers of children who either witnessed violence or were themselves victims (Martin, Kupersmidt & Harter, 1996). Large percentages of the children in the study exhibited emotional and behavioral problems. Many children are forced to leave school to work in the fields and have little more than a sixth-grade education. This limits their opportunities and forces them to repeat the life cycle of their parents. In addition, bilingual children often become negotiators for their parents. This stressful role requires skills well beyond their years. Finally, adult roles are forced on migrant children early. Girls are viewed as adults when they are capable of taking care of the household and can bear children, whereas boys are considered men as soon as they start earning as much as their fathers (see Voices From the Community).

Living in cramped, dirty, and unsanitary quarters often leads to domestic violence. Physical and sexual abuse of women and children occurs, and migrant women are more susceptible to domestic and intimate partner violence than the general population. Lacking access to health services and fearing deportation and isolation, these women often have no choice but to endure the violence (Migrant Clinicians Network, 1997). One migrant woman related that while sharing one room with her husband, infant, and five single men, her husband became increasingly violent and unpredictable. He began to beat her and the baby, and she was unable to predict what would initiate a violent attack. She finally fled when one of the men living with them also began beating her. She attributed the aggressive behavior to the powerlessness felt by the men (National Advisory Council on Migrant Health, 1995). The Violence Against Women Act of 1994 affords protection for undocumented battered women and children by allowing them to seek legal immigration status without the help of their abusers (Camacho, 1998) (see Levels of Prevention).

Deterioration of family values is a concern of some migrant workers who see their children becoming acculturated into mainstream values and becoming less family oriented. Conflicts sometimes erupt when children start to identify with mainstream lifestyles despite parental enforcement of traditional values. Yet, despite concerns that the very fabric of their culture may be threatened by problems with drugs and alcohol, domestic violence, prostitution, and deterioration of family values, the migrant community remains extremely resilient and proud. Families place high premiums on work and self-sufficiency. Family and family structure are highly valued, and migrant families form cohesive units based on language, food, music, religion, social interaction, and beneficial folk health practices.

Voices From the Community

(Page 9) "I am the product of undocumented parents who dared to swim across the Rio Grande so that they could find a better opportunity for themselves and their children. . . . My mother had no prenatal care and none was available to her. . . . I lived in tents, I picked fruit so I could get through school along with my other family members. I have had to deal with not wanting to be Hispanic because of the language and cultural barriers and what it did to women. . . .

"I am the oldest of five children and became my parents' advocate because they could not speak English. . . . Being an advocate at the age of seven when I learned English as a second language, I encountered a system that was not very sensitive to people who had a different cultural and different language. . . . And so, as I picked grapes and I was on my knees spreading those grapes for raisins, I decided that someday I would hope to work in the system. That I would try to change it so that it would be sensitive and poor people would get care with love, . . . dignity, and respect for their cultural barriers.

"I think that it is incumbent on all of us to remember where we came from and turn our face around to the injustices. And that together we make a difference."

A. V., 1996 National Farmworker Health Conference,
Nashville, Tennessee

(Page 34) "First of all, a nurse should expect the unexpected. Because of the migratory way of life . . . they do not always know where they will be next week or next month: therefore we must understand that they do not always have their medical records, immunization records, or income records . . . hours are very irregular. Depending on what time the workers get in from the fields and what time the shifts are. . . . Because of the distances we travel, we work anywhere from eight to twelve hours a day. . . . The most rewarding part of the job is bringing health services to the underserved and uninsured. The people are so gracious and appreciative of whatever services we provide."

J. S., RN, Michigan

(Page 39) "Since farmworkers come to our area for only four months of the year, it is rare that I care for a migrant woman through her entire pregnancy. I may diagnose her pregnancy, I may see her for three or four prenatal visits, or I may meet her only once before she goes into labor and delivers her baby. . . . I struggle with the desire to make a difference in a short period of time and with the disappointment of not being able to follow-through."

C. K., CNM, RN, Pennsylvania

(Pages 40–41) "Encourage clinicians to trust old diagnostic skills of palpation, auscultation, and careful

(continued

listening. Exhaustive laboratory work or radiology studies are not likely to be welcomed by farm workers who seek relief of symptoms so that they may return to work. . . . Be warm and interested in the whole family. If you do not speak Spanish or Creole, work with translators who understand how you work. Use translators as . . . vehicles to get the information out and in. Eye contact and touch are crucial. Learning to be clinically relevant as well as competent utilizing a translator is an art, and takes time and experience to hone. Learning some phrases or some of the most frequently asked questions in the language of the farm worker should be encouraged. Even the attempt to speak the patients' language will build trust and confidence. These harvesters of the nation's food are very bright and resourceful people who travel great distances and undergo severe deprivation in order to work. The nobility of this pursuit is getting short shrift in the press and legislative bodies today, but the sheer enormity of the service [that] this group of oppressed people do for the rest of us needs to be acknowledged and honored by the clinicians who will provide primary health care to them and theirs."

W. H., RN, Michigan

(Pages 32–33) "A new provider is first challenged by a culture with beliefs and practices foreign to their own. . . . Sensitivity, respect and acknowledgment of those beliefs are essential in establishing trust and rapport. The new provider is challenged, secondly, by the living and social situations of our migrant patients. . . . The lack of adequate housing, appropriate sanitary conditions, refrigeration, heat and air conditioning plays an integral part in the complexities of caring for our patients. . . . The third unique aspect is the . . . exposure of our patients to chemicals, pesticides and other toxic materials in the environment. Probably the most dramatic, emotional, and challenging experience I have faced during my career with migrant and seasonal farmworkers occurred during the treatment and follow-up of 84 migrant workers following the largest pesticide accident to occur in Florida and possibly the country. The incident dramatized many of the issues and problems seen by clinicians in migrant health, including lack of education on health issues (protective clothing, food washing, reentering sprayed fields too soon). The deficiencies in our legal system regarding the protection of farmworkers were exemplified by the shortage of investigators and the lack of enforcement of existing laws regarding worker safety and health. . . . I explained that I was here for them, that they were my patients, and were important to me. Then they began to cry. I guess no one had ever taken an interest in their lives, health, and well-being. Had anyone ever related to them as human beings? . . . the lessons learned in working with migrant farmwork-

(continued)

ers are lessons of tolerance and dignity. In short, they are lessons of integrity, lessons of justice, and lessons of life."

D. P., DO, Florida

(From Migrant Clinicians Network [1997]. *Migrant health provider orientation manual.*)

BARRIERS TO HEALTH CARE

When you get sick, you expect to go to a doctor and use your insurance to cover medical expenses. You expect your illness to be understood, and you expect to be treated as a person in need of medical attention. This is not the case with migrant workers. Migrant health clinics often fail to serve migrants by imposing legal, financial, and physical impediments. Many clinics do not account for cultural differences, and some have staff that are unable to speak the clients' language. Understanding why less than 20% of migrant workers use primary care health services is essential in providing better health care to this aggregate. Barriers to primary health care access are isolation, powerlessness, economics, limited health resources, language, and culture.

Isolation and Powerlessness

The rural communities in which migrant workers live generally lack primary care providers, and migrant workers lack the transportation necessary to get to clinics that may be far away from migrant camps. Lack of adequate child care facilities is also a hindrance for working mothers. Because migrant workers will not miss a day's work until their illnesses become dire, migrant clinics are not helpful unless they offer weekend and evening hours. Unfortunately, office hours are normally from 9:00 to 5:00, Monday through Friday—the times that migrant farmworkers spend in the fields (Bechtel et al., 1995) (see The Global Community).

Nomadic lifestyle and poverty render migrant workers politically powerless. Furthermore, they do not stay in their communities long enough to affect local decision-making processes that could improve their working and living conditions. Many state and federal agencies are too understaffed to adequately enforce health regulations and labor laws (Bechtel et al., 1995).

Migrant workers tend to be clannish and suspicious of strangers, and they mistrust outsiders for fear of deportation and job loss. They are even fearful of reporting minor injuries because health care providers may be viewed as having policing power. The Immigration Law of 1986, designed to open up more jobs for American citizens by limiting the hiring of illegal immigrants, increased discrimination against Hispanics, even those who are citizens (Caudle, 1993). Racism and discrimination abuses are pervasive among migrant farmworkers and their families (Perilla et al., 1998).

Suffering discrimination due to their ethnicity and migrant status, many migrant men and women encounter prejudice and racism in medical facilities, grocery stores, shopping centers, restaurants, schools, and even in churches (Perilla et al., 1998).

Economic Barriers and Limited Health Resources

Inability to obtain Medicaid, coupled with lack of health insurance, severely handicaps migrant farmworkers' ability to access health care. Because they are low-wage earners, migrant workers often cannot afford to pay for health care and are not willing to take time off from work when pay depends on each bushel picked (Gwyther & Jenkins, 1998). Migrant farmworkers are usually not covered by health insurance because farm owners, especially those who own smaller farms, cannot afford to provide health insurance for their workers (Castiglia, 1997). Mobility disqualifies migrant families from Medicaid–managed care systems because of the inability to maintain a single primary care provider (Gwyther & Jenkins, 1998). Primary and secondary prevention are almost nonexistent because funds for these services are not available (Bechtel et al., 1995) (see Voices From the Community).

Migrant workers are unable to qualify for basic health and disability benefits such as Workers' Compensation and Social Security because of loopholes in the legal system. Although eligible for public programs such as Medicaid, food stamps, and Women, Infants, and Children Supplemental Food Program (WIC), migrant farmworkers cannot participate. They may fear immigration penalties or be totally unaware of the available benefits. Although many have worked in this country for several years, they are often not U.S. citizens or may be in the country illegally (Castiglia, 1997). Although undocumented immigrants are not eligible for public assistance, they do have protected rights to decent wages, health, safety, and Workers' Compensation (Migrant Clinicians Network, 1997).

Medicaid was enacted to protect and increase health care for vulnerable populations such as the migrant community. However, as a group migrant farmworkers have more difficulty accessing Medicaid than any other population. In the face of constant mobility, Medicaid benefits have little value because they are not transferable from state to state. On one hand, although the low income of migrant workers meets the guidelines for state medical assistance, few families remain in one state long enough for the 30-day residency requirement (Castiglia, 1997). On the other hand, farmworker families may not qualify for Medicaid because, during certain months of the year, they earn more than the state's poverty limits (Stein, 1993). Ironically, migrant workers suffer from preventable and treatable diseases covered under Medicaid but are unable to obtain treatment.

In a New York migrant camp, a group of nurses made obtaining Medicaid a priority and worked to facilitate the Medicaid application process by assisting with the completion of the form, scheduling interviews, gathering appropriate documents, and interpreting as necessary. Although assisting with the Medicaid application was extremely time consuming and labor intensive, it was an important strategy for expediting health care access. This strategy was helpful only if the applications were started as soon as the farmworkers arrived in the area; otherwise, they would be gone before Medicaid benefits started (Poss & Meeks, 1994). Also, if the farmworkers began earning salaries before completing their application, they would make too much money to qualify for Medicaid benefits because income guidelines are based on recent paychecks and not yearly earnings.

Often, the emergency room is the most accessible health care option for migrant families, yet it is the most expensive

Voices From the Community

(Page 5) "Going out into the migrant camps, one of the migrant workers said, 'We expect one of us to die.' I thought, 'Why do you expect that to happen?' They shouldn't have this mentality when they go traveling state to state—that it's a part of life."

(Page 25) "They [women] also need child care. What happens with the children? Go out in the fields. They lay under the trees and there is a residue falling on the children. They are picking grapes, what happens? The sprayers are there with the residue falling on the children."

I. A., health promoter, La Clinica del Carino, Hood River, Oregon, and Representative to the 1991 Farmworker Women's Health Conference, San Antonio, Texas

(Page 6) "What we have to do is reeducate our people and let them know that we have many rights to live and work and to educate and to have health care. And without health care, we cannot have the other three."

Unidentified male farmworker, California

(Page 9) "We're used to working. We don't want to be given things. We just want to be respected and to be paid the salaries."

T. S., California

(Page 9) "They [farmworkers] don't demand to go to the doctor [for medical treatment after injuries] nor do they file any complaints. They feel that if they do not come back to work the next day, they will lose their job. The foremen do not help because they do not want people that will not produce for them."

(Page 17) "Now there are a lot of people who are making a living in the same way but are unable to find adequate housing, consequently having to live under the trees. What's even worse, the foremen even charged them for sleeping under the trees."

T. V., Migrant Health Center Board Member, California

(Page 13) "The pesticides we live in day and night. . . . You go to the fields and you think that it's a foggy day because it's so pretty and it's white, but actually it's the chemicals that have been sprayed."

A. R., California

(Page 18) "I have seen people that work in the fields stay wherever, outside on the edge of their fields, and in their cars and vans. And we have the whole family, they come in their vans and they stay there. Those people just ask for permission to take a bath in some cabin or some field, to be able to take a bath or drink some water and that's all. And that's the way they spend their lives."

E. S., Board member, La Clinica del Carino, Hood River, Oregon

(continued)

> (Page 22) "I'm dealing right now with Hispanic women, migrant workers, who do not have any access to prenatal care, none whatsoever. What I'm doing is creative financing, a lot of begging, a lot of pleading, a lot of being nice to people I don't even want to be nice to because it means that much to me for them to get help. So I find myself in situations that are sometimes uncomfortable, but nonetheless I do it because I feel that as a nurse that's my job. Having been a farmworker myself, I would want someone to do that for my mother, and they did."
>
> *Unidentified female nurse, Idaho Falls, Idaho*
>
> (From Galarneau, C. [Ed.]. [1993]. *Under the weather: farmworker health. A compendium of farmworker testimony before the National Advisory Council on Migrant Health.* Rockville, MD: National Advisory Council on Migrant Health, Bureau of Primary Health Care.)

health care facility for this population. Migrant families even hesitate to use this option because hospitals are viewed with anxiety and mistrust and as a place to die.

Cultural and Language Barriers

Because many migrant workers do not speak or read English, the language barrier makes it difficult for migrant workers to navigate difficulties in communication such as negotiating appointments, applying for insurance, or adhering to medical treatment (Bechtel et al., 1995). Many families do not comprehend the language in which application forms are written. Research shows that increasing the number of bilingual personnel and nurses at migrant centers was crucial for increasing health care access (Piniero, 1994).

Many migrant families are unable to effectively communicate health care needs, and many health care providers lack sensitivity to understand the needs of this culturally diverse population. To become effective health care providers, community health nurses must embrace the notion of **cultural sensitivity,** the awareness of different values, beliefs, and behaviors of others (Jezewski, 1990). To become effective health care providers, you must work on developing the capacity to appreciate differences and value diversity and assess your reactions to different cultures.

In a study conducted in a New York state migrant camp, cultural sensitizing took place on several occasions. Nurses and staff discussed their cultural values and opinions about what was right and good in caring for migrant farmworkers. The sharing of this information sensitized staff members and nurses to migrant value systems and injustices migrant workers endure as a group and also as members of an ethnic group (Jezewski, 1990). To learn about migrant family values, nurses observed behaviors and asked questions, especially about health care behaviors. They also visited migrant camps and interacted socially. Cultural sensitivity enabled the nurses to anticipate culturally based problems that could arise during health care encounters (Jezewski, 1990). Bechtel (1995) conducted a similar study when community health nursing students were taken to migrant camps as part of a summer course requirement. Forced to confront migrant culture, the working conditions, and unique health problems, the students soon learned that although economic, social, and racial issues may divide communities, the basic elements of wanting a better environment and enhancing self-worth transcend all differences.

Culture affects health beliefs. For example, a strong component of Hispanic culture, folklore medicine and rituals, are commonly practiced by many migrant workers (Morrison et al., 1995). Because of limited access to health care and a tendency to distrust mainstream medical personnel, many migrant workers will first seek health care from healers in their own communities (Perilla et al., 1998). Herbal medicines are common, as is seeking advice from **curanderas** (folk healers). If unsuccessful, migrant workers will then seek out medical interventions. In rural areas of Mexico, strong beliefs in folk illnesses, such as the evil eye, require traditional folk remedies. Many Hispanics believe in hot and cold theories of illness. Mexican women may refuse fruits and vegetable during the "hot" postpartum state because these foods are considered "cold" (Caudle, 1993). Many recent Mexican immigrants use needles and syringes to give themselves vitamins, medications, and contraceptives purchased in Mexico. A threat to health, the needles may be shared for these injections, exposing the users to infection and possible HIV (Caudle, 1993).

The Mexican culture is patriarchal, with "machismo" men playing the dominant role in decision-making while women carry out the decisions (Siantz, 1994). Treating disease involves remedies approved by the male head of the household and implemented by the female member of the household. Hispanics also appreciate the qualities of **simpatica** (positive interpersonal relationships) and **personalismo** (pleasant conversation). Although diseases are often viewed with fatalistic acceptance, migrant families expect health care providers to relieve their disease symptoms. Many nurses do not possess an adequate understanding of the impact of the migrant family's cultural beliefs and expectations of the nurse (Bechtel et al., 1995). Migrant families expect to have symptoms relieved quickly and effectively, with nurses using a personal, warm approach. The migrant worker must also be considered in the context of family because family is an important source of emotional and physical support for members who become ill. Community health nurses who are sensitive to cultural beliefs can and do increase the effectiveness of treatment (Gwyther & Jenkins, 1998).

THE ROLE OF COMMUNITY HEALTH NURSES IN CARING FOR A MOBILE WORKFORCE

Beyond the barriers to health care such as lack of health services, language and cultural impediments, inadequate to nonexistent transportation, financial strains, underinsurance, and questionable residency status, which are by themselves formidable obstacles, the migrant lifestyle is fraught with challenges. Because of the insecurity and instability inherent in a mobile lifestyle, long-term health goals are difficult to establish and long-term follow-up of any chronic illness is doubtful (Artemis, 1996). Nonetheless, community health nurses provide much-needed services using community resources, innovative thinking, tenacity, and sensitivity.

Trenchant strategies for improving the health status and resource use of migrant workers and their families can be accomplished by:

Improving existing services
Advocating and networking
Practicing cultural sensitivity
Using lay personnel for community outreach
Utilizing unique methods of health care delivery
Employing information tracking systems

Community health nurses are the major providers of migrant health services and have a crucial role in the development and management of interventions. In response to the growing need for available, accessible, and affordable health care for farmworker families, they are called on not only to understand the migrant lifestyle but also to help migrant families overcome the barriers to health care.

Evaluating and Improving Health Services

No clearly defined leadership to develop policies for migrant workers exists. Because the farmers themselves, under financial constraints, are not traditionally consulted regarding migrant health issues, health care for this population becomes fragmented in the federal domain. Federal appropriations for migrant workers are low, and most existing services exclude them because of residency requirements. The government's funding structure provides incentives for agencies that treat a greater number of clients rather than stressing quality, disease prevention, and continuity of care (Sandhaus, 1998). In addition, an effective tracking system to maximize services is desperately needed.

The National Advisory Council on Migrant Health (1995) recommends universal health coverage for migrant families with Medicaid coverage transferable from state to state. It suggests that migrant health centers provide culturally sensitive health care that includes transportation, translation services, and case management to the diverse and underserved migrant populations. Currently, most translators at health care sites are

clerical support staff. Untrained personnel can impede health care delivery if unable to translate accurately and may be perceived as threats to confidentiality by the clients.

Investigations to improve the health care of migrant workers are needed. Laws regulating safety, wages, sanitation, and employment must be better enforced. All migrant health centers should be funded to provide oral health care. Migrant workers should be included in mental health and substance abuse health services. The Office of Substance Abuse Prevention recommends increased appropriations for migrant-specific health issues (National Advisory Council on Migrant Health, 1995). Assessment, intervention, and evaluation of health care delivery, areas in which community health nurses excel, are needed as well as increased numbers of culturally and linguistically competent nurses. To develop outreach and primary care services, increased federal funding for migrant health projects is essential. Regulations that limit reimbursement, especially for dental and eye examinations, hypertension and diabetes screening, mammograms, and preventive health care, should be reevaluated. Improving public health services, such as providing drinkable water, ensuring sanitation services in the fields, guarding against pesticide exposure, and addressing substandard housing, is crucial to disease prevention.

Advocacy, Networking, and Cultural Brokering

Advocating for the migrant population is an important strategy in facilitating health care. As advocates, community health nurses can effectively intervene when a treatment plan is incongruent with the migrant lifestyle. For example, if a doctor were to prescribe bed rest for a migrant farmworker who injured his leg, that protocol would most likely not be followed because missing a day's work means missing a day's pay. An alternative plan, one more consistent with the migrant lifestyle, would be for the migrant farmworker to stay off the injured leg in the evening when he is not working. In advocating on the behalf of the injured worker, the community health nurse would have to ensure that the leg was elevated and that appropriate pharmaceutical treatments were applied. Although healing would probably take longer, this plan is more realistic.

When community health nursing students, in an experimental learning program, spent a summer in the fields working within a migrant community, they came across a migrant worker suffering from dehydration and nausea (Bechtel, 1995). Through an interpreter, he told the students that the crew leader would not allow the men to interrupt work to go to the bathroom. He also said that the crew leader was withholding his pay. A visit to the worker's trailer revealed that 16 other workers were living in one trailer and that they shared a bathroom with two other families. After advocating to both the crew chief and local officials to collect the wages that were due, the students helped relocate the worker to another camp so he would not to suffer recriminations for reporting the squalid conditions to the authorities. In addition, the students contacted several state and federal agencies to report the unsanitary living conditions and also attended a rural outreach forum to discuss health, labor, and migrant issues.

Community health nurses can obtain health care services for migrant workers through **cultural brokering,** whereby nurses intervene to assist in acquiring needed health care (Jezewski, 1991). Cultural brokering involves facilitating health care for migrant workers who are unable to overcome the barriers of existing health care. This includes negotiating, mediating, and innovating on behalf of migrant workers (Jezewski, 1991). Essential to this role are sensitivity to patient needs, knowledge of the barriers that impede health care, and commitment to facilitate heath care for those who do not have the power to access health care on their own.

Cultural Sensitivity

Community health nurses who have consistent and frequent contact with the migrant community will become aware of migrant families' social and culturally based needs. Intervening with culturally diverse clients and communities must reflect cultural sensitivity such as viewing culture as an enabler to pursue health care rather than a resistant force (Caudle, 1993). Culturally sensitive assessments and interventions must include health, education, income, degree of acculturation, level of participation in traditional culture, and length of time in the United States (Siantz, 1994). Incorporating cultural beliefs in plans of care that stress **familialism** and taking time for pleasant conversation with Hispanic clients, for example, require knowing about their culture, customs, beliefs, and language. Dialogues between the community health nurse and migrant workers should not be patronizing or one-sided but open, with an opportunity to learn and teach. Each time migrant families are helped, they become encouraged and empowered for the common good of the entire community.

Because the traditional mainstream ideal of professionalism may be construed as cold and distant, a warm, accepting attitude and pleasant conversation are cornerstones of effective health care relationships (Rodriguez, 1993). Successful intervention strategies include nonjudgmental communication and the ability to convey respect and genuine affection for the family (Siantz, 1994). This may take time to nurture and develop, but in the end it very much enhances communication with migrant clients. For example, a migrant worker did not finish his prescribed antibiotic (Caudle, 1993). By being less formal, warm, and showing concern and by avoiding criticism and confrontation, the nurse was able to explain the importance of finishing the antibiotic. This resulted in the client becoming more receptive to care and even referring family members to the nurse.

Family is the most important source of support for those who become ill. Decision-making about health matters is a family function. Having family members present during assessment and teaching enhances client satisfaction and compliance. For example, when dealing with drug addiction in a migrant family, the entire family should be included. Fear of being isolated from family may prevent the drug-addicted member from seeking treatment. **Machismo,** or male qualities of dominance, has been described as a cultural reason why Hispanic men attempt to prove their masculinity through substance abuse and use of prostitutes, which carry high risks for AIDS and HIV. True machismo, however, translates into pride, honor, and dignity when men must take responsibility for their families and protect them from harm. By incorporating machismo and familialism into health education programs and stressing that the males are responsible for and capable of protecting their household, the community health nurse will have better success. Love of family and children is so strong that Mexican Americans have shown themselves to be more likely than non-Hispanic whites to quit smoking when they perceive it as a threat to their children (Caudle, 1993).

Being nonjudgmental and nonthreatening provides a framework for communication. Inquiring about folk remedies, for example, should never be broached with direct questioning; rather, a third-person inquiry approach should be used (Pachter, 1994). You should not attempt to dissuade migrant families from their folk remedies if they are harmless but should instead educate them on the importance of medical therapy. Combining folk and medical therapies may help increase compliance because it places medicine within the context of the culture and lifestyle. If a Hispanic mother wishes to give her child a harmless folk potion for asthma or massage the abdomen of a child with viral gastroenteritis as is culturally prescribed, no harm can be done if these remedies are continued along with prescribed medical treatments (Pachter, 1994). Although a Spanish-speaking Hispanic herself, Rodriguez (1993) had a difficult time in her research in getting migrant women to open up about domestic violence. After several failed assessment questions, a new approach was tried. Migrant women were asked what a nurse should tell a woman who might come to her as a result of physical abuse by her partner. This third-person approach met with success when women who had previously denied being physically abused offered information about their handling of abusive situations.

Lay Personnel for Community Outreach

Lay outreach personnel can overcome the language and cultural barriers as well as isolation. Using migrant lay community **outreach** workers who have received basic training in health care and resources is a method of reaching and improving health care. Recognizing the value of family, friends, and the sharing of cultural values, migrant lay personnel are readily accepted within the migrant community, overcoming cultural and language barriers. Despite the stereotypical portrayal of Hispanic women as passive, they are, in fact, a source of strength for family members by maintaining and nurturing strong family ties and loyalty (Olmos, Ybarra & Monterrey, 1999). Many Hispanic women often become involved outside the family sphere in education and community activities as lay workers. **Lay workers** in migrant communities are typically trained and supervised by community health nurses (Gwyther & Jenkins, 1998). Already familiar with life in the migrant community, lay migrant outreach workers create formal and informal links with one another to promote health and provide continuity of care. Perhaps one of the most trenchant advantages of using lay personnel is the sense of empowerment engendered when they believe they can take control in caring for one another.

One successful program using lay migrant women is the North Carolina Maternal and Child Health Migrant Project. This program overcame stringent barriers to health care such as limited transportation, communication difficulties, and lack of child care. Volunteer women in the migrant camps were trained to become lay health advisors providing health education, prescription instruction, and first aid. Bilingual staff also streamlined follow-ups, referrals, and appointments and acted as interpreters. The program used a bus as well as volunteer drivers to transport clients to appointments (National Advisory Council on Migrant Health, 1995).

When 40 migrant women trained as lay health advisors were evaluated in two migrant health centers in North Carolina, they were found to have interacted with 50% to 82% of the 470 migrant women and infants within the year-long study. Mothers who had contact with the lay advisors were more likely to visit health care providers when their children were sick. Furthermore, they had more knowledge about health than did the mothers without contacts to the lay advisors (Watkins et al., 1994).

Another intervention strategy using lay leaders is the Camp Health Aide program. **Camp health aides** who are bilingual and bicultural are recruited to overcome language restrictions and negative stereotyping that prevent the migrant workers from getting proper health care. Camp health aides, usually women and themselves workers, help reinforce positive health values and create a sense of self-esteem and empowerment (Sandhaus, 1998). Recruited in the same manner that lay health advisors are, camp health aides are trained to teach their peers on topics such as hygiene, spread of disease, preventive health care measures, nutrition, prenatal care, pesticides, and availability of health services. Migrant women trained in this manner are able to provide on-site care, which decreases the amount of time lost from work and reduces the complications from inattention to health problems.

The Camp Health Aide Program in Monroe, Michigan, recruits lay workers to teach about nutrition, first aid, prenatal care, well-child care, environmental protection, diabetes, hypertension, sexually transmitted diseases, HIV/AIDS, and mental health. Gaining better access to health care, migrant farmworkers benefit by having illnesses diagnosed and treated sooner in a more cost-effective manner (Health Resources and Services Administration, 1998).

Unique Methods of Health Care Delivery

Because migrant health centers do not adequately meet the health needs of the migrant community, several innovative methods of health care delivery have been developed and implemented by community health nurses. Although changes are often minor and slow to occur in the migrant population, even minute changes are a milestone because the migrant lifestyle does not support any type of health stability. Any progress made must be welcomed with recognition and support (Artemis, 1996).

Mobile health vans traveling directly to migrant camps are an effective strategy for outreach health screening and education (Health Resources and Services Administration, 1998). By going to migrant camps and delivering care to where the clients live and work, especially during nonwork hours such as evenings and weekends, community nurses increase health access and overcome barriers of culture and lack of child care. Mobile van clinics in Maricopa County, Arizona, provide health care for five migrant communities (Stein, 1993). Although migrant families had only received fragmented acute care, the nurses' outreach team succeeded by encouraging migrant farmworkers to prevent illness with immunizations, good nutrition, and healthy lifestyles. A viable alternative to traditional medical clinics, the mobile nursing clinic provides primary care to an underserved population through health promotion, disease prevention, and early treatment.

Other migrant services may include migrant ministries that are ecumenical organizations formed to assist migrant workers with government and state grants as well as donations. For example, a ministry in Florida, supported by local donations, distributes sacks of food staples such as rice, beans, flour, and vegetables, as well as gas for cooking to needy migrant families. Classes in English, basic parenting skills, banking needs, and understanding medicine labels are offered in the evenings (Jorn & Ros, 1999). The ministry has also developed vocational training programs and has goals of developing a day care center for children and educational programs that focus on gang violence and substance abuse prevention.

To streamline enrollment in Medicaid, Wisconsin operates a model Medicaid reciprocity system in which migrant farmworker families with valid medical assistance cards from other states automatically qualify for Medicaid without having to reestablish eligibility again. Wisconsin also uses average annual income rather than monthly earnings to qualify families for Medicaid, because migrant farmworker earnings vary considerably from month to month and a single higher-income month could disqualify the worker from Medicaid eligibility (Health Resources and Services Administration, 1998). To help access primary care, vouchers can be implemented in areas that do not make separate services economically feasible. For example, in Colorado voucher programs have evolved into migrant health programs that are trenchant strategies to meet health needs. Whereas migrant health care centers provide direct service, **migrant health programs** depend on referrals and vouchers to address gaps in health care services (Castro, 1999). A migrant health program in Colorado maintains formal agreements with medical, dental, and pharmacy providers that accept reduced fees. With an identification card, migrant workers can directly access primary medical services themselves. Responding to the needs of the migrant workers, evening hours are maintained with bilingual community health nurses who also advocate for migrant workers to ensure that services are accessible and appropriate. A model worthy of replication, the Colorado migrant health program promotes health care advocacy, empowerment, continuity of care, improvement of living and working environments, and accountability to the community.

Resources

Community health nurses involved with migrant families benefit from using federally funded resources such as the National Advisory Council on Migrant Health, Midwest Migrant Health Information Office, Farmworker Health Services, Farmworker Justice Fund, and Health Resources and Services Administration Bureau of Primary Care. Promoting health, social services, education, and employment, these agencies also are important networking sources.

Information Tracking Systems

Mobility impedes continuity of care, and the inadequate system of medical record keeping for the migrant population is particularly frustrating (Weinman, 1999). Data information systems are vital components for monitoring the health status of individual farmworkers as they migrate. Furthermore, these data are essential for generating research and follow-up care as well as long-range health planning. They will also help justify appropriation of monies to migrant health agencies (Gwyther & Jenkins, 1998). Many proposals for data tracking systems have required the implementation of expensive and complicated computer systems that present almost insurmountable barriers to their widespread use. The HEART FAX, a simple and secure system for retrieving medical records using only telephones and fax machines, was initially developed to track cardiac patients who are part-time residents of Florida. HEART FAX functions as a medical database clearinghouse with continuous service via a toll-free telephone number. All instructions for accessing records are provided in both English and Spanish. This data retrieval system would improve continuity of care, especially for pregnant women and children who are most at need (Weinman, 1999).

Migrant children are susceptible to medical feast or famine and may be either overtreated or undertreated simply because their medical histories are unknown to current providers. One method for tracking the health status of migrant school-aged children is through the Migrant Student Record Transfer System (MSRTS), a computerized system that collects and maintains health and academic records for migrant children.

Records of more than half a million migrant children collected by school nurses include data on personal and family history; immunization status; visual, auditory, or dental problems; nutritional status; and general physical condition (Castiglia, 1997). Although this tracking system does serve to enhance the health of migrant children, many migrant children may or may not attend school or do so only on a sporadic basis. The ability to track these children in the migratory lifestyle from work location to work location is often minimal. Early intervention for migrating children is unlikely, although it has proved to greatly improve outcomes. The creation of a national database for information on the health status of migrant workers that parallels the information included in the MSRTS has also been suggested (Piniero, 1994).

Health Goals

The challenge of providing a uniform strategy of care for a highly mobile population prompted the development of a compilation of goals by the National Migrant Resource Program and Migrant Clinicians Network (1997). These goals include the promotion of better health, fewer risk factors, increased awareness, and improved services. Objectives are to improve nutrition, immunization, occupational safety, prenatal care, dental health, preventive services, and medical records; and to reduce drug and alcohol abuse, violent behavior, mental illness, adolescent pregnancy, and HIV transmission (Display

---

DISPLAY 33–2. Migrant-Specific Health Objectives

1. Reduce alcohol and other drug abuse.
2. Improve nutrition.
3. Improve mental health and prevent mental illness.
4. Reduce environmental health hazards.
5. Improve occupational safety and health.
6. Prevent and control unintentional injuries.
7. Reduce violent and abusive behavior.
8. Prevent and control HIV infection and AIDS.
9. Immunize against and control infectious diseases.
10. Improve maternal and infant health.
11. Improve oral health.
12. Reduce adolescent pregnancy and improve reproductive health.
13. Prevent, detect, and control chronic diseases and other health disorders.
14. Improve health education and access to preventive health services.
15. Improve surveillance and data systems.

(From National Migrant Resource Program and Migrant Clinicians Network [1996]. *Migrant and seasonal farmworker health objectives for the year 2000.* Austin, TX: U.S. Department of Health and Human Services, National Center for Farmworker Health, Inc.)

33–2). These objectives both complement and enhance the health objectives for the nation for the year 2010 to increase years of healthy life and eliminate health disparities (U.S. Department of Health and Human Services, 1997).

The transience of the migrant workforce also makes it difficult to ascertain its numbers. A specific goal for the immediate future is to improve research data on migrant workers. Toward this end, community health nurses can gather information concerning changes in family relationships and acculturation to mainstream values to be used in designing health programs. Because few researchers have studied migrant health needs, status, and behavior, this would ensure that health services closely match the needs of specific migrant cultures. Continued efforts must be made to conduct research assessing risks and hazards, especially those of pesticide exposure. Many government publications document the despair and isolation of migrant workers, yet very little has been done to address the living and working environments that contribute to diminished health. Although difficult to study as a mobile population, migrant workers are important as an integral part of our economy and because infectious disease in their sector increases health risks for all (Halcon, 1997).

Community health nurses can become involved in politics and educate the public on the importance of migrant workers to the American economy and their compromised health and living conditions. Community health nurses can influence and implement improvements in public health policy, especially increasing funding to provide greater insurance coverage and better health care to migrant farmworkers. Health interventions, however, must reflect cultural sensitivity and language differences as well as environmental risks. Adequate follow-up and referrals and transferable medical records are crucial for continuity of care. To impact on migrant health issues, community health nurses must advocate to fund training for lay health advisors, promote law enforcement to ensure safe environments, and educate community leaders regarding the special needs of migrant farmworkers (see Research: Bridge to Practice).

SUMMARY

An aggregate at risk, migrant workers suffer higher frequency of illness, more complications, and more long-term debilitating effects. Diseases, often resembling those of a Third World country, are due to poor nutrition, neglect and inadequate treatment, and occupational hazards and conditions arising from poverty and migration. Exacerbated by a magnitude of environmental and work stressors, the health of migrant families is also compromised by limited access to health care, mobility, language and cultural barriers, low educational levels, and few economical and political resources.

Because migrant health needs are largely manageable within community settings, community health nurses are ideal health providers. Implementing health education at migrant camps, training lay health workers, and providing clinic hours to accommodate late workdays are successful interventions. Learning the language of the migrant workers and their unique cultures will also be helpful in reaching this population. Community health nurses must advocate for the health of migrant workers who have very little economic or political power and also guide them through the complexities of a changing health care system. Although many resources and programs exist to help the migrant families, the needs are still overwhelming. By aligning with the goals of *Healthy People 2010* to improve the health of one of our most underserved populations, the health of the nation as a whole will be improved.

The abysmal conditions and health needs of migrant workers have changed little in the past 40 years. However,

RESEARCH Bridge to Practice

Bechtel, G. 1998. Parasitic infections among migrant farm families. *Journal of Community Health Nursing, 15* (1), 1–7.

The author conducted a retrospective study of 422 migrant farmworkers and their families in a migrant camp located in the southeastern United States to determine the prevalence of parasitic infections as an indicator of health, social, and economic conditions. Prevalence of parasitic infestation was 11.4%, and the most significant predictors of infestation were the mother's years of schooling and the presence of other parasitic infections within the family. A low level of education among mothers was associated with infestation. Significant differences were not found between infected and noninfected migrant workers and their families regarding country of origin, time spent in the United States, father's years of schooling, sex, or age.

Because the mother's level of education was the strongest predictor of parasitic infection, developing education programs for parents that are aimed at mothers is imperative to ensure healthy families and communities. Furthermore, informal community-based programs with trained bilingual and bicultural female leaders as educators and caregivers have been shown to be effective in providing primary health care (Bechtel et al., 1995). The fact that the number of years that the mother attended school was significantly associated with the incidence of parasites supports the premise that women provide the framework for health education programs in Hispanic families (Caudle, 1993). Hence, promoting mother's schooling, in addition to educating about hygiene and health practices, can be effective in reducing parasitic infections. The author concludes that efforts to promote education, especially among mothers, may be the single most important factor in raising the health and social well-being of vulnerable populations everywhere.

new needs are arising in the migrant community. In the past, migrant workers traveled primarily in organized crews; they are now traveling in family units with women and children. Added attention must be given to family members exposed to the hazards of the migrant lifestyle. Even as many migrant workers settle into communities, the cycle of poverty continues as others arrive from impoverished countries. With a paucity of health resources, the community health nurse is sometimes the only health provider able and willing to care for this population. Providing care for the migrant workers presents a challenge to

be innovative and go beyond the boundaries of traditional health services.

Community health nurses are charged with the challenge to break the cycle of poverty by providing a voice for those who are not seen or heard. Migrant workers and their families, vital contributors to the American economy, can barely afford the produce that their grueling, underpaid labor provides. Awareness of this plight drives community health nurses to ensure that migrant worker families come to enjoy the harvest of bounty along with improved health and living conditions.

CLINICAL CORNER | Migrant Workers

As you looked at your reflection in the mirror this morning, you said to yourself, "It's finally here . . . the day I've been waiting for the past 6 years." You are now a public health nurse working with migrant farmworkers in the maternal–child program of the county health department! You are excited but somewhat anxious. You can hardly believe this moment has arrived. The years of Spanish courses, along with your already challenging nursing coursework . . . two years working on the medical–surgical unit of your local hospital . . . then, resumes, interview . . . You've finally made it!

After a brief orientation to your new workplace and introductions to new colleagues, your supervisor hands you a chart. "This is the first client we'll be seeing today," she tells you. "I'd like you to review the record and tell me what you think we ought to do during our home visit today." Okay, here goes!

The record indicates a referral from the family planning clinic after a positive pregnancy test. Your client is Angelica, a 23-year-old, monolingual Spanish-speaking woman who came to this country 5 years ago from El Salvador. Angelica is married to Hector, a 38-year-old migrant farmworker from the same village in El Salvador. They have a 4-year-old daughter, Esperanza.

As you read through Angelica's chart, you note the following significant information:

■ Angelica had gestational diabetes with her previous pregnancy. She sought prenatal care at 7 months' gestation after presenting in the emergency room with complaints of dizziness. Esperanza weighed 11 lb, 13 oz at birth.

■ The family has expressed concerns about the fact that they are "undocumented." They are concerned about deportation, and, although they seem to trust the health department staff, they seem reluctant to use other available services.

■ Angelica is at approximately 16 weeks' gestation.

Questions
1. What issues have you identified as priorities for your visit this morning? How do you

plan on addressing those issues with the client?

Your supervisor advises you that the Spanish-speaking community health worker contacted the family yesterday and told them you would be visiting this morning.

You feel excited and confident as you drive to the family's home.

The home is a two room shack in a complex for migrant field workers. After entering the home, you greet Angelica. She advises you that Hector has gone to work but hopes to come home early from working in the field so he may participate in the visit as well. You see Esperanza watching a small television, drinking a bottle of chocolate milk. Angelica invites you to sit on the couch and asks you if you'd like a soda.

2. What will you do in the first few minutes of your visit to develop rapport with your client?

Angelica tells you, "I am glad to have you as my nurse and I am happy that you came to my home. I don't like going to that doctor's office. They always tell me I weigh too much and that I have to stop eating the food that is good for my baby."

After several minutes, Hector comes in from working in the fields and says, "Let me wash my hands. . . . I've been spraying 'chemicos' (chemicals) in the field all morning."

3. Considering the information you garnered from the chart, along with the information obtained thus far during the home visit, discuss your plan for the remainder of today's visit. Present ways in which you will implement your plan.

4. What issues will you identify on subsequent visits? How have you prioritized those issues?

5. What issues does this situation elicit for you regarding:
   Fears and anxiety in dealing with this family
   Lack of immediate resources (supervisor)
   Building partnerships with families, communities, and area resources

ACTIVITIES TO PROMOTE CRITICAL THINKING

1. On the website at http://www.ncfh.org (March, 1999), the following quotation from Paula Diperna appeared: "Justice in the fields slips through the fingers like a handful of soil." Considering what you have read in this chapter about social justice and migrant workers and undocumented immigrants, explain how these words express the inequities this aggregate endures regarding working and living conditions and health.

2. Download migrant workers' educational material from the National Center for Farmworker Health, Inc., at http://www.ncfh.org. Explain why the topics, which include diabetes, healthy eating, alcohol, teen sex, work injuries, family planning, high blood pressure, skin emergencies, care of teeth, and tips to reduce stress, are appropriate for this population. All these teaching materials can also be downloaded in Spanish. Considering language barriers and lack of health care knowledge, discuss the need for using simplicity and pictures in teaching these topics to migrant families. Perhaps, if you live near a migrant camp, you could organize a project with groups of students to implement much-needed teaching strategies using this educational material.

3. The Hispanic Stress Inventory—Brief Version tool displayed in Display 33–1 lists migrant-specific stressor items. How are these items unique to the migrant lifestyle? How are they different from yours?

4. Changes in the structure of health care and social services greatly impact on farmworkers' access to care. Many states are choosing to limit both legal and undocumented immigrants' access to social and health services. For example, federal food stamps were discontinued for hundreds of thousands of legal immigrants in Texas without plans for alternatives (Migrant Clinicians Network, 1997). Many migrant farmworkers return to Texas after 6 months of working in the northern states but cannot find work in the off season. During this time, the migrant workers rely on food stamps. Without food stamps, many migrant families will go hungry in the winter. Suggest ways to advocate for this group, and discuss implementing methods to ensure that health and nutritional needs can be met.

5. Compare and contrast health, living, and working concerns between migrant workers and recent immigrants. Discuss how many recent immigrants from places such as Asia and Kosovo experience the same hardships as migrant workers do. How does nomadic lifestyle affect and differentiate the needs of migrant workers and recent immigrants? (See Clinical Corner.)

REFERENCES

Anderson, P. (1998). Nursing the nomads. *Nursing Times, 27,* 42–43.

Artemis, L. (1996). Migrant health care: Creativity in primary care. *Advanced Practice Nursing Quarterly, 2*(2), 45–49.

Barat, L. (1999). Management of the febrile migrant farmworker. *Streamline: The Migrant Health News Source, 4*(6), 1–4.

Bechtel, G. (1998). Parasitic infections among migrant farm families. *Journal of Community Health Nursing, 15*(1), 1–7.

_____. (1995). Community health nursing in migrant farm camps. *Nurse Educator, 20*(4), 15–18.

Bechtel, G., Shepherd, M., & Rogers, P. (1995). Family, culture, and health practices among migrant farmworkers. *Journal of Community Health Nursing, 12*(1), 15–22.

Camacho, L. (1998). Battered women and U.S. immigration policy: The Violence Against Women Act. *Streamline: The Migrant Health News Source, 4*(1), 2–3.

Castiglia, P. (1997). Health needs of migrant children. *Journal of Pediatric Health Care, 11,* 280–282.

Castro, J. (1999). Migrant health programs: Essential component in health care [online]. *Migrant Health Newsline, 16*(l). Available: http://www.ncfh.org.

Caudle, P. (1993). Providing culturally sensitive health care to Hispanic clients. *Nurse Practitioner, 18*(12), 40–51.

Centers for Disease Control and Prevention. (1992). HIV infection, syphilis, and tuberculosis screening among migrant farm workers. *Morbidity and Mortality Weekly Report, 41,* 723–725.

Cole, A., & Crawford, L. (1991). Implementation and evaluation of the health resource program for migrant women in the Americus, Georgia area. In A. Bushy (Ed.), *Rural nursing,* (Vol. 1, pp. 364–374). Newbury Park: Sage.

Dever, G. (1991). Profile of a population with complex health problems [online]. *Migrant Health Newsline, 8*(2). Available: http://www.ncfh.org.

Health Resources and Services Administration. (1998, April). *Fact sheet: Health care access for farmworker children* [online]. Available: http://www.hrsa.dhhs.gov/.

Furomoto, K. (1993, May). Viva La Causa! Cesar Chavez remembered [online]. *Diatribe of People of Color News Collective, 2*(4). Available: http://www.The city.sfsu.edu/ccipp/remembered.htm.

Garcia, D. (1997). Assessing stress among migrant and seasonal farmworkers. *Streamline: The Migrant Health News Source, 3*(5), 1–5.

Gargas, D., & Sheery, B. (1998). Vitamin A needs of children of farm worker families. *Streamline: The Migrant Health News Source, 4*(5), 1–2.

Gwyther, M., & Jenkins, M. (1998). Migrant farmworker children: Health status, barriers to care, and nursing innovations in health care delivery. *Journal of Pediatric Health, 12*(2), 60–66.

Halcon, L. (1997). Migrant farmworkers and infectious diseases: A review of the literature. *Streamline: The Migrant Health News Source, 3*(3), 1–4.

Jezewski, M. (1990). Culture brokering in migrant farmworker health care. *Western Journal of Nursing Research, 12*(4), 497–513.

Jorn, E., & Ros, R. (1999). Bethel mission serves farmworkers in Florida [online]. *Migrant Health Newsline, 16*(l). Available: http://www.ncfh.org.

Lambert, M. (1995). Migrant and seasonal farmworker women. *Journal of Obstetric, Gynecologic and Neonatal Nursing, 24*(3), 265–268.

Marier, A. (1996). A health education program for migrant children. *American Journal of Public Health, 86,* 590–591.

Martin, S., Kupersmidt, J., & Harter, K. (1996). Children of farm laborers: Utilization of services for mental health problems. *Community Mental Health Journal, 32*(4), 327–339.

Migrant Clinicians Network. (1997). *Migrant health provider orientation manual.* Austin, TX: Author.

Morrison, S., Rienzo, B., & Frazee, C. (1995). Developing health education for Hispanic migrant preschool youth. *Journal of Health Education, 26*(94), 207–210.

National Advisory Council on Migrant Health. (1995). *Losing ground: The condition of farmworkers in America. Recommendations of the National Advisory Council on Migrant Health.* Bethesda, MD: Author.

National Migrant Resource Program and Migrant Clinicians Network. (1996). *Migrant and seasonal farmworker health objectives for the year 2000.* Austin, TX: U.S. Department of Health and Human Services, National Center for Farmworker Health.

Olmos, E., Ybarra, L., & Monterrey, M. (1999). *Americanos: Latino life in the United States.* Boston: Little, Brown.

Pachter, L. (1994). Culture and clinical care: Folk illness beliefs and behaviors and their implications for health care delivery. *Journal of the American Medical Association, 271*(9), 690–694.

Perilla, J., Wilson, A., Wold, J., & Spencer, L. (1998). Listening to migrant voices: Focus groups on health issues in South Georgia. *Journal of Community Health Nursing, 15*(4), 251–263.

Piniero, O. (1994). *The use of health services in Pennsylvania by the children of migrant and seasonal farmworkers.* Unpublished doctoral dissertation, Penn State University, University Park, PA.

Poss, J. (1998). The meaning of tuberculosis for Mexican migrant farmworkers in the United States. *Social Science and Medicine, 47*(2), 195–202.

Poss, J., & Meeks, B. (1994). Meeting the health care needs of migrant farmworkers: The experience of the Niagara County Migrant Clinic. *Journal of Community Health Nursing, 11*(4), 219–228.

Rodriguez, R. (1993). Violence in transience: Nursing care of battered women. *AWHONN's Clinical Issues, 4,* 437–440.

Sandhaus, S. (1998). Migrant health: A harvest of poverty. *American Journal of Nursing, 98*(9), 52–54.

Sansing, S. (1999). Did you know column [online]. *Migrant Health Newsline, 15*(3). Available: http://www.ncfh.org.

Siantz, M. de Leon. (1994). The Mexican-American migrant farmworker family. *Nursing Clinics of North America, 29*(1), 65–72.

Snyder, J. (1998). *Tuberculosis among migrant farmworkers in Northeastern Colorado.* Available: http://www. HI-_CAHS.com.

Stein, L. (1993). Health care delivery to farmworkers in the southwest: An innovative nursing clinic. *Journal of the American Academy of Nurse Practitioners, 5*(3), 118–124.

U.S. Department of Health and Human Services, Office of Disease and Health Promotion. (1997). *Developing objectives for Healthy People 2010.* Washington, DC: U.S. Government Printing Office.

Vasquez, M. (1999). Saludando salud [online]. *Migrant Health Newsline, 15*(3). Available: http://www.ncfh.org.

Watkins, E., Harlan, C., Eng, E., Gansky, S., Gehan, D., & Larson, K. (1994). Assessing the effectiveness of lay health advisors with migrant farmworkers. *Family and Community Health, 16,* 72–78.

Weinman, S. (1999). Heart Fax makes migrant patient records available worldwide [online]. *Migrant Health Newsline, 15*(3). Available: http://www.ncfh. org.

SELECTED READINGS

Anderson, W., & Kelley, J. (1998). Immigration and ethnicity: Implications for holistic nursing. *Journal of Holistic Nursing, 16*(3), 301–319.

Brown, N., & Barton, J. (1992). A collaborative effort between a state migrant health program and a baccalaureate nursing program. *Journal of Community Health Nursing, 9*(3), 151–159.

Camacho, L. (1998). Privacy, confidentiality and security in the transfer of health data. *Streamline: The Migrant Health News Source, 4*(4), 2–3.

Davis, S. (1998). Restrictions of welfare reform law begin to bite. *Streamline: The Migrant Health News Source, 4*(1), 1–3.

Farmer, P. (1997). Social scientists and the new tuberculosis. *Social Science and Medicine, 44,* 347–358.

Haraldson, S. (1994). Reflections on nomadic and scattered populations. *Journal of Community Health, 19*(5), 303–306.

Hogan, P. (1995). Community care: Temporary address, permanent care. *Nursing Standard, 9*(33), 20–22.

Koday, M. (1998). Children's dentistry and the general dentist. *Streamline: The Migrant Health News Source, 4*(5), 3–7.

Liebman, A. (1999). A program to provide safe drinking water. *Streamline: The Migrant Health News Source, 4*(6), 2–3.

McCurdy, S. (1997). Tuberculosis among agricultural workers. *Streamline: The Migrant Health News Source, 3*(1), 1–2.

Miller, M., & Keifer, M. (1998). Cholinesterase monitoring as a predictor for overexposure to pesticides. *Streamline: The Migrant Health News Source, 4*(3), 1–2.

Retzlaff, C., & Hopewell, J. (1996). Puntos de Vista: Primary eye care in migrant health: Eye care needs assessment. *Migrant Clinicians Network Monograph Series,* 1–12.

Rose, V. (1993). On the road. *Nursing Times, 16*(3), 30–31.

Unterberger, A., Medrano, B., & Leon, L. (1997). The role of migrant farmworker men in family planning decision making. *Streamline: The Migrant Health News Source, 3*(2), 1–4.

Washington, G. (1998). After the flood: A strategic primary health care plan for homeless and migrant populations during an environmental disaster. *Nursing and Health Care Perspectives, 19*(2), 65–71.

Weekers, J., & Siem, H. (1997). Is compulsory screening of migrants justifiable? *Public Health Reports, 112,* 397–402.

Weissman, A. (1994). Preventive health and screening of Latin American immigrants in the United States. *The Journal of the American Board of Family Practice, 7,* 310–323.

Clients With Mental Health Issues

KEY TERMS

- Burden of disease
- Community mental health
- Community mental health center
- Community support programs
- Deinstitutionalization
- Disability-adjusted life year (DALY)
- Halfway house
- Insanity
- Mental health
- Mental health promotion
- Mental illness
- Neurosis
- Psychosis
- Serious and persistent mental illness (SPMI)
- Serious mental illness (SMI)
- Stigma

LEARNING OBJECTIVES

Upon mastery of this chapter, you should be able to:

- Discuss the historical evolution of mental health care.
- Explain the obstacle of stigma in community mental health.
- Discuss the incidence and prevalence of mental illness in the U.S.
- Describe the risk factors affecting the mentally ill population.
- Discuss the needs of and treatment approaches for the mentally ill population.
- Identify and describe community mental health resources.
- Describe preventive interventions for the mentally ill population at each level of the public health prevention model.
- Define health promotion and discuss health-promoting interventions for community mental health.
- Describe six aspects of the nurse's role in community mental health.

On your way to school this morning, you notice a group of people picketing on the sidewalk in front of an attractive, three-story Victorian home. As you drive by, you notice one sign reads, "Not in our neighborhood!" and another says, "Protect our children!" You tune your radio to the local news station and learn that a neighborhood group is protesting the purchase of the home by a private health care agency for use as a halfway house for the mentally ill. What are some of the concerns—both legitimate and misconceived—that might have sparked such a protest? What is the place of the mentally ill in the wider community, and who is included in this population? Can a community health nurse contribute to preventing or treating mental illness? What is the nurse's role in promoting mental health or advocating on behalf of the mentally ill? These are some of the questions we explore in this chapter.

This chapter provides you with an opportunity to examine the needs of a vulnerable population in the community—those with mental disorders. It also describes how epidemiologic information about this population becomes a roadmap to guide community mental health nursing practice in community mental health services, mental illness prevention, and mental health promotion.

COMMUNITY MENTAL HEALTH IN PERSPECTIVE

In the past century, research and public health innovations in the United States and worldwide have contributed to significant improvements in health and treatment of disease.

Once-dreaded diseases, such as cancer and HIV/AIDS, are increasingly survivable and even curable. The average American's lifespan has nearly doubled and the physical health of Americans, overall, has never been better. However, the picture has been different for mental health, which has remained a low national priority, and for mental illness, which has been mostly feared and misunderstood.

Only recently has mental health begun to receive the attention it needs and deserves. Speaking of the overall health and well-being of our nation, Donna Shalala, Secretary of Health and Human Services, commented, "We are coming to realize . . . that mental health is absolutely essential to achieving prosperity" (Substance Abuse and Mental Health Services Administration [SAMHSA], 1999, p. 1). It is now recognized that worldwide, 4 of the 10 leading causes of disability for persons 5 years and older are mental disorders (World Health Organization [WHO], 1999). Furthermore, depression is the leading cause of disability in all developed nations, including the U.S. Mental disorders also tragically lead to death; suicide is one of the main preventable causes of death in the U.S. and globally. Addressing these concerns, much research was conducted in the 1990s, declared the "Decade of the Brain" by the U.S. Congress, to gain understanding of mental functioning and mental illness (SAMHSA, 1999). *Healthy People 2010,* published by the U.S. Department of Health and Human Services, includes mental health among the top ten leading indicators of health. The Surgeon General's Report on Mental Health underscores that mind and body are inseparable and that "mental health is fundamental health" (SAMHSA, 1999, p. 2).

Mental health, as defined in *Healthy People 2010,* "is a state of successful mental functioning, resulting in productive activities, fulfilling relationships, and the ability to adapt to change and cope with adversity" (U.S. Department of Health and Human Services [USDHHS], 2000, p. 37). Mental health, although a somewhat elusive and value-driven concept, clearly undergirds successful performance in life. On the other hand, **mental illness** "refers collectively to all diagnosable mental disorders (which) are health conditions that are characterized by alterations in thinking, mood, or behavior (or some combination thereof) associated with distress and/or impaired functioning" (SAMHSA, 1999, p. 8). Mental illness and mental health are not polar opposites but rather can be viewed as points along a health continuum. Mental disorders vary in severity and manifest through specific, distinguishing characteristics. They may arise without regard to age, gender, or ethnicity, as a product of genetic, biological, environmental, social, physical, or behavioral factors acting alone or in combination.

Serious mental illness (SMI) refers to any mental illness that has compromised both the clients' level of function and their quality of life. **Serious and persistent mental illness (SPMI)** is the preferred term for serious mental illness of a chronic nature. For example, schizophrenia is usually classified as an SPMI.

Neurosis is a general term commonly used to describe any of a variety of mental or emotional disorders involving anxiety, phobia, or other abnormal behavioral symptoms. It is considered less severe than **psychosis,** which is a mental disorder characterized by partial or complete withdrawal from reality.

Finally, the word **insanity** is a legal term reserved for mental impairment that may relieve a person from the legal consequences of his or her actions. Tests for insanity are usually conducted by psychiatrists who try to determine whether or not the individual can distinguish right from wrong, or whether his or her reason was overpowered by irresistible impulses when committing the criminal act.

Evolution of Community Mental Health

The way mental health and illness were viewed down through the ages dictated how people with mental disorders were treated. It is helpful for you, as a community mental health nurse, to understand how those views have changed and how that influences the field now. Here, we will examine the historical evolution of mental health services up to the present time.

MENTAL ILLNESS IN ANCIENT CIVILIZATIONS

The common term *lunacy* (from the Latin *luna,* moon) has its basis in the ancient belief that the moon has the power to drive people insane; people were once supposed to have become insane by being exposed to the full moon (see Research: Bridge to Practice). Many ancient civilizations be-

RESEARCH Bridge to Practice

Barr, W. (2000). Lunacy revisited: The influence of the moon on mental health and quality of life. *Journal of Psychosocial Nursing and Mental Health Services, 38*(5), 28–35.

The idea that the stars and planets may influence human health and behavior can be traced to at least Roman times, and research suggests a high proportion of health professionals continue to hold this belief. Nevertheless, evidence for the supposed influence of the moon on human behavior has proved particularly elusive, and research has tended to suffer from weaknesses in methodology and data analysis.

This article reports findings drawn from a re-analysis of data from a research study into the functioning of a sample of mentally ill people living in the community. The mental health and quality of life of a sample of 100 people were assessed on four occasions during a 30-month period. Data were aggregated to represent the span of 1 lunar month, with scores being allocated to the relevant week of the lunar cycle during which each assessment was made. Comparison of mean values across the weeks of the lunar cycle was performed using the ANOVA. Results showed significant change at the time of the full moon only in subjects with a diagnosis of schizophrenia ($n = 56$), where deterioration was observed in three areas of psychopathology and one area of quality of life. Some implications for nursing practice are discussed, and it is suggested that future research into the possibility of a lunar effect on human life should focus on the direct measurement of functioning in people with schizophrenia.

lieved that mental illness was caused by possession, either by an evil spirit or a divine power. In some ancient societies, the mentally ill were believed to possess special powers of divination and healing and were supported and revered by the community.

In ancient Greece, Hippocrates (460–377 BC), called the Father of Medicine, was the first to attempt to explain diseases on the basis of natural causes (Bennett, 1978). He combined bedside observations with the speculations of the philosphers of medicine. He was the first to recognize the brain as man's most important organ, although he believed that if the brain were plagued by heat, cold, or excessive moisture, madness would ensue. Hippocratic physicians first classified mental illness and described the symptoms of melancholia, which we call depression, believing that such conditions were caused by an accumulation of black bile.

Mental illness was considered nonexistent in ancient Chinese culture. The Chinese family was traditionally very large and hierarchical in structure, and individuals had little chance to express themselves. The family system along with the teachings of Confucius interfered with an individualistic concept of life. Much later in the 20th century, the influence of Mao and Marxism redefined any sign of mental illness as reflections of guilt toward socialism and society. Thus, depression, mania, and neurosis were viewed as expressions of guilt rather than symptoms of mental illness.

Egyptian beliefs in ancient times were influenced both by Oriental mysticism and by African views of nature. In 525 BC Imhotep was named a god of medicine, and his temple at Memphis became a medical school and hospital. Here the Aesculapian priests developed a form of psychotherapy using incubation sleep. Patients were encouraged to occupy themselves with recreational activities such as painting, drawing, or concerts, which were believed to have therapeutic value. Egyptian medicine influenced Moses as well as Hippocrates. Egyptian physicians were as knowledgeable in their observations as they were magical in their explanations and esoteric in their teachings.

INFLUENCE OF THE CHURCH
THROUGH THE MIDDLE AGES

Medieval European society was dominated by the church. Thus, in a religious society, madness or any deviant behavior was viewed as demonic possession and the work of Satan (Rosen, 1968). Such beliefs existed before the 13th century and led to extensive witch hunts resulting in the Inquisition. Deviants, or witches, were believed to be heretical agents of Satan from whom people needed protection. The protector was the inquisitor. Furthermore, the Church regarded women, especially midwives, as evil so that women were persecuted as members of an inferior, sinful, and dangerous class of individuals. Physicians and priests were both involved in witch hunts, utilizing various methods to distinguish between those who were witches and those who were truly ill. Witches, like involuntary mental patients, were cast into a degraded and deviant role against their will, subjected to certain diagnos-

tic procedures, and finally deprived of their liberty or their lives, supposedly for their own benefit.

EMERGENCE OF THE SCIENTIFIC VIEW

Toward the end of the Middle Ages, a pattern of hospital care for the insane began to emerge. The famous English hospital of Saint Mary of Bethlehem, commonly called "Bedlam," was founded in 1450 as an institution for those who had "fallen out of their wit and their health." Nevertheless, the mentally ill were more likely to be housed in jails or poorhouses than hospitals. Almost 200 years would pass before a foundation was constructed for a scientific interpretation of insanity that would come to replace supernatural and religious interpretations.

In the mid-17th century, the work of natural scientists, such as Sir Francis Bacon and Sir Isaac Newton, placed science at the forefront of human achievement. The universe was thought to be a complex mechanism similar to a clock whose structure and function could be examined, categorized, and understood. This approach influenced investigations of the human body, and was buoyed by the English physician William Harvey's demonstration of the function of the heart and circulatory system. Also at this time, the French philosopher Descartes proclaimed the preeminence of rational thinking as proof of existence, and the physician Thomas Willis, who is considered the father of neuroanatomy, placed the brain at the center of human action and disease.

By the early 18th century, the English physicians Thomas Wright and Robert Burton stressed the psychological causes and cures of insanity. In the "age of reason," madness stood out as a dark challenge. During this century, physicians discovered that the insane were amenable to medical intervention. Modern psychiatry began in 1775 when the French physician Philippe Pinel, chief physician at an asylum for women in Toulouse, removed the chains from the inmates. In a famous essay published in 1809, he advocated humane treatment of the mentally ill and a more empirical study of mental disease. By recognizing categories of mental illness and promoting symptom identification, Pinel revolutionized psychiatric medicine (Kiple, 1995).

ADVANCES IN THE NINETEENTH CENTURY

In the first half of the 19th century, the treatment of mental illness was marked by asylum-building (Grob, 1991). Originally, asylums were designed as centers for "moral treatment" of the mentally ill—places where troublesome persons would be subjected to occupational therapy and moral persuasion. Chains were replaced by admonitions, physical tasks, and distractions; however, treatment was still coercive and primitive (Gamwell & Tomes, 1973).

As the 19th century progressed, medical professionals turned increased attention on mental illness and the brain, some claiming care of the mentally ill as their special domain. With the formal development of the human sciences within and across disciplines, significant attention was devoted to the study of the human brain and human behavior.

Not only physicians but also nurses, social reformers, and spiritual leaders became increasingly interested in humane treatment of the mentally ill. Dorothea Lynde Dix worked ceaselessly for humane treatment, health care, and social services for the mentally ill, and by the close of the century many of her reforms had been implemented in the U.S. and Europe.

THE TWENTIETH CENTURY AND THE IMPACT OF MANAGED CARE

During the early decades of the 20th century, the modern profession of psychiatry was born. Medical schools began to offer instruction in the medical treatment of insanity, and the Freudian model of psychoanalysis became increasingly popular. Psychiatric hospitals and long-term care facilities were constructed, and individuals with severe disorders were increasingly institutionalized, removed from their families and communities. Although institutionalization was intended to produce humane and effective treatment and care of the mentally ill, in reality conditions were often inhumane. Overcrowding, overmedicating, sporadic or inexpert care, physical restraint, and even beatings were reported in many institutions. Additionally, once admitted, most patients remained in the institution for the rest of their lives, in part because the inadequate and even callous care did not effect an improvement in their conditions, and in part because the community had no resources for assisting recovery from mental illness.

Around the 1950s the reform movement began. The quality and efficacy of institutional care came under attack, and new policies were implemented that sought to provide more humane treatment for the mentally ill (Grob, 1994). It was thought that people with mental disorders would fare better if living in the community. Community mental health centers were built to provide community-based services. With a large number of patients moving into community settings, the need for state-owned mental institutions declined, and many were closed. The process of transferring the mentally ill from public institutions to community-based care settings was called **deinstitutionalization**. During the Reagan Administration the effects of deinstitutionalization were felt. Many mentally ill individuals who formerly would have been institutionalized in a secure and ordered residential setting were left to wander the streets, unable to sustain employment or function adequately in a stressful and confusing world. Their feelings of abandonment, loneliness, and fear only exacerbated their mental disability. Stigmatization further jeopardized the health of this population. Misperceptions and fears of the general public caused the mentally ill to become even more socially isolated and cut off from needed support. In response to criticisms that the community mental health centers were not meeting the needs of the deinstitutionalized chronically ill client, community support programs were created. Funded by the federal government, community support programs offered an array of services, including vocational training, crisis services, transportation, housing, and employment.

In the late 20th century, the advent of managed care again altered treatment approaches for mental illness. Initially, managed care was heralded as a solution to spiraling health care costs, but disadvantages have also become evident. In order to control costs, most managed care plans severely restrict treatment for mental illness. These restrictions include limitations on the length of treatment and the choices of medications that can be prescribed. In addition, certain hospitals or clinics that are the sole designated providers of mental health care may be geographically inaccessible to the populations most in need of services. Finally, more funding is often allocated for in-patient care than for out-patient care, a policy that promotes crisis care as the preferred vehicle of treatment.

Community Mental Health Today

As is evident from this historical view, we have come a long way in our understanding of mental illness and mental health, yet many challenges remain. The treatment of mental illness today still remains controversial. Whereas some see mental illness as primarily a physiological disorder and advocate pharmacologic therapy, others see it as a crisis of meaning, development, or cognition that requires primarily "talk therapy" with a skilled psychotherapist. Others view mental illness as a spiritual crisis requiring spiritual guidance, meditation, prayer, and a supportive community. All of these views have been prominent in different societies at different historical periods, and all still have some validity today.

Traditionally mental health services have focused primarily on treatment of the mentally ill. However, in an era of greater enlightenment, the significance of prevention and health promotion are influencing community mental health to start expanding its range of services. Today, **community mental health** is a field of practice that seeks to address the needs of the mentally ill, prevent mental illness, and promote the mental health of the community. With a new national commitment for mental health, with advances in research, and with improved treatment modalities, it would seem that the future for promotion of mental health and treatment of mental disorders looks promising.

THE OBSTACLE OF STIGMA

However, the Surgeon General's Report emphasizes that "a formidable obstacle to future progress" remains and "that obstacle is stigma" (SAMHSA, 1999, p. 5). **Stigma** is an unjustified mark of shame and discredit attached to mental illness. It is the result of myths and misunderstandings that have been perpetuated down through the ages as illnesses of the mind remained a mystery and a threat. Stigma toward mental illness is largely attributable to ignorance and misconceptions. Until recently society has lacked knowledge about the mind, how it works, why mental illness occurs, and how to successfully recover from it. In addition, most people have experienced some form of mental health problem that

THE GLOBAL COMMUNITY

The "Burden of Disease"

With rapid changes in disease patterns, both in the U.S. and worldwide, new ways of measuring the health status of populations are needed. Noncommunicable diseases, such as depression and heart disease, are beginning to pose a greater threat than the traditional infectious diseases of the past. This is particularly true in developing countries, where infectious diseases and malnutrition have previously been the leading causes of disability and premature death. Furthermore, the World Health Organization projects that by 2020, injuries, both intentional and unintentional, may pose as great a threat to ill health worldwide as infectious diseases (WHO, 1999). No longer is it enough to simply quantify the number of deaths caused by a disease; instead, we need to be able to measure how populations are affected by premature death and disability.

Various measures have been developed in different countries to measure the health status of populations. Some are variants of the Quality-Adjusted Life Year (QALY), which measures the usefulness of interventions. However, the **Disability-Adjusted Life Year (DALY)** was developed to measure the impact of premature death and disability on populations (SAMHSA, 1999).

DALYs were initially developed and assessed in 1993 by the World Bank collaborating with the World Health Organization and Harvard University (Murray & Lopez, 1996). For any given population studied, DALYs measure how many years of life are lost to premature death and how many years are lived with a disability, adjusted for the severity of the disability. In other words, each DALY equals a year of healthy life lost, whether to premature death or to disability. The researchers defined "premature death" as death occurring before that person's expected survival age if that person were part of a standardized model population whose life expectancy at birth equalled the world's longest living population, which is Japan. DALYs measure the **burden of disease;** which refers to "the gap between a population's health status and some reference status" (WHO, 1999, p. 15).

An estimate of global disease burden for 1998 showed that nearly 43% of all DALYs were due to noncommunicable diseases, 39% in low- and middle- income countries and 81% in high income countries. Of these noncommunicable diseases, neuropsychiatric conditions, particularly depression, made up 10% of the disease burden for low- and middle-income countries and 23% of the disease burden in high-income countries (WHO, 1999).

This improved method of measuring the burden of disease with DALYs has brought new information to light and underscores the magnitude of the burden that mental illness poses. Previous measures focusing on mortality underestimated the impact of mental disorders, but with DALYs measuring time lived with disability the disease burden of mental illness becomes visible and significant. Furthermore, the burden of disease from depression is estimated to be increasing worldwide, both in developed and developing countries (WHO, 1999).

is similar to the symptoms of mental illness and assume one can get over it. They greatly underestimate the difficulty of dealing with a painful, disabling SMI. Stigma is also attributable to fear—fear that is spawned by ignorance. People fear what they do not understand, and they do not understand the aberrant, sometimes socially deviant, even hostile or violent behavior exhibited with some mental disorders (Angermeyer & Matschinger, 1996). Consequently, it is easy to label such behavior as shameful and to shun and discredit those who are the victims. Persistence of this stigma and fear is a destructive force that prevents this population from receiving the health services it needs.

Fortunately, as discussed earlier, the tide is turning. The purpose of the Surgeon General's Report is, in part, to dispel the myths and stigma surrounding mental illness. The White House Conference on Mental Health in 1999 promoted a national antistigma campaign, and mental health has become a higher priority nationally as evidenced in *Healthy People 2010*. Finally, the Global Burden of Disease study (WHO, 1999) has shown that mental illness is surprisingly significant in its contribution to the world's burden of disease (see The Global Community). As these efforts spawn new information, expanded research, and more effective policies and programs, there will be increasing opportunities, particularly for community mental health nurses, to educate the public and start eradicating the obstacle of stigma (Jones, 1998).

EPIDEMIOLOGY OF MENTAL DISORDERS

Epidemiologic information about mental illness, which describes its occurrence and distribution in the community, provides a road map that guides community mental health nursing practice. Such information helps you determine what, where, and for whom services are needed. However, in the past, to epidemiologically measure the incidence and prevalence of mental illness in the community was not easy. Mental illness has not been a reportable condition by law; thus, only those individuals housed in mental hospitals or asylums could be accurately counted. Yet an even larger number of persons, either receiving treatment through mental health centers and in private practice or untreated and living in the community, were unknown to public health policy makers and program planners. Then, in 1952 the American Psychiatric Association first published its *Diagnostic and Statistical Manual of Mental Disorders (DSM),* which listed and described 17 categories of mental disorders. The DSM has become a source of diagnostic information for clinical practice, research, and education, in addition to providing a language for communicating about mental illness with other service providers and policy makers. For epidemiologic purposes, the DSM made it possible to more consistently define mental disorders and estimate their occurrence in the community. A later version of this manual, DSM-IV, reviews 17 categories of mental disorders (American Psychiatric Association, 1994):

- substance-use disorders
- delirium
- dementia and other cognitive disorders
- psychotic disorders
- medication-induced movement disorders
- sleep disorders
- mood disorders
- late luteal phase dysphoric disorders
- anxiety disorders
- personality disorders
- psychiatric system interface disorders
- sexual disorders
- learning disorders
- pervasive developmental disorders
- conduct disorders
- multiaxial system
- family/relational problems and cultural issues

Incidence and Prevalence of Mental Disorders

Every year, one out of five Americans, or more than 51 million, experience a diagnosable mental disorder. Of this group, more than 6.5 million, including 4 million children and adolescents, are disabled by an SMI (SAMHSA, 1999). More than 19 million Americans over the age of 18 will suffer from a depressive illness at some time during their lives, and many of these individuals will be incapacitated for significant lengths of time by their illness. Over two-thirds of suicides in the U.S. each year are caused by major depression, which is also the leading cause of disability. More than 2.3 million Americans 18 or older, about 1% of the population, suffer from bipolar disorder; typically, as many as 20% of those suffering from this disorder commit suicide. Indeed, almost all people who kill themselves have a diagnosable mental disorder.

Studies focusing on prevalence of mental illness are limited and sometimes inconclusive; however, the poor, the poorly educated, and the unemployed typically experience higher rates of mental illness than the general population. A large portion of the mentally ill population, many of whom are the homeless, remains untreated in the community.

Age influences the patterns of mental illness in the community. Each year about one out of five children and adolescents has the signs and symptoms of a DSM-IV disorder. The most commonly occurring conditions among U.S. children ages 9 to 17 years are anxiety disorders, disruptive disorders, mood disorders, and substance use disorders. Attention-deficit/hyperactivity disorder (ADHD) occurs in 3% to 5% of U.S. school-aged children, with boys four times more likely to have it than girls. Autism, a developmental disorder, has a prevalence among children of 10 to 12 per 10,000 population (Bryson & Smith, 1998). For American adults the most preva-

lent mental disorders are anxiety disorders, followed by mood disorders, especially major depression and bipolar disorder. Anxiety, depression, and schizophrenia present special problems for this age group—anxiety and depression because they contribute to such high rates of suicide and schizophrenia because it is so persistently disabling. For the growing number of older adults there is increased incidence of Alzheimer's disease, major depression, substance abuse, anxiety, and other disabling mental disorders (SAMHSA, 1999). Particular problems arise with dementia, which causes significant dependency and costly long-term care; with depression, which contributes to high suicide rates among males in this group; and with the disabling effects of schizophrenia.

Gender differences also arise in the prevalence of certain mental disorders. Anxiety disorders and mood disorders, including major depression, occur twice as frequently in women as in men. Women of color, women on welfare, poor women, and uneducated women are more likely to experience depression than women in the general population. Eating disorders also affect more women than men. Three percent of young women have one of the three major eating disorders, either anorexia nervosa, bulimia nervosa or binge-eating disorder (Becker, 1999). Women attempt suicide more frequently than men, but completed suicides are more common in men.

Adding to the heavy toll that mental illness takes on our country is the financial burden it creates. Costs associated with treatment of mental disorders, poor productivity, lost work time, and disability payments are astronomical. The direct and indirect costs of mental illness and addictive disorders in the U.S. are over $273 billion annually. Furthermore, the cost to society when treatment is *not* provided for these illnesses is three times the cost of direct treatment (Office of Women's Health, 2000). Certainly this has policy implications and suggests the need for greater preventive and mental health promoting efforts.

Risk Factors Influencing the Mentally Ill Population

As a community health nurse concerned about the mentally ill, you have examined some of the epidemiologic information about this population. What are some of the causative factors contributing to the at-risk status of the mentally ill? Using a vulnerability model, it is helpful to consider four categories of factors that influence their at-risk status: biological, behavioral, sociocultural, and environmental factors.

BIOLOGICAL FACTORS

Certain biological factors can place people at increased risk for mental illness. Neurobiological and genetic mechanisms play a significant role, usually in combination with other factors. An example is autism, which is due to structural brain abnormalities and genetic predisposition (Bryson & Smith, 1998). Although no single gene has been found to cause a specific mental disorder, variations in multiple genes can disrupt healthy brain function and, under certain environmental conditions, lead to mental illness. Age is another factor since many mental illnesses appear to have their origins in early childhood, or even in the way the brain develops prenatally, but lie dormant until adulthood.

Biological risk factors for children for developing a mental disorder include:

- prenatal damage from exposure to alcohol, illegal drugs, and tobacco
- low birth weight
- inherited predisposition to mental disorder
- physical problems (such as abnormalities of the central nervous system affecting behavior, thinking or feeling, caused by infection, injury, poor nutrition or environmental toxins)
- intellectual disabilities such as retardation (SAMHSA, 1999)

Some individuals may acquire mental impairment from traumatic brain injuries or illnesses that cause tissue damage or anoxia. Birth defects and injuries sustained at birth may also contribute to risk.

BEHAVIORAL FACTORS

Behavioral factors also influence the vulnerability of this population. Psychological stress connected with employment, financial worries, family problems, death of a loved one, and other life events can contribute to mental illness when individuals affected have not developed healthy coping patterns. Neglect and abuse during childhood place individuals at greater risk for various mental disorders, and dysfunctional family life can predispose to conduct disorders and antisocial personality disorders. Low self-esteem also seems to accompany poor mental functioning. Alcohol and drug abuse can lead to chemical dependence, physiologic damage, and mental impairment; also, a family history of mental and addictive disorders is a risk factor for children (SAMHSA, 1999).

SOCIOCULTURAL FACTORS

Economic hardship affects the mental health of many individuals. Anxiety over such things as inadequate income and housing, increasing debt, or unemployment can create emotional stress with which some people cannot cope. Multigenerational poverty continues to place individuals at greater risk for mental disorders.

Data on racial and ethnic distribution among the mentally ill are limited and inconclusive. A higher proportion of minorities appear among the impoverished mentally ill in the community. However, mental health problems and mental disorders exist in families of all social classes and cultural backgrounds; no one is immune.

Inadequate mental health services in the community, lack of adequate community support systems, and little emphasis on prevention are major sociocultural factors increasing vulnerability to mental illness. Overall, research is demonstrating that most mental disorders are caused by some combination of genetic, biological, and/or psychosocial influences (SAMHSA, 1999).

ENVIRONMENTAL FACTORS

Geographic environmental factors play a lesser role in affecting vulnerability to mental illness. Nonetheless, climate and geography can cause severe stresses with the threats of frequent hurricanes, tornadoes, floods, or earthquakes. Some individuals are affected by absence of natural sunlight during long, grey winters. They experience a type of depression called *seasonal affective disorder* (SAD), which is far more common in northern regions. Additionally, many of the conditions in urban areas are anxiety-producing; these include transportation problems, excessive noise, crowded streets, inadequate sanitation, high crime rates, and impersonal services.

Lead poisoning continues to be a serious public health problem contributing to mental impairment. Children are especially vulnerable to lead poisoning, whose sources include peeling paint in older homes and workplaces, exhaust fumes, drinking water channeled through lead pipes, the glaze on ceramic mugs or bowls that have not been properly fired, and crystal glassware whose lead has leaked after repeated dishwasher use. Figure 34–1 summarizes factors influencing vulnerability to mental illness.

INTERVENTIONS FOR COMMUNITY MENTAL HEALTH

Epidemiologic data and information about risk factors help to guide the community mental health nurse in planning for community mental health services. Such services, to be truly comprehensive, should encompass the entire range of prevention levels—primary, secondary, and tertiary. The majority of community mental health services in the past have focused their efforts on addressing the needs of the mentally ill. Although this population must continue to be a priority, it is now becoming clear that community mental health efforts must also focus to a much greater degree on preventing mental illness and promoting mental health. These latter two emphases hold the key to a healthier future for the nation and the world.

In this section we first review the *Healthy People 2010* national objectives for mental health, which suggest certain service priorities. Then we focus on services to the mentally ill population, their needs, and various treatment approaches and community resources that help in addressing those needs. Next we examine ways to prevent mental illness in the community, and finally we explore the important topic of promoting mental health in the community. Nurses play an important role throughout all these aspects of intervention for community mental health.

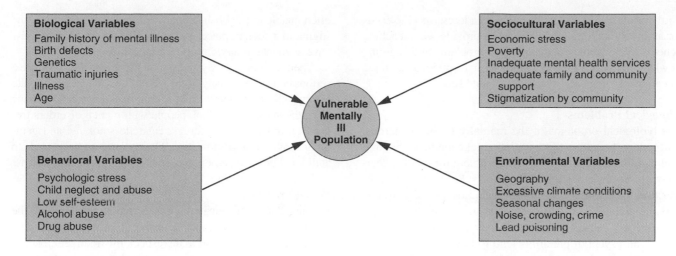

FIGURE 34–1. Factors that influence the vulnerability of the mentally ill population.

Healthy People 2010 Objectives for Mental Health

For the focus area of mental health and mental disorders, *Healthy People 2010* states the goal: "Improve mental health and ensure access to appropriate, quality mental health services" (USDHHS, 2000). Fourteen objectives were developed to accomplish this goal to be completed by the year 2010. They are:

MENTAL HEALTH STATUS IMPROVEMENT

1. Reduce the suicide rate.
2. Reduce the rate of suicide attempts by adolescents.
3. Reduce the proportion of homeless adults who have serious mental illness.
4. Increase the proportion of persons with serious mental illnesses who are employed.
5. Reduce the relapse rates for persons with eating disorders, including anorexia nervosa and bulimia nervosa.
6. Increase the number of persons seen in primary health care who receive mental health screening and assessment.
7. Increase the proportion of children with mental health problems who receive treatment.
8. Increase the proportion of juvenile justice facilities that screen new admissions for mental health problems.
9. Increase the proportion of adults with mental disorders who receive treatment.
10. Increase the proportion of persons with co-occurring substance abuse and mental disorders who receive treatment for both disorders.
11. Increase the proportion of local governments with community-based jail diversion programs for adults with serious mental illnesses.

STATE ACTIVITIES

12. Increase the number of States and the District of Columbia that track consumers' satisfaction with the mental health services they receive
13. Increase the number of States, Territories, and the District of Columbia with an operational mental health plan that addresses cultural competence.
14. Increase the number of States, Territories, and the District of Columbia with an operational mental health plan that addresses mental health crisis interventions, ongoing screening, and treatment services for elderly persons.

Clearly these objectives emphasize the reduction and prevention of suicide, better access to and utilization of services, early detection of mental illness, and improved functioning for persons with mental disorders in the community. All levels of prevention—primary, seconday and tertiary—are included.

Serving the Mentally Ill Population

In order to design appropriate services for the mentally ill population, it is important for you to build on your knowledge of epidemiologic data, risk factors, and other information, then work in concert with other health team members for planning and implementing services. To begin with, it is important to know the needs of people with mental disorders.

NEEDS OF THE MENTALLY ILL

As you assess the needs of this population, you will find they have various health-related problems. The nature of these problems, as well as the degree to which they are preventable, varies with the type and severity of the mental disorder, whether or not the affected individuals are receiving and complying with needed treatment, and the degree of independence with which they can function in the community. Although the mentally ill population is disparate in terms of its wide range of diagnoses and conditions, there are nonetheless many problems shared by members of this group.

Furthermore, interventions designed to address specific needs for an individual or a group can often provide wide-reaching benefits to the whole population. The problems of this group, as with other vulnerable populations, can be divided into three categories: biological, psychological, and social.

Biological Problems

The biological problems of the mentally ill are numerous. Since many people in this population take medications for a prolonged period of time, a major problem for them is dealing with serious medication side effects. Prolonged tranquilizer use, for example, can cause tardive dyskinesia, an irreversible condition in which damage to the cerebral cortex from the drug leads to tremors and loss of motor control. Clients on psychotropic drugs tend to have increased problems with constipation and regular elimination. They frequently have sleep disturbances that lead to sleep deprivation and make them vulnerable to other physical health problems. Poor compliance in taking prescribed medications is an additional problem for this population. Many forget to take their medications or do not value their importance; others lose track in moving from one group home or living situation to the next. Psychotropic medications can affect clients' vision, making it difficult to read or even decipher medication label instructions. Generally, the medications are needed to enable mentally ill individuals to function and live independently. When treatment protocols are not followed consistently, many are at risk for exacerbation of symptoms and even violent behavior (Swartz, Swanson, & Burns, 1998).

Poor nutrition is another serious concern with the mentally ill population, particularly those living on their own. Eating disorders and poor eating habits are prevalent in this group. Because of their impaired function and/or limited finances, many are unable to shop, prepare food for themselves, or make appropriate food choices. A high-fat, high-carbohydrate, "junk food" diet leads to obesity for many in this population, as well as promoting greater risk for coronary artery disease, diabetes, and dental problems. The mentally ill are also vulnerable to liver disease, heart disease, and cancer because of their high dependency—particularly among males—on alcohol, drugs, and cigarette smoking.

As a population, the mentally ill are vulnerable to a number of communicable diseases, including sexually transmitted diseases, HIV/AIDs, and tuberculosis. Varying with the extent of mental dysfunction, they also face problems associated with limited motor coordination and self-care ability, including personal hygiene, particularly for those with SMIs.

Psychological Problems

The psychological problems of the mentally ill vary depending on the type and severity of their disorder. The stresses of coping with daily living, compounded by the complexities of city life for most, create such responses as confusion, depression, frustration, and anger. Psychological isolation, loneliness, and poor self-esteem are interrelated problems for most people with mental disorders. People with these conditions are often unable to establish supportive relationships and feel the stigma that society places on mental illness. In addition, few have adequate, if any, family or friendship supports.

Chemical dependency and/or other forms of addiction are a serious concern for many of the mentally ill. Lacking adequate coping skills to deal with daily life and seeking relief or escape from the stresses they feel, people with mental disorders frequently turn to alcohol, drugs, cigarette smoking, and gambling, singly or in combination. Dependence on these leads to additional physical, emotional, social, and financial problems.

Social Problems

Stigma, discussed earlier, poses a major problem for the mentally ill. Fear and misunderstanding of mental disorders by the larger society lead to disrespect, mistreatment, lack of acceptance, and social isolation, which in turn reduce this population's already limited resources. Without needed support from family, friends, and community, the mentally ill are further handicapped and even more vulnerable.

System inadequacies cause another set of problems for the mentally ill. Income for these individuals is limited, and finding and sustaining employment is difficult given their disabilities. If they have worked, they are eligible in the U.S. for Social Security Disability income; if they have never worked, they can receive supplemental income under the Social Security Act. However, in both cases this allows only a subsistence level of living. Many have unstable housing, which creates mobility with additional problems. A further problem is limited finances for treatment or health care benefits. The Mental Health Parity Act of 1996 limits mental health coverage as compared with non-mental health conditions. It has resulted in increased numbers of the poor going without their prescribed psychotropic medications and psychotherapy because they do not have the means to pay for them. It has also resulted in several high-visibility crimes committed by individuals with SPMI who were without treatment at the time of the crime. Services for the mentally ill are often fragmented and inadequate; improved services and collaboration between providers who serve this population are needed. A summary of these problems is listed in Table 34–1.

SERVICE INTERVENTIONS FOR THE MENTALLY ILL POPULATION

The needs of the mentally ill are addressed primarily through either biomedical or psychotherapeutic approaches. Often a combination of both is found to be effective.

Biomedical Approaches

Biomedical therapy for persons with mental disorders involves the use of medications or electroshock therapy.

Pharmacotherapy. Historically, the treatment of the mentally ill consisted of isolation, restraint, ice packs, insulin shock therapy, electroconvulsive therapy, brain surgery, and minimal drug use. The most common drugs in use were paraldehyde, chloral hydrate, and barbiturates. In the early 1950s the first tranquilizer, thorazine, was prescribed, ushering in a

TABLE 34–1. Health-Related Problems of the Mentally Ill

Physical Problems	Psychological Problems	Social Problems
Medication side effects	Depression	Low income
Loss of motor control	Confusion	Unemployment
Constipation	Anger/frustration	Physical isolation
Sleep disturbances	Lack of motivation for compliance with treatment	Unstable housing
Poor nutrition	Anxiety	System does not foster independence
Dental problems	Low self-esteem	Disjointed and inconsistent mental health services
Obesity	Unable to establish relationships	Stigma
Chronic diseases (coronary artery disease, diabetes, heart disease, liver disease, cancer)	Feelings of stigmatization	Parity problems
Limited self-care ability	Psychological isolation	
Communicable diseases (STDs, AIDS, Tbc)	Neuroses	
	Psychoses	
	Addictive behaviors	

new wave of pharmacologic treatment for mental illness. Psychotropic medications not only have resulted in relief of symptoms but also have significantly improved the quality of life for millions of clients worldwide. Many clients previously held in long term psychiatric facilities are now treated in community mental health centers or group homes or access out-patient facilities from their homes. The successful addition of medications to the treatment regimen of mental illness has promoted the position that mental illness is often biologically based or responsive to biologic treatment.

Electroconvulsive Therapy. Electroconvulsive therapy (ECT), also called *shock therapy,* uses electrically induced seizures primarily to treat severe depression. It has been proved a safe and effective therapy and is often used for clients who have not responded to drug therapies, with the elderly, and with highly suicidal clients, where there is not time to wait for the onset of the effects of antidepressants (Haber et al., 1997).

Psychotherapy

Psychotherapy refers to the treatment of mental or emotional disorders through psychologically based interventions. These interventions may be used alone, in combination with pharmacotherapies, or with complementary therapies such as yoga, relaxation exercises, or visualization.

Common Psychotherapeutic Strategies. Psychotherapeutic strategies include the following:

- *Art therapy* is used as a means for expression through drawings, sculpture, or music. It is particularly effective with children or clients whose verbal skills are limited.
- *Behavior therapy* aims to reduce or eliminate certain behaviors through concentrated, specific guidelines. Smoking cessation and weight-loss groups are examples of behavior-modification approaches.
- *Client-centered therapy* focuses on enabling clients to identify and actualize their own internal resources to work through their concerns.

- *Cognitive behavioral therapy* focuses on clients' beliefs and actions and on reducing these beliefs and actions into more positive moods.
- *Insight-oriented therapy* assists clients to improve their functioning through insight into themselves and their situation.
- *Interpersonal therapy* focuses on clients' ability to gain insight into their psychological distress in relation to disturbed interpersonal relationships.
- *Group therapy* uses the interaction of several clients sharing an interest in a common issue, such as anxiety, panic, depression, or eating disorders. Therapy groups may also be used for survivors of sexual assault, sexual abuse, or domestic violence, as well as many other topics.

Psychotherapy, sometimes called "talk therapy," uses one or more of the strategies described above. It is offered in a variety of settings and is available either individually or in groups. Private psychotherapy services can be accessed through referral or word-of-mouth for clients who are financially able to pay. Managed care organizations often restrict the number of therapy visits, posing a challenge to both clients and therapists. Clients with limited funds may access individual and group therapies through mental health clinics or community agencies.

In addition to the above therapies, there are community resources that enhance primary treatment. They are discussed in the next section.

Community Mental Health Resources

A variety of resources exist in the community to promote mental health, prevent mental illness, and serve the needs of the mentally ill. They include sources for education, advocacy, treatment, support, referral, rehabilitation, financial assistance, case management, and more. Community mental health centers, halfway houses, support programs, mobile crisis teams, self-help groups, and private mental health services are discussed next.

COMMUNITY MENTAL HEALTH CENTERS

Community mental health centers (CMHC) provide comprehensive, publicly funded services to the mentally ill population. CHMCs provide 10 required services (Price-Hoskins, 1997):

- services for children and the elderly
- consultation and education services
- alcoholism and drug abuse services
- outpatient care
- inpatient care
- emergency care
- partial hospitalization
- screening before admission to state hospitals
- transitional housing
- follow-up care for discharged clients

Some of the services of CHMCs are 24-hour, whereas others are day programs. They are staffed by a multidisciplinary team who provide the on-site services listed above. The community mental health nurse is an important member of this team. CHMCs were initially funded by the federal government but now are supported through state and local funds.

HALFWAY HOUSES

A **halfway house** is a residential program for individuals with SPMI that, in addition to housing, offers supervision, treatment, safety, socialization, recreation, and support. One of the difficulties many clients with mental illness experience is an inability to form attachments or have meaningful interactions with others. Halfway houses offer an opportunity to work within a framework of social support. The benefits include:

- learning from the experiences of others
- observing social interventions
- feeling a sense of belonging
- drawing on the strengths of others
- learning new strategies for problem-solving

Halfway houses provide the seriously mentally ill with the opportunity to function in a setting with their peers. Although they often cause some initial concern in neighborhoods in which they are located, problems anticipated by the neighboring residents are rarely seen. They may be part of a CHMC or located elsewhere in the community.

COMMUNITY SUPPORT PROGRAMS

Community support programs are a publicly funded set of services designed to assist persons with SPMIs. These services include crisis intervention; mental health treatment integrated with medical care; psychosocial rehabilitation; support services for living, work and family; case management; assistance with applications and referrals; advocacy; and protection of rights (Price-Hoskins, 1997).

Community support programs may be found within a CHMC or housed separately; they are supported by state and local funds wherever the funds are available.

MOBILE CRISIS TEAMS

A mobile crisis team is a group of multidisciplinary clinicians who travel to the scene of a crisis or critical event. They provide on-site evaluation of both the individual(s) involved in the crisis and the circumstances surrounding the incident. Although the immediate goal of this method of intervention is crisis management, education and facilitation of community support are also important objectives.

SELF-HELP GROUPS

A self-help group is a group of individuals who meet regularly with or without a professional leader or consultant to work on personal problems and issues. Leadership is frequently facilitated by the members, who rotate responsibilities. The goals of self-help groups usually include:

- instillation of hope—that solutions to the problem are possible
- imparting of information—that resources for help are available
- increasing feelings of universality—that the individual is not alone with the problem
- increasing feelings of altruism—that others can be trusted to care

Alcoholics Anonymous (AA) is a classic example of a self-help group that works (see Chapter 35). Codependents Anonymous (CODA) is a self-help group for individuals struggling with issues of self-esteem and dysfunctional families. It assists individuals who grew up in homes where either violence, substance abuse, neglect, or child abuse occurred and compromised the individuals' abilities to relate to others.

PRIVATE MENTAL HEALTH SERVICES

Many different independent mental health treatment options are available in the community. Examples include individual, group, or family therapy with a psychiatrist, a psychologist, a nurse with advanced training in mental health, or a psychiatric social worker. Payment for these services may come from clients themselves, from managed care or other insurance, or through community assistance funds.

Preventing Mental Disorders

With the burden of disease imposed by mental disorders, both nationally and worldwide, there is a growing urgency felt in the field of public health to put more effort into prevention. This is evident in the Surgeon General's Report on Mental Health (SAMHSA, 1999), which seeks to promote greater understanding of mental health and mental illness. The World Health Report, underscoring the increasing threat of mental disorders, calls them a "rising burden" (WHO, 1999) and points out the need for research and policy changes.

We currently have much more scientific information on the treatment of mental illness than we do on how to prevent it. To enhance preventive intervention efforts, we need more clarity on the causes of mental illness, whom to target, and more accurate measures for evaluating program effectiveness. Yet there is still much that can be done.

MODELS FOR PREVENTING MENTAL DISORDERS

Some models have proved useful in approaching the prevention of mental disorders. We examine two here: the Public Health Model and the Mental Health Intervention Spectrum Model.

The Public Health Model

Early efforts to prevent illness used the public health model of prevention, originally designed to control infectious diseases. This model includes three levels of prevention: primary prevention keeps a health problem from occurring; secondary prevention seeks to detect a health problem at its earliest stage and keep it from getting worse; and tertiary prevention aims to reduce the disability associated with the health problem. Applying the public health model to the mentally ill population, Gerald Caplan (1964), in his classic work using this model, proposed population interventions at three prevention levels.

- *Primary prevention* activities with a population would decrease the number of new cases (incidence) of a mental disorder or reduce the rate of their development.
- *Secondary prevention* activities would lower the number of existing cases of a mental disorder, thereby reducing its rate (prevalence). Examples of secondary prevention activities would be screening, early case finding, and early treatment.
- *Tertiary prevention* activities would decrease the severity of a mental disorder and its associated disabilities through rehabilitation. An example would be a program of intensive case management and social skills training for schiziphrenics.

Mental health prevention efforts in the U.S. have used this model for many years in addressing the range of prevention levels. However, its application, in terms of funding and support, has been strongest in the area of secondary prevention.

The Mental Health Intervention Spectrum Model

In recent years, research has enhanced our understanding of risk factors and their association with health outcomes in relation to mental disorders. As a result, in 1994 the Institute of Medicine's Committee on Prevention of Mental Disorders developed a comprehensive model called the Mental Health Intervention Spectrum Model (MHISM) (Institute of Medicine, 1994).

The MHISM model presents a range of interventions for mental illness that includes prevention, treatment, and maintenance. The prevention aspects of the model are most relevant to our discussion here.

The prevention section of the MHISM model lists three types of interventions: universal, selective, and indicated. *Universal* preventive interventions target a whole population group or the general public who are not identified as being at risk for a specific mental disorder. This approach is useful for planning large-scale preventive interventions, such as a comprehensive program of prenatal services that could promote healthy brain development with a subsequent reduction in the incidence of schizophrenia.

The second type, *selective* preventive interventions, targets selected at-risk groups or individuals within a population. These are individuals or groups who have been identified as having a much higher risk of developing a mental disorder. An example of a selective preventive intervention is a support group and bereavement counseling for elderly persons who have lost a spouse to prevent the onset of or lessen the degree of depression.

The third type, *indicated* preventive intervention, targets high-risk individuals who show signs of a beginning mental disorder or who have other evidence of a predisposition for a mental disorder. An example is parenting training and support for young mothers who were abused as children, especially if they show early signs of repeating that abuse with their own children.

Both the Public Health Model and the MHISM provide useful perspectives for designing preventive interventions and continue to be used today.

PREVENTIVE INTERVENTIONS

Prevention is a fundamental role of the community health nurse working with mentally ill clients or with communities attempting to respond to the problems of mental disorders. Here we discuss primary, secondary, and tertiary prevention activities.

Primary Prevention Activities

With primary prevention the goal is to both anticipate potential threats and prevent the actual development of a mental disorder. Combining the public health model with "universal" preventive intervention from the MHISM, you can design an intervention for a population or group using the following steps:

- *Select a mental disorder*—one that epidemiologic data have shown to be a significant problem for intervention, e.g., adolescent alcoholism.
- *Identify the target population for intervention,* e.g., all adolescents in a given community.
- *Determine causes and risk factors that contribute to the disorder.* From research data in the literature, identify factors that appear to contribute to teenagers wanting to use and abuse alcohol.
- *Design, implement, and evaluate an intervention.* Conduct an educational program in the schools that addresses peer pressure, signs of early addiction, dangers of alcoholism, being "cool" in other ways, etc.

Other examples of primary prevention include support groups for children of divorced parents and spouses considering divorce, safe-housing projects, programs to prevent substance abuse, suicide prevention programs, and parenting classes. Informing parents of developmental milestones, age-related behaviors, and stress-reducing strategies can significantly reduce the risk of abuse. Other opportunities for primary prevention include supportive care for teenage mothers, well-baby classes, and stress-management classes.

Secondary Prevention Activities

Secondary prevention efforts attempt to reduce the prevalence of mental disorders in the community or the severity of disorders in affected individuals. Health screening for mental illness is an important secondary prevention strategy to detect illness in its earliest stages. National Anxiety Screening Day, National Depression Screening Day, and similar programs are community-based examples and should be promoted in local media, clinics, libraries, schools, churches, welfare offices, and even on bulletin boards in supermarkets.

Also, the community health nurse provides secondary prevention through monitoring medications. It is essential that the nurse be familiar with medications that clients are taking, with particular attention to drug interactions and contraindications. This is particularly true for elderly clients who may be taking medications for physical conditions as well. The nurse may be the primary person to identify breakthrough symptoms, noncompliance, or failure of clients or family members to fill prescriptions. As we will discuss later, the nurse's advocacy role can enable the client or family to negotiate systems that may be interfering with medication compliance.

Secondary prevention efforts also include case-finding and referral for primary or follow-up care. This means alertness and vigilance to find people in the community who show early signs of problems developing. Examples are developing a support program for family caregivers of Alzheimer's patients and an educational and support program for parents of autistic children. The facilitation of a self-help group, depending on its precise nature and goals, can also be an effective secondary prevention measure.

Tertiary Prevention Activities

The goal with tertiary preventive intervention is to decrease the amount of disability associated with mental disorders. You can design a tertiary preventive program for a population or group, combining the Public Health Model and the MHISD described earlier. First, select a significant mental disorder, such as attention-deficit/hyperactivity disorder (ADHD), which occurs in 3% to 5% of school-aged children. Second, identify the target population for intervention; with the above example, it would be schoolchildren with diagnosed ADHD or with symptoms that suggest the onset of this disorder. Third, identify the causes and risk factors that contribute to ADHD; it is known that boys are four times more likely to have ADHD than girls, that it is found in all cultures,

that it runs in families so that inheritance appears to play a part, and that multimodal therapies (combination of psychosocial and pharmacologic) are most effective with ADHD (SAMHSA, 1999). Finally, design, implement, and evaluate an intervention, such as a combined individual and group therapy program for these children.

Psychiatric rehabilitiation, in which the intervention goal is to promote clients' functioning and independence, is another means of accomplishing tertiary prevention. An example is a rehabilitation program for depressed clients who have attempted suicide. Tertiary preventive activities seek not only to reduce symptoms and the overall disabling effects of the disorder but also to improve clients' quality of life. These interventions include activities such as focusing on clients' strengths, increasing their coping skills, helping them develop better support systems, providing skill coaching for new settings, and encouraging self-determination (Hauenstein, 1998).

Resocialization programs for people with SMIs are another form of tertiary prevention. These include sheltered workshops, development of life skills, and recreational programs with social events that work to enable clients to improve the quality of their lives and have more meaningful contact with society.

Finally, a tertiary preventive intervention of great significance is stigma eradication. Stigmatizing the mentally ill has resulted in lost opportunities for individuals to seek treatment, to improve, or to recover.

Discrimination and social isolation only exacerbate the problems of the mentally ill; reversing this process could reduce their disabilities and enhance the quality of their lives. Widespread public education and information programs about mental disorders help to erase the obstacle of stigma. The community mental health nurse may promote stigma eradication through involvement in educational programs for the public, by serving on committees and boards in the community, and by influencing community leaders, lawmakers, and health policy development.

MENTAL HEALTH PROMOTION

As the field of mental health has matured through advances in epidemiologic methods, research, and treatment, there has been an increasing interest in illness prevention and health promotion (SAMHSA, 1999). Treating and preventing mental illness are important and ongoing priorities in community mental health, but promoting mental health, which is essential to healthier people for the future, needs greater emphasis.

What Is Mental Health Promotion?

Mental health promotion refers to interventions that enhance well-being and strengthen life-sustaining and life-enhancing activities (Griffin-Francell, 1997). Well-being means a state of being happy, healthy, or prosperous, which is subjective but measurable, to a degree, when one examines people's life styles and behavior. Life-sustaining and life-enhancing activities include a wide range of life style behaviors that ultimately influence our state of well-being.

Another way to think about health promotion intervention is to review the definition of mental health. It is a successful performance of mental function that results in (1) productive activities, (2) fulfilling relationships, (3) the ability to adapt to change, and (4) the ability to cope with adversity. Targeting these areas becomes a way of prioritizing in planning for health-promoting interventions. In other words, it would be useful to design programs in community mental health that encourage productive activities such as sports or hobbies, fulfilling relationships such as foster grandparenting, adapting to change such as volunteering, and coping with adversity such as preparing developmental crises.

Interventions for Mental Health Promotion

Several different approaches can be used while designing interventions for mental health promotion. We will discuss two: to develop interventions to protect people potentially at risk for mental disorders, and to promote healthy activities and life styles in the public.

RISK-PROTECTIVE ACTIVITIES

Epidemiologic data, along with the results of a growing body of other kinds of research, provide the community mental health nurse with increasing information about the factors that place people at risk for mental disorders. Targeting these individuals with health promotion interventions gives them the resources needed to raise their own levels of health and protects them from mental disorders. We know, for example, that alcohol, illegal drugs, and tobacco taken during pregnancy can damage the fetus. Consquently, extensive prenatal education and support programs can promote parental health and reduce this risk for the next generation. We also know that abuse and neglect during childhood are risk factors for certain mental disorders. Promoting healthy parenting and stress-reducing activities through classes, group work, and other means can promote the health of parents and protect the health of their children.

LIFE STYLE AND BEHAVIOR ACTIVITIES

To promote the well-being of the public we can plan health promotion interventions that are both life-sustaining and life-enhancing. Life-sustaining activities include proper nutrition and exercise, healthy sleep patterns with adequate rest, healthy coping with stress, and the ability to use family and community supports and resources. Health promotion programs in the community may address any or all of these. An example is educating school children about the food pyramid and encouraging the provision of healthy snacks and well-balanced meals in the home. Other examples include fitness programs for all ages, promotion of community playgrounds and walking/biking trails, and establishing networks of support in the community such as Meals on Wheels and other volunteer programs.

Life-enhancing activities include meaningful work, whether through or outside of employment, creative outlets, interpersonal relationships, recreational activities, and opportunities for spiritual and intellectual growth. Again, mental health promotion interventions can address any or all of these areas. For example, arts and crafts classes and fairs encourage creative expression, community sports events promote social outlets, elder hostels and other kinds of learning experiences promote spiritual and intellectual stimulation, volunteer programs encourage community participation, and classes to develop new skills can promote meaningful vocation.

ROLE OF THE COMMUNITY MENTAL HEALTH NURSE

The nurse's role is multifaceted in community mental health; this has been evident throughout the chapter. First of all, the nurse must be able to *access and use epidemiologic data* in order to understand and serve the mentally ill population. This means identifying the incidence and prevalence of mental disorders, examining the causes and risk factors associated with mental illness, and identifying the needs of people with mental disorders. Nurses sometimes serve as part of the epidemiologic investigative team to conduct surveys and assist with data collection.

Next, an important part of the nurse's role with the mentally ill is *advocacy*. In this role the nurse seeks to increase client access to mental health services, to reduce stigma and promote improved public understanding of this population, and to work for improved services in community mental health (Christoffel, 2000). The advocacy role requires being politically involved by serving on decision-making boards and committees, lobbying for legislative changes, and helping to influence mental health policy development that will better serve this population. Membership in state and national nursing organizations can be helpful in establishing collaborative partnerships to benefit the mentally ill. Membership in the National Alliance of the Mentally Ill or other advocacy groups can also effect positive change. In any of these venues, the vision and expertise of the community mental health nurse can be used to advocate for the enhancement of existing services, the development of new services, and increased access for the mentally ill to all services.

Another aspect of the nurse's role is *education*. The community mental health nurse teaches clients individually and in groups about their mental health conditions, their treatment protocols, ways to function more independently in the community, prevention and health-promoting strategies, and much more. The nurse also teaches the public through community education programs and has an educational role with caregivers, family and community members, and health care decision makers by providing information for service planning.

Case management of persons with SMIs is also part of the community mental health nurse's role. This includes screening, assessment, care planning, arranging for service delivery, monitoring, reassessment, evaluation, and discharge. It is often offered within the context of a community mental health center. Case management helps the person with an SMI to access services and live as independently as possible.

The nurse's role also involves *case-finding and referral*. This means early identification of persons with mental disorders who are in need of treatment and then referring those persons to the appropriate resources for treatment. The purpose of this role is secondary prevention since early identification and treatment help to ameliorate the severity of the mental disorder and promote a speedier recovery.

Finally, the nurse's role includes *collaboration*. Whether serving individual clients, groups, or populations, the nurse is part of the larger community mental health team and works in collaboration with many people to accomplish the goals of community mental health. The composition of the team—made up of clients, psychiatric nurses, physicians, social workers, nutritionists, epidemiologists, psychologists, health planners, and many more—is diverse and varies depending on the community health nurse's work setting. Collaboration allows for a pooling of professional expertise that enhances the quality and effectiveness of services for the mentally ill.

When working with the mentally ill, the nurse must be aware of issues of personal safety. Although most mentally ill clients are no more prone to violence than the population at large, conditions involving paranoia, hallucinations, and mania can increase clients' tendency toward physical violence. Unfortunately, there are many cases in which social workers, physicians, or nurses have been harmed by psychotic clients.

Thus, nurses working with this population must use caution in any situation that suggests danger and take action immediately to protect themselves and their clients. This may require the nurse to take self-defense classes or assertiveness training or to carry protective gear. It may help to use an escort from a security service, collaborate with the police, or establish a "buddy system" in which two nurses work together in isolated or dangerous homes or areas. Additionally, the public health agency may consider hiring risk-management consultants to examine dangerous situations and recommend actions to preserve safety.

In conclusion, the nurse serving in community mental health plays many roles. These are practiced in a variety of settings in collaboration with other members of the community mental health team. It is the challenge of this role and the opportunity to assist in raising the level of mental health for individuals and communities that make this field of practice so rewarding.

SUMMARY

Although there have been significant improvements with some diseases, mental illness remains a serious, persistent, and even an increasing problem, both in the U.S. and globally. Mental health has become a growing priority nationally for research and services.

Community mental health has evolved through several phases of development. In early times the mentally ill were misunderstood and badly treated. This mistreatment persisted from ancient times, through the Middle Ages, and into the scientific era. Even with advances in treatment in the 19 century, little was known about the causes of mental disorders, and inadequate services for this population continued well into the 20th century. Deinstitutionalization left many mentally ill persons adrift in the community; a broader range of services in community mental health began. Community mental health today focuses on treatment of the mentally ill, prevention of mental illness, and promotion of mental health for the community. Stigma is a major obstacle to accomplishing this goal.

Epidemiologic information provides a road map for community mental health nursing practice. These data describe the incidence and prevalence of mental disorders nationally and worldwide. They show that a considerable portion of the burden of disease in the U.S. and globally is attributable to mental disorders. A variety of biological, behavioral, sociocultural, and environmental risk factors influence the vulnerability of the mentally ill population.

Most community mental health efforts have focused on treatment of the mentally ill, with only a recent growing emphasis on prevention and health promotion. The national *Healthy People 2010* objectives particularly target suicide and serious mental illnesses but include some prevention objectives as well. Knowing the needs of the mentally ill population assists in planning services. Their needs include biological, psychological, and social problems. Services for the mentally ill use either biomedical or psychotherapeutic approaches. Various therapies are included under these two approaches. Many resources exist in the community to serve the mentally ill population. Among them are community mental health centers, halfway houses, and community support programs. Two models for preventing mental illness are the Public Health Model and the Mental Health Intervention Spectrum Model. Separately or combined, they provide a focus for designing preventive interventions at the primary, secondary, and tertiary levels.

Mental health promotion seeks to promote well-being through strengthening life-sustaining and life-enhancing activities. Interventions for mental health promotion include risk-protecting activities and healthy life style and behavior activities.

The nurse's role in community mental health includes being able to use epidemiologic data; engaging in advocacy, education, case management, case-finding, and referral; and collaborating with the mental health team.

CLINICAL CORNER   Clients with Mental Health Issues

Scenario 1

You are a community health nurse in Smithville. Today you will begin following a new client, Emmit. Emmit is a 50-year-old man who lives with his 83-year-old mother, Alice, in rural Smithville. Emmit is a veteran of the Vietnam War. His diagnoses include:

- paranoid schizophrenia with delusions
- hypertension
- CAD (coronary artery disease)
- peripheral neuropathy
- hypertension

Emmit receives home health nursing services in order to monitor compliance with medications and for assessment of complications related to his multiple diagnoses. Since the nearest Veteran's Hospital is located in Capitol City, Emmit's physician determined that home health services would provide the most cost-effective means of ongoing care. Emmit's case is currently under review for possible benefits related to Agent Orange exposure leading to peripheral neuropathy.

Emmit's daily medication regimen includes seven drugs prescribed TD or BID and nitroglycerin prn. He receives home health nursing visits three to four times each week for the purposes of:

- assessment and education about compliance with medications
- physical assessment, including cardiovascular and pulmonary
- assessment of mental health status and adequacy of caregiver support
- follow-up on complaints of fatigability with ADLs
- assessment and referrals about caregiver support
- foot care

Prior to your initial visit with Emmit, you discuss the case with his previous nurse, James. James informs you that he has provided home health nursing services to Emmit for over 2 years. He states that Emmit is pleasant, but that he frequently exhibits inappropriate behavior and adds "You'd better be ready to deal with it." Primarily, Emmit's behavior focuses on expressing his anger about issues in the news. James reports that Emmit keeps abreast of political and other news events and that he has a propensity to become loud and angry when expressing his views. Emmit is also very insistent that he is capable of living independently. Despite numerous complications due to inappropriate self-medicating, Emmit has stated repeatedly, "I don't want any help from anyone, I don't mind you all visiting us, but I can take care of myself and my mother just fine."

James informs you that Alice seemed very resistant to his intervention during the first year of the home visitation but that she "came around" eventually. Due to Emmit's inconsistency in self-medicating, Alice has assumed responsibility for administering all medications. She has made formal requests to Emmit's physician and the Veteran's Hospital to receive daily home health visits as well as a live-in support person. In re-

viewing previous notations in the chart, you see that Alice relates an inability to pay "with my pension"; besides, she added, "they messed up his mind . . . they should pay to take care of him." She informed James that "if something happens to me they'll just let him die . . . we have no other family to take care of him." She has frequently stated that the responsibility of caring for Emmit "is taking its toll on me."

Given the information available to you, you identify the goals of the involved parties:

Agency goals: assessment, monitoring, and education of existing medical conditions. Caregiver support.

Veteran's Hospital and physician goals: maintenance of ongoing care needs in a cost-effective manner.

Caregiver goals: emotional and financial support, increased level of supportive services.

Client goals: increased independence.

Questions

1. Based on this information, what are *your goals* for the initial visit with this family?
2. If you were to approach this situation with the goal of accomplishing all of the agency's goals each visit, what do you anticipate would occur during your initial visit? Why?
3. Conversely, what do you predict the outcome of the visit would be if you attempted to address only the issues that Emmit and Alice felt were important?
4. How will you "sell" yourself and your services in this situation?
5. Prioritize your goals and objectives:

    #1:

    #2:

    #3:

    #4:

After working with Emmit for 6 months, you attend a case conference held at the V.A.. In attendance at the case conference with you are Emmit's V.A. physician, a medical social worker, and the V.A. benefits specialist. During the course of your discussion with the other health care professional after the case conference, you realize that there are many families in your community who are in situations similar to that of Emmit and his mother.

The group decides that, given your success in working with Emmit and Alice, they would like you to begin a support group in Smithville for veterans and family members/support persons who are dealing with mental illness.

Questions

6. What more do you need to know about your aggregate?
7. How will you go about getting this information?
8. How will you define your aggregate (criteria . . .)?

(continued)

CLINICAL CORNER (Continued)

9. Brainstorm about a program that would offer a holistic approach to medical and psychosocial support for your aggregate, the veterans, and their families.

10. How will you outreach to your aggregate?
11. Where might you begin to obtain assistance in your endeavors? How will you solicit funding, volunteers, donations of meeting space and foot, etc.?

ACTIVITIES TO PROMOTE CRITICAL THINKING

1. As a community health nurse, you have been asked to design and present a 2-hour program on suicide to the entire student body of the local high school. This activity is representative of which level of prevention? What are some of the considerations involved in planning this program in order to promote optimal success? How might you measure the effectiveness of this intervention?

2. John is a 26 year-old Asian male who has been diagnosed with schizophrenia for 5 years. He lives with his parents who moved to the U.S. from China 10 years ago. He participates in a resocialization program at the local YWCA. He told the nurse that his parents do not want him to take medication and believe he is not sick at all. What cultural influences should be considered in this situation? How can the community health nurse assist this client and his family in order to prevent further exacerbation of the client's symptoms? What other services might be helpful in this situation?

3. You are part of a multidisciplinary team whose goal is to identify families in your city who are at risk for crisis (e.g., single parent, divorce, teen pregnancy, loss of job) and develop a set of interventions. How would you determine who these families are? What interventions would be appropriate to meet their needs? What level of prevention would you be targeting?

4. Susan is a 38-year-old high school teacher who, along with three of her students, was attacked by a student with a gun who was threatening to kill all of them. The teacher and students are hysterical, sobbing, and screaming about the fear and terror they had experienced. The school nurse has been called to the scene and has contacted the mobile crisis unit to report to the school. What priorities would the school nurse establish? What plan would be the most realistic? What interventions would be most applicable under these circumstances?

5. You have met a few elderly men in your area who live alone and are widowed, and you have heard that there are others. Assuming your advocacy role in community mental health, you decide to take some action to ensure that their needs are being met. How would you determine the risks and needs for this group? What interventions would be appropriate to meet their needs?

6. Select a problem that places people at risk for mental disorders (such as child abuse and neglect or drug abuse) and do a search on the Internet to learn all you can about it. What is the incidence and prevalence of this problem? What interventions are most effective in addressing it? What can be done to prevent it? (See Clinical Corner.)

REFERENCES

American Psychiatric Association (1994). *Diagnostic and statistical manual of mental disorders* (4th ed.) (DSM-IV). Washington DC: American Psychiatric Press.

Angermeyer, M.C. & Matschinger, H. (1996). The effect of violent attacks by schizophrenic persons on the attitude of the public towards the mentally ill. *Social Science Medicine, 43,* 1721–1728.

Becker, A.E., Grinspoon, S.K., Klibanski, A., & Herzog, D.B. (1999). Eating disorders. *New England Journal of Medicine, 340,* 1092–1098.

Bennett, S. (1978). *Mind and madness in ancient Greece.* New York: Cornell University Press.

Bryson, S.E. & Smith, I.M. (1998). Epidemiology of autism: Prevalence, associated characteristics, and service delivery. *Mental Retardation and Developmental Disabilities Research Reviews, 4,* 321–329.

Caplan, G. (1964). *Principles of preventive psychiatry.* New York: Basic Books.

Christoffel, K.K. (2000). Public health advocacy: Process and product. *American Journal of Public Health, 90*(5), 722–726.

Gamwell, L. & Tomes, N. (1973). *Madness in America: Cultural and medical perceptions of mental illness before 1914.* New York: Cornell University Press.

Griffin-Francell, C. (1997). Health promotion and maintenance and preventive interventions. In J. Haber, B. Krainovich-Miller, A. MacMahon, & P. Price-Hoskins. *Comprehensive psychiatric nursing* (5th ed.). St. Louis: Mosby–Year Book.

Grob, G.N. (1991). *From asylum to community: Mental health policy in modern America.* Princeton, NJ: Princeton University Press.

Grob, G.N. (1994). *The mad among us: A history of the care of America's mentally ill.* New York: Free Press.

Haber, J., Krainovich-Miller, B., McMahon, A., & Price-Hoskins, P. (1997). *Comprehensive psychiatric nursing* (5th ed.). St.Louis: Mosby–Year Book.

Hauenstein, E.J. (1998). Case-finding and care in suicide: Children, adolescents, and adults. In M.A. Boyd & M.A. Nihart (Eds.). *Psychiatric nursing: Contemporary practice.* Philadelphia: Lippincott Williams & Wilkins.

Institute of Medicine (1994). *Reducing risks for mental disorders.* Washington, DC: National Academy Press.

Jones, A.H. (1998). Mental illness made public: Ending the stigma? *Lancet, 352,* 1060.

Kiple, K.F. (1995). *The Cambridge world history of human disease.* Cambridge: Cambridge University Press.

Murray, C.J.L., & Lopez, A.D. (Eds.). (1996). *The global burden of disease. A comprehensive assessment of mortality and disability from diseases, injuries, and risk factors in 1990 and projected to 2020.* Cambridge, MA: Harvard School of Public Health.

National Institute of Mental Health. *The invisible disease— Depression: Fact sheet* (*www.nimh.nih.gov/publicat/invisible.cfm*). Bethesda, MD: U.S. Department of Health and Human Services, National Institutes of Health.

Office of Women's Health (2000). *Costs of mental and addictive disorders.* The National Women's Health Information Center. Washington, DC: US Department of Health and Human Services, June. (*www.4woman. gov/owh/pub/mental/fscost.htm,* June 2000).

Price-Hoskins, P. (1997). Psychiatric nursing in community settings. In J. Haber, B. Krainovich-Miller, A. MacMahon, & P. Price-Hoskins. *Comprehensive psychiatric nursing* (5th ed.). St. Louis: Mosby–Year Book.

Rosen, G. (1968). *Madness in society.* Chicago: University of Chicago Press.

Swartz, M.S., Swanson, J.W., & Burns, B.J. (1998). Mental disorder, substance abuse, and community violence: An epidemiological approach. In J. Monahan & H.J. Steadman (Eds.). *Violence and mental disorder: Developments in risk assessment.* Chicago: University of Chicago Press.

Substance Abuse and Mental Health Services Administration (1999). *Mental health: A report of the Surgeon General.* Rockville, MD: U.S. Department of Health and Human Services, National Institutes of Health. (*www.surgeongeneral.gov/library/mentalhealth/*)

U.S. Department of Health and Human Services (2000). *Healthy people 2010: Understanding and improving health* (Chapter 18). Washington, DC: U.S. Department of Health and Human Services, Government Printing Office. (*www.health.gov/healthypeople/Document/*)

World Health Organization (1999). *The World Health Report 1999* (Chapter 2). Geneva, Switzerland: WHO. (*www.who.int/whr/1999/en/report.htm*)

INTERNET RESOURCES

Bazelon Center for Mental Health Law: *www.bazelon.org/*

Center for Research on Services for People with Severe Mental Disorders: www.nimh.nih.gov/grants/research/9294.htm

Epidemiology of Mental Illness: www.nimh.nih.gov.mhsg

Mental Health Patient's Bill of Rights: www.apa.org/pubinfo/rightshtml, www.nimh.nih.gov/mhsgrpt/pofs/c2pdf

National Institutes of Mental Health: www.nimh.nih.gov

Practitioners Research Reports and Current Information on the Daignosis and Treatment for Mental Disorders: www.nimh.gov/practitioners/

RECOMMENDED READINGS

Adams, S.M., Dolfie, E.K., Feren, S.S., Love, R.A., & Taylor, S.W. (1999). Mental health disaster response: Nursing interventions across the life span. *Journal of Psychosocial Nursing and Mental Health Services, 37*(11), 11–19.

Badger, F. & Nolan, P. (1999). General practitioners' perceptions of community psychiatric nurses in primary care. *Journal of Psychiatric Mental Health Nursing, 6*(6), 453–459.

Baker, C. (1999). From chaos to order: A nursing-based psycho-education program for parents of children with attention-deficit hyperactivity disorders. *Canadian Journal of Nursing Research, 31*(2), 71–75.

Barker, E., Robinson, D., & Brautigan, R. (1999). The effect of psychiatric home nurse follow-up on readmission rates of patients with depression. *Journal of the American Psychiatric Nurse Association, 5*(4), 116–119.

Chaudry, R.V., Polivka, B.J., & Kennedy, C.W. (2000). Public health nursing directors' perceptions regarding interagency collaboration with community mental health agencies. *Public Health Nursing, 17*(2), 75–84.

Eronen, M., Angermeyer, M.C., & Schulze, B. (1998). The psychiatric epidemiology of violent behavior. *Social Psychiatry and Psychiatric Epidemiology, 33*(Suppl. 1), S13–S23.

Frank, R. G., McGuire, T.G., Normand, S.L., & Goldman, H.H. (1999). The value of mental health services at the system level: The case of treatment for depression. *Health Affairs, 18,* 71–88.

Gibson, D.M. (1999). Reduced rehospitalizations and reintegration of persons with mental illness into community living: A holistic approach. *Journal of Psychosocial Nursing and Mental Health Services, 37*(11), 20–25.

Hanson, K.W. (1998). Public opinion and the mental health parity debate: Lessons from the survey literature. *Psychiatric Services, 49,* 1059–1066.

Kessler, R.C., Nelson, C.B., McKinagle, K.A., Edlund, M.J., Frank, R.G., & Leaf, P.J. (1996). The epidemiology of co-occurring addictive and mental disorders: Implications for prevention and service utilization. *American Journal of Orthopsychiatry, 66,* 17–31.

Link, B., Phelan, J., Bresnahan, M., Stueve, A., & Pescosolido, B. (1999). Public conceptions of mental illness: Labels, causes, dangerousness and social distance. *American Journal of Public Health, 89*(9), 1328–1333.

Malone, J. (1998) Concepts for the rehabilitation of the long-term mentally ill in the community. *Issues in Mental Health Nursing, 19,* 121–135.

Pelletier, L. R. (1998). Eye on Washington: Update on mental health parity. *Journal of Child and Adolescent Psychiatric Nursing, 14,* 159.

Penn, D.L., & Martin, J. (1998). The stigma of severe mental illness: Some potential solutions for a recalcitrant problem. *Psychiatric Quarterly, 69,* 235–247.

Secker, J. (1998). Current conceptualizatons of mental health and mental health promotion. *Health Education Research, 13,* 57–66.

Wald, A. (1998). Psychiatric home care builds effective treatment bridges. *Nursing Spectrum, 10A*(12), 4–5.

Yurkovich, E. & Dean, S.T. (1999). Maintaining health: Proactive client-oriented community day treatment centres for the chronic mentally ill. *Journal of Psychiatric Mental Health Nursing, 6*(1), 61–69.

Clients Living With Addiction

KEY TERMS

- Addiction
- Chemical dependence
- Detoxification
- Polysubstance use and abuse
- Relapse
- Substance abuse
- Tolerance
- Triggers
- Withdrawal symptoms

LEARNING OBJECTIVES

Upon mastery of this chapter, you should be able to:

- Define terms commonly used to describe addiction and addictive behaviors.
- Discuss the history and current incidence and prevalence of addiction in the U.S.
- Compare and contrast various theories on the etiology of addiction.
- Clarify your own assumptions and beliefs regarding clients living with addiction.
- Identify the *Healthy People 2010* goals for reducing addiction in the U.S.
- Discuss a variety of physical, psychosocial, and economic problems of clients, families, and communities struggling with addiction.
- Compare and contrast the preventive measures appropriate to clients addicted to alcohol, tobacco, other depressants, stimulants, and gambling.
- Describe the role of the nurse in caring for clients, families, and communities struggling with addiction.

This might not be an easy chapter to read. It may stir thoughts of a loved one who is struggling with an addiction or challenge you to rethink your assumptions about people with addictions. Perhaps you will learn that the problem of addiction is more widespread and complex than you had previously believed. Why should community health nurses be concerned about addiction anyway? In what sense does it threaten the health of communities? What are the global implications? Is there anything a community health nurse can do to help individuals, families, and communities cope with addictions? These are some of the questions we will address in this chapter. We will also describe some of the most common addictions and the preventive measures that are most often used in approaching clients with addictions.

AN OVERVIEW OF ADDICTION

Community health nurses have encountered populations with addiction problems for decades. Consider, for example, the rural nurse who serves a Native American population with a high rate of fetal alcohol syndrome, or the school nurse who sees an increasing number of adolescents reporting experimentation with marijuana and cocaine. Sometimes the nurse has no idea what to do or where to turn to help clients begin to maintain healthful lifestyles. Before we can discuss assessment, interventions, or resources for addiction, we need to clarify the terms commonly used when characterizing the problem and review the history and demographics of addiction. Also, since you may have personal issues to overcome before you are able to intervene in a therapeutic manner, we will assist you with values clarification as it relates to addiction.

Terminology of Addiction

The term **addiction** is defined as a compulsive use and impaired control over using a substance, preoccupation with obtaining and using the drug, and continued use despite adverse consequences. It also describes a compulsion to participate in and a preoccupaton with a certain activity, such as gambling or binge eating. Notice that the word compulsive indicates that the addictive behavior is beyond the individual's self-control; thus, addictions are very difficult to treat.

Several terms relate specifically to the abuse of chemical substances. **Chemical dependence** is a strong, overwhelming preoccupation with and desire to have a drug. It is often described as a *craving*. Chemical dependence usually accompanies addiction, but does not necessarily signify the presence of addiction. **Detoxification** is a term used to describe the process of ridding the body of harmful substances. **Relapse** refers to continuing to use a chemical or participate in an activity after a period of abstinence. **Substance abuse** refers to excessive and prolonged use of some chemical (alcohol, tobacco, drugs) that leads to serious physical, emotional, and social problems. Thus, an individual may face a problem of substance abuse without actually being chemically dependent or addicted. Approximately 10% of the population that consumes alcohol meet the criteria for alcohol dependence, and an additional 7% meet the diagnostic criteria for alcohol abuse. **Polysubstance use and abuse** occurs when a person is using or abusing more than one chemical. Typical combinations of drugs include alcohol and marijuana, alcohol and cocaine, cocaine and marijuana, and alcohol with antianxiety medications. Addiction to chemicals is characterized by **tolerance,** a need for increasing amounts of a substance to achieve the desired effects, or a significantly diminished effect with continued use of the same amount of the same substance (American Psychiatric Association, 1995). **Triggers** are events and activities that may cause a person to continue addictive activities. When the addicted individual does not use the substance for a certain period of time, he or she may experience **withdrawal symptoms,** physical and psychological symptoms such as tremors, lethargy, anxiety, or depression that are typically opposite to the effects of the addictive substance.

This chapter will focus primarily on chemical addictions to alcohol, tobacco, and other drugs, which together are commonly referred to as *ATOD.* The "other drugs" usually include caffeine, marijuana, cocaine, central nervous system (CNS) depressants and stimulants, hallucinogens, opiates, over-the-counter drugs, prescription drugs, and inhalants (Allen, 1996). We will also briefly discuss non-substance addictions, such as addiction to gambling.

History of Addictive Behavior in the US

A look at the U.S. history of taxation and legislation regarding alcohol, tobacco, and other drugs reveals that most of these substances were not regulated until fairly recently. As early as 1600, tobacco, introduced to European settlers by Native Americans, had become a cash crop in North Carolina. A federal tax was imposed on tobacco in 1862 to help finance the Civil War. In 1864 the first federal cigarette excise tax was imposed. This began a long history of taxing cigarettes.

Cocaine is derived from the coca plant. Cocaine was first extracted from coca leaves in the 1800s. Coca is grown in South America and was chewed as early as 3000 BC. In 1862, the pharmaceutical company Merck produced a fourth of a pound of cocaine. In the 1870s Parke, Davis manufactured a fluid extract of coca. Freud published *On Coca* in 1884, in which he recommended the use of cocaine to treat various conditions. That same year cocaine was being used as a local anesthetic in eye surgery.

Opium has been imported, albeit illegally, for many years. Opium was used by the Sumerians as early as 3000 BC. In the 1700s opium-tobacco mixtures began to be used in the East Indies, and their use spread to Formosa and the South China coast. The Chinese emperor prohibited the sale of opium and the operation of smoking houses. In the mid-1700s Hong Kong merchants served as intermediaries between the foreigners and the Chinese authorities. Patent medicines were readily available in the United States without restrictions. Many people used opium instead of alcohol because it was cheaper. This caused many people to be addicted. In 1800 it was legal to smoke opium and cocaine, and in 1900 patent medicines, tonics, and elixirs commonly included significant amounts of opium, cocaine, and alcohol. Not surprisingly, then, by 1914 many U.S. citizens were addicted to one or more of these substances. Although the Harrison Act was passed by Congress in 1914, requiring that narcotics dealers register with the Internal Revenue Service, no attempt was made at that time to criminalize the trade in or use of narcotics. It was not until the 1930s that the federal government established the first treatment programs for narcotics addiction; these were located in Lexington, Kentucky and Fort Worth, Texas (Allen, 1996).

The Women's Christian Temperance Union was established in 1874 to decrease the consumption of alcohol and cigarettes. Federal legislation prohibiting the manufacture and sale of alcohol did not take effect until 1919. Prohibition has been seen as a failed experiment for many reasons: it spawned illegal trafficking in liquor, which in turn resulted in increasing rates of violent crime, and it did not significantly decrease the consumption of alcohol, in part because it did not stop people from making their own spirits.

Until the early 20th century, no treatment was available for addiction to alcohol. In 1935, a stockbroker named Bill Wilson and a physician, Robert Smith, both alcoholics, founded Alcoholics Anonymous (AA) to help themselves and others struggling with alcohol addiction. AA is still an important treatment option for those struggling with alcohol abuse. This self-help model is the basis for many other groups that help people deal with addictions.

In the last 30 years, Presidents Richard Nixon and George Bush declared a "war on drugs," First Lady Nancy Reagan tirelessly promoted an anti-drug campaign called "Just Say No," and President Bill Clinton signed the "three strikes" crime bill, calling for life imprisonment after three convictions for drug offenses. Despite these efforts, substance abuse and chemical addiction remain serious national problems. Indeed, as we will see shortly, the incidence and prevalence of addiction to certain drugs actually increased in the final decades of the 20th century.

Population Statistics

Drug abuse is found among all socioeconomic classes, age groups, races, and genders. Recent data show that 76 million Americans experience alcoholism in their families. Alcohol is the most widely used (51%) and abused (7%–10%) drug of choice among all age groups.

INCIDENCE AND PREVALENCE

The prevalence of alcohol and drug use varies according to gender, age, and race/ethnicity. Young adults are more likely to binge drink (five or more drinks on one occasion during the past 30-day period) or drink heavily (at least five drinks on the same occasion on at least 5 different days in the past month). In the 18- to 25-year-old age group, over half of current drinkers were binge drinkers and nearly one quarter were heavy drinkers. Men are more likely to drink than women (59% versus 45%). They are also more likely to binge drink and more likely to drink heavily, according to the 1999 National Household Survey.

Trends in adolescent drug abuse and use have been measured for the past two decades in grades 8, 10, and 12. The three most prevalent drugs of abuse by adolescents are alcohol, cigarettes, and marijuana. The overall rate of drug use among adolescents has declined since 1975, although marijuana and cigarette use among students at all three grade levels actually increased during the 1990s. From 1991 to 1997, marijuana use rose from 3.2% to 9.7% among 8th graders; among 10th graders marijuana use rose from 8.1% to 20.5% from 1992 to 1997. There was also a change in the attitudes of adolescents during the 1990s; there was a decline in the percentage of students who believed that marijuana is harmful and disapprove of its use.

Almost one third of heavy drinkers were also current illicit drug users. By comparison, only 1.7% of non-drinkers were illicit drug users.

DEMOGRAPHICS

Drug abusers are individuals, primarily adolescents and young adults, who try drugs on an experimental and impulsive basis, often because of peer pressure. Repeated use in many cases leads to addiction. Some individuals are well-adjusted and become addicted as a result of over-prescription of medications for treating insomnia, pain, obesity, or other medical reason. Others are having trouble coping with the stresses of life or may have personal problems. Recently there has been an increase in the number of senior citizens who are suffering from addiction problems. Senior citizens often suffer from medical problems, loneliness, loss, and grief from which they seek relief through alcohol and drugs. There are individuals who become addicted as they repeatedly seek escape or release through illicit drug use. Individuals in certain professions tend to have higher rates of alcohol and drug abuse than in others. Nurses have been plagued by addiction problems, probably because of the easy access to drugs and the stresses related to the profession.

Community health nurses will want to be particularly alert to aggregates that appear to be more at risk than others. One of the populations at greater risk for abusing chemicals is the adolescent. Adolescents are particularly vulnerable to peer pressure and have a tendency to be impulsive. Older populations also are vulnerable because they often have medical problems that require medication, have pain, may be lonely or depressed, and are often suffering from grief and loss. Some medications can cause people to forget when they have taken them, or they have not received the relief they expected from their medication; thus, they may be over-medicating, which can cause addiction problems.

Etiology of Addiction

There is no consensus about the causes of alcohol and drug addiction. Research approaches to studying the population of substance abusers have pointed to a variety of possible causal factors, some physiological, some social, and some psychological. There is evidence, for example, that certain individuals using alcohol seem to "need" more, even at the onset of their drinking, suggesting a chemical predisposition leading to addiction. Other evidence points to psychological factors such as low self-esteem, or behavioral patterns such as drug experimentation, promoting use and abuse. Social factors, too, such as over-prescription and drug advertising, influence use and abuse. Also, the environmental milieu surrounding certain individuals, such as peer pressure, dysfunctional families, and societal attitudes about drugs—both "good" and "bad" drugs—can promote use and eventual dependence. There seem to be few, if any, single causes but rather an interaction of multiple factors operating to influence substance abuse.

Biological causative factors include a family history of alcoholism or drug abuse. Although there is little conclusive evidence that genetic predisposition is an actual cause, there is reason to believe that in some cases, individuals who begin using alcohol or certain drugs are more readily susceptible to addiction. Neurobiological theory research is beginning to identify the affects that alcohol has on the neurotransmitters in the brain. Drugs inhibit, stimulate, or change the release or action of neurotransmitters in the brain. The disease theory was first described by Jellink in 1946 and later by Vaillant in 1983. The rationale behind the disease theory was that alcoholism had a biological cause and that there was a predictable natural history to the disease. The disease is progressive and fatal. Regardless, the belief that alcohol or drug dependence and addiction are diseases has a basis in fact when one considers the effect on the health of substance abusers.

The behavioral/psychological causative factors are varied. For children and adolescents, trying new and risky things is part of normal developmental behavior; this often includes experimentation with drugs, alcohol, and tobacco. Peer pressure for adolescents is a major influence and, when combined with drug experimentation, can lead to dependence. Even people who are relatively well adjusted emotionally turn to alcohol or drugs as a way to relieve stress from such things as divorce, death of a loved one, chronic pain, job loss, work pressures, family conflict, or simply a life that is too fast paced. Drug choices may range from excessive coffee consumption and smoking, to self-medication with over-the-counter medications such as tranquilizers, to the use of illicit drugs. Social activities incorporating alcohol consumption are commonplace, and even illicit drugs such as marijuana or cocaine are encouraged in some social groups. When these patterns persist, tolerance and dependence can result. People with low self-esteem are at greater risk for substance abuse, as are those with personality disorders or other psychological disturbances who may be seeking thrills or defying authority through drug use. Their mental impairment contributes to maladaptive coping patterns, prompting some in society to unfairly label substance abuse as a "moral failing."

Sociocultural factors form another set of variables influencing substance abuse. Substance abusers include all ages, sexes, race, and economic levels, but the poor and minorities are often more vulnerable because they lack the education and resources to cope with life stresses and find needed assistance. Many individuals do not realize the danger inherent in certain drugs or do not know how to use drugs safely. They may drink alcohol when taking tranquilizers, which can be lethal. Misleading information is another factor. Over-the-counter drugs are often not considered drugs, and their ready access and heavy advertising promotion leads to abuse. Examples are the excessive use of diet pills, cold remedies, and nonprescription painkillers. Over-prescription of medications, such as morphine for pain or valium for anxiety, can also lead to addiction. The quality of illegal drugs cannot be controlled so that many drugs, such as heroin and cocaine, may be poorly mixed and have unpredictable dosages; an example is marijuana, which is now twenty times more potent than it was in the 1960s and 1970s. Social values that promote competition, productivity, and involvement in too many activities further contribute to stress that can lead to alcohol and drug abuse. Drug laws labeling users as criminals often prevent these individuals from seeking appropriate help that might prevent addiction or treat dependence. Some cultural groups promote moderate substance use or even abstention, but in the U.S. these influencing variables generally are not present.

Environmental factors related to the physical and social milieu can influence substance abuse. Dysfunctional families and abusive relationships contribute to both alcohol and drug use leading to dependence. Peer pressure, with a desire for social acceptance among adolescents and young adults especially, is a strong contributing factor. Availability of legal and illegal drugs, particularly in highly populated urban settings, further promotes use. Widespread public misconceptions about which drugs are dangerous to one's health can influence abuse; many people feel that alcohol, tobacco, and over-the-counter and prescription drugs are acceptable because they are legal. A summary of these influencing factors is shown in Figure 35–1.

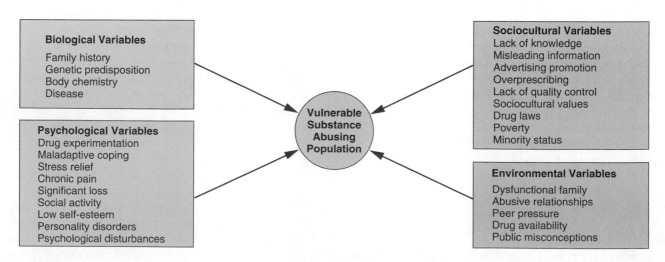

FIGURE 35–1. Factors that influence the vulnerability of the substance-abusing population.

Public Health Model

Since public health is dedicated to attaining the highest level of wellness for the greatest number, addictions are a grave public health concern. The nurse can apply the traditional public health model of host-agent-environment, described in Chapter 14, to ATOD addiction in the following way: The *host* is the individual or population affected. One must consider their ethnicity, race, gender, age, and occupation, as well as the biochemical, physiological, and psychological aspects of the disease. The disease-causing *agent* is the substance of use. The *environment*, which may foster the substance abuse, includes the values, beliefs, and norms of the culture, community, and society (Fig. 35–2). This includes governmental and non-governmental organizations, faith communities, volunteer groups, peer groups, schools, and local, state, and federal governments. Even other nations must be considered part of the environment of addiction; since many substances that are illegal in the U.S. are smuggled in from other countries, it is essential that policy-making with foreign governments supports activities to eliminate international trafficking in drugs.

Common Assumptions About Clients Living With Addiction

Our society holds conflicting views about addictions. The moralistic view proposes that individuals should simply "stop the behavior"; if individuals would only exercise their willpower, they could cease the abuse and overcome the addiction. This view is grounded in the belief that substance abuse, even when accompanied by chemical dependence and addiction, is a choice.

On the other hand, as we have discussed, the overwhelming evidence of scientific research in the 20th century indicates that addiction, especially chemical addiction, is a disease. Thus, proponents of the scientific view advocate the same level of compassionate assessment and intervention that would be appropriate for clients with physical disorders. Community health nurses must look at the reasons behind their own beliefs and values so that they can establish a therapeutic relationship with the clients involved. Some questions you might ask yourself are listed in Display 35–1.

Healthy People 2010 Goals

The U.S. Department of Health and Human Services has identified goals to help our nation become healthier. These goals can provide community health nurses with some guidelines for their practice in the community. The main goals are to reduce the average annual alcohol consumption, decrease

---

DISPLAY 35–1. Values Clarification

Some questions you might ask yourself include:
- What do I believe about chemical dependency?
- Is it a disease, or is it a choice people make?
- Did I have close contact with someone (mother, father, sibling, husband) who had an addiction?
- How did I feel about this person and their behavior?
- Do my religious beliefs influence my attitudes toward addictions?
- How do I ask questions about the individual and his or her use?
- Am I uncomfortable asking assessment questions?
- If I am uncomfortable, what are the reasons for this?
- Is it that I might have to intervene?
- What are my feelings when I'm making a home visit to a mother who is using chemicals?
- Do I relate to her with empathy or disdain?
- Do I distrust this mother when she states she will quit using chemicals, or do I find support systems for her and encourage her to seek help?
- How do I feel about the mother who is living with a man who is chemically dependent and abusive to her?
- Do I get annoyed that she won't leave?
- Do I understand why she stays with him?
- Do I suspect emotional and/or physical abuse?
- How do I feel about women and men who are in abusive relationships?
- How do I ask the questions to assess whether she is being abused without offending her?
- How do I assess whether he is being abused?
- What is my role if I suspect both parents are addicted?
- Are the children safe? How can I protect the children from harm?
- Am I looking at the clients' strengths?

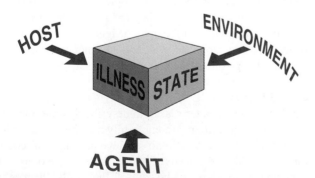

FIGURE 35–2. Epidemiologic triad. Epidemiologists study the causal agent, the susceptible host, and environmental factors that contribute to an illness state (or a wellness state). Intervention may focus on any of these three to prevent the spread of illness or to improve health in a population.

the proportion of persons engaging in binge drinking, and reduce the cost of lost productivity in the workplace due to alcohol and drug use. (Data showed that in 1995 the economic costs were $276 billion and the productivity costs were $196 billion.)

The goals related to substance abuse include decreasing the number of emergency room visits related to drugs and alcohol. In 1996 drugs and alcohol accounted for 2.4% of emergency department visits. Motor vehicle deaths related to drugs and alcohol were 6.1 per 100,000 in 1997. Goals related to these data are to decrease the number of deaths and injuries caused by alcohol and drugs and to reduce the proportion of adolescents who report the use of drugs and alcohol and engage in risky behavior, such as driving while intoxicated.

Several goals relate to decreasing tobacco use by all populations. These include an increase in smoking-cessation programs, an increase in work-site smoking policies that prohibit smoking, and an increase in the enforcement of laws prohibiting sale of tobacco products to minors (U.S. Department of Health and Human Services, 2000).

PROBLEMS RELATED TO ADDICTION

Addiction is typically accompanied by a variety of other problems, many of which affect the addict's family and community. Each substance or addictive activity has its own particular side effects and possible consequences; these are listed more specifically in Table 35–1. As we consider the overall health needs of this at-risk population, we can group these problems into four categories: physical, psychosocial, economic, and problems of the fetus, newborn, and children of addicted parents.

Physical Problems

Serious physical health problems can arise from substance abuse. Damage to organs and other body parts is common from most drugs and includes damage to the liver, brain, central nervous system, heart, kidneys, skin, ligaments and tendons, bowel, and lungs. Disease resulting from substance abuse includes cirrhosis of the liver with alcohol abuse, heart disease and liver cancer with abuse of steroids, AIDS and hepatitis from needle sharing with narcotics, and lung cancer with tobacco and marijuana abuse. Abuse of steroids can cause impotence and sterility in men and menstrual problems for women, and marijuana abuse can lead to infertility in both women and men. Other physical problems include headaches, malnutrition, severe withdrawal symptoms from addiction, memory disorders with marijuana, pulmonary edema with narcotics, convulsions, respiratory arrest, heart failure, suffocation, unconsciousness, and, with overdose, coma and death. Polysubstance use and abuse can also lead to serious results from multiple drug interactions.

Psychosocial Problems

Social problems resulting from substance abuse cover a broad area affecting individual abusers, their families, and the community. Monetary and social costs to the individual of maintaining a drug habit can lead to poverty, unemployment, social stigma, and punishment for crime. Alcohol and drug abuse creates family disruption, neglect, and abuse and depletes financial and emotional resources. For the community, problems include an increased incidence of violence, traffic accidents and deaths, homicides, and crime related to obtaining money or possessing illicit drugs. Further problems for the community come from added costs of law enforcement, welfare programs, drug abuse surveillance, and drug treatment and rehabilitation services (Table 35–2).

PSYCHOLOGICAL DEPENDENCE
Psychological dependence occurs when the user perceives the need for a substance to maintain his or her optimal state of well-being, interpersonal relationships, or skill performance. Often the person does not recognize that he or she may have an addiction to the drug. This is common when people are using anti-anxiety drugs; the drugs may have been prescribed, but the user will increase the dose as he or she experiences increased problems coping. Other problems experienced by substance abusers include anxiety and depression with inhalants; agitation, hyperactivity, and hallucinations with hallucinogens; and neuroses, psychoses, violence, and suicide.

DEPRESSION AND SUICIDE
Depression is a common disorder associated with chemical use and abuse. Many of the drugs used and abused are CNS depressants. People who experience clinical depression and other psychological disorders use drugs to self-medicate or to help diminish their symptoms. Some people are suicidal when they use drugs or alcohol. It is important for nurses to assess the level of depression, previous suicide attempts, and suicide ideation. It is not uncommon for people who are intoxicated to talk about suicide and when they are sober deny any suicide ideation. These symptoms cannot be ignored. It is a myth that people who are intoxicated will not or cannot commit suicide. People who are intoxicated often commit suicide.

CO-DEPENDENCE
Co-dependence is a term used to describe dysfunctional behaviors that are evident among family members. It describes individuals who are able to achieve a sense of control through fulfilling the needs of others. An example of a co-dependent person is a wife who controls the family finances and gives her alcoholic husband an allowance to prevent him from spending his money on alcohol. People who are co-dependent are unable to meet their needs for autonomy and self-esteem and feel a sense of powerlessness.

There is no criterion available to describe this behavior as a psychiatric condition. Some of the behaviors seen in

TABLE 35–1. Drugs Involved in Substance Abuse

Drug Type	Facts	Possible Signs of Use/Abuse	Possible Health Risks of Use/Abuse
CANNABIS Hashish (hash, herb, kif) Hashish oil (hash oil, honey) Marijuana (grass, weed, dope, ganja, reefer, pot, Acapulco gold, Thai sticks)	Cannabis is made from the hemp plant, *Cannabis sativa*. When smoked or ingested produces mild euphoria, relaxation, and intense sensory perception. Users may develop tolerance and physical dependence. Sinsemilla is a highly potent form of marijuana.	Relaxation and euphoria Altered perceptions of time and space Hallucinations or anxiety attacks with Sinsemilla use	Damage to heart and lungs Damage to brain nerve cells Memory disorders Temporary loss of fertility Psychological dependence
DEPRESSANTS Alcohol (brew, juice, liquor) Barbiturates (downers, barbs) Benzodiazepines (Valium, Librium, tranquilizers) Chloral hydrate (knockout, Mickey Finn) Glutethimide (Dorden) Methaqualone (Quaalude, Ludes) Other Depressants (Equanil, Miltown, Noludar, Placidylm, Valmid)	Depressants depress or slow down the central nervous system by relaxing muscles, calming nerves and producing sleep. Alcohol is a depressant. Depressants are composed of sedative-hypnotic and tranquilizer drugs. Depressants are addictive. Users of depressants develop a tolerance to the drugs, meaning larger doses must be taken each time to produce the same effect.	Relaxation and drowsiness; lack of concentration; disorientation; loss of inhibitions; lack of coordination; dilated pupils; slurred speech; weak and rapid pulse; distorted vision; low blood pressure; shallow breathing; staggering; clammy skin; fever, sweating; stomach cramps; hallucinations, tremors; and delirium	Liver damage; convulsions; addiction with severe withdrawal symptoms; coma; death due to overdose. For pregnant women: the newborn may be dependent and experience withdrawal or suffer from birth defects and behavioral problems
HALLUCINOGENS Lysergic acid diethylamide (LSD) Phencyclidine (PCP, angel dust) Mescaline and peyote (Mexc., buttons, cachaus) Psilocybin (mushrooms) Amphetamine variants (MDMA/Ecstasy, MDA/Love Drug, TMA, DOM, DOB, PMA, STP, 2.5-DMA) Phencyclidine analogues (PCE, PCPy, TCP) Other Hallucinogens (Bufotenine, Ibogaine, DMT, DET, Psilocybin)	Hallucinogens are psychedelic, mind-altering drugs that affect a person's perception, feelings, thinking, self-awareness, and emotions. A "bad trip" may result in the user experiencing panic, confusion, paranoia, anxiety, unpleasant sensory images, feelings of helplessness, and loss of control. A "flash back" is a reoccurrence of the original drug experience without taking the drug again.	Dilated pupils, increased body temperature, heart rate, and blood pressure; sweating; loss of appetite; sleeplessness; dry mouth; tremors; hallucinations; disorientation; confusion; paranoia; violence; euphoria; anxiety; and panic	Agitation; extreme hyperactivity; psychosis; convulsions; mental or emotional problems; death

continued

TABLE 35–1. Drugs Involved in Substance Abuse (Continued)

INHALANTS Amyl Nitrate (poppers, snappers) Butyl Nitrate (rush, bolt, bullet) Chlorohydrocarbons (aerosol sprays, cleaning fluids) Hydrocarbons (solvents, airplane glue, gasoline, paint thinner) Nitrous Oxide (laughing gas, whippets)	Inhalants are substances that are breathed or inhaled through the nose. Inhalants are depressants and depress or slow down the body's functions. Inhalants are normally not thought of as drugs because they are often common household or industrial products. However, inhalants are often the most dangerous drugs per dose.	Euphoria and lightheadedness; excitability; loss of appetite; forgetfulness; weight loss sneezing; coughing; nausea and vomiting; lack of coordination; bad breath; red eyes; sores on nose and mouth; delayed reflexes; decreased blood pressure; flushing (skin appears to be reddish); headache; dizziness; and violence	Depression; damage to the nervous system and body tissues; damage to liver and brain; heart failure; respiratory arrest; suffocation; unconsciousness; seizures; heart failure; sudden sniffing death
NARCOTICS Codeine (school boy) Heroin (H. harry, junk, brown sugar, smack) Meperidine (doctors) Methadone (dollies, methadose) Morphine (morpho, Miss Emma) Opium (Dovers Powder) Other narcotics (Percodan, Talwin, Lomotil, Darvon, Numorphan, Percocet, Tylox, Tussionex, Fentanyl)	Narcotics are composed of opiates and synthetic drugs. Opiates are derived from the seed pod of the Asian poppy. Synthetic drugs called opoids are chemically developed to produce the effects of opiates Initially, narcotics stimulate the higher centers of the brain, but then slow down the activity of the central nervous system. Narcotics relieve pain and induce sleep. Narcotics, such as heroin, are often diluted with other substances (i.e., water, sugar) and injected. Other narcotics are taken orally or inhaled. Narcotics are extremely addictive. Users of narcotics develop a tolerance to the drugs, meaning larger doses must be taken each time to produce the same effect.	Euphoria; restlessness and lack of motivation; drowsiness; lethargy; decreased pulse rate; constricted pupils; flushing (skin appears to be reddish); constipation; nausea and vomiting; needle marks on extremities; skin abscess at injection sites; shallow breathing; watery eyes; and itching	Pulmonary edema; respiratory arrest; convulsions; addiction; coma; death due to overdose. For users who share or use unsterile needles to inject narcotics: tetanus, hepatitis, HIV/AIDS. For pregnant women: premature births; stillbirth, and acute infections among newborns

STEROIDS			
Anabolic-Androgenic (roids, juice, d-ball)	Steroids may contribute to increases in body weight and muscular strength. The acceleration of physical development is what makes steroids appealing to athletes and young adults. Anabolic-androgenic steroids are chemically related to the male sex hormone testosterone. Anabolic means to build up the muscles and other tissues of the body. Steroids are injected directly into the muscle or taken orally.	Sudden increase in muscle and weight; increase in aggression and combativeness; violence ("'roid rage"); hallucinations; jaundice; purple or red spots on body, inside mouth, or nose; swelling of feet or lower legs (edema); tremors; and bad breath. For women: breast reduction, enlarged clitoris, facial hair and baldness, deepened voice. For men: enlarged nipples and breasts, testicle reduction, enlarged prostate, baldness.	Acne, high blood pressure; liver and kidney damage; heart disease; increased risk of injury to ligaments and tendons; bowel and urinary problems; gallstones and kidney stones; liver cancer. For men: impotence and sterility. For women: menstrual problems. For users who share or use unsterile needles to inject steroids: hepatitis, tetanus, AIDS
STIMULANTS			
Amphetamines (uppers, pep pills) Cocaine (coke, flake, snow) Crack (rock) Methamphetamines (ice, crank, crystal) Methylphenidate (Ritalin) Phenmetrazine (Preludin, Preludes) Other stimulants (Adipex, Cylert, Didrex, Ionamin, Melfiat, Plegine, Sanorex, Tenuate, Tepanil, Prelu-2)	Stimulants stimulate the central nervous system, increasing alertness and activity. Users of stimulants develop a tolerance, meaning larger doses must be taken to get the same effect. Stimulants are psychologically addictive.	Increased alertness; excessive activity; agitation; euphoria; excitability; increased pulse rate, blood pressure, and body temperature; insomnia; loss of appetite; sweating; dry mouth and lips; bad breath; disorientation; apathy; hallucinations; irritability; and nervousness	Headaches; depression; malnutrition; hypertension; psychosis; cardiac arrest; damage to the brain and lungs; convulsions; coma; death

(From Spradley, B.W., & Allender, J.A. [1996]. *Community health nursing* [4th ed.]. Philadelphia; Lippincott-Raven.)

TABLE 35–2. Health-Related Problems of the Substance-Abusing Population

Physical Problems	Psychological Problems	Social Problems
Physical damage (liver, brain, heart, central nervous system, kidneys, skin, ligaments and tendons, bowel, lungs)	Psychological dependence	Poverty
	Anxiety	Unemployment
	Depression	Stigma
Disease (heart, lung cancer, AIDS, cirrhosis of liver, hepatitis)	Agitation	Punishment for crimes committed to support habits
	Hyperactivity	
Exposed newborns (low birth weight, birth defects, addiction, stillbirth, premature birth, infections)	Hallucinations	Family disruption
	Neuroses	Family neglect/abuse
	Psychoses	Depleted family resources
Polysubstance interactions	Violence	Increased violence in community
Sterility	Suicide	Homicide
Headaches		Crime
Malnutrition		High cost of drug treatment and rehabilitation
Addiction and withdrawal		
Memory disorders		
Pulmonary edema		
Convulsions		
Respiratory arrest		
Cardiac arrest		
Suffocation		
Unconsciousness		
Coma and death		

(From Spradley, B.W., & Allender, J.A. [1996]. *Community health nursing* [4th ed.]. Philadelphia; Lippincott-Raven.)

people who are co-dependent are controlling or attempting to control others; assuming responsibility for meeting others' needs; exhibiting anxiety and boundary distortions; and being enmeshed in relationships, especially with people who have personality disorders, are chemically dependent, or are also co-dependent. It is not uncommon for people who are chemically dependent to seek help for their own issues of co-dependency. Several resources are available to help people overcome some of the problems related to co-dependency; the most available and widely used is Al-Anon, a self-help organization designed on the principles of Alcoholics Anonymous. Groups are available in most communities.

FAMILY DISRUPTION, NEGLECT, AND ABUSE

Families are almost always adversely affected when someone in the family is using and/or abusing drugs or alcohol. There are often family secrets and abuse, both physical and emotional. Children do not bring friends home for fear of being embarrassed by the behavior of the person in the household who is chemically dependent. There is often poverty, related to the amount of money that goes for drugs or alcohol. Children may have to go without food because there is no money for groceries. It is not uncommon to see bruises on family members that are hard to explain. The toll that gambling takes on a family is especially difficult. Family members are usually the last to know there is a gambling problem.

COMMUNITY PROBLEMS

There is a high cost to communities related to addiction problems. Children miss school because no one is available to get

them off to school. States are increasing jail and prison space to house more and more people who are convicted of drug-related crimes. Communities are often spending more tax dollars on jails than on schools. In many communities parents are afraid to let their children play outside because of their fears that they may be caught in the crossfire of rival drug-dealing gangs or may be approached by drug dealers. Children often are living in deplorable situations in a "crack house" because the caregiver is an addict. These conditions are often very unsafe as children may have access to drugs, needles, and weapons. Many people are leaving inner city communities to avoid the problems related to poverty, drug and alcohol abuse and related crimes, and poor school systems. This leaves less of a tax base for prevention programs in many communities.

Economic Problems

Many economic problems are associated with addiction. Clients often are poor as a result of their inability to keep a job; they may end up working for temporary agencies or at low-paying jobs. It is not uncommon for people to move frequently because they are unable to pay rent or are evicted because of their destructive behavior. Often people have lost their families because of their addiction. Legal problems often are encountered by the addict. These problems may be a result of stealing money to support their habit. There are endless costs in disability, treatment programs, unemployment, and low productivity on the job, as well as welfare costs when a family loses a breadwinner. The gambling addict has often mortgaged the house and spent all the savings, and the bill collectors are at the door before the family is aware of the problem. This causes a great deal of anger among the family members toward the addict. There is a high divorce rate among gambling addicts.

Problems of the Fetus, Newborn, and Children of Addicted Parents

The problem of alcohol use during pregnancy has led to a significant amount of research, covering all ages of women of childbearing age. A study done by the Centers for Disease Control and Prevention (CDC) found a substantial increase in alcohol use among pregnant women ages 18 to 44 years from 1991 to 1995 (*MMWR*, 1997). This has warranted several goals in *Healthy People 2010*. One goal that relates to pregnant women who may use or abuse drugs during pregnancy is to increase abstinence from alcohol, cigarettes, and illicit drugs among pregnant women. Another goal is to decrease the incidence of fetal alcohol syndrome. Prenatal use of alcohol causes many birth defects, and there is a wide window of opportunity during pregnancy for alcohol to affect the central nervous system of the fetus. It is not known what affect alcohol has on the sperm or on the woman prior to pregnancy. Adolescents are becoming sexually active at an earlier age and consequently are becoming pregnant. Teenage sexual promiscuity and teenage pregnancy have been linked to adolescent substance abuse (Winters, 1999). Many women are drinking alcohol before they know they are pregnant, which can cause problems during fetal development. Primary prevention information can be disseminated throughout a community through the schools, public service announcements, doctors' offices, fliers, and newspaper articles.

ALCOHOL ADDICTION

One of the most widely available and deadly chemicals is alcohol. It has been used for thousands of years for "recreational purposes," that is, to induce relaxation, disinhibition, or euphoria. Alcohol has also been used as a beverage when water supplies were contaminated, as a medicine, for pain relief and sedation, and in religious ceremonies to promote visions or feelings of community or ecstasy. Even today a community's social, cultural, and religious values influence the level of alcohol use observed in that community.

Community health nurses have an opportunity to implement appropriate prevention strategies once they become informed about the uniqueness of the community they serve. Thus, community assessment is the first activity that should be accomplished. What does the population look like, in terms of age, level of education, ratio of families to singles, employment, and so on? What local statutes or programs focus on preventing alcohol abuse? What resources are cur-

rently available? The community health nurse is in a unique position to facilitate community-wide coalitions to address alcohol abuse, dependence, and addiction.

Preventive Measures

Since experimentation with alcohol commonly begins in the early teen years, prevention strategies work best if they are begun with young children. Also, a multidimensional approach that includes the family, social groups, school, church, local community, and local media is also important at all stages of prevention.

PRIMARY PREVENTION
Primary prevention is extremely important to help decrease the multitude of problems associated with alcohol use and abuse. Primary prevention methods in alcohol addictions need to take into consideration the theories of addiction that are now understood—for example, the probability of a genetic predisposition. It is important that the community health nurse include this aspect in presentations to the community. Since many people begin using alcohol by junior high school or before, primary prevention must begin before junior high school (see Research: Bridge to Practice).

SECONDARY PREVENTION
Secondary prevention strategies begin with individuals who have been assessed and are seen to be at risk of developing an addiction. The nurse will assess the amount of use; the impact the use is having on the family, job, and other relationship; and the safety of the family if the alcoholic is violent when drinking. Binge drinking must also be assessed, as it is a very common phenomenon among young adults. Many people do not think they have a problem with alcohol if they "just drink on weekends."

Many tools have been developed to assist with screening people for alcohol addiction problems. Using the *Diagnostic and Statistical Manual of Mental Disorders* (DSM-IV) criteria and the CAGE screening tool will help you assess the severity of the drinking problem. The CAGE screening tool, developed in 1984, is simple, easy to use, and widely applied (Ewing, 1984) (Display 35–2).

Once a problem is identified, the nurse will have to assess the readiness of the individual for treatment and the kind of intervention that is most appropriate. The progression from substance abuse or dependence to recovery has been researched extensively by Prochaska and colleagues (1992). Five stages of change in addictive behaviors have been identified. The first stage is precontemplation, when there is no intention to change behavior in the foreseeable future. At this stage the individual may be denying a problem; family and friends either are not aware of the problem or may also deny it. The next stage is the contemplation stage; the person is seriously thinking about overcoming the problem but has not yet made a commitment to take action. In the preparation stage, the individual makes a

RESEARCH Bridge to Practice

Sieving, R.E., Perry, C.L., & Williams, C.L. (2000). Do friendships change behaviors, or do behaviors change friendships? Examining paths of influence in young adolescents' alcohol use. *Journal of Adolescent Health, 26*(1), 27–35.

What causes adolescents, especially young adolescents, to consume alcohol? In this study, the researchers postulated that young adolescents would use alcohol if their friends did and that they would choose friends whose drinking behaviors were the same as their own.

To test these ideas, the researchers conducted a longitudinal study of 1804 adolescents in Minnesota while they were in grades 7, 8 and 9. They used a self-report survey instrument to determine such things as the students' alcohol use history, drinking patterns, parental expectations, family practices, and friends' drug use and offers.

The study findings showed that the friends' higher level of drug use (alcohol, tobacco, and marijuana) led to the participants' increased alcohol use. It also showed that the participants' alcohol use and their friends' alcohol and drug use remained stable over time.

As a result of their findings, the researchers concluded that peer influence, more than peer selection, appears to change adolescents' drinking behavior. The implications of this study suggest that alcohol use prevention programs in the community should address peer influence as an essential element. Adolescents should be exposed to peers who "model, reinforce, and expect health-enhancing alternatives to alcohol use" (p. 34). Prevention programs can also arm adolescents with skills to resist and counter peer influence to use alcohol and other drugs. Finally, since the alcohol and drug use behaviors of the students in the study were stable over time, the researchers concluded that prevention programs should begin at an early age, before patterns of behavior become fixed. They also recommended "multicomponent approaches" targeting alcohol use standards involving parents, schools, the community, and adolescents to reduce and/or prevent the adolescent population's use of alcohol.

DISPLAY 35–2. CAGE Screening Tool

C Have you felt you ought to **cut down** on your drinking?

A Have people **annoyed** you by criticizing your drinking?

G Have you felt bad or **guilty** about your drinking?

E Have you ever had a drink first thing in the morning—an **eye opener**—to steady your nerves or get rid of a hangover?

Note: More than one positive response indicates a probable drinking problem. (Ewing, J.A. [1984]. Detecting alcoholism: The CAGE questionnnaire. *Journal of the American Medical Association, 252*(14), 1905–1907.)

commitment to change and prepares for action. The action stage is when individuals modify their behavior to overcome alcohol use. The maintenance stage involves work to prevent relapse (Prochaska et al., 1992).

Once the problem has been identified, the nurse will explore the most appropriate kind of intervention. Alcoholics Anonymous (AA) is an excellent referral resource that is available in most communities. The meetings are anonymous because many people are afraid they will be looked down on, lose their jobs, or be isolated from family or friends if their addiction is found out. Since the mid-20th century there has been a proliferation of treatment programs for people with alcohol problems. Employers began to recognize that alcoholism was costing them money due to accidents on the job, lost time from work because of employees using alcohol on weekends, and other problems. Many corporations began to set up or contract with agencies to provide counseling to employees and their families. These programs are generally called Employee Assistance Programs (EAP). Counseling often includes issues surrounding the substance abuse, family relationships, anger management, and financial management.

The nursing assessment must include a determination of whether the individual is experiencing withdrawal symptoms. Withdrawal symptoms include increased anxiety, diaphoresis, tremors, increased vital signs, nausea and vomiting leading to dehydration, seizures (if not given immediate medical attention), delirium tremens, and ultimately death. Individuals often self-medicate with alcohol when the withdrawal symptoms appear, thus continuing the vicious circle of alcoholism. The nurse will have to be supportive and assist the individual in accessing detoxification services. Detoxification services are available in most communities and provide medical intervention, which includes giving the client medications that will decrease the withdrawal symptoms.

The next step after detoxification is to get the client into a treatment program or AA. Many treatment programs are conducted on an outpatient basis. For most people who are addicted to alcohol, abstinence is the only option for sobriety. Sobriety is difficult for many people because they must change their life style, old habits, and way of thinking, and dealing with life's problems besides dealing with physiological withdrawal such as cravings.

TERTIARY PREVENTION

The most important aspect of tertiary prevention is to help the individual remain drug free. There should be rapid intervention if the client relapses. Interventions implemented before the relapse will help the client build his or her self-esteem and to feel positive about the ability to stay sober. Growing evidence shows that memories of places and events, while using alcohol, can cause cravings and can trigger a relapse in people who have some sobriety. Helping the client identify the triggers that precipitate his or her use is very helpful so that those situations can be avoided. It is especially important that the client be able to talk about and work through these feelings with nonjudgmental, sober people.

Another aspect is helping the client who has residual health problems as a result of his or her former alcohol abuse maintain as active and healthy a life style as possible. Health prob-

Voices From the Community

I guess I always thought drinking was "cool." In junior high school my friends and I would sneak beer from our refrigerator and drink it out behind the garage. I don't think my parents knew. Then in high school we got hold of the hard stuff for our weekend parties. There were a lot of times when I passed out cold. My family and friends got concerned about me, so in college I kept my drinking less obvious and hid a bottle of vodka in my dorm room and drank after my roommate went to sleep. I guess that got me started on drinking secretively. After I married John, and even after the kids were in school, I'd hide bottles around the house and be drunk before noon.

It took me a long time to admit I had a problem. Even when my neighbors wouldn't let me drive the carpool, I denied anything was wrong. Finally, I hit bottom. My family did an "intervention" and got me into treatment. I've been sober for 8 years now and I go to my AA meetings every week. I'll tell you, I like myself a lot better now and so does my family!

Marie, 42, mother of two

lems can cause depression, which can cause the individual to relapse into using alcohol again.

Role of the Community Health Nurse

The community health nurse plays a vital role in working with clients, their families, and communities. The nurse will provide the community with prevention information and work with other agencies to provide prevention programs to pregnant women, adolescents, and other high-risk populations. Because the community health nurse has access to individuals and families, he or she can provide information and assess the level of the alcohol addiction problem and assist in the referral process. One of the most important aspects of intervention is the support the nurse can provide to the client and family during very difficult times. The nurse should work with the family to ensure that a safety plan is in place if there is a possibility of violence. The nurse knows the referral resources in the community for the family as well as the client and can facilitate appropriate referrals (see Voices From the Community).

TOBACCO ADDICTION

The first report on the detrimental effects of tobacco on the health of individuals was the Surgeon General's Report to Congress in 1964. Since that time, there has been an increasing awareness of the impact of tobacco on the health of the nation. Specifically, smoking or using other forms of nicotine, such as snuff and chewing tobacco, increases the risk of coronary artery disease, chronic obstructive pulmonary disease, and cancers of the mouth, throat, and lungs.

Nicotine is also highly addictive, providing both relaxation and an increase in energy. When smoked, it reaches the brain in just 7 seconds, and one pinch of chewing tobacco produces the effects of three to four cigarettes. Finally, because it is legal, widely available, relatively inexpensive, and socially acceptable in many peer groups, tobacco is often the first substance to which adolescents form an addiction.

Preventive Measures

All health care workers see the effects of tobacco use daily. For the elderly client facing surgery for lung cancer, even tertiary measures may be of little consequence. Prevention measures are most effective before tobacco use begins and are also moderately successful in achieving long-term cessation before the onset of addiction.

PRIMARY

There appears to be a set of stages that adolescents go through when beginning to use tobacco. In the *preparatory stage,* the adolescent develops attitudes about smoking. In the *trying stage,* he or she tries a few cigarettes. The *experimental stage* is marked by repeated but irregular use of tobacco. This stage often advances to the *regular use* stage and then to *addiction,* with physiological dependence on tobacco (U.S. Dept. of Health and Human Services, 1994).

Given this information, it is important for the community health nurse to use aggressive primary prevention strategies. As usual, a multidimensional approach is the most effective, with families, schools, neighborhood groups, and governmental agencies working together. The earlier that information is disseminated to parents and children, the more likely that tobacco use will never start. Teaching should include the problems nicotine can cause to the health of the individual, the effects of second-hand smoke, and the highly addictive nature of nicotine, including chewing tobacco and snuff. Teaching strategies for children could employ colorful pictures, simple language, and role-playing and other interactive games.

In many communities, law-enforcement officials and citizens monitor cigarette machines to prevent underage smoking. Cigarette machines are being discouraged and merchants are being encouraged to keep cigarettes and smokeless tobacco behind the counter and require some identification before purchasing these products.

SECONDARY PREVENTION

Secondary prevention includes identifying people who are using tobacco or who are addicted. There are four stages that people go through when trying to quit using tobacco. The first stage is when the client is not thinking seriously about quitting; in the next stage there is serious thinking about quitting; in the third stage the client is actively trying to quit; and the in fourth stage the person has quit and is trying to maintain abstinence from nicotine. Understanding which stage the client is in can help the nurse identify appropriate interventions. Some of the resources available for clients who are addicted are health insurance plans that offer education materials and support groups. The American Cancer Society and the American Lung Association have excellent materials; state and local health departments often have developed materials to help people quit using tobacco. The community health nurse can help the client identify triggers that cause him or her to want to use tobacco.

Pregnant women who use tobacco are at high risk of causing harm to the fetus. The community health nurse can be very helpful and supportive to this population. Useful materials are available, and in some cases nurses have established support groups in the community. Parents who smoke are exposing their children to problems such as asthma, poor performance in language skills and visual/spatial abilities, and more behavior problems (Lambers & Clark, 1996).

TERTIARY PREVENTION

Many people who have smoked are suffering from the long-term effects of their addiction. The health problems can be numerous and life-threatening and include emphysema, lung cancer and other forms of cancer, and heart disease. Many people who have diseases related to tobacco use continue to use tobacco; some will quit or have quit tobacco use. You must provide encouragement to those who have quit to help them maintain a tobacco-free lifestyle. Those individuals who continue to smoke can be encouraged to quit the use of tobacco. The nurse may provide care to individuals who are suffering from life-threatening diseases caused by tobacco use. It may be helpful for you to again evaluate your own attitudes about addictions (see Display 35–1).

Role of the Community Health Nurse

Community health nurses play a significant role in working with communities to prevent tobacco addiction. The community may need to be educated about the addictive qualities of tobacco, and the nurse may work with educators to help prevent students from beginning to use tobacco. The nurse plays an important role in helping pregnant women to quit using tobacco to prevent the problems related to low-birth-rate infants and other medical problems associated with tobacco use. The nurse can provide the support and resources necessary to help people addicted to tobacco to quit. In the community, the nurse can work with law enforcement agencies and community members to ensure that laws regarding sales to minors are enforced.

OTHER CENTRAL NERVOUS SYSTEM DEPRESSANTS

Marijuana is the most widely used illicit drug. It is widely available, easy to grow and relatively inexpensive, and used by all age groups. There is considerable disagreement about the medicinal effects of marijuana use to decrease the nausea associated with chemotherapy, AIDS, and other disorders. There is also disagreement about the addictive qualities of marijuana. Marijuana affects the CNS, cardiovascular system, and the respiratory system. It causes intoxication, euphoria, relaxation, impaired judgment, memory failure, increased heart rate, reddened eyes, and dry mouth.

Other depressants used by people are the benzodiazepines, opiates, and sedatives/hypnotics. The benzodiazepines that are the most widely used and abused are diazepam (Valium), chlordiazepoxide (Librium), lorazepam (Ativan), clonazepam (Klonopin), and alprazolam (Xanax). They are addictive, and withdrawal is similar to the withdrawal from alcohol. Almost all CNS depressants cross the blood–brain and placental barriers, so women who are pregnant should not be prescribed these medications. Withdrawal symptoms include drowsiness, slurred speech, unsteady gait, mood lability, lack of coordination, impaired judgment, memory failure, and seizures. It is important to assess the person for suicidal tendencies, anxiety, depression, and alcoholism.

Sedatives/hypnotics are the drugs of choice for people who have other addictions. These drugs include the barbiturates secobarbital (Seconal), phenobarbital, pentobarbital (Nembutal), amobarbital (Amytal), tuinal, and other barbiturate-like drugs. The toxic effects of these drugs cause similar symptoms as the benzodiazepines. They cause drowsiness, euphoria, emotional lability, poor judgment, and decreased blood pressure, respirations, temperature, pulse, and urinary output. Respiratory and cardiac failure can occur with an overdose. Accidental overdoses are fairly common as the individual cannot remember how much or when he or she has taken the drug.

Opiates are commonly used analgesics and are often abused and cause addiction. The most commonly abused opiates are morphine, heroin, hydromorphone (Dilaudid), methadone, and, more recently, designer drugs. They affect the CNS receptors, respiratory system, and peripheral nervous system.

Preventive Measures

People who use and abuse depressants are usually obtaining the drugs through illegal methods. Preventive measures can be effective when the drugs are prescribed and education is provided to the client about the effects and side effects. Working with law enforcement agencies can help curb some of the illegal drug activity.

PRIMARY PREVENTION

Primary prevention methods used in preventing abuse of and addiction to depressants are similar to those used with other chemicals. It is important that the community health nurse assess the amount of use and the availability of the drugs in the community. Sources of information include emergency rooms, police departments, drug and alcohol counselors, and drug treatment programs. Benzodiazepines are prescribed for people suffering from anxiety, panic attacks, and other mental health problems. Educating the client regarding the importance of taking the medication as prescribed and the potential of the addictive quality of the medication is useful. The client should feel free to contact the prescribing physician if the medication is not working, rather than increase the dose or begin self-medicating. Pregnant women should be educated about the problems that can be caused by ingesting CNS depressants. These problems include the fact that the fetus will experience the same effects that the woman experiences. It is especially important for the community health nurse to be vigilant with older people, who often forget when they have taken their medication. They may also have adverse effects from the medication, which include confusion.

SECONDARY PREVENTION

Nurses often are confronted with problems associated with clients whom they suspect of having, or who have, problems of addiction to CNS depressants. If the nurse believes that a client is abusing any of the depressants, it is important that the client be medically withdrawn and detoxified from the chemical. Benzodiazepine withdrawal is similar to alcohol withdrawal. The withdrawal symptoms are anxiety, tremors, diaphoresis, increased vital signs, and possible seizures. Withdrawal from opiates causes "flulike" symptoms, including nausea, vomiting, muscle aching and cramping, rhinorrhea, diaphoresis, dilated pupils, piloerection, diarrhea, fever, insomnia, yawning, irritability, increased sensitivity to pain, and "craving." Gradual tapering of the chemical may be indicated but is more safely done in a medical facility than on a self-monitored outpatient basis, which can be risky for the client and the family. It is relatively easy to access chemicals illegally, so it is important that treatment be started immediately after the withdrawal is completed.

TERTIARY PREVENTION

Tertiary prevention includes ongoing support groups and staying away from places and people who might cause the client to remember past use and cause cravings. The family will need ongoing support. The individual must be encouraged to share with his or her physician and care providers that he or she once had a substance abuse problem so that they will not inadvertently be given a prescription for their drug of choice, thus starting the cycle over again. There may be long-term health problems related to the addiction, including hepatitis, AIDS, lung problems, heart problems, and other systemic disorders. Community health nurses will provide nursing care to clients with these long-term problems.

Role of the Community Health Nurse

Many people do not know what can be done for someone who is addicted to depressants. The community health nurse is in a unique position to provide education and information about the effects and side effect of these drugs and can help assess the level of use and/or abuse. Helping the family or client access appropriate referral sources and giving the client and family support are important activities of the nurse.

STIMULANTS

People use stimulants for a variety of reasons: for recreational purposes to "get high," for weight loss to decrease the appetite, and to increase energy levels. Chemicals used include methylphenidate (Ritalin), cocaine, and crack (the solid form of cocaine). Crack and cocaine are used and abused by all age and income groups. Because cocaine costs more than crack, cocaine is most likely to be used and abused by people with higher income levels. Cocaine and crack stimulate the CNS, peripheral nervous system, and cardiovascular system. Cardiac arrest and heart failure are not uncommon side effects of cocaine and crack use. Cocaine blocks reabsorption of the neurotransmitter dopamine by nerve cells, or neurons, in one of the brain's key pleasure centers. There is buildup of dopamine in the space between the nerve cells, which causes stimulation of the receiving neurons (*NIDA Notes,* 1999).

Most people who use cocaine or crack also use either marijuana or alcohol to counteract the effects of cocaine. Crack and cocaine are particularly life-threatening when first administered and the "rush" occurs. Nurses need to identify what depressant the client is using to counteract the impact of the cocaine. If the client uses alcohol, there is a chance that alcohol withdrawal symptoms will appear. The addicting feature of crack and cocaine is the need of the addict to increase the dose to intensify and prolong the euphoric effects.

Cocaine appears to affect the fetus, causing children to have problems with attention, alertness, and intelligence (Zickler, 1999). Longitudinal studies are under way to identify the long-term impact of cocaine on the fetus and, subsequently, on children born to mothers who were using cocaine. There are problems with the samples because most cocaine users also use other drugs; researchers have trouble deciding which drugs cause some of the CNS problems in children.

More individuals are using amphetamines and methamphetamines. They are readily available, fairly inexpensive, and easy to manufacture in unsophisticated laboratories. These stimulants produce euphoria, grandiosity, increased energy, suppressed appetite, aggressive feelings, and paranoia. They increase the blood pressure and heart and respiration rates, cause pupils to dilate, and cause depression after the initial rush. Amphetamines and methamphetamines are used at "rave parties," among college students and others. Methamphetamine is referred to by various street names, including "ice," "crystal," "glass," and "crank." It is stronger in its effects than amphetamines. Methamphetamines are being used more and more by youth and young women as a weight-loss agent. There has been a significant increase in the number of young people referred for treatment in the last few years.

It is very difficult to keep track of all the drugs that are used by various people or groups of people. Immigration not only brings new people into the country, it also brings drugs that are not familiar in this country. One such drug that has entered the scene is "Khat" (pronounced "cot"), which is grown in East Africa, southern Arabia, and the Middle East. It is used socially and medicinally for its stimulant properties. Cathinone is the active ingredient and is only found in the fresh Khat leaves. It must be shipped promptly and wrapped in plastic or fresh banana leaves (Falkowski, 1998).

It is often very difficult for the nurse to get accurate information from an individual when he or she is using these drugs. The only thing a nurse might be able to assess is the level of consciousness, the affect, and the mood the individual is displaying.

Preventive Measures

Stimulants are usually received by the addict from illegal sources. Some of these drugs are manufactured in unsophisticated laboratories. Prevention includes working with law enforcement agencies and communities to force drug dealers out of neighborhoods by exposing their activities and by arresting the dealers. Education of the community about the dangers of various stimulants can decrease the sale of these drugs by preventing youth from engaging in drug use and sales.

PRIMARY PREVENTION
Community health nurses working with other community agencies can identify high-risk populations and can provide information about stimulants. Parents and community members should be informed about the availability of stimulants in their communities. They should be educated to identify the effects of stimulants. Young people in the community are especially vulnerable as they experiment with stimulants. Another aspect that the community will have to deal with is the illegal dealing of drugs. Drug dealers often recruit young people to sell drugs on the streets. The lure for young people is easy money, which is not available through jobs in poor neighborhoods.

The community health nurse can be alert to possible drug dealing and crack houses in the neighborhoods where he or she is visiting clients. Working closely with the police can help to eliminate some of the dangers of drugs in communities. Community health nurses can work with other community agencies to help provide job opportunities to youth. These efforts are working in many neighborhoods where youth are providing much-needed services, such as doing work for the elderly. These activities help to maintain the elderly in their homes longer while providing youth with meaningful activities and preventing them from getting involved in illegal activities.

Another primary prevention activity focuses on providing a "sense of belonging," which many youth feel is lacking in their lives. This makes gang membership very attractive as the gang provides the sense of belonging. Faith communities and community centers provide activities that help youth feel a sense of belonging and are excellent referral sources for the community health nurse. Parenting courses are available in many communities to help parents and adolescents communicate more effectively and will help prevent youth from feeling alienated from their parents. In many communities the community health nurse provides parenting classes.

SECONDARY PREVENTION
Stimulants are extremely addicting. People who are addicted to stimulants, especially crack and cocaine, have a difficult time staying drug free. The community health nurse will find that addicts spend more and more money on the drug of choice. The effects of crack and cocaine are so short-lived that the addict rapidly increases his or her daily dosage. The addict's days are filled with activities that are directed at getting the next "fix." The addict is often malnourished because all his or her money goes for drugs. People are often driven into prostitution and other illegal activities to support their habit.

The nursing assessment must be comprehensive, including questions about sexual practices, sexually transmitted diseases, and safe sex practices. It is also important to assess how the children are being cared for when the mother is away from home. Are the children left alone? Are they left with someone the mother knows and trusts? Assessing the situation for safety and the nutritional status of the mother and children is a high priority. The nurse assesses for bruising or any other signs of abuse or neglect. If there are concerns about child abuse and/or neglect, you are required to report these findings to the child protection agency (see Chapters 25 and 27).

One of the problems with individuals who are addicted to crack and cocaine is that there are often children living in very unsafe situations. Community health nurses often receive referrals to these residences to assess the health of children. The safety of the children and the nurse must be assessed. It may be necessary to do joint visits with other nurses, child protection workers, or police officers. There is always a dilemma: should the nurse attempt to establish a trusting relationship with the mother who is living in the crack house, or is it so unsafe that it is better to involve the police immediately and have the children removed from the home? These are hard decisions for the community health nurse because often the mother will view the nurse as safe and a helper. It is also possible to negotiate with the mother to meet her someplace other than her residence, which may allow for better communication and safety. It is especially important to try to get the pregnant mother into prenatal care as early as possible and into treatment. Many more treatment programs are now available for pregnant women who have children. These may be outpatient programs that provide day care or inpatient programs with facilities for day care and some kind of communal living for mothers and their children.

TERTIARY PREVENTION
Relapse, or returning to drug use, is very common among individuals who are addicted to crack and cocaine. To stay drug free the individual will have to change his or her life style, which includes developing friendships with people who are sober; he or she may have to move away from the neighborhood because there are too many triggers or reminders that

cause cravings. Much is still not understood about the causes of relapse, but it is known that abstinence is the only way to ensure recovery.

Many people suffer from the residual effects of their drug use. These individuals may be referred to the community health nurse to administer care related to a medical problem. Some clients have had seizures, heart attacks, or gunshot wounds due to their drug activity. Some of these individuals have adjusted to their disability, whereas others are angry and have made poor adjustments. Often these individuals are young adults who are not able to lead a normal life due to their disability. Medication compliance, rehabilitation, sober social support systems, relapse programs, and aftercare groups are all important factors in helping the addict remain sober and lead as normal a life as possible.

The Role of the Community Health Nurse

There are various activities the community health nurse can perform related to persons addicted to stimulants. The nurse can provide the community with information about the availability of stimulants and the signs and symptoms of stimulant intoxication, as well as work to provide youth with activities that help them feel they belong to the family and community. Nurses can work with women to help them obtain access to drug treatment and prenatal services. Children are often in need of safe housing; by working with other community agencies the nurse can help provide safety for children. The nurse is often called on to provide nursing care to people who have health problems related to their drug use.

GAMBLING

Over the last two decades gambling has become a large-scale issue and is recognized as being potentially addictive. The etiology of gambling appears to be somewhat more evasive to researchers than the etiology of substance abuse. Some theories suggest that there are sociological, biological, and psychological processes interacting with respect to the etiology of problem gambling (Henry, 1994). Researchers are studying the affect that gambling has on the brain and the neurotransmitters. It appears that many people experience a rush, which seems to be associated with the "process" rather than the "win." Often people will "chase," which means they will return the next day to win back losses. Until recently, most studies of gambling behavior had been conducted on the male population. One study conducted on 40 problem gamblers in an outpatient treatment program suggested that the reasons for gambling were a desire for excitement or to win; risk-taking; an attempt to change mood states, especially boredom or depression; an escape; and to relieve physical pain (Specker et al., 1996). Female gamblers have a higher percentage of psychiatric hospitalizations and suicide attempts than male gamblers. It appears that men seek treatment more than women. In one outpatient program, 80% of the clients were men and 20% were women. One study conducted in New Jersey high schools showed that of over 800 students, 91% had gambled at least once in their lifetime, 86% had gambled in the past year, and 32% gambled once a week. Over 5% showed signs of pathological gambling.

There has been an increase in problem gambling with the increased availability of gambling opportunities. The elderly and poor populations are often the target of gambling establishments through advertisements and free bus transportation to casinos. Gambling provides older adults with an opportunity to fill their idle time, socialize with other people, and possibly win some money to supplement their incomes.

Preventive Measures

There has been increasing concern about problem gambling and the affect it has on individuals, families, and communities. Some state lottery organizations have begun placing advertisements warning people to be cautious when buying lottery tickets. Many people buy numerous tickets in the hope that they will have a better chance at winning the lottery. Public education is helpful to warn people of the potential dangers of gambling. Education should start with youth, who are gambling at greater rates than ever before.

PRIMARY PREVENTION
When doing the community assessment, you will need to identify the opportunities for people to gamble. Are there many opportunities to play the lottery? Are there casinos near the community with easy access such as free transportation? Are there pull-tabs in the bars and restaurants? Then you will have to identify at-risk populations. Are there large numbers of idle elderly and poor people in the population? Are there buses of people bound for casinos? What other activities are being provided for high-risk populations?

Gambling is not just a problem of the elderly and the poor populations. Data may be available from state gambling organization, treatment programs, and the court system to help with your community assessment. This information will help you focus your primary prevention strategies on at-risk populations. Excellent educational material is available, and in some communities speakers are available to discuss their own experiences with a gambling problem.

SECONDARY PREVENTION
When the nurse assesses the family or individual, it is important to assess for all addictions, including gambling. In one study of 30 people recruited through advertising, 67% reported a gambling problem, 60% had a lifetime mood disorder, and 64% had a lifetime substance-use disorder (Black & Moyer, 1998).

Skills for the nurse include observation, assessment, and careful attention to the client's history. Duncan has identified

10 key points to help in assessing whether gambling has become a problem (Duncan, 1996) (Display 35–3). Another assessment tool that might be helpful is the South Oaks Gambling Screen (SOGS), developed by Dr. Sheila Blume and Henry Lesieur (Lesieur & Blume, 1987). Depending on the individual, the community health nurse may want to leave an assessment tool with the client; this will provide for more privacy, and the client may feel less shame and fill out the tool more honestly. It is very important for the nurse to maintain a non-judgmntal attitude, allowing the individual to be more open and honest. The assessment must include a suicide and chemical dependency assessment. Lesieur states that, "Gambling did not replace alcohol abuse, it joined it" (Lesieur & Blume, 1987).

There is a high rate of suicide among problem gamblers, particularly women who are also using substances. The client may need help both with the gambling addiction and with other mental health issues. It will be important for you to work with the client to obtain the appropriate help. Gamblers Anonymous (GA), a self-help group based on the principles of Alcoholic Anonymous, is available in most communities. There are now more programs available, both inpatient and outpatient, for problem gamblers.

Withdrawal from gambling poses some of the same symptoms as withdrawal from chemicals. Some of the symptoms that have been reported are restlessness, irritability, and "cravings." It is important for the family to be aware of these symptoms as they are common during withdrawal.

DISPLAY 35–3. Nine Key Indicators of Pathological Gambling

Skills in identifying compulsive gambling revolve around observation, assessment, and careful attention to detail in a client's history. The following nine key points help in establishing whether the person's gambling behavior is pathological:

- Preoccupation with gambling and dreaming of the "big win"
- Concealment of gambling behavior; loss of money and defaults
- Increasing the frequency and quantity of bets to get a buzz
- A history of failed attempts at controlling or curtailing gambling
- "Withdrawal-like" symptoms such as headache, irritability, restlessness, agitation, and feeling on edge when reducing or curtailng gambling
- Relief gambling to ease feelings of anxiety, tension, depression, and guilt
- Criminal activities sponsor gambling
- "Chasing," that is, betting in an attempt to recoup past and future losses and come good again
- A history of loss of friends', relatives', colleagues' support, employment and career opportunities, and social contact

(Duncan, S. [1996]. Just a flutter. *Nursing Standard, 10*(48), 22–23.)

Unlike with chemical dependency, the family of the gambler may be the last to know there is a problem. It is common for the gambler to keep his or her activities hidden from other family members for a long time. When the family discovers the gambling problem, they are often very angry and not supportive of the individual.

The family will find out that bills have not been paid; there may be legal problems or huge debts that the family is ill prepared to handle. It is important that the nurse understand and work with the family to help them cope with their anger in appropriate ways. It may be necessary for the family to seek financial counseling. There may be irreparable damage to relationships, so additional family counseling may be necessary.

TERTIARY PREVENTION

Considerations in providing tertiary care are the emotional and financial drain on the problem gambler and the family. The community health nurse will have to provide ongoing support to the client and family. It will be especially important if the gambler also has had a chemical dependency problem, as alcoholics are more likely to relapse when they have a gambling problem. After the client has been through treatment, it is important to provide support to the client so that he or she will maintain abstinence from gambling. There are as many opportunities to gamble as there are to use substances, so it will be necessary for the client to establish relationships with people who do not gamble and who are in recovery. The client will most likely be faced with large debts, possible legal problems, and fragile relationships with family and old friends. Attending Gamblers Anonymous will be critical to maintaining abstinence.

OTHER ADDICTIONS

Community health nurses need to be aware of other types of addictions that can inhibit an individual's ability to lead a healthy lifestyle. There are many addictions that can affect a person's quality of life, including work, exercise, shopping, sex, food (often classified in the literature as eating disorders), and in recent years television, video games, the Internet, and—last but not least—day trading on the stock market via the Internet. The community health nurse will include in a comprehensive assessment information about numerous types of addictions.

GLOBALIZATION OF ADDICTION PROBLEMS

Addiction problems are not unique to the U.S. There has been concern about gambling in other countries, including England and Canada, where research is being conducted on the reasons people become addicted to gambling. Much of the research currently being conducted looks at the physiological aspects, including a possible genetic link or a predisposition to addictions. Many countries are struggling with chemical addiction problems and laws governing the use, sale, and availability of chemicals. History has shown that many countries have outlawed certain drugs, but they are still being imported illegally.

There are many issues involved in the use and abuse of drugs. Few incentives are available for the people of Colombia who raise coca to replace their cash crop with something else; any other crop would not produce the same income. The farmers are often very poor but are enticed by drug lords to continue growing coca. There is so much corruption related to drugs, especially cocaine, that many people working in governments are also involved in the illegal activities of selling and distributing drugs. Curbing drug traffic from country to country is very difficult, and it is costly to enforce drug laws. Countries have different laws regarding legal and illegal drugs, so there is inconsistency among these laws. This makes drug enforcement next to impossible. The U.S. spends much money on trying to curb drug trafficking across the borders and at airports; this expenditure has still not made a dent in the illegal drugs coming into our country. Poor countries do not have the sophistication or the resources to fight drug trafficking.

SUMMARY

Many clients the community health nurse will encounter will have some kind of an addiction problem. It is important for the community health nurse to assess clients for their use of addictive substances and for addictive behaviors. Some of these behaviors include addiction to chemicals, food, sex, gambling, computer games, the Internet, and day trading on the stock market. There are also certain people and populations who are at high risk for addiction problems. Various factors may contribute to addictions. Among them are a family history of drug or alcohol abuse, drug experimentation, stress relief, chronic pain, psychological disturbances, advertising of substances and gambling opportunities, poverty and minority status, abusive relationships, and peer pressure. Addiction problems are a significant public health problem affecting all ages and socioeconomic levels that often result in serious health and social consequences.

The most common addictions are chemical addictions. Drugs used by people with chemical addiction problems fall into several categories: depressants (such as alcohol and benzodiazepines) slow down the central nervous system; hallucinogens (such as LSD) stimulate the central nervous system; inhalants (such as paint and paint thinner) provide stimulation, then cause depression; narcotics (such as heroin) depress the central nervous system, relieving pain and inducing sleep; steroids build muscle and body tissue; stimulants (such as caffeine or cocaine) stimulate the central nervous system; and marijuana promotes euphoria and sensory perception.

Gambling has become another major community health problem, causing legal and financial problems for the individual and the family. More gambling opportunities are available in communities; thus, there is an increase in the number of people who become addicted. Data show that more adolescents are becoming involved in gambling.

The community health nurse will want to access the resources in the community that are available for people with addiction problems. People who have addiction problems experience many health and social problems. Among them are various organ (heart, lung, liver) diseases and cancer, depression, psychoses, poverty, unemployment, family disruption, stigma, homelessness, violence, and crime. The community health nursing actions aim at primary, secondary, and tertiary prevention. They accomplish this through educational programs, assessing the needs of clients and families, assisting them to find healthier ways to cope, and working collaboratively with other professionals to improve existing services and develop needed ones.

ACTIVITIES TO PROMOTE CRITICAL THINKING

1. Describe the possible political connections between the repeal of Prohibition and the economy of the nation.
2. Discuss answers to the following questions:
   a. What were the issues the nation was facing during Prohibition?
   b. What are some reasons alcohol and tobacco are not restricted like other chemicals?
   c. Why is it so hard to control cocaine production and trafficking?
   d. Why are people (adults) admitted to chemical dependency programs covered under strict federal confidentiality laws?
   e. What are the economic and social ramifications of legalizing all drugs?
   f. What are the economic and social ramifications of gambling?
3. Using the Internet, locate local and regional substance abuse treatment programs. Download to keep a file as a resource for clients.

REFERENCES

Allen, K.M. (1996). *Nursing care of the addicted client.* Philadelphia: Lippincott-Raven.

American Psychiatric Association. (1995). Diagnostic criteria. From *Diagnostic and statistical manual of mental disorders* (4th ed.). Washington, D.C.: American Psychiatric Association.

Anderson, A. (1990). The postoperative client in withdrawal on a general medical-surgical unit. In L. Jack (Ed.). *Nursing care planning with the addicted client, Vol. II* (pp. 147–165). Skokie, IL: Midwest Educational Associates.

Baer, J., Barr, H., Bookstein, F., Sampson, P., & Streissguth, A.P. (1998). Prenatal alcohol exposure and family history of alcoholism in the etiology of adolescent alcohol problems. *Journal of Studies on Alcohol, 59*(5), 533.

Black, D.W., & Moyer, T. (1998). Clinical features and psychiatric comorbidity of subjects with pathological gambling behavior. *Psychiatric Services, 49*(11), 143–149.

Brustuen, S. & Gabriel, G. (1991). *Pathological gambling and chemical dependency: Similarities and unique characteristics.* Granite Falls, MN: Project Turnabout/Vanguard.

Centers for Disease Control. (1997). Alcohol consumption among pregnant and childbearing-aged women: United States, 1991 to 1995. *MMWR, 46*(16), 346–350. http://www.cdc.gov/epo/mmwr/preview/mmwrhtml/00047306.htm

Duncan, S. (1996). Just a flutter. *Nursing Standard, 10*(48), 22–23.

Ewing, J. (1984). Detecting alcoholism: The CAGE questionnaire. *Journal of the American Medical Association, 252*(14), 1905–1907.

Falkowski, C. (1998). *Drug abuse trends: Minneapolis/St. Paul.* Center City, MN: Hazelden Institute, Butler Center for Research and Learning.

Hanson, G., & Venturelli, P. (1995). *Drugs and society* (4th ed.). Boston: Jones and Bartlett.

Jellinek, E.M. (1946). Phases in the drinking history of alcoholics: An analysis of a survey conducted by the official organ of Alcoholics Anonymous. *Quarterly Journal of Studies on Alcohol, 7,* 188.

Johnston, L.D., O'Malley, P.M., & Bachman, J.G. (1999). *National survey results on drug use from the Monitoring the Future study, 1975–1998. Volume I: Secondary school students* (NIH Publication No. 99–4660). Bethesda: National Institute on Drug Abuse: http://www.isr.umich.edu/src/mtf/

Lambers, D., & Clark, K. (1996). The maternal and fetal physiological effects of nicotine. *Seminars in Perinatology, 20*(2), 115–126.

Leavell, H. R. & Clark, E. G. (1965). *Preventive medicine for the doctor in your community.* New York: McGraw-Hill.

Lesieur, H., Blume, S., & Zoppa, R. (1986). Alcoholism, drug abuse and gambling. *Alcoholism: Clinical and Experimental Research, 10*(1), 33–38.

Lesieur, H., & Blume, S. (1987). The South Oaks Gambling Screen (SOGS): A new instrument for identification of pathological gamblers. *American Jourrnal of Psychiatry, 144,* 1184–1188.

Merriam Webster's collegiate dictionary (10th ed.). Springfield, MA: Merriam Webster.

Moreno, I., Suiz, R.J., & Lopez-Ibor, J.J. (1991). Serotonin and gambling dependence. *Human Psychopharmacology: Clinical and Experimental, 6*(Suppl.), 912.

Morse, R., & Flavin, D. (1992). The definition of alcoholism. *Journal of the American Medical Association, 268*(8), 1012–1014.

National Clearinghouse for Alcohol and Drug Information (NCAD) (1999). *Straight facts about drugs and alcohol.* Rockville, MD: National Clearinghouse for Alcohol and Drug Information. http://www.health.org/pubs/strafact/straight.htm

NIDA Notes (1999). New report provides information on cocaine abuse and treatment. *NIDA Notes, 14*(3). http://165.112.78.61/NIDANotes/NNVoll4N3/Tearoff.html

Prochaska, J.P., & DiClemente, C.C. (1992). Stages of change in the modification of problem behaviors. In M. Hersen, R.M. Eisler,& P.M. Miller (Eds.). *Progress in behavior modification* (pp. 184–214). Sycamore, IL: Sycamore Press.

Specker, S.M., Carlson, G.A., Edmonson, K.M., Johnson, P.E., & Marcotte, M. (1996). Psychopathology in pathological gamblers seeking treatment. *Journal of Gambling Studies, 10,* 67–81.

U.S. Department of Health and Human Services (2000). *Healthy People 2010 objectives* (conference edition in two volumes). Washington, D.C.: U.S. Government Printing Office.

U.S. Department of Health and Human Services, Centers for Disease Control and Prevention. (1994). *Preventing tobacco use among young people: A report of the Surgeon General.* Washington, D.C.: U.S. Government Printing Office.

Vaillant, G. (1983). *The natural history of alcoholism.* Cambridge, MA: Harvard University Press.

Winters, K.C., Latimer, W.W., & Stinchfield, R.D. (1999). *Screening and assessing adolescent substance involvement.* Minneapolis, MN: Department of Psychiatry, University of Minnesota.

Zickler, P. (2000). NIDA studies clarify effects of prenatal cocaine exposure. *NIDA Notes, 14*(3), 1–4. http://165.112.78.61/NIDANotes/NNVoll4n3/Prenatal.html

SUGGESTED READING

Addiction's path. (1997). *Brain Briefings* [on-line]. http://www.sfn.org/briefings/addiction.html

Blume, S.B. (1988). Current trends explored in compulsive gambling. *Psychiatric Times: Medicine and Behavior, 28.*

Butler, C., Rollnick, S., & Stott, N. (1996). The practitioner, the patient and resistance to change: Recent ideas on compliance. *Canadian Medical Association Journal, 154*(9), 1357–1362.

Chang, G., Wilkins-Haug, L., Berman, S., Goetz, M.A., Behr, H., & Hiley, A. (1998). Alcohol use and pregnancy: Improving identification. *Obstetrics and Gynecology, 91*(6), 892–989.

Ciliska, D., Hayward, S., Thomas, H., Mitchell, A., Dobbins, M., Underwood, J., Rafael, A., & Martin, E. (1996). A systematic overview of the effectiveness of home visiting as a delivery strategy for public health nursing interventions. *Canadian Journal of Public Health, 87*(3), 193–198.

Coles, C.D., Russell, C.L., & Schuetze, P. (1997). Maternal substance use: Epidemiology, treatment outcome, and developmental effects: An annotated bibliography, 1995. *Substance Use and Misuse, 32*(2), 149–168.

Council on Child and Adolescent Health (1998). American Academy of Pediatrics: The role of home-visitation programs in improving health outcomes for children and families. *Pediatrics, 101*(3), 486–489.

Curry, M.A. (1998). The interrelationships between abuse, substance use, and psychosocial stress during pregnancy. *Journal of Obstetrical, Gynecologic, and Neonatal Nursing, 27,* 692–699.

DiClemente, C.C. (1993). Changing addictive behaviors: A process perspective. *Current Directions in Psychological Science, 2*(4), 101–106.

Faden, V.B., Graubard, B.I., & Dufour, M. (1997). The relationship of drinking and birth outcome in a U.S. national sample of expectant mothers. *Pediatric and Perinatal Epidemiology, 11,* 167–180.

Garwick, A.W., Kohrman, C., Wolman, C., & Blum, R.W. (1998). Families' recommendations for improving services for children with chronic conditions. *Archives of Pediatric Adolescent Medicine, 152,* 440–448.

Gruenewald, P.J. (1998). Community-based prevention programs. *The National Clearinghouse for Alcohol and Drug Information* [on-line]. http://www.health.org/nasadad2.htm

Hutchins, E., & Dipietro, J. (1997). Psychosocial risk factors associated with cocaine use during pregnancy: A case-control study. *Obstetrics and Gynecology, 90*(1), 142–147.

Jones, H.E., & Balster, R.L. (1998). Inhalant abuse in pregnancy. *Substance Abuse in Pregnancy, 25*(1), 153–167.

Keitner, N.L. (1997). Catastrophic consequences secondary to psychotropic drugs, parts I and II. *Psychopharmacology Update, 35*(5), 41–50.

Kindt, J.W. (1994). The negative impacts of legalized gambling on businesses. *University of Miami Business Law Journal, 14*(2), 93–124.

Lesieur, H.R., Cross, J., Frank, M., Welch, M., White, C.M., Rubenstein, G., Moseley, K., & Mark, M. (1990). *Gambling and pathological gambling among university students.* Paper presented at the International Conference on Gambling and Risk Taking, London, England, August 1990.

Lesieur, H.R., & Klein, R. (1987). Pathological gambling among high school students. *Addictive Behaviors, 12,* 129–135.

Lesieur, H.R., & Rosenthal, R.J. (1991). Pathological gambling: A review of the literature (prepared for the American Psychiatric Association Task Force on DSM-IV Committee on Disorders of Impulse Control Not Elsewhere Classified). *Journal of Gambling Studies, 7*(1), 5–39.

Lesieur, H.R., & Rothschild, J. (1989). Children of Gamblers Anonymous members. *Journal of Gambling Behavior, 5*(4), 269–281.

Mattson, S.N., & Riley, E.P. (1998). A review of the neurobehavioral deficits in children with fetal alcohol syndrome or prenatal exposure to alcohol. *Alcoholism: Clinical and Experimental Research, 22*(2), 279–294.

Miller, W. (1986). Individual outpatient treatment of pathological gambling. *Journal of Gambling Behavior, 2*(2), 95–107.

Mosher, J.F. (1996). A public health approach to alcohol and other drug problems: Theory and practice. In F.D. Scutchfield & C.W. Keck (Eds.). *Principles of public health practice* (pp. 243–260). Albany, NY: Delmar Publishers.

National Association for Children of Alcoholics. *Children of alcoholics: Important facts. The National Clearinghouse for Alcohol and Drug Information* [On-line]. http://www.health.org/pubs/coa/impfacts.htm

Rollnick, S. (1996). Behavior change in practice: Targeting individuals. *International Journal of Obesity, 20*(Suppl. 1), S22–S26.

Sherman, D.K., McGue, M.K., & Iacono, W.G. (1997). Twin concordance for attention deficit hyperactivity disorder: A comparison of teachers' and mothers' reports. *American Journal of Psychiatry, 154*(4), 532–535.

Smith, B.A. (1998). The problem drinker's lived experience of suffering: An exploration using hermeneutic phenomenology. *Journal of Advanced Nursing, 27*(1), 213–222.

Sprauve, M.E., Lindsay, M.K., Herbert, S., & Graves, W. (1997). Adverse perinatal outcome in parturients who use crack cocaine. *Obstetrics and Gynecology, 89*(5), 674–678.

Streissguth, A.P., Bookstein, F.L., Barr, H.M., Press, S., & Sampson, P.D. (1998). A fetal alcohol behavior scale. *Alcoholism: Clinical and Experimental Research, 22*(2), 325–333.

Sumner, M.L. (1994). Clinical assessment of problem gamblers using the advanced integrated model of addition treatment. Paper presented at the National Conference on Gambling Behavior, Rimrock Foundation, Billings, Montana, July 1994.

Svikis, D., Henningfield, J., Gazaway, P., Huggins, G., Sosnow, K., Hranicka, J., Harrow, C., & Pickens, R. (1997). Tobacco use for identifying pregnant women at risk of substance abuse. *Journal of Reproductive Medicine, 42*(5), 299–302.

Teagle, S.E., & Brindis, C.D (1998). Substance use among pregnant adolescents: A comparison of self-reported use and provider perception. *Journal of Adolescent Health, 22,* 229–238.

Travers, K.D. (1997). Reducing inequities through participatory research and community empowerment. *Health Education and Behavior, 24*(3), 344–356.

Volberg, R.A., & Abbott, M.W. (1997). Gambling and problem gambling among indigenous peoples. *Substance Use and Misuse, 32*(11), 1525–1538.

Weinberg, N.Z. (1997). Cognitive and behavioral deficits associated with parental alcohol use. *Journal of the American Academy of Child and Adolescent Psychiatry, 36*(9), 1177–1187.

Werner, M.J., Walker, L.S., & Greene, J.W. (1996). Concurrent and prospective screening for problem drinking among college students. *Journal of Adolescent Health, 18,* 276–285.

Wiemann, C.M., & Berenson, A.B. (1998). Factors associated with recent and discontinued alcohol use by pregnant adolescents. *Journal of Adolescent Health, 22,* 417–423.

Young, N.K. (1997). Effects of alcohol and other drugs on children. *Journal of Psychoactive Drugs, 29*(1), 23–42.

Clients in Correctional Facilities

- Correctional facility
- Felony
- Forensics
- Jail
- Inmates
- Literacy
- Maximum security
- Minimum security
- Penitentiary
- Prison
- Recidivism

LEARNING OBJECTIVES

Upon mastery of this chapter, you should be able to:

- Define a variety of terms associated with correctional health care and correctional institutions.
- Describe the correctional culture and environment.
- Describe the history of correctional health care.
- Identify the key issues and challenges of correctional health care.
- List and describe at least four organizations associated with inmates of correctional facilities.
- Identify the communicable diseases and physical and mental health disorders commonly seen in correctional populations.
- Discuss the special areas of concern for nurses working with incarcerated women.
- Describe the role of the community health nurse while working with populations in correctional facilities.

Have you ever been inside a jail, prison, or other correctional facility? Do you know anyone who is incarcerated? Do you even know where your city or county's correctional facility is located? Have you ever considered a career in correctional nursing? If you answered "no" to all of these questions, you are not alone. To most people, correctional facilities, incarcerated populations, and the nurses who serve them are invisible. With our Western ideals of independence, we tend to dislike even thinking about those who have had their freedoms taken away from them. Nurses working with incarcerated clients thus face multiple challenges: the challenge of working in a physically and emotionally stressful environment, the challenge of working with a client population that most people would rather ignore, and the challenge of invisibility within their profession.

Nevertheless, correctional nursing can be an exciting opportunity to practice compassionate community health nursing. As we will see, the majority of prisoners have a history of poverty, substance abuse, physical and emotional abuse, and mental illness with episodic health care. Indeed, incarceration may represent the first time an inmate has received comprehensive, continuous health care or has had the opportunity to develop a therapeutic relationship with a nurse (Maeve, 1997). Correctional nursing also gives nurses an opportunity to apply the principles of public health and **forensics**—the science of health care jurisprudence where legal argument advocates for offenders—while practicing all their skills, including the therapeutic use of self (Miller, 1999).

In this chapter, we first examine basic concepts and terminology in correctional health care and describe the facilities' environment and inmates. We then review the history of correctional health care and explore the issues and challenges of correctional nursing. We also describe the health care concerns most common among inmate populations and take an in-depth look at the health care issues of women prisoners. Finally, we examine the roles of educator, client advocate, and discharge "bridge" that are so vital to community health nursing with the incarcerated population.

BASIC CONCEPTS IN CORRECTIONAL HEALTH CARE

Because most people have had little if any exposure to correctional issues, environments, or populations, we begin by reviewing some basic terminology and concepts.

Terminology of Corrections

A **correctional facility** is one whose primary objective is to provide safety to the public by incarcerating those who have committed crimes and who are deemed a threat to their community. People detained in correctional facilities are called **inmates** or offenders. More progressive institutions are moving toward the latter term. As indicated by the term correction, a correctional facility also ideally serves to improve inmates, to give them new perspectives and options so that upon their release they can begin to live as productive citizens. For many people, however, this ideal of improvement seems frivolous; they see correctional facilities as warehouses for "undesirable elements" and programs to improve inmates' physical and mental health, literacy, and employability as a waste of public funds.

Jails, also called *detention centers* or *holding cells,* are facilities where people accused of committing a crime await arraignment, the summons to appear in court to answer charges. Jails also confine individuals both before and after sentencing for minor offenses, called *misdemeanors,* and parole violations. In addition, in some communities it is not uncommon for intoxicated individuals to be put in jails overnight to "dry out." Incarceration for detainees generally ranges between a month and a year, although some stay fewer than 3 weeks; thus, jails often have a high turnover rate.

State departments of corrections (DOC) detain individuals convicted of crimes against the state. State DOC facilities are usually referred to as **prisons,** which are assigned a security level ranging from **minimum security** to **maximum security,** depending on the type of prisoners housed there. For example, prisoners who have committed **felonies,** serious crimes such as murder, rape, or burglary, are typically housed in maximum-security prisons.

The Federal Department of Corrections detains individuals who have committed crimes against the United States Government, as well as individuals who have committed interstate crimes. Most federal correctional facilities are called **peni-** **tentiaries** and are commonly referred to among prisoners as "the big house." Like state prisons, federal penitentiaries have a security level ranging from minimum to maximum.

Most states and counties also have prison camps that are available to minimum security-risk criminals. Such camps usually have a rehabilitative or work-related focus.

The Correctional Environment

The environment within which correctional nurses perform their duties differs greatly from that of the hospital, clinic, or home setting. In addition to a variety of unfamiliar rules and restrictions, the nurse in a correctional setting must adapt to constant security monitoring that may be unnerving for the novice. The nurse must also work to inspire hope in an atmosphere often filled with despair.

Overcrowding is another aspect of the typical correctional environment that the nurse must cope with. Indeed, 1998 became the year that the U.S. incarcerated 1 million nonviolent prisoners (Irwin, 2000). This statistic represents a threefold increase in prison and jail populations over the previous two decades and is a direct result of more stringent sentencing laws (described later in this chapter). In any environment where large numbers of people live together in small, confined quarters, the rapid spread of infectious diseases emerges as a public health concern. In addition, the increased rates of incarceration lead to increases in staffing needs, health care costs, and fragmentation of families and communities.

The "chain of command" within correctional institutions also differs greatly from that of traditional health care settings. Nurses generally report directly to the administrator of the correctional institution and, as employees, are bound to the rules of the institution, which are often made by non–health care personnel. A statement commonly heard from prisoners and staff within correctional facilities is, "This is the warden's house." The warden, or chief administrator, sets the rules that are to be followed. Thus, ethical dilemmas may arise when an inmate's health care needs require actions that challenge the institution's standard policies and procedures. In some situations, advance practice nurses report to a managed care agency specializing in correctional health care. This situation can allow nurses greater freedom to provide nursing care according to professional nursing standards. Even when the nurse is employed by the correctional facility, however, strict adherence to state nursing practice guidelines as well as to the ANA's *Scope and Standards of Nursing Practice in Correctional Facilities* (1995) will provide the foundation within which to accomplish the most therapeutic outcomes (Display 36–1).

Profile of the Inmate

Although precise numbers are difficult because of the high turnover rate, in 1999 there were approximately 600,000 peo-

DISPLAY 36–1. Guidelines for Correctional Nursing Practice

In the correctional health setting, the nurse:
1. Adapts to an environment of strict rules, regulations, and monitoring where client custody is of primary importance.
2. Expands the scope of nursing practice to meet the unique needs and demands of a prison population with a variety of physical and mental health conditions.
3. Utilizes the nursing process to assess, plan for, implement, and evaluate treatment, prevention, and health promotion services to individuals and groups of inmates.
4. Seeks to establish a trusting professional relationship and carry out needed teaching and counseling activities as inmates' length of incarceration permits.
5. Recognizes that health services are the nurse's sole responsibility and refrains from involvement in security or correctional procedures.
6. Seeks to ensure inmates' human rights and the provision of equitable health care, both in prison and upon release, through advocacy and collaborative efforts.
7. Exercises care to maintain professional conduct and personal safety.

ple incarcerated in city and county jails in the United States. In addition, the U.S. Bureau of Justice (1999) identified a combined state and federal prison population of over 1.2 million. Over 140,000, or approximately 10%, of these are federal prisoners (Federal Bureau of Prisons, 2000). Of these,

- 92% are male
- the average age is 37 years
- 34% are in high- or maximum-security institutions
- 40% have a sentence of 10 or more years
- 58% were convicted for drug trafficking or possession

Although European Americans make up the majority of federal prisoners (58%), African Americans are represented in numbers disproportionate to their prevalence in the population as a whole—39% in the 1999 study. Asian and Native American inmates make up roughly 2% each of the remaining federal prisoners. African American women are an especially over-represented minority: although they make up only 14.5% of the total U.S. population, they represent 52% of women incarcerated in jails, prisons, and penitentiaries (Human Rights Watch, 1996).

Many incarcerated individuals have a prior history of abuse, neglect, or other troubling circumstances in childhood. For example, children arrested for a violent crime had a history of abuse four times greater than that of the general population. A recent study demonstrated that exposure to childhood sexual abuse "conveys a greater risk for experi-

encing other violence, psychologic and physical morbidity, and high-risk behaviors" (Cohen et al., 2000, p. 564). Approximately 50% of juveniles incarcerated had a parent who was also incarcerated, and one-third were living in families without fathers when arrested.

Approximately 75% of prisoners incarcerated today are nonviolent offenders. Their offenses include drug trafficking and possession, robbery, arson, extortion, fraud, bribery, immigration offenses, and other nonviolent crimes. As noted earlier, violent felons who have committed crimes such as murder, rape, kidnapping, armed robbery, aggravated child molestation, aggravated sodomy, and aggravated sexual battery are usually incarcerated in different institutions from nonviolent offenders.

In many prison populations, there is a hierarchy of "prestige" related to the type of offense committed. In particular, sex offenders represent a broad and diverse segment of the correctional population often stigmatized by other inmates. Child molesters are even more discriminated against. Because crimes against children are considered by most inmates as the most despicable, child molesters are not only excluded from recreational activities and friendships but also are often harmed by fellow prisoners. Thus, the correctional nurse may need to take on an additional role as protector when caring for a child molester, for example, by scheduling appointments to avoid confrontations with other inmates. For both sex offenders and child molesters, outcome-based interventions designed with a clear understanding of the characteristics of the offender can play an important role in rehabilitation and secondary prevention.

EVOLUTION OF CORRECTIONAL HEALTH CARE

How health care is delivered within a correctional institution is often a reflection of the social and political milieu of the time. Understanding the history of prison health care as well as the development of legislation and professional organizations related to prisoners will provide insight into the current challenges of correctional nursing.

Historical Overview

Until recently prisons were designed to be punitive, and prisoners were considered to have forfeited all rights. Consequently, incarcerated individuals were often mistreated, tortured, and malnourished; denied exercise, sanitation, and the means for basic hygiene; and had no rehabilitative care or health care. Because of these deplorable conditions, prisoners historically have been at high risk for plagues, sexually transmitted diseases, tuberculosis, typhus, gangrene, and scurvy.

The history of corrections in the U.S. is tied to that of England and Europe. In 1775 an epidemic of typhus hit the U.S.

and Europe, prompting reforms in hygienic practices in institutions, including poor houses, hospitals, and prisons. Delousing upon arrival to prisons, issuing clean clothing, and being examined by a physician were practices that originated during this time, along with crusades to improve prisoners' diets.

In the 1800s mortality attributable to the social and health conditions of prisons was again examined. For the first time, epidemiologic studies of prisoners were conducted. In particular, the work of Louis René Villerme led to reduced crowding in prisons, exercise, increased lighting and ventilation, provision of fresh foods, opportunities for productive work, and fair treatment of prisoners. It was believed that these reforms would improve prisoners' mental outlook and that this would contribute to their rehabilitation.

It was also at this time that physicians began to treat prisoners with more regularity and to re-examine them just prior to their release, a practice that has continued to this day. Additionally, reform-minded physicians noted that medical under-staffing was contributing to a severe lack of health education among prisoners.

In 1929 the U.S. published 15 reports that eventually gave rise to correctional care as it is practiced today: the report of the National Society on Penal Information and the 14 reports of the Wickersham Commission, appointed by President Herbert Hoover. These reports were the first national and comprehensive survey of the American criminal justice system and recommended changes in parole, probation, and incarceration treatments that laid the foundation for significant correctional care reform.

In 1955 the First United Nations Congress on the Prevention of Crime and the Treatment of Offenders adopted a set of international standards for the treatment of incarcerated persons. These standards, which were updated in 1977, provide guidelines on food, clothing, exercise, health care, discipline, books, religion, contact with the outside world, and many other aspects of prison life. The fundamental thread throughout this document is respect for the humanity and dignity of all prisoners and detainees regardless of race, religion, color, creed, political affiliation, gender, or economic status.

In 1975 the National Institute of Law Enforcement and Criminal Justice published another report that directly addressed the issues of health care within correctional institutions (Brecher & Della Penna, 1975). *The Prescriptive Package: Health Care in Correctional Institutions* was a landmark document calling for significant social and medical reforms and providing guidance on organizing medical services within prisons and jails (King, 1998). In particular, it advocated the following actions:

- Utilization of outside health care agencies in an effort to increase the variety of services offered, decrease costs, and decrease the isolation of health care personnel within correctional facilities
- Collaboration with community liaisons in all aspects of correctional care, including ties to medical and nursing schools and to professional organizations
- Development of a high-quality, consistent, and

reliable system of health care as the antidote for numerous class-action suits plaguing prison administrations
- Improvements in medical record systems

The *Prescriptive Package* has resulted in more humane and expert health care of prisoners. It has also increased the utilization of health care agencies, which in turn has increased health care workers' autonomy to provide quality care. On the other hand, the *Prescriptive Package* has been criticized for its lack of emphasis on rehabilitative and mental-health care, issues that were found in the 1929 reports.

Correctional health care today continues to improve, but many problems remain. The relationship between health care provider agencies and correctional institutions is still undefined. Overcrowding has increased in the last decade, as has the number of HIV-infected prisoners. Perhaps the greatest problem is correctional care workers' lack of a united professional voice, leading to a lack of comprehensive standards of care for incarcerated persons. The bureaucracy of federal, state, and local policies and procedures in the different correctional facilities further compounds this fragmentation.

Legislation Affecting Correctional Health Care

The Eighth Amendment to the Constitution guarantees the right of prisoners to a safe and humane environment. The 1976 U.S. Supreme Court *Estelle v. Gamble* decision further clarified that correctional facilities could not deliberately show indifference to serious medical needs of prisoners (Anno & Spencer, 1998). This decision opened the door to questions about what constitutes a minimum standard of health care for prisoners. As a result, community standards for health care began to be applied within correctional institutions.

In 1987, as part of the "War on Drugs," Congress passed legislation enacting stiffer prison sentences for trafficking in or possessing drugs. A further refinement of this law was the 1994 Violent Crime Control and Law Enforcement Act, commonly called the Crime Bill. It calls for mandatory sentencing for certain drug offenses, including a mandatory prison sentence for first-time possession of crack cocaine. These laws have contributed to the escalation in incarcerations seen in the last decade and the resulting overcrowding of correctional facilities across the country.

The 1994 Crime Bill also empowered the Federal Department of Justice to enforce the constitutional rights of incarcerated individuals through civil suits. This provision enables the Department to investigate and bring legal action against state institutions when there is a question of civil rights violations. This provision was weakened in 1996, however, with the Prison Litigation Reform Act. This newer law significantly decreases the ability of the federal courts, non-governmental organizations, and individuals to intervene in class-action suits pertaining to prison conditions. It does, however, require correctional institutions to be responsible for the quality of health care delivered to individuals while incarcerated.

Professional Organizations Affecting Inmates

Integral to correctional health care are many professional organizations and agencies. The official federal law enforcement agency is the National Institute of Law Enforcement and Criminal Justice, currently referred to as the National Institute of Justice (NIJ). Professional organizations contributing to correctional health care standards include the International Association of Forensic Nurses, the American Nurses Association, the American Public Health Association's Jail and Prison Health Council, the American Correctional Health Care Services Association, and the National Commission on Correctional Health Care. In addition, organizations such as the World Health Organization, United Nations, Amnesty International, and the Human Rights Watch Women's Rights Project monitor human rights of incarcerated persons internationally.

ETHICAL ISSUES IN CORRECTIONAL HEALTH CARE

The priority of the correctional system is confinement and security. The priority of the nurse is caring. Thus, correctional nurses often get caught in ethical dilemmas when security policies of the institution require actions that threaten the therapeutic nurse–client relationship. These actions include body searches (called "pat downs"), body-cavity searches, collection of forensic evidence, use of restraints and force, and writing up inmates' behavior or complaints. Many professional organizations suggest that, whenever possible, the primary caregiver who has developed a relationship of trust and respect with an inmate not be required to discipline that inmate or perform any of the above actions. Alternatively, performing such procedures with respect, sensitivity, and compassion can make them less traumatic for the inmate. Any procedure having to do with "chain of evidence" is done by outside health agencies, such as drawing blood for blood alcohol levels, which is done by a contractor who is not a jail medical department employee.

An ethical dilemma may also surface around the conflict between the imposition of a death penalty or life sentence versus the nursing goal of rehabilitation. At present, 38 states have death penalties, and over 400 executions have occurred in the last 25 years. Yet most professional health care organizations prohibit their members from participating in executions. The ANA states that it is "inappropriate for nurses practicing in corrections to participate in disciplinary decisions or committees or to participate directly or indirectly in executions by lethal injection" (ANA, 1995, p. 3). This situation prompts a variety of ethical questions for correctional nurses. Who will ensure compassionate care at the time of execution? Who will ensure that appropriate doses of medications are administered? Who will certify the death?

Confidentiality is another difficult issue, as privacy virtually does not exist within correctional institutions. For example, in many prisons care to inmates with HIV is provided in special HIV clinics; everyone knows who attends these clinics, yet the nurse must be careful not to reveal the name of anyone attending the clinic to any non-authorized person. However, the person in charge of the facility, the commander or warden, must be notified of all HIV-positive inmates in the facility. As in any setting, it is the responsibility of the nurse to be careful of where and when she or he speaks about confidential issues.

It may also be difficult for some nurses to remain objective and provide compassionate care while knowing the prisoner's criminal history. This may be especially true when the nurse cares for inmates who have committed murder, rape, or crimes against children. In most cases it is best and easiest to not know the charges. As we have emphasized earlier, strict adherence to state practice guidelines and nursing standards, coupled with outcome-oriented interventions, will help the nurse in these situations to provide appropriate, compassionate care.

Correctional nurses may also be required to provide care to inmates who exhibit a personal or sexual interest in them. It may help the nurse to remember that incarcerated adults have the same sexual needs and desires as the population at large; at the same time, the nurse must recognize that the prisoner's behavior is innapropriate. The importance of maintaining strict and specific boundaries without compromising the nurse–client relationship cannot be stressed enough. Inmates have poorly developed coping skills, often seek methods to hold staff hostage emotionally, and may have difficulty acknowledging the nurse's boundaries or limits. The best approach is to treat the inmate with respect and to avoid showing partiality or accepting gifts and favors from offenders.

These are just a few of the ethical issues that arise in correctional nursing. Resolving these issues and continuing to practice within corrections can be very difficult; however, active involvement in professional nursing associations and development of a support system of colleagues within correctional nursing can be extraordinarily beneficial in helping the nurse face these complex concerns.

In addition, correctional nurses should maintain accurate information regarding laws that influence their practice. Among the resources available are state bar association publications, state codes, publications of the state's Office of the Attorney General, federal and state registers, and case law. The computerized search tool called "Lexis" and a service from the Library of Congress called "Scorpio" are also helpful legal resources for nurses.

HEALTH CARE CONSIDERATIONS

The health care needs of incarcerated individuals pose a myriad of concerns. Prior to incarceration, prisoners may have had poor access to health care and unmet or unrecognized health care needs, including chronic systemic illnesses, traumatic injuries, substance abuse, mental illness, sexually transmitted diseases, and/or a history of physical or sexual abuse. In addition, because the prison population is aging, correctional nurses must address increased incidences of the acute and chronic illnesses common to all aging populations, as well as exacerbations of those illnesses that may be related to long-term incarceration.

Communicable Diseases in Correctional Facilities

It is difficult to ascertain the exact rates of communicable disease within correctional facilities because most do not require mandatory testing. This may be in part because mandatory testing can be considered an infringement of human rights; however, another factor is that if the facility has not identified a health problem, it has no obligation to treat it. For these reasons, diligent assessment, surveillance, and reporting are key tasks of the correctional nurse. These activities can assist not only in the detection and prevention of the spread of communicable disease but also in the development of educational programs and other initiatives for inmates and staff.

TUBERCULOSIS

Tuberculosis (TB) rates peaked in 1991 within correctional facilities in the U.S., then declined in the mid-1990s. It now appears to be on the rise again, particularly among border states, due to the entrance of illegal aliens from Third World countries. Tuberculosis remains the single most important communicable disease within correctional facilities today (Hammett, Harmon, & Maruschak, 1999). Confinement to relatively small areas assists in its spread by aerosol droplets. Multi-drug resistant TB (mTB) is an even more serious concern: currently, mTB is reported at a 7% level in state and federal prisons and 10% in jails.

Testing for TB is mandatory in 73% of all types of correctional facilities and occurs in 92% of state and federal prisons and 51% of jails upon admission. Thereafter, annual PPD screening for TB is mandated in 91% of state and federal prisons and 41% of jails. Health education regarding testing, identification, management, and policies for TB within correctional institutions for both inmates and staff are important roles for the correctional nurse. Investigation and follow-up on release are essential. Many non–English-speaking inmates have particular dilemmas with continuing treatment; the correctional nurse is their link to ongoing treatment and community health resources.

SEXUALLY TRANSMITTED DISEASES

Rates of sexually transmitted diseases (STDs) in prisons and jails are nearly double that of the population in general. Syphilis, gonorrhea, and chlamydia may be screened for upon admission to correctional facilities. The majority of prisons are in a difficult position with respect to sexual behavior and STDs: sex between inmates or between inmates and staff is a punishable crime in many jurisdictions, yet if sex is prohibited, the use of condoms is prohibited. Most prison officials consider condoms contraband that can be used to hide drugs or other illegal substances or objects. They also fear that condoms promote the message that sex among prisoners is acceptable. However, the prohibition of condoms is under review in many prison systems because of high rates of STDs and rising rates of HIV infection among prisoners.

HIV/AIDS

Only 16 states require mandatory testing for human immunodeficiency virus (HIV) upon admission to correctional facilities; however, many more states have voluntary testing, testing after an incident, or testing with medically related problems.

Prevalence rates vary widely around the U.S. Data from 1997 indicate that approximately 2.6% of state prisoners and 0.7% of federal prisoners are HIV-positive. These rates are significantly higher than in the general population (0.09%). AIDS was responsible for 29% of inmate deaths in state prisons in 1995 and is currently the leading cause of death for female inmates (CDC, 1999; Hammett, Harmon, & Maruschak, 1999).

HIV-infected inmates have the same health care needs as HIV-infected individuals in the general population, but those needs, because of their incarceration, may be more complex. Many inmates did not have continuous health care before they entered prison, and so their viral loads are often higher and they are generally sicker. Prisoners not on highly active anti-retroviral therapy (HAART) with elevated viral loads are also more susceptible to opportunistic infections (OI), including tuberculosis. They also have reduced treatment outcomes; are potentially more contagious to others during sexual intercourse, needle exchanges, and violent altercations (including biting); and are at higher risk for end-of-life complications. Finally, they may be more likely to miss their medications, take their medications improperly, or be unable to meet the complex dietary needs that many HIV medications require. Indeed, educating prison staff and inmates regarding the importance of strict compliance with all aspects of HIV medication administration is an essential responsibility of the correctional nurse. In addition, the nurse must address these issues:

- How to get offenders to volunteer for testing
- How to ensure that prisoners have HAART available during lockdowns and transfers
- How to ensure that prisoners have a pre-release plan that includes housing, employment, HIV clinic appointments, and medications for a month

Confidentiality is difficult to maintain within a prison. Many prisons contract out for HIV care, and leaving the institution to attend an outside HIV clinic instantly identifies a prisoner as HIV-positive. Such a label carries tremendous stigmatization from other inmates. Additionally, prisoners are often taken in shackles to these outside HIV clinics, where they feel that both their HIV-positive status and their status as a prisoner are "on display." Finally, prisoners may fear the loss of their partner or children outside the prison if their HIV status becomes known. Rather than endure such stigmatization, humiliation, and loss, many inmates will not disclose their HIV status, if known, or will not complain of symptoms that they fear will lead to a diagnosis of AIDS.

Other ethical issues related to the care of HIV-infected prisoners include the following:

- Notification of sexual partners or those who share needles
- Disclosure of status
- Methods for halting transmission via sexual intercourse or injecting drug use
- Post exposure
- Pregnancy and vertical transmission
- Access to medicines from clinical trials
- Discharge planning to provide for the optimal health of the client and the safety of the community

HEPATITIS

There is no mandatory testing in any state for hepatitis C virus (HCV), which often accompanies HIV. Currently, the vaccine available for HCV is unproved and not widely available; however, the Occupational Safety and Health Administration recommends that correctional staff receive hepatitis B vaccine. Once the hepatitis A and C vaccines have proven efficacy rates, they should be required of correctional staff. Hepatitis C threatens to become a growing problem in terms of both treatment costs and poor compliance. Health legislators will need to develop guidelines soon as the affected population is growing quickly.

Mental Illness in Correctional Facilities

Correctional care nursing includes caring for the mentally ill. The entire range of mental illnesses, including depression, bipolar disorder, post-traumatic stress disorder (PTSD), behavioral disorders, and schizophrenia, may be seen in the prison population as in the population at large. The risk of suicide attempts and completions is also of significant concern, and clients withdrawing from alcohol or drugs also have significant treatment needs. The nurse can oversee the development of written policies and guidelines for risk assessment and management of these inmates and assist with proper referal and transportation to medical facilities when needed. Nurses in correctional care, then, must be prepared to perform the assessments and interventions appropriate for nurses in psychiatric facilities (see Research: Bridge to Practice).

Correctional facilities have large populations of mentally ill persons whose mental health needs are often poorly addressed (Jordan, Schlenger, Fairbank, & Caddell, 1996). These people are incarcerated for behavior that generally results from their mental illness, and when they are released without adequate treatment or community follow-up the cycle tends to be repeated. It is a dangerous situation for the

RESEARCH Bridge to Practice

Keaveny, M.E., & Zauszniewski, J.A. (1999). Life events and psychological well-being in women sentenced to prison. *Issues in Mental Health Nursing, 20*(1), 73–89.

Women who are sentenced to serve time in prison are often severely depressed and anxious. The researchers in this study postulated that the women inmates' coping skills and events in their lives leading up to incarceration might influence their level of depression while in prison.

The researchers conducted a descriptive correlational study using a convenience sample of 62 incarcerated female offenders. The inmates being studied were all single, in their early 30s, unemployed, and receiving various kinds of financial support. The inmates were asked to identify events in their lives for the 12 months prior to incarceration that caused stress and required adaptation. On average, they reported 10 life events and an accumulated average of 354 life change units.

The study demonstrated a positive correlation between the number of life events the inmates experienced and their high levels of depression and anxiety. The researchers concluded that, at the time offenders were admitted to a correctional facility, nursing interventions to assist with coping and to offset offenders' feelings of loss, inadequacy, and powerlessness could help prevent serious levels of depression.

mentally ill as well as for the community. Mentally Ill Offenders' Diversion programs are slowly being developed in many states as well as in other countries to address this problem. These programs team mental health nurses and other mental health workers with the police to monitor and assist mentally ill offenders who are living in the community.

Family Considerations

The importance of providing support to the parents, partners, and children of inmates cannot be emphasized strongly enough. Assisting families to grieve over the loss of their loved one, deal with the embarrassment and humiliation that surrounds incarceration, and provide for the inmate's needs for love and belonging is an essential component of compassionate and effective nursing care. Inmates who receive no visitors or communication from "outside the walls" are at risk for suicidal behaviors, depression, and violence. When transportation or financial issues interfere with visitation, the correctional nurse can suggest community resources to assist the family.

The impact on children of incarceration of a parent is immeasurable. First, the loss of the parent's physical presence can create anxiety, fear, sadness, and anger. Explaining the absence to friends and schoolmates can cause the child deep humiliation. The child's attitude toward people in authority, including teachers and law-enforcement officials, may become fearful or resentful. These factors may influence the child to run away from home; engage in self-destructive behaviors such as drinking, drug use, sexual promiscuity, or suicide attempts; or commit petty crimes. As we noted earlier, many of the children of incarcerated parents go on to become criminals themselves. In consideration of these effects, the correctional nurse may wish to develop support groups for the partners and children of inmates, which can provide participants with a safe forum for dealing with their feelings, thoughts, and experiences following the incarceration. On a broader scale, nurses can advocate for the elimination of poverty conditions that spawn violence and crime.

WOMEN IN PRISON

There are approximately 138,000 women currently incarcerated in U.S. jails and prisons (Human Rights Watch, 1996). This number represents a 100% increase over a decade ago. About 85% of these women are mothers, the overwhelming majority of whom have children under the age of 18. An average of 6% to 10% of women enter prison pregnant, and there are 1300 live births and 900 miscarriages or abortions annually among female inmates (Richardson, 1998).

Some Gender Differences in Corrections

More women live in poverty, earning just 75¢ to every dollar that men earn (Census Bureau, 2000). Economic power buys better legal advice, which translates into reduced sentences for crimes. Women also tend to lack comprehensive knowledge about crimes in which they have participated. Thus, they have little information to trade for reduced sentences. This lack of power extends into the prison system, especially with male prison guards. Studies have shown that anxiety and depression are escalated during incarceration because of this perceived powerlessness, combined with fear of retribution such as sexual assault for speaking out.

Violence Against Women in Prison

Most women enter prison with a history of domestic violence and/or sexual assault. One study estimates that 75% have experienced sexual abuse as children or adults (Browne, Miller, & Maguin, 1999); another suggests that 44% were beaten by one or both parents (Bond & Seman, 1996); and many estimate that 90% have come from homes where hitting, slapping, and striking were commonplace (Bond & Seman, 1996; Browne, Miller, & Maguin, 1999; Fogel & Belyea, 1999).

Physical and sexual abuse continues to be problematic for women within prison (Davis, 1998). Although the Fourth Amendment to the Constitution provides protection against sexual abuse while incarcerated, 23 states currently have no laws prohibiting sexual abuse and misconduct in correctional facilities. In 1999, Amnesty International released a report called *Not Part of My Sentence,* which detailed numerous instances of sexual assault and inappropriate conduct of male guards against female prisoners (U.S.A. Rights for All, 1999). The findings of this report were so appalling that two television networks, ABC and CNN, followed up with investigations into sexual assault and misconduct against women in U.S. prisons. Some women "consent" to sexual relations with guards; this is commonly called "trading favors." However, consent between a prisoner and a guard is legally impossible (as between a minor and an adult); it typically reflects the woman's overwhelming sense of powerlessness and her fear that she will not be able to survive within the system unless she consents. Indeed, retribution by guards against women for withholding sex has been documented to include putting feces in prisoners' food, urinating on prisoners, refusing prisoners medical care, and even forced hanging.

Reproductive and Family Issues

Women in prison have the same reproductive and family issues as women in the population at large. Those who are mothers are as concerned about their children's welfare and safety as any mother who is separated from her child anywhere. Some children are left with fathers who are abusive, with uncaring relatives, or in foster care. Some imprisoned women lose their children to adoption. Even those children who remain at home with loving fathers or grandparents may be unable, because of financial constraints or their geographical distance from their mother's prison, to visit more often than once every few months. Thus, many imprisoned women suffer from the "empty nest syndrome" and are almost unbearably lonely.

The correctional nurse can do much in this area. Support groups allowing women to express their feelings regarding their families and providing techniques for healing these wounds can be tremendously beneficial. For instance, the nurse can offer suggestions as to how to begin to heal the pain of their loss and to reach out to the children they have harmed. Alleviation of incarcerated mothers' shame and guilt can spur them to connect more meaningfully with their loved ones (see Voices From the Community).

As we have noted, approximately 6% to 10% of women entering prison are pregnant. Some miscarry, others choose abortion, and others carry their babies to term only to lose them immediately after birth to foster care. New York State's Bedford Hills is one of only a few programs allowing women prisoners to keep their babies following childbirth. It provides comprehensive prenatal care, parenting classes, and counseling to mothers in an attempt to break the cycle of crime, violence, and substance abuse that typically contributes to women's incarceration.

Gynecologic exams can be part of the admission process to screen for STDs, pregnancy, and concealed contraband or weapons. This can be a difficult experience for a woman with a history of sexual abuse, as it may trigger memories of the incident and cause her extreme anxiety or tears. A gentle,

Voices From the Community

I worked in a psychiatric hospital on the campus of a large women's prison. It was perhaps the most challenging job I will ever have! Among other assignments, I facilitated a group for an hour each afternoon. The issues we discussed were similar to those most women struggle with in the "real world": self-esteem, family concerns, interpersonal relationships, loneliness, and many more. However, here when a woman spoke of concern for her child, it was that she would never see it again—"Will my child ever remember me?" or even, "Where is my child and who has her?" Loneliness was profound. One inmate told me with tears in her eyes, "Ms. Lind, I know I can do one life term but I don't think I can do two." Her sentences ran back to back.

The group remained relatively stable the year I was there. Some women would improve and leave the acute unit and return to a general population. Many cycled through on a regular basis, and a few remained acute the whole time.

The reward for the nurse working in this type of setting is great. These women have so few resources or coping skills that you can have tremendous impact on their ability to find some inner strength or peace to cope with their dismal future.

Barbara Lind, RN

stepped process of providing gynecologic care to traumatized inmates is described in Dole (1996, 1999). Taking the additional time with traumatized inmates is imperative if the painful wounds of sexual abuse are ever to heal. The prison environment affords the correctional nurse this opportunity, as many inmates are incarcerated for several years.

ROLE OF THE COMMUNITY HEALTH NURSE

According to the Federal Bureau of Prisons (2000), nurses constitute 19% of the federal prison health services population. In some settings, nurses work with health care trained custody staff as partners in delivering care. The nurse working with the prison population assumes a variety of roles similar to those in the outside world; in particular, we explore the correctional nurse's role in education, advocacy, and providing a bridge for inmates into the community.

Educational and Literacy Issues

Literacy is defined as an ability to read and write to an extent that allows the individual to function in daily life. Low literacy levels have been associated with increased rates of

incarceration, possibly in part because literacy is usually a requirement for employment.

Screening for illiteracy among prisoners is important both in combating recidivism and in ensuring that written health education materials are understood. In addition, poor readers are typically ill-informed and hold many misconceptions about their bodies, illness, and health care. However, screening can be difficult; many individuals who are illiterate have learned to compensate for this shortcoming and hide it very well (Doak, Doak, & Root, 1996). When asked directly, most will deny their inability to read. Suggested questions for ascertaining literacy might include the following: "Some people find it hard to understand what they read. Is this true for you?" "Do you like to read?" or "What have you read recently?" (Wheeler, 1997).

Correctional nurses can be helpful not only in identifying illiteracy but also in encouraging improvement in literacy and health knowledge among prisoners. Almost all correctional facilities have educators and existing educational programs, including health education programs and materials. The nurse works with educational staff to ensure that health-education materials are comprehensible to all inmates. For example, videos and cartoon-like instructional materials with vivid pictures and few words can be utilized effectively. The nurse also utilizies informal opportunities to provide health education to inmates, such as during "sick call" contacts.

In addition, correctional nurses have an opportunity to provide inmates with an increased understanding of their bodies, their disease, or their medications. Often the nurse is the first person to ever offer this information. Health education in these areas empowers inmates and improves their outcomes, ultimately benefiting the institution as well. Educating prisoners about the medication system and sick-call procedures is mandated. Additionally, education to correctional staff about use of universal precautions, transmission of communicable disease, reporting changes in inmates' health conditions, monitoring for depression and suicide risk, and not withholding medications as punishment is an important responsibility of the correctional nurse.

Advocacy

An important role of the correctional nurse is that of advocate and activist. Inmates have essentially no power and often experience abusive and health-damaging treatment from fellow prisoners as well as custody personnel. Nurses can and must advocate for prisoners when they suspect improprieties. However, they need to understand that they may be labeled a "snitch" by inmates or a "trouble-maker" by staff or administrators. Advocacy and empowerment are not highly valued by most prison authorities, who fear that prisoners will become agitated and cause riots or other behavior problems. Nonetheless, although advocacy for prisoners' health care may be met with resistance, the nurse must remain undaunted. Custody staff and custody administration understand chain of command and authority. Thus, the nurse must earn respect of custody personnel and act with authority, using the chain of command with impunity.

The nurse's advocacy role can be enhanced significantly by consulting with or using a forensic nurse when one is available. Forensics allows for legal argument to be used to advocate for the health and well-being of clients.

Bridge Programs With the Community

As prisoners are released into the community, the correctional nurse again plays a vital role. Unless prisoners are prepared and their release plans coordinated, **recidivism,** which refers to a relapse into criminal behavior with subsequent incarceration, will likely occur. Recidivism is highest in the first 24 hours and the earliest days of release; its rates vary but are generally about 35%. Comprehensive pre-release programs can decrease recidivism by half (Freudenberg, Wilets, Greene, & Richie, 1998). They require attention to issues of housing, employment, and continuity of medical care. Providing these necessities actually decreases public costs because of the corresponding decrease in recidivism. Some correctional facilities use peer education programs to provide inmates with information and beginning skills for application outside (Boudin et al., 1999).

Some pre-release programs bring health care providers into the prison before the inmate's release for a first appointment. Most prisoners have difficulty maneuvering within the health care system outside the prison, and this allows them to make a meaningful contact with their health care provider prior to release (Mitty et al., 1998). It is helpful to arrange for a "drop-in" policy for inmates initially and to schedule an appointment for the second week post-release. This gives prisoners a sense that someone cares about them and is invested in their successful transition to post-prison life. Providing them a business card and encouraging them to call for any problem also increases their confidence and provides a safety net for social and health care support. Prisoners are typically anxious upon their release and must deal with many life stressors concurrently. Having a safe place to drop into may mean the difference between success and a return to a life of crime.

Preparing inmates for release is an expanded role for the correctional nurse. Re-entering a community that may be hostile poses significant challenges, both in terms of successful reintegration and the avoidance of a return to criminal behaviors. Substance abuse, self-destructive behavior, or recidivism commonly occur when released inmates are shunned by their communities or denied employment or housing. Thus, the correctional nurse must work with community liaisons to design discharge plans that will result in positive outcomes for the client. Nursing practice at its most comprehensive level will benefit clients, society, and the system within which it occurs.

In discharge planning, the nurse must remember to consider the needs of the inmate's family. While the inmate is incarcerated, the family has adjusted to his or her absence and has reorganized the family system to fill the roles and responsibilities

of the missing member. The return home of an ex-convict can thus create upheaval and conflict. Family therapy and support throughout the reintegration process can result in a smoother adjustment. Long-term support rather than brief intervention is more effective in enabling family members to begin communicating and interacting in a positive manner, and thus to resolve their anger, disappointment, humiliation, and grief.

Personal Safety, Stress Reduction, and Self-Care

Working within the confines of the prison system poses significant stress for the nurse. Stressors include the following:
- An environment fraught with rules, restrictions, and constant monitoring
- A philosophically conflicting culture that poses ethical dilemmas
- An unknown, often unstable, and potentially dangerous client population
- A setting where nursing decisions often must be made in isolation, without immediate access to other health team members or resources

Self-care, stress reduction, relaxation and planned "time-out" are essential for the success of your practice within the correctional system. Personal safety issues must be addressed and incorporated into daily practice. This includes avoiding health risks though immunization, safety precautions around inmates with infectious diseases, and close proximity of correctional officers when working with potentially dangerous clients. Avoidance of "vicarious traumatization" is essential in order to prevent burnout and the development of significant emotional distress. Correctional nurses face additional concerns in terms of personal relationships and their ability to separate the multifaceted stressors associated with their professional responsibilities and maintain a positive and healthy personal life. Establishing a peer support group both within the correctional care team and with other correctional nurses can reduce the sense of professional isolation that can accompany this particular area of specialization.

SUMMARY

Serving clients in correctional facilities poses unique challenges and opportunities for community health nurses. To understand the prisoner population and the issues affecting their health, the nurse must be familiar with the correctional environment; know its rules, restrictions, and strict chain of command; adapt to security monitoring; and recognize the problems associated with an atmosphere of overcrowding, despair, and numerous health problems.

Inmates in the U.S. are growing in numbers; the majority are white males, many have a history of abuse or neglect in childhood, and about three-fourths of them are nonviolent offenders. Generally they tend to be poor, undereducated, and at risk for many chronic and infectious diseases.

Historically, prisoners were mistreated and the condition of correctional facilities was deplorable. Reforms in the 1700s and 1800s gradually improved conditions until international standards were adopted in 1955 that promoted respect for inmates' humanity and rights. Correctional health care today has greatly improved, but many problems remain.

Various laws enacted in the past 25 years have improved prison conditions, standards, and inmates' rights. Some laws, intended to curb drug trafficking and other offenses, have contributed to an escalation in the number of prisoners with resultant overcrowding of correctional facilities.

A variety of professional organizations and agencies influence the incarcerated population's living conditions, rights, and policies that govern their treatment.

Ethical dilemmas arise in correctional health care, such as death penalties conflicting with nursing goals of rehabilitation. The need to preserve client confidentiality and privacy poses additional problems. Furthermore, it is difficult for the nurse to practice objectively with offenders who have committed heinous crimes or to deal with inmates who make sexual advances.

The incarcerated population has many health problems and needs. Communicable diseases are a major problem, particularly tuberculosis, sexually transmitted diseases, and HIV/AIDs, along with hepatitis and other associated illnesses. Caring for an incarcerated population with these health problems is more complex since treatment compliance, confidentiality, and follow-up after discharge are difficult to ensure. Mental illness affects a large portion of the prison population and leads to a vicious circle of recidivism if not treated adequately. Inmates' families, particularly children, suffer in many ways as a result of the inmate's incarceration and need support.

Women are a minority of the prison population but have many special health care needs because of their vulnerability and powerlessness. Many were abused as children and again as adults and suffer from depression, loneliness, and misconduct on the part of guards. Inmates who are mothers suffer loss and the grief of separation from their children.

The correctional health nurse can make a significant difference with the incarcerated population and plays various roles. In particular, the nurse serves as health educator to combat illiteracy and ignorance, as advocate to correct improprieties and promote inmates' health, and as a "bridge" to assist with predischarge planning and preparation of inmates for release into the community.

Finally, correctional health nurses must protect their own personal safety, take measures to cope with a stressful work environment, and find needed outlets and support (see Clinical Corner).

CLINICAL CORNER | **Improving the Health of an Incarcerated Population**

Scenario

You have been working as a nurse in a large prison outside Metropolis for 4 years. Recently you were promoted to the role of supervisor. You are now responsible for analysis of health care services for the prison. You look forward to the opportunity to address some of the suboptimal health practices that you have observed in your time as a staff nurse working in the system. You feel strongly that previous supervisors have been remiss in failing to address serious health issues facing the prison population. You plan to implement policies and programs that will address these issues and lead to a healthier environment for the inmates and staff.

The health issues that you plan to address include:
- substance use among inmates
- noncompliance with medications
- unsafe sex among inmates

Demographics of Prison Population
- Gender: all male inmates and guards
- Number: 700–900 inmates on average

Staff
- Guards are employees of the state correctional department.
- Health care providers are employees of the local health department.
- Health care staff consists of one male physician, one male and one female nurse practitioner, and four female and two male registered nurses.

Substance Abuse Among Inmates

The problem of substance abuse among inmates in Metropolis Prison has been identified and discussed by previous administrators. Attempts have been made to address the issue. Interventions have included group education, counseling by local drug diversion program staff, and weekly AA/NA meetings. Although some inmates have expressed interest in these approaches, the problem of substance abuse remains rampant.

You have gathered anecdotal information from health service staff, correctional officers, and inmates regarding the extent of the problem and believe that the drug-using population in this facility comprises a demographically mixed subculture of about 30% of the total population. It is generally believed that the most common drugs being utilized by prisoners include "crack" cocaine or heroin. Needles and syringes are valuable commodities and are used in the underground bartering system. It is highly likely that these IV drug "works" are being shared by inmates without cleaning between users.

Question

1. Discuss your application of the nursing process to address the issue presented above. Use information available to you given the scenario and extrapolate when information is unknown.

Assessment:

ACTIVITIES TO PROMOTE CRITICAL THINKING

1. You are treating several women incarcerated in a medium-security prison for post-traumatic stress disorder. All of these inmates have been sexually abused or assaulted. They express significant distress at the constant monitoring of all their activities day and night by male guards. How would you handle this? What are the issues inherent in this case?

2. John S., age 58, was recently incarcerated for the second time for armed robbery. He has been monitored for suicidal risk and is being treated for hypertension. He reported to the nurse that he is not being given his medications at night because the guards "don't like him." This inmate has been labeled a trouble maker. How would you handle this situation? What are some of the issues inherent in this case?

3. You are responsible for examining the health issues affecting the incarcerated population at your all-male facility. In particular, you learn that unsafe sexual practices among inmates is a major problem that is emotionally charged and that no one has been willing to address. You learn that:

   sexual acts are used in the underground bartering system

   sexually transmitted diseases often go untreated during the period of incarceration

   non-consensual sexual violence occurs frequently, yet is rarely reported to staff

   one inmate informed you that, by his estimate, more than 30% of inmates are practicing unsafe sex

   condoms are not available to inmates

   previous attempts to make condoms available to inmates were unsuccessful because the Department of Corrections felt that they would encourage illegal activities (such as sodomy and drug smuggling)

   With a group of your classmates, discuss how you would apply the nursing process to these issues, using the information given above and extrapolating when information is unknown. Identify the host/agent/environment factors in the epidemiologic triad that are present in this situation. Develop a plan for primary, secondary, and tertiary prevention for unsafe sex, sexual abuse, and STDs with this population.

4. Assume that you are a correctional nurse researching information about a health problem that affects your inmates. Search at least two Web sites for information on this problem. Summarize what you learn about the problem and describe its application to your practice.

REFERENCES

American Nurses Association (1995). *Scope and standards of nursing practice in correctional facilities*. Washington, DC: American Nurses Publishing.

Anno, J. & Spencer, S. S. (1998). Medical ethics and correctional health care. In M. Puisis, *Clinical practice in correctional medicine* (pp. 32–40). St. Louis: Mosby.

Bond, L. & Seman, S. (1996). At risk for HIV infection: Incarcerated women in a county jail in Philadelphia. *Women and Health, 24*(4), 27–45.

Boudin, K., Carrero, I., Clark, J., Flournoy, V., Loftin, K., Martindale, S., Martinez, M., Mastroieni, E., & Richardson, S. (1999). ACE: A peer education and counseling program meets the needs of incarcerated women with HIV/AIDS Issues. *Journal of the Association of Nurses in AIDS Care, 10*(6), 90–98.

Brecher, E. M. & Della Penna, R. D. (1975). *Health care in correctional institutions*. Washington, DC: National Institute of Law Enforcement and Criminal Justice, U.S. Department of Justice.

Browne, A., Miller, B., & Maguin, E. (1999). Prevalence and severity of lifetime physical and sexual victimization among incarcerated women. *International Journal of Law and Psychiatry, 22*(3–4), 301–322.

Census Bureau (2000). *Men still make more*. Washington, DC: Census Bureau.

Centers for Disease Control and Prevention (1999). Decrease in AIDS-related mortality in a state correctional system—New York, 1995–1998. *Mortality and Morbidity Weekly Report, 47*(51), 1115–1117. Available: www.mmwrq@cdc.gov

Cohen, M., Deamant, C., Barkan, S., Richardson, J., Yound, M., Holman, S., Anastos, K., Cohen, J., & Melnick, S. (2000). Domestic violence and childhood sexual abuse in HIV-infected women and women at risk for HIV. *American Journal of Public Health, 90*(4), 560–565.

Davis, A. Y. (1998). Public imprisonment and private violence: Reflections on the hidden punishment of women. *New England Journal on Criminal and Civil Confinement, 24*(2), 339–351.

Doak, C. C., Doak, L. G., & Root, J. H. (1996). *Teaching patients with low literacy skills* (2nd ed.). Philadelphia: J.B. Lippincott.

Dole, P. (1999). Examining sexually traumatized incarcerated women. *HEPP News* [HIV Education Prison Project, Brown University], June. Available: ccg@ccgnetwork.com

Dole, P. J. (1996). Centering: Reducing rape trauma syndrome anxiety during a gynecologic examination. *Journal of Psychosocial Nursing, 34*(10), 32–37.

Federal Bureau of Prisons (2000). *Public information: Facts and statistics, April 27, 2000*. Washington, DC: Office of Public Affairs. Available: www.bop.gov

Fogel, C. I. & Belyea, M. (1999). The lives of incarcerated women: Violence, substance abuse, and at risk for HIV. *Journal of the Association of Nurses in AIDS Care, 10*(6), 66–73.

Freudenberg, N., Wilets, I., Greene, M. B., & Richie, B. E. (1998). Linking women in jail to community services: Factors associated with rearrest and retention of drug-using women following release from jail. *Journal of the American Medical Women's Association, 53*(2), 89–93.

Hammett, T. M., Harmon, P., & Maruschak, L. M. (1999). *1996–1997 update: HIV/AIDS, STDs, and TB in correctional facilities*. Washington, DC: U.S. Department of Justice.

Human Rights Watch Women's Rights Project (1996). *All too familiar: Sexual abuse of women in U.S. state prisons.* New York: Human Rights Watch. Available: http://www.hrw.org

Irwin, J. (2000). *America's one million nonviolent prisoners.* Washington, DC: Justice Policy Institute. Available: cjcj.org/jti/one million

Jordon, K., Schlenger, W. E., Fairbank, J. A., & Caddell, J. M. (1996). Prevalence pf psychiatric disorders among incarcerated women. *Archives of General Psychiatry, 53,* 513–519.

Justice Works Community (1999). *Breaking silence: Voices of mothers in prison.* Brooklyn, NY: Author. Available: www.justiceworks.org

King, L. N. (1998). Doctors, patients, and history of correctional medicine. In M. Puisis, *Clinical practice in correctional medicine* (pp. 3–11). St. Louis: Mosby.

Maeve, M. K. (1997). Nursing practice with incarcerated women: Caring within mandated alienation. *Issues in Mental Health Nursing, 18,* 495–510.

Miller, S. K. (1999). New directions for nurse practitoners: Correctional health care. *Patient Care for the Nurse Practitioner, 2*(11), 53.

Mitty, J. A., Holmes, L., Spaulding, A., Flanigan, T., & Page, J. (1998). Transitioning HIV-infected women after release from incarceration: Two models for bridging the gaps. *Journal of Correctional Health Care, 5*(2), 239–254.

Richardson, S. Z. (1998). Preferred care of the pregnant inmate. In M. Puisis, *Clinical practice in correctional medicine* (pp. 181–187). St. Louis: Mosby.

United States of America Rights for All (1999). "*Not part of my sentence*": *Violations of the human rights of women in custody.* New York: Amnesty International USA. Available: www.amnesty-usa.org (rights for all)

U.S. Bureau of Justice (1999). *Sourcebook of criminal justice statistics.* Washington, DC: Author. Available: www.albany.edu/sourcebook/

Wheeler, L. (1997). Nurse-midwifery handbook: A practical guide to prenatal and postnatal care (pp. 145–147). Philadelphia: J. B. Lippincott.

RESOURCES

A sister's story (free comic book for female offenders about HIV, available in Spanish and English. Bristol-Meyers Squibb.

Cell wars (comic book on HIV in prison populations). Bristol-Meyers Squibb.

Get tested (video on HIV in correctional facilities). Glaxo Wellcome.

HIV Inside: A Quarterly Newsletter for Correctional Professionals. New York: World Health CME, 1-212-481-8534. (Free subscription supported by a grant from Glaxo-Wellcome.)

Inmate Adherence Videotape Series: A strategy to increase HIV/AIDs medication adherence in correctional settings. Albany Medical Center (518-262-6864) or santosm@mail.amc.edu.

Peternelj-Taylor, C. A., & Johnson, R. *Custody and caring: A challenge for nursing* (video documentary).

Reeder-Bey, V. & Wilburn, A. M. *My Grandma has*

AIDS: Annisha's story. Agouron Pharmaceuticals, Inc. (1-888-847-2237).

INTERNET RESOURCES

Amnesty International: www.amnesty-usa.org(rights for all)

Association of Nurses in AIDS Care: www.anacnet.org

Clinician's Educational Resource: www.hivline.com

HEPP News, Brown University HIV Education Prison Project: www.hivcorrections.org

Human Rights Watch: www.hrw.org

Justice Policy Institute: www.cjcj.org/jti/one million

Justice Works: www.justiceworks.org

Medscape (operated by UCLA; has a range of HIV articles updated regularly): http://hiv.medscape.com/medscape/hiv/clinicalmgmt/cm.v09/public/index-cm.v09.html

National Commission on Correctional Health Care: www.ncchc.org

National Internet Listserver Resources for Correctional Health Care Professionals: majordomo@hypoxia.uchsc.edu

The Bureau of Justice Statistics: http://www.ojp.usdoj.gov/bjs

The Corrections Connection Network: http://www.corrections.com

SUGGESTED READINGS

Canadian HIV-AIDS Legal Network (1997–1998). Prisoners and HIV/AIDS. *Canadian HIV-AIDS Policy and Law Newsletter, 3*(4)/*4*(1).

Centers for Disease Control and Prevention (1999). High prevalence of chlamydial and gonococcal infection in women entering jails and juvenile detention centers—Chicago, Birmingham, and San Francisco, 1998. *Mortality and Morbidity Weekly Report, 48*(36), 793–796.

Clark, C. C. (1997). Posttraumatic stress disorder: How to support healing. *American Journal of Nursing, 97*(8), 26–33.

Coombes, R. (1999). Men get raped too. *Nursing Times, 95*(8), 12.

DeGroot, A. S., Hammett, T. M., & Scheib, R. G. (1996). Barriers to care of HIV-infected inmates: A public health concern. *AIDS Reader,* May/June, 78–87.

Draucker, C. B., & Madsen, C. (1999). Women dwelling with violence. *Image: Journal of Nursing Scholarship, 31*(4), 327–332.

Dubik-Unruh, S. (1999). Peer education programs in corrections: Curriculum, implementation, and nursing interventions. *Journal of the Association of Nurses in AIDS Care, 10*(6), 53–62.

El-Bassel, N., Ivanoff, A., Schilling, R. F., et al. (1995). Preventing HIV/AIDS in drug-abusing incarcerated women through skills building and social support enhancement: Preliminary outcomes. *Social Work Research, 19*(3), 129–192.

Fergusson, D. M., Horwood, L. J., & Lynskey, M. T. (1997). Childhood sexual abuse, adolescent sexual behaviors and sexual revictimization. *Child Abuse and Neglect, 21*(8), 789–803.

Flanigan, T. P. (1999). *HIV behind bars: The challenge of providing comprehensive care.* Women and HIV Conference, Los Angeles, CA, October 12, 1999.

Frank, L. (1999). Prisons and public health: Emerging issues in HIV treatment adherence. *Journal of the Association of Nurses in AIDS Care, 10*(6), 25–31.

Gollub, E. B. (1999). Human rights is a US problem too: The case of women and HIV. *American Journal of Public Health, 89*(10), 1476–1485.

Grinstead, O. A., Zack, B., & Faigles, B. (1999). Collaborative research to prevent HIV among male prison inmates and their female partners. *Health Education and Behavior, 26*(2), 225–238.

Heritage, C. H. (1998). Working with childhood sexual abuse survivors during pregnancy, labor, and birth. *Journal of Obstetrics, Gynecology, and Neonatal Nursing, 27*(6), 671–677.

Holman, J. (1997). Prison care: Our penitentiaries are turning into nursing homes: Can we afford it? *Modern Maturity, 40*(3), 30–36.

Kantor, E. (1998). AIDS and HIV infections in prisoners. *HIV Knowledge Base, HIV InSite,* May. Available: http://www.insite.ucsf.edu

Keamy, L. (1998). Women's health care in the incarcerated setting. In M. Puisis, *Clinical practice in correctional medicine* (pp. 188–205). St. Louis: Mosby.

Keaveny, M. E., & Zauszniewski, J. A. (1999). Life events and psychological well-being in women sentenced to prison. *Issues in Mental Health Nursing, 20,* 73–89.

Koppel, T. (1999). Crime and punishment: Women in prison (six-part series). *Nightline.* Available at ABCNewstore.com or 1-800-CALL-ABC for transcripts.

Kupers, T. A. (1999). *Prison madness: The mental health crisis behind bars and what we must do about it.* San Francisco: Jossey-Bass.

May, J. P. (2000). *Building violence.* Thousand Oaks, CA: Sage Publications.

Morrill, A. C., Mastroieni, E., & Leibel, S. R. (1998). Behavioral HIV harm reduction programs for incarcerated women: Theory and practice. *Journal of Correctional Health Care, 5*(2), 225–235.

Romeo, C. (1998). Catch the Hope Program at Massachusetts Correctional Institution—Framingham: A model for providing critical services to incarcerated pregnant women. *New England Journal on Criminal and Civil Confinement, 24*(2), 417–425.

Shaylor, C. (1998). "It's like living in a black hole": Women of color and solitary confinement in the prison industrial complex. *New England Journal on Criminal and Civil Confinement, 24*(2), 385–416.

Snider, W. G. (1998). Banishment: The history of its use and proposal for its abolition under the First Amendment. *New England Journal on Criminal and Civil Confinement, 24*(2), 455–509.

Sowbik, L., & Frank, L. (1999). Peer education program educates inmates with HIV. *CorrectCare.* National Commission on Correctional Health Care, pp. 8, 13.

Stevens, J., Zierler, S., Cram, V., et al. (1995). Risks for HIV infection in incarcerated women. *Journal of Women's Health, 4*(5), 569–577.

Vicini, J. (2000). Supreme Court upholds segregation of HIV-infected inmates. *Reuters Medical News on Medscape,* January 18. Available: www.hiv.medscape.com

Vigilante, K. C., Rich, J. D., et al. (1997). The women's HIV prison prevention program: Reduction of prison recidivism may suggest HIV risk reduction. *Programs and Abstracts of the 4th Conference on Retroviruses and Opportunistic Infections,* January, Abstract 524, Washington, DC.

Zeidenberg, J., Irwin, J., & Schiraldi, V. (1999). *America's one million nonviolent offenders.* Washington, DC: Justice Policy Institute.

Clients in Home Health, Hospice, and Long-Term Care Settings

KEY TERMS

- **Assisted living**
- **Durable medical equipment**
- **Formal caregivers**
- **Home health care**
- **Home health nursing**
- **Homebound**
- **Homemaker agency**
- **Hospice**
- **Hospital-based agency**
- **Informal caregivers**
- **Long-term care**
- **Ombudsman**
- **Palliative care**
- **Respite**
- **Skilled nursing facility (SNF)**
- **Skilled nursing services**
- **Terminally ill**

LEARNING OBJECTIVES

Upon mastery of this chapter, you should be able to:

- Describe the home care, hospice, and long-term care populations.
- Discuss standards and credentialing for home care, hospice, and long-term care nursing.
- Provide an overview of the evolution of home care, hospice, and long-term care nursing.
- Identify a variety of home care and long-term care agencies.
- Explain the roles and responsibilities of the various members of the home health, hospice, and long-term care team.
- Describe the reimbursement systems common to home health, hospice, and long-term care.
- Describe the role of the community health nurse in meeting the health care needs of the homebound population.
- Describe the role of the community health nurse in meeting the health care needs of the hospice family.
- Describe the role of the community health nurse in meeting the health care needs of clients in long-term care settings.

Have you ever sat with a frail, elderly gentleman with chronic obstructive pulmonary disease receiving oxygen at home and listened to his stories of the "good old days" when he was young, full of vigor, and taking on the world? Have you ever tried to comfort a middle-aged woman dying of cancer and fearful for the welfare of her teenage daughter after she is gone? Have you ever provided nursing care to an older adult on a respirator in a skilled nursing facility? These are just three of the myriad of experiences that make up the daily lives of nurses who work in homes, hospices, and long-term care facilities. Indeed, nursing within these setting allows us to practice what some see as the very heart of compassionate nursing care.

In this chapter, we discuss home care and hospice nursing as domains of practice. As you read these sections, you might want to refer back to Chapters 24 and 30 in which we discussed how to plan for, implement, and evaluate the family visit at home; issues of personal safety; and the older adult. Finally, we turn to nursing care within the wide variety of long-term care settings that have burgeoned in the United States in the past decade.

AN OVERVIEW OF HOME CARE

The need for health care at home has been growing steadily in the last two decades. Drastic changes in financing, provider roles, and increasing client acuity have contributed to this trend. For example, early hospital discharges resulting from third-party payers' efforts toward cost containment have forced clients back into their homes to recuperate from surgeries and severe illnesses far more quickly than 20 years ago. Moreover, third-party payers are now requiring that certain procedures be performed only on an outpatient basis. As a result, such complex procedures as intravenous chemotherapy, parenteral nutrition, and mechanical ventilation, all of which were once only provided in hospitals or skilled nursing care facilities, are today routinely provided and maintained in the client's home. Hospital stays for mothers and newborns have been shortened to an average of 24 to 48 hours, requiring postpartum and infant home care (Madigan, 1997). Advances in technology have led to the development of machines that can provide dialysis, pain control, and ventilatory care in the client's home. In addition, terminally ill clients — those with less than 6 months to live — find the supportive services of hospice care allow them to live as fully as possible and die at home rather than in a hospital. Finally, there are now simply more elderly people in the U.S. than there were two decades ago; this means a corresponding increase in clients with chronic illnesses, many of whom prefer to be cared for in their homes.

As a result, many community health nurses are spending more of their time caring for clients in their homes. Thus, it is important for us to take a look at the terminology of home care, the demographics of the home care population, and the standards and credentials associated with home care nursing.

Terminology of Home Health Care

Home health care, broadly defined, refers to all the services and products provided to clients in their homes to maintain, restore, or promote their physical, mental, and emotional health. Its purpose is to maximize clients' level of independence and to minimize the effects of existing disabilities through noninstitutional services. Its primary goal is to use these supportive services to decrease rehospitalization and prevent or delay institutionalization (Acampora, 1997; Jackson, 1997).

There is a distinct difference between the professional and technical home care services provided to clients. Professional home care services are practice-driven; that is, the boundaries of practice are determined by standards based on scientific theory and research. Professional home care is provided by professionals with licenses, certification, or specific qualifications. These professionals typically work for home care agencies that have internal and external standards that guide the provision of their services. Nurses, social workers, physical therapists, and home health aides are examples of professional home-care practitioners.

Technical home care services are product-driven and thus do not always consider what is best for the client. Providers of technical home care do not necessarily have standards or regulations that govern how they serve clients. **Durable medical equipment** (DME) includes the equipment that is used for a long period of time and can be used again by others, such as wheelchairs, walkers, hospital beds, ventilators, IV poles, and so forth. Such suppliers, oxygen providers, and other equipment home delivery providers make up the majority of providers in this category (Allender, 1998).

Home health nursing is a specialized area of nursing practice with its roots firmly placed in community health nursing (American Nurses Association [ANA], 1999). The provision of home health nursing is to acute, chronic, and terminally ill clients of all ages in their home while integrating community health nursing principles that focus on the environmental, psychosocial, economic, cultural, and personal health factors affecting a client's and family's health status and well-being. It is thus a unique field of nursing practice. It requires a synthesis of community health nursing principles with the theory and practice of medical/surgical, maternal-child, geriatric, and mental health nursing. Home care nurses care for clients who have procedures and treatments conducted in their homes and for those who wish to live out the final days of their lives in their homes rather than in an institution.

The focus of home care nursing is the treatment of human responses. Home health nursing demands that the varied human responses seen in home care clients be addressed in a holistic framework so that the client and family can be assisted to reach their goals.

The Home Care Population

The client cared for in home care nursing is the individual patient, the family, and any significant others. Thus, the nurse must consider numerous factors related to the client's family, community, culture, society, and religion. The nurse must consider how the environmental, psychosocial, economic, cultural, and personal health-related factors affect the client's illness and ability to meet the goals outlined in the plan of care.

In 1998, it was estimated that more than 8 million people received home care services for acute illnesses, long-term health conditions, permanent disability, or terminal illness (National Association for Home Care, 1999). The demographics of home care clients in the U.S. reveal a predominantly female (66.8%) and European American (65.5%) population. The majority (72.4%) of home care clients are 65 years of age or older, although home care is provided to clients of all ages, from birth to death.

The most common diagnoses for home care clients are shown in Display 37–1. Notably absent from Display 37–1

DISPLAY 37–1. Most Common Diagnoses for Home Care Clients

- Heart disease
- Musculoskeletal and connective tissue disease
- Diabetes mellitus
- Diseases of the respiratory system
- Injury
- Poisoning

---

are cancer diagnoses. A primary diagnosis of malignant neoplasm represents only 4.7% of home care clients, whereas it accounts for 58.3% of hospice clients (Haupt, 1998).

The majority of clients receiving home care are registered with urban home care agencies (Haupt, 1998). As reimbursements for home care nursing continue to decrease, the costs of visiting clients in geographically remote areas have forced many rural home care agencies to close, limiting home care access for populations in rural regions.

Although home care nursing is provided to a large number of people in the U.S., it still represents a small percentage of the national health care expenditures. Whereas hospital care consumed 40% of health care dollars in 1996 and physician services consumed 22%, home care represented

only 3% of health care spending. This statistic supports many researchers' observations of the cost-effectiveness of home care practice.

Standards and Credentials in Home Care Nursing

The American Nurses Association (ANA, 1999) has developed the *Scope and Standards of Home Health Nursing Practice* (Display 37–2). These 14 standards guide professional nursing practice in home care settings and are based on the association's work in 1986 and 1992. Since there are several types of home care agencies (discussed later in this chapter), these standards are designed to assist nurses in providing a level of service that meets a minimal expectation while being appropriate to clients, regardless of the home care agency from which they receive services.

In addition to standards of practice, home care nurses can hold advanced credentials and belong to professional organizations in order to enhance skills in this practice area.

The American Nurses' Credentialing Center (ANCC) credentials nurses in many specialty areas, including home care nursing. This credential can be granted after the required years of home care practice and passing a nationally administered test.

Membership in a specialty organization, such as the Na-

DISPLAY 37–2. Scope and Standards of Home Health Nursing Practice

Standards of Care

Standard I Assessment
The home health nurse collects client health data.

Standard II Diagnosis
The home health nurse analyzes the assessment data in determining diagnoses.

Standard III Outcome Identification
The home health nurse identifies expected outcomes to the client and client's environment.

Standard IV Planning
The home health nurse develops a plan of care that prescribes intervention to attain expected outcomes.

Standard V Implementation
The home health nurse implements the interventions identified in the plan of care.

Standard VI Evaluation
The home health nurse evaluates the client's progress toward attainment of outcomes.

Standards of Professional Performance

Standard I Quality of Care
The home health nurse systematically evaluates the quality and effectiveness of nursing practice.

Standard II Performance Appraisal
The home health nurse evaluates his or her own

nursing practice in relation to professional practice standards, scientific evidence, and relevant statutes and regulations.

Standard III Education
The home health nurse acquires and maintains current knowledge and competency in nursing practice.

Standard IV Collegiality
The home health nurse interacts with and contributes to the professional development of peers and other health care practitioners as colleagues.

Standard V Ethics
The home health nurse's decisions and actions on behalf of clients are determined in an ethical manner.

Standard VI Collaboration
The home health nurse collaborates with the client, family, and other health care practitioners in providing client care.

Standard VII Research
The home health nurse uses research findings in practice.

Standard VIII Resource Utilization
The home health nurse assists the client or family in becoming informed consumers about the risks, benefits, and cost of planning and delivering client care.

(Reprinted with permission from American Nurses Association [1999]. *Scope and standards of home health nursing practice.* Washington, DC: American Nurses Publishing, American Nurses Foundation/American Nurses Association.)

---

tional Association of Home Care (NAHC), gives a bevy of direct services to members, including the publication *Caring* and monthly newsletters. Such focused organizations give their members the most recent information in their specialty area. Hospice nursing and community health nursing organizations also prove to be a useful resource to the home care nurse.

AGENCIES, PERSONNEL, AND REIMBURSEMENT

The types of agencies engaged in providing home care services have changed drastically as reimbursement policies have changed and as specializations in various domains of health care have evolved. We look at these agencies, personnel, and reimbursement structures next.

Types of Home Care Agencies

Currently, many types of agencies provide home care to clients. In the early days of home care most providers worked in visiting nurses associations (VNAs). In some parts of the U.S. this continues to be true, but in most parts of the country the mix of home care agencies includes voluntary agencies, proprietary agencies, hospital-based agencies, official agencies, homemaker agencies, and hospices. Official, voluntary, and proprietary agencies are discussed more fully in Chapter 6 but are reviewed here for clarity. Table 37–1 lists the number of Medicare-certified home care agencies by type in the U.S. over the last 30 years.

VOLUNTARY AGENCIES
A *voluntary agency* is a home health agency that does not depend on state and local tax revenues, but instead is financed with non-tax funds such as donations, endowments, United Way contributions, and third-party provider payments. Voluntary agencies are usually governed by a voluntary board of directors and are considered community-based because they provide services within a well-defined geographic location.

An example of a voluntary agency system is the visiting nurse agencies (VNAs). They are non-profit agencies with a charitable mission. Like all non-profits, VNAs are exempt from paying taxes. Whereas in the past VNAs were assured of receiving almost all of the home care referrals in their community, the proliferation of other agencies has eroded their traditional base and put them in a competitive mode; VNAs are therefore expanding their services to appeal to a broader market.

PROPRIETARY AGENCIES
A private, for-profit home health agency is known as a *proprietary agency*. Although proprietary agencies can be governed by individual owners, many are part of large, national chains that are administered through corporate headquarters.

TABLE 37–1. Number of Medicare-Certified Home Care Agencies by Auspice, for Selected Years, 1967–1999

| Year | Freestanding Agencies | | | Facility-Based | |
	VNA	PUB	PROP	HOSP	TOTAL
1967	549	1,228	0	133	1,753
1970s	474	985	1,884	1,486	5,695
1980s	575	1,182	3,951	2,470	9,120
1999	452	918	3,192	2,300	7,747

VNA: Visiting Nurse Associations are freestanding, voluntary, nonprofit organizations governed by a board of directors and usually financed by tax deductible contributions as well as by earnings.

PUB: Public agencies are government agencies operated by a state, county, city, or other unit of local government having a major responsibility for presenting disease and for community health education.

PROP: Proprietary agencies are freestanding for-profit home care agencies.

HOSP: Hospital-based agencies are operating units or departments of a hospital. Agencies that have working arrangements with a hospital, or perhaps are even owned by a hospital but operated as separate entities, are classified as freestanding agencies under one of the categories listed above.

(From National Association for Home Care [2000]. *Basic statistics about home care*. Washington, DC: Author. Reprinted with permission.)

Proprietary agencies are expected to turn a profit on the services they provide, either for the individual owners or for their stockholders. Although some participate in the Medicare program, others rely solely on "private pay" clients.

HOSPITAL-BASED AGENCIES
A hospital may operate a separate department as a home health agency. This agency would then be governed by the sponsoring hospital's board of directors or trustees. The referrals to such **hospital-based agencies** usually come from the hospital staff itself, and the missions of the agency and the sponsoring hospital are similar.

OFFICIAL AGENCIES
Governmental home health agencies are called *official agencies*. They are created and empowered through statutes enacted by legislation. Services are frequently provided by the nursing divisions of state or local health departments and may or may not combine care of the sick with traditional public-health nursing services, including health promotion, illness prevention, communicable disease investigation, environmental health services, and maternal-child care. Administrative support for these agencies is the responsibility of the

city, county, and/or state government. Funding comes from taxes and is usually distributed on the basis of a per-capita allocation.

HOMEMAKER AGENCIES

Homemaker agencies provide homemaker aides who perform services such as cooking, cleaning, and shopping, and/or home health aides who perform personal client care such as bathing, dressing, feeding, assistance in ambulating, companionship, etc. These agencies are usually private and derive their funding from direct payment by the client or from private insurers. They may be governed by individual owners or by corporations.

HOSPICES

Hospice care "signifies a care perspective that recognizes that death is inevitable and near and that cure is not within present human capacity" (Burke & Walsh, 1997, p. 564). Hospice services are comprehensive and delivered by an interprofessional team, including volunteers, that focuses on "care" rather than "cure." The caregiving team has physician leadership, and care can be provided on an in-patient basis or through home health care where the client lives.

Hospices have received certification from the federal government to provide end-of-life care to the terminally ill in the community. Some hospices are free-standing and serve only hospice clients, whereas others are part of a larger organization such as a VNA. Various long-term care settings can apply for a "hospice waiver" and be reimbursed for end-of-live caregiving to a person in the last months of life. This enables them to achieve a more peaceful death by dying "at home" rather than being transferred to different surroundings with a medical and curative focus.

Types of Home Care Personnel

Home care providers are usually characterized as either informal or formal caregivers.

INFORMAL CAREGIVERS

Informal caregivers are family members and friends who provide care in the home and are unpaid. It is estimated that almost three quarters of the elderly with multiple co-morbidities and severe disabilities who receive home care rely on family members or other sources of unpaid assistance. Most of the estimated 18 million family caregivers in the United States are women, and 10% to 17% of the working public also care for an elderly relative (Sultz & Young, 1999). The type of care they provide ranges from routine custodial care such as bathing and feeding to sophisticated skilled care, including tracheostomy care and IV medication administration.

Informal caregivers assume a considerable physical, psychological, and economic burden in the care of their significant other in the home. When layered on top of existing responsibilities, caregiver tasks compete for time, energy, and attention.

As a result, caregivers often describe themselves as emotionally and physically drained and may very much need information about resources to assist them (D'Amico-Panomeritakis & Sommer, 1999). Home care nurses can teach caregivers how to manage clients successfully at home following these guidelines:

APPROACH

- Keep a positive attitude that is focused on abilities, not limitations, of the caregivers.
- Keep safety at the forefront of all interventions.
- Include all family members and caregivers in the plan.
- Choose an area to teach first that the client is motivated to learn to help keep caregiver frustration low.

THINGS TO INCLUDE

- Provide tips on energy conservation for the caregiver and client.
- Include how to manage and maintain equipment.
- Provide resources for support, information, equipment, and assistance.
- Help the family develop a home emergency escape plan.

The economic cost of providing home care places a significant burden on informal caregivers. Out-of-pocket expenditures include medications, transportation, home medical equipment, supplies, and respite services. These costs may be non-reimbursable and are often invisible, but they are very real to families struggling to provide care on a fixed income. In addition, often the primary informal caregiver is an elderly spouse who is physically and emotionally involved (D'Angelo, 1999).

FORMAL CAREGIVERS

Formal caregivers are professionals and para-professionals who are compensated for the in-home care they provide. In 1998, it was estimated that there were 662,000 persons employed in home health agencies. Nurses represent 36% of formal caregivers in Medicare-certified agencies. Home health aides account for 33% (Bureau of Labor Statistics, 1999). Table 37–2 lists the range of formal home care providers in home health agencies.

In addition to the personnel described in the table, the business-office staff of a home health agency is critical to the agency's ability to deliver services to clients. Home health nurses must acquire an understanding of the financial aspects of their clients' care and provide this information to the business-office staff so that reimbursement can be obtained for the services provided.

Reimbursement Systems in Home Care

Home health services are reimbursed by both corporate and governmental third-party payers as well as by individual clients and their families. Corporate payers include insurance companies, HMOs, preferred provider organizations, and

TABLE 37–2. **Types of Providers in Home Care**	
Type of Provider	**Role and Responsibilities**
NURSES	
Registered nurses	Deliver skilled care to clients in the home under the direction of the physician. Considered the coordinator of care.
Licensed practical nurse	Deliver routine care to clients under the direction of a registered nurse
Advanced practice nurse	Provide total client care to complex clients, supervise other nurses in difficult cases related to their speciality, and direct a special program
THERAPISTS	
Physical therapist	Deliver skilled care that includes assessment for assistive devices in the home. Perform therapy procedures with the client and teach the client and family to assist in treatment. Assist client to improve mobility.
Occupational therapist	Focus on improving physical, mental and social functioning. Rehabilitation of the upper body and improvement of fine motor ability.
Speech therapist	Rehabilitation of clients with speech and swallowing problems.
Respiratory therapist	Provide support to clients using respiratory home medical equipment such as ventilators. Perform professional respiratory therapy treatments.
OTHER CLINICAL STAFF	
Social workers	Help clients and families identify needs and refer to community agencies. Assist with applications for community-based services and provide financial assistance information.
Dieticians	Provide diet counseling to clients with special nutritional needs. *Direct service of a dietician is not a reimbursable service in home care.*
PARA-PROFESSIONALS	
Home-health aide	Perform personal care, basic nursing tasks (as opposed to skilled), and incidental homemaking.
Homemaker	Perform housekeeping and chores to ensure a safe and healthy home care environment.

case-management programs. Government payers include Medicare, Medicaid, CHAMPUS, and the Veterans Administration system. These governmental programs have specific conditions for the coverage of services that are often less flexible than those of corporate payers. For a general description of these reimbursement systems, please see Chapter 7.

MEDICARE CRITERIA FOR HOME CARE SERVICES

Medicare is the largest single payer for home care services in the U.S. and has set the standard in establishing reimbursement criteria for other payers (Humphrey & Milone-Nuzzo, 1996; Waid, 1997). Thus, it is essential that home care nurses understand Medicare and its criteria for determining eligibility for home care services. A client must meet all five criteria to be eligible for reimbursement by Medicare (Display 37–3).

MEDICARE'S PROSPECTIVE PAYMENT SYSTEM

The number of home health agencies grew approximately 10% a year during the 1990s. This pattern of increased uti-

lization was a source of increasing concern for government agency officials, policy analysts, and some members of Congress (*Nursing Trends and Issues,* 1999). As part of the Balanced Budget Act of 1997, Congress adopted changes in payment for home health services. These include implementation of a prospective payment system (PPS). During the transition period in the year 2000, the use of an interim payment system (IPS) was used. The PPS system bases reimbursement on an episode of illness. Clients are assigned to one of approximately 80 reimbursement schemes depending on their clinical and functional characteristics. Theoretically, the more clinically and functionally complex the case, the greater the potential reimbursement.

Once admitted to the agency, the client receives the necessary care to assist in achieving clinical outcomes. If the agency is efficient and the client achieves the identified goals in a few visits, the overall expenses for the client might be less than the Medicare reimbursement and the agency might realize a profit. However, if the client has problems in the course of treatment and requires unanticipated visits, the agency must assume the financial burden of this care. Because of the PPS system, agencies have become very careful about the amount and type of services they provide to Medicare clients. Each home health care encounter must be carefully designed to assist clients to achieve their clinical goals.

Because of the PPS approach to reimbursement, many home health agencies went out of business in the late 1990s.

DISPLAY 37–3. Medicare Criteria for Reimbursement

1. Services provided must be reasonable and necessary. This refers to the type of services provided and the frequency. The decision as to whether or not this criterion has been met is based on a review of the client's medical record and plan of care and the client's current health status. For example, daily visits may not be deemed reasonable for a client who requires weekly blood-glucose monitoring. Also, if a care plan has been ineffective with a client over a long period of time, continuation of that care plan would not be considered reasonable. Therefore, comprehensive documentation is essential to validate that the provided care was both reasonable and necessary.

2. The client must be **homebound**. This means that the client leaves the home with difficulty in mobility and only for medical appointments or adult day care related to the client's medical care.

3. The plan of care must be entered onto specific Medicare forms (HCFA forms 485, 486, and 487). These forms require very specific information regarding the client's diagnosis, prognosis, functional limitations, medications, and types of services needed. The home health nurse often has the primary responsibility for ensuring that these forms are completed appropriately.

4. The client must be in need of a skilled service. In the home, skilled services are provided only by a nurse, physical therapist, or speech therapist. **Skilled nursing services** include skilled observation and assessment, teaching, and performing procedures requiring nursing judgment.

5. Services must be intermittent and part-time. It is anticipated that clients requiring more than intermittent, part-time care could be cared for more cost-effectively in a setting other than the home, such as a skilled nursing facility.

The law affected Medicare's 39 million recipients as well as insurers, providers, suppliers, physicians, and home health agency staff, including nurses, by reducing projected federal government spending on the program by $116 billion between 1998 and 2002 (Harris, 1998).

AN OVERVIEW OF HOSPICE CARE

The concept of hospice care is relatively new to the United States, with programs no more than 25 years old. Even more recently, hospice services have been recognized by insurance companies as legitimate services for which the third-party payers assume the costs. It was not unusual for hospice programs in the early 1980s to be supported by sponsoring institutions or private-pay clients or to fail, due to a lack of steady reimbursement sources. In 1995 Medicare paid for 74% of hospice care in the United States, while private health plans paid for about 12% (HCFA, 1999).

Hospices have a unique philosophy and serve a population who are not best served in the acute-care setting, which focus on cure and have technology, services, and personnel geared toward diagnosis, treatment, and recovery. The dying client needs a focus on care rather than cure. Community health nurses often work in hospice programs or with hospice personnel in the community.

The Philosophy of Hospice Care

Hospices focus on providing holistic, family-centered care to the terminally ill person, with death being accepted as a human experience. Holistic care is delivered to terminally ill people who are in the final phase of their illness, are expected to die, and are not receiving curative treatment. Any activities or services that will enhance the comfort and well-being of the hospice client are employed. Hospice care goals can be achieved in the client's home or, if needed or desired, in an in-patient hospice program (see Voices From the Community).

The hospice philosophy is a caregiving philosophy that does not depend on the setting but on the holistic nature of caring, delivered through an interprofessional team, that encompasses the family and client values. Hospices rely heavily on family members and volunteers who work in collaboration with a broad range of professional caregivers. The nurse is a key member of the caregiving team who works with the primary care provider, pharmacy, clergy, social services, family, volunteers, and other support personnel to orchestrate well-coordinated caregiving services.

Voices From the Community

Hospice nursing, even more than home health nursing, gives me such a full feeling of satisfaction. I know I make a difference in these family's lives when they allow me into the most personal aspect of their lives during the dying of a loved one. They accept me as a family member and I cry with them as I feel their pain and laugh with them as they recall happier days. This kind of nursing is everything I always thought nursing would be.

Ann, RN, BSN, hospice nurse

Precepts underlying hospice care are essential principles for all end-of-life care (Display 37–4). These precepts are in accord with the International Council of Nurses' mandate that nurses have a unique and primary responsibility for ensuring that individuals at the end of life experience a peaceful death (International Council of Nurses, 1997).

The Hospice Population

The hospice population can include any person diagnosed with an illness that cannot be cured, who chooses not to continue active treatment and has less than 6 months to live. Since the time of death cannot be precisely determined, it is the decision of the health care provider responsible for the client to determine hospice status.

Traditionally, the largest number of hospice-eligible clients have been diagnosed with cancer and are over the age of 65. Increasingly, clients have been diagnosed with AIDS, heart disease, end-stage renal and respiratory disease, and a variety of other diseases with terminal diagnoses. Some hospice programs focus caregiving programs on clients with AIDS. Such hospices are often affiliated with community outreach services for gay communities and are located where there is the greatest need and close to the client's support systems.

THE EVOLUTION OF HOSPICE CARE

The concept of hospice is derived from medieval Europe, when hospice was a place where travelers on long and arduous journeys could stop to rest and replenish themselves before they moved onward. As early as the 19th century, hospices in England evolved to provide palliative care in hospitals and in homes. **Palliative care** is comfort care directed at the alleviation of pain and other symptoms. Dying, like birthing,

has always been known as a natural process that was most effectively managed in the home with the assistance of family and friends. As health care became more complex, these natural events were shifted from the home to the hospital.

England has been a leader in the modern hospice movement, with nurse Dame Cicely Saunders being the visionary guide at St. Christopher's Hospice in the 1960s (Schroeder & Towle, 1999). The first American hospice, in Connecticut, was created as a freestanding in-patient hospice in the 1970s. After this initial endeavor, hospices began to emerge throughout the U.S. Once reimbursement systems were actualized for this care in the mid-1980s, the hospice movement expanded to over 2000 separate programs sharing the same philosphy of care. Most major cities in the country have an in-patient hospice program for short-term admissions and respite care. In addition, all communities with home care services have the potential to receive in-home hospice services through the home care agency.

HOSPICE SETTINGS, TEAM MEMBERS, AND REIMBURSEMENT

As mentioned earlier, hospice is not a place but a philosophy. As part of that philosophy, skilled and volunteer team members deliver care. In addition, there is a well-developed reimbursement system for hospice clients on Medicare.

In-Patient Hospices

The prototype for an in-patient hospice is a freestanding hospice. This is a small in-patient setting not associated with an acute-care facility. In some communities an in-patient hospice is created in a large house or a renovated existing building, or built to meet community preferences. They are usually small, accommodating 6 to 30 clients. They have a large volunteer staff and a professional staff of registered nurses who demonstrate the primary caregiving model of nursing care. Each nurse has a small group of clients to be responsible for as the primary nurse—ideally, three to four clients. Volunteers are used extensively to assist with personal care. Alternative or complementary care methods are integrated with traditional Western medical practices to alleviate pain and provide comfort. Imagery, biofeedback, massage, and music are just a few of the care methods used in addition to medications, positioning, and bathing.

In-patient hospices, as well as in the home, are free of most high-tech equipment seen in the acute-care setting. All clients have a no-code status, and technology is present for comfort alone. Oxygen is available to ease difficult breathing. IVs are used to deliver pain medication or alleviate symptoms of nausea or diarrhea, not to hydrate the client. Suction equipment is used to clear the airway of a client with

---

DISPLAY 37–4. Precepts of Hospice Care

- Individuals live fully until the moment of death.
- Care offered until death may be offered by a variety of professionals, family members, and volunteers.
- Care is coordinated, sensitive to diversity, and offered around the clock, and respects client's dignity and worth.
- Care gives attention to the physical, psychological, social, and spiritual concerns of the client and the client's family.

(From American Association of Colleges of Nursing [1998]. *Peaceful death: Recommended competencies and curricular guidelines for end-of-life nursing care.* Washington, DC: Author; and Schulkin, V. [1999]. Providing palliative care for the dying elderly client. In S.M. Zang & J.A. Allender, *Home care of the elderly* [pp. 486–505]. Philadelphia: Lippincott Williams & Wilkins.)

throat or neck cancer who is unable to swallow. There are no crash carts or diagnostic equipment. The environment is as homelike as possible.

The typical routines of acute-care facilities are forfeited to meet the client's wishes. The type of arrangement that is more typical of an in-patient hospice may be a client who chooses to have his wife help to bathe him in the evening, eat eight small meals a day of home-cooked foods and have a beer or glass of wine, sleep with all the lights on and with music playing, and have his wife and pet dog snuggle in bed with him.

Clients come into in-patient hospices for a variety of medical and/or social reasons. Hospice clients are usually cared for through in-home hospice services but may come into an in-patient hospice for pain management, symptom control, family respite, or to die. Family members who give care 24 hours a day, 7 days a week, may need **respite,** or a break from the intensity of caregiving. They may plan a week-end trip or just want to rest and care for themselves for a few days. Such respite is not a luxury; it is a necessity.

In some situations the family has been able to manage the dying family member's care well, but during the final days of life they are unable to see the person die at home. They may have culturally based feelings that would make the home difficult to live in if a family member dies in it, or they may feel uncomfortable or inadequate in dealing with the actual death experience at home. Home health hospice nurses work closely with the family, primary care provider, and in-patient hospice staff to accommodate client and family wishes in such situations.

In-Home Hospices

Most hospice care is provided to clients and families in their homes. People generally want to remain in familiar surroundings, in the comfort of their own bed, and prefer to die at home. This decision should be assessed early in the hospice care services and planned for throughout the care. At times the decision to die in an acute-care setting or in-patient hospice may be made near the end of the client's life, and the nurse should be prepared for this change in plans. It may be a serious decision or a fleeting fear of what to expect; the nurse needs to provide the support needed to help the family and client make either decision.

Home health hospice nurses provide the support the family needs throughout the hospice care, but especially at the time of death. The nurse encourages a relationship with the family in which the nurse is notified if the client's condition changes, regardless of the time of day or night. The hospice nurse talks to the family or comes to be with the client and family if desired. He or she assists with providing comfort measures, terminal caregiving needs, and immediate bereavement care to family members when death occurs.

There are legal aspects of care at the time of death. In many states hospice nurses can pronounce a person deceased and call to arrange for the body to be removed from the home by the selected funeral parlor or cremation society. In other states the community ambulance service is called for the body to be transported to an emergency room to be pronounced by a physician. This does not end the hospice services to the family. The nurse often attends the funeral or traditional ceremony or memorial service selected by the family. The nurse keeps in contact with the family, providing support and bereavement care and counseling long after the client's death. Many hospice programs have annual memorial services to which they invite family members of deceased clients in the year following the death, continuing a holistic approach as they deliver hospice care to an entire family.

Skilled Team Members

The skilled hospice team includes a broad array of professionals, each providing a unique service that the hospice client and family needs. The primary care provider, nurse, and social worker are core team members. For hospice clients, the team is broader and includes the pharmacist, clergy member, and psychologist.

Medically ordered combinations of medications, or "cocktails," can be provided in liquid form by the pharmacist to alleviate pain, nausea, syncope, constipation or diarrhea, edema, anxiety, and shortness of breath. Given these medications orally, in combination, eliminates injections and IVs and the need to swallow multiple pills. In addition, large doses of narcotics are delivered in smaller amounts of IV fluids. At times a pharmacist may need to provide 2000 mg of morphine in 500 mL of fluid. With pain and discomfort from other symptoms a major concern for the terminally ill client, the pharmacist becomes a valuable team member.

A clergy member is frequently available in hospice programs to provide support for the clients, family, and staff. Professional and volunteer staff members become emotionally involved with hospice clients, and regular support or debriefing sessions help the staff cope with their own feelings when providing such intimate and emotional care. In addition, the team members may work with the client's own clergyperson. For clients not involved in an organized religion, the clergyperson on staff is an important resource and works with all clients as desired, or he or she can work collegially with a religious leader the client prefers.

Some hospice programs have the services of a psychologist. This team member provides one-on-one or group meeting support to staff and to clients and families. The psychologist works with clients who are having difficulty with their disease progression and with family members who are having a hard time coping with the impending loss of a family member or the stress of caregiving. Clerical and psychological services are often part-time appointments and can be shared by in-patient and in-home hospice programs on a part-time basis. Sometimes these professionals may volunteer their time to hospice programs.

Volunteer Team Members

Volunteerism is the backbone of a succesful hospice program. Volunteers fill an important need in both in-patient and in-home hospice programs. They act as companions to the client when the family must be somewhere else or away for short respite. They run errands for family members, organize hot meals prepared by friends and neighbors, babysit children in the family—the list can go on and on. In-patient volunteers may act like nursing assistants and assist the nurse with personal care by helping to hold or position clients during treatments, bathing, or dressing. They cook foods the client feels like eating. Most in-patient hospices have a kitchen available for the staff and family to use. Client appetites often tend to be small and selective, so nurses, volunteers, and family members become "short- order" cooks. One in-patient hospice volunteer recalls caring for a 23-year-old man with an inoperable brain tumor who rarely had an appetite. One day he asked for an egg, fried in the middle of a piece of bread with a hole in it for the egg to sit, covered in catsup and served with a warm bottle of beer. The volunteer was so excited that he had an appetite that she worked very hard to make his choice to perfection—and even warmed the refrigerated beer in a pan of hot water.

Reimbursement Systems in Hospice Care

As mentioned earlier, hospice care to people on Medicare is a covered service. In fact, services are covered more fully for in-patient and in-home hospice care than for home health clients in general. Display 37–5 compares criteria and benefits of home care and hospice according to Medicare reimbursement.

Most private insurers cover costs for clients not on Medicare. For clients with no health insurance and not eligble for Medicare, there are voluntary agencies that will assist with covering the costs of caregiving. For instance, the American Cancer Society provides dressings and assists with the costs of medications for up to 3 months. Local churches and disease-specific agencies have funds available to support people during the terminal phase of an illness. In addition, hospices reserve a certain number of beds for the medically indigent so that no one needing hospice care is refused care.

AN OVERVIEW OF LONG-TERM CARE SETTINGS, POPULATION, AND PERSONNEL

Long-term care settings are residences for people unable to physically care for themselves independently due to physical or cognitive alterations. These settings have changed dramatically over the last 20 years and especially in the last decade. At one time the only choice was the skilled nursing facility, generally called "the nursing home." Some people have a negative image of the nursing home and the care delivered there. It has been pictured as being a warehouse for the elderly, who are mistreated by an ill-prepared and uncaring staff and abandoned by family members. Unfortunately, a few nursing homes have earned such a reputation, giving the long-term care industry as a whole a negative image. This image needs to be changed. The aging population is increasing, and the diversity of the population makes their needs different today. Therefore, in an effort to be proactive, many types of living settings with minimal to maximum services and assistance are available.

Long-Term Care Settings

Long-term care options are changing and facilities are being designed to meet a variety of needs presented by the older population. Choices encompass independent (for adults over 55 only) apartment or mobile home living, congregate living, assisted living centers, Alzheimer's centers, continuing care centers, and skilled nursing centers. These choices are also covered in Chapter 30.

Assisted Living Centers

"**Assisted living** is a special combination of housing, personalized supportive services, and health care designed to respond to the individual needs of those who require help with activities of daily living" (Assisted Living Foundation of

DISPLAY 37–5. Home Care and Hospice—Medicare Benefits

Criteria	Home Care	Hospice
Client must be homebound	Yes	No
Skilled need required	Yes	No
Prognosis of 6 months to live	No	Yes
Short in-patient stay and respite available	No	Yes
Supplies and equipment covered	With limitations	No limitations
Chaplain, volunteers, bereavement support	No	Yes
Medications covered	No	Yes (pain and symptom management only)

America [ALFA], 1998, p. 35). Assisted living care promotes maximum independence and dignity for each resident. Staff is available 24 hours a day to meet both expected and unexpected needs. Assisted living residences may be called residential care facilities, adult congregate living facilities, or personal care homes (see Chapter 30). Each community refers to them by locally recognized names.

There is no typical type of assisted living residence. Clients' needs, preferences, and resources vary; thus, there are assisted living centers that span the gamut of amenities and opulence, from small six-resident homes to large, high rise apartment–like complexes with 200 or more residents. Personal space may be a one-room studio apartment up to a two- or three-bedroom apartment.

Medicare or Medicaid does not pay for the care in assisted living residences. People must have their own resources or long-term care insurance policies, as costs for such care can be over $30,000 a year. Long-term care insurance policies are fairly new, and many people are not aware of them. The policy cost is more reasonable the younger the policy holder; however, there is a screening process and all applicants are not accepted. Therefore, it is something to consider when you are a young to middle-aged healthy adult. A policy that costs about $600 a year for a person in their late 40s, and that pays for a place in an assisted living center that costs $30,000 a year, may give a sense of security to someone for whom this type of residence is appealing. Services available in assisted living are shown in Display 37–6.

Skilled Nursing Centers

Skilled nursing facilities (SNF) are designed to meet the caregiving needs of society's frailest citizens who need long-term rehabilitative, recuperative, or custodial care that includes the

---

DISPLAY 37–6. Services Available in Assisted Living

- Three meals a day served in a common dining room
- Housekeeping services
- Transportation to medical appointments and social activities
- Assistance with eating, bathing, dressing, toileting, and walking
- Access to health and medical services
- 24-hour security and staff availability
- Emergency call systems for each resident's unit
- Health promotion and exercise programs
- Medication management
- Personal laundry services
- Social and recreational activities

(From Assisted Living Foundation of America [1998]. Assisted living residence checklist. *Assisted Living Today, 5*(4), 35–37.)

---

need for skilled procedures and equipment. These facilities are changing as the nursing home resident changes (Stanford & Schmidt, 1995–1996). Providers are adapting the environment to accommodate individuals with lifestyles and expectations that are very different from what was provided a decade ago.

Today there is a trend toward specialization in nursing care facilities. Two of the newest additions are Alzheimer's and dementia special care units and rehabilitation and subacute care services (Mor, Banaszak-Holl, & Zinn, 1995–1996). We mentioned earlier the rise in hospice services; these are also considered new long-term care settings and services. The specialized facility offers quality care to the elder needing continuous care, either short term or long term.

The 84-year-old woman needing rehabilitation after a hip replacement can go to a skilled nursing facility where a portion of the bed space is reserved for clients needing subacute or rehabilitative care. There are active physical therapy, occupational, and speech therapy programs, with Medicare covering these rehabilitative services. For older adults with negative attitudes about nursing homes, the limited stay for recuperation and a focus on rehabilitation is an acceptable alternative, especially when they realize that hospitals no longer keep clients for the full recovery phase of illness or post-surgery and they know they are not well enough to return home.

An 81-year-old man with Alzheimer's disease, who was cared for at home by his wife until her death, finds a loving and safe home environment in an Alzheimer's living center. The facility provides ongoing care and appropriate activities by capable staff (Stang, 1998). They are especially trained to deal with clients who suffer from memory loss and degenerative physical functioning. These facilities have a low staff-to-client ratio because of the intense caregiving and supervisory needs of these clients (Hewett & Chang, 1998).

The Long-Term Care Population

The long-term care population is growing, getting older, and staying healthier. Fifteen years ago the average age of residents in skilled nursing facilities was 85. This is now the average age of residents in assisted living centers. The many community-assisted living choices and the ability of functionally independent older adults to manage caring for themselves in their own home postpone the need for admission to a skilled nursing facility.

People needing a skilled nursing facility are the frailest of the older adults. They may be suffering from chronic and degenerative diseases and need nursing care on a regular basis. This may include high-tech treatments, complex wound care, continuous respiratory assistance, or assistance with total personal care. Unfortunately, the reimbursement for a skilled nursing facility is very limited through the Medicare program as it exists today. Medicare will cover a limited number of days at full coverage and another set of days at partial coverage, but skilled nursing care is long-term care, given for years, for many older adults. They must use their resources to pay for their care until their resources are depleted, at which point they may become eligible for Medicaid.

Skilled nursing facilities have a limited number of beds for use by Medicaid clients, and it is possible that the resident may have to be moved to a different facility when his or her resources are depleted if a Medicaid bed is not available. This is an example of a major barrier in our health care delivery system for older adults.

Long-Term Care Personnel

The type of caregiving needs required by people needing long-term care promotes the hiring of paraprofessionals rather than a professional staff. Since care focuses on assistance with personal care, certified nursing assistants provide much of the care. Licensing requirements for assisted living centers and skilled nursing centers are different. Assisted living centers do not have to hire professional nursing staff. If a medical emergency arises, 911 is called and residents are transported to an appropriate service or acute-care facility. However, a registered nurse is often employed by large assisted living centers to coordinate all care to residents and health promotion programs and to provide in-service programs to assistive staff.

In skilled nursing facilities, licenced vocational (practical) nurses are hired for each shift to manage medications, assess clients' health, and assist with caregiving with the complex client. Large facilities have registered nurses on staff each shift; smaller facilities have one registered nurse on the day shift. As consumers demand higher quality of services and demonstrate a willingness and an ability to pay for additional services, the trend to hire more nurses will continue. Just as the acute-care setting has more acutely ill clients, so do skilled nursing facilities accepting clients for rehabilitation, convalescence, and high-tech custodial care. Many of the people that once occupied skilled nursing facility beds are now in assisted living centers.

THE EVOLUTION OF LONG-TERM CARE NURSING

Long-term care has come a long way since 1980. In that year, Bruce Vladeck wrote the groundbreaking book *Unloving Care,* documenting serious problems in both the quality and financing of long-term care. Subsequently, there have been advances and improvements in the long-term care industry. Two milestones in this progress are the Institute of Medicine's 1986 report *Improving Quality of Care in Nursing Homes* and the Omnibus Budget Reconciliation Act of 1987 (OBRA)—a major nursing home reform act that paved the way for improvement in standards for quality of care, resident rights, quality of life, and innovations in resident assessment (Wetle, 1995–1996).

More recently, innovative approaches to the design of long-term care environments and the demographic transitions of nursing home populations have created an expanding array of settings that meet the long-term care needs of people from their 60s to the expert elders—the centenarians.

Older adults are remaining physiologically capable of independence longer than in the past. Regardless of the age and functional level of the older adult, there is a role for the long-term care community health nurse (see Research: Bridge to Practice).

RESEARCH Bridge to Practice

Freedman, V.A. & Martin, L.G. (1998). Understanding trends in functional limitations among older Americans. *American Journal of Public Health, 88*(10), 1457–1462.

With increasing longevity there is a need to know whether the proportion of elders who are disabled might also be increasing. Answers to this question have an impact on planning for medical and social services for the older population.

The researchers had two goals as they conducted this study. They looked at recent trends in functional limitations among older Americans and used this information to shed light on possible explanations for the changes. What they found among the almost 26,000 participants was large declines in the prevalence of functional limitations, especially for adults 80 years old and older. However, among the 65- to 79-year-old group, if mobility-related device use was considered for difficulty walking, significant improvements in functioning remained. However, upon analysis of the survey design, role expectations, and living environments, they did not feel that this alone accounted completely for improvements in functioning. They infer that changes in underlying physiologic capability—whether real or perceived—are likely to underlie such trends.

Some interesting information they found during their data analysis was that within each of the three age groups they used (50–64, 65–79, and 80 and over), the highest prevalence of reported functional limitation was among the oldest, women, the unmarried, Hispanics, the least educated, and those without liquid assets. African-Americans reported more functional limitations than white participants, and regional differences among those studied were also evident.

Their results have important public health implications. They found that older people are likely to be better educated than they were just a decade ago, and this trend will continue. The increased education will likely be associated with beneficial changes in lifestyle, access to care, ability to comply with health care provider instructions, and the ability to modify one's environment. They also represent a more diverse mix of racial and ethnic groups. In addition, the researchers found that improvements in functioning have been greatest among those 80 and older, and that these patients are benefiting as much as others, if not more, from assistive device use, a practice that may be instrumental in helping the aged live longer independently. Finally, the researchers feel there is a need to learn more about specific interventions and behavioral changes that most likely underlie the trend of changes in physiological capability and focus on aspects of adult health that promote positive changes.

With healthier lifestyles, medications to keep chronic illnesses at bay or enable clients to live with them, and increasing longevity, older adults in their 60s and 70s remain at home, care for themselves, and enjoy a healthy and busy retirement or continue to work full- or part-time. Many people in this age group care for grandchildren or great-grandchildren and have altogether different needs (Goldberg-Glen et al., 1998). The community health nurse focuses on these population groups by offering such services as health screening at senior or community centers; organizing health fairs in shopping malls; planning for adult education and recreation services such as computer literacy, yoga, tai-chi, exercise, and water aerobics; the outreach services of parish nursing; home care services when illness or injury occurs; and hospice services if a disease has a terminal diagnosis.

As older adults become affected by functional or cognitive limitations, congregate or assisted living centers are popular choices for elders in their 80s and 90s. Independence and mobility are reinforced through the physical design of the facilities and the services offered. Community health nurses are often on staff to coordinate a wellness program for the population. The nurse works with a team of professionals, including physical therapists, activity directors, social workers, administrators, and assistive personnel, with the common goal of providing a safe environment to promote wellness and enhance the quality of life.

ROLE OF THE COMMUNITY HEALTH NURSE IN HOME, HOSPICE, AND LONG-TERM CARE

Community health nurses working in home, hospice, and long-term care settings have aspects to their caregiving that are similar. Caregiving includes direct care; detailed Medicare- and Medicaid-specific documentation; supervision of other professional, family, and volunteer caregivers; and client advocacy.

Direct Care

Direct care always involves client assessment of physical or psychosocial status and client and/or family education. However, in these roles direct care includes the performance of a skilled procedure. We have discussed family assessment in Chapter 23 and assessment of clients at various developmental stages in Chapters 26 to 30. In addition, we discussed the community health nurse's role in client education in Chapter 9. Some of the other skilled and technological procedures more commonly performed by home care, hospice, and long-term care nurses are shown in Display 37–7.

DISPLAY 37–7. Procedures Performed by Home Care, Hospice, and Long-Term Care Nurses

1. Intravenous services—initiating, monitoring, and teaching family members to monitor and maintain.
2. Wound care—can be simple or complex and includes old and new pressure ulcers, burns and surgical wounds, clean or sterile wet or dry dressings, irrigations and treatments.
3. Oxygen therapy—assessing the need for, use of, and safe use of oxygen delivery systems.
4. Phlebotomy—skillful drawing, storage, and transportation of blood from client veins or arteries as needed to perform ordered blood tests.
5. Ventilators—operating and monitoring stationary and portable units based on client need.
6. Pumps—setting up, monitoring, and in-home care; teaching clients to deliver client-controlled pain medication, insulin, and antibiotics.
7. Nutritional supplementation—setting up, monitoring, and teaching clients and families about TPN or nasal and gastric feeding tubes.
8. Elimination techonology—teaching, initiating, and/or monitoring, dialysis methods, biofeedback for incontinence, indwelling catheters, suprapubic catheters, obtaining sterile urine specimens from catheters or clean-catch urine specimens, enemas to treat elimination problems and for medication instillation as a treatment.
9. New or experimental therapies—in-patient and in-home care for clients with specific diagnoses, such as AIDS and cancer clients receiving state-of-the-art treatments, and portable in-home phototherapy for infants with hyperbilirubinemia.

(From Allender, J.A. [1998]. *Community and home health nursing.* Philadelphia: Lippincott-Raven.)

INFECTION CONTROL

As hospital stays have shortened, clients with communicable diseases and multiple invasive devices are now being cared for in the home or in long-term care settings. There are two major concerns for the nurse in caring for these clients:

- How to prevent infection in clients who are debilitated and may be immunocompromised
- How to protect the nurse, family, and community from a client who has an infectious or communicable disease

The home setting poses special challenges for the nurse in preventing the spread of infection or protecting the immunocompromised client from pathogens. For example, the primary caregivers, usually family members, are often untrained in procedures and know little about aseptic technique. The home may also lack facilities to care for the client under optimal conditions. In some homes there may not be access to running water, a heating unit to boil equipment, or adequate facilities to dispose of contaminated equipment. These conditions may necessitate the development of unique solutions to control infection. To guide the nurse, agencies have developed policies and procedures that deal with infection control; these typically are based on national policies, such as the Centers for Disease Control and Prevention's universal blood and body fluid precautions.

Infection control in long-term care settings is similar to that in the acute care setting, with some exceptions. This facility is home for many of the clients. When a large group of clients with compromised immune systems related to old age and debilitating illnesses live together, communicable diseases can become epidemic. Good handwashing technique for the staff and residents offers a first line of defense to avoid the spread of communicable diseases. Flu and pneumonia vaccines should be given on yearly and 5-year schedules. Tuberculosis skin tests and chest x-rays, if indicated, should be administered upon admission and at regular intervals throughout the client's stay in a long-term care setting. Nuisance diseases such as scabies and pediculosis may infect residents and staff alike. Good staff and client hygiene, proper bedding change and cleaning techniques, and client assessment will help to keep such annoying diseases to a minimum.

CLIENT EDUCATION

Most care provided in the home is the responsibility of someone other than the nurse. Teaching, then, becomes the most common intervention performed by home care nurses. Nurses are responsible for providing the client and family with the necessary information and skills to provide safe and effective care between home visits and following discharge from the home care agency.

In assisted living centers and skilled nursing facilities, the community health nurse's role focuses on in-service teaching of the staff and coordinating wellness programs for the residents. This includes teaching healthy living activities and exercise/water aerobics programs. The nurse may need to conduct one-on-one teaching if a client is diagnosed with a new disease, such as diabetes, or is to receive a new medication or treatment for an existing condition, such as asthma or arthritis. Family members are an integral part of home care, hospice care, and long-term care. Depending on the client's condition and cognitive ability, family members may become the primary contact with whom the nurse teaches and interacts.

Documentation

Accurate and thorough documentation is a critical component of home care, hospice, and skilled nursing care services.

In addition to conveying the clinical course of care for the client, documentation must address reimbursement and regulatory requirements. Not only will the payer inspect the record for the number of home care visits made or the health status of a client in a skilled nursing facility, they may also examine the types of services provided to determine whether the services were appropriate to meet the determined goal. As an indication of the magnitude of the task of documenting in home care, the National Association for Home Care has developed a task force of administrative and clinical experts to examine methods for reducing the paperwork burden for home care providers. Many agencies already have developed strategies to reduce the amount of time a nurse spends on documentation: these include the use of dictaphones, computerized care plans, and flow sheets or standardized care plans.

Similar concerns occur in skilled nursing facilities. Since OBRA regulations were enacted in 1987, the amount of paper work required in skilled nursing facilites has increased. Minimun data sets and standardized health records with concise flow sheets have been initiated to streamline the documentation process. Hospice documentation follows the home care trends if the care is in-home and is similar to acute-care documentation in in-patient hospice facilities.

Supervision and Case Management

The home care and skilled nursing facility nurse is responsible for coordination of the other professionals and para-professionals involved in the client's care. Additionally, the nurse is the primary contact with the client's physician, both reporting changes in the client's condition and securing changes in the plan of care.

As the home care case manager, the nurse conducts case conferences among team members to share information, discuss problems, and plan actions to effect the best possible outcomes for the client. Medicare mandates such case conferences every 60 days in home care. Additionally, the nurse must have the knowledge to refer clients to community resources for services not provided by the agency. Finally, the nurse manager supervises the para-professionals, such as home health aides, who also serve the homebound client. This may entail visiting the client at a time when the home health aide is present to observe the care provided.

Supervisory responsibilities are key roles for community health nurses in assisted living, in-patient hospices, and skilled nursing centers. Assisted living and skilled nursing facilities may have a minimum number of professional registered nurses on staff, while licensed vocational nurses and certified nursing assistants provide the physical caregiving that is needed. The registered nurse is the case manager for each resident and follows through with all the functions identified as part of the case manager's role. In hospices the staff is primarily professional and volunteers, and nurses function as case managers for the clients they have as their primary clients.

Two additional responsibilities of the nurse as case manager in home health care include determining financial coverage and determining frequency and duration of home care services.

DETERMINING FINANCIAL COVERAGE

A unique aspect of the role of the home health nurse as case manager is involvement in securing and maintaining reimbursement for the client's care. The home care nurse must know who is going to pay for services from the first visit to the time of discharge from the agency. If the client does not have a source of payment for the care that is needed, the agency must determine whether the client will receive the care free of charge or at a reduced rate. Many agencies have a sliding fee scale, which means that the charge for the services is based on the client's ability to pay. Nurses who deliver in-home hospice care have similar responsibilities. In skilled nursing facilities the nurse tracks caregiving days to inform the primary care provider of Medicare coverage dates and works closely with billing departments, social workers, and ombudsmen so that arrangements can be made for clients who continue to need care after insurance coverage comes to an end.

DETERMINING FREQUENCY AND DURATION OF SERVICES

The home care nurse is also responsible for determining the frequency and duration of the client's care. Will home visits be made twice weekly, once weekly, or once a month? For how long will visits continue? As the care is provided and the client's condition improves, the home care nurse, in collaboration with the physician, determines whether the frequency of visits should be reduced or whether the client can now be discharged.

Advocacy

Although the role of advocate is not unique to home care, hospice, and skilled nursing care services, the way in which the nurse advocates for the client requires unique knowledge and skills. One of the most common advocacy issues is helping the older client to negotiate the complex medical care reimbursement system. This may involve assisting clients to interpret bills from previous hospitalizations, organizing their receipts for submission to their insurance company, or informing them of the services of hospice programs or rehabilitation services provided in a skilled nursing facility. Although this may not seem significant, nurses must be aware that the stress of financial worries can interfere with the client's recovery, rehabilitation, or peaceful death.

Advocacy in assisted living and skilled nursing facilities is important to the quality of care the residents and clients receive. There needs to be a system of resident leadership in the facility through a resident advisory board and an **ombuds-**

man, who speaks for the client and acts as an advocate in all matters concerning the client stay in the facility. The nurse can ensure that these systems are in place and are not just symbols but active and integral components of the services and functioning of the agency.

SUMMARY

Community health nurses have an important role in working with elders who receive home care or hospice services or reside in a variety of long-term care settings. As our population continues to age, the need for additional nurses to work with older adults where they choose to live during their final years and days will only increase.

Home care services comprise the entire array of health care and nursing care services brought to a person's home. Rapid discharge from acute-care settings does not allow the client to completely recover in that setting, which puts demands on family members if the client goes home or on skilled nursing facilities that provide rehabilitative and convalescence services.

Most home care clients are over 65, female, and predominantly white. Health monitoring, medication instruction, client advocacy, and teaching about disease or treatment processes to the client and/or family members are the focus of the home health nurse's role. Whatever the caregiving needs are, they must be conducted with goals achieved in a few home visits if Medicare is reimbursing for the care given. This has become even more important since the legislative changes restricting the numbers of home visits brought about by the Balanced Budget Act of 1997. If the client pays for the visits or has a private insurance policy, more visits may be available to achieve the goals.

There are many types of home care agencies: voluntary, proprietary, hospital-based, official, homemaker, and hospices. Care is provided by formal and informal caregivers—professional staff members, such as nurses, social workers, therapists, and certified nursing assistants, in collaboration with family members, and friends and neighbors in some situations.

Hospice is a fairly new concept in the United States but has a strong long-term history in England. Medicare covers hospice care without the restrictions experienced by non-hospice home care clients. Hospice programs provide holistic care to clients during the last 6 months of life. Many programs are home-based and are often a service of a home health agency. In addition to in-home hospices, there are inpatient hospices. These can be a free-standing building, part of a skilled nursing facility, or in a section of an acute-care facility. What is different is the focus of care—it is not curative and employs holistic caregiving practices that involve family members, professionals, and volunteers.

The traditional nursing home or skilled nursing facility as

the main choice of residence or caregiving center for the frailer and less independent older adult has given way to a bevy of assisted living choices. The choices, price ranges, and locations of the more than 2000 assisted living centers and additional smaller family-type homes can meet the needs of a large segment of today's aging community members who are unable to provide all the care they need for themselves.

Skilled nursing facilities are expanding their services to accommodate clients who need short-term rehabilitation and convalescence. In addition, some are providing services just for special groups of elders, such as those with dementia and Alzheimer's disease.

Community health nurses have opportunities to focus their attention on this fast-growing population by working in or with these agencies. The nurse provides direct physical nursing care in some settings, teaches clients and staff, supervises, and case manages in all settings. Assessing clients to determine health status and eligibility for additional services and acting as a client advocate occurs in all settings. Determining the frequency and duration of services occurs in home care. In all settings the nurse must become familiar with the requirements of documentation to promote continuity of care and ensure reimbursement. (See Clinical Corner.)

CLINICAL CORNER | Community Health Nursing in the Long-Term Care Setting

Scenario
Sunny Acres is a skilled nursing facility with 49 beds. The staffing pattern for the agency is as follows:
- 1 RN per shift
- 1 LVN for every eight clients
- 1 medical assistant for every two LVNs

The facility is part of a group of homes owned and operated by three retired dentists.

Clients range in age from 42 to 98 and have varied psychological and medical problems. Common medical conditions affecting clients include:
- COPD and CHF
- Organic brain syndrome and dementia
- Peripheral neuropathy
- Osteoporosis
- Post CVA
- Depression

There are 49 residents at Sunny Acres. Eighty percent of the residents of Sunny Acres have Medicare as their sole means of payment. Fifteen percent have Medicare and Medicaid, and 5 % are private pay clients.

Sunny Acres is located in Smithville and offers the following services to its clients:
- Three meals per day
- Nutritionist consults once every 2 weeks
- Social hour (singing, etc.) 9–10:00 AM and 3–4:00 PM
- Physical and occupational therapy weekly
- Assistance with activities of daily living, including feeding and bathing
- Administration of medications
- Volunteers daily (ie, animals brought by local animal shelter volunteers, drama productions by local elementary schools)

In your role as the program manager supervising the adult health programs for the local health department, you have been approached by several family members of the residents of Sunny Acres. The families have become concerned about what they perceive to be inadequate provision of basic hygiene services to the clients at Sunny Acres. As examples, they cite instances of ingrown toenails, dirty and overgrown fingernails, dermatitis of the scalp, and scabies. They report having sought assistance from the owners, to no avail.

They have been advised by the operators of the facility that if they would like additional services for their family members, they will be required to provide services themselves or pay extra to have such service contracted. Although the family members would like to pursue this matter or move residents to another facility, there are no other skilled nursing facility options available in the Smithville area for clients with Medicare as their sole funding source.

Your program has some funding available to provide education to clients and staff of skilled nursing facilities. You are concerned, however, about the fact that previous attempts by your staff to provide this service have been declined by the operators of Sunny Acres.

Questions
1. Discuss additional assessment data needed and how you will go about gathering these data.
2. Present host, agent, and environmental factors, based on data presented in this scenario.
   Host
   Agent
   Environment
3. Describe educational interventions that you will perform.
4. Analyze issues related to social justice for this aggregate.
5. How will you go about building partnerships to assist in your role as educator?
6. How will you evaluate the effects of your interventions?
7. How will you disseminate the information you obtain in order to advance the cause of globalization of community health?

REFERENCES

Acampora, T. (1997). Types of referrals and purpose of home care. In S.M. Zang & N.C. Bailey. *Home care manual: Making the transition* (pp. 3–21). Philadelphia: Lippincott-Raven.

Allender, J.A. (1998). *Community and home health nursing*. Philadelphia: Lippincott-Raven.

American Association of Colleges of Nursing (AACN) (1998). *Peaceful death: Recommended competencies and curricular guidelines for end-of-life nursing care*. Washington, DC: Author.

American Nurses Association (1999). *Scope and standards of home health nursing practice*. Washington, DC: American Nurses Foundation/American Nurses Association.

Assisted Living Foundation of America (ALFA) (1998). Assisted living residence checklist. *Assisted Living Today, 5*(4), 35–37.

Bureau of Labor Statistics (1999). *Employment statistics: Home health care agencies*. Washington, DC: Author.

Burke, M.M. & Walsh, M.B. (1997). *Gerontological nursing: Holistic care of the older adult*. St. Louis: Mosby–Year Book.

D'Angelo, A.M. (1999). Effectively managing the elderly client in the community. In S.M. Zang & J.A. Allender. *Home care of the elderly* (pp. 3–16). Philadelphia: Lippincott Williams & Wilkins.

D'Amico-Panomeritakis, D. & Sommer, J.K. (1998). Promoting and maintaining mobility in the homebound elderly client. In S.M. Zang & J.A. Allender, *Home care of the elderly* (pp. 78–97). Philadelphia: Lippincott Williams & Wilkins.

Freedman, V.A. & Martin, L.G. (1998). Understanding trends in functional limitations among older Americans. *American Journal of Public Health, 88*(10), 1457–1462.

Goldberg-Glen, R., Sands, R.G., Cole, R.D, & Cristofalo, C. (September-October, 1998). Multigenerational patterns and internal structres in families in which grandparents raise grandchildren. *Families in Society: The Journal of Contemporary Human Services, 79*(5), 477–489.

Harris, M.D. (1998). The impact of the Balanced Budget Act of 1997 on home health care agencies and nurses. *Home Healthcare Nurse, 16*(7), 435–437.

Haupt, B. (1998). *An overview of home health and hospice care patients. 1996 Home and Hospice Care Survey*. Washington, DC: National Center for Health Statistics.

Health Care Financing Administration (HCFA) (1999). *Medicare and you 2000* (Publication No.HCFA-10050). Baltimore: U.S. Department of Health and Human Services, HCFA.

Hewett, L.J. & Chang, F. (1998). Alzheimer's disease, a hopeful note for the closing of a century: Challenges for the new millennium. In J.A. Allender & C.L. Rector, *Readings in gerontological nursing* (pp. 484–502). Philadelphia: Lippincott-Raven.

Humphrey, C. & Milone-Nuzzo, P. (1996). *Manual of home care nursing orientation*. Gaithersburg, MD: Aspen.

International Council of Nurses. (1997). *Basic principles of nursing care*. Washington, DC: American Nurses Publishing.

Jackson, N. (March 1997). Health care on the home front. *Workforce, 77*(3), 30–35.

Kane, R. (1995–1996). Transforming care instituitions for the frail elderly: Out of one shall be many. *Generations, 19*(4), 62–68.

Madigan, E.A. (1997). An introduction to pediatric home health care. *Journal of the Society of Pediatric Nurses, 2*(4), 172–178.

More, V., Banaszak-Holl, J., & Zinn, J. (1995–1996). The trend toward specialization in nursing care facilities. *Generations, 19*(4), 24–29.

National Association for Home Care (1999). *Basic statistics about home care*. Washington, DC: Author.

——— (2000). *Basic statistics about home care*. Washington, DC: Author.

Nursing Trends and Issues (1999). Home health payments— Turbulent times. *Nursing Trends & Issues, 4*(2). Available: http://www.nursing world.org/products/9909nti.htm

Schroeder, B. & Towle, S.M. (1999). Care of the terminally ill patient at home. *NurseWeek, 12*(7), 32–34.

Schulkin, V. (1999). Providing palliative care for the dying elderly client. In S.M. Zang & J.A. Allender, *Home care of the elderly* (pp. 486–505). Philadelphia: Lippincott Williams & Wilkins.

Stanford, E. P. & Schmidt, M.G. (1995–1996). The changing face of nursing home residents: Meeting their diverse needs. *Generations, 19*(4), 20–23.

Stang, M. (1998). Keys to quality Alzheimer's care. *Assisted Living Today, 5*(4), 42–45.

Sultz, H.A. & Young, K.M (1999). *Health care USA: Understanding its organization and delivery* (2nd ed.). Gaithersburg, MD: Aspen.

Waid, M.O. (1997). *Brief summaries of Medicare and Medicaid: Title XVII and Title XIX of the Social Security Act*. AHCAG, Health Care Financing Administration, DHHS. Available: http://www.hcfa.gov/medicare/ormedmed.html

Wetle, T. (1995–1996). The nursing home: Are these the golden years? *Generations, 19*(4), 5–7.

Williams, S.J. & Torrens, P.R. (1999). *Introduction to health services*. Albany: Delmar Publishers.

RESOURCES AND INTERNET SITES

American Cancer Society: *www.acs.org*

Assisted Living Federation of America (ALFA): *www.alfa.org*

Complementary Therapies: *www.wholenurse.com/*

Family Caregiver Alliance: *www.caregiver.org*

The Agency for Health Care Policy and Research (AHCPR): *www.AHCPR.gov/clinic*

The Heart Failure Society of America (HFSA): *www.hfsa.org*

Medicare: 1–800–633–4227; *www.medicare.gov*

National Eldercare Locator: 1–800–677–1116

SELECTED READINGS

Abrams, N.M. (1998). Leading a parent to assisted living. *Assisted Living Today, 5*(4), 9–10.

Chan, C. & Chang, A., (1999). Managing caregiver tasks among family caregivers in cancer patients in Hong Kong. *Journal of Advanced Practice Nursing, 29*(2), 484–489.

Collins, C. E., Butler, F. R., Gueldner, S. H., & Palmer, M. H. (1997). Models for community-based long-term care for the elderly in a changing health system. *Nursing Outlook, 45,* 59–63.

Folbrecht, D.W. (1997). Separate and equal: Hospice and home health care. *Home Health Care Management and Practice, 9*(5), 1–9.

Jacob, S.R. (1996). The grief experience of older women whose husbands had hospice care. *Journal of Advanced Nursing, 24,* 280–286.

Jensen, B, Hess-Zac, A. Johnstone, S.K., et al. (1998). Restraint reduction: A new philosophy for a new millennium. *Journal of Nursing Administration, 28*(7/8), 32–38.

Jones, D.H. (1997). The new hospice condtions of participation: Meeting the challenge, keeping the values. *Home Health Care Management and Practice, 9*(5), 10–15.

Klebanoff, N.A. & Smith, N.M. (1997). *Lippincott's guide to behavior management in home care.* Philadelphia: Lippincott-Raven.

Mace, N.L. & Rabins, P.V. (1999). *The 36-hour day* (3rd ed.). Baltimore: Johns Hopkins University Press.

Morris, R.I., & Christie, K.B. (1995). Initiation hospice care. *Home Healthcare Nurse, 13*(5), 21–26.

Neal, L.J. (1998). Current functional assessment tools. *Home Healthcare Nurse, 16*(11), 766–772.

Pearce, B.W. (1998). *Senior living communities.* Baltimore: Johns Hopkins University Press.

Sankar, A. (1999). *Dying at home: A family guide for caregiving* (revised and updated edition). Baltimore: Johns Hopkins University Press.

Schwarz, B. & Brent, R. (1999). *Aging, autonomy, and architecture: Advances in assisted living.* Baltimore: Johns Hopkins University Press.

Seeber, S. & Baird, S.B. (1996). The impact of health changes on home health care. *Seminars in Oncology Nursing, 12*(3), 179–187.

Turkel, M., Tappen, R.M., & Hall, R. (1999). Moments of excellence: Nurses' response to role redesign in long-term care. *Journal of Gerontological Nursing, 25*(1), 7–12.

Yuan, J.R. (1998). Using standards and gudelines in your daily practice. *Home Healthcare Nurse, 16*(11), 753–759.

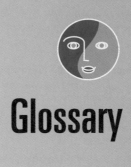

Glossary

Accommodation—being sufficiently mature so that previously unsolved problems can now be solved.

Acquired immunodeficiency syndrome (AIDS)—a severe, life-threatening condition representing the late clinical stage of infection with HIV in which there is progressive damage to the immune and other organ systems.

Active immunity—a long-term resistance to a specific disease-causing organism, acquired naturally or artificially.

Active listening—the skill of assuming responsibility for and understanding the feelings and thoughts in a sender's message.

Adaptation—the ability to cope with the demands of the environment.

Addiction—a compulsive use or impaired control over using a substance, preoccupation with obtaining and using a drug, and continued use despite adverse consequences.

Adult—anyone between the ages of 18 and 64.

Advocate—someone who pleads clients' causes or acts on their behalf.

Affective domain—learning that involves changes in emotion, feeling, or affect.

Ageism—stereotyping older adults and perpetuating false information and negative images and characteristics about them.

Agent—a factor that causes or contributes to a health problem or condition.

Aggregate—a mass or grouping of distinct individuals who are considered as a whole and who are loosely associated with one another.

Alcoholics Anonymous (AA)—a self-help program designed to keep alcoholics sober one day at a time and based on the "12-step" model that includes a belief in a higher power.

Al-Anon—a self-help organization designed around the principles of Alcoholics Anonymous and intended for family members and close friends of an alcoholic.

Ala-Teens—a self-help organization modeled after Al-Anon, designed around the principles of Alcoholics Anonymous, and intended for older children and teenagers affected by an alcoholic in the family.

Alzheimer's disease—a progressive dementia affecting older adults in increasing numbers as people age. Judgment and reasoning are lost, eventually affecting the person physically with increased weakness, wasting, and immobility.

Analytic epidemiology—seeks to identify associations between a particular human disease or health problem and its possible cause(s).

Anorexia nervosa—an eating disorder of emotional etiology that is characterized by a body image disturbance, an intense fear of becoming fat or gaining weight, and a refusal to maintain an adequate body weight.

Anticipatory guidance—a process of assisting the client in preparing for a future role or developmental stage.

Arson—the deliberate burning of buildings.

Assault and battery—the threat to use force against another person, and the accomplishment of that threat.

Assessment—gathering and analyzing information that will affect the health of the people to be served.

Assets assessment—an assessment that focuses on the strengths and capacities of the community rather than on the problems alone.

Assimilation—reacting to new situations by using skills already possessed.

Assisted living—a special combination of housing, supportive services, personalized assistance, and health care designed to respond to the individual needs of those who need help with activities of daily living and instrumental activities of daily living.

Assurance—those activities that make certain that services are actually provided.

Attention deficit disorder (without hyperactivity) (ADD)—a cluster of problems related mainly to inattention, poor motivation, and disorganization.

Attention deficit hyperactivity disorder (ADHD)—a cluster of problems related to hyperactivity, impulsivity, and inattention.

Audit—an organized effort whereby practicing professionals monitor, assess, and make judgments about the quality and appropriateness of nursing care provided by peers as measured against professional standards of practice.

Autocratic leadership style—an authoritarian style in which leaders use their power to influence their followers.

Autonomous leadership style—a facilitative style of leadership that encourages group members to select and carry out their own activities and function independently.

Autonomy—freedom of choice and the exercise of people's rights.

Baby boomers—those people born after World War II, between 1946 and 1964.

Battered child syndrome—the collection of injuries sustained by a child as a result of repeated mistreatment or beatings.

Benchmarking—studying another's processes in order to improve one's own processes.

Beneficence—doing good or benefiting others.

Bilateral agencies—agencies that usually deal directly with other individual governments, such as the U.S. Agency for International Development, the Peace Corps, and the U.S. Centers for Disease Control and Prevention.

Biostatistics—the science of statistically measuring population health conditions.

Bioterrorism—the use of living organisms, such as bacteria, viruses, or other organic materials, to harm and/or intimidate others in order to achieve political ends.

Blended family—a family in which single parents marry and raise the children from each of their previous relationships together.

Brainstorming—an idea-generating process that encourages group members to freely offer suggestions.

Bulimia—an eating disorder characterized by recurrent episodes of binge eating with repeated compensatory mechanisms to prevent weight gain, such as causing vomiting or taking laxatives.

Burden of disease—the impact of premature death and disability on a population's health status; assessed by measuring the gap between the population's health status and some reference status.

Camp health aides—bilingual and bicultural individuals, usually women, who help reinforce positive health values and create a sense of self-esteem and empowerment among migrant farm workers.

Capitation rate—a fixed amount of money paid per person by the health plan to the provider for covered services.

Case management—a systematic process by which a nurse assesses clients' needs, plans for and coordinates services, refers to other appropriate providers, and monitors and evaluates progress to ensure that clients' multiple service needs are met in a cost-effective manner.

Casualty—a human being who is injured or killed during or as a direct result of an accident.

Causal thinking—relating disease or illness to its cause.

Causality—the relationship between a cause and its effect.

Change—any planned or unplanned alteration of the status quo in an organization, situation, or process.

Channel—the medium through which the sender conveys the message.

Chemical dependence—a strong, overwhelming preoccupation with and desire to have a drug.

Child abuse—the maltreatment of children including any or all of the following: physical, emotional, medical, or educational neglect; physical punishment or battering; or emotional or sexual maltreatment and exploitation.

Chronic disease—a set of diseases occurring mainly among adults and including degenerative diseases, diseases of the circulatory system, cancer, and diabetes.

Client myth—the belief that the primary clients in community health nursing are individuals and families.

Clinician—a nursing role in the community that ensures that health services are provided to individuals, families, groups, and populations.

Coalition—an alliance of indiviudals or groups working together to influence outcomes of a specific problem.

Co-dependence—dysfunctional behaviors that are evident among family members.

Cohabiting couples—the forming of a family alliance outside of marriage or through a private ceremony not legally recognized as marriage.

Cohort—a group of people who share a common experience in a specific time period.

Cognitive domain—the area of leaning that involves the mind and thinking processes.

Collaboration—working together in cooperation with other team members, coordinating services and addressing the needs of population groups.

Collaborator—a role in which the nurse works jointly with others in a common endeavor.

Common-interest community—a collection of people who, although they are widely scattered geographically, have an interest or goal that binds them together.

Commune family—a group of unrelated, monogamous couples living together and collectively rearing their children; considered a nontraditional family.

Communicable disease—a disease that can be transmitted from one person to another.

Communication—transferring meaning and enhancing understanding.

Community—a collection of people who interact with one another and whose common interests or characteristics form the basis for a sense of unity or belonging.

Community as client—the concept of a community-wide group of people as the focus of nursing service.

Community-based—a term used to describe the setting for nursing care delivery.

Community collaboration—the ability of the community to work together as a team of citizens, professional and lay people alike, in order to meet an identified need in the community.

Community development—the process of collaborating with community members to assess their collective needs and desires for a positive change and to address these needs through problem solving, use of community experts, and resource development.

Community diagnoses—nursing diagnoses about the community's ineffective coping ability and potential for enhanced coping.

Community health—the identification of needs and the protection and improvement of collective health within a geographically defined area.

Community health advocacy—efforts aimed at creating awareness of and generating support for meeting the community's health needs.

Community health nursing—a field of nursing combining nursing science with public health science to formulate a practice that is community-based and population-focused.

Community mental health—a field of practice that seeks to address the needs of the mentally ill, prevent mental illness, and promote the mental health of the community.

Community mental health centers (CMHC)—sites that provide comprehensive, publicly funded services to the mentally ill population.

Community needs assessment—the process of determining the real or perceived needs of a defined community of people.

Community of solution—a group of people who come together to solve a problem that affects all of them.

Community-oriented, population-focused care—care that is shaped by the characteristics and needs of a given community and employs population-based skills.

Community subsystem assessment—an assessment that focuses on a single dimension of community life, such as churches or schools.

Community support programs—a publicly funded set of services designed to assist persons with serious and persistent mental illness (SPMI).

Commuter family—a family in which both partners work but have jobs in different cities; one parent raises the children in the "home" city while the second partner lives in the other city and commutes home for weekends or less frequently, depending on the distance.

Competition—a contest between rival health care organizations for resources and clients.

Comprehensive assessment—an assessment that seeks to discover all relevant community health information.

Conceptual model—a framework made up of ideas for explaining and studying a phenomenon of interest, conveying a particular perception of the world.

Conceptual skills—the mental ability to analyze and interpret abstract ideas for the purpose of understanding and diagnosing situations and formulating solutions.

Concurrent review—an assessment of care while in the process of being given that is often combined with a retrospective review.

Confidant—a close friend; someone in whom an older adult can confide, reflect on the past, and trust.

Contaminant—organic or inorganic matter that enters a medium, such as water or food, and renders it impure.

Contemporary family—emerging family patterns that did not exist a few years earlier, such as the "loose shirt" family in which parent(s) work from home via the computer and Internet.

Continuing care center—often referred to as a total life center; a type of housing facility for older adults that provides a home-like setting for people at all levels of functioning, from total independence to those most dependent on skilled nursing care, offering older adults a home for life.

Continuous needs—populations in all age groups with birth-to-death developmental health care needs.

Contracting—negotiating a working agreement between two or more parties in which they come to a shared understanding and mutually consent to the purposes and terms of the transaction.

Control group—randomly assigned subjects in a research study who are not receiving the intervention.

Control of communicable disease—the point at which a specific disease has ceased to be a public health threat.

Controller—a management function of the community health nurse in which the nurse monitors the plan and ensures that it stays on course.

Coping—those actions and ways of thinking that assist people in dealing with and surviving difficult situations.

Core public health functions—three areas that include assessment, policy development, and assurance and that encompass a wide variety of activities.

Corporal punishment—violence against a child as a form of discipline.

Correctional facility—one whose primary objective is to provide safety to the public by incarcerating those who have committed crimes and who are deemed a threat to the community.

Cost sharing—a cost-containment strategy in which consumers pay a portion of health care costs.

Crew leader—a person who acts as a mediator between the group of migrant laborers, called crews, and the farmer, with the farmer often paying the crew leader who pays the laborers.

Crisis theory—a body of knowledge that helps to explain why people respond in certain ways; it is useful to predict the phases that people will go through in a crisis of any kind.

Critical incident stress debriefing (CISD)—a mechanism for providing victims emotional reconciliation following a disaster, ideally between 24 and 72 hours after the event.

Critical pathway—written plans and outcomes for patient care with a timetable; a term used synonymously with clinical pathway.

Cross-sectional study—exploring a health condition's relationship to other variables in a specific population at a certain point in time.

Culture—the beliefs, values, and behavior that are shared by members of a society and that provide a design or "map" for living.

Cultural assessment—obtaining health-related information about a designated cultural group concerning their values, beliefs, and practices.

Cultural brokering—facilitating health care for migrant workers who are unable to overcome the barriers of existing health care.

Cultural diversity—a variety of cultural patterns that coexist within a designated geographic area.

Cultural relativism—recognizing and respecting alternative viewpoints and understanding values, beliefs, and practices within their cultural context.

Cultural self-awareness—recognition of one's own values, beliefs, and practices that make up one's culture.

Cultural sensitivity—recognizing that culturally based values, beliefs, and practices influence people's health and life styles.

Culture shock—a state of anxiety that results from cross-cultural misunderstanding and an inability to interact appropriately in the new context.

Curanderas—Mexican folk healers.

Custodial care—personal care that is considered non skilled, such as bathing, dressing, feeding, and assisting with mobility and recreation.

Cycle of violence—the repetitive cyclical pattern of abuse seen in domestic violence situations.

Dating violence—physical, sexual, emotional, and/or verbal abuse between persons who are or have been in a casual or serious dating relationship.

Decoding—translating a message into understandable form.

Deforestation—the clearing of tropical and temperate forests for cropland, cattle grazing, or urbanization.

Deinstitutionalization—the process of transferring the mentally ill from public institutions to community-based care settings.

Delphi technique—a method of arriving at group consensus through a systematic pooling of separate individuals' judgments by written questionnaire and suggestions.

Demographic entrapment—the effect of a population that exceeds the ability of its ecosystem to either support it or acquire the support needed, or when it exceeds its ability to migrate to other ecosystems in a manner that preserves its standard of living.

Department of Health and Human Services (DHHS)—the federal level of five primary agencies concerned with health and organized under the umbrella of the DHHS: the Public Health Service, the Office of Human Development

Services, the Health Care Financing Administration, the Family Support Administration, and the Social Security Administration.

Descriptive epidemiological study—a study that examines the amount and distribution of a disease or health condition in a population by person, place, and time.

Descriptive epidemology—investigations that seek to observe and describe patterns of health-related conditions that naturally occur in a population.

Descriptive statistics—describe in quantitative or mathematical terms the data collected.

Desertification—the conversion of fertile land into desert that is unable to support crop growth or wildlife.

Detoxification—the process of ridding the body of harmful substances.

Developmental crisis—periods of disruption that occur at transition points during normal growth and development.

Developmental disability—a broad scope of limitations that include intellectual limitations and the inability to perform certain activities of daily living, which is identified before age 22.

Developmental framework—studies families from a life-cycle perspective by examining members' changing roles and tasks in each progressive life-cycle stage.

Diagnostic-related groups—a billing classification system based on 23 major diagnostic categories and 467 diagnosis-related groups that provides fixed Medicare reimbursement to hospitals.

Direct transmission—immediate transfer of infectious agents from a reservoir to a new host.

Direct victim—people who experience an event, whether a fire, volcanic eruption, war, or bomb.

Disabling injury—an injury that results in restriction of normal activities of daily living beyond the day on which the injury occurred.

Disability-Adjusted Life Year (DALY)—the combination of years of life lost due to premature mortality and years of life lived with disability adjusted for the severity of disability; developed to compare across conditions and risk factors.

Disaster—any event that causes a level of destruction that exceeds the abilities of the affected community to respond without assistance.

Disenfranchised—someone who does not have full privileges and rights as a citizen.

Displaced persons—people forced to leave their homes to escape the effects of a disaster.

Distributive health policy—promotes non-governmental activities thought to be beneficial to society as a whole.

Distributive justice—a belief that benefits should be given first to the disadvantaged or those who need them the most.

District nursing—the formal organization of visiting nursing, known as district nursing in England; the period in the history of community health/public health nursing from the mid-1800s to 1900.

Domestic violence—morbidity and mortality attributed to violence within the home setting.

Dominant values—the beliefs and sanctions of the dominant or majority culture.

Drug dependent—a person who physically and psychologically requires use of drugs to function and, if pregnant, gives birth to an infant exhibiting withdrawal symptoms.

Drug exposed—a person who uses drugs intermittently and, if pregnant, gives birth to a drug-exposed infant.

Durable medical equipment (DME)—the equipment used for a long period of time in a person's home that can be used again by others, such as wheelchairs, walkers, hospital beds, ventilators, and IV poles.

Ecological perspective—a viewpoint about the community of living organisms and their interrelated physical and chemical environments.

Eco-map—a diagram of the connections between a family and the other systems in its ecological environment; originally devised to depict the complexity of the client's story.

Ecosystem—a community of living organisms and their interrelated physical and chemical environments.

Educator—the role of health teacher; a major function of the community health nurse.

Egalitarian justice—a system that promotes decisions based on equal distribution of benefits to everyone, regardless of need.

Elder abuse—the mistreatment or exploitation of older adults.

Electronic meetings—a method of meeting that applies nominal group technique combined with computer technology.

Elimination—a reduction of prevalence to a level below one case per million population in a given area.

Elite-old—those over age 100, or centenarians.

Emotional abuse—psychological mistreatment and/or neglect, such as when caregivers or family members do not provide the normal experiences producing feelings of being loved, wanted, secure, and worthy.

Empathy—the ability to communicate understanding and vicariously experience the feelings and thoughts of others.

Empirical-rational change strategies—strategies used to effect change based on the assumption that people are rational and when presented with empirical information will adopt new practices that appear to be in their best interest.

Employee assistance programs—programs cooperatively sponsored by employers and bargaining agencies with the intent to promote the mental health of the employee by providing an outlet for employee concerns.

Empowerment—a process of developing knowledge and skills that increase one's mastery over the decisions that affect one's life.

Encoding—the sender's conversion of a message into symbolic form.

Enculturation—learning one's own culture through socialization with the family or significant group.

Endemic—the continuing presence of a disease or infectious agent in a given geographic area.

Energy exchange—materials or information that families exchange with their environment.

Environment—all the external factors surrounding the host that might influence vulnerability or resistance.

Environmental health—assessing, controlling, and improving the impact people make on their environment and the impact of the environment on them.

Environmental impact—the effect of positive or negative changes on the environment and on the people, animals, and plants living in it.

Environmental justice—a movement that has sought to ensure that no particular part of the population is disproportionately burdened by the negative effects of pollution.

Epidemic—a disease occurrence that clearly exceeds normal or expected frequency in a community or region.

Epidemiology—the study of health, disease, and injury determinants and distribution in populations.

Episodic needs—populations with one-time, specific negative health events, such as illness or injury, that are not an expected part of life.

Equity—being treated equally or fairly.

Eradication—the interruption of person-to-person transmission and a limitation of the reservoir of infection such that no further preventive efforts are required.

Ergonomics—a field of study in occupational health concerned with the design of workplaces, tools, and tasks to match the physiological, anatomical, and psychological characteristics and capabilities of the worker; sometimes called human engineering.

Ethical decision making—making a choice that is consistent with a moral code or that can be justified from an ethical perspective.

Ethical dilemma—a decision involving a potential conflict between moral values.

Ethics—a set of moral principles or values; a theory or system of moral values.

Ethnic group—a collection of people with common origins and with a shared culture and identity.

Ethnicity—that group of qualities that mark a person's association with a particular ethnic group.

Ethnocentrism—the belief and feeling that one's own culture is best.

Evaluation—the process by which a practice is analyzed, judged, and improved according to established goals and standards.

Evaluator—a management function in which the nurse compares and judges performance and outcomes against previously set goals and standards.

Evolutionary change—change that is gradual and requires adjustment on an incremental basis.

Experimental design—a research method in which the investigators institute an intervention and then measure its consequences.

Experimental epidemology—follows and builds on information gathered from descriptive and analytic approaches; used to study epidemics, the etiology of human disease, the value of preventive and therapeutic measures, and the evaluation of health services.

Experimental group—randomly assigned subjects who are receiving the intervention in a research study.

Experimental study—a study in which the investigator controls or changes factors suspected of causing a condition and observes the results.

Extinction—the loss of a species from the earth forever.

Familialism—taking responsibility for one's own family and protecting them from harm.

Familiarization assessment—studying data already available on a community, and gathering a certain amount of firsthand data, in order to gain a working knowledge of the community; sometimes called a "windshield" survey.

Family—two or more individuals who share a residence or live near one another; possess some common emotional bond; engage in interrelated social positions, roles, and tasks; and share a sense of affection and belonging.

Family crisis—a stressful and disruptive event, or series of events, that comes with or without warning and disturbs the equilibrium of the family.

Family culture—the acquired knowledge that family members use to interpret their experiences and to generate behaviors that influence family structure and function.

Family functioning—those behaviors or activities by family members that maintain the family and meet family needs, individual member needs, and society's views of family.

Family health—how well the family functions together as a unit.

Family map—a diagram that illustrates the pattern of interactions and interdependence between family members.

Family nursing—a kind of nursing practice in which the family is the unit of service.

Family structure—comprises the characteristics of individuals who make up a family unit: age, gender, and number.

Family system boundary—the greater concentration of energy that exists within the family than between the family and its external environment.

Family violence—action by a family member with the intent to cause harm to or control another family member.

Feedback loop—the receiver indicating that the message has been understood (decoded) in the way that the sender intended (encoded).

Felony—a serious crime such as murder, rape, or burglary, for which the criminal is typically housed in a maximum-security prison.

Feminization of poverty—the growing numbers of women who have fallen into poverty due to weakening of the nuclear family as more women head households alone, low-wage jobs for unskilled work, and the dismantling of social programs for women.

Fetal alcohol effects (FAE)—a combination of birth anomalies characterized by some, but not all, of the symptoms of fetal alcohol syndrome.

Fetal alcohol syndrome (FAS)—a combination of birth anomalies characterized by structural abnormalities of the head and face including microcephaly and flattening of the maxillary area, intrauterine growth retardation, decreased birth weight and length, developmental delays, intellectual impairment, hyperactivity, altered sleep pattern, feeding problems, perceptual problems, mood problems, and language dysfunction; caused by maternal alcohol consumption during pregnancy.

Fidelity—keeping one's promises.

Force field analysis—a technique for examining all the positive and negative forces influencing a change situation.

Forensics—the science of medical or health care jurisprudence in which legal argument advocates for offenders.

Formal caregivers—professionals and para-professionals who are compensated for in-home care they provide.

Formal contracting—a process in which all parties negotiate a written contract by mutual agreement, sign the agreement, and sometimes have it witnessed or notarized.

Foster families—families who have had formal training and are licensed to accept non-related children into their homes to raise temporarily while their families of origin resolve their problems.

Frail elderly—those older than age 85 who need assistance in attending to activities of daily living.

Frontier area—sparsely populated places with six or fewer persons per square mile.

Gang—a loose-knit organization of individuals between the ages of 14 and 24 that has a name, is usually territorial or claims a certain territory as under its exclusive influence, and is involved in criminal acts.

Generalizability—the ability to apply research results to other similar populations.

Genetic engineering—gene manipulation in a laboratory setting.

Genocide—the killing of a group of people because of their racial, political, or cultural differences.

Genogram—a display of family information in a graphic form that provides a quick view of complex family patterns.

Geographic community—a community defined by its geographic boundaries.

Geriatrics—the medical specialty that deals with the physiology of aging and with the diagnosis and treatment of diseases affecting the aged.

Gerontology—a broad, interdisciplinary practice that includes all aspects of the aging process, including economic, social, clinical, and psychological, and their effect on the older adult and society.

Gestalt-field—a family of cognitive theories that assumes that people are neither good nor bad; they simply interact with their environment, and their learning is related to perception.

Gestational diabetes—glucose intolerance of variable degree with onset or first recognition during pregnancy.

Global Burden of Disease (GBD)—disparities, verified with quantifiable data, in the burden of disease worldwide among the developing countries, especially among children.

Global economy—international trade, investment, travel, and ownership of information and ideas.

Global nursing—paid employment or volunteer nursing in foreign/developing countries in a variety of nursing positions based on interest, experience, skills, and credentials.

Global warming—the trapping of heat radiation from the earth's surface that increases the overall temperature of the world, causing a "greenhouse" effect.

Goals—broad statements of desired end results.

Gross national product—the total value of all goods and services produced in the United States economy in 1 year.

Group homes—homes designed to meet the needs of specific populations, such as the mentally ill, developmentally disabled, the elderly, or people with Alzheimer's disease.

Group-marriage family—several adults who share a common household, consider that all are married to one another, and share everything, including sex and child rearing.

Group-network family—nuclear families not related by birth or marriage but bound by a common set of values, such as a religious system, who share goods, services, and child-rearing responsibilities.

Halfway house—a residential program for individuals with SPMI that, in addition to housing, offers supervision, treatment, safety, socialization, recreation, and support.

Head Start—federally funded preschool programs for 3- to 5-year-old children from low-income families in disadvantaged communities.

Health—a holistic state of well-being that includes soundness of mind, body, and spirit.

Health care economics—a branch of the science that describes and analyzes the production, distribution, and consumption of health care goods and services.

Health continuum—a range of degrees from optimal health at one end of a spectrum to total disability or death at the other end.

Health for all—a major social goal of governments and the WHO—the attainment by all people by the year 2000 of a level of health that would allow them to lead a socially and economically productive life; initially declared at Alma-Ata, 1978.

Health maintenance organizations (HMOs)—systems in which participants prepare a fixed monthly premium to receive comprehensive health services delivered by a defined network of providers to plan participants.

Health policy—any policy that constitutes the governing framework for providing health services on a local, state, national, or even international level.

Health promotion—efforts that seek to move people closer to optimal well-being or higher levels of wellness.

Hearty elderly—people older than 65 who maintain a level of wellness and activity well above current expectations for that age.

Hebrew hygienic code—possibly the first written code in the world, which serves as a prototype for personal and community sanitation.

Herd immunity—the immunity level present in a particular population of people.

High-risk families—families exhibiting the symptoms of potentially abusive or neglectful behavior or who are under the types of stress associated with abuse or neglect.

High-risk infant—an infant whose mother has not received adequate nutrition or care during pregnancy due to a lack of proper prenatal care, economic disadvantage, or disease exposure.

Home care nurse—a community health nurse who provides skilled nursing services focusing on physical nursing care needed by family members who are ill, injured, or in the acute or terminal phase of a disease process.

Home health care—all the services and products provided to clients in their homes to maintain, restore, or promote their physical, mental, and emotional health.

Home health nursing—the provision of nursing to acute, chronic, and terminally ill clients of all ages in their home while integrating community health nursing principles that focus on the environmental, psychosocial, economic, cultural, and personal health factors affecting a client's and family's health status and well-being.

Home visit—visiting a family where they live in order to assist them to achieve as high a level of wellness as possible.

Homebase—a migrant farmworker's permanent address.

Homebound—as defined by Medicare, a person who can only leave the home with difficulty in mobility and only for medical appointments or adult day care related to the client's medical care; as a general definition, a person who can only leave the home under great difficulty, for short periods of time, and with assistance.

Homemaker agency —provides homemaker aides who perform services such as cooking, cleaning, and shopping, and/or home health aides who perform personal client care such as bathing and dressing.

Homeless family —families who find themselves without permanent shelter due to a lack of marketable skills, negative economic changes, or chronic mental health problems.

Homicide —any action taken to cause non–war-related death to another person.

Hospice —a philosophy of care that recognizes that death is inevitable and near and that a cure is not within current human reach.

Hospice care —a philosophy of holistic caregiving to families with a dying family member; the purpose is to make the dying process as dignified, free from discomfort, and emotionally, spiritually, and socially supportive as possible.

Hospital-based agencies —outreach services, including home health care, provided by an acute-care facility with similar missions of the sponsoring hospital.

Host —a susceptible human or animal who harbors and nourishes a disease-causing agent.

Human immunodeficiency virus (HIV) —a retrovirus that attacks the body's immune system; transmitted through sexual contact, sharing of HIV-contaminated needles and syringes, blood and blood byproducts, and from infected mother to child during the perinatal period.

Human skills —the ability to understand, communicate, motivate, delegate, and work well with people.

Illness —a state of being relatively unhealthy.

Immunity —the host's ability to resist a particular infectious disease-causing agent.

Immunization —the process of introducing some form of disease-causing organism into a person's system in order to cause the development of antibodies that will resist that disease.

Implementation —putting a plan into action and carrying out the activities delineated in the plan.

Incest —sexual abuse among family members who are blood related.

Incidence —all new cases of a disease or health condition appearing during a given time.

Incubation period —the time interval between exposure and onset of symptoms.

Indigent —people who are impoverished and deprived of basic comforts.

Indirect transmission —occurs when the infectious agent is transported within contaminated inanimate materials such as air, water, or food.

Indirect victim —the relatives and friends of direct victims.

Individualism —a belief that the interests of the individual are or ought to be paramount.

Infant —child from birth to 1 year old.

Infectious —capable of producing infection.

Inferential statistics —making inferences about features of a population based upon observations of a sample.

Informal caregivers —family members and friends who provide care in the home and are unpaid.

Inmates —people detained in correctional facilities.

Insanity —a legal term reserved for mental impairment that may relieve a person from the legal consequences of his or her actions.

Instrument —the specific tool, often a questionnaire or interview guide, used to measure the variables in a study.

Instrumental values —codes of conduct, such as confidentiality, keeping promises, or being honest.

Integrated management of childhood Illness (IMCI) —an intervention that promotes wider immunization coverage, rapid referral of serious cases, prompt recognition of secondary conditions, and improved nutrition.

Intensity —the physical or emotional level of something; in a disaster, the level of destruction and devastation.

Interaction —reciprocal exchange and influence between people.

Interactional framework —describes the family as a unit of interacting personalities and emphasizes communication, roles, conflict, coping patterns, and decision-making processes.

Intermediate care —a level of caregiving at which the amount and type of skilled care given is decreased.

Intrafamilial sexual abuse —sexual activity between family members not related by blood.

Intrarole functioning —playing several roles at the same time, such as when one woman is a wife, mother, grandmother, aunt, teacher, volunteer, author, neighbor, and friend.

Isolation —separation of infected persons or animals for the period of communicability in order to limit the transmission of the infectious agent to susceptible others.

Jail—a facility where people accused of committing a crime await arraignment, the summons to appear in court to answer charges; also called a detention center or holding cell.

Justice—treating people fairly.

Key informants—persons who know much about their community and are willing to share their information with the community health nurse.

Kin-network—several nuclear families who live in the same household, or near one another, and share goods and services.

Lay workers—migrant camp members who are trained and supervised by community health nurses and who form formal and informal links with the community to promote health and provide continuity of care.

Leader—a function of the community health nursing role in which the nurse directs, influences, or persuades others to effect change that will positively affect people's health and move them toward a goal.

Leadership—an interpersonal process in which one person influences the activities of another person or group of persons toward accomplishment of a goal.

Learning—the process of assimilating new information that promotes a permanent change in behavior.

Learning disability—a genetic, environmental, or cultural influence that affects a child's ability to learn; it is estimated that 2% to 10% of school-age children have some type of learning disability.

Life expectancy—the average number of years that an individual member of a specific cohort (usually a single birth year) is projected to live.

Literacy—the ability to read and write to an extent that allows the individual to function in daily life.

Lobbying—the process by which an individual or group acts on behalf of others to influence specific decisions of policy makers, such as legislators.

Location myth—community health nursing described in terms of where it is practiced—in a specific setting or location such as outside of the hospital.

Location variables—a profile of the community that includes community boundaries, location of health services, geographic features, climate, flora and fauna, and the human-made environment.

Long-term care—an assortment of settings that are residences for people unable to physically care for themselves independently due to physical or cognitive alterations.

Looting—stealing goods.

Low birth weight—babies weighing less than 2500 g at birth.

Lynching—executing without due process of law.

Machismo—male qualities of dominance that include pride, honor, and dignity.

Macroeconomic theory—concerned with the broad variables that affect the status of the total economy.

Mandated reporters—people who have the responsibility for the welfare of children, such as nurses, doctors, teachers, counselors, and certain other professionals.

Managed care—a broad system under which case management exists, which is designed to be a cost-containing system of health care administration.

Managed competition—combining market competition to achieve cost savings with government regulation to achieve expanded coverage.

Manager—a nursing role in which the nurse exercises administrative direction toward the accomplishment of specified goals by assessing clients' needs, planning and organizing to meet those needs, directing and leading to achieve results, and controlling and evaluating the progress to ensure that goals are met.

Marginalized—people who live on the margins, or edges, of society, rather than in the mainstream.

Maximum security—a correctional facility with the highest security level, generally housing prisoners who have committed violent crimes.

Medicaid—known as Title XIX of the Social Security Act Amendments of 1965; provides medical assistance for certain individuals and families with low incomes and resources.

Medically indigent—those unable to pay for and totally lacking in medical services.

Medicare—known as Title XVIII of the Social Security Act Amendments of 1965; provides mandatory federal health insurance for adults age 65 and over and certain disabled persons.

Mental health—a state of successful mental functioning, resulting in productive activities, fulfilling relationships, and the ability to change and cope with adversity.

Mental health promotion—interventions that enhance well-being and strengthen life-sustaining and life-enhancing activities.

Mental illness—collectively, all mental disorders; health conditions that are characterized by alterations in thinking, mood, or behavior (or some combination thereof) associated with distress and/or impaired functioning.

Message—an expression of the purpose of communication.

Meta-analysis—a research method that allows researchers to evaluate the results of many similar quantitative research studies in an attempt to integrate the findings.

Metropolitan—counties including one or more cities of 50,000 or more residents and a total population of 100,000 or greater.

Microcultures—systems of cultural knowledge characteristic of subgroups within larger societies.

Microeconomic theory—concerned with the supply and demand of goods and services as these relate to consumer income allocation and distribution.

Migrant farm workers—farmworkers who travel to find agricultural work throughout the year, usually from state to state with the seasons.

Migrant health programs—health programs for migrant workers that depend upon referrals and vouchers to address gaps in health care services.

Migration—the act of moving from one region or country to another, often temporarily or seasonally.

Minimum security—a correctional facility with a minimum level of security, generally housing prisoners who have committed nonviolent crimes.

Minority group—a part of the population that differs from the majority and often receives differential and unequal treatment.

Model—a description or analogy used as a pattern to enhance understanding of some reality.

Moral—conforming to a standard that is right and good.

Moral evaluations—judgments that conform to standards of what is right and good.

Morbidity rate—the relative incidence of disease in a population.

Mortality rate—the relative death rate or the sum of deaths in a given population at a given time.

Multigenerational family—several generations within one family, such as the aged mother of the husband, wife, teen-age children, and one teen's infant.

Multilateral agencies—multinational agencies that support development efforts of governments and organizations in less developed nations of the world, such as the United Nations, the World Health Organization, and the World Bank.

Munchausen syndrome by proxy—a psychological disorder in which clients bring medical attention to themselves by injuring or inducing illness in their children; they fabricate the symptoms of a disease in order that their children undergo medical tests, hospitalization, or even medical or surgical treatment.

Mutual goals—goals that the family and the nurse plan and take action on together.

National health insurance (NHI)—a solution to the high cost and inaccessibility of health services whereby health insurance coverage would be provided for all citizens through a single-payer system.

Natural history—events preceding a disease's development, during its course, and during its conclusion.

Neglect—a state in which the physical, emotional, or educational resources necessary for healthy growth and development are withheld or unavailable.

Neurosis—a general term denoting any of a variety of mental or emotional disorders involving anxiety, phobia, or other abnormal behavioral symptoms.

New and emerging diseases—diseases not know previously and diseases that were previously thought to be under control.

Nominal group technique—a group decision-making method that pools face-to-face group ideas after members initially think and write down their ideas independently.

Non-experimental design—a research design used to describe and explain phenomena or examine relationships among phenomena; also called a descriptive design.

Non-governmental organizations (NGO)—organizations not under government sponsorship or control; also called private voluntary organizations (PVO).

Non-metropolitan—counties that do not have a city of 50,000 residents within their borders.

Non-maleficence—avoiding or preventing harm to others as a consequence of one's own choices and actions.

Non-traditional family—family patterns that have not traditionally been socially acceptable, such as a single-parent household headed by a woman.

Nonverbal messages—messages that are conveyed without words and that constitute nearly two-thirds of the messages transmitted in normal communication.

Normative-reductive change strategies—strategies used to influence change that not only present new information but also directly influence people's attitudes and behaviors through persuasion.

Nuclear family—a mother, father, and child(ren) (biological, adopted, or both) living together, separate from others.

Nuclear-dyad family—husband and wife.

Nursing bag—a carry-all nurses take on home visits that contains supplies needed on the visits.

Nursing informatics—a term for the collective technological sciences available to nurses in the health care delivery system today for the delivery of nursing care.

Objectives—specific statements of desired outcomes stated in behavioral terms that can be measured and include target dates.

Occupational disease—any condition or disorder caused by an exposure that resulted from employment.

Occupational health—a specialty health practice that focuses on the health and well-being of the working population, including both paid and unpaid laborers, thus covering most of the country's well adults.

Occupational health nurse—a nurse employed to ensure that the work force is, and remains, healthy and productive.

Official health agencies—health care agencies publicly funded and operated by federal, state, or local government supported by taxes.

Ombudsman—a person hired through the Area Agency on Aging (AAA) or agency, who serves the residents of assisted living or skilled nursing facilities by speaking for them and acting as an advocate in all matters concerning the residents' stay in the facility.

Operationalizing—putting ideas or concepts into words that can be used.

Opposition defiant disorder (ODD)—a set of "externalizing" behavior problems, including noncompliance, temper tantrums, and other socially provocative behaviors first diagnosed in the preschool years.

Organizer—a function of the community health nurse's manager role that involves designing a structure within which people and tasks can function to reach desired objectives.

Osteoporosis—a systemic skeletal disease characterized by low bone mass and microarchitectural deterioration of bone tissue, leading to increased bone fragility and a consequent increase in fracture risk.

Outcome criteria—measurable criteria the community will work toward and measure their success by as they attempt to improve the health of their community.

Outcome evaluation—the assessment of change in the family's (client's) health status based on mutually agreed upon activities.

Outmigration—the phenomenon of young and middle-age adults leaving their rural homes for a more urban environment.

Palliative care—comfort care directed at the alleviation of pain and other symptoms.

Pan American Health Organization (PAHO)—an arm of the World Health Organization that serves as the central coordinating organization for public health in the Western hemisphere.

Pandemic—an epidemic that is worldwide in distribution.

Paraphrasing—stating back to the sender what you thought you heard.

Participative leadership style—a democratic style in which leaders involve followers in the decision-making process.

Partnerships—agreements between people and agencies to benefit a joint purpose.

Passive immunity—short-term resistance to a specific disease-causing organism that may be acquired naturally or artificially through inoculation with a vaccine that gives temporary resistance.

Passive smoking—exposure to tobacco smoke from other people smoking in one's environment.

Peer review—an organized system by which peer professionals assess the quality of care being delivered.

Penitentiary—a federal correctional facility, commonly referred to among prisoners as "the big house," which may have a minimum or maximum security level.

Personal-care homes—homes that offer basic personal care, such as bathing, grooming, and social support, but provide no skilled nursing services.

Pediculosis (pediculus humanus capitis; head lice)—parasites that live and feed on the human scalp; considered a nuisance disease and affecting one in four elementary school–age children.

Pedophile—an adult whose main sexual interest is a child.

Personalismo—the quality of pleasant conversation appreciated by Hispanics.

Physical abuse—the intentional harm to someone by another person that results in pain, physical injury, or death.

Planned change—a purposeful, designed effort to effect improvement in a system with the assistance of a change agent.

Planner—a function in the management process that requires the nurse to set goals and direction for the organization or project and determine the means for achieving them.

Planning—a logical, decision-making process of designing an orderly, detailed program of action to accomplish specific goals and objectives.

Pluralistic medical systems—consist of traditional healing systems, lay practices, household remedies, transitional health workers, and Western medicine.

Polarization—the process by which a group is split into two or more factions over a political issue.

Policy—an authoritatively stated course of action that guides decision making.

Policy analysis—the systematic identification of causes or consequences of policy and the factors that influence it.

Policy development—formulating local and state health policies and directing resources toward those policies with information gathered during assessment.

Policy system—an entity that receives input from external sources and has legal authority to generate or revise policies governing or managing the constituents it represents.

Political action—actions taken by an individual or group to influence the political decisions of others toward issues or policies beneficial to the welfare of the individual or group.

Political action committee (PAC)—a group or organization that endorses and financially back its candidates and supports the group's position on issues.

Political empowerment—a conscious state in which an individual, group, or organization becomes recognized as influential in determining policy.

Politics—an interactive process of influencing others to make decisions that favor a person's or group's chosen position and the allocation of scarce resources to support that position.

Pollution—the contamination of natural resources such as air, water, and soil, making them foul and unfit for human use.

Polysubstance use and abuse—when a person uses or abuses more than one chemical, such as alcohol and marijuana or cocaine with antianxiety medications.

Population—all the people occupying an area or all those sharing one or more characteristics.

Population-focused—the concern for the health status of population groups and their environment.

Population variables—the size, density, composition, rate of growth or decline, cultural characteristics, social class, and mobility of people within a designated community.

Poverty threshold—an income line below which people are defined as poor.

Power—the ability to influence or control other people's behavior to accomplish a specific purpose.

Power bases—knowledge or skills the powerholder possesses that enable him or her to exert influence over others.

Power sources—the qualities or situations from which the power holder gains a power base.

Power-coercive change strategies—use of coercion based on fear to effect change.

Preferred provider organizations (PPOs)—a model of managed or coordinated care that is a network of physicians, hospitals, and other health-related services that contract with a third-party payer organization to provide comprehensive health services to subscribers on a fixed fee-for-service basis.

Preschooler—a child aged 3 or 4 years.

Prevalence—all people with a health condition existing in a given population at a given point in time.

Primary health care—in developed countries, the partnership between health professionals and communities; in most developing countries, a voluntary health service created at the village level.

Primary prevention—measures taken to keep illness or injury from occurring.

Primary relationship—two or more people interacting in a continuing manner within the greater environment.

Prison—a state Department of Corrections facility that may be assigned a security level ranging from minimum to maximum.

Private voluntary organizations (PVO)—organizations not under government sponsorship or control: also know as non-governmental organizations.

Problem-oriented assessment—an assessment that begins with a single problem and then assesses the community in terms of that problem.

Proprietary health services—privately owned and managed health care services.

Prospective payment—a payment method based on rates derived from predictions of annual service costs that are set in advance of service delivery.

Prospective study—looking forward in time to find a causal relationship.

Psychomotor domain—visible, demonstrable performance skills that require some kind of neuromuscular coordination.

Psychosis—a mental disorder characterized by partial or complete withdrawal from reality.

Public health—the science and art of preventing disease, prolonging life, and promoting health and efficiency through organized community efforts for the sanitation of the environment, the control of communicable infections, the education of the individual in personal hygiene, the organization of medical and nursing services for the early diagnosis and preventive treatment of disease, and the development of the social machinery to ensure everyone a standard of living adequately for the maintenance of health, so organizing these benefits as to enable every citizen to realize his or her birthright of health and longevity.

Public health nursing—the term describing community health nursing from 1900 to 1950; replaced by the term community health nursing to better describe where the nurse practices. In this text the terms are used interchangeably.

Public Health Services (PHS)—a federal umbrella organization concerned with the broad health interests of the country.

Public policy—decisions made by government at the local, state, or federal level that affect the public.

Qualitative research—emphasizes subjectivity and the meaning of experiences to individuals.

Quality assurance—initial setting of standards, formal auditing, and peer review in the health care delivery system to ensure quality.

Quality care—the state in which services provided match the needs of the population, are technically correct, and achieve beneficial results.

Quality circles—a participative management approach in which employees and managers share the responsibility for decision-making and problem solving in client care.

Quality improvement—studying the impact of intervention and instituting tighter controls on the delivery of specific community health nursing services.

Quality indicators—quality-focused objectives used as markers to determine whether a goal has been achieved and to measure client outcomes or process outcomes.

Quality measurement—the ability to identify services and programs that best serve the needs of the community.

Quantitative research—concerns data that can be quantified or measured objectively.

Quarantine—a period of enforced isolations of persons exposed to a communicable disease during the incubation period to prevent spread of the disease should infection occur.

Quasi-experiment—a research method that lacks one of the elements found in a true experiment, such as the randomization of the subjects.

Race—a biologically designated group of people whose distinguishing features are inherited.

Randomization—the systematic selection of research subjects so that each one has an equal probability of selection.

Rape—an act of sexual aggression in which the perpetrator is motivated by a desire to dominate, control, and degrade the victim.

Rates—a statistical measure expressing the proportion of persons with a given health problem among a population at risk.

Rationing—limiting the provision of adequate health services in order to save costs, but in so doing jeopardizing the well-being of some groups of people.

Receiver—the person(s) to whom the message is directed and who is (are) its actual recipient.

Recidivism—an inmate's relapse into criminal behavior following release, with subsequent incarceration.

Referral—a request for service from another agency or person.

Refugee—a person who is forced to leave his or her homeland because of war or persecution.

Regulation—mandated procedure and practice affecting health services delivery that is enforced by law.

Regulatory health policy—policy that attempts to control the allocation of resources by directing those agencies or persons who offer resources or provide public services.

Rehabilitation—efforts that seek to reduce disability and, as much as possible, restore function.

Relapse—continuing to use a chemical after a period of nonuse.

Relationship-based care—care that incorporates the values of establishing ad maintaining a reciprocal, caring relationship with the community.

Reliability—how consistently an instrument measures a given research variable within a particular population.

Research—the systematic collection and analysis of data related to a particular problem or phenomenon affecting community health and community health practice.

Researcher—a role of the community health nurse in which the nurse engages in systematic investigation, collection, and analysis of data for the purpose of solving problems and enhancing community health practice.

Reservoir—any person, animal, or substance in which an infectious agent normally lives and multiplies and then is transmitted from its source to a susceptible host.

Resource directory—a published source of community services developed for professionals and the broader community.

Respect—treating people as unique, equal, and responsible moral agents.

Respite care—a break for caregivers from the intensity of caregiving in which they can care for themselves for a few days; not a luxury but a necessity for successful caregiving.

Restorative justice—a belief that benefits should primarily go to those who have been wronged by prior injustice, such as victims of crime or racial discrimination.

Retrospective payment—reimbursing for a service after it has been rendered.

Retrospective review—a quality assessment process that examines patterns of care over a specified period of time in health records of care given in the past.

Retrospective study—looking backward in time to find a causal relationship.

Revolutionary change—change that is rapid, drastic, and threatening and that may completely upset the balance of a system.

Riot—a violent disturbance created by a large number of people assembled for a common purpose.

Risk—the probability that a disease or other unfavorable health condition will develop.

Risk assessment—the process of identifying factors that lead to negative events.

Roles—the assigned or assumed parts that members play during day-to-day family living; they are bestowed and defined by the family.

Rural—communities with fewer than 10,000 residents and a country population density of fewer than 1,000 persons per square mile.

Sanitation—the promotion of hygiene and prevention of disease by maintaining health-enhancing (sanitary) conditions.

School-based health centers (SBHC)—clinics on school sites that provide ready access to health care for large numbers of children and adolescents during school hours, making absences from school due to health care appointments unnecessary.

School nurse—a specialty branch of professional nursing that serves the school-age population.

School nurse practitioner—a registered nurse with advanced academic and clinical preparation and experience in physical assessment, diagnosis, and treatment, who provides primary care to school-age children.

Scope—the range of effects.

Screening—delivering a testing mechanism to detect disease in groups of asymptomatic, apparently healthy individuals.

Seasonal farm worker—a farm worker who lives in one geographic location and labors in the fields of that particular area.

Secondary prevention—efforts that seek to detect and treat existing health problems at the earliest possible stage when disease or impairment already exists.

Self-care—the process of taking responsibility for developing one's own health potential.

Self-care deficit—when people's ability to continue self-care activities drops below their need.

Self-determination—a person's exercise of the capacity to shape and pursue personal plans for his or her life.

Self-help group—peers who come together for mutual assistance to satisfy a common need, such as overcoming a handicap or life-disrupting problem.

Self-interest—the fulfillment of one's own desires without regard for the greater good.

Sender—the person(s) conveying a message.

Senility—a term widely used by health professionals and lay people alike to denote deteriorating mental faculties associated with old age.

Serious and persistent mental illness (SPMI)—the preferred term for serrious mental illness of a chronic nature.

Serious mental illness (SMI)—any mental illness that has compromised both the client's level of function and the quality of life.

Setting priorities—assigning rank or importance to clients' needs to determine the order in which goals should be addressed.

Sexual abuse—includes acts of sexual assault or sexual exploitation of a person; may consist of many acts over a long period of time or a single incident.

Sexual exploitation—includes conduct or activities related to pornography depicting people in sexual explicit situations.

Shaken baby syndrome—the intentional abusive action of violently shaking an infant or toddler, usually less than 18 months old.

Shattuck Report—a landmark document, written in 1850 and called the "Report of the Sanitary Commission of Massachusetts," that described public health concepts and methods upon which much of today's public health practice is based.

Simpatica—the quality of positive interpersonal relationships appreciated by Hispanics.

Single-adult family—one adult living alone either by choice to remain single or because of separation from spouse and/or children because of divorce, death, or distance from children.

Single-parent family—a mother or father, but not both, and child(ren).

Single-payer system—an approach to health care that emphasizes universal health insurance coverage through a stronger role played by government.

Situational crisis—a stressful disruption event arising from an external event that occurs suddenly, often without warning, to a person, group, aggregate, or community.

Skilled-nursing facilities (SNF)—residences designed to meet the caregiving needs of the frailest of society's citizens who need long-term rehabilitative, recuperative, or custodial care, which includes the skilled procedures and equipment.

Skilled nursing services—includes skilled observation and assessment, teaching, and performing procedures needing nursing judgment.

Skills myth—a belief that community health nurses employ only the skills of basic clinical nursing when working with community clients.

Smokeless tobacco products—tobacco exposure from snuff or chewing tobacco, without exposure to smoke.

Social class—the ranking of groups within society by income, education, occupation, prestige, or a combination of these factors.

Social status—a person's ranking or standing in society, which can be affected by gender, age, and race.

Social support—the quality of interpersonal ties between individuals and the strength and extent of these personal ties.

Social support network map—a detailed display regarding the quality and quantity of social connections.

Social system variables—the various parts of a community's social system that interact and influence the system.

Special interest group—any group of people sharing a common goal who are politically active in attempting to influence policy makers to support their goal.

Spousal abuse—acts of violence against an intimate partner.

Stages of change—the three sequential steps leading to change that include unfreezing, changing, and re-freezing; first described by Lewin, they have become a cornerstone for understanding the change process.

Standards of care—desired goals that can help plan and evaluate nursing practices.

Stigma—an unjustified mark of shame and discredit attached to mental illness.

Strengthening—a communication technique in which, either verbally or in writing, the nurse lists positive points about an otherwise negative situation.

Structural-functional framework—describes the family as a social system relating to other social systems in the external environment, such as church, school, work, and the health care system.

Subcultures—relatively large aggregates of people within a society who share separate distinguishing characteristics.

Substance abuse—excessive and prolonged use of some chemical (alcohol, tobacco, drugs) that leads to serious physical, emotional, and social problems.

Suicide—taking action that causes one's death.

Surveillance—the continuous scrutiny of all aspects of occurrence and spread of a disease that are pertinent to effective control.

Survey—an assessment method in which a series of questions is used to collect data for analysis of a specific group or area.

Tacit—a guide for human interaction that is mostly unexpressed and at the unconscious level.

Teaching—a specialized communication process in which desired behavior changes are achieved.

Technical skills—the ability to apply special management-related knowledge and expertise to a particular situation or problem.

Technology—the application of science for changing processes of production or industry.

Telehealth—electronically transmitted clinician consultation between the client and the health care provider.

Temporary Aid to Needy Families (TANF)—the restructuring of Aid to Families with Dependent Children in 1996, which created federal funding to be channeled to individual states; each state has great latitude in setting up programs, with support limited to 5 years in a person's lifetime.

Tenet—any principle or doctrine held as true.

Terminal values—end-states of existence, such as spiritual salvation, peace of mind, or world peace.

Terminally ill—people with less than 6 months to live.

Terrorism—the unlawful use of force or violence against persons or property to intimidate or coerce a government or civilian population in the furtherance of political or social objectives.

Tertiary prevention—attempts to reduce the extent and severity of a health problem to its lowest possible levels so as to minimize disability and restore or preserve function.

Theory—a set of systematically interrelated concepts or hypotheses that seek to explain or predict phenomena.

Third-party payments—monetary reimbursements made to providers of health care by someone other than the consumer who received the care.

Toddler—a child just out of infancy, from age 1 to 2 years.

Tolerance—a need for increasing amounts of a substance to achieve the desired effects, or a significantly diminished effect with continued use of the same amount of the same substance.

Total quality management (TQM)—a comprehensive term referring to the systems and activities used to achieve all aspects of quality care within a given agency.

Toxic agent—a poisonous substance in the environment that produces harmful effects on human, animal, or plant health.

Traditional family—the family structures that are most familiar and that are most readily accepted by society.

Traditional health care systems—ancient, ethno-cultural-religious health beliefs and practices that have been handed down through generations.

Transactional leadership—a process in which leader and followers engage in a reciprocal transaction whereby the roles and tasks of the followers are clarified and assigned as the group works to accomplish its goals.

Transcultural nursing—culturally sensitive nursing service to people of an ethnic or racial background different from that of the nurse.

Transformational leadership—leadership that inspires followers to high levels of commitment and effort in order to achieve group goals.

Triage—the process of sorting multiple casualties in the event of a war or major disaster.

Triggers—events and activities that may cause a person to continue addictive activities.

True experiment—characterized by instituting an intervention or change, assigning subjects to groups in a specific manner, and comparing the group of subjects who experience the manipulation to the control group.

Unintentional injuries—injuries resulting from unintended exposure to physical agents, including heat, mechanical energy, chemicals, or electricity; usually referred to as accidents.

United Nations International Children's Emergency Fund (UNICEF)—organized in 1946 as a temporary emergency program to assist children of war-torn countries after World War II; now promotes child and maternal health and welfare globally through programs and services.

United States Agency for International Development (USAID)—an agency that provides economic and humanitarian assistance overseas.

Universal coverage—providing health care coverage to all citizens through one system, replacing the 1500 health insurance companies currently involved in reimbursing for health care coverage.

Unsafe condition—any environmental factor, either social or physical, that increases the likelihood of an unintentional injury.

Vaccine—a preparation made either from killed, living attenuated, or living fully virulent organisms and administered to produce or artificially increase immunity to a particular disease.

Validity—the assurance that an instrument measures the variables it is supposed to measure.

Value—a notion or idea designating relative worth or desirability.

Value systems—organizations of beliefs that are of relative importance in guiding individual behavior.

Values clarification—a process that helps one identify the personal and professional values that guide actions by prompting one to examine what one believes about the worth, truth, or beauty of any object, thought, or behavior, and where this belief ranks compared with one's other values.

Vector—a non-human carrier of disease, such as an animal or insect

Veracity—telling the truth.

Verbal messages—communicated ideas, attitudes, and feelings transmitted by speaking or writing.

Violent crimes—those involving physical or psychological injury or death, or the threat of injury or death.

Very low birth weight—babies weighing less than 1500 g at birth.

Voluntary health agencies—privately funded and operated health care agencies without support from tax dollars.

Wellness—includes the definition of health but incorporates the capacity to develop one's potential to lead a fulfilling and productive life; one that can be measured in terms of quality of life.

Well-being—a state of positive health or a person's perception concerning positive health.

Wetlands—natural inland bodies of shallow water, such as marshes, ponds, river bottoms, and flood plains, that filter contaminated surface waters and support wildlife reproduction and growth.

Wider family—a family that emerges from lifestyle, is voluntary, and is independent of necessary biological or kin connections.

Withdrawal symptoms—physical and psychological symptoms, such as tremors, lethargy, anxiety, or depression, that typically are opposite to the effects of the addictive substance and that occur when an addicted individual does not use the substance for a certain period of time.

World Bank (WB)—a major international health-related agency founded in 1944 with a goal of "a world free of poverty."

World Health Organization (WHO)—the body that promotes health on a global basis, with 191 member countries; its mandates include acting as the directing and coordinating authority on international health work.

Internet Resources and Useful 800 Numbers

CHAPTER 1: OPPORTUNITIES AND CHALLENGES OF COMMUNITY HEALTH NURSING

www.medscape.com
www.ebscohost.com
www.altavista.com
www.healthcentral.com
www.healthlinkusa.com
www.aacn.nche.edu

CHAPTER 2: EVOLUTION OF COMMUNITY HEALTH NURSING

American Nurses Association: www.nursingworld.org

CHAPTER 3: ROLES AND SETTING FOR COMMUNITY HEALTH NURSING PRACTICE

Health Web: www.healthweb.org
National Institutes of Health: www.nih.gov
National Library of Medicine:
    www.nlm.nih.gov/nlmhome. html
NurseWeek/HealthWeek: www.nurseweek.com

CHAPTER 4: TRANSCULTURAL NURSING IN THE COMMUNITY

Chinese American Medical Society:
    www.camsociety.org
Minority Health Professions Foundation:
    www.minorityhealth.org
National Association of Hispanic Nurses:
    www.incacorp. com/nahn
National Association of Black Nurses:
    www.bronzeville. com/nbna/default.htm
Office of Minority Health: www.omhrc.gov
Transcultural Nursing Society: 1-888-432-5470;
    e-mail: barnes@smtt.munet.edu

CHAPTER 6: STRUCTURE AND FUNCTION OF COMMUNITY HEALTH SERVICES

California State Health Department information:
    www. dhs.cahwnet.gov/index.htm
CARE: www.care.org
Figuring out the health care system:
    www.healthgrades. com

CHAPTER 7: ECONOMICS OF HEALTH CARE

California State budget (demographics, employment, fiscal
    information for state agencies):
    www.dof.ca.gov/dofhome. htm

Health Insurance Association of America: www.HIAA.org;
   800-879-HIAA
Kaiser Family Foundation: www.kff.org
Medicare: www.medicare.gov
Health Care Financing Administration (HCFA):
   www.hcfa.gov
Joint Commission on Accreditation of Healthcare Organi-
   zations (JCAHO): www.jcaho.org
National Committee for Quality Assurance (NCQA):
   www.ncqa.org

CHAPTER 9: HEALTH PROMOTION THROUGH EDUCATION

American Botanical Council: www.herbalgram.org;
   800-373-7105
Ask the Dietician: www.dietian.com
FDA Home Page: www.fda.gov
Mayo Clinic Health Oasis: www.mayohealth.org
Recipes/nutrition facts: www.mealsforyou.com
Healthy eating and living: www.prevention.com
Health games/chat rooms: www.thriveonline.com
Online medical dictionary: www.graylab.ac.uk/omd
Family Doctor: www.familydoctor.org
National Highway Traffic Safety Administration:
   www. nhtsa.dot.gov
FDA 800 Numbers
Seafood Hotline
   800-332-4010
Vaccine Adverse Event Reporting System
   800-822-7967
Mammography Information Service
   800-322-8615

CHAPTER 11: RESEARCH

National Institute of Nursing Research:
   www.nih.gov/ninr
American Nurses Foundation: www.nursingworld.org/anf
Sigma Theta Tau International Registry of Nursing
   Research www.stti.iupui.edu/library/registry.html
AIDS Clinical Trials Information Service (ACTIS):
   800-TRIALS-A

CHAPTER 14: EPIDEMIOLOGY IN COMMUNITY HEALTH CARE

Association for Professionals in Infection Control and Epidemiology, Inc.: www.apic.org

Centers for Disease Control and Prevention:
   www.cdc.gov
U.S. Census Bureau: www.census.gov

CHAPTER 15: COMMUNICABLE DISEASE CONTROL

CDC National AIDS Clearinghouse: 800-458-5231
National Vaccine Injury Compensation Program:
   800-338-2382
World Health Organization: www.who.org
WHO Network for Global Influenza Surveillance:
   www.whoinfluenza@who.cl
National AIDS Fund: www.aidsfund.org
National Association of People with AIDS:
   www.napwa.org
Public Health Service AIDS Hotline: 800-342-AIDS (for the
   general public); 800-933-3413 (for health professionals)

CHAPTER 16: ENVIRONMENTAL HEALTH AND SAFETY

Environmental Defense Fund: www.edf.org
Consumer Product Safety Commission: www.CPSC.gov
Greenpeace: www.greenpeace.org
National Institute of Environmental Health Sciences:
   www. niehs.nih.gov
American Association of Occupational Health Nurses:
   www.aaohn.org

CHAPTER 20: COMMUNITIES IN CRISIS: DISASTERS, GROUP VIOLENCE, AND TERRORISM

Mothers against handguns: www.handguncontrol.com
Organ and tissue donation: www.unos.org
American Red Cross: www.redcross.org
U.S. Department of Justice: www.usdoj.gov

CHAPTER 24: PLANNING, INTERVENING, AND EVALUATING HEALTH CARE TO FAMILIES

Preventing heart disease: www.amhrt.org
Prevention Magazine: www.prevention.com

CHAPTER 25: FAMILIES IN CRISIS: DOMESTIC VIOLENCE AND ABUSE

American Humane Association (Children's Division):
800-227-4645
Children's Defense Fund:
www.cdf@info@childrensdefense.org
National Clearinghouse on Child Abuse and Neglect:
www.nccanch@calid.com; 800-393-3366
National Council on Child Abuse and Family Violence:
800-422-4453
National Center for Missing and Exploited Children:
800-843-5678
National Runaway Switchboard (24 hours):
800-621-4000
National Committee to Prevent Child Abuse:
www.childabuse.org
Parents Anonymous: 909-621-6184
Shelter Aid Hotline: 800-333-SAFE

CHAPTER 26: MATERNAL, PRENATAL, AND NEWBORN POPULATIONS

The Alliance of Genetic Support Groups: 800-336-GENE
American Medical Association: www.jama.ama-assn.org
Association of Birth Defects in Children: 800-313-2232
March of Dimes Birth Defects Foundation: ww.modimes.org
National Center for Education in Maternal and Child
Health: www.info@ncemcg.org
Planned Parenthood Federation of America, Inc.: 800-829-7732

CHAPTER 27: PROMOTING AND PROTECTING THE HEALTH OF INFANT, TODDLER, AND PRESCHOOL POPULATIONS

Parent education: www.kidshealth.org/parent
Poison Control Center: www.poison.org
American Dental Association: www.ada.org
Children with disabilities:
American Juvenile Arthritis Organization: 800-433-5255
Asthma and Allergy Foundation of America: 800-7ASTHMA
Children's Hospice International: 800-FIGHT-CF
Developmental Disabilities Nurses Association:
800-888-6733
Epilepsy Foundation of America: www.EFA.org;
800-332-1000
Federation for Children with Special Needs:
www.fcsninfo@fcsn.org; 800-331-0688
Muscular Dystrophy Association: 800-572-1717

National Center for Youth with Disabilities:
www.peds.umn. edu/centers/ihd
National Easter Seal Society: www.seals.com; 800-221-6827
United Cerebral Palsy Association, Inc.: 800-USA-5UCP

CHAPTER 28: PROMOTING AND PROTECTING THE HEALTH OF SCHOOL-AGE AND ADOLESCENT POPULATIONS

Learning Disabilities Association of America: 888-300-6710

CHAPTER 29: PROMOTING AND PROTECTING THE HEALTH OF ADULTS AND THE WORKING POPULATION

American Heart Association: 800-AHA-USAI
American Lung Association: www.lungusa.org;
800-LUNG-USA
Sleep problems: www.sleepfoundation.org
Coping with death and dying: www.worldnet.att.net
Skin Cancer Zone: www.skin-cancer.com
Exercise and nutrition: www.netsweat.com
Menopause: www.menopause.org
National Osteoporosis Foundation: www.nof.org
Diabetes: www.diabetes.org
Health, nutrition, and fitness: www.pbs.org
Interactive Nutrition Program:
www.medeorinteractive.com
National Women's Health Resource Center:
www.healthywomen.org
Clearinghouse for Occupational Safety and Health:
www. PUBSPASP@CDC.gov; 800-35-NIOSH
Job opportunities:
www.careermosaic.com
www.hotjobs.com
www.joboptions.com
www.monster.com
www.nationjob.com
www.mysearch.com
Adults with disabilities:
Access/abilities: www.aceassabil.com
Accent on Living: 800-787-8444
Brain Injury Association: www.biavsa.org; 800-444-6443
Disability Rights Center: www.ghsl.nwu.edu/healthweb
Job Accommodation Network: 800-526-7234
National Multiple Sclerosis Society: www.NMSS.org;
800-344-4867
National Rehabilitation Information Center and Clearing-
house on Disability Information: 800-346-2742
National Stroke Association: www.stroke.org;
800-787-6537

Paralyzed Veterans of America:
   www.pvs.org; 800-424-8200
President's Committee on Employment of People with
   Disabilities: www.infor@pcbd.gov
President's Committee on Employment of the
   Handicapped: 800-772-1213
Spinal Cord injuries: www.spinalcord.org

CHAPTER 30: PROMOTING AND PROTECTING THE HEALTH OF THE OLDER ADULT POPULATION

National Hearing Aid Helpline: 800-521-5247
Older Women's League: 800-825-3695

CHAPTER 31: RURAL CLIENTS

Appalachian Regional Commission:
   www.CREA@ARC. gov
Indian Health Services: www.home.HIS.gov
National Congress on American Indians:
   www.NCAI.org
National Rural Electric Cooperative: www.NRECA.org
WAMI Rural Health Research Center: www.fammed.wash-
   ington.edu/wamirhrc
Rural Information Center: www.nal.usda.gov.ric;
   800-633-7701
Florida Rural Health research Center: www.hpe.ufl.edu
University of Minnesota Rural Health Research Center:
   www.hsr.umn.edu/centers/rhrc/rhrc.html

CHAPTER 32: CLIENTS LIVING IN POVERTY

Center for Law and Social Policy (CLASP):
   www.clasp.org
Homelessness: www.csf.colorado.edu/homeless
National health care for the homeless:
   www.nashville. net/nhch
Streetkid-L Resource Page: www.jbu.edu/business/sk.html
U.S. Department of Veteran Affairs: www.VA.gov

CHAPTER 33: MIGRANT WORKERS

National Center for Farm Worker Health: 800-531-5120

CHAPTER 34: CLIENTS WITH MENTAL HEALTH ISSUES

Anxiety disorders: www.freedomfromfear.org

CHAPTER 35: CLIENTS LIVING WITH ADDICTION

National Clearinghouse for Alcohol and Drug Information:
   www.health.org; 800-729-6686
National Alcohol and Drug Helpline: 800-821-4357

CHAPTER 36: CLIENTS IN CORRECTIONAL FACILITIES

HIV/AIDS: www.hivpositive.com

CHAPTER 37: CLIENTS IN HOME HEALTH, HOSPICE, AND LONG-TERM CARE SETTINGS

Alzheimer's Disease and Related Disorders Association,
   Inc.: 800-621-0379
American Association of Homes and Services for the
   Aging: www.aahsa.org; 800-675-9253
Assisted Living Federation of Homes & Services for the
   Aging: www.alfa.org
Caretaking of elders: www.careguide.com
Cancer: www.cancernet.nci.nih.gov
Compare nursing homes: www.medicare.gov
Eldercare locator: www.aoa.dhhs.gov/elderpage/locator.
   html; 800-677-1116
Medicare: www.medicare.gov; 1-800-633-4227
Medicaid information:
   www.hcfa.gov/medicaid/mcaicnsm.htm
Family Caregiver Alliance: www.caregiver.org
National Alliance for Caregiving: www.caregiving.org
National Association for Home Care: www.nahc.org
National Citizens' Coalition for Nursing Home Reform:
   www.nccnhr.org
National Hospice Organization: 800-658-8898
National Institute of Adult Day Care: www.NCOA.org;
   800-424-9046
Visiting Nurse Association of America: 888-862-9693

Suspected Child Abuse Report

SUSPECTED CHILD ABUSE REPORT
To Be Completed by Reporting Party
Pursuant to Penal Code Section 11166

A. CASE IDENTIFICATION

TO BE COMPLETED BY INVESTIGATING CPA

VICTIM NAME: _____

REPORT NO./CASE NAME: _____

DATE OF REPORT: _____

B. REPORTING PARTY

NAME/TITLE

ADDRESS

PHONE ( )   DATE OF REPORT   SIGNATURE

C. REPORT SENT TO

☐ POLICE DEPARTMENT   ☐ SHERIFF'S OFFICE   ☐ COUNTY WELFARE   ☐ COUNTY PROBATION

AGENCY   ADDRESS

OFFICIAL CONTACTED   PHONE ( )   DATE/TIME

D. INVOLVED PARTIES

VICTIM

NAME (LAST, FIRST, MIDDLE)   ADDRESS   BIRTHDATE   SEX   RACE

PRESENT LOCATION OF CHILD   PHONE ( )

SIBLINGS

	NAME	BIRTHDATE	SEX	RACE		NAME	BIRTHDATE	SEX	RACE
1.					4.				
2.					5.				
3.					6.				

PARENTS

NAME (LAST, FIRST, MIDDLE)   BIRTHDATE   SEX   RACE   NAME (LAST, FIRST, MIDDLE)   BIRTHDATE   SEX   RACE

ADDRESS   ADDRESS

HOME PHONE ( )   BUSINESS PHONE ( )   HOME PHONE ( )   BUSINESS PHONE ( )

E. INCIDENT INFORMATION

IF NECESSARY, ATTACH EXTRA SHEET OR OTHER FORM AND CHECK THIS BOX. ☐

1. DATE/TIME OF INCIDENT   PLACE OF INCIDENT   (CHECK ONE)   ☐ OCCURRED   ☐ OBSERVED

IF CHILD WAS IN OUT-OF-HOME CARE AT TIME OF INCIDENT, CHECK TYPE OF CARE:

☐ FAMILY DAY CARE   ☐ CHILD CARE CENTER   ☐ FOSTER FAMILY HOME   ☐ SMALL FAMILY HOME   ☐ GROUP HOME OR INSTITUTION

2. TYPE OF ABUSE: (CHECK ONE OR MORE)   ☐ PHYSICAL   ☐ MENTAL   ☐ SEXUAL ASSAULT   ☐ NEGLECT   ☐ OTHER

3. NARRATIVE DESCRIPTION:

4. SUMMARIZE WHAT THE ABUSED CHILD OR PERSON ACCOMPANYING THE CHILD SAID HAPPENED:

5. EXPLAIN KNOWN HISTORY OF SIMILAR INCIDENT(S) FOR THIS CHILD:

SS 8572 (Rev. 1/93)

INSTRUCTIONS AND DISTRIBUTION ON REVERSE

DO NOT submit a copy of this form to the Department of Justice (DOJ). A CPA is required under Penal Code Section 11169 to submit to DOJ a Child Abuse Investigation Report Form SS-8583 if (1) an active investigation has been conducted and (2) the incident is **not** unfounded.

Police or Sheriff-WHITE Copy;   County Welfare or Probation-BLUE Copy;   District Attorney-GREEN Copy;   Reporting Party-YELLOW Copy

Medical Report—
Suspected Child Abuse

DOJ 900   84 89220

MEDICAL REPORT—SUSPECTED CHILD ABUSE	HOSPITAL

INSTRUCTIONS: ALL PROFESSIONAL MEDICAL PERSONNEL ARE REQUIRED BY SECTION 11166 OF THE PENAL CODE TO COMPLETE THIS FORM IN CONJUNCTION WITH THE SS 8572 SUSPECTED CHILD ABUSE REPORT WHERE CHILD ABUSE, AS DEFINED BY SECTION 11165 OF THE PENAL CODE, IS SUSPECTED. THE REPORTS, DOJ 900 AND SS 8572, MUST BE SUBMITTED TO A POLICE OR SHERIFF'S DEPARTMENT, OR A COUNTY PROBATION OR WELFARE DEPARTMENT WITHIN 36 HOURS. PROFESSIONAL MEDICAL PERSONNEL MEANS ANY PHYSICIAN AND SURGEON, PSYCHIATRIST, PSYCHOLOGIST, DENTIST, RESIDENT, INTERN, PODIATRIST, CHIROPRACTOR, LICENSED NURSE, DENTAL HYGIENIST OR ANY OTHER PERSON WHO IS CURRENTLY LICENSED UNDER DIVISION 2 (COMMENCING WITH SECTION 500) OF THE BUSINESS AND PROFESSIONS CODE. EACH PART OF THE FORM MUST BE COMPLETED UNLESS INAPPLICABLE. IN FILLING OUT THIS FORM, NO CIVIL LIABILITY ATTACHES AND NO CONFIDENTIALITY IS BREACHED.

I. GENERAL INFORMATION   Print or type

PATIENT'S NAME   HOSPITAL ID NO.

ADDRESS   CITY   COUNTY   STATE   PHONE

AGE	BIRTHDATE	RACE	SEX	DATE AND TIME OF ARRIVAL	MODE OF TRANSPORTATION	DATE AND TIME OF DISCHARGE

ACCOMPANIED TO HOSPITAL BY: NAME   ADDRESS   CITY   STATE   RELATIONSHIP

PHONE REPORT MADE TO   ID NO.   DEPARTMENT   PHONE   RESPONDING OFFICER/AGENCY

NAME OF: ☐ FATHER   ☐ STEPFATHER   ADDRESS   CITY   COUNTY   HOME PHONE   BUS. PHONE   AGE/DOB

NAME OF: ☐ MOTHER   ☐ STEPMOTHER   ADDRESS   CITY   COUNTY   HOME PHONE   BUS. PHONE   AGE/DOB

SIBLINGS: LAST NAME, FIRST   DOB   LAST NAME, FIRST   DOB   LAST NAME, FIRST   DOB

II. MEDICAL EXAMINATION

A. History	1. EXPLANATION OF INJURIES BY PARENT OR PERSON ACCOMPANYING CHILD (LOCATION; DATE, TIME AND CIRCUMSTANCES)

2. PATIENT'S STATEMENT EXPLAINING INJURY (PARAPHRASE)

3. PATIENT'S EMOTIONAL REACTION TO EXAMINATION (SUBMISSIVE, COMPLIANT, ETC.)

4. PREVIOUS HISTORY OF CHILD ABUSE (IF KNOWN)

B. Sexual Assault	Perform exam only if necessary.

1. ACTS COMMITTED: NOTE—COITUS, FELLATIO, CUNNILINGUS, SODOMY

2. DURING ASSAULT
☐ VAGINAL PENETRATION (HOW)   EJACULATION: ☐ VAGINAL ☐ ORAL ☐ ANAL ☐ OTHER:

☐ ANAL PENETRATION (HOW)   ☐ CONDOM USED   ☐ VOMITED   ☐ LOSS OF CONSCIOUSNESS   ☐ OTHER:

3. AFTER ASSAULT:
☐ WIPED/WASHED   ☐ BATHED   ☐ DOUCHED   ☐ VOMITED   ☐ CHANGED CLOTHES   ☐ BRUSHED TEETH   ☐ DEFECATED   ☐ OTHER:

C. Physical Examination	DATE AND TIME OF EXAM	DATE AND TIME OF ASSAULT	BP	PULSE	RESP.	TEMP

HEIGHT	WEIGHT	HEAD CIRCUM	LAST TETANUS	KNOWN ALLERGIES	CURRENT MEDICATION

DIAGNOSTIC DATA

Check if indicated and incorporate results in written examination at left

☐ X-rays (skull, chest, longbone, full skeletal)

☐ Bleeding, coagulation, tourniquet, tests

☐ Funduscopic

☐ Other

DOJ 900

DATE	HOSPITAL ID NO.	HOSPITAL

PHYSICAL EXAMINATION (CONTINUED) LOCATE AND DESCRIBE IN DETAIL ANY INJURIES OR FINDINGS: TRAUMA, BRUISES, ERYTHEMA, EXCORIATIONS, LACERATIONS, WOUNDS. TRACE OUTLINE' USED AND INDICATE LOCATION OF WOUNDS/LACERATIONS USING 'X' FOR SUPERFICIAL, 'O' FOR DEEP; SHADE FOR BRUISES OR BURNS. BESIDE EACH INJURY INDICATED NOTE COLOR, SIZE, PATTERN, TEXTURE, AND SENSATION. WRITE OVER UNUSED OUTLINES. DESCRIBE IN DETAIL SHAPE OF ARM OR OTHER BRUISES WHICH MAY INDICATE FORCE.

D. PELVIC — A PELVIC EXAMINATION SHOULD NOT BE PERFORMED UNLESS THE PARENT, GUARDIAN OR MINOR CONSENT OR UNLESS NECESSARY AS PART OF TREATMENT. SEE DEPARTMENT OF HEALTH REGULATIONS TITLE 22, DIVISION 2, VICTIMS OF SEXUAL ASSAULT. SAME INSTRUCTIONS AS GENERAL PHYSICAL; IN ADDITION, NOTE PUBIC HAIR COMBINGS WHERE INDICATED, DRIED SECRETIONS AND RECENT INJURIES TO HYMEN, TRACE AND OUTLINE AS ABOVE.

V. SPECIMENS

STAINS/FOREIGN MATERIALS (WHEN INDICATED)

LOOSE HAIR	____	FINGERNAIL SCRAPINGS	____
BLOOD	____	DIRT OR GRAVEL	____
THREADS	____	VEGETATION	____
GRASS	____	CLOTHING	____
DRIED SECRETIONS	____		

	SLIDES	SWABS
VAGINAL	____	____
RECTAL	____	____
ORAL	____	____
ASPIRATES/ WASHINGS	____	
BITE MARKS	____	____
OTHER:	____	____

PATIENT'S SAMPLES. TIME OF COLLECTION AT MD DISCRETION

BLOOD	____
HAIR FROM HEAD	____
SALIVA	____
HAIR FROM PUBIC AREA	____

III. DIAGNOSTIC IMPRESSION OF TRAUMA AND INJURIES

IV. TREATMENT/DISPOSITION OF PATIENT

A. ☐ GC CULTURE ☐ VDRL ☐ PREGNANCY TEST ☐ POST COITAL ESTROGEN ☐ VD PRO-PHYLAXIS ☐ OTHER:

☐ MOTILE SPERM: ☐ PRESENCE ☐ ABSENCE ☐ NOT TAKEN ☐ FAMILY ASSESSMENT BY: ☐ NOT ORDERED

B. ORDERS:

C. DISPOSITION: ☐ ADMIT TRANSFERRED TO:

☐ RELEASED ACCOMPANIED BY: NAME ADDRESS RELATIONSHIP

D. FOLLOW-UP WITHIN:

☐ MEDICAL
____ HRS ____ DAYS

☐ SOCIAL SERVICES
____ HRS ____ DAYS

☐ PRIVATE MD
____ HRS ____ DAYS

☐ OTHER
____ HRS ____ DAYS

I HAVE RECEIVED THE INDICATED ITEMS AS EVIDENCE AND A COPY OF THIS REPORT.

OFFICER: ID NO.: DATE:

NURSE SIGNATURE OF EXAMINATION PHYSICIAN

Domestic Violence Screening/Documentation Form

DOMESTIC VIOLENCE SCREENING/DOCUMENTATION FORM

DV SCREEN
- ☐ Screened
  - ☐ Yes
  - ☐ No
  - ☐ Probable/Suspected DV
- ☐ Not Screened

Routinely Screen at each visit
"Because violence is so common in women's lives, I've begun to ask about it routinely".

Ask Direct Questions
"I'm concerned that your injuries/symptoms may have been caused by someone hurting you? Is this what happened to you?"

-OR-

"Has you intimate partner or ex-partner ever physically hurt you? Have they ever *threatened* to hurt you or someone close to you?"

Assess Patient Safety

- ☐ Yes ☐ No Is patient afraid to go home?
- ☐ Yes ☐ No Has physical violence increased in severity over past years?
- ☐ Yes ☐ No Have threats of homicide been made?
- ☐ Yes ☐ No Have threats of suicide been made?
- ☐ Yes ☐ No Is alcohol or substance abuse also a problem?
- ☐ Yes ☐ No Is there a gun in the house?
- ☐ Yes ☐ No Is patient afraid of their partner?
- ☐ Yes ☐ No Was safety plan discussed?

Referrals
- ☐ hotline number given
- ☐ legal referral made
- ☐ shelter number given
- ☐ in-house referral made
- ☐ discharge instructions given

Date _____   Patient ID#_____
Patient Name _____
Provider Name _____
Patient Pregnant? Yes ____ No ____

Describe frequency and severity of present and past abuse (use direct quotes as much possible)

_____
_____
_____
_____
_____
_____

Describe location and extent of injury

_____
_____
_____
_____
_____
_____

Indicate where injury was observed

- ☐ Yes ☐ No Photographs taken?
- ☐ Yes ☐ No Consent to be photographed?

(Attach Photographs) + Appropriate Form

Index

Note: Page numbers followed by d indicate display material; those followed by f indicate figures; those followed by t indicate tables.

Abuse. *See* Child abuse; Family violence
Acceptance, as family function, 437
Access to health services
  barriers to, for migrant workers, 670–673
  in communicable disease control, 303
  economic forces and. *See* Health care economics, access to health services and
  poverty and, 648
  in rural areas, 633–634
Accidents
  of adults, 584, 584t
  of children, 540–541, 557
  global concern about, 420
Accommodation, 158
Accreditation
  of health care organizations, 211–212
  of nursing schools, 210–211, 211d
Acid rain, 320
Acne, in adolescents, 565
Acquired immunodeficiency syndrome (AIDS). *See* HIV/AIDS
Active immunity, 256, 277
Active listening, 140
Acute respiratory infections (ARIs)
  global battle against, 418
  prevention of, 419
Adames, Jackie, 651
Adaptability, of nursing process, 384f, 385
Adaptation, 158
Adaptation model, 344
Adaptive behavior, of families, 430
Addiction, 701–719
  to alcohol, 711–713
    community health nurse's role and, 713
    prevention of, 711–712
  assumptions about clients living with, 705, 705d
  to central nervous system depressants other than alcohol, 714–715
    community health nurse's role and, 715, 717
    prevention of, 714–715, 716–717
  etiology of, 703–704, 704f
  to gambling, 717–718
    prevention of, 717–718
  globalization of, 718–719
  Healthy People 2010 goals for, 705–706
  historical background of, 702–703
  population statistics for, 703
  problems related to, 706, 707t–709t, 710–711
    economic, 710–711
    of fetus, newborn, and children of addicted parents, 711

physical, 706
psychosocial, 706, 710, 710t
public health model of, 705, 705f
to stimulants, 715–717
terminology of, 702
to tobacco, 713–714
  community health nurse's role and, 714
  prevention of, 713–714
Adolescents
  alcohol use by, research on, 712
  health-compromising behaviors in, 563
  health problems of, 562–565
    emotional, 562
    poor nutrition and eating disorders as, 565
    sexually transmitted diseases as, 564–565
    substance abuse as, 563–564
    suicide as, 562
    violence and, 562–563
  health services for, 565–570
    health promotion programs, 569–570
    health protection programs, 567–569
    preventive health programs, 566–567
    school-based health clinics, 570
  as parents, 439
  research on, 564
  pregnancy in, 520–521, 564
Adolph Coors Company, 591
Adult(s), 582–586
  definition of, 581
  demographics of, 582, 583t
  developmental tasks of, 583–584
  health problems of, 584–585
    accidents as, 584, 584t
    cancer as, 584–585
    cardiovascular disease as, 585
    HIV/AIDS as, 585
    suicide as, 585
  health promotion for, 585–586
  immunization of, 281, 285t
  life expectancy of, 582–583, 583t, 584t
  older. *See* Older adults
  physical profile of, 582, 582d
Adult learning theory of Knowles, 159, 160d
Advanced disease stage, 257, 257f
Advance directives, 611
Adverse drug effects, in older adults, 608–609
Advocacy. *See also* Community health advocacy
  as community health nurse's role, 43–44
    actions and, 43–44
    in community mental health, 695
    in correctional health care, 730–731
    goals and, 43
    in home care, hospice care, and long-term care, 750

maternal-infant health and, 529–530
  migrant workers and, 674
Aesthetics, 313–314
Affection, as family function, 436–437
Affective domain of learning, 155–156, 156t
Affiliation, as family function, 437
Africa
  community health nursing in, 31
  health care systems in, 410
African Americans, 64–66
  health beliefs and practices of, 65–66
  health problems of, 65, 65d
  population characteristics and culture of, 65
African trypanosomiasis, global battle against, 272
Age. *See also specific age groups*
  poverty and, 644
  of rural population, 627
Ageism, 602–604
Agency for International Development, 103
Agents
  disasters and, 393
  in epidemiology, 251
Aggregates, 5–6
  interaction with, 377
  targeting meaningful health messages to, 276
Aging, successful, research on, 382
Agricultural Labor Relations Act of 1975, 660
AIDS. *See* HIV/AIDS
Aid to Dependent Children, 645
Aid to Families with Dependent Children (AFDC), 645
Airborne transmission, 275
Air pollution, 318–321, 319f
  acid rain due to, 320
  dusts, gases, and naturally occurring elements contributing to, 319–320
  government control of, 320–321
  nurse's role with, 321
  ozone depletion and global warming due to, 320
Alaskan natives, 63
Alcoholics Anonymous (AA), 692, 712
Alcohol use/abuse
  addiction and, 711–713
    community health nurse's role and, 713
    prevention of, 711–712
  by adolescents, research on, 712
  during pregnancy, 517–518
Aluminum exposure, 330
Alzheimer, Alois, 612
Alzheimer's disease (AD), 612–613
Ambulatory service settings, as community health nursing settings, 50